AO SPINE Textbook

AO SPINE Textbook

Comprehensive Overview on Surgical Management of the Spine

AO
SPINE

Editors

Michael P Steinmetz MD
William P and Amanda C Madar Endowed Professor and Chair
Department of Neurological Surgery
Cleveland Clinic Lerner College of Medicine
Neurological Institute
Cleveland, Ohio, USA

Jeffrey C Wang MD
Chief, Orthopedic Spine Service
Co-Director, USC Spine Center
Professor of Orthopedic Surgery and Neurosurgery, USC Spine Center
Los Angeles, California, USA

Thomas E Mroz MD
Director, Center for Spine Health
Director, Spine Research Lab
Center for Spine Health
Departments of Orthopedic and Neurological Surgery
Cleveland Clinic
Cleveland, Ohio, USA

Forewords

Edward C Benzel
S Rajasekaran

JAYPEE

JAYPEE BROTHERS MEDICAL PUBLISHERS
The Health Sciences Publisher
New Delhi | London

Jaypee Brothers Medical Publishers (P) Ltd

Headquarters

Jaypee Brothers Medical Publishers (P) Ltd
4838/24, Ansari Road, Daryaganj
New Delhi 110 002, India
Phone: +91-11-43574357
Fax: +91-11-43574314
E-mail: jaypee@jaypeebrothers.com

Overseas Office

JP Medical Ltd
83 Victoria Street, London
SW1H 0HW (UK)
Phone: +44 20 3170 8910
Fax: +44 (0)20 3008 6180
E-mail: info@jpmedpub.com

Website: www.jaypeebrothers.com
Website: www.jaypeedigital.com

AO Spine Textbook: Comprehensive Overview on Surgical Management of the Spine

First Edition: **2020**

ISBN: 978-93-86056-95-5

Printed at Sanat Printers

Dedication

I would like to dedicate this book to my wife and two children.
Editing such a text is a tireless and time consuming endeavor.
Much of this time is taken away from family events.
This is no lost on me as an editor and
this finished product is a statements to their love and support.

Michael P Steinmetz

I would like to dedicate this book to my late father,
who was an educator and a scholar in the area of political science.
He lead, educated, and brought together stakeholders
by being the prime example of being the best, and
what we all should strive to be. He was the most amazing person
to ever influence and guide my life.

Jeffrey C Wang

I would like to thank my family
who has supported my career with love and
inspiration over past 15 years.

Thomas E Mroz

Contributors

A Jay Khanna MD MBA
Vice Chair and Professor
Department of Orthopedic Surgery,
Neurosurgery and Biomedical Engineering
Johns Hopkins University
Bethesda, Maryland, USA

Abhishek Ray MD
Neurosurgeon
Department of Neurological Surgery
University Hospitals Cleveland
Medical Center
Cleveland, Ohio, USA

Adam L Wollowick MD MBA
Senior Director
Business Development
Stryker Spine
New York City, New York, USA

Ahmet Alanay MD
Professor
Department of Orthopedics and
Traumatology
Acibadem University School of Medicine
Istanbul, Turkey

Ajit A Krishnaney MD FAANS
Vice Chair
Department of Neurosurgery
Patient Safety Officer
Neurological Institute
Cleveland Clinic
Cleveland, Ohio, USA

Alexandra Paraskos MD
Physician
Cleveland Clinic
Columbus, Ohio, USA

Ankit I Mehta MD FAANS
Assistant Professor of Neurosurgery
Director of Spinal Oncology
University of Illinois at Chicago
Chicago, Illinois, USA

Anthony A Scaduto MD
Orthopedic Surgeon
UCLA Medical Center
Santa Monica
Los Angeles, California, USA

Brian K Kwon MD PhD FRCSC
Canada Research Chair in Spinal Cord Injury
Professor
Department of Orthopedics
University of British Columbia
Vancouver, British Columbia, Canada

Caglar Yilgor MD
Associate Professor
Department of Orthopedics and
Traumatology
Acibadem University School of Medicine
Istanbul, Turkey

Casey Fisher MD
Interventional Pain Specialist
Pain Relief Solutions
San Diego, California, USA

Christopher Bonsignore MD
Spine Surgery Fellow
Texas Back Institute
Plano, Texas, USA

Christopher P Ames MD
Professor of Clinical Neurological Surgery
and Orthopedic Surgery
Director of Spinal Deformity and Spine
Tumor Surgery
Co-Director, Spinal Surgery and UCSF
Spine Center
Director, California Deformity Institute
Director, Spinal Biomechanics Laboratory
Department of Neurological Surgery
University of California, San Francisco
San Francisco, California, USA

Colin G Crosby MD
Orthopedic Spine Surgeon
Centennial Medical Center
St Thomas Hospital
Nashville, Tennessee, USA

Daniel G Hoernschemeyer MD
Chief of Pediatric Orthopedics
MU Women's and Children's Hospital
Associate Professor
Department of Orthopedic Surgery
University of Missouri
Columbia, Missouri, USA

Daniel K Resnick MD MS
Professor and Vice Chairman
Department of Neurosurgery
University of Wisconsin School of
Medicine and Public Health
Madison, Wisconsin, USA

Daniel Lubelski MD
Resident
Department of Neurosurgery
Johns Hopkins University
Baltimore, Maryland, USA

Darrel S Brodke MD
Louis and Janet Peery Presidential
Endowed Chair
Professor and Executive Vice Chair
Department of Orthopedics
University of Utah
Salt Lake City, Utah, USA

David E Fish MD MPH
Associate Professor
Department of Orthopedics
Physical Medicine and Rehabilitation
The UCLA Spine Center
David Geffen School of Medicine at UCLA
Los Angeles, California, USA

David Gurd MD
Attending Pediatric Orthopedic Surgeon
Head, Pediatric Spinal Deformity Surgery
Cleveland Clinic Foundation
Cleveland, Ohio, USA

David T Anderson MD
Orthopedic Spine Surgeon
OrthoCarolina
Monroe, North Carolina, USA

Douglas Orr MD
Orthopedic Surgeon
Cleveland Clinic Spine Institute
Luthern Hospital
Cleveland, Ohio, USA

Edward C Benzel MD
Emeritus Chair of Neurosurgery
Cleveland Clinic
Cleveland, Ohio, USA

Emiliano Vialle MD
Spine Surgeon
Cajuru University Hospital
Catholic University of Parana
Curitiba, Parana, Brazil

Emmanuel Menga MD
Assistant Professor
Department of Orthopedics and Rehabilitation
University of Rochester Medical Center
Rochester, New York, USA

Faiz Ahmad MD MCh
Assistant Professor
Department of Neurosurgery
Emory University
Atlanta, Georgia, USA

Fernando Techy MD
Director of Spine Surgery
Department of Orthopedic Surgery
ClinTech Center for Orthopedics and Spine Health
Fort Collins, Colorado, USA

Gabriel Widi MD
Neurosurgeon
Miami Brain and Spine Center
Miami, Florida, USA

Geoffrey Stricsek MD
Neurosurgery Spine Fellow
Emory University
Atlanta, Georgia, USA

George Rymarczuk MD
Staff Neurosurgeon
Division of Neurosurgery
Landstuhl Regional Medical Center
Landstuhl, Germany
Assistant Professor of Surgery
Uniformed Services University of the Health Sciences
Bethesda, Maryland, USA

Ghaith Habboub MD
Neurosurgery Resident
Cleveland Clinic
Cleveland, Ohio, USA

Graham C Calvert MD
Neck and Back Specialist
Mississippi Sports Medicine Orthopedic Center
Jackson, Mississippi, USA

Gregory R Trost MD
Professor, Vice Chair
Director, Spinal Surgery Program
Department of Neurological Surgery
University of Wisconsin School of Medicine and Public Health
Madison, Wisconsin, USA

Haariss Ilyas MD
Resident Physician
Cleveland Clinic Foundation
Cleveland, Ohio, USA

Hillard T Spencer MD
Orthopedic Surgeon
Los Angeles, California, USA

Howard S An MD
The Morton International Endowed Chair
Professor of Orthopedic Surgery
Director, Spine Fellowship Program
Midwest Orthopedics at Rush University
Chicago, Illinois, USA

Isador H Lieberman MD MBA FRCSC
Orthopedic and Spinal Surgeon
Texas Back Institute
Plano, Texas, USA

Jacob Enders BS
Medical Student
Cleveland Clinic Lerner College of Medicine
Cleveland, Ohio, USA

James D Kang MD
Chairman
Department of Orthopedic Surgery
Brigham and Women's Hospital
Boston, Massachusetts, USA

James S Harrop MD FACS
Professor
Department of Neurological and Orthopedic Surgery
Director, Division of Spine and Peripheral Nerve Surgery
Neurosurgery Director of Delaware Valley SCI Center
Thomas Jefferson University
Philadelphia, Pennsylvania, USA

Jason D Berk MD
Mid-Atlantic Permanente Medical Group
Rockville, Maryland, USA

Jason I Liounakos MD
Resident
Department of Neurological Surgery
University of Miami
Miami, Florida, USA

Jean Paul Wolinsky MD
Professor of Neurosurgery and Orthopedic Surgery
Vice Chairman of Neurosurgery
Strategic Planning and Finance
Director of Spinal Oncology
Department of Neurosurgery
Northwestern University
Feinberg School of Medicine
Chicago, Illinois, USA

Jens R Chapman MD
Spine Surgeon
Swedish Neuroscience Institute
Seattle, Washington, USA

Jessica A Tang MD
Resident Physician
Department of Otolaryngology
Temple University
Philadelphia, Pennsylvania, USA

Joel Kolmodin MD
Resident
Cleveland Clinic Foundation
Cleveland, Ohio, USA

Juliann Kwak Lee MD
Assistant Professor
Department of Orthopedic Surgery
University of Southern California
Los Angeles, California, USA

Justin K Scheer MD
Resident Physician, PGY-4
Department of Neurological Surgery
University of California
San Francisco, California, USA

K Daniel Riew MD
Professor of Orthopedic Surgery
Columbia University
Chief, Cervical Spine Surgery and Co-Director, Spine Division
Co-Director, Columbia University Spine Fellowship
New York City, New York, USA

Kaine C Onwuzulike MD PhD
Assistant Professor
Department of Neurological Surgery,
CCLCM CCAG
Section Head
Pediatric Spine and Fetal
Myelomeningocele Repair
Center of Pediatric Neurosciences S-60
Cleveland, Ohio, USA

Karthikeyan E Ponnusamy MD MSE
Orthopedic Surgeon
Pinnacle Orthopedics
Woodstock, Georgia, USA

Keith Bachmann MD
Resident
Cleveland Clinic Foundation
Cleveland, Ohio, USA

Kelly Krohn MD
Clinical Associate Professor
Department of Orthopedic Surgery
University of Arizona College of Medicine
Phoenix, Arizona, USA

Kevin Hines MD
Resident
Department of Neurosurgery
Thomas Jefferson University
Philadelphia, Pennsylvania, USA

Luiz Roberto Vialle MD PhD
Professor
Department of Orthopedics
School of Medicine
Pontifical Catholic University
Cajuru Hospital, Spine Group
Curitiba, Paraná, Brazil

Mari L Groves MD
Neurosurgeon
Johns Hopkins Bayview Medical Center
Baltimore, Maryland, USA

Marzena Buzanowska MD
Physician
Cleveland Clinic
Cleveland, Ohio, USA

Mauricio Silva MD
Clinical Professor
Orthopedic Institute for Children
University of California, Los Angeles
Los Angeles, California, USA

Melissa Nadeau MD MPH FRCSC
Spine Surgeon
Surrey Comprehensive Orthopedics
Surrey, British Columbia, Canada

Michael D Daubs MD
Orthopedic Spine Surgeon
Professor and Chairman
Department of Orthopedic Surgery
University of Nevada, Las Vegas
Las Vegas, Nevada, USA

Michael G Fehlings MD PhD FRCSC FACS
Professor
Department of Neurosurgery
University of Toronto
Toronto, Ontario, Canada

Michael J Beebe MD
Orthopedic Trauma Surgeon
Campbell Clinic
Germantown, Tennessee, USA

Michael J Lee MD
Professor
Orthopedic Spine Surgery
University of Chicago
Chicago, Illinois, USA

Michael P Kelly MD MSc
Associate Professor
Department of Orthopedic and
Neurological Surgery
Director, Adult and Pediatric Spine
Fellowship
Director, Spine Research
Washington University School of Medicine
St Louis, Missouri, USA

Michael P Steinmetz MD
William P and Amanda C Madar Endowed
Professor and Chair
Department of Neurological Surgery
Cleveland Clinic Lerner College of
Medicine
Neurological Institute
Cleveland, Ohio, USA

Michael T Modic MD FACR
Professor of Radiology and Radiologic
Sciences
Senior VP Population Health
Vanderbilt University
Nashville, Tennessee, USA

Michael Y Wang MD FACS
Professor, Neurological Surgery and
Rehab Medicine
Spine Fellowship Director
Chief of Neurosurgery
University of Miami Hospital
University of Miami Miller School of
Medicine
Miami, Florida, USA

Natalie L Leong MD
Assistant Professor
Department of Orthopedic Surgery
University of Maryland School of Medicine
Baltimore, Maryland, USA

Orlando Colina

Paul E Kaloostian MD FAANS FACS
Neurosurgeon
Riverside Community Hospital
Riverside, California, USA

Perry Dhaliwal MD MPH FRCSC
Assistant Professor of Neurosurgery
Section of Neurosurgery
Department of Surgery
University of Manitoba
Manitoba, Canada

Richard E Bowen MD
Co-Director, Spinal Deformity Center
Orthopedic Institute for Children
Clinical Professor
Department of Orthopedic Surgery
David Geffen School of Medicine at UCLA
Los Angeles, California, USA

Robert A Hart MD
Spine Surgeon
Swedish Neuroscience Institute
Seattle, Washington, USA

Ryan Goodwin MD
Surgeon
Cleveland Clinic Foundation
Cleveland, Ohio, USA

S Tim Yoon MD PhD
Professor
Department of Orthopedic Surgery
Emory University
Atlanta, Georgia, USA

Safdar N Khan MD
The Benjamin R and Helen Slack Wiltberger Endowed Chair in Orthopedic Spine Surgery
Associate Professor and Chief of Division of Spine
Department of Orthopedics
Adjunct Associate Professor
Department of Integrated Systems Engineering
Clinical Faculty, Spine Research Institute
The Ohio State University Wexner Medical Center
Columbus, Ohio, USA

Sajeel R Khan MD
Assistant Professor
Department of Neurosurgery
Marshall University
Huntington, West Virginia, USA

Sandeep N Gidvani MD
Orthopedic Spine Surgeon
OrthoNorcal
Los Gatos, California, USA

Scott D Daffner MD
Professor
Department of Orthopedics
West Virginia University
Morgantown, West Virginia, USA

Sean Barry MD MA FRCSC
Assistant Professor
Dalhousie University
Halifax, Nova Scotia, Canada

Shah-Nawaz M Dodwad MD
Assistant Professor
Division of Spine
Department of Orthopedics
University of Texas Health Science Center
Houston, Texas, USA

Shaleen Vira MD
Combined Neurological and Orthopedic Spine Surgery Fellow
Cleveland Clinic
Cleveland, Ohio, USA

Siddharth A Badve
MD MBBS MS(Orthopedics)
Attending Spine Surgeon
Carolina Pines Regional Medical Center
Hartsville, South Carolina, USA

Sohrab S Virk MD MBA
Spine Fellow
Division of Spine
Department of Orthopedics
Hospital for Special Surgery
New York City, New York, USA

Stephen Dechter DO
Benton Franklin Orthopedic Associates
Kennewick, Washington, USA

Sumit K Gupta MD
Associate Professor
Department of Orthopedic Surgery
University of Missouri
Columbia, Missouri, USA

Theodore J Choma MD
Professor of Orthopedic Surgery
Director, Spine Division
University of Missouri
Columbia, Missouri, USA

Todd M Emch MD
Staff Neuroradiologist
Cleveland Clinic
Cleveland, Ohio, USA

Tom D Cha MD MBA
Associate Professor
Chief of the Spine Section
Department of Orthopedics
Massachusetts General Hospital
Boston, Massachusetts, USA

Vikram Mehta MD MPH
Neurosurgery Resident Physician
Duke University Medical Center
Durham, North Carolina, USA

Vincent J Miele MD
Clinical Associate Professor
Department of Neurosurgery
University of Pittsburgh Medical Center
Pittsburgh, Pennsylvania, USA

Wellington K Hsu MD
Clifford C Raisbeck Distinguished Professor of Orthopedic Surgery
Director of Research
Professor
Department of Orthopedic and Neurological Surgery
Northwestern University Feinberg School of Medicine
Chicago, Illinois, USA

Xiaobang Hu PhD
Research Director
Texas Back Institute
Plano, Texas, USA

Yi Lu MD PhD
Assistant Professor
Department of Neurosurgery
Harvard University
Boston, Massachusetts, USA

Yonatan G Keschner MD
Resident Physician
Massachusetts General Hospital–Brigham and Women's Hospital
Boston, Massachusetts, USA

Yu-Po Lee MD
Clinical Professor
University of California, Irvine
Irvine, California, USA

Zachary L Gordon MD
Assistant Professor
Department of Orthopedics
Case Western Reserve University School of Medicine
Cleveland, Ohio, USA

Ziya L Gokaslan MD FAANS FACS
Julius Stoll, MD Professor and Chair
Department of Neurosurgery
The Warren Alpert Medical School of Brown University
Neurosurgeon-in-Chief
Rhode Island Hospital and the Miriam Hospital
Clinical Director
Norman Prince Neurosciences Institute
President
Brown Neurosurgery Foundation
Providence, Rhode Island, USA

Foreword

Within the pages that follow, lies a wonderful contribution to the spine literature—a contribution masterfully crafted by Drs Malhotra, Mroz, Wang, and Steinmetz. The editors of the *AO Spine Textbook* have gathered a who's who list of spine experts who collectively 'blanket' the field of spine care by addressing nearly all relevant aspects of the field. Such was eloquently accomplished, leaving very few, if any, gaps. They have, as would a conductor of an orchestra, played to the strengths of each of the chapter authors—leading them, in a way, to create a first class performance that leaves jaws dropping.

The book is beautifully illustrated. The illustrations are not only well-done, but are used in a manner that is very educational and enlightening. The chapters are placed in an orderly manner, with the book flowing nicely as one peruses the pages. The *AO Spine Textbook* can be used as a textbook to be read from cover to cover or as a reference for the busy spine practitioner. Though, once a reader initially thumbs through the text, he/she may be compelled to keep on reading. The book may indeed be very difficult to put aside for many of its readers.

Although the book covers many nonoperative topics, the focus in general is surgical. It is written, though, to be of interest and significant value to surgeons and nonsurgeons alike.

I am proud to have been a part of this project. The end result is truly remarkable. Please enjoy this well-orchestrated gem of a book. It will occupy a place on the book shelves of many for years to come.

Edward C Benzel MD
Emeritus Chair of Neurosurgery
Cleveland Clinic
Cleveland, Ohio, USA

Foreword

Spine surgery is not only one of the fastest growing subspecialties in orthopedic surgery but is also a very challenging one. Arriving at a perfect diagnosis, ordering and interpreting appropriate investigations, choosing the perfect management pathway without erring on over or undertreatment still remains a major challenge in the field of spine surgery. An error at any one of these decisions can lead to poor outcome commonly termed as 'failed back syndrome' the incidence of which is quoted from 3 to 18% in literature. In the event of such an unfortunate situation, it is a miserable scenario for the patient, his family members and the treating surgeon team.

The rapid progress that the last decade has witnessed a tremendous progress in all fields of spine surgery. The practising surgeon can often be confused with the numerous and often untested options in diagnostic techniques and surgical procedures. Often literature points to many successful methods to approach and manage a problem and the surgeon has to choose appropriately a solution suited for the patient from the large number of 'arrows in the quiver'. This book will surely help the surgeon in this process as it is a comprehensive overview of the entire spectrum of spine surgery. There is a good focus on the physical examination, nonoperative and surgical treatment from leading orthopedic and neuro spine surgeons from international institutions. The contributors are renowned spine surgeons and the textbook naturally carries a huge amount of collective wisdom from all over the world. The book is also excellently illustrated to make reading and understanding easier.

I would like to congratulate the Editors, Michael P Steinmetz, Jeffrey C Wang and Thomas E Mroz for this outstanding textbook. The book will certainly help to achieve AOSpine's aim of improving spine surgery education throughout the world and I am confident that this will be a welcome addition to the library of all institutions and spine surgeons across the world.

S Rajasekaran MS FRCS MCh PhD
International Chair—AO Spine

Preface

We are proud to present the *AO Spine Textbook: Comprehensive Overview on Surgical Management of the Spine*. This comprehensive text covers the surgical treatment of the spine from 'head-to-toe'. The text serves as a state-of-the-art one stop shop for the reader. It is appropriate for students, trainees or seasoned veterans.

The book begins in the cervical region, ends at the sacrum, while the last chapter focuses on the future of spine care and surgery. Each section begins with a discussion of pathology and pathophysiology. This is followed by diagnostic workup and then surgical management. Specialty chapters focus on disease specific issues such as scoliosis, deformity and oncology.

Each chapter is written by a true expert in the field. They are able to bring in up-to-date evidence and combine this with years of experience. Each section will provide a complete discussion of management of simple to the most complex pathologies.

Michael P Steinmetz
Jeffrey C Wang
Thomas E Mroz

Acknowledgments

We like to first thank the authors for taking this journey with us. It has been a long road, but we are very proud of the final product. We thank M/s Jaypee Brothers Medical Publishers (P) Ltd, New Delhi, India. We thank Ms Nedup Denka Bhutia for her tireless efforts in the completion of this text as well as Ms Chetna Malhotra Vohra. We also thank the AO for support and aid in the completion of this text. Lastly, we would like to acknowledge our mentors, trainees and, present and past partners, and collaborators.

Contents

Section 1: General Topics

Section 2: Pediatric Spine

Section 4: Thoracic

Section 5: Lumbosacral

Section 6: Future Trends in Spine Surgery

SECTION

1

General Topics

CHAPTER 1 Relevant Surgical Anatomy

Graham C Calvert, Michael J Beebe, Darrel S Brodke

OVERVIEW

The normal human spine is segmented into 7 cervical vertebrae (C1–7), 12 thoracic vertebrae (T1–12), 5 lumbar vertebrae (L1–5), 5 fused sacral vertebrae (S1–5), and 3 or 4 fused coccygeal vertebrae. The spine has four distinct sagittal curves, lordosis (concave posterior curvature) in the cervical and lumbar regions, and kyphosis (concave anterior curvature) in the thoracic and sacral/coccygeal regions. Sagittal balance should be such that, on a standing film, a line drawn vertically downward from the center of the C7 vertebral body intersects the posterior edge of the S1 superior endplate. Sagittal balance is also dependent on the shape of the pelvis and the takeoff of the sacrum (sacral slope) combined with the tilt of the pelvis, which when added together results in the fixed measurement of pelvic incidence. The coronal alignment of the normal human spine is straight. Various congenital, environmental, idiopathic, and degenerative changes can result in deviation from this normal anatomy. Understanding these relationships is paramount when managing spinal deformity.

CORRELATIVE ANATOMY

When performing surgery on the spine and planning incisions, particularly during anterior approaches, it is important to have an understanding of the particular spinal levels that correspond to externally identifiable structures. While these relationships are somewhat variable, they remain an important guide to the underlying spine. Anteriorly, the angle of the mandible overlies the C1–2 level, the hyoid pinpoints the C3 level, the thyroid cartilage overlies the C4–5 level, and the cricoid cartilage and carotid tubercle identifies the C6 level. The vertebral prominens posteriorly corresponds to the C7 vertebra. The T3 level is in line with the manubrium anteriorly and the spine of the scapula posteriorly. The T7 level corresponds to the xiphoid process anteriorly and tip of the scapula posteriorly. The umbilicus overlies the T10 level anteriorly, while the iliac crest overlies the L4 level posteriorly. Other important correlations include the end of the spinal cord and beginning of the conus medullaris at the L1 level, the aortic bifurcation at the L3–4 level, and the bifurcation of the vena cava just below this at the L4 level.

OSTEOLOGY OF THE SPINE

Cervical Osteology

The cervical spine is composed of seven vertebrae, C1 through C7, stacked vertically in a lordotic alignment from the base of the skull to the thoracic spine. The primary function of the cervical spine is to provide support and motion to the cranium while allowing protective passage of the spinal cord, exiting nerve roots, and vertebral arteries. C1 and C2, termed the atlas and axis, respectively, possess unique anatomic characteristics and functions. C3 though C7 form the subaxial region of the cervical spine and are more uniform, possessing classic cervical vertebral anatomy, though C7 may vary slightly with respect as it transitions to the thoracic spine.

The atlas is the most cephalad vertebra forming the junction between the occiput and cervical spine. It uniquely lacks both a vertebral body and spinous process. It is composed of an anterior arch, left and right lateral masses, transverse processes, and a posterior arch. The posterior arch is the first structure encountered during posterior approach and can be absent in up to 5% of the population.[1] The posterior ponticulus (aka ponticulus posticus), a boney extension of the posterior arch that surrounds the vertebral artery, may be present in 12–19% of the population.[2-4] Preoperative imaging must be examined prior to surgery at this level to rule out these abnormalities and avoid inadvertent breach of both the thecal sac and vertebral artery. The posterior arch contains the posterior tubercle, site of attachment of the ligamentum nuchae, and provides for the wide surface area of the spinal canal at this level with an average sagittal diameter of 23 mm.[5] The transverse processes of the atlas have both anterior and posterior tubercles that serve as cervical musculature origins and insertions, respectively. They also contain a foramen transversarium, which serves as a conduit for passage of the ascending vertebral artery. The lateral masses superiorly contain two concave superior facets that articulate proximally with the occipital condyles to form the atlanto-occipital (AO) joint. The inferior surfaces of the lateral masses contain two inferior facets that articulate with the corresponding superior facets of the axis to form the atlantoaxial (AA) joint. The anterior arch contains the anterior tubercle, site of attachment of the anterior longitudinal ligament (ALL), and longus colli. The anterior ring possesses a posteriorly facing facet covered with hyaline cartilage, which articulates with the dens of axis.

The axis is the second cervical vertebra and has a more typical vertebral body with disk and facet joint articulation caudally with C3, and a cranial extension, the odontoid process (dens), which along with lateral masses, articulates with C1. The spinous process is the first structure encountered at this level from the posterior approach. It is typically large, bifid, and sometimes palpable through the skin. The laminae at this level are also large and slope laterally and caudally to the lateral masses. The pars interarticularis is formed from the junction of the lateral mass and superior aspect of the lamina. It is confluent with the pedicle of the axis, angling 30° medial and 20° cephalad to attach the posterior boney elements to the vertebral body.[6] The pars interarticularis is particularly prone to fracture at this level with a hyperextension load, termed the "hanged man's fracture". The transverse processes are abbreviated at this level and contain transverse foramina for the traversing vertebral arteries, which take a tortuous path through the pars region, as detailed later in this chapter. The location of the transverse foramen within the processes can be variable and careful examination

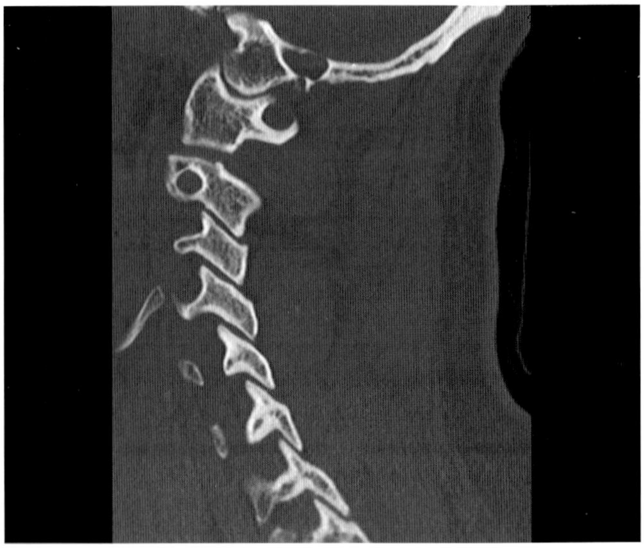

Fig. 1: High riding vertebral artery.

of preoperative imaging to rule out a medial or "high-riding" vertebral artery is paramount before placing instrumentation (Fig. 1). The lateral masses contain two superior concave and inferior convex facets to allow for rotation with respect to atlas and flexion and extension with respect to C3.

The subaxial cervical spine has typical and uniform vertebral anatomy (Fig. 2). Two distinguishing features of cervical anatomy that differ from more caudal vertebra are transverse foramina and uncinate processes. Transverse foramina in the transverse processes of C3–C6 serve as a conduit for the ascending vertebral artery. The uncinate processes are craniolateral extensions of the superior endplates of the vertebral bodies that articulate with the inferior endplate of the next more superior vertebral body. The anteroinferior edge of the vertebral body typically overhangs the anterior edge of the intervertebral disk at each level and may be removed for improved access to the disk space during anterior discectomy procedures. The lateral masses contain the superior and inferior articular processes and are bordered by the pedicle anteriorly and lamina posteriorly, serving as common instrumentation sites for the posterior cervical spine. The pedicles bridge the posterior boney elements to the vertebral body. The spinous processes of the subaxial cervical spine are small, bifid, and not generally externally palpable. They are directly behind their corresponding vertebrae and project posteriorly and slightly inferiorly.

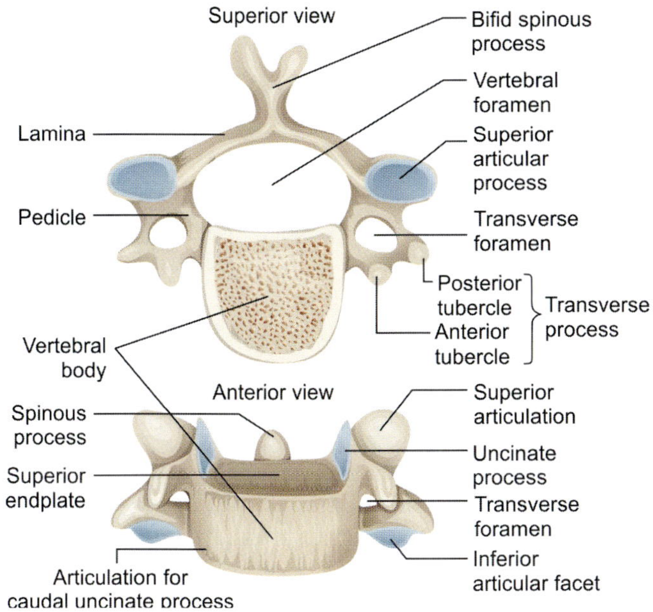

Fig. 2: Typical subaxial cervical vertebra.

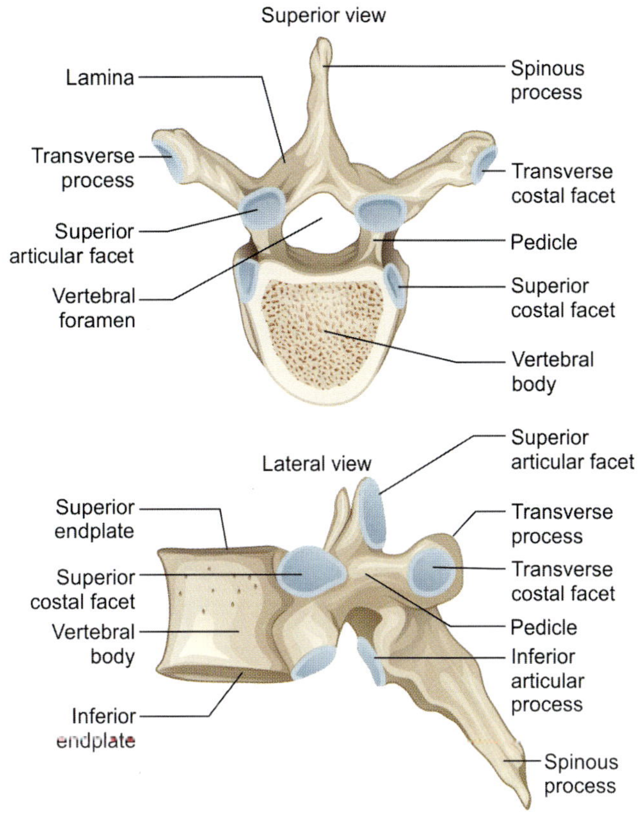

Fig. 3: Typical thoracic vertebra.

The seventh cervical vertebra is a transitional segment with slight variations from the above. It has a more prominent and usually palpable spinous process referred to as vertebral prominens. It also has more steeply inclined articular processes similar to thoracic vertebrae. The C7 pedicles are larger in diameter than the other cervical vertebrae and angle posteromedially and inferiorly. The transverse processes of C7 are shorter and typically have rudimentary transverse foramina that generally do not contain the vertebral arteries. Occasionally the anterior projection of the transverse process will develop into an anterior costal projection referred to as a cervical rib.

Thoracic Osteology

The thoracic spine is composed of 12 vertebrae, T1 through T12, arranged in a kyphotic alignment that possesses costal facets for diarthrodial articulation with ribs. In general, the thoracic spine is stiffer than the cervical or lumbar spine because of these extra articulations. T2–T8 are considered typical thoracic vertebra and have more uniform characteristics. T1 and T9–T12 are considered transitional vertebra having some features of cervical and lumbar vertebra, respectively. The thoracic spine functions to provide anchoring support to the rib cage, protection to the traversing spinal cord, and transmittal of axial loads.

The vertebral body of a typical thoracic vertebra is kidney-shaped with a larger anteroposterior than medial lateral diameter (Fig. 3). The left side of the vertebral body may take on a flattened appearance due to pulsations from the aorta. The dimensions of the vertebral bodies increase moving down the spinal column. The posterosuperior margins give rise to the thoracic pedicles, while the posterolateral margins of the upper thoracic vertebral bodies contain corresponding superior and inferior costal demifacets for articulation with rib heads. The T11 and T12 bodies, however, possess only one costal facet on each side.

The thoracic pedicles have an oval cross-sectional appearance with the height being greater than the width and the height increases in the more caudal segments. The widths of the pedicles, however, do not follow this pattern, which is important from a fixation standpoint. The T1 and T2 pedicles have relatively large widths along with T11 and T12. The pedicles with the smallest transverse width are found at levels T3–T6. Scoles classically documented the distribution of pedicle widths in a study of 50 cadaveric spines, identifying T6 as having the smallest transverse diameter, with a mean of 3.0 mm in males and 3.5 mm in females. T1 had mean diameter of 6.4 mm in females and 7.3 mm in males. T12 was the largest with a diameter of 7.2 mm in females and 7.4 mm in males.[7] The axial plane angulation of the pedicles decreases moving down the spinal column. T1 has a medial angulation of approximately 25°, T2 15°, T3–T10 5–7°, and T11 and T12 have little to no medial angulation. The cortical wall of the medial pedicle is slightly thicker than the lateral wall.

The spinous processes of the thoracic spine arise from the lamina and project posteriorly with caudal angulation. T1 and T2 have longer, more palpable spinous processes than the remaining vertebrae of the thoracic spine. The transverse processes of the thoracic spine possess a concave facet along the anterior margin, which articulates with the tuberculum of the same rib that also articulates with the superior costal facet of the vertebra. The vertebral canal in the thoracic spine takes on a more rounded appearance compared to the typical oval appearance of the cervical and lumbar spine. The diameter of the vertebral canal is also much smaller in thoracic spine measuring only 15–17 mm throughout.[8] For this reason, small changes in dimensions of this space from trauma, space occupying lesions, or disk herniations can cause severe spinal cord injuries.

The superior articular facets are oval-shaped structures with a slightly convex surface and project from the junction of the superior lamina and pedicle. They face dorsal and slightly superolateral. The inferior facet manifests from the inferior lamina with a complimentary surface to that of the superior facet, overlapping it in a shingle-like manner. The coronal and slightly oblique orientation of the thoracic facets contribute to resistance to intervertebral shear forces, compressive forces, and intervertebral torsion.[9,10] It is also advantageous for lateral bending and accommodates flexion, while limiting rotation.[11]

Lumbar Osteology

The lumbar spine is normally composed of the five most caudal mobile vertebrae, L1 through L5, occupying the region between the rib bearing vertebrae of the thoracic spine and the fused sacral vertebrae. While spinal segmentation is generally consistent in humans, there is some variation in the transitional regions of T12/L1 and L5/S1. Approximately 12% of the population shows variation in the normal transitional anatomy from L5 to S1, with around 1.8% of humans displaying complete

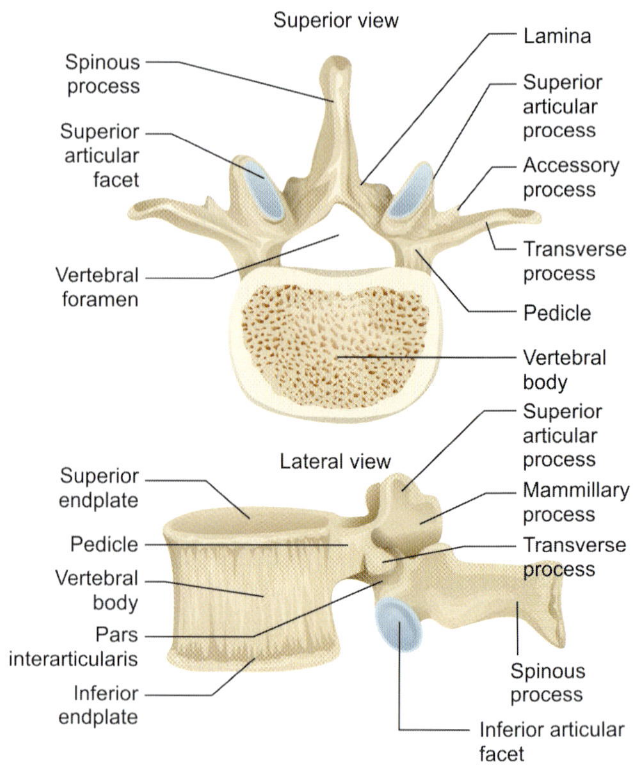

Fig. 4: Typical lumbar vertebra.

lumbarization of the S1 segment (sometimes referred to as L6), while others display sacralization of the L5 segment.[12,13] At the cranial aspect, in the region of the thoracolumbar transition, some patients will also display a rudimentary rib arising from the L1 segment.

The normal lumbar spine assumes a lordotic curvature of around 42–45° in the supine position and 50–53° in the standing position beginning at the superior endplate of S1. The convex anterior curvature of the lumbar spine is especially apparent at the lumbosacral junction; where the wedge-shaped L5–S1 disk and L5 body contribute an average of 16° of lordosis.

Characterized by their lack of transverse foramina, costal facets, or intersegmentary fusion, the lumbar vertebrae are the largest and strongest of the dynamic, presacral spine (Fig. 4). Each vertebra consists of a substantial vertebral body with a posteriorly based neural arch for protection of the conus medullaris and cauda equina. The neural arch is formed by a pair of pedicles, a pair of laminae, four articular processes, two transverse processes, and one spinous process. While this is true of a normal vertebra, lumbar vertebrae frequently display any number of congenital or developmental variations due to genetic or environmental factors.

The vertebral body of the lumbar spine is substantially larger than that in the cervical or thoracic spine. Viewed in the axial plane, the body has the shape of a kidney bean, with a convex anterior surface and a concave posterior. When viewed in the axial plane, the width of each body is larger than the depth, with the mediolateral to anteroposterior ratio increasing from around 1.22 at the L1 level to 1.43 at the L5 level.[14] The average width of the vertebral body in the coronal plane increases at each level from L1 to L5, while the width of the superior endplate of each segment is less than that of the inferior endplate.[14,15] The anteroposterior depth of the vertebral body similarly increases from L1 to L5, with the depth of the inferior and superior endplates of a single segment remaining similar when viewed in the sagittal plane. The lateral and anterior cortices between the inferior and superior endplates are concave in shape, while the posterior cortex gives rise to the neural arch.

The superior and inferior endplates of the vertebral body, as in all nonfused vertebrae, are covered in hyaline cartilage with strong subchondral bone. The edge of each endplate is marked with an area of cartilage free bone, referred to as the ring apophysis, a secondary ossification center of the vertebral body. The ring apophysis serves as the anchoring sight of the Sharpey's fibrils from the disk. The posterior surface of the vertebral body is marked by one or more nutrient foramina, the site of arterial entrance and basivertebral venous exit.

Near the cephalad border of the posterolateral body of each lumbar vertebrae arise a pair of stout pedicles, which form the base of the neural arch. The pedicles contain the strongest bone in the lumbar spine, with the cortical bone of the medial wall being 1.5–2 times thicker than that of the lateral.[16] The concave inferior cortex of the pedicle serves as the cephalad border of the intervertebral foramen for the segment's respectively labeled nerve root while the superior cortex of the pedicle serves as the caudal border of the foramen above.

It is crucial to understand the dimensions, orientation, and relationship of the lumbar pedicles to the surrounding osseous features for safe free-hand placement of pedicle screw fixation. In the past, perforation rates have been reported as occurring in 1.8–54.7% of screws placed, with resultant neurologic changes seen in 0–7% of patients.[17] Knowledge of the morphologic features will allow the

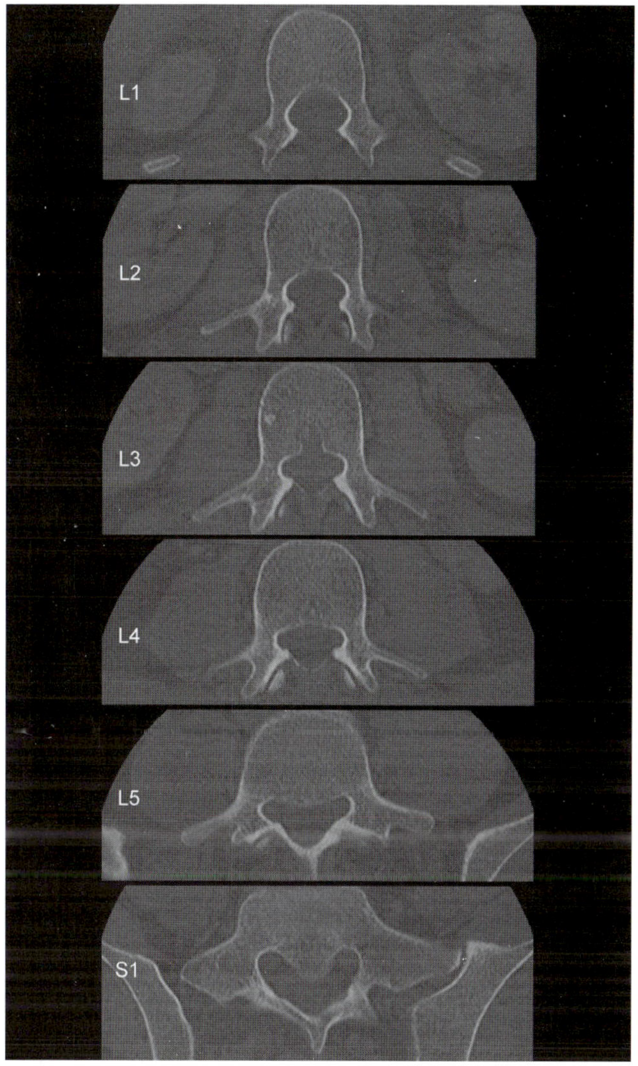

Fig. 5: Lumbar pedicle orientation.

surgeon to select the correct screw starting point, screw length, diameter, and orientation, and thus minimize the occurrence of misplacement.

The lumbar pedicles are generally the widest in the presacral spine. The average width of the L1 pedicle's outer cortex along the short axis (isthmic width) is 8.5 mm increasing to 13.3 mm at L5.[18-21] Inner cortical isthmic width likewise increases from 4.6 mm at L1 to 7.9 mm at L5.[16] This generally allows for placement of a 6.0 to 7.5 mm pedicle screw in all lumbar pedicles.

The pedicles of the L1 segment have an average medial inclination angle of around 7°.[16,21] The posterolateral orientation of the pedicles increases to 8°, 13°, 20°, and 32° at L2, L3, L4, and L5, respectively (Fig. 5). The sagittal pedicle inclination angle decreases only slightly from 2.4° to 1.8° from L1–L5, allowing surgeons to use the endplates on a lateral fluoroscopic image for predictable direction of the pedicle screw in craniocaudal plane.[21] The pedicle inclination must be considered, particularly in the convergent lower lumbar pedicles, as lack of adequate medialization will commonly lead to a lateral breach. Furthermore, appropriate convergent angulation of the pedicle screw increases pullout strength by more than 28%.[22]

The depth from the start point of the pedicle to the anterior cortex of the vertebral body (pedicle chord length) averages around 51 mm, a distance varying greatly amongst patients, but only slightly across the lumbar vertebrae of a single subject.[16,20,21] While the lumbar pedicle itself only contributes 15–25 mm of this depth, it provides as much as 80% of the caudocephalad stiffness and approximately 60% of the pullout strength.[14,16]

Many authors have described methods for determining the center of the pedicle in relation to the superficial structures of the neural arch in the lumbar spine.[18,23-25] This is vitally important for safe free-hand placement of interpedicular fixation. Authors have recommended starting the screw at a point in line with the articulation of the facet joint at the midpoint of the transverse process,[23] at the "nape of the neck," defined as the lateral and inferior corner of the superior articular facet,[25] or at the lateral border of the superior articular process and the midline of the transverse process.[24] Recently, Su et al. has recommended surgeons start at a point in line with the most medial aspect of the lateral pars in the horizontal plane and 1 mm superior to the midpoint of the transverse process in the vertical plane.[18]

Posterior to the pedicle, forming the roof of the neural arch, the lamina of the lumbar spine are short and wide with less overlap than is seen in the thoracic vertebrae. Appreciation of this feature by the surgeon is crucially important to avoid inadvertent penetration into the interlaminar space and resultant dural injury during dissection.

From the superior aspect of each lamina where it adjoins its respective pedicle, arises a superior articular process with a small mammillary process on the posterior border. Emerging from the inferolateral aspect of the lamina is the inferior articular process. In approaching the posterior lumbar spine, it is important for the surgeon to keep in mind the orientation of each vertebra's articular processes to avoid unintended capsular disruption and subsequent destabilization. The superior articular processes exhibit vertical concave articular facets facing posteromedially, while the inferior articular processes exhibit a convex articular surface facing anterolaterally. Together, the ipsilateral inferior and superior articular facets from two adjoining vertebrae form a single facet joint.

The portion of lamina lying between a single vertebra's ipsilateral superior and inferior facet joints and connecting to the pedicle, known as the pars interarticularis, is subjected to considerable bending forces as the energy transmitted by the lamina undergoes a change of direction into the pedicle. To withstand these forces, the cortical bone of the pars interarticularis is generally thicker than other laminar bone in the lumbar spine.[26,27] However, in 4–6% of individuals, despite this cortical thickening, the bone is insufficient to withstand the transmitted forces resulting in fatigue and stress fractures of the pars interarticularis.[28-30]

Arising from the posteromedial meeting point of a lumbar vertebra's laminae is a quadrangular spinous process. In the lumbar spine, the spinous process is aimed almost directly dorsal with little caudal slope and it is thickened along its posterior and inferior borders.[31] The spinous processes of the cranial four lumbar vertebrae are similar, with the fifth being the smallest, baring a rounded and down-turned apex.

Protruding laterally from the junction of a pedicle and its respective lamina is a flat, rectangular transverse process. The transverse processes of the first three lumbar segments are thin and long, projecting laterally and slightly posterior, increasing in length at each level. Conversely, the fourth lumbar transverse process decreases in length when compared to its cranial brethren. The fifth differs significantly from the superior four transverse processes, in that it passes laterally and then superolaterally to a blunt tip and the whole process presents a greater dorsal inclination than the others.[31] Near its attachment to the pedicle, each transverse process bears on its posterior surface a small, irregular bony prominence known as Luschka's accessory tubercle, or the accessory process.[27,32] The accessory processes vary in form and size from a simple bump on the back of the transverse process to a more definitive pointed projection of capricious length.[27] The accessory process is identifiable as the only bony projection from the posteroinferior root of each transverse process and lays slightly inferolateral to the mammillary process, separated by a space known as the mamilla-accessory notch. Between the accessory and the mammillary process, on the dorsolateral facet, runs a ligament known as the mammilloaccessory ligament, which forms the roof of a tunnel through which the medial branches of the posterior primary ramus course.

As in the cervical and thoracic spine, the lumbar spinal canal is bounded dorsally by the lamina and ligamentum flavum, ventrally by the vertebral body, intervertebral disk, and posterior longitudinal ligament (PLL), and laterally by the pedicles and intervening foramina. The shape of the intervertebral canal of the lumbar spine is ellipsoid proximally and gradually becomes triangular at the caudal levels. While the majority of the canal is filled with the thecal sac, the epidural space is principally filled by a thin layer of connective tissue, sometimes referred to as the epidural membrane. The normal lumbar spinal canal has a mid-sagittal height of around 18–20 mm and a cross-sectional area of around 200–225 mm^2, a value that increases by approximately 24 mm^2 in flexion and decreases by 26 mm^2 in extension.[33,34] Symptomatic stenosis has been proposed by Schonstrom et al. to occur at areas of less than 100 mm^2 or mid-sagittal height less than 10 mm.[35]

The radicular canal is the lateral gutter of the spinal canal containing the nerve root, from its emergence through the thecal sac to its exit out the intervertebral foramen.[36] It is formed by a bony concavity, initially directed toward the midline then inferior, that houses the nerve as it exits the spinal canal. The radicular canal can be divided into three parts: retrodiscal, parapedicular, and foraminal. The retrodiscal segment refers to the zone wherein the traversing nerve crosses the disk above its foraminal exit. The second section, the parapedicular segment, commonly known as the lateral recess, runs the entire height of the medial pedicle. Finally, the foraminal portion of the radicular canal is formed by the inferior pedicle as the nerve exits the intervertebral foramen.

In cadaveric studies of lumbar foramina, reported foraminal dimensions vary significantly.[34,37,38] Foraminal height averages around 18–20 mm, while sagittal depth averaged 8–9 mm superiorly and 3–4 mm inferiorly. Together these parameters contributed to an osseous cross-sectional area of around 70–130 mm^2, which is significantly larger than that of the nonosseous area, even in the normal spine.[38] While Hasegawa reported that significant stenosis was noted in 4 of 5 specimens with a foraminal height below 15 mm and 8 of 10 with a posterior disk height below 4 mm,[37] only the latter holds true in a similar study by Inufusa et al.[34] They reported significant stenosis in those cadavers with decreased posterior disk height, midforaminal width, and foraminal cross-sectional area.

Sacral and Coccygeal Osteology

Triangular in nature and formed by five fused vertebrae, the sacrum functions to transmit loads from the dynamic presacral spine to the pelvic girdle and subsequently the lower extremities. While the sacrum is generally a single fused structure, it is important for the surgeon to continue to appreciate the unique markers of each sacral segment to avoid inadvertent nerve injury.

Anteriorly, a longitudinal protuberance represents the fused sacral bodies, the superior most portion of which is known as the sacral promontory. Along this protuberance, transverse apices represent the ossified or vestigial disks. Terminal fibers of the anterior and posterior longitudinal ligaments are attached to the ventral and dorsal surfaces of the first sacral body.[31] Posteriorly a series of midline prominences represent the successively smaller spinous processes. The laminae of each level fuse medially, while laterally the transverse processes fuse to form the lateral mass. Between the fused laminae and transverse processes a set of anterior and posterior foramina arise, which transmit the ventral and dorsal rami, respectively (Fig. 6).

Near the inferomedial edge of each posterior foramen, a small articular tubercle is noted, representing the fused zygapophyseal joint.[27] The consecutive series of articular tubercles constitutes the intermediate crest of the sacrum. Far laterally, the lateral crest of the sacrum is formed by a longitudinal series of transverse tubercles, representing the tip of each fused transverse process.

The superior border of the sacrum is of particular interest to the spine surgeon as many constructs extend to the S1 segment. The superior sacral surface presents a set of posterior facing and coronally oriented articular surfaces, the intact superior articular processes of the S1 segment. In conjunction with the inferior processes of the L5 vertebrae, these form the L5–S1, or lumbosacral articulation. Superolaterally, the transverse processes of the S1 segment extend further lateral than those of the subsequent sacral segments to form the sacral ala.

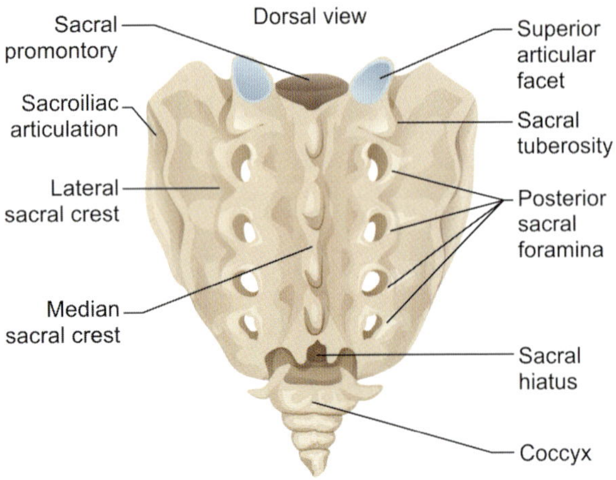

Fig. 6: Sacrum.

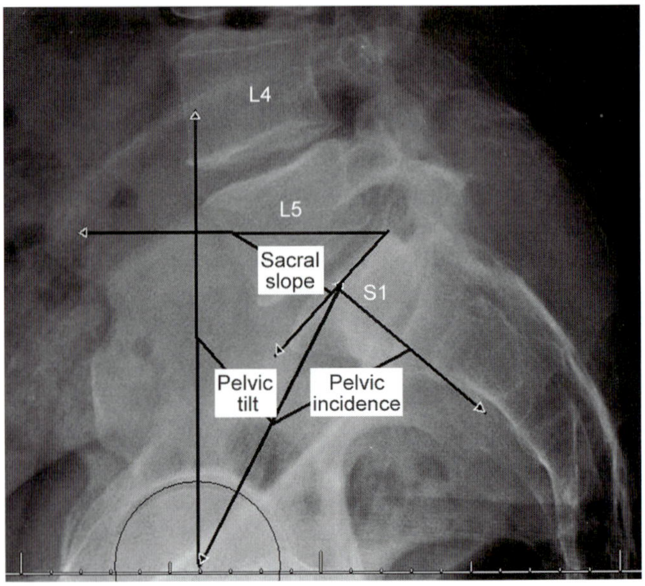

Fig. 7: Pelvic parameters.

The laminae of the fifth sacral segments fail to fuse at the midline, forming the sacral hiatus. At the lateral edges of the sacral hiatus, the inferior articular processes of the S5 segment form the cornua, which articulate with the three to four fused coccygeal segments.

On the ventral surface, the lateral aspect of the ala forms an attachment point for the medial aspect of the iliacus. The lateral mass of the second through fourth segments serves as the origin of the piriformis. The lateral edge of the fifth segment supports the origin of the coccygeus.

On the dorsal surface, the lateral aspects of the fourth and fifth segments serve as an attachment point for the medial aspect of gluteus maximus. Medial to and between the first through fourth dorsal foramina, the multifidus seats its sacral origin. Around the edge of the multifidus origin, the erector spinae aponeurosis attaches.

The sacrum plays a critical role in terms of the overall sagittal alignment of the spine. It is important for the surgeon to have a good understanding of both normal and pathologic alignment of the sacrum in order to assess and treat global sagittal deformity. Three important parameters need to be assessed for complete understanding of sacral alignment: sacral slope, pelvic tilt, and pelvic incidence (Fig. 7). Sacral slope is the angle between the S1 superior endplate and the horizon. Pelvic tilt is the angle between a vertical line and a line connecting the center axis of the femoral heads and the center of the S1 superior endplate. These two parameters are variable and have an inverse relationship with one another. Pelvic incidence is the angle formed between a line perpendicular to the S1 superior endplate and a line between the center axis of the femoral heads and the center of the S1 superior endplate. Pelvic incidence is a morphologically fixed parameter and can be calculated as the sum of the sacral slope and pelvic tilt. Normal pelvic incidence in the asymptomatic adult population is 55° ± 10.6°. The correlation between pelvic incidence and lumbar lordosis has been well described.[39] In general, those patients with high pelvic incidence typically have a vertical sacrum and a high lumbar lordosis. Conversely, those with low pelvic incidence typically have a more flat sacrum and less lumbar lordosis. Consideration of these relationships is the key to assess global sagittal balance prior to any deformity procedure.

While the coccyx provides no structural support, it serves as an attachment for multiple muscles. The gluteus maximus attaches to the dorsal surface, while the levator ani and sphincter ani attach to the tip, and the coccygei attach to the lateral edges.

ARTHROLOGY OF THE SPINE

Special Articulations of the Cervical Spine

The AO articulation is responsible for allowing 25° or up to 50% of the total flexion and extension motion of the cervical spine.[6] The rounded occipital condyles form a ball and socket configuration with the cup-shaped superior articular surface of atlas. The lateral aspect of the articular surface of the atlas is steep to provide containment of the occipital condyles and prevent lateral displacement.

The AA articulation is composed of two lateral joints and one median joint and is responsible for up to 50% of rotatory motion of the cervical spine. The median joint is referred to as a double joint: the anterior odontoid articulation with the posterior surface of the anterior atlas arch and the anterior surface of the transverse ligament articulation with the posterior surface of the odontoid. The transverse ligament of the atlas is the principal stabilizer of the AA joint. It spans the posterior arch of the atlas and possesses superior and inferior extensions referred to as the cruciform ligament. The transverse ligament is on average 21.9 mm in length, 6–7 mm in height, and able to withstand a 350 N load.[40-42] A fibrocartilaginous surface coats the anterior surface of the ligament to facilitate a dynamic pivot interaction with the odontoid. Traumatic rupture of this ligament can lead to AA instability and migration of the dens toward the brain stem. The ligament is prone to congenital laxity in diseases such as Down's syndrome and chronic laxity in diseases such as rheumatoid arthritis.

The secondary stabilizers of the AA articulation are the alar ligaments and tectorial membrane. The alar ligaments are a pair of ligaments that attach the superior aspect of the odontoid to the skull base. They not only stabilize but also limit rotation and lateral bending to the contralateral side of the AA articulation. These ligaments become the primary stabilizers of the AA articulation should the transverse ligament rupture, and have the ability to withstand a 200 N load.[42]

The tectorial membrane is a broad, layered ligament that lies dorsal to the cruciform ligament attaching to the skull base cranially and continuous with the posterior longitudinal ligament caudally. It too is a secondary stabilizer to the AA joint able to withstand a 76 N load before failure.[43] The facet joints of the AA joint are made up of the inferior, caudally projecting medial to lateral articular processes of atlas and the corresponding superior, cephalad projecting lateral to medial articular processes of axis. The surfaces are rounded with respect to each other to allow rotatory motion between them (Fig. 8). The capsules of these joints also act as stabilizers of AA motion.

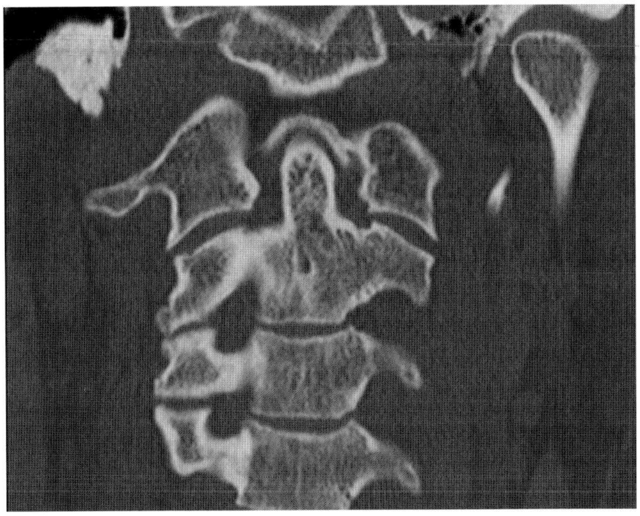

Fig. 8: Atlantoaxial joint.

Intervertebral Joint and Disk

At the junction of any two vertebrae, three joints control movement: the intervertebral joint (the disk /endplate complex), and the bilateral zygapophyseal or facet joints. The first, and most sizeable, is the intervertebral joint between the two vertebral bodies. The intervertebral joint is decidedly specialized, not only permitting multidirectional motion between vertebral segments, but also absorbing and transmitting sizeable, repetitive loads. A single intervertebral joint consists of two vertebral endplates and a single intervertebral disk. Between the two endplates, the intervertebral disk consists of two major components, the nucleus pulposus and the annulus fibrosus, each highly differentiated in both form and function. The posteriorly-eccentric, central component of an intervertebral disk is the proteoglycan-rich nucleus pulposus, constituting the central 50–60% of the diameter, while the peripheral component, the collagen-rich annulus fibrosus, comprises the remaining 40–50%.[44] The major constituent of the in vivo intervertebral disk is water, making up 66–86% of the volume, with maximal concentration in the nucleus and decreasing concentration toward the periphery of the annulus.[44,45] Most of the remaining disk is composed of extracellular matrix, primarily collagen and proteoglycans. Fibroblasts and chondrocytes make up approximately 1% of the disk.[46] Nerves and vessels, while present in the disk, only extend into the outer few millimeters of the annulus.[47]

The annulus fibrosis, the outer band of tissue of the intervertebral disk, offers high tensile strength due to its highly organized structure. It is made up of a series of 15–25 concentric lamellar rings.[48] Each lamella is 0.1 to 0.5 mm thick and composed of parallel collagen fibrils arranged 60° off the vertical axis and alternating left to right in a crisscross pattern between adjacent lamellar rings. The majority of the outer annulus is composed of type I collagen with some of the collagen fibers inserting into the endplate, while others merge with the periosteum and fibers of the ALL and PLL. In the inner annulus, the transitional zone, there is a shift to type II collagen before reaching the nucleus.[49] These transitional collagen fibrils of the inner annulus insert into the mineralized endplate.[50] Functioning in conjunction with the collagen fibrils of the lamellae to absorb radial loads, elastin fibrils make up around 2% of the dry weight of the annulus, with increasing density in the outer margin.[51] Elastin fibrils not only run in parallel with the collagen fibrils of the lamellae, but also connect the adjacent lamellae helping to prevent delamination with torsional loads.[52] Finally, the annulus contains a large assortment of various other structural glycoproteins, such as fibronectin, laminins, and tenascins.[53]

The nucleus pulposus forms the less organized, amorphous-appearing center of the intervertebral disk. Unlike the cells of the annulus, which produce both type I and II collagen in a systematic pattern, the cells of the nucleus produce only type II collagen in an irregular pattern, which serve to link the proteoglycan aggregates.[49] Proteoglycan aggregates are formed from glycosaminoglycan (GAG) chains of chondroitin sulfate and keratan sulfate covalently bonded to a polypeptide core protein.[54] The negatively charged GAG side chains attract cations, which in turn contribute to a high level of water retention.[53] These negatively charged chains also interact with other matrix molecules and soluble factors. The irregular pattern of collagen and proteoglycans within the nucleus pulposus allows for absorption of large axial loads through deformation. Much of this force's vector is converted from an axial direction to a radial direction and dispersed into the annulus. The radial dissipation of the energy by the intervertebral disk results in a load of 60–80 kg/cm^2 across the posterior annulus, putting in place optimal conditions for the commonly occurring tears of the posterior annulus and subsequent herniation of the pulposus.[55]

The vertebral endplate consists of cortical bone covered by a thin layer of hyaline cartilage, on average around 0.6 mm thick and thinner toward the center.[56] The endplate is essential to disk health as the majority of the disk, other than the outer edge of the annulus, receives nutrients from diffusion through the endplate.[47,57] Obstruction of this diffusion, as seen in calcification of the chondral layer in the older population, has been linked to relative nutrient deficiency in the disk resulting in degeneration.[57] The endplate is also vital to joint stability in both traction and rotation. The ring apophysis, at the periphery of the endplate, is the most stable lamellar insertion from the annulus into the vertebra. In the cervical spine, the inferior endplates are concave in the coronal plane while the corresponding superior endplates are convex. In the thoracic and lumbar spine, the superior and inferior endplates are both slightly concave. This is important to understand when performing discectomy work in preparation for fusion or replacement.

The interbody joints of the lumbar spine have a higher axial area than those of the prelumbar spine, an essential characteristic to absorb the large loads transmitted across the lumbar intervertebral disks.[27] Nachemson et al., in a series of studies, showed that the lumbar disks are subjected to loads of around three times the patient's upper body weight in the sitting position.[55,58] These loads were about 30% less in the standing position, about 50% less in the reclining position, and about 30% greater in the forward leaning position. Miller et al. showed that these loads result in histologically notable disk degeneration first appearing in the second decade of life in males and third decade in females.[59] By the age of 50, more than 97% of all lumbar disks are degenerated, even in asymptomatic patients.

With aging, the boundary between the annulus fibrosis and nucleus pulposus becomes less distinct. The nucleus pulposus gradually loses its proteoglycan content, becomes fibrotic, and loses its water retaining properties.[60] Likewise, the collagen within the lamella of the annulus fibrosis becomes less organized resulting in irregular interdigitation of collagen and elastin networks making them prone to cleft formation and fissuring. These processes account for changes in loading characteristics of the disk with a tendency to lose height and bulge under axial loads.[61] They can progress to pathologic conditions such as radial tears in the annulus fibrosis with herniation of the nucleus pulposus or chronic disk bulging with encroachment on the spinal canal.

Zygapophyseal Joints

The zygapophyseal joints (facet joints) of the subaxial spine are diarthrodial joints made up of cephalad projecting, anterior facing inferior articular processes articulating with superior projecting, posterior facing superior articular processes with a surrounding capsule and intervening disk. Anatomic studies demonstrate an average facet joint width of 11 mm with a cartilage thickness ranging from 0.4 mm to 0.9 mm with females having thinner measurements.[62,63] This difference has been postulated to have clinical effects in traumatic situations. The facet joints of the cervical spine are typically angulated 45° in the sagittal plane from the transverse process with a tendency to move toward the horizontal at more caudal levels. The facet capsules are robust and play a large role in cervical stability with the ability to withstand a 61 N load before failure.[64] White and Panjabi classically demonstrated that sectioning the posterior facet capsules produced instability with translation of the vertebral bodies greater than 3.5 mm under normal physiologic loads.[65]

Similar to those of the cervical spine, the facet joints of the thoracolumbar spine are true synovial joints with hyaline cartilage on the articular surfaces and a joint space enclosed by a fibrous capsule. On the superior and medial aspects, the facet capsule blends with the ligamentum flavum. Along the dorsal aspect of the joint, the capsule is about 1 mm thick with the outermost fibers of the capsule attaching about 2 mm from the edge of the articular cartilage.[66,67] This dorsal capsule is also reinforced by some of the deep fibers of the multifidus muscle.[27] Both superiorly and inferiorly, the capsule is more capacious creating subcapsular pockets, which in the intact joint are filled with fat.[68]

Functionally, the facet joints of the lumbar spine have been found to carry 3–35% of the static compressive load and up to 33% of the dynamic load.[69-72] The orientation of the facet, along with the concavity of the superior articular process and convexity of the inferior surface, also plays an important role in allowing flexion and extension, but limits rotation and forward translation of the superior vertebrae on its inferior mate. The inferior facets of a lumbar vertebra lock themselves between the superior facets of the next caudal vertebra. Generally, the facet joints of the lumbar spine are oblique when viewed through an axial cut, with the shape of the joint assuming a "C" or "J" shape with the concavity pointing posteromedial. The angle of the facet joints become increasingly less sagittal and more coronal from L1–2 to L5–S1, with angles off the sagittal plane averaging 25°, 28°, 37°, 48°, and 53° for L1–2 through L5–S1, respectively.[73-75] When the joint takes on a more sagittal orientation it may diminish the protection it offers against forward translation, particularly following surgical decompression, becoming a risk factor for the development of spondylolisthesis and isolated facet arthritis.[76-79] Likewise, greater interfacet width, shorter interfacet height, and shorter, narrower articular facets, have all been shown to be independent risk factors for development of spondylolysis.[80]

Spinal Ligaments

Each functional spinal unit is connected by seven unique ligaments from C2 to the sacrum: the anterior longitudinal ligament, the posterior longitudinal ligament, the ligamentum flavum, the interspinous ligament, the bilateral intertransverse ligaments, the ligamentum nuchae that gives rise to the supraspinous ligament, and the bilateral capsular ligaments (Fig. 9).[81] The spinal ligaments are primarily collagenous except for the ligamentum flavum, which is comprised mainly of elastin.[27]

The ALL originates at the base of the occiput and extends the length of the spine along the anterior aspect. In dissection, the ALL is wider at the level of the vertebral body and narrower at the disk level. Fibers of the ALL incorporate into the periosteum and anterior vertebral bodies of each vertebra, as well as to the annulus of each intervertebral disk.[82] The deep fibers of the ALL connect only a single level, while those of the superficial level may connect 3–5 levels. Functionally, the ALL is a strong, thick

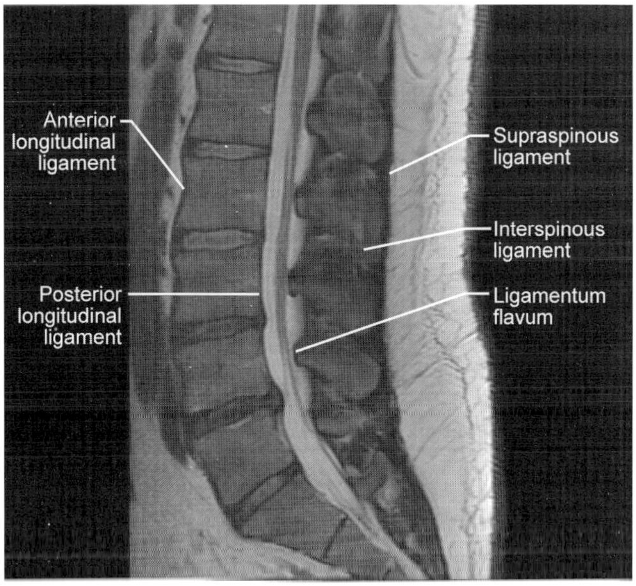

Fig. 9: Spinal ligaments.

ligament that resists hyperextension with a load to failure of around 590 N.[83]

The PLL extends the length of the spine along the posterior aspect of each vertebral body, anterior to the spinal cord. Opposite the ALL, the PLL has a wider attachment at the disk level and narrower attachment at the level of the body.[81] The PLL is less adherent to the posterior body than the ALL is to the anterior and bowstrings across the vertically concave posterior body. At the level of the disk, the PLL is intimately associated with the posterior medial fibers of the annulus but this attachment thins laterally toward the uncinate process resulting in the most common site for a cervical disk herniation. The PLL is prone to abnormal calcification in the cervical spine resulting in a dysfunction termed ossification of the posterior longitudinal ligament (OPLL). Tsuyama has reported the incidence of OPLL as 2.4% in Asian populations with 0.16% in non-Asian populations.[84] The disease process is a known cause of cervical myelopathy and controversy exists over the approach to the cervical spine when this disease process is present.

The ligamentum flavum (LF), Latin for "yellow ligament", lies immediately posterior to the thecal sac. It originates bilaterally on the anteroinferior aspect of the lamina of the superior vertebra and inserts on the posterosuperior aspect of the lamina of the inferior vertebra. It is often difficult to appreciate the bilateral nature of the ligamentum flavum during surgical dissection, as it appears as one ligament across midline. It is composed largely of elastic fibers that decrease with age, resulting in hypertrophy and occasionally infolding toward the spinal cord leading to stenosis of the vertebral canal. This ligament has been shown to have a load to failure of 353 N in the cervical spine.[83]

The interspinous ligament (IL) is a thin, weak membranous ligament that lies interposed between the spinous processes. It functions in resistance of hyperflexion and is easily torn in traumatic situations. The bilateral intertransverse ligaments are likewise interposed between the transverse processes and are usually encountered and preserved during dissection for a posterolateral fusion.

The ligamentum nuchae exists in the cervical spine and lies posterior to the spinous processes and confluent with the supraspinous ligament. It possesses two layers, a dorsal raphe, and a ventral midline septum. The dorsal raphe is a thick strip of collagenous tissue formed by intervening fibers of the upper trapezius, splenius capitis, and rhomboid minor. It is firmly attached to the external occipital protuberance cephalad and the C7 spinous process caudad. This portion has a small attachment to the C6 spinous process but no attachments to the more cephalad spinous processes. The ventral midline septum consists of a thin strip of connective tissue that extends anterior from the dorsal raphe and attaches to the more proximal C2–C6 spinous processes and confluent with the interspinous ligaments and AA, AO membranes.[85]

The supraspinous ligament originates from the ligamentum nuchae at C7. It is the bipedal equivalent of the paxwax ligament in quadrupeds, and extends the length of the spine connecting the posterior apices of the spinous processes. Finally, the capsular ligaments surround each facet joint. The SL, IL, and capsular ligaments are part of the posterior ligamentous complex, which plays an important role in spinal stability with respect to trauma.

NEURAL ELEMENT ANATOMY AND RELATIONS

The spinal cord runs in the vertebral canal throughout the spine giving 31 pairs of nerve roots throughout its course. In total, there are 8 pairs of cervical nerve roots, 12 thoracic, 5 lumbar, 5 sacral, and 1 coccygeal pair. The nerve roots exit the vertebral canal through the intervertebral neuroforamina. The neuroforamen is shaped like a funnel with a narrow medial entrance and wider lateral exit. The nerve root is made up of dorsal and ventral roots within the dural sheath and comprises approximately one quarter to one-third of the cross-sectional diameter of the neuroforamen.[86] In the cervical spine the nerve roots exit the vertebral canal above the corresponding pedicle or ring for which they are named. For example, the C1 nerve roots exits above the C1 ring, the C2 nerve roots exits above the C2 pedicle, and so on. The C8 nerve root is the exception, exiting above the T1 pedicle, as there are only seven cervical vertebrae. The remaining roots of the mobile thoracic and lumbar spine exit below the pedicle for which they are named. For example, the T1 nerve root exits below the T1 pedicle, the T2 exits below the T2 pedicle, and so on to L5.

While the conus medullaris, the caudal aspect of the intact cord, may terminate anywhere between T12 and L3, it usually ends between the first and second lumbar vertebrae, with average being at the level of the middle third of L1.[87] The conus medullaris of females, African-Americans, and elderly tends to terminate, on average, slightly more distal than those of young, white males.[88]

Distal to the conus, the rootlets of the cauda equina do not lie randomly, but are held in position by invaginations of arachnoid.[89,90] The rootlets in the thecal sac lie in a reproducible, layered pattern, analogous to the laminar configuration of the nerve fibers in the tracts of the spinal cord, with the sacral rootlets at the dorsomedial surface and those contributing to the next exiting root most lateral. Each nerve root is formed by 2 to 12 nerve rootlets within the thecal sac.[27,91] The nerve roots from L1 to L5 emerge from the lateral aspect of the thecal sac sequentially, within a dural sleeve, at an inferolateral angle of about 40° from vertical. At the first sacral level, there is an abrupt increase in the acuity of the takeoff to around 22°, with each lower sacral root increasing acuity even further. This is thought to be due to the ascensus medullae spinalis, the cranial migration of the lower cord due to increased growth of the osseous spine in comparison to the cord during development.[92]

As the dorsal and ventral roots of a given level exit the thecal sac, they closely hug the inferomedial surface of the pedicle. The dorsal root ganglia can be found directly inferior to the pedicle as the nerve passes through the foramen, sometimes even overlying the lateral aspect of the disk.[93] At the lateral aspect of the pedicle, the roots converge to form a spinal nerve and then immediately diverge into a larger ventral ramus and a smaller dorsal ramus as they exit the foramen.

Within the vertebral canal, the thecal sac and the nerve root sleeves are secured to the vertebrae by thickenings of the epidural fascia known as dural ligaments or meningovertebral ligaments.[27] These ligaments hold the thecal sac to the ventral surface of the canal until its termination, the filum terminale, which generally occurs at the upper third of the S2 body; although the level of termination can range from the lower third of L3 to the upper third of S5.[87]

The pelvic sympathetic trunk is formed by four of five interconnected sacral ganglia. Superiorly, it is connected to the lumbar sympathetic trunk and inferiorly it terminates in the ganglion impar anterior to the coccyx, which can be treated with an injection or nerve block to potentially relieve coccydynia.[94] Branches from the first two sacral ganglia form the inferior hypogastric plexus, which connects to the superior hypogastric plexus through the hypogastric nerve. Several other branches form a plexus on the median sacral artery.

VASCULAR ANATOMY

Cervical Spine

The vertebral artery is the major blood supply to the brainstem and cerebellum, contributing to the Circle of Willis and providing for the blood supply to the remainder of the brain should the carotids become compromised. It is divided into four sections: V1–V4.[95] The V1 portion spans the take-off point from the subclavian artery to the C6 transverse foramen. The V2 portion spans the C6 transverse foramen to the C1 transverse foramen. The V3 portion spans the exit point of the C1 transverse foramen to the entry point into the foramen magnum. The V4 portion is the intracranial portion where the artery pierces the dura, joins the contralateral artery, and forms the basilar artery. When performing anterior cervical procedures, it is important to have a good understanding of the V2 portion of the vertebral artery. Throughout this section, the vertebral artery lies lateral to the uncinate process just anterior to the nerve root at the middle third level of the vertebral body. An anatomic study by Russo demonstrated an average 1.3 mm gap between the vertebral artery and uncinate process from C3–C6.[96] From C6 to C3 the vertebral artery ascends medially with an angle of 4° referenced to midline and it lies slightly more posterior at C3 than at C6.[97] Therefore, one should exercise caution with anterolateral decompression at more caudal levels. At the C6–7 level, the vertebral artery lies between the transverse process and longus coli before entering the C6 transverse foramen. At this level, extensive lateral dissection of the longus coli could risk injury. In summation, when performing anterior surgery it is paramount to examine preoperative imaging to identify the entry point and course of the vertebral arteries as they are variable. It is also crucial to identify the uncinate process when doing disk preparation work and stay within the confines of this structure.

At the AA level, the artery takes a series of tortuous turns before entering the foramen magnum. In 80% of the population, the vertebral artery takes an acute lateral bend in the lateral mass of C2 under the superior articular process.[98] This bend can occur very high and medial within the lateral mass in some individuals, termed a "high-riding vertebral artery", and is prone to injury during C2 pedicle screw, pars screw, or C1–2 transarticular facet screw placement. Studies have shown that 18–20% of the population has a "high riding vertebral artery".[99,100] Just after emerging from the C1 foramen transversarium, the

CHAPTER 1

vertebral artery takes another turn 90° medial and runs horizontal within the groove of C1 toward the medial edge of the posterior ring before once again turning cephalad toward the foramen magnum. In this area, the artery is at particular risk of injury during exposures for decompressive or fusion procedures. Ebraheim suggested that one should limit lateral dissection of the posterior ring of C1 to 12 mm posterior along the ring and 8 mm along the superior aspect of the ring to avoid vertebral artery injury.[101] A bridge of bone termed the Ponticulus Posticus (Latin for "little posterior bridge") can envelope the vertebral artery as it traverses the groove at C1. This anomaly exists in about 15% of the population and is important to recognize on preoperative imaging as it can be mistaken as a widened posterior arch during exposure, resulting in injury to the vertebral artery during C1 lateral mass instrumentation.[3]

When performing cervical spine procedures, it is also important to understand the anatomy of the carotid artery, the major blood supply to the head and neck. They run vertically in the neck and within the carotid sheath, which also contains the internal jugular vein and vagus nerve. The artery bifurcates into the external carotid artery and internal carotid artery (ICA) around the C3 or C4 level. During an anteromedial approach to the cervical spine pulsations of the carotid artery within the sheath are palpable, helping to identify this structure so it can be retracted laterally to avoid injury. The ICA is particularly prone to injury during C1, C2 transarticular, and C1 lateral mass fixation because of its proximity to the anterior aspect of these levels. In an anatomical study, Currier et al. defined the closest distance between C1 and the internal carotid artery as 2.8 mm.[102]

Blood Supply to the Thoracic Spine

The thoracic aorta runs on the left side of the thoracic spine in an anterolateral position, spanning the T4–T12 segments in straight spines. Kuklo et al. documented a slight movement of the descending aorta toward midline at the more caudal levels of T11 and T12 with a 2.8 mm average distance from the T11 body.[103] They went on to demonstrate that in spinal deformity the descending aorta takes on a more posterolateral position to the left of the vertebral body at the apex of the curve (right thoracic curves), but quickly moves toward midline at the T11 and T12 levels perhaps creating a tethering effect as it traverses the aortic hiatus of the diaphragm. The position of the thoracic aorta is important to understand in both straight and spinal deformity patients when performing instrumentation at these levels.

The thoracic aorta gives off paired intercostal arteries at each level with the right intercostal artery being longer than the left given the left-sided position of the aorta. The intercostal arteries further branch into a posterior and spinal branch before coursing around the thoracic spine and lying posterior to each rib. The posterior branch further divides into the internal branch, which supplies the paraspinal muscles, and the external branch, which supplies the skin. The spinal branch enters the vertebral foramina and branches into anterior and posterior radicular arteries that run with the ventral and dorsal rootlets, respectively. The anterior radicular arteries persist and coalesce to form the anterior segmental medullary artery that anastomoses with the anterior spinal artery. The anterior spinal artery runs vertically in the central sulcus of the spinal cord, providing for the anterior two-thirds of its blood supply. The posterior radicular arteries feed the right and left posterior spinal arteries, which also run vertically along the posterolateral aspect of the spinal cord providing the posterior one-third of its blood supply.

The artery of Adamkiewicz is the largest of the anterior segmental medullary arteries and provides the greatest contribution to the anterior spinal artery. It arises most commonly on the left side at the T7 to T12 level with T10 being the most common.[104] Although it is only one of many segmental arteries, due to its size, compromise of this vessel alone can result in anterior spinal cord syndrome.

Blood Supply to the Lumbar Spine

Discussed earlier in this chapter, the blood supply of L1 through L4 is typical, in that each segment receives its blood supply from a pair of lumbar segmental arteries directly branching from the aorta. However, the blood supply to L5 and the sacrum, from the iliolumbar artery and the median and lateral sacral arteries, is unique and deserves special attention.

The iliolumbar artery arises as the first branch of the dorsal division of the internal iliac artery. Its path begins as it heads superiorly dorsal to the obturator nerve and ventral to the lumbosacral trunk, the connection between the lumbar and sacral plexuses.[105] As it reaches the medial border of the psoas at the inferior margin of the L5–S1 disk, it divides into an iliac and a lumbar branch.

The iliac branch descends to supply the iliacus muscle. Its anastomosis with the obturator artery supplies the bone of the ilium, while also giving off distributing branches to the gluteal and abdominal muscles. It then further anastomoses with the superior gluteal artery, iliac circumflex artery, and the lateral circumflex femoral artery.

The lumbar branch continues its ascent on the posterolateral surface of the L5–S1 disk, supplying the psoas and quadratus lumborum along its path.[106] Cranially, the lumbar branch anastomoses with the L4 segmental artery and in conjunction they supply the spinal vessel to the L5–S1 foramen.

The median sacral artery arises from the dorsal aorta proximal to its bifurcation. It descends in the midline in front of the L4 and L5 vertebral bodies giving off branches, which anastomose with the lumbar branch of the iliolumbar artery as well as the lateral sacral arteries.

The lateral sacral arteries are a bilateral set of superior and inferior arteries. In 93% of specimens, the lateral sacral arteries arise as the second dorsal division of the inferior iliac arteries, with the other 7% arising directly from the internal iliac.[107] In 51% of specimens, the arteries arise as a common trunk then further dividing into superior and inferior branches, while in 47% of specimens they represent two completely distinct arteries.[108] The superior lateral sacral artery anastomoses with branches from the median sacral artery and together they enter the first or second anterior sacral foramen. The inferior branch travels across the front of the piriformis and sacral nerves to the medial side of the anterior sacral foramina where it then descends supplying branches to the third and fourth anterior sacral foramina. The branches from both the superior and inferior lateral sacral arteries, which enter the anterior foramina, supply nutrients to the contents of the sacral canal, then exit through the posterior sacral foramen to supply the muscles on the dorsum of the sacrum and finally anastomose with the superior and inferior gluteal arteries. In their path, the lateral sacral arteries also supply branches to the piriformis and coccygeus muscles, the sacral plexus, and the rectum.

REFERENCES

1. Gehweiler JA, Daffner RH, Roberts L. Malformations of the atlas vertebra simulating the Jefferson fracture. AJR Am J Roentgenol. 1983;140(6):1083-6.
2. Hong JT, Lee SW, Son BC, et al. Analysis of anatomical variations of bone and vascular structures around the posterior atlantal arch using three-dimensional computed tomography angiography. J Neurosurg Spine. 2008;8(3):230-6.
3. Young JP, Young PH, Ackermann MJ, et al. The ponticulus posticus: implications for screw insertion into the first cervical lateral mass J Bone Joint Surg Am. 2005;87(11):2495-8.
4. Hasan M, Shukla S, Siddiqui MS, et al. Posterolateral tunnels and ponticuli in human atlas vertebrae. J Anat. 2001;199(Pt 3):339-43.
5. Ebraheim NA, Lu J, Yang H. The effect of translation of the C1-C2 on the spinal canal. Clin Orthop Relat Res. 1998; 351:222-9.
6. Xu R, Nadaud MC, Ebraheim NA, et al. Morphology of the second cervical vertebra and the posterior projection of the C2 pedicle axis. Spine (Phila Pa 1976). 1995;20(3):259-63.
7. Scoles PV, Linton AE, Latimer B, et al. Vertebral body and posterior element morphology: the normal spine in middle life. Spine (Phila Pa 1976). 1988;13(10):1082-6.
8. Masharawi Y, Salame K. Shape variation of the neural arch in the thoracic and lumbar spine: characterization and relationship with the vertebral body shape. Clin Anat. 2011;24(7):858-67.
9. Adams MA, Hutton WC. The effect of posture on the role of the apophysial joints in resisting intervertebral compressive forces. J Bone Joint Surg Br. 1980,62(3).358-62.
10. Adams MA, Hutton WC. The mechanical function of the lumbar apophyseal joints. Spine (Phila Pa 1976). 1983;8(3):327-30.
11. Masharawi Y, Rothschild B, Dar G, et al. Facet orientation in the thoracolumbar spine: three-dimensional anatomic and biomechanical analysis. Spine (Phila Pa 1976). 2004;29(16):1755-63.
12. Bron JL, van Royen BJ, Wuisman PI. The clinical significance of lumbosacral transitional anomalies. Acta Orthop Belg. 2007;73(6):687-95.
13. Mahato NK. Morphological traits in sacra associated with complete and partial lumbarization of first sacral segment. Spine J. 2010;10(10):910-5.
14. Panjabi MM, Goel V, Oxland T, et al. Human lumbar vertebrae: quantitative three-dimensional anatomy. Spine. 1992;17(3).
15. Masharawi Y, Salame K, Mirovsky Y, et al. Vertebral body shape variation in the thoracic and lumbar spine: characterization of its asymmetry and wedging. Clin Anat. 2008;21(1):46-54.
16. Li B, Jiang B, Fu Z, et al. Accurate determination of isthmus of lumbar pedicle: a morphometric study using reformatted computed tomographic images. Spine (Phila Pa 1976). 2004;29(21):2438-44.
17. Sedory DM, Crawford JJ, Topp RF. The reliability of the ball-tipped probe for detecting pedicle screw tract violations prior to instrumenting the thoracic and lumbar spine. Spine. 2011;36(6):E447-53.
18. Su BW, Kim PD, Cha TD, et al. An anatomical study of the mid-lateral pars relative to the pedicle footprint in the lower lumbar spine. Spine (Phila Pa 1976). 2009;34(13):1355-62.

19. Robertson PA, Stewart NR. The radiologic anatomy of the lumbar and lumbosacral pedicles. Spine (Phila Pa 1976). 2000;25(6):709-15.
20. Chadha M, Balain B, Maini L, et al. Pedicle morphology of the lower thoracic, lumbar, and S1 vertebrae: an Indian perspective. Spine (Phila Pa 1976). 2003;28(8):744-9.
21. Zindrick MR, Wiltse LL, Doornik A, et al. Analysis of the morphometric characteristics of the thoracic and lumbar pedicles. Spine. 1987;12(2):160.
22. Barber JW, Boden SD, Ganey T, et al. Biomechanical study of lumbar pedicle screws: does convergence affect axial pullout strength? J Spinal Disord. 1998;11(3):215-20.
23. Roy-Camille R, Saillant G, Mazel C. Internal fixation of the lumbar spine with pedicle screw plating. Clin Orthop Relat Res. 1986;203:7-17.
24. Magerl FP. Stabilization of the lower thoracic and lumbar spine with external skeletal fixation. Clin Orthop Relat Res. 1984;189:125-41.
25. Weinstein JN, Spratt KF, Spengler D, et al. Spinal pedicle fixation: reliability and validity of roentgenogram-based assessment and surgical factors on successful screw placement. Spine (Phila Pa 1976). 1988;13(9):1012-8.
26. Krenz J, Troup JD. The structure of the pars interarticularis of the lower lumbar vertebrae and its relation to the etiology of spondylolysis, with a report of a healing fracture in the neural arch of a fourth lumbar vertebra. J Bone Joint Surg Br. 1973;55(4):735-41.
27. Bogduk N. Clinical anatomy of the lumbar spine and sacrum. UK: Churchill Livingstone; 2005.
28. Hadley LA. Fatigue fracture of the fifth lumbar neural arch; is spondylolysis a stress fracture? Clin Orthop. 1955;6:110-3.
29. Cavalier R, Herman MJ, Cheung EV, et al. Spondylolysis and spondylolisthesis in children and adolescents: I. Diagnosis, natural history, and nonsurgical management. J Am Acad Orthop Surg. 2006;14(7):417-24.
30. Fredrickson BE, Baker D, McHolick WJ, et al. The natural history of spondylolysis and spondylolisthesis. J Bone Joint Surg Am. 1984;66(5):699-707.
31. Standring S. Gray's anatomy. UK: Churchill Livingstone; 2008.
32. Louyot P. [Comments on the accessory tubercle of the lumbar costiform apophysis (author's transl)]. J Radiol Electrol Med Nucl. 1976;57(12):905.
33. Ullrich CG, Binet EF, Sanecki MG, et al. Quantitative assessment of the lumbar spinal canal by computed tomography. Radiology. 1980;134(1):137-43.
34. Inufusa A, An HS, Lim T-H, et al. Anatomic changes of the spinal canal and intervertebral foramen associated with flexion-extension movement. Spine. 1996;21(21):2412-20.
35. Schonstrom NS, Bolender NF, Spengler DM. The pathomorphology of spinal stenosis as seen on CT scans of the lumbar spine. Spine (Phila Pa 1976). 1985;10(9):806-11.
36. Vital JM, Lavignolle B, Grenier N, et al. Anatomy of the lumbar radicular canal. Anat Clin. 1983;5(3):141-51.
37. Hasegawa T, An HS, Haughton VM, et al. Lumbar foraminal stenosis: critical heights of the intervertebral discs and foramina. A cryomicrotome study in cadavera. J Bone Joint Surg Am. 1995;77(1):32-8.
38. Hasue M, Kikuchi S, Sakuyama Y, et al. Anatomic study of the interrelation between lumbosacral nerve roots and their surrounding tissues. Spine. 1983;8(1):50.
39. Vialle R, Levassor N, Rillardon L, et al. Radiographic analysis of the sagittal alignment and balance of the spine in asymptomatic subjects. J Bone Joint Surg Am. 2005;87(2):260-7.
40. Heller JG, Amrani J, Hutton WC. Transverse ligament failure: a biomechanical study. J Spinal Disord. 1993;6(2):162-5.
41. Dickman CA, Mamourian A, Sonntag VK, et al. Magnetic resonance imaging of the transverse atlantal ligament for the evaluation of atlantoaxial instability. J Neurosurg. 1991;75(2):221-7.
42. Dvorak J, Schneider E, Saldinger P, et al. Biomechanics of the craniocervical region: the alar and transverse ligaments. J Orthop Res. 1988;6(3):452-61.
43. Tubbs RS, Kelly DR, Humphrey ER, et al. The tectorial membrane: anatomical, biomechanical, and histological analysis. Clin Anat. 2007;20(4):382-6.
44. Iatridis JC, MacLean JJ, O'Brien M, et al. Measurements of proteoglycan and water content distribution in human lumbar intervertebral discs. Spine (Phila Pa 1976). 2007;32(14):1493-7.
45. Antoniou J, Steffen T, Nelson F, et al. The human lumbar intervertebral disc: evidence for changes in the biosynthesis and denaturation of the extracellular matrix with growth, maturation, ageing, and degeneration. J Clin Invest. 1996;98(4):996-1003.
46. Roberts S, Evans H, Trivedi J, et al. Histology and pathology of the human intervertebral disc. J Bone Joint Surg Am. 2006;88 Suppl 2:10-4.
47. Brodin H. Paths of nutrition in articular cartilage and intervertebral discs. Acta Orthop Scand. 1955;24(3):177-83.
48. Marchand F, Ahmed AM. Investigation of the laminate structure of lumbar disc anulus fibrosus. Spine (Phila Pa 1976). 1990;15(5):402-10.
49. Chelberg MK, Banks GM, Geiger DF, et al. Identification of heterogeneous cell populations in normal human intervertebral disc. J Anat. 1995;186 (Pt 1):43-53.
50. Nosikova YS, Santerre JP, Grynpas M, et al. Characterization of the annulus fibrosus-vertebral body interface: identification of new structural features. J Anat. 2012;221(6):577-89.
51. Smith LJ, Fazzalari NL. Regional variations in the density and arrangement of elastic fibres in the anulus fibrosus of the human lumbar disc. J Anat. 2006;209(3):359-67.
52. Yu J, Fairbank JC, Roberts S, et al. The elastic fiber network of the anulus fibrosus of the normal and scoliotic human intervertebral disc. Spine (Phila Pa 1976). 2005;30(16):1815-20.
53. Chan WC, Sze KL, Samartzis D, et al. Structure and biology of the intervertebral disk in health and disease. Orthop Clin North Am. 2011;42(4):447-64, vii.
54. Jahnke MR, McDevitt CA. Proteoglycans of the human intervertebral disc. Electrophoretic heterogeneity of the aggregating proteoglycans of the nucleus pulposus. Biochem J. 1988;251(2):347-56.
55. Nachemson ALF, Morris JM. In vivo measurements of intradiscal pressure discometry, a method for the determination of pressure in the lower lumbar discs. J Bone Joint Surg Am. 1964;46(5):1077-92.

56. Roberts S, Menage J, Urban JP. Biochemical and structural properties of the cartilage end-plate and its relation to the intervertebral disc. Spine (Phila Pa 1976). 1989;14(2):166-74.
57. Urban JP, Smith S, Fairbank JC. Nutrition of the intervertebral disc. Spine (Phila Pa 1976). 2004;29(23):2700-9.
58. Nachemson A. The effect of forward leaning on lumbar intradiscal pressure. Acta Orthop. 1965;35(1-4):314-28.
59. Miller JA, Schmatz C, Schultz AB. Lumbar disc degeneration: correlation with age, sex, and spine level in 600 autopsy specimens. Spine (Phila Pa 1976). 1988;13(2):173-8.
60. Buckwalter JA. Aging and degeneration of the human intervertebral disc. Spine (Phila Pa 1976). 1995;20(11):1307-14.
61. Frobin W, Brinckmann P, Kramer M, et al. Height of lumbar discs measured from radiographs compared with degeneration and height classified from MR images. Eur Radiol. 2001;11(2):263-9.
62. Yoganandan N, Knowles SA, Maiman DJ, et al. Anatomic study of the morphology of human cervical facet joint. Spine (Phila Pa 1976). 2003;28(20):2317-23.
63. Francis CC. Variations in the articular facets of the cervical vertebrae. Anat Rec. 1955;122(4):589-602.
64. Lee DJ, Winkelstein BA. The failure response of the human cervical facet capsular ligament during facet joint retraction. J Biomech. 2012;45(14):2325-9.
65. Panjabi MM, White AA, Johnson RM. Cervical spine mechanics as a function of transection of components. J Biomech. 1975;8(5):327-36.
66. Varlotta G, Lefkowitz T, Schweitzer M, et al. The lumbar facet joint: a review of current knowledge: part 1: anatomy, biomechanics, and grading. Skeletal Radiol. 2011;40(1):13-23.
67. Cyron B, Hutton W. The tensile strength of the capsular ligaments of the apophyseal joints. J Anat. 1981;132(Pt 1):145.
68. Giles LGF. Human lumbar zygapophyseal joint inferior recess synovial folds: A light microscope examination. Anat Rec. 1988;220(2):117-24.
69. Nachemson A. Lumbar intradiscal pressure. Experimental studies on post-mortem material. Acta Orthop Scand Suppl. 1960;43:1-104.
70. Grobler LJ, Robertson PA, Novotny JE, et al. Etiology of spondylolisthesis. Assessment of the role played by lumbar facet joint morphology. Spine (Phila Pa 1976). 1993;18(1):80-91.
71. Lorenz M, Patwardhan A, Vanderby R, Jr. Load-bearing characteristics of lumbar facets in normal and surgically altered spinal segments. Spine (Phila Pa 1976). 1983;8(2):122-30.
72. Yang KH, King AI. Mechanism of facet load transmission as a hypothesis for low-back pain. Spine (Phila Pa 1976). 1984;9(6):557-65.
73. Taylor JR, Twomey LT. Age changes in lumbar zygapophyseal joints. Observations on structure and function. Spine (Phila Pa 1976). 1986;11(7):739-45.
74. Van Schaik JP, Verbiest H, Van Schaik FD. The orientation of laminae and facet joints in the lower lumbar spine. Spine (Phila Pa 1976). 1985;10(1):59-63.
75. Ahmed AM, Duncan NA, Burke DL. The effect of facet geometry on the axial torque-rotation response of lumbar motion segments. Spine (Phila Pa 1976). 1990;15(5):391-401.
76. Nagaosa Y, Kikuchi S, Hasue M, et al. Pathoanatomic mechanisms of degenerative spondylolisthesis: a radiographic study. Spine. 1998;23(13):1447-51.
77. Dai L. Orientation and tropism of lumbar facet joints in degenerative spondylolisthesis. Int Orthop. 2001;25(1):40-2.
78. Grobler LJ, Robertson PA, Novotny JE, et al. Etiology of spondylolisthesis. Assessment of the role played by lumbar facet joint morphology. Spine. 1993;18(1):80.
79. Fujiwara A, Tamai K, An HS, et al. Orientation and osteoarthritis of the lumbar facet joint. Clin Orthop Relat Res. 2001;385:88-94.
80. Masharawi Y, Dar G, Peleg S, et al. Lumbar facet anatomy changes in spondylolysis: a comparative skeletal study. Eur Spine J. 2007;16(7):993-9.
81. White AA, Panjabi MM. Clinical Biomechanics of the Spine. Philadelphia: Lippincott-Raven; 1990.
82. Francois RJ. Ligament insertions into the human lumbar vertebral body. Acta Anat (Basel). 1975;91(3):467-80.
83. Devin Leahy P, Puttlitz CM. The effects of ligamentous injury in the human lower cervical spine. J Biomech. 2012; 45(15):2668-72.
84. Tsuyama N. Ossification of the posterior longitudinal ligament of the spine. Clin Orthop Relat Res. 198;(184):71.
85. Mercer SR, Bogduk N. Clinical anatomy of ligamentum nuchae. Clin Anat. 2003;16(6):484-93.
86. Tanaka N, Fujimoto Y, An HS, et al. The anatomic relation among the nerve roots, intervertebral foramina, and intervertebral discs of the cervical spine. Spine. 2000;25(3):286-91.
87. Soleiman J, Demaerel P, Rocher S, et al. Magnetic resonance imaging study of the level of termination of the conus medullaris and the thecal sac: influence of age and gender. Spine (Phila Pa 1976). 2005;30(16):1875-80.
88. Needles J. The caudal level of termination of spinal cord in American whites and American negroes. Anat Rec. 1935;63:417-24.
89. Nauta HJ, Dolan E, Yasargil MG. Microsurgical anatomy of spinal subarachnoid space. Surg Neurol. 1983;19(5):431-7.
90. Wall EJ, Cohen MS, Massie JB, et al. Cauda equina anatomy. I: Intrathecal nerve root organization. Spine (Phila Pa 1976). 1990;15(12):1244-7.
91. Bouchard JM, Copty M, Langelier R. Preoperative diagnosis of conjoined roots anomaly with herniated lumbar disks. Surg Neurol. 1978;10(4):229-31.
92. Villiger E, Piersol GA. Brain and spinal cord: a manual for the study of the morphology and fibre-tracts of the central nervous system. Philadelphia: J. B. Lippincott & Co.; 1918.
93. Cohen MS, Wall EJ, Brown RA, et al. Cauda equina anatomy. II: Extrathecal nerve roots and dorsal root ganglia. Spine (Phila Pa 1976). 1990;15(12):1248-51.
94. Foye PM, Buttaci CJ, Stitik TP, et al. Successful injection for coccyx pain. Am J Phys Med Rehabil. 2006;85(9):783-4.
95. Heary RF, Albert TJ, Ludwig SC, et al. Surgical anatomy of the vertebral arteries. Spine. 1996;21(18):2074-80.
96. Russo VM, Graziano F, Peris-Celda M, et al. The V2 segment of the vertebral artery: anatomical considerations and surgical implications. J Neurosurg Spine. 2011;15(6):610-9.

CHAPTER 1

97. Lu J, Ebraheim NA, Georgiadis GM, et al. Anatomic considerations of the vertebral artery: implications for anterior decompression of the cervical spine. J Spinal Disord Tech. 1998;11(3):233-6.
98. Neo M, Matsushita M, Iwashita Y, et al. Atlantoaxial transarticular screw fixation for a high-riding vertebral artery. Spine. 2003;28(7):666-70.
99. Paramore CG, Dickman CA, Sonntag VKH. The anatomical suitability of the C1-2 complex for transarticular screw fixation. J Neurosurg. 1996;85(2):221-4.
100. Madawi AA, Solanki G, Casey ATH, et al. Variation of the groove in the axis vertebra for the vertebral artery implications for instrumentation. J Bone Joint Surg Br. 1997;79(5):820-3.
101. Ebraheim NA, Xu R, Ahmad M, et al. The quantitative anatomy of the vertebral artery groove of the atlas and its relation to the posterior atlantoaxial approach. Spine (Phila Pa 1976). 1998;23(3):320-3.
102. Currier BL, Maus TP, Eck JC, et al. Relationship of the internal carotid artery to the anterior aspect of the C1 vertebra: implications for C1-C2 transarticular and C1 lateral mass fixation. Spine (Phila Pa 1976). 2008;33(6):635-9.
103. Kuklo TR, Lehman RA, Lenke LG. Structures at risk following anterior instrumented spinal fusion for thoracic adolescent idiopathic scoliosis. J Spinal Disord Tech. 2005;18 Suppl:S58-64.
104. Hyodoh H, Shirase R, Kawaharada N, et al. MR angiography for detecting the artery of Adamkiewicz and its branching level from the aorta. Magn Reson Med Sci. 2009;8(4):159-64.
105. Hassen-Khodja R, Batt M, Michetti C, et al. Radiologic anatomy of the anastomotic systems of the internal iliac artery. Surg Radiol Anat. 1987;9(2):135-40.
106. Ratcliffe J. The anatomy of the fourth and fifth lumbar arteries in humans: an arteriographic study in one hundred live subjects. J Anat. 1982;135(Pt 4):753.
107. Parsons F, Keith A. Sixth Annual Report of the Committee of Collective Investigation of the Anatomical Society of Great Britain and Ireland, 1895-96. J Anat Physiol. 1896;31(Pt 1):31.
108. Poynter CWMC. Congenital Anomalies of the Arteries and Veins of the Human Body: With Bibliography. University of Nebraska; 1922.

CHAPTER 2 Clinical Biomechanics of the Spine: The Nuts and Bolts of Spinal Instrumentation

Fernando Techy, Edward C Benzel

INTRODUCTION

The determination of spine stability and instability is difficult and it can depend on the definition of the anatomical elements involved and the determination of the extent to which they are injured. Instability of the spine can be caused by degeneration, tumor, infection, trauma or iatrogenic etiologies. The study of the biomechanics of the spine encompasses many controversial topics and continues to evolve. This chapter is divided in two parts. First it explores the fundamental biomechanical principles of the intact and diseased spine. Secondly, it analyzes multiple biomechanical and clinical studies regarding different techniques of cervical and thoracolumbar instrumentation. The final goal is to assist the treating physician in crafting the optimal strategy for the management of unstable spine conditions.

THE CERVICAL SPINE

Cervical Spine Biomechanics

Arguably, the most important concept to understand when studying the biomechanics of the spine is the definition of clinical instability. In their classic biomechanics textbook, White and Panjabi introduced the most widely accepted definition of clinical spine instability—"Clinical instability is the loss of the ability of the spine, under physiologic loads, to maintain relationships between vertebrae in such a way that there is neither initial or subsequent damage to the spinal cord or nerve roots, and in addition, there is neither development of incapacitating deformity nor severe pain."[1] Instability of the spine may be caused by degeneration, trauma, infection, tumor or iatrogenic resection or destruction of spinal elements. Multiple clinical and biomechanical studies have been performed in an attempt to define the stability of the spine segment in question and to analyze the properties of different fixation systems, to ultimately aid in the crafting of clinically relevant and appropriate treatment plans.

Upper Cervical Spine: Stability Principles and Biomechanical Evidence

The stability of the upper cervical spine is affected by the unique nature of the osseous and ligamentous regional anatomy. Heller tested the isolated biomechanical properties of the transverse ligament of C1 by simulating an anteroposterior (AP) shear injury mechanism. Two specimens failed by bony avulsion and 11 failed in the mid-substance of the ligament. The mean load to failure was 692 N (range 220–1590 N) and the mean displacement to failure was 6.7 mm (2–14 mm). The study concluded that AP translation of the C1 transverse ligament in relation to the C2 dens is essential for its fracture; and that the rate of loading affects the type of injury (the greater the rate, the more probable a ligamentous injury as opposed to a fracture).[2] When the transverse ligament-dens complex fails, either by mid-substance tear or dens fracture, the greatest increase in instability is in flexion/extension (F/E) (42% or 22°), then lateral bending (24% or 8°), and the least in axial rotation (5% or 5°).[3] The alar ligaments have been extensively studied. Functionally, they predominantly limit axial rotation. A complete injury increases contralateral axial rotation by about 15%. Analogous to the transverse ligament, the rupture of the alar ligaments is rate dependent. They failed at 13.6 N-m at 4°/sec and at 27.9 N-m at 100°/sec.[4] Radiographically, occipito atlantal instability should be considered when there is more than 2 mm of translation or 5° of rotation between the occiput and C1. It is emphasized that significant variability exists from patient to patient, and that patients with rheumatoid arthritis perhaps should be assessed by more lenient parameters. Radiographic instability is observed between C1 and C2 when the atlanto-dens interval (ADI) is greater than 3 mm in adults and 5 mm in children. It is accepted that when the ADI is greater than 5 mm, the transverse ligament is ruptured, and when the ADI is greater than 9 mm, both the transverse and alar ligaments are not capable to provide stability. More than 50% of rotation between C1 and C2 is also considered a radiographic sign of instability.[5]

Subaxial Cervical Spine: Stability Principles and Biomechanical Evidence

Several clinical and biomechanical studies have been performed in order to understand subaxial cervical spine stability. In 1978, Panjabi axially loaded cadaveric necks in increments of 5 kg until failure of the specimen. Dorsal and ventral soft tissue injuries were created. His criterion for instability, after ventral destabilization, was displacement greater than 3.3 mm at the disk level or rotation greater than 3.8°. Likewise, dorsal injuries, resulting in 27 mm of interspinous space widening or an increase in angulation greater than 30° with the axial loading, were considered unstable.[6]

The laminae and spinous processes serve as insertion points for important dorsal stabilizers (the supra and interspinous ligaments and the ligamentum flavum). In a cadaveric study, Goel had reported a 10% increase in the F/E motion after multilevel cervical laminectomy.[7] In another cadaveric model, no instability was observed after multilevel laminoplasty, while a significant increase in motion in all planes was seen after multilevel laminectomy with 25% bilateral facetectomy.[8] Clinical studies have shown that resection of the dorsal elements causes cervical spine instability in children and adults.[9,10] In a recent clinical series, instrumentation was not performed after multilevel cervical laminectomy for resection of intramedullary tumors. No instrumentation was used to avoid implant-related imaging interference on the postoperative MRI in order to more accurately monitor the disease. Cervical deformity developed in 52% of patients and cervical instability in 36%. 16% had moderate to severe disabling neck pain. Risk factors for instability development were laminectomy of C2 ($p = 0.02$) and old age at time of surgery ($p = 0.05$). Multiple surgeries were associated with greater neck pain related disability ($p = 0.01$). The study concluded that only 12% of patients will develop clinical instability and all will need postoperative MR imaging. They recommended that stabilization should only be performed in those who develop clinical instability.[9]

In a 162-patient retrospective case series with a minimum of 5 years follow-up, Jane[107] has looked at the incidence of cervical instability and loss of lordosis after a single level cervical foraminotomy. Instability, as identified by F/E radiographs, was observed in 8 patients (4.9%). Only one patient was symptomatic and needed an anterior cervical discectomy and fusion (ACDF). Loss of lordosis (10°) was seen in 30 patients (20%). Nine were symptomatic and four required further surgery.[11]

The cervical facet joint and its capsule are very important for the stability of the cervical spine. In classic cadaveric studies, Zdeblick has shown that the resection of more than 50% of bilateral facets[12] or more than 50% of the bilateral facet joint capsule in the cervical spine will result in instability.[13] In a Finite Element Model (FEM) study, Voo confirmed that instability, indeed, begins to develop when more than 50% of both cervical facet joints at the same level are resected.[31] When evaluating unilateral facetectomy, even resection of 75% or 100% of one facet joint was more stable than resecting 50% of both joints, tested in flexion and extension. Unilateral complete and 75% facet resection was more unstable than bilateral 50% resection in lateral bending and axial rotation. Unilateral 50% facetectomy was more stable than 50% bilateral facetectomy in all planes of range of motion (ROM).[14] When performing unilateral and bilateral complete cervical facetectomy, the authors of this cadaveric study found that bilateral facetectomy reduces the stability of the joint in 53% and that unilateral complete facetectomy results in a stability reduction of 32%.[15]

Our group has performed a biomechanical study on cadavers to analyze the effects of sequential unilateral facet resection in the cervical spine. It was the first study to look at this variable. The instability effect of sequential bilateral facetectomies or resection of its capsules is well known in the literature and often times, is extrapolated to unilateral cervical facet resection. We found that even a complete unilateral facet resection does not cause any instability in F/E. In lateral bending (LB), unilateral facetectomy remains stable up to the point where 75% of

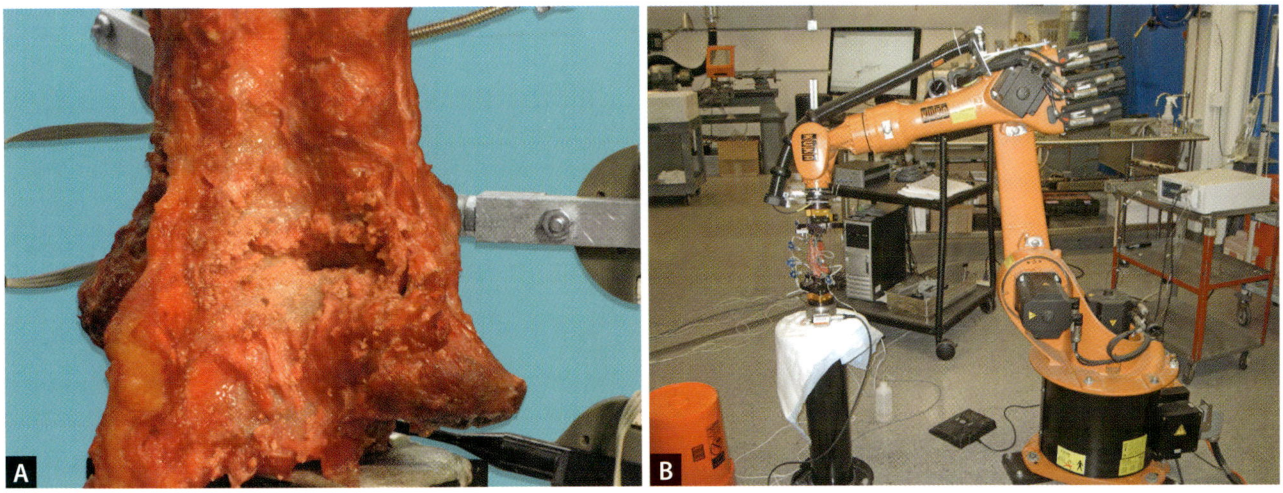

Figs. 1A and B: (A) A specimen with 75% of unilateral facet resection. (B) A 6° of freedom robot used for the biomechanical testing. A six-axis robotic system is a multi-jointed mechanism cable of motion in six different directions. These multiple axes enable better simulation of spinal motion because the additional degrees of freedom. The robotic system comes with a six-axis force/moment sensor which is used to measure the three forces in the principal directions (Fx, Fy, and Fz) as well as moments about these principal directions (Mx, My, and Mz).

the facet is resected. In lateral bending, instability is seen at 100% resection. When analyzing the axial rotation (AR), resection of 75% of the facet caused an 18% increase in the ROM but that difference was not statistically significant (Figs. 1A and B). Resection of 100% of the facet joint was statistically significant in AR. In conclusion, the cervical spine, as assessed by FEM, is not significantly affected by unilateral facet resection. However, significantly higher cervical spine mobility can occur following unilateral facet resection of 75% and above in lateral bending and axial rotation. Our findings suggest that unilateral facet resections are not as destabilizing to the cervical spine as bilateral facetectomies, and up to 75% of unilateral facet resection did not bring any instability to the spinal segment in any plane of motion.[16]

Although ventral discectomy without fusion has been performed for many years, ultimately it was determined that the ventral elements also play a role in spine stability, and anterior fusion after a complete ventral discectomy has become the gold standard of treatment. After a 1-level discectomy (C5–6), Shulte has shown an increase in ROM between vertebral bodies (66% in flexion, 69% in extension, 41% lateral bending, and 40% for axial rotation).[17]

Biomechanics of Cervical Spine Instrumentation

Dorsal C1–2 Instrumentation

Classically, the dorsal fixation of C1–2 was performed with dorsal wiring techniques. More rigid modern constructs have improved the stability and achieved high fusion rates. Biomechanically, transarticular C1–C2 screws, using the Magerl technique, have had a 10-fold increased rotational stiffness and similar lateral bending stiffness to that of dorsal wiring techniques.[18,19] Melcher has performed a cadaveric biomechanical study comparing the stability of different instrumentation techniques for C1–C2 posterior fusion. He concluded that C1 lateral mass and C2 pars constructs have been shown to have superior biomechanical stability characteristics in lateral bending and axial rotation, when compared to dorsal wiring techniques. This same study also found no difference in stability between C1 lateral mass with C2 pars fixation and C1–C2 transarticular screws.[20] Another biomechanical study found that the addition of a dorsal tension band (wires) to the transarticular C1–2 construct improved F/E stability,[21] thus making this combination a popular choice when transarticular screws are selected and the posterior elements were preserved.

C2 Dens Screw Fixation

Odontoid fixation for fixation of the C2 dens has been used since the early 1980's. Initially, the use of two screws was advocated, with the theoretical advantage of increased stability, especially antirotational properties. However, due to the difficulty of placing two screws, as well as the fact that subsequent studies have shown no biomechanical stability difference or difference in the fusion rate when

CHAPTER 2

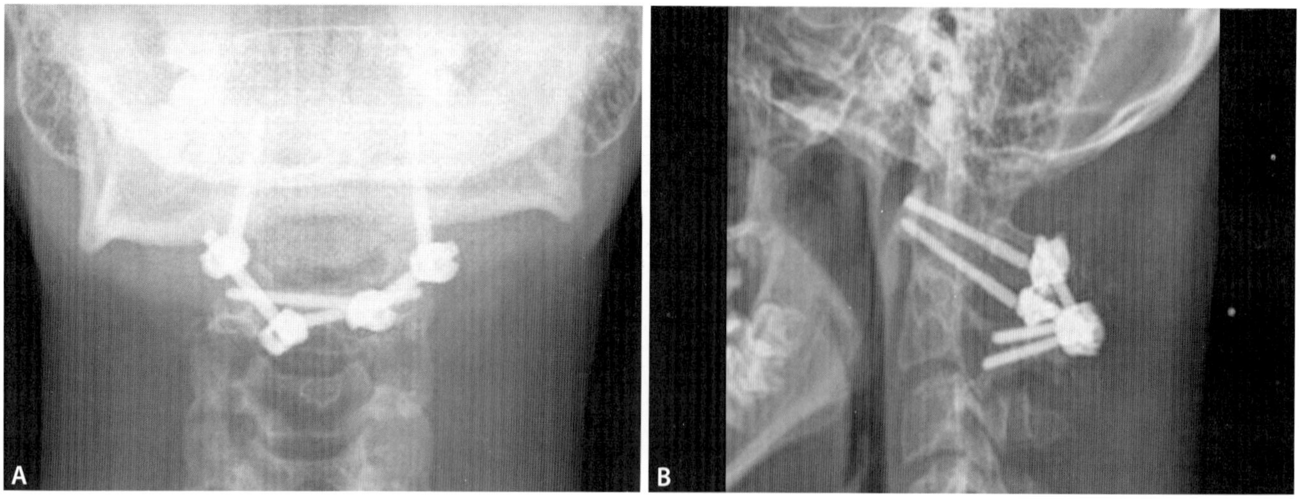

Figs. 2A and B: C1 lateral mass with C2 intralaminar screw fixation. The C2 intralaminar fixation provides equivalent strength as other screw fixation techniques at C2. It, however, obviates the risk of vertebral artery, sympathetic ganglia, and nerve root injury.

using one or two screws,[22] the current standard of practice is to use one screw only.

Dorsal Instrumentation of the Subaxial Cervical Spine

Wire constructs for stabilizing the subaxial cervical spine have been used for decades. In a biomechanical study, Cusick has shown that either facet-lamina or interfacet wiring is able to partially restore (20% of the intact joint strength) the stability of unilateral or bilateral complete facet joint resection.[15] Currently, one of the most popular techniques among spine surgeons for dorsal subaxial cervical instrumentation is the use of lateral mass screws. This relatively easy, quick, and reproducible technique has a low complication rate and overall excellent results. Biomechanically, the fixation strength of lateral mass screws is very good at C1 and from C3–C6. The lateral mass fixation at C2 and C7 is often jeopardized by lack of high quality and sizable lateral masses, and typically other fixation techniques are utilized at these levels. Biomechanically, pedicle screws are superior to lateral mass fixation in any level of the cervical spine. They have demonstrated a significantly lower rate of loosening at the bone-screw interface, greater strength after fatigue testing, and greater pull-out strength when compared to lateral mass screws.[23] Their insertion technique is, however, technically demanding and not free of complications. Cervical pedicle screw insertion has been considered too risky and maybe unnecessary, except at the C2 and C7 levels.

Intralaminar Screw Fixation for the Upper and Lower Cervical Spine

The use of intralaminar screws for the fixation of C2, C7, T1, and T2 has become increasingly popular in the past few years. Low complication rates and high fusion rates have been reported when using laminar screws for constructs at C2 and C7.[24] Intralaminar screws from C3–C6 are not recommended because the laminar thickness of these segments is usually less than 3.0 mm, which is typically too small to safely accept a 3.5 or 4.0 mm screw.[25] Lamina screws are also not usually employed at C3 to C6 due to anatomical limitations of these bones to accept this instrumentation. C2 intralaminar screw fixation has been shown to be biomechanically equivalent to more traditional C2 screw fixation techniques, while decreasing the risk of the vertebral artery injury[26,27] (Figs. 2A and B). Moreover, this type of intralaminar screw fixation has also been used as an alternative technique for patients with intact dorsal elements who need fixation at the upper thoracic spine and the C7 vertebra. At these levels, pedicle screw insertion is possible but can be risky, and the lateral mass bone quality and size is not typically optimal.[28,29]

When extending the dorsal cervical construct to the upper thoracic spine, skipping the C7 vertebra is also a very popular choice. This strategy, however, is usually employed for ease of insertion reasons. Placement of screw in either the pedicle or lateral mass of C7 can usually be accomplished in such constructs, if desired.

Biomechanically, laminar screws in T1 and T2 were only slightly less stable than pedicle screws at those levels, when used in long cervicothoracic constructs (in the cervical portion, lateral mass screws from C4–C6 were used).[30]

Ventral Instrumentation of the Cervical Spine

It is well accepted that the fusion rate after ACDFs has increased once surgeons began using rigid plates to enhance stability. Excessive motion is known to impede fusion, but the absolute elimination of motion can also retard bone growth (stress shielding). There is an exact amount of stability (i.e. restriction of motion or stiffness) that can be called optimal for the fusion to develop. Rigid plate fixation for ACDFs provides a clear advantage regarding stability augmentation and improved fusion rates. It, however, is also associated with a biomechanical drawback regarding the reduction of load sharing through the bone graft. Therefore, a reduction of the stresses applied to bone and the resultant elimination of micromotion at the graft-endplate interface may have an adverse effect on bone healing. The more rigid the plate, the greater the unloading effect on the bone graft. In a cadaveric study, the authors performed a C5 corpectomy, and found that the rigid plates saw 23% of the load as opposed to 9% in dynamic plates ($P < 0.05$).[31] Other biomechanical studies have demonstrated that rigid plates bear even more load when the graft initially subsides, thus acting as a distraction device that can further interfere with the fusion.[31,32]

In order to address concerns related to excessive plate stability and the stress shielding of bone healing, dynamic plates were developed. When considering their use, one must decide how much stability is desired from a construct.

The reconstruction of multilevel corpectomies is a much more complex biomechanical scenario than is plate fixation of an anterior cervical discectomy and fusion. Standalone ventral plating for the stabilization of long strut-graft possesses unfavorable biomechanical activities. Several clinical series report high complication rates of implant fixation failure and graft migration.[33,34]

One study has shown that under fatigue loading (1,000 cycles), 3-level corpectomy constructs significantly loosen after the initial achievement of stability, while the 1-level constructs remain stable.[35] DiAngelo has demonstrated that the addition of a rigid plate to a multilevel corpectomy reconstructed with a long strut graft may paradoxically reverse load transfer through the graft. Normally, the unplated graft would be loaded in flexion and unloaded in neck extension. The plate acts as a tension band placed ventral to the spine. The instantaneous axis of rotation (IAR), in these circumstances, moves from the region of the graft to the region of the plate, thus explaining such findings. The graft then becomes loaded with neck extension and unloaded in flexion. The forces created within this construct can be sufficient to overcome the strength of the endplates and lead to their fracture.[36] Therefore, when reconstructing multilevel corpectomies, particularly those greater than 2 levels, strong consideration should be given to supplemental dorsal fixation, or to perform a more stable, hybrid corpectomy/ACDF construct, when possible.

A ventral cervical plate functions as a ventral cantilever fixation device. A cantilever is a beam supported on only one end (like a flagpole bolted to a wall, or in the case of spine instrumentation, a screw connected to a plate). Cantilever systems can be further divided into fixed moment arm cantilever beam systems and nonfixed moment arm cantilever beam systems (Figs. 3A to C). Fixed moment arm cantilever beam constructs are those in which the screws are rigidly secured to the plate, thus not permitting toggling of the screws to accommodate subsidence. This is called a fixed angle device and is the most rigid of constructs. Therefore, they are the most prone to potential complications associated with excessive stability, i.e. stress shielding and screw fracture (Fig. 3B). Virtually all modern dorsal spine instrumentation constructs are fixed moment arm cantilevers, in which the screw is locked at a fixed angle with the rod.

Nonfixed moment arm cantilever beam systems are those in which the screws are not locked into the plate. Screw toggling can take place and will accommodate subsidence to a moderate degree. These constructs are less rigid than the fixed variant.

True axially dynamic ventral cervical plates permit axial implant subsidence. Mechanisms include implant shortening and slotted holes for screws.

All implants respond differently to various loading conditions. Under axial loading conditions, ventral

CHAPTER 2

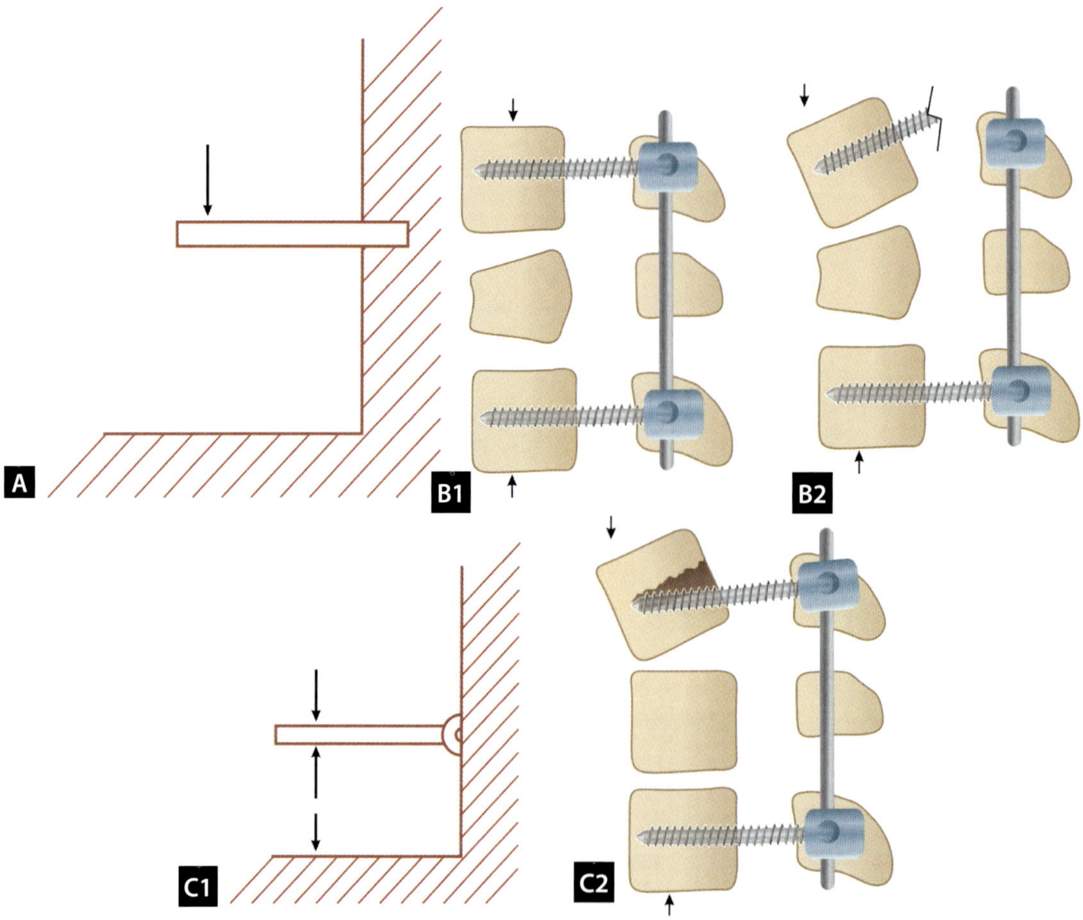

Figs. 3A to C: (A) A fixed moment arm cantilever beam. In this case, the cantilever beam is rigidly affixed to the wall. Note the lack of need for an accompanying applied force vector during the bearing of a load (arrow). (B) The stress realized by a fixed moment arm cantilever beam during load bearing is often maximal at the screw-plate or screw-rod interface (B1). This may result in construct failure at his location following the bearing of an axial load (B2) (arrows). (C) A non-fixed moment arm cantilever beam. In this case the cantilever beam is fixed by a hinge to the wall (C1). Note the requirement for an accompanying applied force vector (opposed arrows) during the bearing of a load (single arrow). Non-fixed moment arm cantilever beam constructs may fail by screw pullout, as depicted (C2).

implants resist compression and, hence, function as a distraction device (similar to interbody spacers). In extension, a ventral implant resists extension, and functions as a compression device. The same happens to dorsal implants with cervical flexion.

An implant can resist three-point bending forces, without an intervening fixation anchor if the spine comes in contact with the longitudinal member. Ventral plates are extremely effective in resisting axial loads and spinal extension. Supplemental dorsal fixation may be necessary to preserve stability in flexion, especially with unstable long anterior constructs.[37]

THE THORACIC AND LUMBAR SPINE

Entire books can be written on biomechanics and instrumentation of the thoracic and lumbar spine. This section focuses on studies that address surgically relevant issues in the treatment of degenerative disease of the thoracic and lumbar spine and the principles of instrumentation techniques.

Adequate decompression of lumbar central and foraminal stenosis without causing iatrogenic instability is certainly one of the many important skill sets required of a spine surgeon. The necessary amount of compressive tissue to be resected (bone, ligamentum, hypertrophied facets) varies with each case. Iatrogenic instability depends not only on the amount of tissue resected, but also on characteristics of the lumbar spine of the patient. In a biomechanical study, the authors suggest that factors such as—(1) low bone mineral density, (2) small intervertebral disks, and (3) absence of osteophytes could predict the development of postoperative instability following lumbar laminectomy.[38] Factors not tested in biomechanical studies, but that very likely play a role in possibly creating instability, are patient weight, age, and level of activity. Abumi performed an in vitro experiment using human lumbar functional spinal units. Range of motion was not affected by the division of the supraspinous/interspinous ligaments in all loading modes. In flexion, the ROM increased slightly after unilateral medial facetectomy. In right axial rotation, ROM increased after left unilateral total facetectomy. Range of motion in extension and lateral bendings was not affected, even by bilateral total facetectomies. The authors concluded that medial facetectomy does not affect lumbar spinal stability, and total facetectomy, even when performed unilaterally, makes the lumbar spine unstable.[39]

Zander has performed a finite element analysis to test lumbar spine stability after resection of different posterior elements. The results indicated that a unilateral hemifacetectomy increases intersegmental rotation in axial rotation. Performing a bilateral hemifacetectomy increases intersegmental rotation even more, while further resection up to a bilateral laminectomy has only a minor additional effect. Hemilaminectomy and laminectomy only differ in their effect on flexion and muscle-supported forward bending. Two-level laminectomy increases the intersegmental rotation only for standing. Degenerated disks result in smaller intersegmental rotations and higher disk stresses at respective levels. Decompression procedures affect the biomechanical parameters less in degenerated than in intact disks. Resection of dorsal bony or ligamentous elements has a stronger influence on the amount than on the distribution of stresses and deformations in a disk. It has a minor effect on the biomechanical behavior of the adjacent region. Spinal stability is decreased after a one-level laminectomy in forward bending, and after a two-level laminectomy for standing. For axial rotation, spinal stability is decreased even after a unilateral hemifacetectomy. The authors concluded that core muscle strengthening and avoiding those ranges of motion that promote instability is probably good after decompression of the spine.[40]

Instrumentation of the Thoracic and Lumbar Spine

During the past few decades, pedicle screw-rod instrumentation has become the gold standard for all fixation methods in the thoracic and lumbar spine. Pedicle screw insertion is time consuming, sometimes very challenging (i.e. cases in which there is a loss of landmarks due to deformity, instability or degeneration), and presents risks to neurological and other adjacent structures. The open technique for pedicle screw insertion also requires a significant amount of stripping of the musculature, and can lead to complications, as bleeding and formation of scar tissue where once healthy muscle was present. Despite the excellent stability provided by pedicle screw/rod constructs, all the aforementioned cited disadvantages continue to cause surgeons to search for easier, faster, lesser invasive and safer ways to instrument the spine. Unfortunately, there are few clinical studies, and all with short follow-up, that provide data regarding technique selection.

Cortical Screw Purchase and Technique

This technique has recently ben advocated by a few authors. The main advantage is related to less muscle stripping, since the entry point for pedicle screw placement is located more medially. Pull out strength is greater than traditional pedicle screw techniques, most likely due to "quality of fixation". In addition, this method also allows the use of shorter screws, diminishing the risk to adjacent structures.

Very few studies have been published on this method. Recently, Santoni et al.[41] suggested that inserting a screw in a more lateral and cephalad direction, from a more caudal and medial entry point than the classic lumbar pedicle screw, provided a 30% greater pull out strength. This is likely due to the fact that it encompasses more cortical bone than the classical pedicle screw trajectory. Others found similar results.[42] Advantages of this method, in addition to improved pull out strength, include—(1) the use of screws with less risk to neural and visceral structures; and (2) a more medial entry point, thus diminishing the need for extensive muscle stripping.

Perez-Orribo et al. performed a study in 28 cadavers and concluded that a bilateral cortical screw/rod fixation constructs provided equivalent stability to that provided by pedicle screw/rod fixation, regardless of the presence of interbody axial load bearing support.[43]

Pedicle Screw-based Dynamic Fixation

Pedicle screw based dynamic or semirigid fixation represents a strategy in which the screws are connected by longitudinal members that are less rigid than metal rods. The theoretical benefits include the creation of a less stiff and less rigid construct. Hence, the adjacent levels would not "suffer" as much as they would if they were located adjacent to a solid fusion. Others argue that these systems could provide the exact amount of stability needed for the acquisition of a fusion. A third application for such devices involves the creation of partial stability at an unstable segment, in order to promote pain relief without fusion.

Many biomechanical studies have attempted to address these questions. The amount of stability required for fusion can only be tested in clinical or animal studies that permit the assessment of fusion rates. To date, no study has shown that semirigid systems are superior in achieving fusion than rigid fixation with pedicle screws and metal rods. Schulte et al., however, conducted a biomechanical study on dynamic semirigid implants and found an overall reduction in ROM at the operated level when compared with intact specimens.[44] Strube et al.[45] showed that the ROM at the operated level decreased significantly, while there was a significant increase in adjacent-level ROM following the implantation of semirigid stabilizers.

Niosi et al.[46] demonstrated that implantation of a dynamic stabilization system in an injury model of the lumbar spine caused a decrease in the ROM of the operated level in F/E, lateral bending, and axial rotation when compared with intact specimens. Gedet[47] compared two different dynamic stabilization systems and found that both systems significantly reduced the overall ROM of the operated level in F/E and lateral bending, but axial rotation was associated with no significant difference compared with the intact state. Schmoelz et al.[48] also reported a reduction in ROM at the operated level; in their study, however, the levels adjacent to the dynamically stabilized level did not change significantly when compared with their intact state. Cheng[49] has reported minimal impact on the adjacent levels following a single-level hybrid construct. Our group has also performed a study instrumenting one lumbar level with bilateral pedicle screws and rigid metal rods. We then instrumented the rostral level with a semirigid system (Dynesys, Zimmer, Warsaw, IN) creating a so called "hybrid construct". The working hypothesis was related to the notion that a dynamic stabilized level would create a smoother stress transmission to the adjacent levels. The semirigid instrumented level was practically as rigid as the metal rod fixation level. "Topping off" the construct, hence, acted as an additional level of fusion with increased transmission of stress to the adjacent levels (Figs. 4A and B). This contrast in findings for the latter two studies compared, with our study, may be attributed to the test methodology used for assessing adjacent-level effects. In our study,[50] we used an established hybrid sequence test protocol,[51-54] while the latter two studies used pure moment flexibility tests with no hybrid sequence testing. The pure moment flexibility test is not an appropriate test to evaluate adjacent-level effects because the application of a pure moment results in a uniformly constant moment at all spinal levels. Thus, following a surgical treatment such as fusion, the nonoperated adjacent levels will always remain unaffected.[51] The aforementioned emphases the simple fact that study design is critical and that one should exercise extreme care when evaluating biomechanical studies. One can design a study to "prove" almost anything.

Another problem with biomechanical studies on semirigid systems is related to the fact that implant materials often behave differently at human body temperature than at laboratory room temperature. Schmoelz et al.[48] had custom polycarbonate urethane tubes manufactured in their study, in an attempt to approximate and account for the effects of the temperature difference. No data was presented on how temperature affected this custom material or its equivalence to the standard tubes.

Presently, there is a lack of biomechanical data supporting the solo or hybrid application of dynamic systems. In particular, there is a lack of information regarding the effect of hybrid stabilization on the levels above the dynamically stabilized level. It is possible that dynamic stabilization above a fusion will simply transmit stresses created by the fusion to the motion segment above the dynamic stabilization, accelerating degeneration over a longer segment of the spine. The more levels stabilized, more motion will be transmitted to the fewer mobile adjacent levels. Of note, several clinical studies have focused on dynamic stabilization as a standalone alternative to traditional fusion.

In a multicenter controlled prospective randomized study (FDA IDE to approve Dynesys as a fusion device),

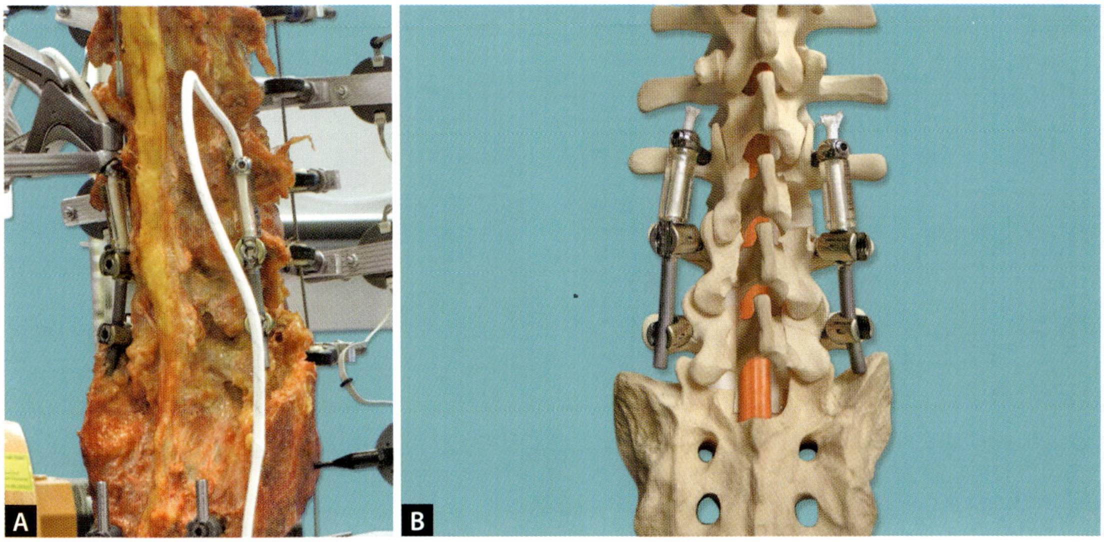

Figs. 4A and B: (A) An illustration of a human cadaveric specimen with the "hybrid" dynamic and rigid lumbar instrumentation construct. The rigid part of the construct is pedicle screw base and connected by titanium rods between L4–L5. The dynamic part is also pedicle screw-based and connected by a system of strings (control flexion) and plastic tubes (control extension) at L3–L4 (Dynesys, Zimmer, Warsaw, IN). (B) Depicts the same construct on a "saw-bones" model.

Welch et al.[55] compared dynamic stabilization to rigid fusion and observed improvement of leg pain, back pain, and Oswestry Disability Index (ODI) in the groups. Follow-up was only 1 year. In a separate study, Kim et al.[56] conducted a 3-year retrospective case series review of 21 patients who underwent lumbar spinal stabilization with dynamic stabilization (standalone) and found a significant decrease in ROM at the operated level and a significant increase in ROM at the adjacent levels. Cakir et al.[57] performed an in vivo retrospective radiographic review of 26 patients with degenerative instability who underwent decompression and standalone dynamic stabilization, compared with decompression and standard fusion. Patients who underwent fusion demonstrated decreased global and segmental ROM, while patients who underwent dynamic stabilization demonstrated preserved global and segmental ROM. In both groups, adjacent-level ROM was unchanged when compared with the preoperative state. Kumar et al.[58] (prospective case series) performed dynamic stabilization in 32 patients, using both standalone (n = 20) and hybrid (n = 12) procedures. Follow-up was performed with 2-year postoperative MRI scans; clinical outcomes were not assessed.

In patients who received a hybrid procedure, the unfused, dynamically stabilized segments demonstrated evidence of additional degeneration in 25% of patients, and the segment above the dynamically stabilized segment demonstrated additional degeneration in 8%. However, interpretation of these hybrid results is limited by the small number of patients involved and the subjective nature of the primary outcome measure. Putzier et al.[59] conducted an in vivo prospective randomized controlled study with initially adequate power. They looked at 60 patients using both standalone (n = 30) and hybrid (n = 30) procedures. A 6-year postoperative follow-up was performed using both radiological (MRI, radiography) and clinical (Oswestry Low Back Pain Disability Questionnaire, visual analog scale, patient satisfaction) evaluations. The study found that the 6 patients who underwent a standalone procedure and 1 patient who underwent a hybrid procedure showed progression of adjacent segment degeneration. The study also found that 4 patients who underwent the hybrid procedure experienced radiological implant failure. Overall, they recommended against dynamically fixating the adjacent level segments with clinically asymptomatic adjacent-level degeneration. Follow-up was up to 5 years and 5/30 from the fusion group and 8/30 of the Dynesys group were lost to follow-up, what unfortunately lowered the quality level for this excellent designed study (Follow-up was less than 80% and the study was underpowered).

Interspinous Process Stabilization

An old site of fusion (interspinous fusion) has regained the interest of many in the past few years due to the development of new instrumentation strategies designed for this purpose. The question that arises in this regard is related to the notion that minimally invasive and easy to use strategies can "bring back" a technique that fell from favor when more stable spine fixation strategies were introduced several decades ago. In 1984 Bostman reported a union rate of 86% using the Daab plate as an interspinous process fusion device. Of note, a dorsolateral fusion (inter-facet and inter-transverse processes) was also performed in conjunction with the interspinous fusion. The indication for the surgery varied substantially (trauma, degenerative, infection, malignancy) as well as the location (3 cervical, 8 thoracic, 12 thoracolumbar, and 20 lumbosacral).[60]

With recent interest in interspinous fixation devices (ISDs), modern biomechanical, animal studies data has emerged regarding this new generation of implants. Wang et al.[61] have found that the Medtronic SPIRE interspinous construct had an equivalent stability to bilateral pedicle screw fixation in F/E, but less unstable in lateral bending and axial rotation after anterior lumbar interbody fusions (ALIFs). The interspinous device was also insufficient to maintain the stability if the anterior column was disrupted. In the end, the authors concluded that the ISD is sufficient to stabilize the segment after an ALIF. Karahalios has found similar stability results when supplementing ALIFs with the Aspen Interspinous Fixation Device from Lanx. They concluded that the acquired stability was greater in flexion and extension (25% of normal motion retained) and much less in axial rotation and lateral bending (71% of normal motion was retained for both ROMs). Nevertheless, the authors concluded that there was no statistically significant difference in stability between bilateral pedicle screws and interspinous devices for the supplementation of ALIFs. They also state that ISDs offer excellent initial stability and are probably stable enough to augment ALIF fusion rates.[62] In our study[63] when using the ISD to supplement transforaminal lumbar interbody fusions (TLIFs), we found similar restrictions in motion of the tested segment (74% for F/E, 5% for lateral bending, and 0.4% for axial rotation). However, our statistical analysis found that bilateral pedicle screws were significantly more stable in axial rotation and lateral bending (bilateral pedicle screws limited the ROM around 70% in every plane in our series).

Bae has created a sheep model to access the interspinous segmental fusion rate when using an ISD. He obtained 100% fusion rate when the device was supplemented with bone graft and bone morphogenic protein (BMP) and 0% of fusion when no BMP was used.[64] Very little is known regarding how this new generation of ISDs will perform clinically in humans. Wang has compared a small group (21 patients) with ISDs to supplement ALIFs to 11 patients with bilateral pedicle screws. He reported no complications, no pseudarthroses, and no hardware failure at approximately 5 months follow-up for both groups.[65]

Biomechanically, our results assessing the stability achieved by the interspinous device after a TLIF are very similar to the other authors' after stabilizing an ALIF. Nevertheless, our conclusions are not necessarily equivalent. One animal study analyzing this issue has shown that when BMP was used, great fusion rates were obtained. This is compared to a fusion rate of 0% when BMP was not used. Clinical data is very limited as well. Older studies were written many years ago when different implants were used and the diagnoses were heterogeneous. All these variables make the comparison of interspinous process fusion devices to more standardized methods of fixation, such as pedicle screws, very difficult. Newer clinical studies currently have very few patients and short follow-up, so that a definite answer on the results of this fixation method is still not available (Figs. 5A to C).

Facet Screws

Two distinct facet fixation techniques have been described in the literature. The Boucher technique (1959) utilizes a facet screw entering into the inferior articular process, just medial to the joint; thus crossing the joint into the ipsilateral articular bone. The second method was described by Magerl. It maximizes the length of the screw by moving the insertion point to the contralateral side of the lamina, through the facet joint.[66,67] Both fixation techniques restrict facet motion, but the length of the screw and angle of insertion are very different.

Facet screws seem to be associated with fewer complications, compared to pedicle screws. The rate of neurological deficit and cerebrospinal fluid leakage associated with translaminar facet fixation has been reported as 25–50% of that associated with bilateral pedicle screw fixation.[68,69] Wound infection rates are also described to be as being 10% that of pedicle screw fixation. Additionally, blood loss, operation time, and surgical

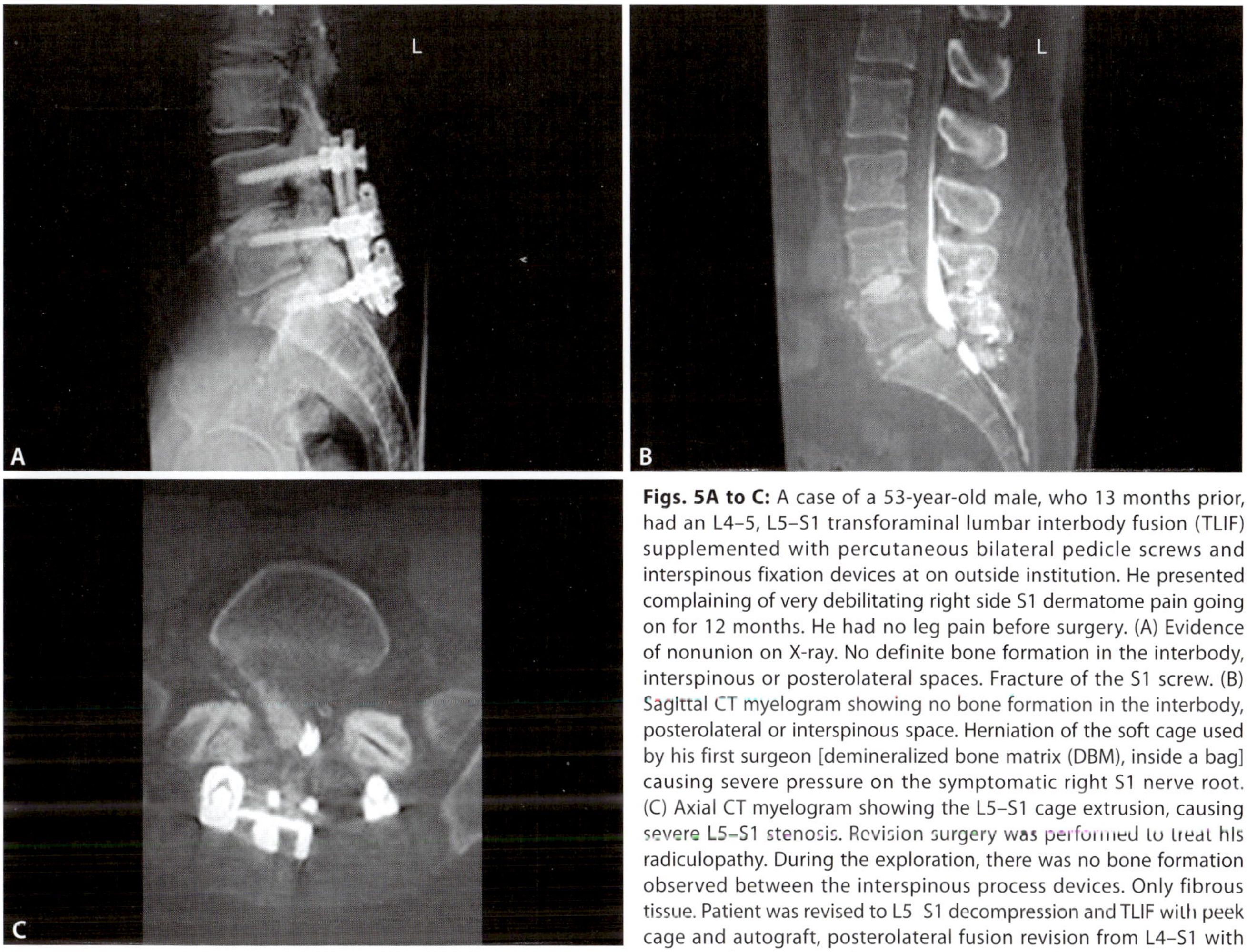

Figs. 5A to C: A case of a 53-year-old male, who 13 months prior, had an L4–5, L5–S1 transforaminal lumbar interbody fusion (TLIF) supplemented with percutaneous bilateral pedicle screws and interspinous fixation devices at on outside institution. He presented complaining of very debilitating right side S1 dermatome pain going on for 12 months. He had no leg pain before surgery. (A) Evidence of nonunion on X-ray. No definite bone formation in the interbody, interspinous or posterolateral spaces. Fracture of the S1 screw. (B) Sagittal CT myelogram showing no bone formation in the interbody, posterolateral or interspinous space. Herniation of the soft cage used by his first surgeon [demineralized bone matrix (DBM), inside a bag] causing severe pressure on the symptomatic right S1 nerve root. (C) Axial CT myelogram showing the L5–S1 cage extrusion, causing severe L5–S1 stenosis. Revision surgery was performed to treat his radiculopathy. During the exploration, there was no bone formation observed between the interspinous process devices. Only fibrous tissue. Patient was revised to L5–S1 decompression and TLIF with peek cage and autograft, posterolateral fusion revision from L4–S1 with removal of hardware and insertion of new screws. His leg pain resolved.

cost are all less than that of pedicle screw fixation.[66] Nevertheless, there exist conflicting long-term patient data when directly comparing facet screw and pedicle fixation clinical outcomes.

Best has found that in a patient pool of 67 patients undergoing 360° fusions of the lumbar spine (24 fixed with pedicle screws and 43 facet screws), 37.5% of pedicle screw cases needed a reoperation, while only 4.7% of facet screws cases required revision surgery.[66] Tuli, however, assessed 77 patients who underwent interbody ALIF or PLIF fusions (33 pedicle screws, 40 facet screws), 27% of pedicle screws cases required a second operation, and 32.5% facet screws required a new surgery. The mean time to reoperation was greater for the pedicle screw group (4.35 years) than for the facet screw patients (2.94 years) cases.[66] The clinical outcomes of transfacet screw fixation, as per the Boucher technique, have not been compared directly to traditional pedicle screw fixation in the literature. The best evidence available are case series, which have reported favorable outcomes. El Masry et al.[70] concluded that 92% of patients had good or excellent results after undergoing posterolateral primary fusion with transfacet fixation. In another similar study, the authors report 91% of patients achieving an excellent final outcome.[71]

There are four biomechanical studies that compare traditional pedicle screw and facet screw technique (Boucher) to supplement ALIFs, and no biomechanical studies looking at this technique as means of primary posterior fixation. Kandziora[72] compared the stability among bilateral pedicle screws and the two techniques for transfacet fixation to diminish ALIFs instability. He found that pedicle screw fixation was stiffer than both transfacet techniques in flexion and rotation, but not in extension and in lateral bending. They concluded that facet screws (both techniques) compensated for the stiffness decrease observed in extension and axial rotation due to the anterior cage placement. In contrast, Beaubien et al.[73] found that both pedicle screws and facet screws (Boucher) significantly reduced ROM at the ALIF level, but that there was no significant difference in the resultant stability for either group.

Similarly Mahar et al.[74] found no differences in anterior column loading and stiffness between pedicle screw fixation and the Boucher transfacet screw construct. In one study, looking at screw pullout strength, the strength necessary was higher for transfacet (694 N) versus pedicle screws (670 N).[75] In a very comprehensive study, Ferrara concluded that facet screw constructs (Boucher) were significantly stiffer than pedicle screw fixation in flexion. No statistical difference was observed in extension, bending, or axial rotation. Moreover, the longevity of the facet screws was tested in that study over 180,000 cycles. It was found that the stiffness remained uncompromised.[67] In a cadaveric study, Agarwala has shown that transfacet pedicle screws (Boucher technique) provided similar fixation to bilateral pedicle screws in primary and circumferential fixations during F/E. In lateral bending and axial rotation, transfacet screw rigidity is, on average, less than bilateral pedicle screws when used alone, but with the addition of additional ventral instrumentation the differences are minimized.[76]

Anterior Lumbar Interbody Fusion

Anterior lumbar interbody fusions are commonly accepted procedures. Most studies, with few exceptions, demonstrate that an ALIF is associated with stability and substantial fusion rates, with or without dorsal fixation. There is no doubt the supplemental fixation with bilateral pedicle screws provides the stiffest of all constructs. Nevertheless, even standalone cages demonstrate excellent fusion rates and clinical results in high quality studies.

In a cadaveric biomechanical study, Gerber has shown that after ALIFs and ventral plating provide the same stability as that provided by pedicle screws in F/E, AR, and AP translation. Pedicle screws were more stable in lateral bending.[77]

Tzermiadinos has found that at L5–S1, pedicles screws are the most stable construct to supplement stability after an ALIF. However, the extent of restriction provided by the ventral plate should also suffice the stability necessary for a fusion.[78] Wang et al.[61] have found that the Medtronic SPIRE interspinous construct achieved an equivalent stability to that of bilateral pedicle screw fixation in F/E, but was less unstable in lateral bending and axial rotation. The interspinous device also proved insufficient to maintain the stability if the anterior column was disrupted. Their final conclusion, though, was that the device is sufficient to stabilize the segment after an ALIF. Karahalios found similar stability results when supplementing ALIFs with the Aspen Interspinous Fixation Device. They concluded that the acquired stability was greater in F/E (25% of normal motion retained) and much less in AR or LB (71% of normal motion was retained for both ROMs). The authors concluded that there was no statistically significant difference in stability between bilateral pedicle screws and interspinous devices to supplement ALIFs in any ROM. They also state that ISDs offer excellent initial stability and are probably stable enough to augment ALIF fusion rates.[62]

Clinically, many have analyzed fusion success following anterior/posterior arthrodesis procedures.[78] Moore et al.[79] performed a study on 58 patients treated with ALIF and posterior instrumentation. His fusion rate was 95%. El Masry[80] reported an overall fusion rate of 97% in 47 patients treated by ALIF, using iliac crest autograft supplemented with posterior pedicle fixation. Sarwat et al.[81] in a study of 43 patients who underwent ALIF with allograft bone followed by a dorsolateral instrumented fusion, reported a radiographic fusion rate of 100% for one-level procedures and 93% fusion rate in two-level operations. Liljenqvist et al.[82] had an overall fusion rate to be 95.2% in a study of 41 patients who were treated with ALIF, using a cortical femoral ring allograft filled with autologous iliac crest bone, and dorsal fusion with translaminar facet screws. These findings are very different from those found by Pradhan et al.,[83] who reported a high rate of graft collapse and pseudarthrosis following "standalone" ALIFs using femoral ring allograft and BMP-2.

Burkus et al., however, reported excellent fusion (95–100%) and clinical results in several prospective randomized controlled studies using standalone cages without plating, filled with either BMP or autograft.[84,85]

Finally, in a retrospective case control study, the authors divided the patients in two groups. Patients would have their ALIFs stabilized either with anterior plates or posterior pedicle screws. They found 100% fusion rate in both groups. Subsidence was greater on the pedicle screw group.[86]

Direct Lateral Interbody Fusion or Extreme Lateral Interbody Fusion

The lateral transpsoas approach for lumbar interbody fusion [direct lateral interbody fusion (DLIF) or extreme lateral interbody fusion (XLIF)] has gained popularity in recent years for a variety of reasons—(1) The technique can be performed using a minimally invasive approach; (2) It provides wide access to the disk allowing extensive discectomy with the possibility of insertion of a large, stable cage; (3) It also facilitates the preservation of the anterior and posterior longitudinal ligaments, annulus and posterior elements, with some authors suggesting that no further stabilization is necessary. Its major disadvantage is the possible injury to the lumbar plexus as the surgeon dissects through the psoas muscle. A larger cage inserted in the interbody space creates a more stable construct. Nevertheless, this will demand a more extensive dissection through the psoas with theoretical higher risk to the lumbar plexus.

When performing a cadaveric biomechanical study, Cappuccino concluded that the extreme lateral interbody construct provided the greatest standalone reduction in ROM compared with literature-reported ALIF and TLIF constructs. Supplemental bilateral pedicle screw-based fixation provided the overall greatest reduction in ROM, similar among all interbody approach techniques. Lateral fixation and unilateral pedicle screw fixation provided intermediate reductions in ROM. Their conclusion was that surgeons may evaluate these comparative results to choose fixation options accordingly.[87]

In another biomechanical study on DLIFs, Pimenta concluded that the larger the cage used for DLIF, the more stable the construct. The 26 mm DLIF cage provided greater stability than the 18 mm XLIF cage with unilateral PS and 11 mm TLIF cage with bilateral PS. The 18 mm XLIF cage with unilateral PS provided greater stability than the 11 mm TLIF cage with bilateral PS. They concluded that wider spacers are biomechanically more stable and, hence, provide the option to be used with less or even no supplemental fixation.[88]

Laws et al. compared DLIF with ALIF. Standalone DLIF was shown to have greater stability than standalone ALIF in all directions.[89]

Standalone interbody constructs have historically been considered unstable in all planes of ROM, whether the technique is ALIF,[90,91] TLIF,[63,91] PLIF,[92] or DLIF with a cylindrical cage.[93] DLIF flat, larger cages seem to be biomechanically sufficient to stabilize a level without deformity or ligamentous instability. This likely holds true because the insertion of the large DLIF cage does not disrupt the posterior elements (like TLIFs and PLIFs) or the anterior longitudinal ligament (like ALIFs).[88]

Clinically, some studies (most by the Pimenta group) report overall good results when using standalone cages for DLIFs[94-96] when no deformity or instability is present. However, cage subsidence impairing the indirect decompression when standalone DLIF cages were used has been reported by the same authors.[96]

During the 2012 Scoliosis Research Society meeting in Chicago, IL, a course on deformity correction using minimally invasive spine surgery (MISS) techniques was presented. The panel was asked if any of them used either standalone cages or lateral plates or rods to instrument their DLIFs. A general consensus was that they absolutely do not recommend standalone or lateral fixation for deformity correction. They also said that standalone or lateral fixation might be sufficient to instrument a one-level DLIF without any or with minimal deformity, however, 100% of the surgeons in the panel, currently, were instrumenting even their one level, no deformity, DLIFs with the most stable construct of all: posterior bilateral pedicle screws.[97]

Transforaminal Lumbar Interbody Fusion

Standalone TLIFs are essentially unstable procedures that require supplemental fixation. Their instability is fundamentally due to two factors. The first is related to the resection of a facet joint to facilitate insertion of the cage. The second is related to the use of a small cage that is inserted through this approach, in order to prevent the harming of adjacent neural structures. Biomechanical studies have shown that even a unilateral complete facetectomy in the lumbar spine causes instability,[97] and that the larger the cage placed in the interbody space, the more stable the construct.[88]

Classically, bilateral pedicle screws, used to supplement the stability after a TLIF, have proven to be the most stable construct of all in biomechanical studies and have become the gold standard of stability to which all other methods of fixation are compared.[63] Clinically, this construct has been shown to be associated with very good results and excellent fusion rates. However, bilateral pedicle screw fixation is reasonably invasive, time consuming and not without risk. For these reasons, other options to supplement stability after TLIFs have been studied and compared to bilateral pedicle screws. Some of them are associated with very similar stability to the gold standard and are likely stable enough to promote fusion of the segment. Other constructs are not so stable and are not recommended. Perez-Orribo et al. performed a study in 28 cadavers and concluded that a bilateral cortical screw/rod fixation construct provided approximately the same stability as pedicle screw/rod fixation regardless of the presence of interbody support (DLIF or TLIF).[43]

Our group compared the stability of an interspinous process fixation device and that of bilateral pedicle screws to supplement a TLIF. The pedicle screw group was much more stable, particularly in axial rotation and lateral bending. The interspinous device was associated with minimal advantage over no instrumentation in lateral bending and axial rotation.[63]

In a cadaveric study, Harris concluded that unilateral pedicle screws are not as stable as bilateral pedicle screws to stabilize TLIFs.[98] In a finite element analysis study, Chen demonstrated that TLIFs with bilateral pedicle screws contributed similar annulus stress at the surgical or adjacent segment; while unilateral screws in the TLIF model showed increased ROM and stresses concentrated on the neighboring pedicle screw, annulus and cage-endplate interface, predominantly in contralateral axial rotation and lateral bending.[99] This may increase the chance for screw breakage, contralateral radiculopathy, cage micromotion, and endplate fracture, as in the reported complications of minimal access TLIF technique using unilateral pedicle screws.[100-104]

In the same study, Chen simulated the insertion of a facet screw in the contralateral facet (TLIF/unilateral pedicle screw model). This new construct provided much better stability and much less stress at the pedicle screws, annulus, and endplates. The authors concluded that the construct with the addition of the facet screw is probably stable enough to promote fusion and better distributes the stresses at the operated level avoiding possible complications. Suk et al. reported comparable clinical results and fusion rates when using unilateral or bilateral pedicle screws in patients undergoing one- and two-level posterolateral lumbar fusions.[105]

Goel demonstrated that unilateral constructs were subject to coupled motions due to construct asymmetry, which probably did not provide enough rigidity after TLIFs.[106,107] Slucky et al. found that unilateral pedicle screw constructs provided only half of the stiffness compared to bilateral constructs after TLIFs.[108]

This chapter is largely based on biomechanical in vitro studies that cannot be classified according to the table of level of evidence for clinical therapeutic, prognostic, diagnostic or economic/decision analysis studies. The clinical studies cited in this chapter were classified accordingly in Table 1.

CONCLUSION

Although the data is confusing, the principles remain the same. A frequent revisit of the principles of spine surgery (which are based on the laws of physics and biomechanics) is, indeed, recommended.

Understanding the anatomy and the biomechanical principles associated with spine instability and spine stabilization is essential regarding the performance of successful spine surgery. The clinician must harbor vast knowledge of the properties and characteristics of the implants available for spine reconstruction. Construct failure rarely takes place due to intrinsic implant failure. It is most often due to the surgeon's inability to correctly understand the biomechanical concepts involved or due to suboptimal surgical technique.

Table 1: Studies on clinical and biomechanical results of spinal instrumentation.

Author	*Type of study*	*Level of evidence*	*Outcome measure*	*Conclusion*
Asthagiri et al.[9]	Prospective case series	IV	Presence of instability after multilevel cervical laminectomy in children	Clinical instability will develop in 12% of patients Deformity will develop in 52% and instability in 36%
Bell et al.[10]	Retrospective case series	IV	Presence of instability after multilevel cervical laminectomy in children	Instability was observed in 56% of patients after multilevel laminectomy for Chiari treatment
Jagannathan et al.[11]	Retrospective case series	IV	Presence of instability after one level unilateral foraminotomy	Instability was seen in 4.9% of patients and loss of at least 10° of lordosis in 20%
Hong et al.[24]	Case series	IV	Early complications and outcomes of intralaminar screws at C2 and C7	Low complication rate (0% associated with screw placement). No hardware failure
Kretzer et al.[28]	Case series	IV	Early complications and outcomes of intralaminar screws at T1 and T2	No complications and no hardware failure
Riew et al.[33]	Retrospective case series	IV	Complications of anterior buttress plate fixation after multilevel corpectomies	N = 14. One graft dislodgement with death. 4 nonunions, 3 requiring posterior surgery
Vaccaro et al.[34]	Retrospective case series	IV	Failure rate of anterior constructs after 2 or 3 level corpectomies	9% of failure for 2-level corpectomies vs. 50% failure for 3-level corpectomies
Welch et al.[55]	Prospective randomized multicenter controlled trial	I-II (follow-up of 1 year only)	Visual Analog Pain Scale, ODI, SF 12	Improvement in leg and back pain for both dynamic stabilization and fusion groups
Putzier et al.[59]	Prospective randomized controlled trial	II (underpowered and follow-up less than 80%)	Radiographic and clinical outcomes of prophylactically stabilizing the adjacent level with semirigid implants	Recommend against it due excessive hardware failure in the treating group
Bostman et al.[60]	Retrospective case series	IV	Fusion rate	The Daab plate (interspinous process) achieved 86% fusion rate in posterolateral fusions
Wang et al.[65]	Case control study	III	Complication rate of pedicle screw vs. interspinous process device to supplement ALIFs	No complications in either group
Best et al.[66]	Case control study	III	Reoperation rate comparing bilateral pedicle screws vs. facet screws	Pedicle screws had a reoperation rate of 37.5% and facet screws only 4.7%
Tuli et al.[68]	Case control study	III	Reoperation rate comparing bilateral pedicle screws vs. facet screws	Reoperation rate was 27% in the bilateral pedicle screw group and 32.5% in the facet screw group
El Marsy et al.[70]	Case series	IV	Clinical outcomes after spinal fusion with facet screws	92% good or excellent outcomes
Margulies et al.[71]	Case series	IV	Clinical outcomes after spinal fusion with facet screws	91% excellent outcome
Multiple authors[78-82]	Case series	IV	Fusion rate after ALIF supplemented by bilateral pedicle screws	Fusion rate from 93–100%

Contd...

Contd...

Author	*Type of study*	*Level of evidence*	*Outcome measure*	*Conclusion*
Pradhan et al.[83]	Case control	III	Comparison of standalone femoral ring allograft filled with either autograft or BMP (fusion rate in ALIFs)	36% nonunion for the autograft vs. 56% nonunion for the BMP group. Massive resorption of the allograft in the BMP group. Study interrupted before statistical significance was reached
Burkus et al.[84,85]	Prospective randomized controlled studies	I	ALIF fusion rate with a standalone metal threaded cage filled with either autograft or BMP	95–100% fusion rate with either group. No statistical difference between groups
Aryan et al.[86]	Case control	III	ALIF fusion rate stabilized with either anterior plate or posterior pedicle screws	100% fusion rate in either group. More graft subsidence with the pedicle screw group
Marchi et al.[94]	Prospective case series	IV	Clinical and radiographic results using standalone DLIF to treat grade 1 spondylolisthesis	Improvement in ODI and VAS, 86% fusion rate
Marchi et al.[95]	Prospective case series	IV	Standalone DLIF cage to treat back pain	Improvement in ODI and VAS, 93% fusion rate. 14% cage subsidence

(ALIF: Anterior lumbar interbody fusion; BMP: bone morphogenic protein ; DLIF: Direct lateral interbody fusion; ODI: Oswestry Disability Index; VAS: visual analog scale)

SECTION 1

REFERENCES

1. White AA, Panjabi MM. Clinical Biomechanics of the Spine, 2nd edition. Philadelphia: JB Lippincott; 1990.
2. Heller JG, Amrani J, Hutton WC. Transverse ligament failure: a biomechanical study. J Spinal Disord. 1993;6(2):162-5.
3. Oda T, Panjabi MM, Crisco JJ 3rd, et al. Multidirectional instabilities of experimental burst fractures of the atlas. Spine. 1992;17(11):1285-90.
4. Panjabi MM, Yue JJ, Dvorak J, et al. Cervical spine kinematics and clinical instability. In: Clark CR (Ed). The Cervical Spine, 4th edition. Philadelphia: Lippincott Williams and Wilkins; 2005.
5. Maak TG, Grauer JN. The contemporary treatment of odontoid injuries. Spine (Phila Pa 1976). 2006;31(11 Suppl):S53-60; discussion S61.
6. Panjabi MM, White AA, Keller D, et al. Stability of the cervical spine under tension. J Biomech. 1978;11:189-97.
7. Goel VK, Clark CR, Harris KG, et al. Kinematics of the cervical spine: effects of multiple total laminectomy and facet wiring. J Orthop Res. 1988;6:611-9.
8. Nowinski GP, Visarius H, Nolte LP, et al. A biomechanical comparison of cervical laminoplasty and cervical laminectomy with progressive facetectomy. Spine. 1993;18:1995-2004.
9. Asthagiri AR, Mehta GU, Butman JA, et al. Long-term stability after multilevel cervical laminectomy for spinal cord tumor resection in von Hippel-Lindau disease. J Neurosurg Spine. 2011;14:444-52.
10. Bell DF, Walker JL, O'Connor G, et al. Spinal deformity after multilevel cervical laminectomy in children. Spine. 1994;19:406-11.
11. Jagannathan J, Sherman JH, Szabo T, et al. The posterior cervical foraminotomy in the treatment of cervical disc/osteophyte disease: a single-surgeon experience with a minimum of 5 years' clinical and radiographic follow-up. J Neurosurg Spine. 2009;10(4):347-56.
12. Zdeblick TA, Abitbol JJ, Kunz DN. Cervical stability after sequential capsule resection. Spine. 1993;18(14):2005-8.
13. Zdeblick TA, Zou D, Warden KE, et al. Cervical stability after foraminotomy. A biomechanical in vitro analysis. J Bone Joint Surg Am. 1992;74:22-7.
14. Voo LM, Kumaresan S, Yoganandan N, et al. Finite element analysis of cervical facetectomy. Spine. 1997;22(9):964-9.
15. Cuisick JF, Yoganandan N, Pintar F, et al. Biomechanics of cervical spine facetectomy and fixation techniques. Spine. 1988;13(7):808-12.
16. Techy F, Tolhurst S, Magewasran P, et al. Effects of Sequential Unilateral Facetectomy on Cervical Spinal Stability. Presented at the 2013 AAOS meeting. Chicago, IL.
17. Schulte KR, Clark CR, Goel VK. Kinematics of the cervical spine following discectomy and stabilization. Spine. 1989;14:1116-21.
18. Grob D, Crisco JJ III, Panjabi MM, et al. Biomechanical evaluation of four different posterior atlantoaxial fixation techniques. Spine. 1992;17:480-90.
19. Montesano PX, Juach EC, Anderson PA, et al. Biomechanics of cervical spine internal fixation. Spine. 1991;16:S10-6.

20. Melcher RP, Puttlitz CM, Kleinstueck FS, et al. Biomechanical testing of posterior atlantoaxial fixation techniques. Spine. 2002;27(22):2435-40.
21. Henriques T, Cunningham BW, Olerud C, et al. Biomechanical comparison of five different atlantoaxial posterior fixation techniques. Spine. 2000;25(22):2877-83.
22. Sasso R, Doherty BJ, Crawford MJ, et al. Biomechanics of odontoid fracture fixation. Comparison of the one- and two-screw technique. Spine. 1993;18:1950-3.
23. Johnston TL, Karaikovic EE, Lautenschlager EP, et al. Cervical pedicle screws vs. lateral mass screws: uniplanar fatigue analysis and residual pullout strengths. Spine J. 2006;6(6):667-72.
24. Hong JT, Yi JS, Kim JT, et al. Clinical and radiologic outcome of laminar screw at C2 and C7 for posterior instrumentation—review of 25 cases and comparison of C2 and C7 intralaminar screw fixation. World Neurosurg. 2010;73(2):112-8.
25. Nakanishi K, Tanaka M, Sugimoto Y, et al. Application of laminar screws to posterior fusion of cervical spine: measurement of the cervical vertebral arch diameter with a navigation system. Spine. 2008;33:620-3.
26. Cassinelli EH, Lee M, Skalak A, et al. Anatomic considerations for the placement of C2 laminar screws. Spine. 2006;31:2767-71.
27. Gorek J, Acaroglu E, Berven S, et al. Constructs incorporating intralaminar C2 screws provide rigid stability for atlantoaxial fixation. Spine. 2005;30:1513-8.
28. Kretzer RM, Sciubba DM, Bagley CA, et al. Translaminar screw fixation in the upper thoracic spine. J Neurosurg Spine. 2006;5:527-33.
29. Xing-guo L, Yun H, Yan Z, et al. Applied anatomy of the lower cervical pedicle screw insertion. Chin J Traumatol. 2007;10:299-305.
30. McGirt MJ, Sutter EG, Xu R, et al. Biomechanical comparison of translaminar screw versus pedicle screws at T1 and T2 in long subaxial cervical constructs. Neurosurgery. 2009;65:167-72.
31. Reidy D, Finkelstein J, Nagpurkar A, et al. Cervical spine loading characteristics in a cadaveric C5 corpectomy model using a static and dynamic plate. J Spinal Disord Tech. 2004;17:117-22.
32. Brodke DS, Gollogly S, Alexander Mohr R, et al. Dynamic cervical plates: biomechanical evaluation of load sharing and stiffness. Spine. 2001;26:1324-9.
33. Riew KD, Sethi NS, Devney J, et al. Complications of buttress plate stabilization of cervical corpectomy. Spine (Phila Pa 1976). 1999;24(22):2404-10.
34. Vaccaro AR, Falatyn SP, Scuderi GJ, et al. Early failure of long segment anterior cervical plate fixation. J Spinal Disord. 1998;11(5):410-5.
35. Isomi T, Panjabi MM, Wang JL, et al. Stabilizing potential of anterior cervical plates in multilevel corpectomies. Spine. 1999;24:2219-23.
36. DiAngelo DJ, Foley KT, Vossel KA, et al. Anterior cervical plating reverses load transfer through multilevel strut grafts. Spine. 2000;25:783-95.
37. Benzel E. Ventral Subaxial Spine Constructs in Biomechanics of Spine Stabilization. New York, NY: Thieme Medical Publishers, 2001. pp. 239-53.
38. Bisschop A, van Royen BJ, Mullender MG, et al. Which factors prognosticate spinal instability following lumbar laminectomy? Eur Spine J. 2012;21:2640-8.
39. Abumi K, Panjabi MM, Kramer KM. Biomechanical evaluation of lumbar spinal stability after graded facetectomies. Spine (Phila Pa 1976). 1990;15(11):1142-7.
40. Zander T, Rohlmann A, Klöckner C, et al. Influence of graded facetectomy and laminectomy on spinal biomechanics. Eur Spine J. 2003;12:427-34.
41. Santoni BG, Hynes RA, McGilvray KC, et al. Cortical bone trajectory for lumbar pedicle screws. Spine J. 2009;9:366-73.
42. Daftari TK, Horton WC, Hutton WC. Correlations between screw hole preparation, torque of insertion, and pullout strength for spinal screws. J Spinal Disord. 1994;7:139-45.
43. Perez-Orribo L, Kalb S, Reyes PM, et al. Biomechanics of lumbar cortical screw-rod fixation versus pedicle screw-rod fixation with and without interbody support. Spine (Phila Pa 1976). 2013;38(8):635-41.
44. Schulte TL, Hurschler C, Haversath M, et al. The effect of dynamic, semi-rigid implants on the range of motion of lumbar motion segments after decompression. Eur Spine J. 2008;17:1057-65.
45. Strube P, Tohtz S, Hoff E, et al. Dynamic stabilization adjacent to single-level fusion: part I. Biomechanical effects on lumbar spinal motion. Eur Spine J. 2010;19:2171-80.
46. Niosi CA, Zhu QA, Wilson DC, et al. Biomechanical characterization of the three-dimensional kinematic behaviour of the Dynesys dynamic stabilization system: an in vitro study. Eur Spine J. 2006;15:913-22.
47. Gédet P, Haschtmann D, Thistlethwaite PA, et al. Comparative biomechanical investigation of a modular dynamic lumbar stabilization system and the Dynesys system. Eur Spine J. 2009;18:1504-11.
48. Schmoelz W, Huber JF, Nydegger T, et al. Dynamic stabilization of the lumbar spine and its effect on adjacent segments: an in vitro experiment. J Spinal Disord Tech. 2003;16:418-23.
49. Cheng BC, Gordon J, Cheng J, et al. Immediate biomechanical effects of lumbar posterior dynamic stabilization above a circumferential fusion. Spine (Phila Pa 1976). 2007;32:2551-7.
50. Mageswaran P, Techy F, Colbrunn R, et al. Hybrid dynamic stabilization: a biomechanical assessment of adjacent and supradjacent levels of the lumbar spine. J Neurosurg Spine. 2012;17(3):232-42.
51. Panjabi MM. Hybrid multidirectional test method to evaluate spinal adjacent-level effects. Clin Biomech (Bristol, Avon). 2007;22:257-65.
52. Panjabi MM, Henderson G, Abjornson C, et al. Multidirectional testing of one- and two-level ProDisc-L versus simulated fusions. Spine (Phila Pa 1976). 2007;32:1311-9.
53. Panjabi MM, Henderson G, James Y, et al. StabilimaxNZ® versus simulated fusion: evaluation of adjacent level effects. Eur Spine J. 2007;16:2159-65.
54. Panjabi MM, Malcolmson G, Teng E, et al. Hybrid testing of lumbar CHARITE discs versus fusions. Spine (Phila Pa 1976) 2007;32:959-67.

CHAPTER 2

55. Welch WC, Cheng BC, Awad TE, et al. Clinical outcomes of the Dynesys dynamic neutralization system: 1 year preliminary results. Neurosurg Focus. 2007;22(1):E8.
56. Kim CH, Chung CK, Jahng TA. Comparisons of outcomes after single or multilevel dynamic stabilization: effects on adjacent segment. J Spinal Disord Tech. 2011;24:60-7.
57. Cakir B, Carazzo C, Schmidt R, et al. Adjacent segment mobility after rigid and semirigid instrumentation of the lumbar spine. Spine (Phila Pa 1976). 2009;34:1287-91.
58. Kumar A, Beastall J, Hughes J, et al. Disc changes in the bridged and adjacent segments after Dynesys dynamic stabilization system after two years. Spine (Phila Pa 1976). 2008;33:2909-14.
59. Putzier M, Hoff E, Tohtz S, et al. Dynamic stabilization adjacent to single-level fusion: part II. No clinical benefit for asymptomatic, initially degenerated adjacent segments after 6 years follow-up. Eur Spine J. 2010;19:2181-9.
60. Böstman O, Myllynen P, Riska EB. Posterior spinal fusion using internal fixation with the Daab plate. Acta Orthop Scand. 1984;55:310-4.
61. Wang CJ, Haid Jr WR, Miller JS, et al. Comparison of CD HORIZON SPIRE spinous process plate stabilization and pedicle screw fixation after anterior lumbar interbody fusion. J Neurosurg Spine. 2006;4(2):132-6.
62. Karahalios DG, Kaibara T, Porter RW, et al. Biomechanics of a lumbar interspinous anchor with anterior lumbar interbody fusion. Laboratory investigation. J Neurosurg Spine. 2010;12:372-80.
63. Techy F, Gilbertson L, Mageswaran P, et al. Comparison of different posterior instrumentation systems in achieving stability to supplement transforaminal lumbar interbody fusions (TLIFs). A Biomechanical cadaver study. Spine J. 2011;11(10S):151S.
64. Bae H, Ashraf N, Kanim LEA. Evaluation of Interlaminar Lumbar Instrumented Fusion (ILIF) in a Sheep Model. Abstract 617 from the 17th IMAST, 2010– Toronto, ON.
65. Wang JC, Spenciner D, Robinson JC. SPIRE spinous process stabilization plate: biomechanical evaluation of a novel technology. Invited submission from the Joint Section Meeting on Disorders of the Spine and Peripheral Nerves, March 2005. J Neurosurg Spine. 2006;4:160-4.
66. Best NM, Sasso RC. Efficacy of translaminar facet screw fixation in circumferential interbody fusions as compared to pedicle screw fixation. J Spinal Disord Tech. 2006;19:98-103.
67. Ferrara LA, Secor JL, Jin BH, et al. A biomechanical comparison of facet screw fixation and pedicle screw fixation: effects of short-term and long-term repetitive cycling. Spine. 2003;28:1226-34.
68. Tuli J, Tuli S, Eichler ME, et al. A comparison of long-term outcomes of translaminar facet screw fixation and pedicle screw fixation: a prospective study. J Neurosurg Spine. 2007;7:287-92.
69. Grob D, Rubeli M, Scheier HJ, et al. Translaminar screw fixation of the lumbar spine. Int Orthop. 1992;16:223-6.
70. El Masry MA, McAllen CJ, Weatherley CR. Lumbosacral fusion using the Boucher technique in combination with a posterolateral bone graft. Eur Spine J. 2003;12:408-12.
71. Margulies JY, Seimon LP. Clinical efficacy of lumbar and lumbosacral fusion using the Boucher facet screw fixation technique. Bull Hosp Joint Dis. 2000;59:33-9.
72. Kandziora F, Schleicher P, Scholz M. et al. Biomechanical testing of the lumbar facet interference screw. Spine. 2005; 30:E34-9.
73. Beaubien BP, Mehbod AA, Kallemeier PM, et al. Posterior augmentation of an anterior lumbar interbody fusion: minimally invasive fixation versus pedicle screws in vitro. Spine. 2004;29:E406-12.
74. Mahar A, Kim C, Oka R, et al. Biomechanical comparison of a novel percutaneous transfacet device and a traditional posterior system for single level fusion. J Spinal Disord Tech. 2006;19:591-4.
75. Liu GY, Xu RM, Ma WH, et al. Biomechanical comparison of cervical transfacet pedicle screws versus pedicle screws. Chin Med J (Engl). 2008;121:1390-3.
76. Agarwala A, Bucklen B, Muzumdar A, et al. Do facet screws provide the required stability in lumbar fixation? A biomechanical comparison of the Boucher technique and pedicular fixation in primary and circumferential fusions. Clin Biomech (Bristol, Avon). 2012;27(1):64-70.
77. Gerber M, Crawford NR, Chamberlain RH. Biomechanical assessment of anterior lumbar interbody fusion with an anterior lumbosacral fixation screw-plate: comparison to stand-alone anterior lumbar interbody fusion and anterior lumbar interbody fusion with pedicle screws in an unstable human cadaver model. Spine (Phila Pa 1976). 2006;31(7):762-8.
78. Tzermiadianos MN, Mekhail A, Voronov LI, et al. Enhancing the stability of anterior lumbar interbody fusion: a biomechanical comparison of anterior plate versus posterior transpedicular instrumentation. Spine (Phila Pa 1976). 2008;33(2):E38-43.
79. Moore KR, Pinto MR, Butler LM. Degenerative disc disease treated with combined anterior and posterior arthrodesis and posterior instrumentation. Spine. 2002;27(15):1680-6.
80. El Masry MA, Badawy WS, Rajendran P, et al. Combined anterior interbody fusion and posterior pedicle screw fixation in patients with degenerative lumbar disc disease. Int Orthop. 2004;28(5):294-7.
81. Sarwat AM, O'Brien JP, Renton P, et al. The use of allograft (and avoidance of autograft) in anterior lumbar interbody fusion: a critical analysis. Eur Spine J. 2001;10(3):237-41.
82. Liljenqvist U, O'Brien JP, Renton P, et al. Simultaneous combined anterior and posterior lumbar fusion with femoral cortical allograft. Eur Spine J. 1998;7(2):125-31.
83. Pradhan BB, Bae HW, Dawson EG, et al. Graft resorption with the use of bone morphogenetic protein: lessons from anterior lumbar interbody fusion using femoral ring allografts and recombinant human bone morphogenetic protein-2. Spine. 2006;31(10):E277-84.
84. Burkus JK, Heim SE, Gornet MF, et al. Is INFUSE Bone Graft Superior to Autograft Bone? An integrated analysis of clinical trials using the LT-CAGE lumbar tapered fusion device. J Spinal Disord Tech. 2003;16(2):113-22.
85. Burkus JK, Dorchak JD, Sanders DL. Radiographic assessment of interbody fusion using recombinant human

bone morphogenetic protein type 2. Spine (Phila Pa 1976). 2003;28(4):372-7.
86. Aryan HE, Lu DC, Acosta FL Jr, et al. Stand-alone anterior lumbar discectomy and fusion with plate: initial experience. Surg Neurol. 2007;68(1):7-13; discussion 13.
87. Cappuccino A, Cornwall GB, Turner AW, et al. Biomechanical analysis and review of lateral lumbar fusion constructs. Spine (Phila Pa 1976). 2010;35(26 Suppl):S361-7.
88. Pimenta L, Turner AW, Dooley ZA, et al. Biomechanics of lateral interbody spacers: going wider for going stiffer. Scientific World Journal. 2012;2012:381814.
89. Laws CJ, Coughlin DG, Lotz JC, et al. Direct lateral approach to lumbar fusion is a biomechanically equivalent alternative to the anterior approach: an in vitro study. Spine (Phila Pa 1976). 2012;37(10):819-25.
90. Beaubien BP, Derincek A, Lew WD, et al. In vitro, biomechanical comparison of an anterior lumbar interbody fusion with an anteriorly placed, low-profile lumbar plate and posteriorly placed pedicle screws or translaminar screws. Spine (Phila Pa 1976). 2005;30(16):1846-51.
91. Ploumis A, Wu C, Fischer G, et al. Biomechanical comparison of anterior lumbar interbody fusion and transforaminal lumbar interbody fusion. J Spinal Disord Tech. 2008;21(2):120-5.
92. Lund T, Oxland TR, Jost B, et al. Interbody cage stabilization in the lumbar spine. J Bone Joint Surg Br. 1998;80(2):351-9.
93. Le Huec J, Liu M, Skalli W, et al. Lumbar lateral interbody cage with plate augmentation: in vitro biomechanical analysis. Eur Spine J. 2002;11(2):130-6.
94. Marchi L, Abdala N, Oliveira L, et al. Stand-alone lateral interbody fusion for the treatment of low-grade degenerative spondylolisthesis. Scientific World Journal. 2012;2012:456346.
95. Marchi L, Oliveira L, Amaral R, et al. Lateral interbody fusion for treatment of discogenic low back pain: minimally invasive surgical techniques. Adv Orthop. 2012;2012:282068.
96. Oliveira L, Marchi L, Coutinho E, et al. A radiographic assessment of the ability of the extreme lateral interbody fusion procedure to indirectly decompress the neural elements. Spine (Phila Pa 1976). 2010;35(26 Suppl):S331-7.
97. Personal communication with panel of specialists at the 2012 Scoliosis Research Society meeting. Chicago, IL.
98. Harris BM, Hilibrand AS, Savas PE. Transforaminal lumbar interbody fusion: the effect of various instrumentation techniques on the flexibility of the lumbar spine. Spine. 2005;30:E562-6.
99. Chen SH , Lin SC, Tsai WC et al. Biomechanical comparison of unilateral and bilateral pedicle screws fixation for transforaminal lumbar interbody fusion after decompressive surgery: a finite element analysis. BMC Musculoskelet Disord. 2012;13:72.
100. Villavicencio AT, Burneikiene S, Bulsara KR, et al. Perioperative complications in transforaminal lumbar interbody fusion versus anterior posterior reconstruction for lumbar disc degeneration and instability. J Spinal Disord Tech. 2006;19:92-7.
101. Potter BK, Freedman BA, Verwiebe EG, et al. Transforaminal lumbar interbody fusion: clinical and radiographic results and complications in 100 consecutive patients. J Spinal Disord Tech. 2005;18:337-46.
102. Ozgur BM, Yoo K, Rodriguez G, et al. Minimally-invasive technique for transforaminal lumbar interbody fusion (TLIF). Eur Spine J. 2005;14:887-94.
103. Holly LT, Schwender JD, Rouben DP, et al. Minimally invasive transforaminal lumbar interbody fusion: indications, technique, and complications. Neurosurg Focus. 2006;20:E6.
104. Peng CWB, Yue WM, Poh SY, et al. Clinical and radiological outcomes of minimally invasive versus open transforaminal lumbar interbody fusion. Spine. 2009;34:1385-9.
105. Suk KS, Lee HM, Kim NH. Unilateral versus bilateral pedicle screw fixation in lumbar spinal fusion. Spine. 2000;25:1843-7.
106. Goel VK, Panjabi MM, Patwardhan AG, et al. Test protocols for evaluation of spinal implants. J Bone Joint Surg Am. 2006;88:103-9.
107. Goel VK, Lim TH, Gwon J. Effects of rigidity of an internal fixation device a comprehensive biomechanical investigation. Spine. 1991;16:S155-61.
108. Slucky AV, Brodke DS, Bachus KN, et al. Less invasive posterior fixation method following transforaminal lumbar interbody fusion: a biomechanical analysis. Spine J. 2006;6:78-85.

CHAPTER 3 Bone and Intervertebral Disk Physiology

Shah-Nawaz M Dodwad, Sohrab S Virk, Safdar N Khan, Tom D Cha, Howard S An

BONE PHYSIOLOGY

Introduction

Bone is the fundamental building block of the skeleton that provides the rigid framework of the body. In the spine, the vertebrae provide the structure of the axial skeleton to support the body. Bone is a dynamic and organized structure that is composed of organic and inorganic components, giving a relatively lightweight structure that has a tensile strength similar to cast iron.[1] About 40% of the dry weight of bone is organic material, composed primarily of collagen, proteoglycans, and other proteins. Collagen is a protein that has a triple helix configuration, composed of two alpha-1 chains and one alpha-2 chain. There are several types of collagen, Type I being most abundant in bone, as well as in ligament, tendon, and meniscus. Collagen abnormalities are the underlying mutations involved in osteogenesis imperfecta and Ehlers-Danlos syndrome. About 60% of the dry weight of bone is inorganic material, composed primarily of hydroxyapatite which contains calcium and phosphate with the molecular formula of $Ca_{10}(PO_4)_6(OH)_2$. These crystals deposit around collagen within the osteoid or unmineralized organic matrix in a specific orientation to allow for rigid bone formation.

Bone Structure

Bone is found primarily in two structural forms: Cortical or dense compact bone, and trabecular or cancellous spongy bone. Trabecular bone has a lattice structure that inherently provides a much larger surface area than cortical bone given this increased porosity. This increase in surface area allows trabecular bone to have eight times the metabolic activity of cortical bone. In the spine, most of the trabecular bone is found within the vertebral body itself. The increased surface area of trabeculae is where the bone marrow is housed to facilitate the metabolic activity in this region of increased surface area. Trabecular bone represents 20% of total bone mass and is primarily responsible for adapting to external stresses to provide support according to Wolff's law which states that bone will react to the stress placed upon it and remodel to resist those stresses.[2] The cortical bone is dense and lines the exterior of cancellous bone. This dense bone provides 80% of total bone mass. The outer layer of bone is covered by a thick fibrous tissue called the periosteum. The inner surface of the bone is lined by the endosteum. The deep surface of the periosteum as well as the endosteum contains the osteoprogenitor cells.

Cells Involved in Bone Metabolism

Three major cells involved in bone metabolism and homeostasis are osteoclasts, osteoblasts, and osteocytes. Bones also contain osteoprogenitor cells as well as hematopoietic cells that reside in the bone marrow and give rise to lymphocytes, granulocytes, monocytes, erythrocytes, and platelets. These osteoprogenitor cells are similar to stem cells but have already been ordained to become bone-forming cells.[3] Osteoclasts are monocyte-derived multinucleated giant cells that have a ruffled border which is in contact with the bone surface. This ruffled border is the site of enzymatic processes that break down and absorb bone. These resorption troughs that are created within the bone are called Howship's lacunae. Osteoclasts are essentially macrophages of bone. Abnormalities of osteoclasts are the underlying abnormalities with osteopetrosis or brittle bone disease. Osteoblasts are mesenchymal-derived mononuclear cells that produce osteoid or the unmineralized organic portion of the bone matrix. 90% of the osteoid is primarily composed of type I collagen. The remaining 10% of osteoid is composed of noncollagenous proteins, carbohydrates, and lipids. The osteoid undergoes mineralization by osteoblasts as well, thus creating the rigid structure of bone. These osteoblasts are responsible for bone deposition as well as indirectly involved in bone resorption through activation of osteoclasts. Osteocytes are also mesenchymal-derived mononuclear cells. Once osteoblasts become entrapped in the osseous matrix they produce, they become osteocytes. Osteocytes comprise 90–95% of all bone cells.[4] These cells reside in bone within spaces called lacunae and have cytoplasmic processes that extend within canaliculi or channels. These canaliculi allow osteocytes to communicate via gap junction and play key role in the regulation of bone resorption, bone formation, and local homeostasis.[4]

Regulation of Bone Metabolism

The complex interaction of these cells with a myriad of molecular proteins creates a homeostasis for bone metabolism that balances bone formation with bone resorption known as bone remodeling. This interplay allows the bone to respond to different stresses by adaptation and also gives bone the ability to heal. Dysregulation of this process leads to various pathologic processes, such as osteoporosis or decreased bone mass and density.[1,5] Of the signaling processes involved in bone metabolism, we will briefly discuss the roles of a few major proteins including receptor activator of nuclear factor kappa-B ligand (RANKL), receptor activator of nuclear factor kappa-B (RANK), and osteoprotegerin. RANKL is a signaling molecule that is bound to the cell membrane of osteoblasts. RANKL production by osteoblasts is stimulated by parathyroid hormone. RANK is a receptor protein found on osteoclast membranes. Osteoclasts differentiate and are activated when RANKL on the osteoblast cell surface binds with RANK on the osteoclast cell surface. RANKL activation has also been involved in metastatic bone disease. Osteoprotegerin is a cell receptor decoy for RANKL that acts as a competitive inhibitor which prevents RANKL from binding RANK and therefore inhibits osteoclast differentiation and activation thus preventing bone resorption. Clinically, osteoprotegerin-like compounds are being used as pharmaceutical target in diseases such as osteoporosis and metastatic bone disease to decrease bone loss.[6]

Calcium Regulation

Bone metabolism plays a role in calcium storage and availability.[7] Several major hormones involved in regulation of bone metabolism are parathyroid hormone, calcitonin, and vitamin D. Parathyroid hormone is secreted from the parathyroid in response to low levels of calcium. Osteoblasts express parathyroid hormone receptors and respond by activating osteoclasts to increase bone resorption to release calcium into the body. Teriparatide or recombinant parathyroid hormone is a medication used for the treatment of osteoporosis as a pulsatile use of parathyroid hormone that more selectively activates osteoblasts more than osteoclasts, thereby increasing bone formation.[1,5,8] The effects of calcitonin are antagonistic to parathyroid hormone. Calcitonin is secreted from the parafollicular C-cells of the thyroid and decrease serum calcium levels. One mechanism involves calcitonin binding to receptors on osteoclasts to inhibit their activity, thereby decreasing the release of calcium into the body.[9] Calcitonin has been used pharmacologically to treat osteoporosis and reduce osteoporotic fractures by decreasing bone resorption.[1,5,10] Vitamin D or the active form of 1,25-dihydroxycholecalciferol plays a complex role in the absorption of calcium from the intestines and regulation of bone metabolism. Vitamin D is used clinically in the treatment of rickets and the prevention and treatment of osteoporotic bone.[11]

Bone Grafts

In the setting of spine surgery, hardware is placed into the spine to provide time zero fixation; however, the ultimate success of fusion surgery is dependent on union of the bone to create a solid bone fusion mass. There is always a race between eventual hardware failure with subsequent instability and bone fusion in the setting of spinal fusion surgery. Bone grafts are used to augment this bone fusion. Three broad categories of bone graft exist and include osteoconductive, osteoinductive, and osteogenic grafts. Osteoconductive grafts are essentially a scaffold that allows the patients' own cells to populate and create new bone growth. Osteoinductive grafts contain bone growth stimulating factors such as bone morphogenetic protein (BMP) that induce or stimulate bone growth. Osteogenic grafts contain viable cells such as osteoblasts, osteocytes, and mesenchymal stem cells needed for bone growth. Autograft or bone graft that is locally harvested from the patient, usually from the spine, ribs, or pelvis is an example of osteoconductive, osteoinductive, and osteogenic graft. The benefits of autograft are that it contains cells and proteins needed for bone production and has no risk of communicable disease transfer as can happen from cadaveric bone or allograft. The problems with autograft involve donor site morbidity and limited supply of bone.[12] Another term used when describing grafts is structural versus nonstructural. Structural grafts provide some rigid support, compared to nonstructural grafts that provide no structural support, for example bone putty. When compared to cortical bone, cancellous bone is preferable for bone grafting as it remodels and incorporates faster into bone in a process called creeping substitution. Cortical bone, however, has the advantage of providing structural support but is slower to incorporate into bone. The graft choice has effects on patient care, surgical outcomes, complications, and cost.

Bone Morphogenetic Protein

Given that BMP has garnered much attention with its use as an osteoinductive protein, a further discussion of this product is warranted. BMPs are a group of cell-signaling proteins that are part of the transforming growth factor beta family.[13] There are about 20 types of BMP. BMP 2, 4, 6, 7, and 9 have been shown to induce bone formation.[14] The only FDA approved BMPs in spine surgery are recombinant BMP2 (rhBMP2) and BMP7 (rhBMP7 or OP-1). However, up to 85% of BMP use is off-label.[15] The goals of BMP are to avoid donor site morbidity from harvesting autograft, as well as to induce more bone formation than the body would normally produce in the setting of spinal fusion. These proteins induce bone formation via osteoblast differentiation. BMPs bind to BMP receptors located on the cell surface which subsequently activates intracellular signaling proteins called SMADs. These proteins go on to induce transcription of specific genes that enhance bone formation.

Bone morphogenetic protein must be used in the appropriate procedure, for the appropriate patient, and at the appropriate concentration. BMP is not to be used in the cervical spine as it may cause massive soft tissue swelling leading to airway compromise. Smucker et al. reported clinically significant soft tissue swelling following anterior cervical decompression and fusion and had an incidence of 27.5% with rhBMP2 use compared to 3.6% without the use of rhBMP2.[16] The incidence of retrograde ejaculation from rhBMP2 use in anterior interbody lumbar surgery was 7.2% of which half (3 out of 6 patients) had resolved by 1 year out from surgery.[17] Other complications of BMP use in the spine include radiculitis, osteolysis, seroma formation, and potential increase in malignancy.[14,18] There are also significant costs with the use of BMP. The difference in total payer expenditure during the 3-month perioperative period following posterolateral spinal fusion averaged $33,860 in the patients that used BMP2 and $37,227 in the patients that used iliac crest bone graft.[19] Although, there are potential risks with BMP use, rate of spinal fusion is enhanced with its use.[20] Recently, the Yale Open Data Access (YODA) project involved a large systematic review and meta-analysis of rhBMP2 data. Interestingly, YODA found substantial evidence of reporting bias with no evidence that rhBMP2 is significantly more effective than iliac crest bone in spinal fusion.[21,22] Additionally, they found that early postsurgical pain is increased with rhBMP2 use and that there is some evidence to suggest a potential increased risk of cancer with rhBMP2 use. They concluded that based on their analysis it is unclear what the exact clinical indications for BMP2 use are. Given the controversy surrounding BMP, a thorough discussion of the risk to benefit analysis must be undertaken with the patient as well as preoperative planning to balance the dose as well as concentration of BMP used.

Physiology of Bone Fusion

Similar to fracture healing, bone fusion in spine surgery is a dynamic process that is influenced by a myriad of factors, including biochemical, biomechanical, cellular, hormonal, and pathological mechanisms.[23] Bone fusion proceeds in a similar fashion as fracture healing. There are three broad categories which are the reactive or inflammatory, reparative, and remodeling phases. After initial surgery, with decortication and bone graft implantation, the reactive phase begins. A hematoma and local inflammatory reaction occurs, resulting in the formation of vascular granulation tissue. Anti-inflammatory medications can impede this inflammatory phase and result in nonunion or delay in fusion.[24] As a result, some surgeons avoid anti-inflammatory medications in the initial postoperative period. The reparative phase involves cartilage and bone formation from osteoblasts, chondroblasts, and precursor cells and their substitution into the bone graft. The resulting tissue is called fracture callus. This fracture with its immature, weak, and poorly organized woven bone is replaced with organized collagen known as lamellar bone. Finally, the lamellar bone undergoes remodeling to become stronger and more organized and complete fusion according to Wolff's law. Other factors that significantly impede the process of fusion include smoking, instability, and malnutrition.[25-27] Smoking is considerably detrimental to the process of bone fusion. The nicotine in cigarettes impedes vascular ingrowth needed for successful fusion.[28] In fact smoking doubled the likelihood of nonunion for two-level lumbar fusion and tripled the likelihood of nonunion for greater than two-level lumbar fusions.[29]

Although there are a myriad of factors involved in bone fusion including patient factors, bone bed preparation, graft selection, and spine immobilization, a basic understanding of bone physiology is needed by any spine surgeon to determine the best treatment options for their patients and to succeed in their surgical interventions.[30]

INTERVERTEBRAL DISK PHYSIOLOGY

Anatomy

The intervertebral disk (IVD) is located between the vertebral bodies of the spine. The IVD is bound superiorly and inferiorly by the cartilaginous endplates. The basic anatomy of the IVD consists of the inner nucleus pulposus (NP) and the outer annulus fibrosus (AF). Cell density in the IVD is as low as 6000 cells/mm^3 as measured by Maroudas et al.[31] The disk is most cellular at the outer edge of the AF. As one moves centrally into the NP, the cell density decreases. Also, the IVD are poorly vascularized structures.

Annulus fibrosus is composed of type-1 collagen while NP is composed of type-2 collagen. The AF cells have an elongated shaped and are fibroblast-like cells. These cells make both type-1 and type-2 collagen even though the AF is primarily composed of type-1 collagen. Under polarized light, 15–25 lamella or bundles of collagen have been found within adult AF. Cells in the NP are chondrocyte-like and oval-shaped. These cells primarily create collagen type 2.[32]

Embryology

The embryonic spine is derived from the notochord and surrounding mesoderm. The vertebral column is induced to develop from the neural tube and notochord at about 4 weeks of gestation. The NP arises from the notochord and the AF comes from mesoderm.[33] Each vertebral body forms from adjacent somites and these vertebral bodies surround the notochord. Cartilage endplates also arise from the notochord.[34] The AF forms from sheets that are aligned and oriented in alternate directions to the vertebral axis.[34,35] These layered sheets create an organized lamellar structure typical of an adult AF. In the embryonic disk, there is a distinct change between the fibrous AF and the more fluid-like NP. The AF is composed of mainly collagen and fibroblast-like cells, while the NP is composed primarily of notochordal cells and proteoglycans.

From the embryo to maturity, the disk composition changes dramatically. The embryologic disk consists of many more cells and is much more vascular than at any other point in the lifetime of the IVD. Immature disks have vascular channels between lamella within the AF. Furthermore, cartilage endplates start off at birth as having large vascular channels and make up 50% of the intervertebral disk height. Soon after birth, extracellular matrix begins to take over space occupied by the vascular channels. The sequential steps in IVD maturation from highly cellular/vascular to acellular/avascular are shown in Figure 1.

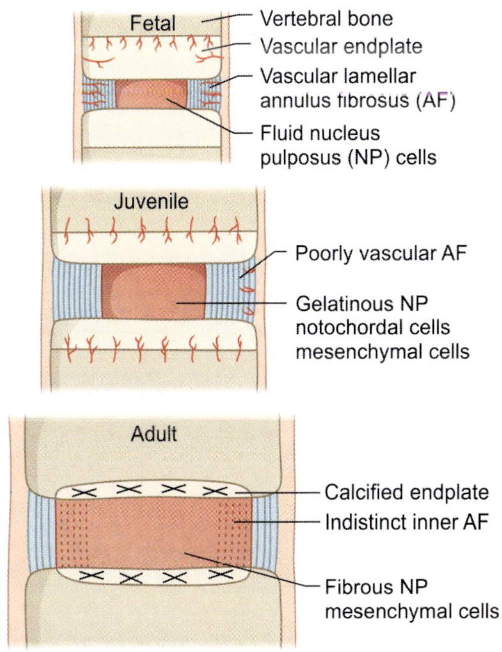

Fig. 1: The changes in disk physiology over time. The vascular supply and the total number of cells decrease dramatically over time from the fetal to juvenile to adult disk.
Source: Roughley PJ. Biology of intervertebral disc aging and degeneration: involvement of the extracellular matrix. Spine (Phila Pa 1976). 2004;29(23):2691-9.

The cartilage endplates also change dramatically during IVD maturation. Prior to skeletal maturity these endplates act like epiphyseal growth plates for vertebral bodies. By skeletal maturity these endplates become hyaline cartilage. During growth and development, the amount that cartilage endplates contribute to disk height decreases. By skeletal maturity the hyaline cartilage is only 0.6 mm thick. At maturation, the hyaline cartilage has fused to the outer rim of the vertebral body.

Biochemical Components

There are three major components of the biochemical makeup of IVDs which include water, collagen, and proteoglycans.[36] The types of collagen and class of proteoglycans vary tremendously based upon location within the IVD, as well as the age and stage of degeneration of a disk. In the AF, 60% of dry weight is collagen while 20% of dry weight in the NP corresponds to collagen.[37] As will be discussed later, certain proteoglycan components play a pivotal role in sustaining the concentration of water in the IVD. Proteoglycans make up 50% of dry weight in the NP and 20% of dry weight in the AF.

The principle components of the collagen framework in IVDs are type-1 collagen and type-2 collagen, although several other collagen types are present within the IVD as well. As mentioned previously, type-1 collagen is more associated with the more fibrous AF while type-2 collagen is more abundant in the more gelatinous NP. Collagen types-5, 11, 12, and 14 all assist in creating narrow hybrid fibrils of type-1 and type-2 collagen. There are also unique components to collagen type-1 and type-2 that are present in the IVD. Type-2 collagen in the NP has increased hydroxylation of proline and lysine which may both limit longitudinal growth of fibrils and make the collagen less susceptible to breakdown from collagenase.[38] Collagenase has an important role to play in the breakdown of cartilage in the disk. Given that collagen in the IVD is highly cross-linked, breakdown by collagenase does not necessarily mean that damaged collagen will be removed. The damaged collagen simply remains in the IVD, weakening the mechanical strength of the tissue.[39]

Aggrecan is the most abundant proteoglycan in the IVD and plays a pivotal role in maintaining water concentration. It consists of keratan sulfate and chondroitin sulfate bound to a core protein.[40] Over time the amount of keratan sulfate and collagen increases while the amount of chondroitin sulfate decreases.[41] This occurs due to the fact that as the aging process progresses there is less blood supply and oxygen delivered to the disks and this oxygen is required for formation of chondroitin sulfate, but not for keratan sulfate. Keratan sulfate, however, does provide a distinct advantage as it is more highly charged and is therefore able to bring more water into the central part of the disk. This allows the disk to increase its pressure and aids the IVD in resisting compressional forces.

During the aging process there is also a gradual increase in nonaggregating proteoglycans, likely from breakdown of aggrecan.[42,43] Furthermore, degradation products of link proteins and hyaluronan also accumulate during the lifetime of IVDs.[44] These products may contribute to disk swelling pressure which would be of benefit, but may also increase the amount of advanced glycation end-products (AGE) which may limit the ability of the disk to swell.[45]

Two matrix proteins have unique functions in disk physiology.[33] Fibronectin plays a role in the interaction between cells and disk matrix. During the aging process, the concentration of fibronectin increases which results in increased proteolysis.[46] These degradation products may augment the breakdown of disk components. Elastin is another matrix protein that assists in allowing the disk shape to deform when under stress. Elastin runs parallel to the collagen lamellae in the AF and is oriented radially and laterally within the NP to counteract forces arising from bending of the spine.[47] The role of elastin in disk physiology is not fully understood and is an active area of research.

Blood Supply and Innervation

The environment of the IVD is characterized as avascular, acellular, and acidic. This is an environment that is isolated and difficult for the body to regenerate when injured. As mentioned above, the vasculature to the IVD decreases from the most vascular period prior of birth to virtually no direct vascular supply as an adult. In a fetus, penetrating vessels provide the IVD with nutrients from the endplates arising above and below.[48] These vessels, however, eventually recede. In order to provide nutrients to the central NP, a diffusion gradient is needed. Over time the end plates themselves calcify making diffusion impossible. The lack of blood supply may also lead

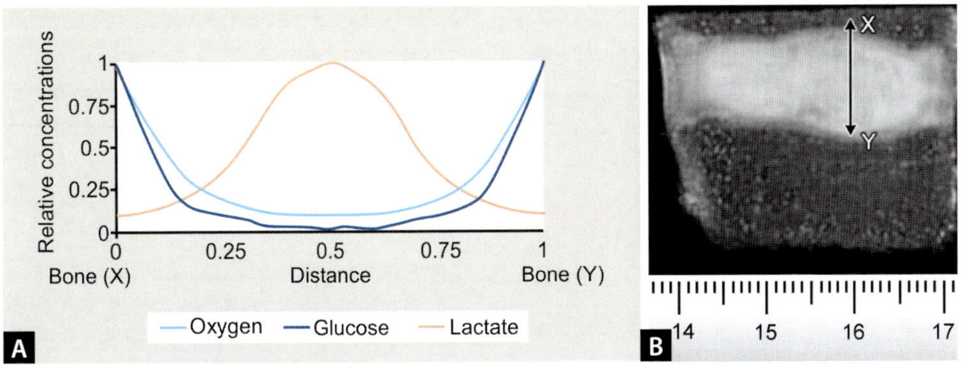

Figs. 2A and B: Elucidates the nutrient gradients in bovine disk cells by showing how glucose, lactate, and oxygen levels change as you move deeper into the disk.[48]

to matrix breakdown. While oxygen is a vital part of maintaining cell viability, it is actually the lack of glucose in an acidic environment that causes cell death within the IVD.[49] Figures 2A and B, from Urbana et al., elucidates the nutrient gradients in bovine disk cells by showing how glucose, lactate, and oxygen levels change as you move deeper into the disk.

Oxygen, glucose and lactate levels move in tandem as one moves from one end of the intervertebral disk to the next. Glucose and oxygen lowers and accordingly lactate increases as you move towards the center.[48]

Innervation to the IVD is limited, but influenced by several IVD chemicals. The IVD is primarily innervated at the outermost layer of the disk at the AF by sinuvertebral nerves from the ventral ramus.[50] Aggrecan slows innervation at both the AF and NP, although aggrecan's effect are more pronounced at the NP.[51] Nerve growth factor (NGF) is a chemical that promotes vascular and neural ingrowth. NGF has been found to be more preferentially expressed in symptomatic disks, potentially suggesting NGF plays a role in disk pathology and perhaps low back pain.[52]

Biomechanical Properties

The biomechanical properties of the IVD allow the spine to better withstand stresses exerted with flexion, extension, and rotation. In particular, they allow load-bearing and mobility between vertebral bodies.[53] The forces exerted on the IVDs over time also play a pivotal role in the changes that occur within their biomechanical properties.

The ability of the AF to resist tensile and shearing loads is based upon its fibrous structure.[53] The type-1 collagen in the AF is organized into concentric lamellae to provide tensile strength to the AF. This strength is based upon the layering of concentric lamellae in parallel and opposing directions. This configuration converts axial spinal loads into tensile hoop stresses.[40]

Hydration also plays an important role in the ability of the IVD to withstand compressive loads.[50] Aggrecan is the most abundant proteoglycan of the NP and it is composed of disaccharide side chains. These side chains are hydrophilic and draw water into the NP. The water fills the small space occupied by the NP creating a swelling pressure which resists compressive loads through the spine. The swelling pressure within the NP is then balanced by the tensile strength of the AF. This interplay of tensile strength of the AF and swelling pressure within the NP creates disk height. When the IVD loses the ability to retain water, the fine balance described above of swelling pressure, compressive loads, and tensile forces breaks down. With aging and loss of water within the IVD, it becomes more difficult for the IVD to resist compressive loads.

Whether or not the IVD plays a role as a shock absorber is somewhat controversial. A portion of studies claim that the IVD has no role as a shock absorber.[54,55] Holmes et al. performed an experiment in which cadaveric lumbar spines with IVD and adjacent vertebral bodies were sequentially compressed. Results showed that the spine could not function as a shock-absorber with compression. Another study by Broberg on loaded IVDs with a constant force noted creep with outflow of fluid from the IVD. The deformation, however, eventually recovered.[56]

CHAPTER 3

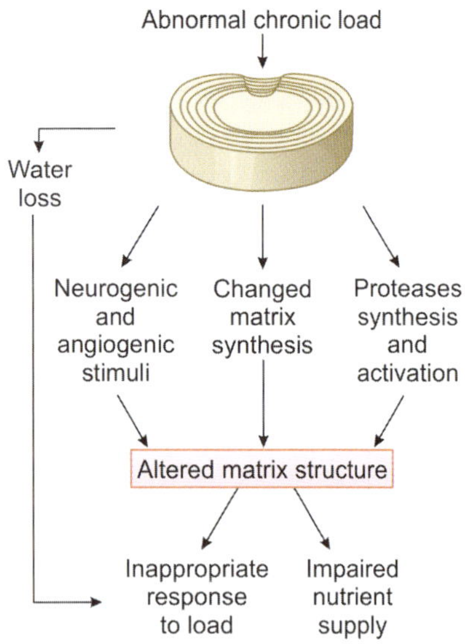

Fig. 3: There are various mechanical and chemical stimuli that influence the structure of each intervertebral disk.[58]

Table 1: The role of enzymes in degenerative disk disease.

Enzyme	*Change in expression in degenerative disk disease*	*Strengthen or weaken IVD?*
Platelet-derived growth factor	Decrease	Weaken
Insulin-like growth factor-1	Decrease	Weaken
Fibroblast growth factor	Decrease	Weaken
Matrix metallo-proteinase-1 (MMP-1)	Increase	Weaken
MMP-8	Increase	Weaken
MMP-13	Increase	Weaken
ADAMTS	Increase	Weaken
Cathepsins	Increase	Weaken

(ADAMTS: A disintegrin and metalloproteinase with thrombospondin motifs)

Mechanical loads on the IVD serve to influence the biochemical structure of the IVD itself. Application of 2 MPa for 20 second leads 2–3 fold increase in production of proteoglycans, collagens, and matrix proteins[57] (refer to Figure 3 for an illustration of how various stimuli influence the creation of matrix composition). Clearly, there is a multifactorial process which creates the homeostatic environment of collagen, protease inhibitors, matrix proteins, and proteoglycans needed for mechanical strength in the IVD.

Chemical Homeostasis

The extracellular matrix and cells within the AF and NP are all balanced by specific biochemical and biomechanical signals. This process is disrupted in disk degeneration.[59] At the cellular level there is increased disk-cell proliferation and cell-cluster proliferation with cell death.[60,61] While these cellular changes occur, there are also changes in the activity of various proteins, including collagen, elastin, fibronectin, amyloid, and others that play a role in disk degeneration.

The loss of type-2 collagen and aggrecan makes it difficult for the aging IVD to handle loads.[62,63] In degenerated disks, there is a loss of the more flexible type-2 collagen and an increase in the relative amount of fibrous type-1 collagen. Not only there are changes in the type of collagen, but there are also collagenases that alter the mechanical properties of the collagen itself.[64] Therefore, the collagen in degenerated disks is less able to bear mechanical loads. As mentioned, aggrecan also decreases which alters the ability of the NP to retain water, which decreases the water content and results in reduced ability of the IVD to create swelling pressure.[65] All these changes diminish the ability of nutrients to diffuse into the disk and also reduce the amount of outflow of waste material from the disk. This may play a role in increased cell loss through apoptosis which can be found in degenerated IVDs.[66]

Along with these changes to collagen and aggrecan, there are also dramatic alterations in the synthesis and production of growth factors and degradative enzymes at the same time that there is an upregulation of inflammatory cytokines. A summary table with changes to degradation enzymes as well as mitogenic factors is seen in Table 1.[67-74] Studies have indicated that matrix metalloproteinases do in fact bind and directly damage the extracellular matrix (ECM). Of note, cathepsins may have a particularly important role in degenerative disk disease given that they work best in the acidic environment of the IVD.

Cytokines play an important role in the inflammatory process that weakens the IVD ECM and triggers apoptosis. Interleukin-1 (IL-1) is upregulated in disks

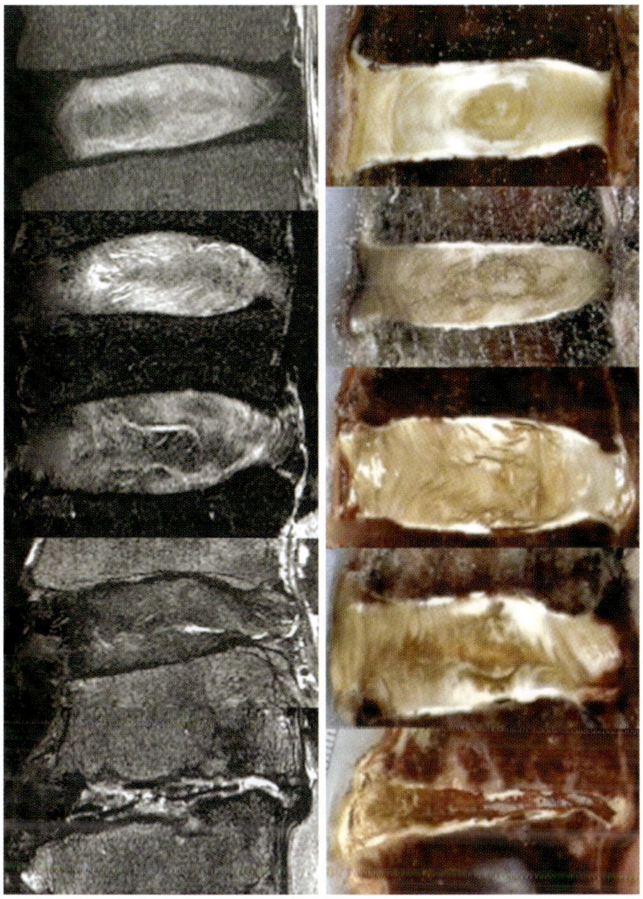

Fig. 4: Pfirrmann classification.[53]

with degenerative disease causing an inhibition of ECM production, as well as sensitizes IVD cells to apoptosis triggers and further upregulates other inflammatory cytokines.[75] During the degenerative disk disease process, the activity of IL-1 increases in part due to the inability of the inhibiting molecule (IL-1 receptor antagonist) to counterbalance IL-1. The upregulation of TNF-alpha within degenerative disk disease may play an important role in the symptoms of low-back pain by encouraging neurogenic growth into degenerated disks and directly irritating afferent nerves.

The chemical processes described above play a dramatic role in the mechanical properties of the degenerated IVD. As mentioned above, the inability for the disk to create swelling pressure makes it difficult for disks to correctly transmit loading forces. The repetitive trauma of unbalanced forces creates weak areas within the disk that could potentially create a fissure in the AF. This fissure can then lead to disk protrusion and back symptomatology. Furthermore, the degenerated disks become stiffer and redirect the applied load to be offset by the posterior elements of the spine, such as the facet joints. The macroscopic changes in the degenerated disk are shown in Figure 4. The figure demonstrates the five levels of disk degeneration as defined by the Pfirrmann classification. This classification system is based upon an MRI study.[76] A brief description of relevant clinical studies can be found in Table 2.

CONCLUSION

There exists a complex interplay between various cells, proteins, and external forces that regulate bone and intervertebral disk physiology. This interaction is fundamental to homeostasis of the body and a critical understanding of its processes aid in the treatment of spinal disease and therapeutic options. Clinical studies (Table 2) continue to focus on the use, efficacy, costs, and complications of different biologic agents in the setting of spine surgery.

REFERENCES

1. Truumees E, Dodwad SN. Osteoporosis and Spine Care, Part 1: General Overview and Medical Management. North American Spine Society SpineLine. 2008.
2. Frost HM. Wolff's Law and bone's structural adaptations to mechanical usage: an overview for clinicians. Angle Orthod. 1994;64(3):175-88.
3. Seaberg RM, van der Kooy D. Stem and progenitor cells: the premature desertion of rigorous definitions. Trends Neurosci. 2003;26(3):125-31.
4. Schaffler MB, Kennedy OD. Osteocyte signaling in bone. Curr Osteoporos Rep. 2012;10(2):118-25.
5. Dodwad SN, Khan SN. Surgical stabilization of the spine in the osteoporotic patient. Orthop Clin North Am. 2013;44(2):243-9.
6. Pageau SC. Denosumab. MAbs. 2009;1(3):210-5.
7. Bauer W, Aub JC, Albright F. Studies of Calcium and Phosphorus Metabolism: V. A Study of the Bone Trabeculae as a Readily Available Reserve Supply of Calcium. J Exp Med. 1929;49(1):145-62.
8. Dempster DW, Cosman F, Parisien M, et al. Anabolic actions of parathyroid hormone on bone. Endocr Rev. 1993;14(6):690-709.
9. Nicholson GC, Moseley JM, Sexton PM, et al. Abundant calcitonin receptors in isolated rat osteoclasts. Biochemical and autoradiographic characterization. J Clin Invest. 1986;78(2):355-60.

CHAPTER 3

Table 2: Level-of-evidence—bone and disk physiology.

Author, journal, year	*Design*	*LoE*	*Topic*	*F/U (m)*	*Measures*	*Main results*
Even, JAAOS, 2012	Systematic Review (SR)	II	Review of BMP efficacy and risks	Variable	Bone fusion, SF-36, complications	BMP induces bone formation, comparable to ICBG. Safety concerns and increased cost exist with BMP and it should not be used routinely on every spine patient. BMP could potentially be used in complex revision fusion surgery where no more ICBG harvest is available or in smokers, diabetics, and nonunions
Ong, Spine, 2010	Retrospective Review (RR)	III	Epidemiologic study of off-label use of BMP	2003–2007	Use of BMP in spine fusion patients	Between 2003 and 2007, the annual number of procedures involving BMP increased by 4.3-fold from 23,900 to 103,194. 85% of principal procedures using BMP were for off-label applications
Smucker, Spine, 2006	Retrospective Comparative	III	To identify if BMP2 is associated with increased clinically relevant postoperative prevertebral swelling in anterior cervical fusions	Within 6 weeks of surgery	Visible swelling of the surgical site, swallowing dysfunction, and/or breathing difficulties, which led to any of the following: (1) delay in discharge; (2) otolaryngological consultation; (3) a premature return to clinic or emergency room; (4) readmission for medical or surgical management of swelling	Off-label use of rhBMP-2 in the anterior cervical spine is associated with an increased rate of clinically relevant swelling events
Carragee, Spine J, 2011	Case Series (CS)	III	Comparing the incidence of RE after ALIF in patients with and without rhBMP-2 use	2002–2004	Occurrences of retrograde ejaculation	There is a higher rate of retrograde ejaculation in ALIF procedures using rhBMP-2. At 1 year, 3 of 6 patients had resolution of their symptoms
Glassman, Spine J, 2008	Prospective Randomized Control	II	Perioperative costs for patients treated with BMP2 as compared with an iliac crest bone graft	3 months	Total cost of admission, physician fees, and rehabilitation	Total cost following posterolateral spinal fusion averaged $33,860 in the patients that used BMP2 and $37,227 in the patients that used iliac crest bone graft, however, the mean hospital cost for the index admission was $24,736 for the BMP2 group and $21,138 for the ICBG group.

Contd...

Contd...

Author, journal, year	*Design*	*LoE*	*Topic*	*F/U (m)*	*Measures*	*Main results*
Fu, Annals of Internal Medicine, 2013	Systematic Review	III	To assess the effectiveness and harms of BMP-2 in spinal fusion and reporting bias in industry-sponsored journal publications	N/A	Fusion rate and complications	BMP-2 has no proven clinical advantage over bone graft and may be associated with important harms, making it difficult to identify clear indications for rhBMP-2
Simmonds, Annals of Internal Medicine, 2013	Systematic Review	III	To evaluate the effectiveness and safety of BMP2	24 months	Primary outcomes were pain (Oswestry Disability Index or Short Form-36), fusion, and adverse events	BMP-2 increased fusion rates, reduce pain by a clinically insignificant amount, and increased early postsurgical pain compared with ICBG. Evidence of increased cancer incidence is inconclusive
Maroudas, J Anat, 1975	CS	IV	Cadaveric study of glucose diffusion and cell density in intervertebral disks (IVD)	N/A	Cell density, glucose concentration	Cell density decreases and glucose diffusion lowers toward the center of the IVD
Yang, Eur J Biochem, 1993	CS	IV	Collagen II in IVD	N/A	Degree of glycosylation and hydroxylation of collagen, diameter of fibrils	Hydroxylation and glycosylation of fibrils, diameter of fibrils increased in annulus fibrosus (AF) compared to articular cartilage (AC)
Hollander, J Orthop Res, 1996	CS	IV	Damage to collagen II in IVD	N/A	Amount of denatured collagen II	Damage to collagen II increased in AF and nucleus pulposus (NP) compared to AC
Verziji, Arthritis Rhem, 2002	CS	IV	Advanced glycation end products (AGEs) in cartilage collagen	N/A	Instantaneous deformation of cartilage, hydration of cartilage	Increased AGE crosslinking resulted in increased stiffness
Oegema, Spine, 2000	CS	IV	Concentration of fibronectin in degenerated IVD	N/A	Fibronectin concentration	Fibronectin is increased in degenerated disks
Johnson, Arthritis Rheum, 2002	CS	IV	Relationship between aggrecan and nerve growth	N/A	Growth of neurites	Disk aggrecan inhibits nerve growth
Holmes AD, Med Eng Phys, 1996	CS	IV	Role of the spine as a shock absorber	N/A	Strain and load-relaxation curves	Spine cannot act as a shock absorber
Gruber, Spine, 1998	Case Control (CC)	III	Rate of apoptosis in IVD	N/A	Extracellular matrix production and distribution of collagen	High incidence of apoptosis in the IVD
Johnson, Connect Tissue Res, 2001	CS	IV	Cell cluster formation in degenerate lumbar IVD	N/A	Proliferating cell nuclear antigen	Disk cell proliferation is associated with disk degeneration causing cell clusters
Cs-Szabo, Spine, 2002	CS	IV	mRNA expression and protein levels of proteoglycans in IVD	N/A	mRNA expression of aggrecan, versican, biglycan, decorin, fibromodulin	NP cells have reduced expression of protein in degenerated IVD

Contd...

Contd...

Author, journal, year	*Design*	*LoE*	*Topic*	*F/U (m)*	*Measures*	*Main results*
Gruber, Spine, 2000	CS	IV	Relationship between insulin-growth factor I (IGF-1), platelet-derived growth factor (PDGF), and apoptosis in AF	N/A	Percent of apoptosis	IGF-1 and PDGF slowed apoptosis
Tolonen, Eur Spine J, 2006	CC	III	Expression of growth factors in degenerated IVD	N/A	Transforming growth factor beta (TGF-B), basic fibroblast growth factor (BFGF), and PDGF expression	BFGF decreases and PDGF decreases in degenerated disks
Tolonen, Spine, 1995	CC	IV	Expression of BFGF in cells and blood vessels of disk herniations	N/A	Immunoreactions of antibodies to BFGF in disks and blood vessels of IVD	Increased expression of BFGF in degenerated IVD when compared to smaller group of controls
Doita, Spine, 1996	CS	IV	Expression of proinflammatory molecules in herniated disks	N/A	Expression of Interleukin-1, intercellular adhesion molecule-1, BFGF	Mononuclear cells at margins of extruded disks express inflammatory mediators and may induce neovascularization
Roberts, Spine, 2000	CS	IV	Expression of matrix metalloproteinases (MMP), tissue metalloproteinases, and proteoglycan degradation products in various disk disorders	N/A	Immunohistochemical staining to find various tissue metalloproteinases, matrix metalloproteinases, and proteoglycan degradation products	Matrix metalloproteinases most active in herniated disks
Weiler, Eur Spine J, 2002	CS	IV	Expression of matrix metalloproteinases in IVD degradation and resorption	N/A	Expression of MMP-1, -2, -3, -9 in IVD of patients of various ages	Younger IVD had less MMPs than older IVD. Also, MMP expression correlated with clefts/tears of IVD
Hatano, Spine, 2006	CS	IV	ADAMTS-4 expression within lumbar disk herniations	N/A	mRNA and protein expression of ADAMTS-4	Macrophages infiltrating granulation and adjacent tissues express ADAMTS-4
Le Maitre, Arthritis Res Ther, 2005	CS	III	Role of Interleukin (IL) -1, IL-1Ra, IL-1RI in IVD degeneration	N/A	Expression of IL-1, IL-1Ra, IL-1RI, IL-1beta-converting enzyme	All interleukins tested were present in normal as well as diseases disk, IL-1 expression correlated with extent of IVD disease
Pfirrmann, Spine, 2001	CS	IV	MRI classification of degenerative disk disease	N/A	Grading of degenerative disk disease by three observers with a grading system developed by authors	T2-weighted MRI can be used to grade degenerative disk disease

10. Martens MG. Risk of fracture and treatment to prevent osteoporosis-related fracture in postmenopausal women. A review. J Reprod Med. 2003;48(6):425-34.
11. Vieth R. The role of vitamin D in the prevention of osteoporosis. Ann Med. 2005;37(4):278-85.
12. Olabisi R. Cell-based therapies for spinal fusion. Adv Exp Med Biol. 2012;760:148-73.
13. Wozney JM, Rosen V. Bone morphogenetic protein and bone morphogenetic protein gene family in bone formation and repair. Clin Orthop Relat Res. 1998;346:26-37.
14. Even J, Eskander M, Kang J. Bone morphogenetic protein in spine surgery: current and future uses. J Am Acad Orthop Surg. 2012;20(9):547-52.
15. Ong KL, Villarraga ML, Lau E, et al. Off-label use of bone morphogenetic proteins in the United States using administrative data. Spine (Phila Pa 1976). 2010;35(19): 1794-800.
16. Smucker JD, Rhee JM, Singh K, et al. Increased swelling complications associated with off-label usage of rhBMP-2 in the anterior cervical spine. Spine (Phila Pa 1976). 2006;31(24):2813-9.
17. Carragee EJ, Mitsunaga KA, Hurwitz EL, et al. Retrograde ejaculation after anterior lumbar interbody fusion using rhBMP-2: a cohort controlled study. Spine J. 2011;11(6):511-6.
18. Tannoury CA, An HS. Complications with the use of bone morphogenetic protein 2 (BMP-2) in spine surgery. Spine J. 2014;14(3):552-9.
19. Glassman SD, Carreon LY, Campbell MJ, et al. The perioperative cost of infuse bone graft in posterolateral lumbar spine fusion. Spine J. 2008;8(3):443-8.
20. Burkus JK, Gornet MF, Dickman CA, et al. Anterior lumbar interbody fusion using rhBMP-2 with tapered interbody cages. J Spinal Disord Tech. 2002;15(5):337-49.
21. Fu R, Selph S, McDonagh M, et al. Effectiveness and harms of recombinant human bone morphogenetic protein-2 in spine fusion: a systematic review and meta-analysis. Ann Intern Med. 2013;158(12):890-902.
22. Simmonds MC, Brown JV, Heirs MK, et al. Safety and effectiveness of recombinant human bone morphogenetic protein-2 for spinal fusion: a meta-analysis of individual-participant data. Ann Intern Med. 2013;158(12):877-89.
23. Kalfas IH. Principles of bone healing. Neurosurg Focus. 2001;10(4).
24. Pountos I, Georgouli T, Blokhuis TJ, et al. Pharmacological agents and impairment of fracture healing: what is the evidence? Injury. 2008;39(4):384-94.
25. Yamaji T, Ando K, Wolf S, et al. The effect of micromovement on callus formation. J Orthop Sci. 2001;6(6):571-5.
26. Day SM, DeHeer DH. Reversal of the detrimental effects of chronic protein malnutrition on long bone fracture healing. J Orthop Trauma. 2001;15(1):47-53.
27. Glassman SD, Anagnost SC, Parker A, et al. The effect of cigarette smoking and smoking cessation on spinal fusion. Spine (Phila Pa 1976). 2000;25(20):2608-15.
28. Riebel GD, Boden SD, Whitesides TE, et al. The effect of nicotine on incorporation of cancellous bone graft in an animal model. Spine (Phila Pa 1976). 1995;20(20):2198-202.
29. Andersen T, Christensen FB, Laursen M, et al. Smoking as a predictor of negative outcome in lumbar spinal fusion. Spine (Phila Pa 1976). 2001;26(23):2623-8.
30. Kaufman HH, Jones E. The principles of bony spinal fusion. Neurosurgery. 1989;24(2):264-70.
31. Maroudas A, Stockwell RA, Nachemson A, et al. Factors involved in the nutrition of the human lumbar intervertebral disc: cellularity and diffusion of glucose in vitro. J Anat. 1975;120(Pt 1):113-30.
32. Oegema TR, Jr. Biochemistry of the intervertebral disc. Clin Sports Med. 1993;12(3):419-39.
33. Roughley PJ. Biology of intervertebral disc aging and degeneration: involvement of the extracellular matrix. Spine (Phila Pa 1976). 1 2004;29(23):2691-9.
34. Roberts S, Evans H, Trivedi J, et al. Histology and pathology of the human intervertebral disc. J Bone Joint Surg Am. 2006;88 Suppl 2:10-4.
35. Rufai A, Benjamin M, Ralphs JR. The development of fibrocartilage in the rat intervertebral disc. Anat Embryol (Berl). 1995;192(1):53-62.
36. Setton LA, Chen J. Cell mechanics and mechanobiology in the intervertebral disc. Spine (Phila Pa 1976). 2004;29(23):2710-23.
37. Buckwalter J. The fine structure of the human intervertebral disc. In: White A, Gordon S (Eds). AAOS Symposium on Idiopathic Low Back Pain. St. Louis: Mosby; 1982. pp.108-43.
38. Yang CL, Rui H, Mosler S, et al. Collagen II from articular cartilage and annulus fibrosus. Structural and functional implication of tissue specific posttranslational modifications of collagen molecules. Eur J Biochem. 1993;213(3):1297-302.
39. Hollander AP, Heathfield TF, Liu JJ, et al. Enhanced denaturation of the alpha (II) chains of type-II collagen in normal adult human intervertebral discs compared with femoral articular cartilage. J Orthop Res. 1996;14(1):61-6.
40. Roughley PJ, Alini M, Antoniou J. The role of proteoglycans in aging, degeneration and repair of the intervertebral disc. Biochem Soc Trans. 2002;30(Pt 6):869-74.
41. Lyons G, Sweet MBE. Age-related changes in proteoglycans of bovine intervertebral disc. S Afr J Sci. 1986;82:151-5.
42. Jahnke MR, McDevitt CA. Proteoglycans of the human intervertebral disc. Electrophoretic heterogeneity of the aggregating proteoglycans of the nucleus pulposus. Biochem J. 1988;251(2):347-56.
43. DiFabio JL, Pearce RH, Caterson B, et al. The heterogeneity of the non-aggregating proteoglycans of the human intervertebral disc. Biochem J. 1987;244(1):27-33.
44. Pearce RH, Mathieson JM, Mort JS, et al. Effect of age on the abundance and fragmentation of link protein of the human intervertebral disc. J Orthop Res. 1989;7(6):861-7.
45. Verzijl N, DeGroot J, Ben ZC, et al. Crosslinking by advanced glycation end products increases the stiffness of the collagen network in human articular cartilage: a possible mechanism through which age is a risk factor for osteoarthritis. Arthritis Rheum. 2002;46(1):114-23.

46. Oegema TR, Jr., Johnson SL, Aguiar DJ, et al. Fibronectin and its fragments increase with degeneration in the human intervertebral disc. Spine (Phila Pa 1976). 2000;25(21):2742-7.
47. Yu J. Elastic tissues of the intervertebral disc. Biochem Soc Trans. 2002;30(Pt 6):848-52.
48. Urban JP, Smith S, Fairbank JC. Nutrition of the intervertebral disc. Spine (Phila Pa 1976). 2004;29(23):2700-9.
49. Bibby SR, Urban JP. Effect of nutrient deprivation on the viability of intervertebral disc cells. Eur Spine J. 2004;13(8):695-701.
50. Kepler CK, Anderson DG, Tannoury C, et al. Intervertebral disk degeneration and emerging biologic treatments. J Am Acad Orthop Surg. 2011;19(9):543-53.
51. Johnson WE, Caterson B, Eisenstein SM, et al. Human intervertebral disc aggrecan inhibits nerve growth in vitro. Arthritis Rheum. 2002;46(10):2658-64.
52. Freemont AJ, Watkins A, Le Maitre C, et al. Nerve growth factor expression and innervation of the painful intervertebral disc. J Pathol. 2002;197(3):286-92.
53. Slikker W, An HS. Pathophysiology of disc degeneration. In: Sharan AD, Tang SY (Eds). Basic Science of Spinal Diseases. New Delhi: Jaypee Brothers Medical Publishers (P) Ltd; 2013. pp. 73-9.
54. Holmes AD, Hukins DW. Analysis of load-relaxation in compressed segments of lumbar spine. Med Eng Phys. 1996;18(2):99-104.
55. Hughes SP, Freemont AJ, Hukins DW, et al. The pathogenesis of degeneration of the intervertebral disc and emerging therapies in the management of back pain. J Bone Joint Surg Br. 2012;94(10):1298-304.
56. Broberg KB. Slow deformation of intervertebral discs. J Biomech. 1993;26(4-5):501-12.
57. Urban JP, Roberts S. Cells of the intervertebral disc: making the best of a bad environment. Biochemist. 2003;25:15-7.
58. Colombini A, Lombardi G, Corsi MM, et al. Pathophysiology of the human intervertebral disc. Int J Biochem Cell Biol. 2008;40(5):837-42.
59. Iannone F, Lapadula G. The pathophysiology of osteoarthritis. Aging Clin Exp Res. 2003;15(5):364-72.
60. Gruber HE, Hanley EN, Jr. Analysis of aging and degeneration of the human intervertebral disc. Comparison of surgical specimens with normal controls. Spine (Phila Pa 1976). 1998;23(7):751-7.
61. Johnson WE, Eisenstein SM, Roberts S. Cell cluster formation in degenerate lumbar intervertebral discs is associated with increased disc cell proliferation. Connect Tissue Res. 2001;42(3):197-207.
62. Herbert CM, Lindberg KA, Jayson MI, et al. Proceedings: Intervertebral disc collagen in degenerative disc disease. Ann Rheum Dis. 1975;34(5):467.
63. Brickley-Parsons D, Glimcher MJ. Is the chemistry of collagen in intervertebral discs an expression of Wolff's Law? A study of the human lumbar spine. Spine (Phila Pa 1976). 1984;9(2):148-63.
64. Monnier VM, Kohn RR, Cerami A. Accelerated age-related browning of human collagen in diabetes mellitus. Proc Natl Acad Sci U S A. 1984;81(2):583-7.
65. Cs-Szabo G, Ragasa-San Juan D, Turumella V, et al. Changes in mRNA and protein levels of proteoglycans of the annulus fibrosus and nucleus pulposus during intervertebral disc degeneration. Spine (Phila Pa 1976). 2002;27(20):2212-9.
66. Gruber HE, Norton HJ, Hanley EN, Jr. Anti-apoptotic effects of IGF-1 and PDGF on human intervertebral disc cells in vitro. Spine (Phila Pa 1976). 2000;25(17):2153-7.
67. Tolonen J, Gronblad M, Vanharanta H, et al. Growth factor expression in degenerated intervertebral disc tissue. An immunohistochemical analysis of transforming growth factor beta, fibroblast growth factor and platelet-derived growth factor. Eur Spine J. 2006;15(5):588-96.
68. Murakami H, Yoon ST, Attallah-Wasif ES, et al. The expression of anabolic cytokines in intervertebral discs in age-related degeneration. Spine (Phila Pa 1976). 2006;31(16):1770-4.
69. Tolonen J, Gronblad M, Virri J, et al. Basic fibroblast growth factor immunoreactivity in blood vessels and cells of disc herniations. Spine (Phila Pa 1976). 1995;20(3):271-6.
70. Doita M, Kanatani T, Harada T, et al. Immunohistologic study of the ruptured intervertebral disc of the lumbar spine. Spine (Phila Pa 1976). 1996;21(2):235-41.
71. Matsui Y, Maeda M, Nakagami W, et al. The involvement of matrix metalloproteinases and inflammation in lumbar disc herniation. Spine (Phila Pa 1976). 1998;23(8):863-8; discussion 868-9.
72. Roberts S, Caterson B, Menage J, et al. Matrix metalloproteinases and aggrecanase: their role in disorders of the human intervertebral disc. Spine (Phila Pa 1976). 2000;25(23):3005-13.
73. Weiler C, Nerlich AG, Zipperer J, et al. 2002 SSE Award Competition in Basic Science: expression of major matrix metalloproteinases is associated with intervertebral disc degradation and resorption. Eur Spine J. 2002;11(4):308-20.
74. Hatano E, Fujita T, Ueda Y, et al. Expression of ADAMTS-4 (aggrecanase-1) and possible involvement in regression of lumbar disc herniation. Spine (Phila Pa 1976). 2006; 31(13):1426-32.
75. Le Maitre CL, Freemont AJ, Hoyland JA. The role of interleukin-1 in the pathogenesis of human intervertebral disc degeneration. Arthritis Res Ther. 2005;7(4):R732-45.
76. Pfirrmann CW, Metzdorf A, Zanetti M, et al. Magnetic resonance classification of lumbar intervertebral disc degeneration. Spine (Phila Pa 1976). 2001;26(17):1873-8.

CHAPTER 4 Preoperative Bone Health Assessment and the Potential use of Systemic Osteoporosis Drugs in Select Patients Undergoing Elective Spine Fusion Surgery

Kelly Krohn

INTRODUCTION

Elective spine fusion surgery in older patients is quite common and likely to increase given the improved technologies and the aging population. More elderly patients want to maintain an active lifestyle and will consider spine surgery to regain function.

There are a number of complications of spine fusion surgery, which are likely in part due to underlying poor bone health. While it is not clear that osteoporosis per se decreases the success of spine fusion there is good evidence that older patients with poor bone health would be more likely to suffer complications such as adjacent segment fracture (proximal junctional kyphosis due to fracture) and failure of the instrumentation such as pedicle screw loosening or interbody cage subsistence. Bone toxins such as chronic glucocorticoid use, smoking, rheumatoid arthritis, and poorly controlled long-standing diabetes contribute to the development of osteoporosis and are potentially associated with reduced spine fusion success and boney complications of spine surgery.

There are several approved systemic drugs used to reduce fracture risk in patients with osteoporosis. This review will summarize the biology of these drugs and highlight the human studies when they are used in the setting of spine fusion. Drugs for osteoporosis should be used in spine fusion surgery patients with documented poor bone health. It is important to consider an evaluation of the patient's bone health in the preoperative period to potentially anticipate bone related complications and also consider perioperative treatment with osteoporosis drugs. Bone health assessment in patients with severe degenerative changes of their spine may present some challenges. This review will suggest an approach to the evaluation of bone health in patients undergoing elective spine surgery and some of the data to support the use of systemic osteoporosis drugs in select patients.

PATHOPHYSIOLOGY OF OSTEOPOROSIS/ BONE LOSS

Peak bone mass is achieved in both men and women at about age 30. A number of factors influence how much bone mass an individual will develop. These include genetic influences, nutrition, mechanical loading of the growing skeleton, hormonal influences, comorbid illnesses, and the exposure to bone toxic drugs such as glucocorticoids.[1] There are studies where interventions such as mechanical loading of the skeleton on children have improved bone mineral density (BMD).[2,3] Once peak bone mass is achieved, there is a slow age-related bone loss in both men and women. However, in women when they go through menopause, estrogen deficiency results in fairly rapid bone loss for several years. Depending on where the woman starts with her peak bone mass, this rapid bone loss can result in bone fragility and associated fragility fractures beginning in her 50's and 60's. Typical early fractures include the distal radius and vertebral fractures. Later in life fractures of the proximal humerus and proximal femur become more common.[4]

Men also achieve peak bone mass at a young age and experience a slow age-related bone loss. Since men generally achieve a higher peak bone mass and do not experience a rapid bone loss related to hormonal deficiency, clinical fragility fracture often do not become significant until their 70's and 80's. If a man survives into his 80's, his risk of fractures including the proximal femur are not rare and can be associated with loss of independence and increased mortality. Men also suffer from vertebral fractures and this increase in prevalence with age. A recent vertebral fracture prevalence study in men and women over the age of 40 in the US showed that men have higher prevalence rate of vertebral fractures than women beginning in the fifth decade.[5] It is hypothesized that not all of these vertebral fractures are fragility fractures and perhaps some are related to high-risk activities that young men are more likely to participate in. With each decade of life, the prevalence of spine fractures increases in both men and women.

Glucocorticoid-induced osteoporosis impacts both men and women and can result in fragility fractures at a very early age. The pathophysiology of chronic glucocorticoid-induced osteoporosis is primarily low-bone formation.[6] The spine is preferentially impacted by glucocorticoid-induced osteoporosis and planning surgery on someone who has been exposed to chronic glucocorticoids should always be a situation where bone health should be assessed preoperatively.

While there are a number of less common causes of bone fragility, typical patients presenting for spine surgery will be at risk for postmenopausal bone loss, age-related bone loss, and glucocorticoid-induced osteoporosis. A preoperative evaluation of bone health should be considered in patients who may be at higher risk for bone health-related complications of spine surgery. While there is no consensus or guidelines, it seems reasonable to consider a bone health evaluation in women over 60 and perhaps men over 70 prior to spine fusion surgery. Any patient who has had chronic glucocorticoid exposure should be evaluated prior to surgery. Since most spine surgery is elective, it seems reasonable to plan the bone health evaluation with the goal of being able to potentially intervene with nutrition and pharmacologic agents prior to elective spine surgery in select patients.

PHARMACOLOGIC AGENTS USED IN OSTEOPOROSIS

There are currently no systemic drugs that are approved to enhance spine fusion or reduce the bone-related complications of spine surgery. There are currently several drugs approved to treat osteoporosis on the basis of reducing vertebral fractures. Some of the drugs have evidence for reduction of nonvertebral fractures but all approved osteoporosis drugs have data to support a reduction in vertebral fractures.

There are two basic families of pharmacologic agents to treat osteoporosis. The majority of drugs are known as antiresorptive agents. These include estrogen, raloxifene, bisphosphonates, calcitonin, and denosumab. While their biology and potency are different they all target the osteoclast, which is responsible for bone resorption/bone loss/bone remodeling. Reducing osteoclastic driven bone resorption stabilizes the skeleton and with reduced bone turnover there is increased mineralization of the existing bone. This increase in mineralization is responsible for most of the increase in BMD as measured by the dual energy X-ray absorptiometry (DXA) machine. More importantly, these drugs effectively reduce vertebral fractures and in some cases nonvertebral fractures. It is likely that the timing of the drug initiation, the duration of treatment, the potency of the drug, and the methodology of determining the "fusion success" outcome may all impact the potential for spine fusion success in the presence of these drugs. While animal studies may be informative, it requires good human data to potentially understand the impact of these drugs on spine fusion surgery.

The other family of osteoporosis drugs is known as anabolic agents. There are two anabolic agents approved for osteoporosis in the US, teriparatide (TPTD) which is the first 34 amino acids of human parathyroid hormone (PTH) 1-84 and abaloparatide which is also a 34 amino acid analog of human parathyroid hormone-related protein (hPTHrP). When given in a pulsatile fashion with a short daily exposure to the PTH receptor, TPTD increases the maturation of stem cells into chondroblasts and osteoblasts.[7] TPTD is an anabolic which accelerates bone remodeling with net increase in true bone mass with each remodeling cycle.[8] Abaloparatide is a synthetic peptide analog of hPTHrP and has recently been approved by FDA. Abaloparatide has been shown to be effective in fracture risk reduction in postmenopausal women.[9] There are differences in anabolic potency between TPTD and abaloparatide. The study by Miller et al. used 80 μg/d of abaloparatide compared with the approved dose of TPTD i.e. 20 μg/d. Abaloparatide results in less increases in the marker of bone resorption compared to TPTD suggesting less of a remodeling biology. There are no published human studies looking at abaloparatide and spine fusion. The third anabolic agent which has considerable human osteoporosis data is romosozumab, which is a monoclonal antibody against sclerostin, an inhibitor of bone formation. The inhibition of sclerostin results in dramatic anabolism. Romosozumab 210 mg/month has been shown to dramatically reduce spine fractures but there was no statistical difference in the development of nonvertebral fractures.[10] The new bone formed under the influence of romosozumab is primarily a result of bone modeling rather than remodeling. The impact of romosozumab on spine fusion in humans is not well studied to date.

PHARMACOLOGIC AGENTS USED IN PATIENT UNDERGOING SPINE FUSION SURGERY

The most studied drug for spine fusion is TPTD. The anabolic nature of TPTD with primarily a remodeling-based biology makes some sense for the biology of promoting successful spine fusion. The fusion mass, much like the callus of fracture healing in long bones, undergoes considerable remodeling and maturation in the several months postoperatively. In addition to the potential impact on the fusion mass, complications such as pedicle screw loosening and adjacent segment fracture would likely benefit from TPTD given the known efficacy of improving bone mass and reducing spine fractures in osteoporosis studies. The preclinical data for the use of TPTD in spine fusion models is robust and generally positive.[11,12] This review will only look at more recent human studies on TPTD and spine fusion.

Ohtori et al. looked at spine fusion success as defined by limited motion on flex/extension X-rays in 57 postmenopausal women with low BMD undergoing posterior lateral fusion of 1–2 levels. Half of the women received daily TPTD 20 μg/d and half received 17.5 mg/week of the oral bisphosphonate, risedronate. The medications were started 2 months before surgery and continued for an average of 8 months postoperatively. The rate of bone union was 82% in the TPTD group and 68% in the risedronate group at 1 year.[13] Ohtori et al. also looked at fusion rates depending upon duration of treatment with TPTD. Those who received TPTD longer (13 months on average) had a higher rate of fusion than the shorter duration of TPTD (5 months on average) or patients who received oral risedronate with fusion rates of 92%, 80%, and 70% respectively.[14]

Ohtori also looked at pedicle screw loosening in postmenopausal women undergoing posterior lateral fusion who received TPTD compared to risedronate and a control group who did not receive any osteoporosis drug. The TPTD group had pedicle screw loosening by X-ray in 7% and by CT in 13% at 12 months. The risedronate and control groups had similar rates of pedicle screw loosening at 12 months with rates of 13% and 15% by X-ray and 26% and 25% by CT, respectively. This data suggests that TPTD may reduce the complications of pedicle screw loosening compared to an oral bisphosphonate and control patients.[15]

In a creative study which supports preoperative use of TPTD for perhaps at least 2 months before surgery, Inoue looked at the insertional torque required to turn in a pedicle screw. Women who received either daily or weekly TPTD (weekly TPTD is approved only in Japan) required a higher torque to turn the pedicle screw than control patients. The women had received TPTD on average of 61 days preoperatively and a minimum of 30 days. This suggests a fairly rapid anabolic effect on the trabecular bone of the vertebral body and the potential for fairly short preoperative treatment with TPTD that may impact the purchase and survival of the pedicle screw.[16]

Yagi et al. studied the vertebral body above the upper instrumented vertebral body in women who received TPTD for 18 months postoperatively compared to controls who did not receive any osteoporosis drugs. As predicted, standard DXA and CT studies showed increases in BMD of the adjacent vertebral body. More importantly perhaps, the patients who received TPTD postoperatively for 18 months had a lower rate of proximal junctional kyphosis due to vertebral fracture compared to controls with 4.6% of the TPTD group and 15.2% in the control group suffering a vertebral fracture.[17]

Since TPTD is limited to 2 year lifetime limit of use, consideration should be given to following a course of TPTD with an antiresorptive drug such as a bisphosphonate. Ohtori and colleagues followed 19 postmenopausal women who underwent posterior lateral fusion (PLF) surgery. All of the women had received TPTD for 2 months preoperatively and at least 8 months postoperatively. Their rate of boney fusion was 95% under the influence of TPTD. After they stopped TPTD, they were given oral risedronate and followed for 3 additional years. The volume of the fusion mass was maintained by the addition of a bisphosphonate after the use of TPTD.[18] This is fairly

CHAPTER 4

standard treatment in the field of osteoporosis where TPTD is given for a maximum of 2 years followed by an antiresorptive osteoporosis drug to maintain the gains in bone mass that have occurred with the anabolic drug.

While there is considerable preclinical data on bisphosphonates and spine fusion there is limited human data. Nagahama et al. studied the use of the oral bisphosphonate alendronate in 40 postmenopausal women undergoing single level PLF fusion utilizing an interbody device. The alendronate group was compared to control patients getting calcium and Vitamin D. The fusion success was determined by radiographic bridging across vertebral levels. The alendronate group appeared to have a slight advantage in visualization of the fusion bridging across levels early on but at 1 year there was not much difference. More importantly perhaps, they showed that the alendronate group had fewer adjacent vertebral fractures (zero) compared to the control group (four). The women receiving alendronate had a single patient with cage subsistence into the vertebral body compared to five women suffering cage subsistence in the control group.[19]

In a very similar study, Chen et al. studied the IV bisphosphonate zoledronic acid compared to saline given 3 days postoperatively in 65 men and women with osteoporosis by DXA undergoing single level fusion. After decompression the disk space was packed with allograph and local bone but there was not an interbody device. Fusion was graded by the visualization of bridging across the vertebral bodies. Early on, the patients with zoledronic acid had better visualization of bone bridging across the vertebral bodies but at 1 year there was no difference. There were 6 patients in the saline group who suffered adjacent vertebral fractures and no patients in the zoledronic acid group. The patients in the zoledronic acid arm had better Oswestry scores which in part may be due to the reduction in adjacent segment vertebral fractures.[20]

Tu et al. studied IV zoledronic acid in 64 patients with osteoporosis undergoing lumbar interbody fusion surgery. 32 were treated with an IV infusion of zoledronic acid (ZOL) 3 days after surgery and a second injection 1 year later, and the other 32 patients did not receive ZOL. At 2-year follow-up, a solid fusion was achieved in 75% of the ZOL group and only 56% of the control group. At final follow-up, the incidence of final subsequent vertebral compression fractures (19% of the ZOL group and 51% of the control group, $P = 0.006$), pedicle screw loosening (18% of the ZOL group and 45% of the control group, $P = 0.03$), and cage subsidence > 2 mm (28% of the ZOL group and only 54% of the control group, $P = 0.04$) were significantly lower in the ZOL group than in the control group. The ZOL group demonstrated improvement in visual analog scale (VAS) (for leg pain VAS, 2/10 for the ZOL group and 5/10 for the control group; for back pain VAS, 2/10 for the ZOL group and 6/10 for the control group) and Oswestry disability index scores (7/25 for the ZOL group and 16/25 for the control group).[21]

It appears that the use of bisphosphonates does not inhibit fusion when given postoperatively. It is important to think about the biology of bisphosphonates which substantially reduce bone remodeling. When a potent bisphosphonate like IV zoledronic acid is given shortly after surgery it is likely that due to the local increased bone activity of the fusion mass that much of the zoledronic acid may preferentially go to the fusion mass. When potent antiresorptive drugs like zoledronic acid reduce bone turnover substantially there in an increase in local mineral apposition. This contributes to the increase in BMD, by DXA with these drugs, when given for osteoporosis. Perhaps, the increase in local mineralization of the fusion mass may make it appear sooner to the eye on X-ray or CT. The fact that after 12 months the rates of fusion are not much different is consistent with this hypothesis. Probably most importantly we can be comfortable that bisphosphonates given after surgery do not appear to reduce the success of spine fusion and they appear to reduce vertebral fractures in the adjacent vertebra. There were no pedicle screw failures in either group in both the alendronate and zoledronic acid trial by Chen. There was significantly less pedicle screw loosening in the study by Tu suggesting a powerful bisphosphonate may help preserve pedicle screw purchase/survival in a high-risk population. There is also some evidence in long-term survival studies of total joints that the use of bisphosphonates may reduce loosening and revision arthroplasty.[22,23] This may make some sense since once loosening begins there is activation of osteoclasts in part due to bone and metal debris. A bisphosphonate may reduce further loosening of the orthopedic device by reduction of local osteoclastic function with less local bone resorption.

It appears that in high risk patients there is reasonable clinical data to support the use of both antiresorptive drugs like bisphosphonates and anabolic drugs like TPTD in patients with poor bone health and at high risk for complications of spine surgery due to bone-related complications. The challenge may be in how do we decide which patients we should treat with systemic bone active agents.

PREOPERATIVE BONE HEALTH ASSESSMENT IN PATIENTS UNDERGOING ELECTIVE SPINE FUSION

There are currently no guidelines on which patients undergoing elective spine fusion should undergo a bone health assessment. It seems reasonable to draw from our guidance about assessment of fracture risk in the general population and the performance of testing such as DXA by organizations such as the International Society of Clinical Densitometry (ISCD).[24] It seems appropriate to also incorporate an understanding of the type of surgery planned and the number of levels that will be fused. The following are the author's suggestions on who should be considered for bone health evaluations before spine surgery. They are somewhat parallel to the guidance for osteoporosis testing for decisions on treatment for osteoporosis:

- Women over the age of 60 especially if there are other risk factors including early menopause or other clinical risk factors for fracture
- Men over age 70
- Any adult over age 50 who has been exposed to chronic glucocorticoid use which is generally defined as at least 5 mg/d for over 90 days
- These suggestions could be modified based upon the type of surgery planned. For example, a 55-year-old woman who is undergoing 10 level fusion for adult spine deformity should perhaps be considered differently than a similar woman undergoing single level fusion.

The simplest way to evaluate bone health of the adult spine is to look for prevalent fractures of the spine. The literature is full of studies that document that a prior fracture is a very important risk factor for a future fracture. Siris et al. looked at about 2,500 women in the placebo arms of two large osteoporosis studies with baseline and 2 year spine X-rays. They looked at the 2 year incidence of spine fractures based upon the fracture status of their baseline spine X-ray and their baseline BMD by DXA. There was a clear relationship between low BMD and the risk of incident spine fracture. The risk was substantially higher, independent of BMD, in women with baseline fractures. The risk was significantly higher depending on the number of baseline fractures and the severity of the vertebral fracture[25] (Figs. 1A to D). The severity of spine fractures on X-ray has also been correlated with the quality of the bone on iliac crest bone biopsy.[26] A recent study by the Center of Disease Control (CDC) National Health and Nutrition Examination Survey (NHANES) group did a population survey of US men and women age 40 and above using the imaging of spine fractures available on the DXA machine, known as vertebral fracture assessment (VFA). This can be done at the point of service when the patient gets a standard BMD assessment by DXA with minimal radiation and just a few extra minutes on the table. The prevalence of spine fractures steadily increases with age in both men and women. Importantly, of patients who reported they had a previous spine fracture, about 80% of them did not have a vertebral fracture on imaging. Of the patients who had a documented vertebral fracture, less than 10% of them were aware of the fracture when asked in a survey before the X-ray was performed.[5] This tells us that spine fractures are very important predictors of bone health of the spine but we must image the thoracic and lumbar spine to identify the fractures.

The technology used most commonly to assess bone health is DXA). Absorptiometry is based upon an X ray energy emitted below the patient on the table with a detector above the patient. Mineral within bone will block the X-ray from the detector. Based upon a known mineral standard and routine calibration of the machine there is an estimation of bone mineral content in the region of interest, such as a vertebral body. The machine then measures the area of the individual vertebral body and an areal BMD (aBMD) is determined. The machines have a built in normative database of healthy men and women. Adults are compared to the average BMD of healthy 30-year-old and assigned a standard deviation above or below the average BMD of a healthy 30-year-old. This is known as a T-score. The World Health Organization (WHO) established that the definition of osteoporosis by DXA as a T-score of at least 2.5 standard deviations below the healthy 30-year-old average. Most clinicians would agree that in the presence of an obvious fragility fracture that a patient can be labeled with clinical osteoporosis even if their BMD does not meet the -2.5 criteria. The advantages of DXA include low radiation, fast acquisition time, low

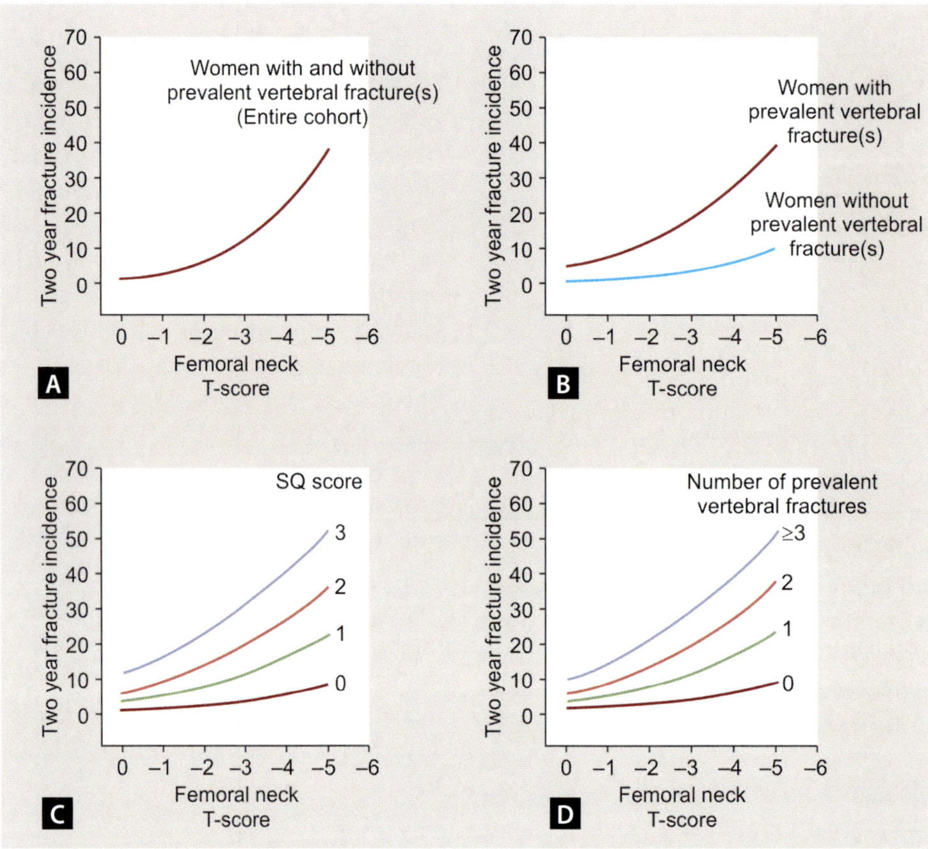

Figs. 1A to D: (A) Relationship of baseline BMD with 2-year fracture incidence; (B) Incidence of incident fractures in women with and without baseline prevalent vertebral fractures; (C) Incidence of vertebral fractures dependent upon the severity of the baseline fracture (0—no fracture, 1—mild fracture, 2—moderate fracture, and 3—severe fracture); (D) Incidence of vertebral fractures dependent upon the number of baseline vertebral fractures.

Source: Adapted from Siris ES, Genant HK, Laster AJ, et al. Enhanced prediction of fracture risk combining vertebral fracture status and BMD. Osteoporos Int. 2007;18(6):761-70.

cost, and availability. However, in patients with significant degenerative changes, DXA of the spine has limitations. Significant degenerative changes of the posterior elements will impact the BMD results but the bone from osteophytes does not add to the strength of the vertebral body. Generally, an experienced clinician reading the DXA images will not allow individual vertebral bodies to be included in the analysis of L1-4 if there are significant degenerative changes. The guidelines ask for at least two vertebral bodies to be free of degenerative changes for a lumbar spine DXA to be used to assess fracture risk. The DXA will also assess BMD at the hip and the forearm which is helpful for overall fracture risk assessment at all sites. However, with spine fusion patients it seems logical that we would like to get a bone health assessment of the spine to guide our management.

An additional software to further analyze the DXA images of the spine is known as trabecular bone score (TBS). This software looks at the distribution of the bone within the vertebral body on a two dimensional image acquired by the DXA machine. A low TBS value has been independently associated with increased fracture risk.[27] Two patients may have the same BMD but the patient with a low TBS value will have a higher fracture risk and perhaps be more vulnerable to bone-related complications of spine surgery (Fig. 2). Populations such as patients on glucocorticoids and patients with long-standing diabetes may be good candidates for TBS evaluation prior to spine fusion surgery. One potential advantage of TBS in addition to standard BMD by DXA is that TBS is not impacted by the presence of osteoarthritis of the spine.[28] Cadaver studies have shown that an increased TBS score is related to increased pull-out strength.[29] TBS is FDA approved but

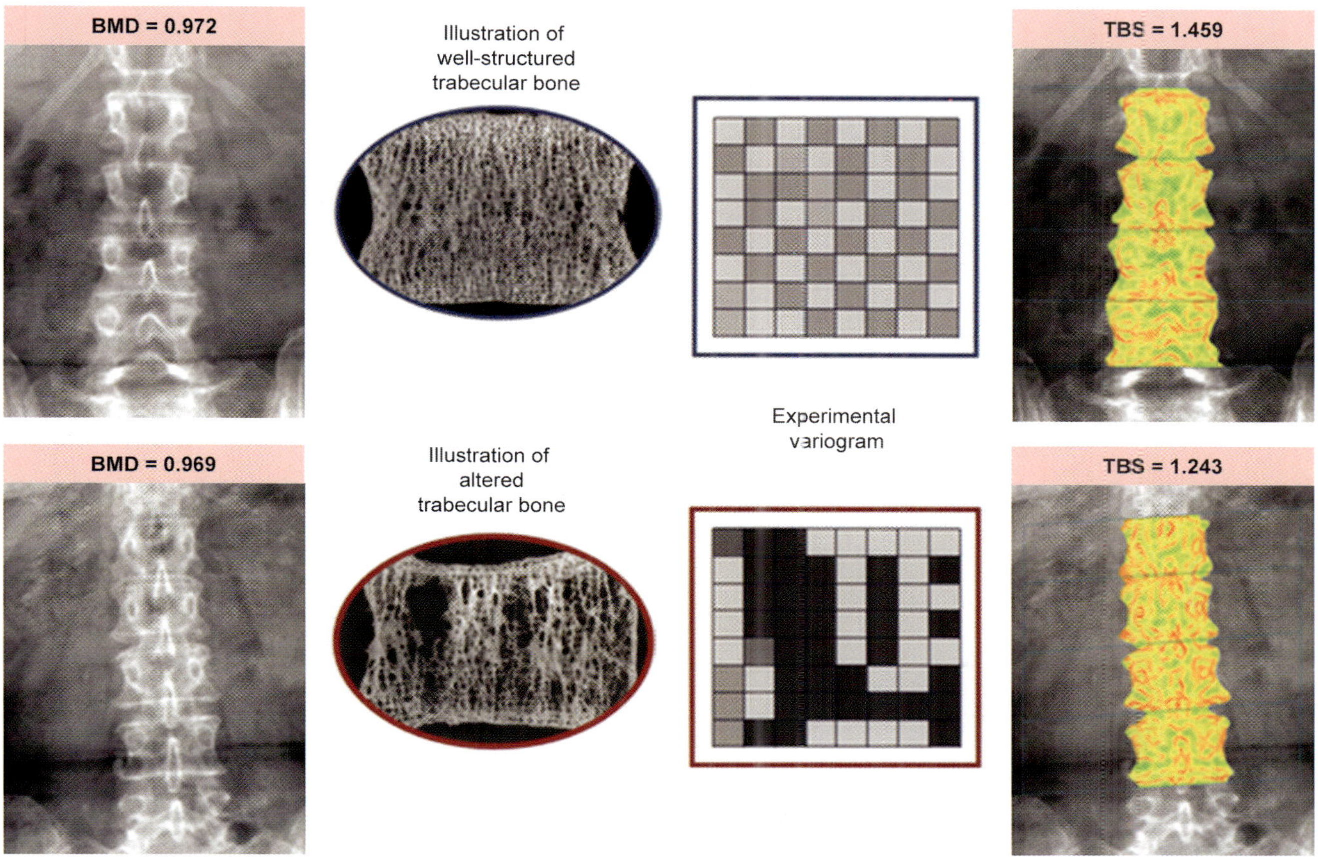

Fig. 2: Trabecular bone score (TBS). These two individuals have essentially the same LS BMD by DXA but due to altered trabecular bone, the patient on the bottom has a significantly lower TBS.

generally not well-reimbursed by insurances in the US at this time.

Many patients will have lumbar spine CT scans as part of their preoperative evaluation. CT images may be used to acquire volumetric BMD. Volumetric BMD may be more sensitive to change but there is less epidemiology data to use it routinely for fracture risk assessment. Finite element analysis (FEA) is a technique of using the CT image of a vertebral body and assigning individual voxels a material property based upon mineral density. Estimates of bone strength can be done for the proximal femur and the vertebra. An axial load is placed upon the vertebral body to the point of virtual fracture (Fig. 3). The algorithm for the software for this assessment required validation with cadaveric vertebral bodies and biomechanical testing. The output of FEA is strength in Newtons. The software will also give the clinician a volumetric BMD. Low vertebral compressive strength estimates by FEA have been shown to predict fracture risk better than standard DXA BMD in an elderly male cohort.[30] The report produced by the company simply labels the strength as normal, low or fragile (Table 1). This may be much less confusing than the historical use of T-scores with DXA. Burch et al. have looked at bone strength in a population of women of ages 50–70 undergoing elective spine fusion using CT-based FEA. They found that 29% were classified as having poor bone quality (either osteoporosis or fragile bone strength) using pre-established validated threshold values to define the presence of osteoporosis (trabecular BMD of 80 mg/cm^3 or lower) and fragile bone strength (vertebral strength of 4,500 N or lower).[31] Work is ongoing to determine if low bone strength by CT-based FEA is predictive of bone-related complications of spine surgery. This may be an attractive technology especially if the patient has already had a lumbar spine CT as part of their workup for spine

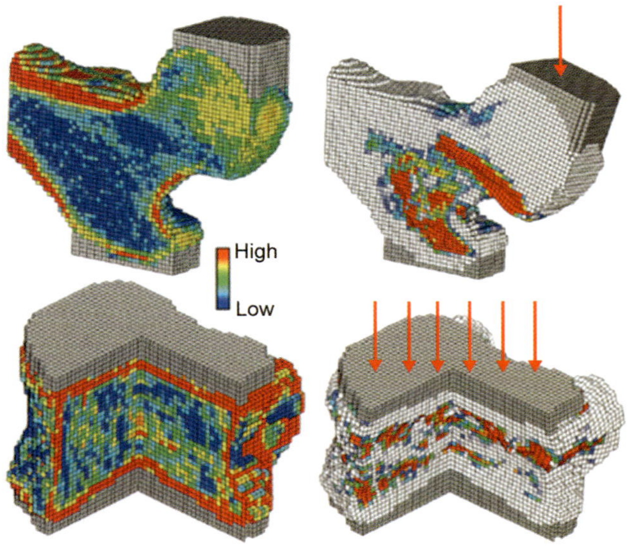

Fig. 3: The VirtuOst bone strength measurements. Left: Sectioned views of finite element models of a proximal femur (sideways fall configuration) and a vertebral body, the colors showing the local material properties as derived from the CT scan. Right: The bones undergo virtual stress testing, the colors depicting where the bone tissue fails (red is more intense failure).
Source: ON Diagnostics.

surgery. Again, FEA is FDA approved but generally not reimbursed by US insurance.

DISCUSSION

Spine fusion surgery on older patients is likely to continue to grow with the aging population and the improvements in spine surgery techniques and instrumentation. Older adults often want to remain physically active and successful spine surgery can be life changing in appropriate patients. It appears that poor bone health is associated with increased bone-related complications such as pedicle screw failure, adjacent segment vertebral fractures and perhaps lower success of spine fusion. There is a growing acknowledgement of the importance of bone health in older patients undergoing elective spine fusion surgery.[32]

While the evidence for use of systemic osteoporosis medications appears to be reasonably solid, the studies were appropriately done in patients with poor bone health and in some studies the patients met the criteria for the diagnosis of osteoporosis. Standard assessments such as DXA are helpful but have limitations in this population of older patients with degenerative changes of the spine.

Table 1: The VirtuOst interventional thresholds for BMD and bone strength. Together with the BMD and bone strength measurements, these thresholds are used to identify osteoporosis and fragile bone strength, respectively.

Interpreting the VirtuOst Report: Summary			
	Spine	*Bone mineral density (BMD)*	*HIP*
Women and men	BMD ≥ 120 mg/cm^3	Normal	BMD T ≥ –1.0
	80 < BMD < 120	Low (osteopenia)	–2.5 < BMDT < –1.0
	BMD ≤ 80	Osteoporosis	BMDT ≤ –2.5*
			** At either femoral neck or total hip regions*
		Bone strength (STR)	
Women	STR ≥ 6000 N	Normal	STR ≥ 4000 N
	4500 < STR < 6000	Low	3000 < STR < 4000
	STR ≤ 4500	Fragile bone strength	STR ≤ 3000
Men	STR ≥ 8500 N	Normal	STR ≥ 5000 N
	6500 < STR < 8500	Low	3500 < STR < 5000
	STR ≤ 6500	Fragile bone strength	STR ≤ 3500

Source: ON Diagnostics.

SECTION 1

Other imaging technologies such as TBS and CT-based FEA may complement standard DXA. Assessment of prevalent spine fractures in the thoracic and lumbar spine seems to be appropriate to preoperatively assess bone health in these patients. Selective use of both anabolic and antiresorptive drugs has the potential to reduce complications and improve fusion success in high-risk patients. Medical doctors who specialize in bone health need to have basic clinical insights into spine fusion surgery and the unique bone-related issues in this population. Spine surgeons likely do not want to oversee the bone health assessment or the prescribing of systemic osteoporosis drugs. It appears to be a great opportunity for medical and surgical specialists to work together to improve the outcome of their patients undergoing spine fusion surgery.

REFERENCES

1. Bonjour J, Theintz G, Law F, et al. Peak bone mass. Osteoporos Int. 1994;4(Suppl 1):7-13.
2. Bradney M, Pearce G, Naughton G, et al. Moderate exercise during growth in prepubertal boys: changes in bone mass, size, volumetric density, and bone strength: a controlled prospective study. J Bone Miner Res. 1998;13(12):1814-21.
3. Fuchs RK, Bauer JJ, Snow CM. Jumping improves hip and spine bone mass in prepubescent children. J Bone Miner Res. 2001;16(1):148-56.
4. van Staa T, Dennison EM, Leufkens HG, et al. Epidemiology of fractures in England and Wales. Bone. 2001;29(6):517-22.
5. Cosman F, Krege J, Looker A, et al. Spine fracture prevalence in a nationally representative sample of US women and men aged ≥40 years: results from the National Health and Nutrition Examination Survey (NHANES) 2013-2014. Osteoporos Int. 2017;28(6):1857-66.
6. Weinstein R. Clinical practice. Glucocorticoid-induced bone disease. N Engl J Med. 2011;365(1):62-70.
7. Jilka R, Weinstein R, Bellido T, et al. Increased bone formation by prevention of osteoblast apoptosis with PTH. J Clin Invest. 1999;104(4):439-46.
8. Langdahl B, Ferrari S, Dempster DW. Bone modeling and remodeling: potential as therapeutic targets for the treatment of osteoporosis. Ther Adv Musculoskelet Dis. 2016;8(6):225-35.
9. Miller PD, Hattersley G, Riis BJ, et al; ACTIVE Study Investigators. Effect of Abaloparatide vs Placebo on New Vertebral Fractures in Postmenopausal Women with Osteoporosis: A Randomized Clinical Trial. JAMA. 2016;316(7):722-33.
10. Cosman F, Crittenden D, Grauer A. Romosozumab treatment in postmenopausal osteoporosis. NEJM. 2017;376(4):396-7
11. Lehman RA Jr, Dmitriev AE, Cardoso MJ, et al. Effect of teriparatide [rhPTH(1-34)] and calcitonin on intertransverse process fusion in a rabbit model. Spine (Phila Pa 1976). 2010;35(2):146-52.
12. O'Loughlin P, Cunningham M, Bukata S, et al. Parathyroid hormone (1-34) augments spinal fusion, fusion mass volume, and fusion mass quality in a rabbit spinal fusion model. Spine (Phila Pa 1976). 2009;34(2):121-30.
13. Ohtori S, Inoue G, Orita S, et al. Teriparatide accelerates lumbar posterolateral fusion in women with postmenopausal osteoporosis: prospective study. Spine (Phila Pa 1976). 2012; 37(23):E1464-8.
14. Ohtori S, Orita S, Yamauchi K, et al. More than 6 months of teriparatide treatment was more effective for bone union than shorter treatment following lumbar posterolateral fusion surgery. Asian Spine J. 2015;9(4):573-80.
15. Ohtori S, Inoue G, Orita S, et al. Comparison of teriparatide and bisphosphonate treatment to reduce pedicle screw loosening after lumbar spinal fusion surgery in postmenopausal women with osteoporosis from a bone quality perspective. Spine (Phila Pa 1976). 2013;38(8):E487-92.
16. Inoue G, Ueno M, Nakazawa T, et al. Teriparatide increases the insertional torque of pedicle screws during fusion surgery in patients with postmenopausal osteoporosis. J Neurosurg Spine. 2014;21(3):425-31.
17. Yagi M, Ohne H, Konomi T, et al. Teriparatide improves volumetric bone mineral density and fine bone structure in the UIV+1 vertebra, and reduces bone failure type PJK after surgery for adult spinal deformity. Osteoporos Int. 2016;27(12):3495-502.
18. Ohtori S, Orita S, Yamauchi K, et al. Does discontinuing teriparatide treatment and replacing it with bisphosphonate maintain the volume of the bone fusion mass after lumbar posterolateral fusion in women with postmenopausal osteoporosis? Asian Spine J. 2017;11(2):272-7.
19. Nagahama K, Kanayama M, Togawa D, et al. Does alendronate disturb the healing process of posterior lumbar interbody fusion? A prospective randomized trial. J Neurosurg Spine. 2011;14(4):500-7.
20. Chen F, Dai Z, Kang Y, et al. Effects of zoledronic acid on bone fusion in osteoporotic patients after lumbar fusion. Osteoporos Int. 2016;27(4):1469-76.
21. Tu CW, Huang KF, Hsu HT, et al. Zoledronic acid infusion for lumbar interbody fusion in osteoporosis. J Surg Res. 2014;192(1):112-6.
22. Khatod M, Inacio MC, Dell RM, et al. Association of Bisphosphonate use and risk of revision after THA: Outcomes from a US Total Joint Replacement Registry. Clin Orthop Relat Res. 2015;473(11):3412-20.
23. Namba RS, Inacio MC, Cheetham TC, et al. Lower total knee arthroplasty revision risk associated with bisphosphonate use, even in patients with normal bone density. J Arthroplasty. 2016;31(2):537-41.
24. Schousboe J, Shepherd J, Bilezikian J, et al. Executive summary of the 2013 International Society for Clinical Densitometry Position Development Conference on Bone Densitometry. J Clin Densitom. 2013;16(4):455-66.
25. Siris ES, Genant HK, Laster AJ, et al. Enhanced prediction of fracture risk combining vertebral fracture status and BMD. Osteoporos Int. 2007;18(6):761-70.

26. Genant H, Delmas P, Chen P, et al. Severity of vertebral fracture reflects deterioration of bone microarchitecture. Osteoporos Int. 2007;18(1):69-76.
27. Martineau P, Leslie W. Trabecular bone score (TBS): method and applications. Bone. 2017;104:66-72.
28. Kolta S, Briot K, Fechtenbaum J, et al. TBS result is not affected by lumbar spine osteoarthritis. Osteoporos Int. 2014;25(6):1759-64.
29. Le Nost P, Kolta S, Lelong C, et al. ASBMR Meeting Atlanta, GA Poster Sessions, Presentation Number: LB-MO0346 Session: Late-Breaking Posters III Monday, September 19, 2016.
30. Wang X, Sanyal A, Cawthon PM, et al; Osteoporotic Fractures in Men (MrOS) Research Group. Prediction of new clinical vertebral fractures in elderly men using finite element analysis of CT scan. J Bone Miner Res. 2012;27(4):808-16.
31. Burch S, Feldstein M, Hoffmann P, et al. Prevalence of poor bone quality in women undergoing spinal fusion using biomechanical-CT analysis. Spine (Phila Pa 1976). 2016;41(3):246-5.
32. Fischer C, Hanson G, Eller M, et al. A systematic review of treatment strategies for degenerative lumbar spine fusion surgery in patients with osteoporosis. Geriatr Orthop Surg Rehabil. 2016;7(4):188-96.

CHAPTER 5 Inflammatory Diseases of the Spine

Yu-Po Lee

RHEUMATOID ARTHRITIS

Epidemiology and Natural History

Rheumatoid arthritis (RA) is a chronic systemic autoimmune disorder. It affects approximately 1–2% of the population and symptoms typically begin between 20 and 45 years of age.[1-3] Females are more prone to develop RA with 70% of patients affected being female.[1-3] A positive rheumatoid factor (RF) is present in about 85% of patients, but it is not specific for RA and may be present in normal individuals.[1-3] In addition, individuals with the human leukocyte antigen–D related 1 (HLA-DR1) or human leukocyte antigen–D related 4 (HLA-DR4) serotypes have an increased risk for developing the disorder.[4,5] RA primarily affects the smaller joints of the appendicular skeleton in symmetric fashion. Progressive joint swelling, pain, and stiffness develop secondary to synovitis. Spine involvement is usually restricted to the cervical spine but patients may develop lumbar pain and the use of corticosteroids may lead to osteoporotic compression fractures.

Disease manifestations are seen in the synovial-lined joints secondary to erosive synovitis.[4,6,7] The destructive synovitis seen in RA is believed to be the result of an autoimmune response to an antigen expressed by the synovial cells. RF is an immunoglobulin G (IgG) that is directed against the antigens of these targeted synovial cells. This antigen-antibody interaction leads to the release of proteolytic enzymes that destroy the joint.[4,6,7] Spinal disease eventually occurs in about 60% of patients with RA.[1-3] Patients with more severe disease and longer duration of disease are at higher risk for cervical spine involvement. Once instability begins, the disease tends to progress to more complex instability patterns. In particular, atlantoaxial subluxation tends to progress toward superior migration of the odontoid. Rheumatoid synovitis may affect the synovial joints around the dens. This leads to erosion of the dens and progressive damage of the transverse, alar, and apical ligaments, leading to atlantoaxial subluxation. Pannus formation posterior to the dens may further contribute to cord compression.[4,6] Superior migration of the odontoid occurs from bony erosion between the occipitoatlantal and atlantoaxial joints or bilateral erosion of the lateral masses. This can result in brainstem compression and vascular compromise to the basivertebral and anterior spinal arteries. Erosion of the facet joints and degeneration of the interspinous ligaments and facet joints may lead to subluxation of the subaxial spine. Multiple level subluxation may lead to a "stepladder" appearance or a kyphotic deformity.[4,6] A positive RF, greater peripheral joint involvement, male gender, and corticosteroid use have been linked to greater cervical involvement.[4,6,7]

Work-up

Symptoms and Signs

The clinical presentation of RA is variable and ranges from asymptomatic patients to those with severe deformity and neurologic compromise.[1-3] Neck pain is the most common initial complaint and is often localized to the upper cervical spine and associated with occipital headaches.[1-3] Greater occipital nerve root irritation (C2) can lead to referred pain in the face, ear, and mastoid regions. Vertebrobasilar insufficiency may cause vertigo, nausea, vomiting, dysphagia, and dysarthria.[1-3] Patients with cord compression will show symptoms of myelopathy. The Ranawat classification is often used for myelopathy classification (Box 1).[8]

Box 1: Ranawat classification.

- Patients have no neurologic deficit
- Patients have subjective weakness, dysesthesias, and hyperreflexia
- Patients have objective signs of weakness and upper motor signs.
  - Patients are ambulatory
  - Patients are nonambulatory.

Laboratory Findings

When RA is clinically suspected, laboratory studies are helpful in confirming the diagnosis. One laboratory study is testing for the presence of RF.[9,10] A negative RF does not rule out RA; rather, the arthritis is called seronegative. This is the case in about 15% of patients.[9,10] During the first year of illness, RF is more likely to be negative with some individuals converting to seropositive status over time. RF is also seen in other illnesses, such as Sjögren's syndrome, systemic lupus erythematosus (SLE), chronic infections and in approximately 10% of the healthy population, therefore the test is not very specific.

Because of this low specificity, new serological tests have been developed, which test for the presence of the anticitrullinated protein antibodies (ACPAs) or anticyclic citrullinated peptide (anti-CCP).[9,10] Like RF, these tests are positive in only a proportion (67%) of all RA cases, but are rarely positive if RA is not present, giving it a specificity of around 95%.[9,10]

Also, several other blood tests are usually done to allow for other causes of arthritis, such as lupus erythematosus. Erythrocyte sedimentation rate (ESR), C-reactive protein, CBC with differential, metabolic panel, liver enzymes, and other immunological tests (such as ANA) are also suggested to rule out other causes of inflammation.

Imaging

Lateral radiographs are the most helpful for initial evaluation of the cervical spine. The posterior atlantodens interval (ADI), anterior ADI, subaxial subluxation, and superior migration of the odontoid should be evaluated. Flexion-extension lateral cervical radiographs are useful for evaluation of dynamic instability (Figs. 1A to D). An anterior ADI greater than 3.5 mm is considered abnormal. But, the posterior ADI was noted to have more prognostic value in one study.[11] An anterior ADI > 9–10 mm or posterior ADI < 14 mm is associated with an increased risk of neurologic injury and usually requires surgery.

Diagnosing superior migration of the odontoid can be difficult. Further evaluation with MRI or CT is recommended. A couple of criteria can be used to evaluate basilar invagination. The first one is the Redlund-Johnell criterion.[12] Here, the distance between the McGregor line and the midpoint of the inferior border of C2 is measured. A measurement less than 34 mm in males and less than 29 mm in females indicates basilar invagination. Another method is to divide the odontoid into three equal parts, the top, the middle, and the bottom. If the anterior ring of the atlas is level with the middle third, basilar invagination is diagnosed. Lastly, there is the Ranawat criterion.[13] Here, the distance between the pedicle of C2 and the ring of C1 is measured. A distance less than 15 mm in males and less than 13 mm in females is indicative of basilar invagination.

Medical Management

Disease-modifying antirheumatic drugs (DMARDs) are administered to reduce the rate of bone and cartilage damage. DMARDs have been found to reduce pain and to delay or halt progression.[14-16] This is important as such damage is usually irreversible. Anti-inflammatories and analgesics improve pain and stiffness but do not prevent joint damage or slow the disease progression.[14-16]

It is now believed that permanent damage to the joints occurs at a very early stage in the disease. In the past, it was common to start with just an anti-inflammatory drug, and assess progression clinically and radiographically. If there was evidence that joint damage was starting to occur then a more potent DMARD would be prescribed. The aim now is to treat before damage occurs.[14-16] DMARDs such as methotrexate, hydroxychloroquine sulfate, and sulfasalazine gold can have a significant impact. Oral steroids are also often used. Agents that target tumor necrosis factor-α (infliximab, etanercept, and adalimumab) and interleukin-1 (anakinra) can be added for patients that do not respond well to the DMARDs.

Surgical Indications and Treatment

Surgery is considered for patients with intractable pain or neurologic deficits. Surgical intervention should be attempted before the onset of Ranawat class III myelopathy because neurologic improvement is limited after this.[17-19] In patients who have limited symptoms or who are asymptomatic, the decision for surgery is more complex. Based on radiographic criteria, three subgroups

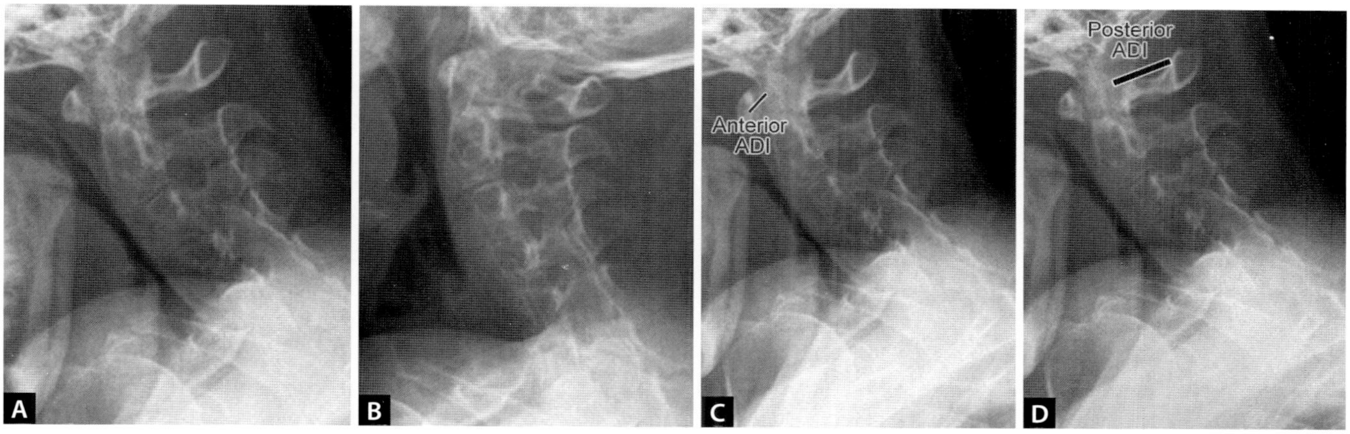

Figs. 1A to D: (A) Flexion of patient with rheumatoid arthritis. Note anterior atlantodens interval (ADI) of 5 mm; (B) Extension of patient with rheumatoid arthritis. Note how anterior ADI corrects to normal; (C) Anterior ADI; (D) Posterior ADI.

have been identified who would benefit from surgery even if they have limited or no symptoms. In the first group, C1-C2 fusion is recommended for patients with a posterior ADI < 14 mm or if there is more than 3.5 mm of segmental mobility.[11,17-19] In one study, patients with neurologic deficits and a posterior ADI of less than 10 mm showed no recovery, whereas those with a posterior ADI of at least 10 mm showed some recovery, and those with a posterior ADI of at least 14 mm had complete neurologic recovery after surgery.[11] Patients with a posterior ADI between 10 and 14 mm had recovery of at least one Ranawat class.

C1-2 Fusion

The goals of surgery are to prevent further neurologic deterioration and alleviate pain by decompression and stabilization of deformity. The traditional method of C1-C2 fusion involves the use of sublaminar wires and bone graft. Gallie first described C1-C2 fusion in 1939 with sublaminar wires and a tricortical H-shaped bone graft taken from the iliac crest.[20] The primary drawback of this technique is that there is only a single, midline point of fixation that is susceptible to rotational forces. Consequently, this is not a very rigid construct and requires a rigid orthosis, preferably a halo, for postoperative immobilization. In addition, concern exists when more than one spinal segment is spanned using sublaminar wires because of the increased risk of injury to the spinal cord. This is particularly significant in cases in which anterior translation of C1 results in a decrease in spinal canal dimensions and a relative spinal canal stenosis. Brooks later modified this technique with bilateral sublaminar wiring and grafting.[21] While better rotational control is obtained with the Brooks technique with bilateral wiring, the Brooks fusion method shares the same disadvantage associated with the Gallie procedure of requiring multisegment sublaminar wires. Heavy-gauge single-strand wires pose a significant danger of causing injury to the spinal cord during their passage. In patients with spinal cord compression and an irreducible atlantoaxial subluxation, the use of posterior C1 arch wires should be avoided and a laminectomy should be performed. Furthermore, a relatively high pseudoarthrosis rate has been noted in a number of studies. In a study by Coyne et al., the authors performed a retrospective review of 32 patients who had either a Gallie or Brooks wiring procedure. Even with halo supplementation, the nonunion rate was 19%.[22] In another study by Farey et al., the authors evaluated 12 patients who had a modified Gallie procedure retrospectively after a mean follow-up of 6.9 years.[23] In this study, the pseudoarthrosis rate was noted to be 42%. Hence, while relatively easier to apply, posterior wiring of C1 and C2 has been noted to have a relatively high pseudoarthrosis rate.

A major advance in posterior C1-2 fixation was described by Magerl in 1986.[24] In this chapter, Magerl describes crossing the C1-C2 joints with a screw. Fixation of the C1-2 lateral masses with transarticular screws provides immediate stabilization. Also, a posterior decompression can be performed if necessary because this method does not require a complete or competent arch of C-1 for a successful fusion. In most cases, an interspinous Gallie style H graft taken from the iliac crest is placed between the posterior arch of C-1 and the posterior spinous process and superior laminar surface of C-2. Careful preoperative planning is required, with thin-cut CT scans and CT reconstructions to confirm that adequate bone exists to allow passage of the screws without injury to the vertebral arteries. The pros of this procedure are that there is immediate stabilization of the C1 and C2 vertebrae and the high fusion rates. In one study by Gluf et al., the authors performed a retrospective review on 191 patients who had a C1-C2 fusion with transarticular screws.[25] The fusion rate was noted to be 98% with a mean time of fusion occurring at 9.5 months. Of note, there were five vertebral artery injuries with one resulting in death. In another study by Dickman et al., the authors performed a retrospective review on 121 patients who had a posterior fusion with either C1-C2 transarticular screws or Gallie wiring.[26] In this study, a 98% union rate was noted with C1-C2 transarticular screws versus 86% with Gallie wiring.

Technique 1

In this procedure, the occiput and the posterior arches of C-1, C-2, and C-3 are exposed subperiosteally. Passage of the wire, drill, and screw require a fairly "flat" angle and, frequently, secondary incisions need to be created in the upper thoracic region to obtain the required angle, thus avoiding the need to perform a much longer cervical incision. Hence, it is necessary to drape down to the lumbar spine. Draping down to the lumbar spine is also advised because a tricortical iliac crest graft is also often used to obtain the fusion. By exposing the superior edge of the C-2 lamina and the isthmus bilaterally, the medial surface of the C-2 pedicle can be palpated using a probe. The drill entrance point is located on the inferior facet of C-2 2–3 mm lateral from the medial edge and 2–3 mm above the caudal edge. With the aid of fluoroscopy, the trajectory is adjusted to exit C-2 at the posterior edge of the superior articular surface, near the entrance of the C-2 pedicle. The lateral mass articulation is crossed so that the subarticular surface is entered at its posterior to middle third. The ideal trajectory orients the drill toward the anterior arch of C-1 (Fig. 2A). Instrumentation can then be placed once satisfactory positioning has been confirmed with fluoroscopy (Figs. 2B and C).

Although transarticular C1-C2 screws provide improved biomechanical strength, they may not be feasible for use in patients with a large or aberrant foramen transversarium in C2 (Fig. 3). In a study by Madawi et al., a retrospective review was performed in 67 patients who underwent C1-C2 transarticular fusion.[27] Evaluation of the CT scans showed that 20% of the patients had narrowing of the C2 pedicle to less than 3.5 mm, thus making the procedure unfeasible or potentially dangerous. In another study by Paramore et al., the authors performed a retrospective review on 94 patients who underwent C1-C2 transarticular screw fixation.[28] The authors noted that the procedure was not feasible in 18% of patients and dangerous or risky in an additional 5%. Hence, fine cut

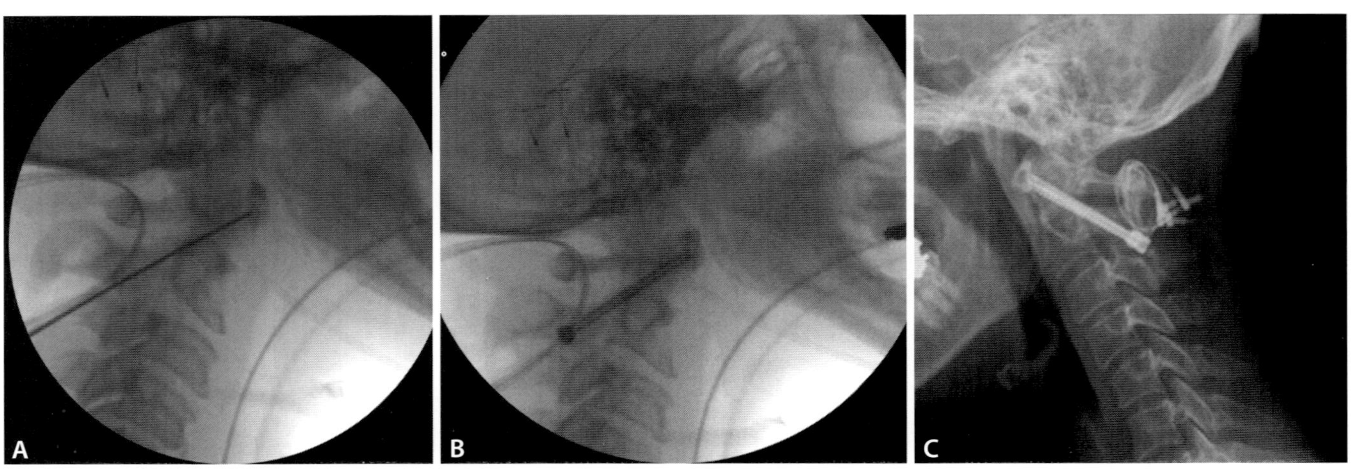

Figs. 2A to C: (A) A guidewire is drilled along the pars of C2 aiming toward the anterior ring of C1 passing the C1-2 joint between posterior and middle third; (B) A cannulated screw is placed along the guidewire; (C) Bilateral C1-2 transarticular screws have been placed with sublaminar wires.

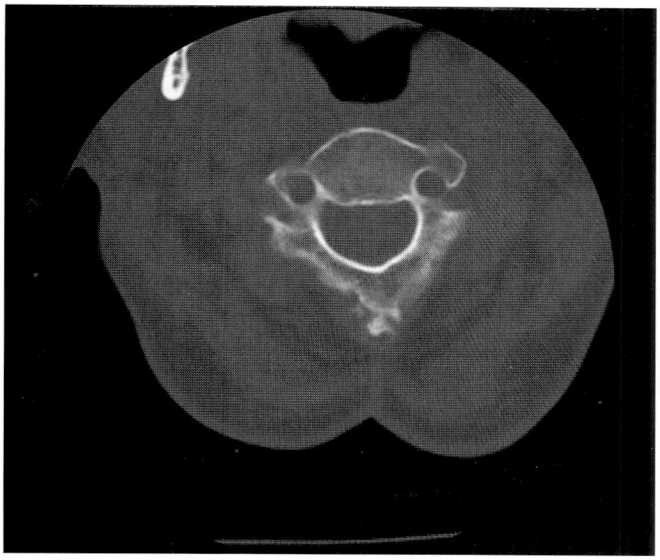

Fig. 3: Note the enlarged foramen transversarium. The pedicle of C2 is too small to accommodate a screw without potential risk of injury to the vertebral artery.

CTs are recommended on all patients prior to considering C1-C2 transarticular fixation to determine feasibility. In the event that the vertebral artery has an injury, do not attempt transarticular fixation of the contralateral side. Instead, place the screw to stop the bleeding and proceed with posterior wiring of the C1-C2 lamina. Leave the contralateral side alone to prevent injury to the contralateral vertebral artery because injury to both vertebral arteries is fatal. In one study by Song et al., the authors retrospectively reviewed 19 patients who had unilateral C1-C2 transarticular screws supplemented with laminar wiring and grafting. The authors noted a solid fusion in 18 patients.[29] Hence, bilateral C1-C2 transarticular screws are not absolutely necessary to obtain a solid fusion and a unilateral construct should be considered if the preoperative CT shows the C2 pedicles are too small for safe passage of the screws or if one vertebral artery has been injured.

In 2001, Harms and Melcher described another method of atlantoaxial stabilization.[30] Polyaxial head screws are inserted into the lateral mass of C-1 and into the pars or the pedicle of C-2. These screws are secured by rods bilaterally. Using this technique, C1-2 fixation can be attained in patients who are not candidates for transarticular screws because of fixed subluxation of C-1 on C-2 as well as in patients in whom the vertebral artery (VA) is in an aberrant location, which would preclude the passage of screws.

Technique 2

In these patients 3.5 mm polyaxial screws are inserted into the lateral masses of C-1 and through the pars interarticularis into the pedicles of C-2. If necessary, a fluoroscopically-guided reduction of the C1-C2 articulation can then be performed prior to the insertion of the 3 cm rods. This is not possible with C1-C2 transarticular screws and is one of the pros of C1-C2 fixation. Cancellous bone graft obtained from the iliac crest can be used for fusion. No structural grafting or wiring is required.

A standard posterior exposure of C1 and C2 is performed from the occiput to C4. There is a venous plexus lateral to the C1 lateral masses and this can bleed profusely. It is recommended to have gelfoam and thrombin and other hemostatic agents available to control this bleeding. Also, when exposing C1, avoid exposing more than 1.5 cm past midline because the vertebral artery may be injured if the exposure is carried too far laterally. The C1-C2 complex is exposed to the lateral border of the C1-C2 articulation. The C2 nerve root is retracted inferiorly to expose the C1 lateral mass. Once the midpoint of the C1 lateral mass has been identified, a drill is inserted and aimed 5–10° medially in the axial plane and in line with the arch of C1 in the sagittal plane. Sometimes, a small portion of the caudal edge of the C1 posterior arch must be removed with a Kerrison punch to be able to align the drill in the correct orientation. Sometimes, it may also be necessary to ligate the C2 nerve root to be able to get adequate exposure of the C1 lateral mass. In a study by Aryan et al., the authors performed a multicenter retrospective review on patients who had ligation of the C2 nerve root.[31] This was performed in 102 patients bilaterally without any significant sequelae with fusion noted in all but two patients. Bicortical purchase is recommended but care must be taken not to advance the drill bit too far anteriorly after the anterior cortex of the C1 lateral mass has been perforated. In a study by Currier et al., the authors performed a CT study on 50 random patients.[32] The authors noted that the internal carotid artery was within 2–3 mm of the C1 lateral masses and if the internal carotid artery is in close proximity to the anterior border of C1, unicortical fixation or a different fusion technique should be considered. When placing the C1 lateral mass screw, a partially threaded screw is used to

CHAPTER 5

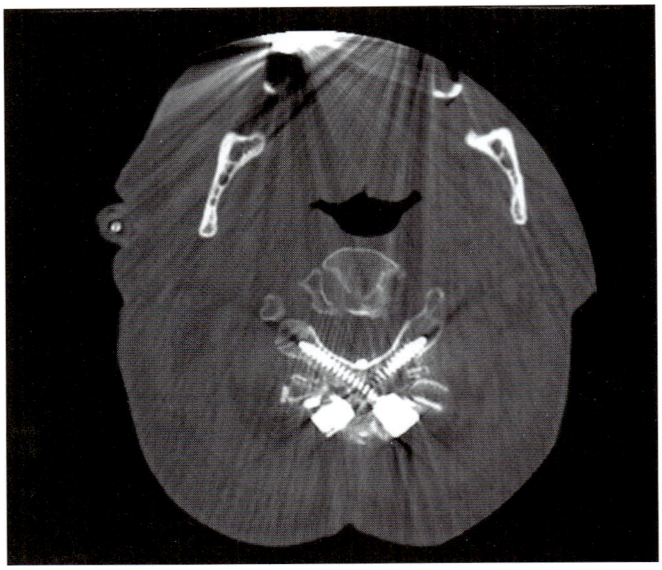

Fig. 4: Translaminar screws have been placed in C2.

minimize irritation of the C2 nerve root. Also, it should be placed approximately 1 cm proud to facilitate connection to the C2 screw.

Once the C1 lateral mass screw has been placed, attention is turned to the C2 screw. A number 4 Penfield can be used to delineate the medial border of the C2 pars interarticularis. A pilot hole is prepared with a drill bit. The ideal spot is at the intersection of the midlines of the C2 lamina and the par interarticularis. The direction of the bit is approximately 20–30° in a convergent and cephalad direction, guided directly by the superior and medial surface of the C2 isthmus. The drill bit is advanced under fluoroscopy and the trajectory adjusted as necessary. A 3.5 mm polyaxial screw of the appropriate length is inserted if imaging shows good positioning.

Alternative techniques include the use of C1 lateral mass screws coupled with C2 laminar screws (Fig. 4). This is a useful technique when a solid fusion is desired but preoperative CTs show that C1-C2 transarticular screws and C1-C2 screws are not feasible or potentially dangerous. In a study by Sciubba et al., the authors performed a retrospective review on 16 patients on whom they attempted C1-C2 fusion with C1 lateral mass screws and C2 laminar screws.[33] The authors noted a solid fusion in all of the patients except for one. When a solid fusion is obtained, the periodontoid pannus tends to regress and slow the progression of cranial settling.[18,19]

If basilar invagination has occurred, an occiput to C2 fusion is recommended. Decompression may be accomplished with a C1 arch removal or transoral odontoid resection. In cases where there is severe settling, cervical traction may be useful to reduce the dens to its normal position and take pressure off of the brainstem/spinal cord prior to occiput to C2 fusion.[34] For patients with subaxial subluxation requiring surgery, a posterior fusion with lateral mass screws is sufficient.

Complications

The main concern with RA is progressive neurologic deterioration. Hence, early diagnosis and intervention is very important. With earlier diagnosis, patients can be started on the DMARDs sooner to halt or slow down deterioration of the spine. As mentioned previously, once degeneration has occurred, the DMARDs do not repair the damage; hence prevention is very important in this case. Once the spine has become affected by RA, monitoring of these patients is very important because intervention before patients have deteriorated to a Ranawat III grade myelopathy may still allow some or complete motor recovery. When surgery is performed, spinal cord injury and vertebral artery injury are concerns since the cervical spine is usually affected more than the lumbar spine. CT scans of the cervical spine are recommended prior to surgery because they are very important in surgical planning and may help prevent injury to the spinal cord or vertebral artery.

Prognosis

The prognosis now for patients with RA is very good. The DMARDs have been shown to be very effective in preventing or slowing down the progression of deterioration. Also, surgical techniques have improved to allow for more effective fusions and have been shown to halt or reverse myelopathy once it starts in many cases.

ANKYLOSING SPONDYLITIS

Epidemiology and Natural History

Ankylosing spondylitis (AS) is a chronic seronegative inflammatory disease of unknown origin that affects the axial spine.[35-39] It begins in the third decade of life, and has a 3:1 male to female predominance. It is a member of the seronegative spondyloarthropathies (inflammatory arthropathies that share similar characteristics, including a negative RF, sacroiliitis with or without spondylitis, peripheral inflammatory arthritis, and a genetic predisposition).[35-39] Members include AS, psoriatic arthritis, Reiter's syndrome, and the enteropathic spondyloarthropathies. AS occurs in about 0.2–0.3% of the US population.[35-39] It is believed that there is a genetic predisposition, although the mode of inheritance remains unknown.

There are a few theories regarding the link of HLA-B27 to AS.[37-39] One includes the binding of HLA-B27 to a peptide in the joint and the resultant stimulation of the pathologic cascade. Another is that HLA-B27 positive individuals are more susceptible to certain microorganisms, such as *Klebsiella pneumoniae*, leading to a disease-producing synovitis.[37,38] Lastly, some believe that autoimmunity against HLA-B27 itself by cytotoxic T cells may also play a role.[37,38]

The seronegative spondyloarthropathies share fundamental differences from RA besides being RF negative. This class of disease affects the entheses (the bony insertions of ligaments and tendons) whereas RA affects the synovial lining. Inflammation of the entheses leads to bony erosions followed by new or reactive bone formation and eventual ankylosing. Inflammation of the annulus fibrosis leads to formation of bridging syndesmophytes. The seronegative spondyloarthropathies tend to affect the entire axial spine, whereas RA is limited primarily to the cervical spine. The spondyloarthropathies are characterized by sacroiliitis and a distinctive pattern of involvement of the appendicular skeleton. In the peripheral skeleton, AS involves the entheses. Patients with psoriatic arthritis have interphalangeal destruction. While Reiter's syndrome affects the synovial joints of the lower extremity. The nonspinal manifestations of AS include large peripheral joint (hip and shoulder) arthritis, acute anterior uveitis, renal amyloidosis, ascending aortic abnormalities (stenosis, aortitis, and regurgitation), and cardiac conduction abnormalities.[35-38]

Work-up

Signs and Symptoms

Most patients present with chronic low-back pain in early adulthood. Pain is often localized to the gluteal and sacroiliac regions initially.[35-38] With further inflammatory changes, back stiffness develops that is exacerbated by periods of inactivity. Patients have decreased chest expansion relative to other people. Any patient with AS who presents with a sudden onset of back or neck pain must be worked up for a fracture.[40,41] These fractures are considered unstable because they extend across all three columns and create two rigid segments with long lever arms that move independent of each other. Rapid neurologic deterioration can occur as a result of spinal instability or hematoma formation. Patients may also present with a kyphotic deformity in their spine. This is due to multiple microfractures that occur over time.[42]

Laboratory Findings

The laboratory test most commonly associated with AS is HLA-B27. Variations of the HLA-B gene increase the risk of developing AS, although it is not a diagnostic test. Patients who develop AS are HLA-B27 positive approximately 95% of the time, but 6–8% of Caucasians who never develop symptoms also test positive for HLA-B27.[35-38] Hence, the HLA-B27 test is a very useful test, but in itself is not diagnostic of AS in a person with back pain

Other blood tests are usually done to check for other causes of inflammation. ESR, C-reactive protein, CBC with differential, metabolic panel, liver enzymes, and other immunological tests (such as ANA) are also suggested.

Radiographic Evaluation

The earliest sign of AS is erosion on the iliac side of the sacroiliac joint.[35-38,42,43] AS has a predilection for bilateral sacroiliitis and marginal thin flowing syndesmophytes leading to the characteristic "bamboo spine" appearance.[35-38,42,43] (Figs. 5A and B) The chin-brow to vertical angle can be measured to determine the degree of deformity. This is the angle between a line connecting the chin and brow and a vertical line. This angle is helpful in determining the amount of correction needed when doing an osteotomy. Other diagnostic modalities include scintigraphy, CT, and MRI. Scintigraphy is sensitive to the inflammation in sacroiliac joints, but lacks specificity. CT detects early bony changes, but is unable to show active inflammation. MRI can detect active inflammation, making it the best for early detection.[42,43]

If a fracture is suspected, fine-cut CT scans with sagittal reconstructions should be ordered in addition to plain radiographs. Fractures can be missed in up to 50% of cases.[40,41] MRI should also be considered to evaluate for hematomas.

Treatment

Medical Management

Physical therapy and exercise, along with medication, are the main forms of treatment for AS.[35-38] Physical therapy that includes a program to improve flexibility and strength should be advised. Bracing can be considered for pain control.

Anti-inflammatory medications are often given to reduce inflammation prior to initiating therapy.[44] NSAIDs have been the mainstay of treatment, but have provided minimal relief. Hence, narcotic analgesics are also given to reduce pain while the NSAIDs reduce the inflammation.

Recent studies have shown promising results with tumor necrosis factor-α blocking agents.[45,46] Short symptom duration and a positive C-reactive protein test at baseline are currently the best predictors for a good response to TNF-blocking agents.

Surgical Indications and Treatment

Any patient with AS and the sudden onset of neck or back pain regardless of how minor should be considered to have a fracture until proven otherwise. Most fractures are located in the midcervical to cervicothoracic junction and at the thoracolumbar junction.[40,41] A fractured ankylosed spine may be very unstable because these fractures extend across three columns, creating two rigid segments with long moment arms that move independently. Stable fractures without neurologic compromise often heal without complications and may be immobilized in an external brace or halo device. Unstable fractures require instrumentation and fusion.[47] Because of the risks of neurologic deterioration and the difficulty with bracing caused by thoracic kyphosis, surgery is often recommended for cervical spine fractures. Most fractures may be treated with posterior instrumentation, but anterior stabilization may also be necessary when patients are osteoporotic.[47-50] When surgery is considered, instrumentation is recommended at least across three segments to prevent instrumentation complication or pullout.[47-50]

For patients with kyphotic deformities of their spine, surgery may be an option. The goals of surgery are restoration of sagittal balance and level of horizontal gaze. Anterior opening osteotomies or pedicle subtraction osteotomies are the preferred surgeries. Osteotomies can be done at the cervical, thoracic, or lumbar spine, depending on the site of the deformity.

Cervical spine osteotomies may be performed in patients with a fixed flexion deformity.[51] In the most severe cases, a "chin-on-chest" deformity is present. Cervical

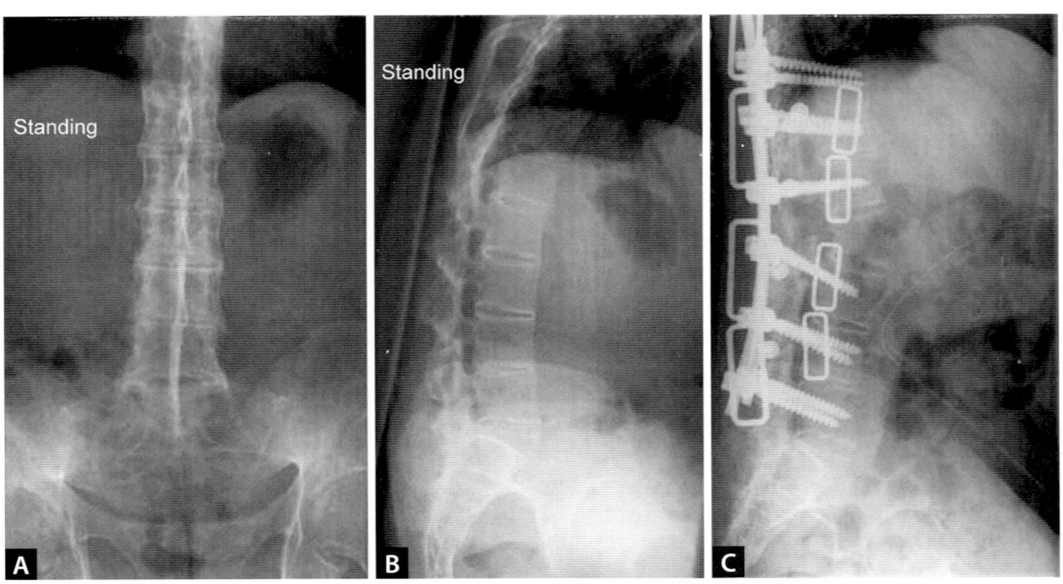

Figs. 5A to C: (A) AP of patient with ankylosing spondylitis. Note the marginal syndesmophytes that give it the characteristic "bamboo spine" appearance; (B) Lateral; (C) Patient after a L2 pedicle subtraction osteotomy.

deformities impair the patient's ability to maintain a forward gaze, cause difficulties with personal hygiene, and lead to swallowing difficulties. This is a high-risk procedure. The osteotomy typically is performed at C7-T1.[51] This is because the vertebral artery normally enters the foramen transversarium at C6 and the spinal canal at C7-T1 is relatively more spacious. Also, injury to C8 would cause less disability than to the other nerve roots.

Thoracolumbar osteotomies can be performed to correct global alignment and gaze alignment (*see* Fig. 5C). Classically, an anterior opening osteotomy that pivots on the posterior edge of the vertebral body has been used. This procedure has an increased risk of major vascular injuries especially in elderly patients with reduced arterial compliance. Vascular complications occurred when the osteotomies were performed at L2 or above the point at which the renal vessels tether the aorta and above the bifurcation.

Another option is to perform a pedicle subtraction osteotomy.[52,53] This may need to be done at more than one level depending on the severity of the kyphotic deformity. These osteotomies involve the removal of the posterior elements above and below the pedicle where the osteotomy will be performed. Then a wedge is removed via a transpedicular decancelization procedure. The posterior wedge is then closed hinging on the anterior cortex. This leads to direct bony apposition and rapid consolidation. Studies have shown that this is a safe and effective method to correct kyphosis and sagittal imbalance. In a study by Chen et al., the authors performed a retrospective review on 78 patients with AS who underwent a single- or two-level pedicle subtraction osteotomy for a fixed flexion deformity.[52] The authors found that there was a mean correction of 34.5° for every level where an osteotomy was performed. Good or excellent results were obtained in 77 patients (98.7%) at the final follow-up. There was no mortality, nor were there any major neurological complications noted. In another study by Kim et al., the authors performed a prospective study on 45 patients who had developed a fixed flexion deformity.[53] The authors noted a mean correction of 34° for every level where an osteotomy was performed. They noted that most of the patients maintained good correction and had good clinical results, but that clinical outcome did not necessarily correlate with radiographic correction.

Technique

Care should be taken in intubating and positioning the patient. It is important to keep in mind that the slightest trauma may cause a cervical or thoracolumbar fracture so once the patient has been intubated, the patient should be gently placed prone in their natural alignment and well padded. A Wilson frame can be helpful here because it is adjustable and in severely kyphotic patients, you may need to start the case in maximal kyphosis. Once the exposure is complete and the levels identified, pedicle screws should be placed. The ideal location for the osteotomy is at L2 and pedicle screws should be placed 3 levels above and below. Next, a laminectomy is performed and the necessary posterior elements are resected. When resecting the posterior elements, the surgeon should start off using hand instruments such as rongeurs to remove the spinous processes. Then, if needed, a high-speed air-drill is used to thin the posterior elements. This may be necessary because there will not be a patent interlaminar space and a burr is needed to enter the spinal canal. Once the spinal canal is entered, Kerrison punches can then be used to complete the laminectomy. If performing a L2 PSO, it is recommended to also perform a laminectomy of L1 and L3. This should provide enough of a decompression so that when the wedge is closed at the end of the case, the nerve roots will not get pinched. Once the laminectomy has been performed, a Smith-Petersen osteotomy both cephalad and caudal to the pedicles on both sides of L2 is performed. This involves exposing the nerve root caudal to the pedicle.

The next step is to decancellate the pedicles and vertebral body. The medial wall of the pedicle is identified, and the thecal sac and the nerve root are retracted with a nerve root retractor to identify the posterior wall of the vertebral body. The pedicle is first decancellated with a high speed burr. The walls of the pedicle can then be removed with a rongeur until the pedicle stump is flush with the posterior wall of the vertebral body.

Care should be taken to retract the neural elements so that the exiting nerve root is not injured during the process. The transverse process is identified and the muscular attachments are released with curettes. The transverse process on both sides can then be removed with Kerrison punches. Then, the cancellous bone of the vertebral body is removed with curettes. The next step is to finish the resection of the posterior wall of the vertebral

CHAPTER 5

body. Working underneath the posterior vertebral cortex, the surgeon thins the cortex as much as possible with curettes. Once the posterior wall of the vertebral body is thin enough, a Woodson elevator or a substantial reverse-angled curette is placed beneath the ventral surface of the dura and gently tamped anteriorly to create a greenstick fracture of the posterior vertebral cortex. The fractured posterior cortex is then removed. The amount of the posterior wall that is removed should be symmetrical.

Next, the lateral walls of the vertebral body are identified and the soft tissues are released with a Penfield 1 elevator. The lateral vertebral cortex should be hugged during the dissection so that the segmental vessel is not injured. Then, a thinner rongeur is used to resect the lateral vertebral body walls down to, but not through, the anterior cortex in the shape of a wedge with the apex anterior.

The final step is to close the osteotomy. The Wilson frame can be let down and pillows may be placed underneath the knees to gently extend the spine. Then the rods are cut and contoured to connect the pedicle screws. AP and lateral images should be taken to ensure that no subluxation anteriorly has occurred or any coronal deformity introduced. When the construct is complete and the osteotomy is closed on both sides, the spinal canal is evaluated again with a Woodson elevator to confirm that there is no dorsal compression of the dural sac. The lateral masses should be squeezed together very tightly to promote stability and osteogenesis.

Complications

The main concern in patients with AS is the risk of fractures. Hence, any patient with AS who complains of the sudden onset of acute pain after any trauma, regardless of how insignificant should be considered to have a fracture until proven otherwise. Radiographs may be negative even though a fracture may be present. So, follow-up evaluation with CT scans or MRI is necessary to truly rule out a fracture. Hematomas may form in these patients and cause neurologic injury so these patients should have frequent neurologic evaluations to make sure that there is not a hematoma forming or a fracture causing instability.

Prognosis

Ankylosing spondylitis can range from mild to progressively debilitating and from medically controlled to refractive. Some patients have times of active inflammation followed by times of remission, while others never have times of remission and have acute inflammation and pain.

With studies on newer medications, it is hopeful that patients may live longer with AS before severe deformities become debilitating.

PSORIATIC SPONDYLITIS

6–48% of patients with psoriatic arthritis develop a spondyloarthropathy.[54] The exact cause remains unknown but there are a number or genetic associations. Of these patients, 70% are HLA-B27 positive.[55] Unlike AS, discovertebral erosions and axial ankylosis occur in a noncontiguous asymmetric pattern with both marginal and nonmarginal syndesmophytes. Patients with psoriatic spondylitis may also have a synovial proliferative process in the cervical spine similar to RA, with a similar clinical presentation. There is no definitive test to diagnose psoriatic arthritis. Diagnosis is based on physical examination, health history, blood tests, and X-rays characteristic of psoriatic arthritis. Factors that contribute to the diagnosis of psoriatic spondylitis are a past medical history of psoriasis or family history of psoriasis, a negative RF, and radiographic images showing joint destruction.[54,56,57] Other symptoms that are more typical of psoriatic arthritis than other forms of arthritis include inflammation in the Achilles tendon or the plantar fascia, and dactylitis (sausage-like swelling of the fingers or toes). Medical treatment is similar to that for patients with RA, with early use of DMARDs and tumor necrosis factor-α blocking agents in addition to NSAIDs.[58-60] Surgical indications are similar to those for patients with RA who have cervical disease or AS and deformity.

REITER'S SYNDROME

Reiter's syndrome is thought to occur as a postinfectious reactive arthritis.[61-63] It typically affects people in the third and fourth decade of life. Symptoms usually occur within 1 month of urethritis or enteritis. The manifestations of Reiter's syndrome include the following triad of symptoms: An inflammatory arthritis of large joints, uveitis, and urethritis in men or cervicitis in women.[61,62] Reiter's syndrome is RF seronegative but there is a link to HLA-B27.[63] Lumbar spine involvement occurs in approximately 50% of patients, but cervical spine involvement is rare. In contrast to AS, asymmetric sacroiliitis and nonmarginal syndesmophytes are seen in patients with spine involvement. Treatment is symptomatic and surgery is rarely necessary.[61,62] The main goal of treatment is to identify and eradicate the underlying infectious source with the appropriate antibiotics, if still present. Otherwise, treatment is symptomatic for each problem. Analgesics particularly NSAIDs, steroids, and immunosuppressants may be needed for patients with severe reactive symptoms that do not respond to any other treatment.[61,62]

ENTEROPATHIC ARTHRITIS

Spondylitis can occur in association with ulcerative colitis or Crohn's disease.[39] The clinical presentation and treatment is identical to that for idiopathic AS. 80% of patients who have spinal involvement are HLA-B27 positive.[39] Spine involvement is independent of the bowel disease course and may even occur before the onset of intestinal symptoms.

DIFFUSE IDIOPATHIC SKELETAL HYPEROSTOSIS

Diffuse idiopathic skeletal hyperostosis (DISH) or Forestier's disease is an enthesopathy of the spine, shoulder, elbow, knee, and calcaneus. It typically occurs in patients who are middle-aged or older. In contrast to AS, DISH patients have large nonmarginal syndesmophytes and do not have involvement of the sacroiliac joints.[64] Four contiguous vertebral bodies must be involved to be classified as DISH. Thoracic and lumbar involvement leads to stiffness and pain, while cervical involvement results in large anterior osteophytes that can cause dysphagia and stridor.[65] Ossification of the posterior longitudinal ligament can lead to myelopathy, whereas large segmental ossification makes the spine vulnerable to fractures like in AS.[66] These fractures are similarly unstable and often require surgery.[67] DISH is more common in patients with diabetes or gout. DISH is associated with extraspinal ossification at several joints, including an increased risk of heterotopic ossification following total hip surgery.[68]

REFERENCES

1. Majithia V, Geraci SA. Rheumatoid arthritis: diagnosis and management. Am J Med. 2007;120(11):936-9.
2. Haraoui B. Assessment and management of rheumatoid arthritis. J Rheumatol Suppl. 2009;82:2-10.
3. Anderson RJ. The diagnosis and management of rheumatoid synovitis. Orthop Clin North Am. 1975;6(3):629-39.
4. Harris ED Jr. Pathogenesis of rheumatoid arthritis. Clin Orthop Relat Res. 1984;(182):14-23.
5. Stastny P. Rheumatoid arthritis: relationship with HLA-D. Am J Med. 1983;75(6A):9-15.
6. Weyand CM, Goronzy JJ. Pathogenesis of rheumatoid arthritis. Med Clin North Am. 1997;81(1):29-55.
7. Mannik M, Nardella FA. IgG rheumatoid factors and self-association of these antibodies Clin Rheum Dis. 1985;11(3):551-72.
8. Ranawat CS, O'Leary P, Pellicci P, et al. Cervical spine fusion in rheumatoid arthritis. J Bone Joint Surg Am. 1979;61(7):1003–10.
9. Tedesco A, D'Agostino D, Soriente I, et al. A new strategy for the early diagnosis of rheumatoid arthritis: a combined approach. Autoimmun Rev. 2009;8(3):233-7.
10. Lee AN, Beck CE, Hall M. Rheumatoid factor and anti-CCP autoantibodies in rheumatoid arthritis: a review. Clin Lab Sci. 2008;21(1):15-8.
11. Boden SD, Dodge LD, Bohlman HH, et al. Rheumatoid arthritis of the cervical spine. A long-term analysis with predictors of paralysis and recovery. J Bone Joint Surg Am. 1993;75(9):1282-97.
12. Redlund-Johnell I, Pettersson H. Vertical dislocation of the C1 and C2 vertebrae in rheumatoid arthritis. Acta Radiol Diagn (Stockh). 1984;25(2):133-41.
13. Riew KD, Hilibrand AS, Palumbo MA, et al. Diagnosing basilar invagination in the rheumatoid patient. The reliability of radiographic criteria. J Bone Joint Surg Am. 2001;83(2):194-200.
14. Saeki Y, Matsui T, Saisho K, et al. Current treatments of rheumatoid arthritis: from the 'NinJa' registry. Expert Rev Clin Immunol. 2012;8(5):455-65.
15. Sen D, Brasington R. Tight disease control in early RA. Rheum Dis Clin North Am. 2012;38(2):327-43.
16. Gramling A, O'Dell JR. Initial management of rheumatoid arthritis. Rheum Dis Clin North Am. 2012;38(2):311-25.
17. Falope ZF, Griffiths ID, Platt PN, et al. Cervical myelopathy and rheumatoid arthritis: a retrospective analysis of management. Clin Rehabil. 2002;16(6):625-9.
18. Matsunaga S, Sakou T, Onishi T, et al. Prognosis of patients with upper cervical lesions caused by rheumatoid arthritis: comparison of occipitocervical fusion between c1 laminectomy and nonsurgical management. Spine (Phila Pa 1976).. 2003;28(14):1581-7.
19. Omura K, Hukuda S, Katsuura A, et al. Evaluation of posterior long fusion versus conservative treatment for the progressive rheumatoid cervical spine. Spine (Phila Pa 1976). 2002;27(12):1336-45.
20. Gallie WE. Fractures and dislocations of the cervical spine. Am J Surg. 1939;46(3):495-9.
21. Brooks AL, Jenkins EB. Atlanto-axial arthrodesis by the wedge compression method. J Bone Joint Surg Am. 1978;60(3):279-84.
22. Coyne TJ, Fehlings MG, Wallace MC, et al. C1-C2 posterior cervical fusion: Long-term evaluation of results and efficacy. Neurosurgery 1995;37(4): 688-92.
23. Farey ID, Nadkarni S, Smith N. Modified Gallie technique versus transarticular screw fixation in C1-C2 fusion. Clin Orthop Relat Res. 1999;(359):126-35.

CHAPTER 5

24. Magerl F, Seemann P-S. Stable posterior fusion of the atlas and axis by transarticular screw fixation. In: Kehr P, Weidner A (Eds). Cervical Spine I. New York, Wien: Springer; 1987. pp. 322-7.
25. Gluf WM, Schmidt MH, Apfelbaum RI. Atlantoaxial transarticular screw fixation: a review of surgical indications, fusion rate, complications, and lessons learned in 191 adult patients. J Neurosurg Spine. 2005;2(2):155-63.
26. Dickman CA, Sonntag VK. Posterior C1-C2 transarticular screw fixation for atlantoaxial arthrodesis. Neurosurgery. 1998;43(2):275-80.
27. Madawi AA, Casey AT, Solanki GA, et al. Radiological and anatomical evaluation of the atlantoaxial transarticular screw fixation technique. Neurosurg. 1997;86(6):961-8.
28. Paramore CG, Dickman CA, Sonntag VHS. The anatomical suitability of the C1-2 complex for transarticular screw fixation. J Neurosurg. 1996;85(2):221-4.
29. Song GS, Theodore N, Dickman CA, et al. Unilateral posterior atlantoaxial transarticular screw fixation. J Neurosurg. 1997;87(6):851-5.
30. Harms J, Melcher RP. Posterior C1-C2 fusion with polyaxial screw and rod fixation. Spine (Phila Pa 1976). 2001;26(22):2467-71.
31. Aryan HE, Newman CB, Nottmeier EW, et al. Stabilization of the atlantoaxial complex via C-1 lateral mass and C-2 pedicle screw fixation in a multicenter clinical experience in 102 patients: modification of the Harms and Goel techniques. J Neurosurg Spine. 2008;8(3):222-9.
32. Currier BL, Maus TP, Eck JC, et al. Relationship of the internal carotid artery to the anterior aspect of the C1 vertebra: implications for C1-C2 transarticular and C1 lateral mass fixation. Spine (Phila Pa 1976). 2008;33(6):635-9.
33. Sciubba DM, Noggle JC, Vellimana AK, et al. Laminar screw fixation of the axis. J Neurosurg Spine. 2008;8(4):327-34.
34. Graziano GP, Hensinger R, Patel CK. The use of traction methods to correct severe cervical deformity in rheumatoid arthritis patients: a report of five cases. Spine (Phila Pa 1976). 2001;26(9):1076-81.
35. Sieper J, Braun J, Rudwaleit M, et al. Ankylosing spondylitis: an overview. Ann Rheum Dis. 2002;61(Suppl 3):iii8-18.
36. Stafford L, Youssef PP. Spondyloarthropathies: an overview. Intern Med J. 2002;32(1-2):40-6.
37. Reveille JD, Arnett FC. Spondyloarthritis: update on pathogenesis and management. Am J Med. 2005;118(6):592-603.
38. Braun J, Sieper J. Ankylosing spondylitis. Lancet. 2007; 369(9570):1379-90.
39. Reveille JD. The genetic basis of spondyloarthritis. Curr Rheumatol Rep. 2004;6(2):117-25.
40. Nakstad PH, Server A, Josefsen R. Traumatic cervical injuries in ankylosing spondylitis. Acta Radiol. 2004;45(2):222-6.
41. Grisolia A, Bell RL, Peltier LF. Fractures and dislocations of the spine complicating ankylosing spondylitis: a report of six cases. J Bone Joint Surg Am. 1967;49(2):339-44.
42. Brophy S, Mackay K, Al-Saidi A, et al. The natural history of ankylosing spondylitis as defined by radiological progression. J Rheumatol. 2002;29(6):1236-43.
43. Grigoryan M, Roemer FW, Mohr A, et al. Imaging in spondyloarthropathies. Curr Rheumatol Rep. 2004;6(2):102-9.
44. Braun J, Sieper J. Biological therapies in the spondyloarthritides-the current state. Rheumatology (Oxford). 2004;43(9):1072-84.
45. Song IH, Maksymowych WP. Therapeutic controversies: tumor necrosis factor α inhibitors in ankylosing spondylitis. Rheum Dis Clin North Am. 2012;38(3):613-33.
46. Sieper J. Developments in therapies for spondyloarthritis. Nat Rev Rheumatol. 2012;8(5):280-7.
47. Taggard DA, Traynelis VC. Management of cervical spinal fractures in ankylosing spondylitis with posterior fixation. Spine. 2000;25(16):2035-9.
48. Payer M. Surgical management of cervical fractures in ankylosing spondylitis using a combined posterior-anterior approach. J Clin Neurosci. 2006;13(1):73-7.
49. Sapkas G, Kateros K, Papadakis SA, et al. Surgical outcome after spinal fractures in patients with ankylosing spondylitis. BMC Musculoskelet Disord. 2009;10:96.
50. Olerud C, Frost A, Bring J. Spinal fractures in patients with ankylosing spondylitis. Eur Spine J. 1996;5(1):51-5.
51. Belanger TA, Milam RA 4th, Roh JS, et al. Cervicothoracic extension osteotomy for chin-on-chest deformity in ankylosing spondylitis. J Bone Joint Surg Am. 2005;87(8):1732-8.
52. Chen IH, Chien JT, Yu TC. Transpedicular wedge osteotomy for correction of thoracolumbar kyphosis in ankylosing spondylitis: experience with 78 patients. Spine. 2001;26(16):354-60.
53. Kim KT, Suk KS, Cho YJ, et al. Clinical outcome results of pedicle subtraction osteotomy in ankylosing spondylitis with kyphotic deformity. Spine (Phila Pa 1976). 2002;27(6):612-8.
54. Day MS, Nam D, Goodman S, et al. Psoriatic arthritis. J Am Acad Orthop Surg. 2012;20(1):28-37.
55. Haroon M, Fitzgerald O. Pathogenetic overview of psoriatic disease. J Rheumatol Suppl. 2012;89:7-10.
56. van Tubergen A, Weber U. Diagnosis and classification in spondyloarthritis: identifying a chameleon. Nat Rev Rheumatol. 2012;8(5):253-61.
57. Amrami KK. Imaging of the seronegative spondyloarthopathies. Radiol Clin North Am. 2012;50(4):841-54.
58. Soriano ER. The actual role of therapy with traditional disease-modifying antirheumatic drugs in psoriatic arthritis. J Rheumatol Suppl. 2012;89:67-70.
59. Richards BL, Whittle SL, van der Heijde DM, et al. Efficacy and safety of neuromodulators in inflammatory arthritis: a Cochrane systematic review. J Rheumatol Suppl. 2012;90: 28-33.
60. Cantini F, Niccoli L, Nannini C, et al. Infliximab in psoriatic arthritis. J Rheumatol Suppl. 2012;89:71-3.
61. Carter JD, Hudson AP. Reactive arthritis: clinical aspects and medical management. Rheum Dis Clin North Am. 2009;35(1):21-44.

62. Kataria RK, Brent LH. Spondyloarthropathies. Am Fam Physician. 2004;69(12):2853-60.
63. Rihl M, Barthel C, Klos A, et al. Identification of candidate genes for susceptibility to reactive arthritis. Rheumatol Int. 2009;29(12):1519-22.
64. Olivieri I, D'Angelo S, Palazzi C, et al. Diffuse idiopathic skeletal hyperostosis: differentiation from ankylosing spondylitis. Curr Rheumatol Rep. 2009;11(5):321-8.
65. Verlaan JJ, Boswijk PF, de Ru JA, et al. Diffuse idiopathic skeletal hyperostosis of the cervical spine: an underestimated cause of dysphagia and airway obstruction. Spine J. 2011;11(11):1058-67.
66. Kim TJ, Kim TH, Jun JB, et al. Prevalence of ossification of posterior longitudinal ligament in patients with ankylosing spondylitis. J Rheumatol. 2007;34(12):2460-2.
67. Paley D, Schwartz M, Cooper P, et al. Fractures of the spine in diffuse idiopathic skeletal hyperostosis. Clin Orthop Relat Res. 1991;(267):22-32.
68. Nilsson OS, Persson PE. Heterotopic bone formation after joint replacement. Curr Opin Rheumatol. 1999;11(2):127-31.

CHAPTER 6 Principles of Spine Trauma and Spinal Cord Injury

Melissa Nadeau, Brian K Kwon

EPIDEMIOLOGY

Traumatic spine injuries and the disabilities that they cause, particularly when associated with a spinal cord injury (SCI), can be devastating for patients and their families, and are a great concern for society as a whole. The average lifetime cost of treating an individual with a traumatic SCI is between C$1.47 million and $3.03 million in Canada, and between US$500 000 and $2 million in the United States. Total annual costs of caring for individuals with traumatic SCI are estimated to be around $2.67 billion in Canada, and over $7 billion in the United States.[1-3] Because they often cause lifelong disability and have significant socioeconomic consequences, an understanding of the epidemiology, demographics, and etiologies of traumatic spinal injuries is important. This may help identify potential risk factors in various populations, direct the development of prevention programs, and guide the distribution of health care resources towards appropriately specialized treatment and rehabilitation facilities.[4]

In North America, the incidence of SCI ranges between 27 and 48.4 cases per million individuals.[5-10] These numbers vary in other parts of the world, from as low as 12.1 in the Netherlands[11] to as high as 57.8 cases per million in Portugal.[12] A recent meta-analysis found large variation in the incidence of SCI from one continent to another—North America had the highest incidence, with 51 SCI per million inhabitants per year, Asia 23.9, Europe 19.4, and Australia 16.8.[13]

Demographics of Spinal Cord Injury

There is a bimodal age distribution for SCI—the first peak is found in young adults (15–29 years) and the second peak in older adults (> 70 years).[6,7,14] The lowest rate of SCI is observed in children younger than 10 years.7 Despite the incidence of SCI remaining stable for the last 30 years or so, the demographic trends in the SCI population are changing. There has been an increase in the mean age at injury from 28.6 years in the 1970s to 41.5 years in 2004.[6,15] While young individuals continue to suffer from SCI, the rise in average age at time of injury is likely due to a bimodal distribution of injuries, where a growing number of elderly individuals are suffering from SCI. This is contributed by the general aging of our population: Canadian individuals older than 65 years increased from 7.7% in 1966 to 14.4% in 2011.[16] In addition, public health measures have been focusing on transport-related injuries, which tend to affect young men and women. In contrast, there has been a lack prevention programs for fall-related SCI,[17] which typically involves elderly individuals.

The ratio of men to women with SCI differ with each age group, with a ratio of 1.5:1 in the youngest (< 10 years) and oldest (> 70 years) age groups, and up to 3.5:1 in the 10–69 years age group.[7] This ratio has recently decreased, probably because women's lifestyles are becoming more similar to that of men with respect to workplace and participation in high-risk sporting activities.

Etiology of Spinal Cord Injury

Between 2005 and 2012 in the United States, motor vehicle collisions (MVC) accounted for 39.2% of reported SCI cases. The next most common cause of SCI is falls (28.3%), followed by acts of violence (14.6%), and lastly sports and recreation (8.3%).[15] These numbers differ slightly in Canada with a larger proportion of injuries attributed to MVC and sports, and a smaller proportion to violence (Table 1).[4,6,14,18]

Table 1: Etiology of adult traumatic spinal cord injury (SCI).

	Incidence (%)	
Cause of Injury	*USA*	*Canada*
MVC	39	53
Falls	28	25
Sports and recreation	8	12
Violence	15	5
Other	10	5

(MVC: Motor vehicle collisions)

Source: Based on data from the National Spinal Cord Injury Statistical Center.[15] Canadian data based on averages from reports in Pirouzmand 2010,[18] Dryden 2003,[6] Lenehan 2012,[4] Pickett 2006.[14]

Leading etiologies differ greatly from one age group to another. Most notably, falling is associated with the oldest mean age, and violence with the youngest.[18] Changing trends in etiology have therefore paralleled changing trends in SCI incidence by age groups, with an increasing proportion of SCI occurring secondarily to falls in the elderly.[19-21] Fall-induced injuries are a major public health concern in North America and other developed countries.[22] Prevention programs should aim their focus toward home safety and avoidance of falls in the elderly. Physicians are encouraged to adopt the use of tools such as the World Health Organization's FRAX algorithm to identify patients at risk and institute more aggressive medical treatment of osteoporosis to help halt this trend.[14,23] There is also an increasing proportion of injuries in thrill-seeking sports such as snowboarding, skiing, mountain biking, rock climbing, parachuting, and hand gliding.[20,24,25] Despite this, the incidence of SCI due to sports in general has decreased over time.[15] For example, the percentage of injuries resulting from diving, a leading cause of SCI in Canada in the 1980s has steadily decreased because of prevention programs and improved swimming pool design.[26-28] Similarly, the average annual number of spinal injuries in ice hockey decreased from an average of 13.0 in 1981–1999 to 6.7 in 2000–2005. This is thought to be the result of the implementation of several educational initiatives and targeted prevention programs, as well as rule changes (e.g. Hockey Canada's "no-checking-from-behind" rule).[29,30] This demonstrates the importance of knowledge about the etiology of SCI to establish awareness and preventive measures that are effective in decreasing injury rates.

According to data collected by the National Spinal Cord Injury Statistical Center between 2005 and 2012, the most frequent neurologic category of patients with SCI in the United States is incomplete tetraplegia (40.8%), followed by complete paraplegia (21.6%), incomplete paraplegia (21.4%), and complete tetraplegia (15.8%). Over the last 15 years, the percentage of persons with incomplete tetraplegia has increased while complete paraplegia and complete tetraplegia have decreased.[15] Acute SCIs are most often seen in cervical spine injuries, accounting for 55–75% of all SCIs.[14,20] 6–15% occur in every other region thoracic (T1–T11), thoracolumbar (T11–L2), and lumbosacral (L2–S1).[14,20] The vulnerability of the cervical spine to SCI is likely due to the increased mobility, smaller vertebrae, and decreased strength of stabilizing soft tissue structures in that region relative to the more caudal areas.[20] Neurologic deficit and level data differ greatly between the two peak age groups for spine injuries. Generally, geriatric patients have fewer cervical and more lumbar fractures, sustain a lower severity of injury, and suffer paralysis less frequently then their adult counterparts.[31]

FIELD RESUSCITATION AND TRANSPORTATION

Over the last 50 years, the neurological consequences of traumatic spine injuries have been decreasing. This is likely the result of improvements in retrieval systems and immobilization during transportation to hospital as well as the quality of immediate care following the injury, which include prompt diagnosis and management, aggressive avoidance of systemic hypotension and hypoxia, as well as improved moving and nursing of patients.[20] This section discusses issues surrounding initial recognition, evaluation, and emergency management of trauma patients with spinal column and SCI.

Recognition

Spinal cord injuries are not always obvious in the multi-traumatized patient. Physicians must maintain a high index of suspicion, as well as perform a careful, comprehensive, and timely initial evaluation in order to initially recognize the presence of a SCI and administer appropriate preliminary treatment. This is of utmost importance to prevent potential deterioration of neurologic function, which can be catastrophic and irreversible. As mentioned in the epidemiology section, high-risk mechanisms

CHAPTER 6

that should raise awareness of a possible spine injury consists of high-energy trauma in young patients such as motor vehicle accidents, and low-energy trauma in the elderly such as falls. Moreover, physicians should have a heightened clinical suspicion in the presence of head injury or facial trauma, which suggest the possibility of high forces at the cervical spine.[32] A recent nationwide review in the United States reported the following rates of concomitant cervical spine injuries: 6.7% in patients with facial fractures, 7.0% in patients with head injuries, and 7.8% in patients with combined facial fracture and head injury.[33] Underlying comorbidities such as osteoporosis or ankylosing spondylitis should also raise awareness about the increased risk of spine injuries.[34] Noncontiguous spine injuries are seen in 10–19% of cases, and therefore the identification of one spinal injury should lead to close scrutiny of the entire spine to rule out others.[35,36]

Pre-Hospital Evaluation and Management

The protection of a potentially injured spine and spinal cord must begin at the accident scene to prevent any further neurologic injury through poor immobilization and improper handling of the spine during extrication and transportation. In previous reports, such neurological change has been shown to occur in up to 25 % of cases.[37] However, more recent care models and protocols to immobilize and protect the spine during extrication and transportation have likely contributed to the increased survival[38] and decrease neurological sequelae of spine-injured patients.[26] Current recommendations for patient immobilization during transport consist of a rigid cervical collar, lateral supports (e.g. sandbags), tape across the forehead and body straps to secure the patient to a hard backboard, thus protecting the entire spine (ATLS book). Because young children have a disproportionally large head relative to their body size, an occipital recess or a mattress placed under the torso needs to be added to the standard backboard to maintain neutral cervical spine alignment and prevent anterior translation and flexion through an injured segment.

A rapid transport time to the definitive care centers is associated with improved neurological function.[26,39] Unstable patients should nonetheless be stabilized at the nearest regional center and be transported, when hemodynamically stable, to a tertiary care center. Studies have demonstrated that air and ground transport are both safe when spinal precautions are taken for transport, with no documentation of any ascending neurological deficits with either modality.[40-42] Therefore, the choice of transportation should depend on availability and rapidity of transport.

It is important to recognize that emergency treatment protocols for the spine-injured patient also have their potential pitfalls. Cervical collars may elevate intracranial pressure[43-45] or cerebrospinal fluid pressure,[46] cause skin ulceration,[47] and increase the risk of aspiration in the elderly.[47,48] The ruling out of cervical injuries with the appropriate clinical and imaging studies must be done as soon as possible so as to allow for collar removal. One should be aware that simply leaving a trauma patient in cervical collar has potentially significant physiologic consequences. In the presence of a confirmed unstable cervical injury, changing the collar from a stiff-neck or Philadelphia collar (typically applied at the scene) to a collar with a lower capillary closing pressure (i.e. Miami-J or Aspen collar) has been shown to decrease skin ulceration.[49,50] Additionally, the detrimental effect of leaving patients for prolonged periods on spine boards has been demonstrated; they may decrease respiratory function[51,52] and cause increased tissue pressures leading to skin necrosis and ulcers at the sacral and occipital regions, especially in SCI patients who lack protective sensation.[53-55] These boards should only be used for extrication and transport; they should be removed once in hospital, aside from when they are being used for transfers.

Initial Emergency Evaluation and Management

Initial evaluation and resuscitation of the polytrauma patient adheres to guidelines set by the American College of Surgeons through their Advanced Trauma Life Support (ATLS) initiatives. They provide a systematic approach to rapidly identify and manage acute life and limb-threatening injuries. The essential first steps of this evaluation include the primary survey—An assessment of airway, breathing, and circulation (A-B-Cs); followed by disability and environmental exposure (D and E).[56] During this entire ATLS process, the presence of a spinal column or cord injury raises important considerations, which will be elaborated upon in this section.

A: Airway

Managing the trauma patient's airway is of paramount importance, and must be done while maintaining the

SECTION 1

cervical spine in a stable position. If urgent intubation is indicated, the possibility of endangering the cervical spinal cord should not be overlooked. Several studies suggest that in the hands of an experienced physician, direct laryngoscopy and orotracheal intubation during in-line immobilization of the cervical spine in neutral position is safe.[57,58] Manual in-line traction is contraindicated due to the risk of causing distraction of an unstable cervical spine injury, particularly at the occipitocervical junction where a ligamentous injury may not be so apparent on initial presentation.

B: Breathing

Cervical SCI render patients vulnerable to breathing difficulties; those with an injury level at C3 or higher will often experience acute respiratory arrest at the scene, requiring urgent intubation and ventilation.[59] Individuals with lower cervical SCI (C3–T1) may have impaired diaphragmatic and intercostal muscle function, causing a more delayed compromise in their breathing due to ventilatory failure.[60] One case series identified three independent risk factors for intubation: Injury severity score >16, SCI above the level of C5, and a complete SCI.[61] Overall, 74% of patients with cervical SCI require intubation.[61-63] Anticipation and close pulmonary function monitoring (e.g. vital capacity, arterial blood gases) are of utmost importance. When any sign of ventilatory failure is observed, preemptive intubation under controlled settings is preferable to an emergent intubation under strenuous conditions, which may exacerbate the neurologic injury.[62] Intubation should also be considered prior to hospital-hospital transfer in any patient with a cervical cord injury as securing the airway and providing ventilatory support in the midst of transport can be extremely challenging.

C: Circulation

Hypotension in the acute trauma patient is assumed to be of a hemorrhagic etiology until proven otherwise. It should, therefore, be initially treated with fluid resuscitation and a source of blood loss should be extensively sought; the chest, abdomen, and pelvis being the commonest areas. If no bleeding source is found and the patient is bradycardic, neurogenic shock is likely to be the diagnosis. Neurogenic shock is typical in SCIs rostral to T4 and occurs in approximately 20–25% of patients with cervical SCI.[64,65] Its mechanism is that of disruption of sympathetic tone on the peripheral vasculature and heart. Although, no universally accepted hemodynamic parameters define neurogenic shock, most studies use a systolic blood pressure less than 100 mm Hg and a heart rate less than 50 beats per minute in patients without any other cause of shock.[66] Absence of cutaneous vasoconstriction (as seen in hemorrhagic shock) is another distinguishing feature.[56]

Regardless of its etiology, hypotension must be aggressively corrected to minimize secondary ischemic damage to the spinal cord. In patients whose blood pressure is unresponsive to crystalloid, universal donor blood group (group O, Rh-negative) is recommended until matched blood products are available. Early administration of blood products is of particular importance in spinal cord-injured patients to maximize the oxygen carrying capacity and thereby minimize the secondary ischemic and hypoxemic injury to the vulnerable cord.[67] Invasive monitoring from arterial and central venous access is imperative to guide interventions. Once the patient is normovolemic, a mean arterial pressure of 85–90 mm Hg has been recommended for 5–7 days, although it is recognized that the clinical evidence to support this target MAP is relatively weak.[68-70] Ongoing hypotension can be managed with vasopressors such as dopamine, norepinephrine, or phenylephrine, whose agonist activity raises the systemic vascular resistance. This can be followed by the oral agonist midodrine, which can be weaned over a couple of weeks as hemodynamic stability is achieved. Low cardiac output resulting from persistent bradycardia can be treated with atropine. If recalcitrant, temporary diaphragmatic pacing may be required.[69]

D and E: Disability and Exposure

After addressing the ABCs and all life-threatening injuries, it is important to document the patient's level of consciousness and establish the presence or absence of voluntary movement in the four extremities after exposing the patient fully. The presence of any appendicular skeleton and pelvic injuries should be examined for as well.

Log rolling the patient to inspect and palpate the spine is essential. In addition to localizing potential injuries, the presence of tenderness, swelling, or a step deformity can suggest the presence of posterior ligamentous injury and warrants advanced imaging.[71] The physician must individualize the extent and interpretation of this part of the examination to the clinical context. For example, a patient with a known unstable cervical spine based on radiographs should not have his collar removed for cervical spine palpation. Similarly, patients with complete cervical SCI and a thoracolumbar spine injury are unlikely to have tenderness or pain below the neck and thus, such noncontiguous injuries need to be ruled out with complete spinal imaging.

The final component of the log roll is the digital rectal examination. This is arguably the most important component of the neurologic examination in a spinal cord-injured patient. Perianal and anal sensation, anal tone and voluntary contraction, as well as the bulbocavernosus reflex (BCR) should all be documented. If the BCR is absent, this means that "spinal shock" is still present, and the true extent of the neurologic impairment may not be fully measurable. The end of spinal shock is heralded by the return of the BCR (usually within 48–72 hours from the injury) and at that time, the diagnosis of a "complete" SCI can be made.

SPINAL CORD INJURY SYNDROMES

After the trauma patient is stabilized, the neurologic examination is performed according to the International Standards for Neurologic Classification of Spinal Cord Injury (ISNCSCI), which was formerly referred to as the "ASIA Examination". This defines the extent of neurologic impairment in terms of motor power in 10 key myotomes of the upper and lower extremities, light touch and pin prick sensation throughout 28 dermatomes, and the extent to which the lowest sacral roots are spared based on voluntary anal contraction and perianal sensation (Box 1). Incomplete SCI may further be characterized, based on their clinical presentations, by one of six different clinical syndromes: Central cord syndrome (CCS), Brown-Séquard syndrome (BSS), anterior cord syndrome (ACS), posterior cord syndrome (PCS), conus medullaris syndrome (CMS), and cauda equina syndrome (CES), the latter not being a "true" SCI, but rather a peripheral nerve injury. 21% of all SCI patients have one of these syndromes (Fig. 1).[72] Optimal treatment, degree of recovery, and functional outcomes vary for each syndrome and therefore identifying them is clinically relevant for physicians and patients.[73]

Box 1: The American Spinal Cord Association Impairment Scale (AIS), based on the International Standards for Neurological Classification of Spinal Cord Injury.

- **A = Complete**. No sensory or motor function is preserved in the sacral segments S4–S5
- **B = Sensory incomplete**. Sensory but not motor function is preserved below the neurological level and includes the sacral segments S4–S5 [light touch, pin prick at S4–S5; or deep anal pressure (DAP)], and no motor function is preserved more than three levels below the motor level on either side of the body.
- **C = Motor incomplete**. Motor function is preserved below the neurological level**, and more than half of key muscle functions below the single neurological level of injury (NLI) have a muscle grade less than 3 (Grades 0–2).
- **D = Motor incomplete**. Motor function is preserved below the neurological level**, and at least half (half or more) of key muscle functions below the NLI have a muscle grade ≥ 3.
- **E = Normal**. If sensation and motor function as tested with the ISNCSCI are graded as normal in all segments, and the patient had prior deficits, then the AIS grade is E. Someone without an initial. SCI does not receive an AIS grade.

**For an individual to receive a grade of C or D, i.e. motor incomplete status, they must have either (1) voluntary anal sphincter contraction or (2) sacral sensory sparing with sparing of motor function more than three levels below the motor level for that side of the body. The standards at this time allows even non-key muscle function more than 3 levels below the motor level to be used in determining motor incomplete status (AIS B versus C).

Note: When assessing the extent of motor sparing below the level for distinguishing between AIS B and C, the motor level on each side is used; whereas to differentiate between AIS C and D (based on proportion of key muscle functions with strength grade 3 or greater) the single neurological level is used.

Source: American Spinal Injury Association. [online] Available from http://www.asia-spinalinjury.org/elearning/ISNCSCI_Exam_Sheet_r4.pdf. [Last accessed July, 2019]

Central Cord Syndrome

Traumatic cervical CCS presents with disproportionate motor loss in the distal upper extremities relative to the lower extremities, bladder dysfunction (usually urinary retention), and a variable degree of sensory impairment below the level of injury.[74] It was long believed that the neuroanatomic reason for the distal upper limbs being most affected was based on locations of the arm and leg fibers within the corticospinal tract.[75] However, this somatotopic organization theory has been challenged by recent studies.[76,77] An alternative theory is that the corticospinal tracts within the lateral columns of the cervical spine in mammals, that have acquired an upright posture and complex hand function, supply mainly the

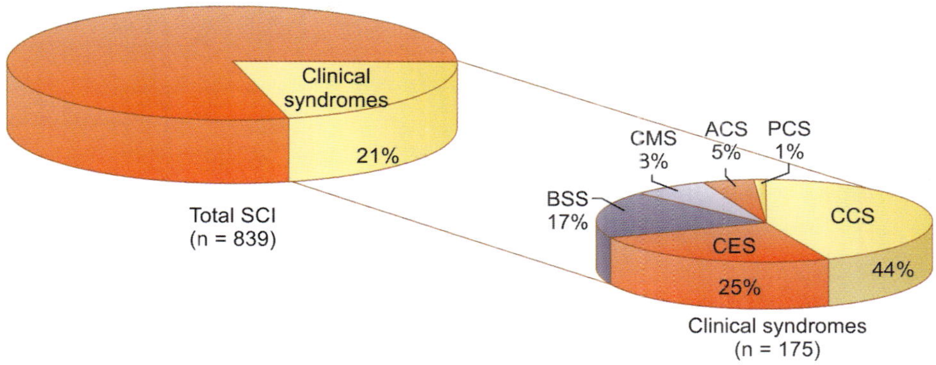

Fig. 1: Incidence of SCI clinical syndromes.
Source: Adapted from McKinley 2007.

distal upper limb musculature[78-80] Of note, this syndrome is seen exclusively in patients with injuries at the cervical spine level.[72]

It is the most common of the SCI syndromes, accounting for 44–50% of them, and 9% of all traumatic SCIs.[72,81] ASIA Impairment Scale (AIS) grade D is the most frequent impairment classification for these patients.[72] The classic mechanism of injury is that of hyperextension during a fall in an elderly person's spondylotic canal, where cord compression occurs between osteophytes at the posterior vertebral bodies and buckling ligamentum flava in an already stenotic canal. There is often no skeletal injury present, or a relatively stable extension-type injury may be present (Figs. 2A and B).[74,82] The term "centrAl cord syndrome", however, is not synonymous with elderly patients, as this pattern of neurologic impairment can also occur in young patients after severe cervical spinal cord trauma or anterior disk herniation.[83-85]

Central cord syndrome generally has a favorable prognosis for functional return. This begins in the lower extremities, followed by the bladder, proximal upper extremities, and lastly hand function, which unfortunately may not recover at all and is often the source of considerable ongoing disability.[85] The surgical management of patients with CCS but without significant spinal instability is extremely controversial. A recent systematic review and ambispective analysis of observational data[86] concluded that early surgical decompression (at < 24 hours post-injury) is reasonable and safe, particularly when the patient's neurologic deficit is profound (AIS grade C). Patients with less severe deficits (AIS grade D) can be treated initially with observation, with late surgery being considered if they reach a neurologic plateau with significant remaining dysfunction or if they deteriorate neurologically.[86] Functional status has been shown to positively correlate with a higher AIS grade at the time of injury, formal education, absence of comorbidities, absence of spasticity, and younger age. Bowel and bladder continence was achieved in 81% of patients and independent ambulation in 86%.[87] The rate of recovery of all three of these functions has been shown to strongly inversely correlate with patient age.[84,86] In addition, the absence of abnormal cervical spinal cord signal on MRI is another significant predictor of full neurologic recovery.[83]

Brown-Sequard Syndrome

Brown-Sequard syndrome (BSS) presents clinically as ipsilateral weakness and loss of proprioception and vibratory sensation, with contralateral pin prick, pain and temperature sensation deficits below the level of the lesion. It is caused by injury to one-half of the cord, where disruption of the descending lateral corticospinal tracts cause the ipsilateral motor impairment, and the ascending lateral spinothalamic tracts cause the contralateral sensory symptoms, as these tracts decussate one to two segments above the dorsal root entrance, rather then at the medulla oblongata as the corticospinal tracts do.[88] The most common cause of traumatic BSS is penetrating trauma from a knife or bullet (Figs. 3A and B). Most of these patients are classified as AIS grade D.[72] It is difficult to estimate the frequency of BSS, but they have been reported in the literature as accounting for approximately 2–4% of the traumatic SCI.[72,81]

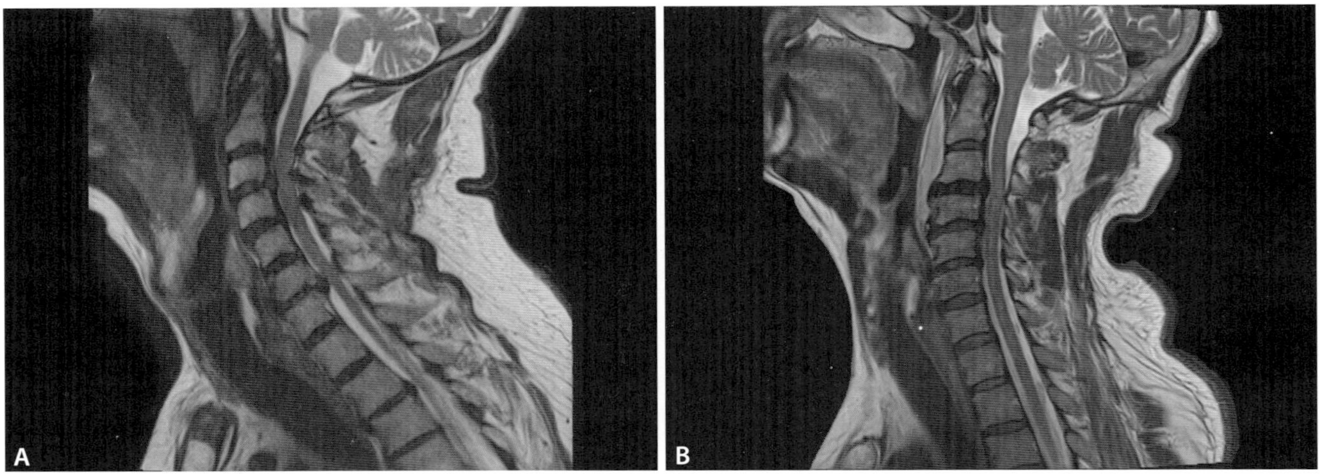

Figs. 2A and B: Sagittal cervical spine MRI images of patients who presented with clinical features of CCS. (A) An elderly man who sustained a hyperextension injury to his neck when falling from his own height. Note the underlying stenotic spinal canal and degenerative spine, most notably the retrolisthesed C4. A hyperextension injury further narrows the spinal canal and causes the spinal cord injury that presents as CCS, and is reflected on this image by the spinal cord signal change seen from the C2–3 disk space to C6. (B) A man in his late 40s who sustained a fall from his own height. The level of injury is demonstrated by cord signal change from C2 to C3, where there is as well a disk herniation and buckling of the ligamentum flavum into the canal, causing further stenosis than seen at the levels below.

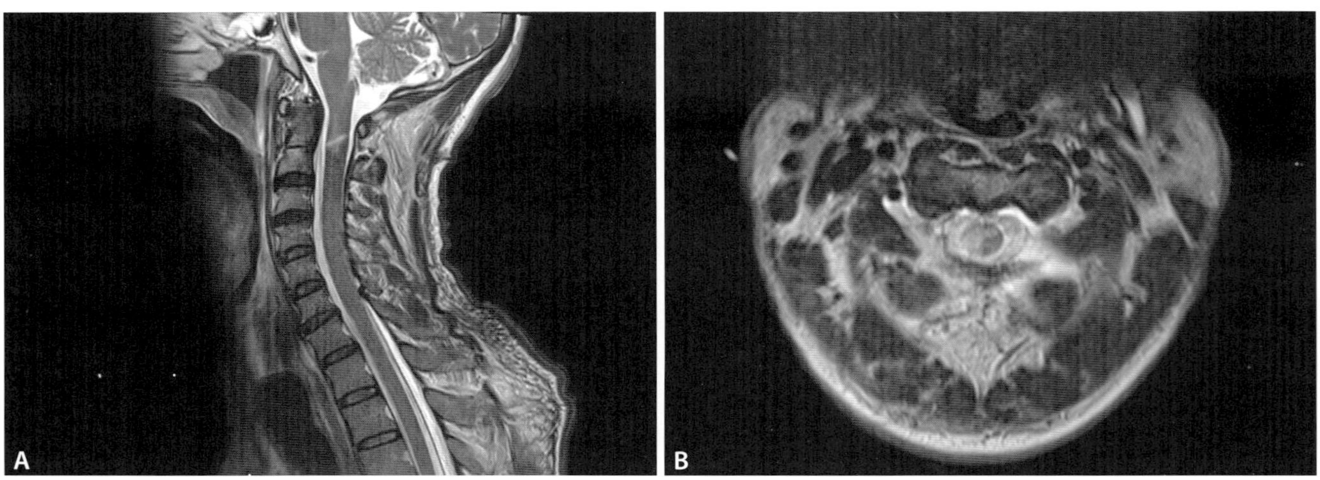

Figs. 3A and B: (A) Sagittal; and (B) Axial MRI images of a patient who was stabbed by a knife and presented with ipsilateral hemiparesis and partial contralateral hemi hypoanesthesia. The cord signal change reflective of the knife injury is visible on both images.

A pure presentation of BSB is rare, and therefore the term "Brown-Séquard plus" syndrome is used to describe the more common patients who presents with asymmetric paresis and hypoalgesia more severe on the less paretic side.[89] Patients with BSS or BSSP generally have excellent outcomes and return to near preinjury lifestyles.[85,90] In a small series of such patients, approximately three-fourth were able to ambulate independently, two-third were able to ultimately care for themselves independently, and one-third eventually were employed again.[85]

Anterior Cord Syndrome

The ACS is characterized by a lesion that affects the anterior two-thirds of the spinal cord while preserving the posterior columns.[91] This presents clinically as variable motor and pain and temperature sensation loss, with a relative preservation of light touch, deep-pressure sensation, and proprioception below the level of injury.[73] Its reported incidence is 2.7% of all traumatic SCIs[81] and 5% of all incomplete spinal cord syndromes.[72] It has been associated with flexion injuries, direct damage to the anterior cord by bone fragment or disk compression, or occlusion of the anterior spinal artery leading to vascular insufficiency of the cord.[81,92,93] Most patients (62.5%) with this diagnosis present with an AIS grade C. This syndrome carries a poor prognosis for functional improvement. Even in those with some recovery, muscle power and coordination remains quite poor.[72]

Posterior Cord Syndrome

Posterior cord syndrome is the least common of the SCI clinical syndromes, with an incidence of less than 1% of all incomplete syndromes. It is described as a selective lesion of the posterior columns and therefore presents as a loss of proprioceptive and vibration sense below the level of injury, but preservation of all other motor and sensory functions. Almost all of these patients are classified as AIS grade D.[72,73] Etiologies include neck hyperextension injuries, posterior spinal artery occlusion, tumors, disk compression, and vitamin B_{12} deficiency.[72,94]

Conus Medullaris Syndrome

Strictly speaking, the CMS refers to an injury to the distal tip of the spinal cord, where the sacral nerve roots emerge. As the conus typically resides between T12 and L2, it is vulnerable to injury in thoracolumbar burst fractures. This syndrome often presents as a mixed neurologic picture of conus and cauda impairment with both upper and lower motor neuron deficits. This typically consists of saddle anesthesia, areflexic bladder and bowel functions (with absent bulbocavernosus reflex), and mild lower extremity weakness.[72,95] CMS accounts for only 1.7% of all syndromes seen in trauma patients, and patients with this syndrome tend to have a high degree of neurologic impairment: 21% are classified as AIS grade A and 36% as AIS grade B.[72] Although, there is a lack of prospective studies on the treatment of these injuries, surgical decompression is generally recommended to optimize the potential for neurologic recovery.[95,96] Patients with CMS from blunt trauma improve on average by 1.5 AIS grades, and bladder function improvement is seen in 64% of patients of which approximately half have complete bladder function recovery.[97]

Cauda Equina Syndrome

Cauda equina syndrome is not considered a true SCI and is not assigned an American Spinal Injury Association score because the level of injury is distal to the spinal cord, at the level of the lumbosacral nerve roots within the cauda equina.[72,95] It presents as a pure lower motor neuron injury with saddle anesthesia, bladder and bowel dysfunction, sexual dysfunction, and/or variable lower extremity deficiency (sensory/motor, hyporeflexia), which is typically asymmetric. It is primarily a clinical diagnosis and must be made in a timely fashion based on a detailed history, thorough physical examination, and high index of suspicion. Key features of the physical exam are decreased perineal sensation to pin prick, decreased rectal tone and voluntary contraction, absent BCR and anal wink reflexes, absent or diminished deep tendon reflexes, and suprapubic distention.[95] Imaging is necessary to confirm the diagnosis. Traumatic causes of CES usually consist of low lumbar burst fractures.

Cauda equina syndrome is believed to have a better prognosis for neurological recovery than injuries at the level of the spinal cord because peripheral nerves tend to regenerate much more robustly than those of the central nervous system. Decompressive surgery is recommended, and timing of it remains a matter of controversy.[98-100] Randomized control studies to clarify this question do not exist as it would be difficult to randomize patients to delayed surgery, and it is usually difficult to determine the time of onset of the syndrome when the etiology is nontraumatic. Despite this, most investigators have recommended emergent surgical decompression for CES.[101,102]

NEUROPROTECTION AFTER ACUTE SPINAL CORD INJURY

When a traumatic SCI occurs, the spinal cord undergoes two types of insults referred to as the primary and secondary injuries. The primary injury sustained from the initial trauma and resulting spinal cord compression initiates a cascade of local and systemic factors that lead to ischemia, loss of autoregulation, inflammation, production of free radicals, increase in membrane permeability, and

CHAPTER 6

pathologic electrolyte shifts, all of which can profoundly modulate the extent of injury from the initial mechanical stress.[103] This cascade of events is known as the secondary injury. It develops over minutes to weeks following trauma, and is where the opportunity for neuroprotection and attempt at therapeutic intervention lie.[103,104]

Methylprednisolone

One of the most extensively studied pharmacological neuroprotective agents is intravenous methylprednisolone sodium succinate (MPSS). This steroid has been studied extensively in animal models, and has been reported to act through a number of different mechanisms including the reduction of lipid peroxidation, improvement in spinal cord blood flow, and attenuation of inflammation.[103,105-110] The administration of MPSS to acute SCI patients was tested in three large-scale prospective randomized double-blinded multicenter clinical trials, reported as the National Acute Spinal Cord Injury Studies (NASCIS) I, II, and III.[111-113] The first study failed to reveal any neurological improvements with MPSS, and it was later suggested from animal studies that this was due to the administration of subtherapeutic doses. In the NASCIS II trial, the dose was increased to a 5.4 mg/kg bolus followed 45 minutes later by a 24-hour infusion of 30 mg/kg. This study reported that patients treated within 8 hours from the time of injury experienced significant motor and sensory improvements. The NASCIS III study refined the administration protocol by reporting greater motor and functional improvement when the infusion was extended to a 48-hour period in patients whose treatment was initiated at 3–8 hours post-injury (24-hour infusion was shown to be equivalent for those treated at less than 3 hours post-injury). The longer infusion time, however, increase the incidence of severe sepsis and severe pneumonia.

The NASCIS trials have subsequently been heavily criticized for inadequacies in randomization (e.g. large difference in severity of neurologic deficits for patients in each treatment arms), deficiencies in statistical analysis (e.g. arbitrary 8-hour time window suspected to have been decided after a post-hoc analysis), and poorly defined clinical end points (scoring of motor improvements not clinically relevant).[114-117] Numerous societies have performed exhaustive reviews of the NASCIS trials and other smaller human SCI studies and have concluded that MPSS should not be considered a standard of care, but rather a treatment option.[118-120] The majority of Canadian surgeons have since abandoned the use of MPSS, although its use in the United States continues, in large part due to the medicolegal climate and fears of litigation.[121] This issue, therefore, is not resolved and remains somewhat controversial.

TIMING OF SURGICAL DECOMPRESSION

Based on the pathophysiology of secondary injury after acute SCI, it is intuitive to think that early decompression of the spinal cord would be an effective neuroprotective strategy. Many animal studies have demonstrated that early decompressive surgery diminishes the extent of secondary injury and improves neurological outcomes, although the majority of these studies have utilized models of low velocity compression rather than high velocity contusion.[122-125] Some have even noted that this benefit is inversely proportional to the time from injury to decompression.[122,126] Despite this, it has been difficult to demonstrate in clinical studies of human SCI a significant neurologic benefit after early surgical decompression. There are many potential reasons for this. Firstly, human injuries occur with considerably higher and faster biomechanical forces than are simulated in animal studies, and hence the primary injury in humans is likely to be more severe and leave less tissue amenable to the neuroprotective benefits of surgical decompression. Secondly, the definition of what constitutes an "early surgical decompression" has not been well-established and even today there remains wide variability in the time to which SCI patients have surgery. Finally, there are large practical difficulties in designing and executing a study in which timing of surgery can be evaluated as most clinicians would be unwilling to randomize a patient to a later decompression. In an international survey of spine surgeons, over 80% of the respondents indicated a preference to surgically decompress the spinal cord within 24 hours. In fact, for an incomplete cervical SCI, 72.9% of respondents felt that decompression should be achieved within 6 hours, while 46.2% felt that this time to decompression should be achieved for complete cervical SCI as well.[127]

Recently, the Surgical Timing in Acute Spinal Cord Injury Study (STASCIS) was published[128] and represents the largest prospective multicenter cohort study comparing the neurologic outcomes of patients with cervical SCI receiving "early" (less than 24 hours) versus "late" (over 24 hours) surgical decompression. The 313 patients enrolled were not randomized to a specific treatment arm. Instead, the decision of surgical timing was left to the enrolling surgeons and was often dependent on the individual's circumstances (time for transfer to hospital, time required to obtain adequate imaging, and discretion of the attending spinal surgeon). 19.8% of patients in the early decompression cohort showed a ≥2 AIS grade improvement compare to 8.8% in the late decompression group. After a multivariate analysis was performed to account for preoperative neurological status and steroid administration in both groups, the odds of having two or more AIS grades of improvement were 2.8 times higher in those who were decompressed early. The secondary outcomes consisted of inhospital postoperative complication rates and mortality; the early group experienced a complication rate of 24.2% compared to 30.5% in the late surgery group. When the complications data is looked at more closely, "construct failure requiring surgery" is reported to have occurred in 6.3 versus 2% of cases in early versus late surgery respectively, which likely relates to the lack of specific equipment and experienced personnel when surgery is expedited. One mortality occurred in each group in the 30-day post-injury period. Of note, the STASCIS study excluded patients with severe concomitant injuries and was restricted to cervical injuries.[128]

SPINAL CORD REHABILITATION

Rehabilitation begins in the hospital setting, preferably in a specialized spinal cord unit, where an integrated team of health care professionals can provide initial optimal SCI-specific care, preventing and/or treating medical complications as well as addressing new physical needs, social issues, and emotional stresses that spinal cord injured patients experience. This setting provides a strong framework for early initiation of SCI-specific rehabilitation. Delaying this has been shown to adversely affect functional outcome and lead to prolonged rehabilitation stay.[129,130]

The first big step into the rehabilitation phase is acceptance of the injury and realization that life with a SCI can be fulfilling. It is immensely helpful to have an interdisciplinary approach which includes and fully engages the patient and family in an education process that will optimize their level of independence and ability to cope after discharge. Frequent team conferences with early evaluation from the physical medical rehabilitation physicians, and home and equipment evaluation should be performed.[131]

Rehabilitation plans are based on the projected functional outcome for every individual case of SCI. This depends on the AIS grade and level of SCI, as well as on the patient's age, medical status and comorbidities, motivation, and social support. Generalized projected outcomes for different motor complete injury levels have been published to help guide the goals of rehabilitation based on injury level (Tables 2 and 3). This should serve as a guide only, as individual patient factors may alter their rehabilitation potential. Once a patient's projected functional outcome is determined, short and long-term functional goals can be formulated and a therapy prescription established. Of note, patients with motor levels at or above C3 will usually require long-term mechanical ventilation, whereas patients with levels at C4 or lower can eventually be weaned off and breathe independently.[131]

Ambulation

Prognosis for ambulation is dependent on the initial injury level and the AIS classification. Oleson et al.'s results have also demonstrated that baseline lower-extremity pinprick preservation as well as sacral pinprick preservation at 4 weeks post-injury are both associated with an improved prognosis for ambulation.[132] Statistics show that at 1 year post-injury, 46% and 14% of patients with incomplete tetraplegia are community and household ambulators respectively. This compares to 76% of incomplete paraplegics and 5% of complete paraplegics achieving community ambulation. More patients with incomplete tetraplegia achieve community ambulation than patients with incomplete paraplegia with equivalent lower-extremity motor strength, because the upper-extremity deficiencies in the latter groups make it much more difficult to use assistive devices for ambulation. As mentioned in the Spinal Cord Rehabilitation section, community ambulation requires antigravity strength (grade 3/5 motor score or more) in hip flexors bilaterally and in one knee extensor.[131]

Table 2: Projected functional outcomes for motor complete spinal cord injury (SCI) at 1 year post-injury, by injury level (C1–T1).

Measure	*C1–4*	*C5*	*C6*	*C7*	*C8–T1*
Feeding	Dependent	Independent with adaptive equipment after setup	Independent with/ without adaptive equipment	Independent	Independent
Grooming	Dependent	Minimal assistance with equipment	Some assistance to independent with adaptive equipment	Independent with adaptive equipment	Independent
UE dressing	Dependent	Requires assistance	Requires assistance	Independent	Independent usually
LE dressing	Dependent	Dependent	Independent	Some assistance to independent with adaptive equipment	Independent
Bathing	Dependent	Dependent	Some assistance to independent with equipment	Some assistance to independent with equipment	Independent with equipment
Bed mobility	Dependent	Requires assistance	Requires assistance independent	Independent to some assistance	Independent
Weight shifts	Independent in power chair with power tilt or recline mechanism	Requires assistance unless in power chair	Some assistance to independent on level surfaces	Independent	Independent
Transfers	Dependent	Requires maximum assistance	Independent with manual	Independent with or without board for level surfaces	Independent
Wheelchair propulsion	Independent with power chair; dependent in manual wheelchair	Independent with power chair; independent to some assistance in manual wheelchair with adaptations on level surfaces	Wheelchair with coated rims on level surfaces	Independent, except for curbs and uneven terrain	Independent in car hand controls or adapted van
Driving	Unable	Independent with adaptations	Independent with adaptations	Independent in car with hand controls or adapted van	Independent in car with hand controls or adapted van

(LE: lower extremity; UE: upper extremity)
Source: Adapted from Kirshblum 2007 (Adapted with permission on February 6th, 2013).

Table 3: Potential functional outcomes at 1 year post-injury for complete paraplegia, by injury level (T2–S5).

Measure	*T2–9*	*T10–L2*	*L3–S5*
ADLs (grooming, feeding, dressing, bathing)	Independent	Independent	Independent
Bowel/bladder	Independent	Independent	Independent
Transfers	Independent	Independent	Independent
Ambulation	Standing in frame, tilt table, or standing wheelchair; exercise only	Household ambulation with orthoses; can trial ambulation outdoors	Community ambulation is possible
Braces	Bilateral KAFOs with forearm crutches or walker	KAFOs with forearm crutches	Possibly KAFO or AFOs, with canes or crutches

(ADLs: activities of daily living; AFOs: ankle-foot orthoses; KAFO: knee-ankle-foot orthoses)
Source: Adapted from Kirshblum 2007.

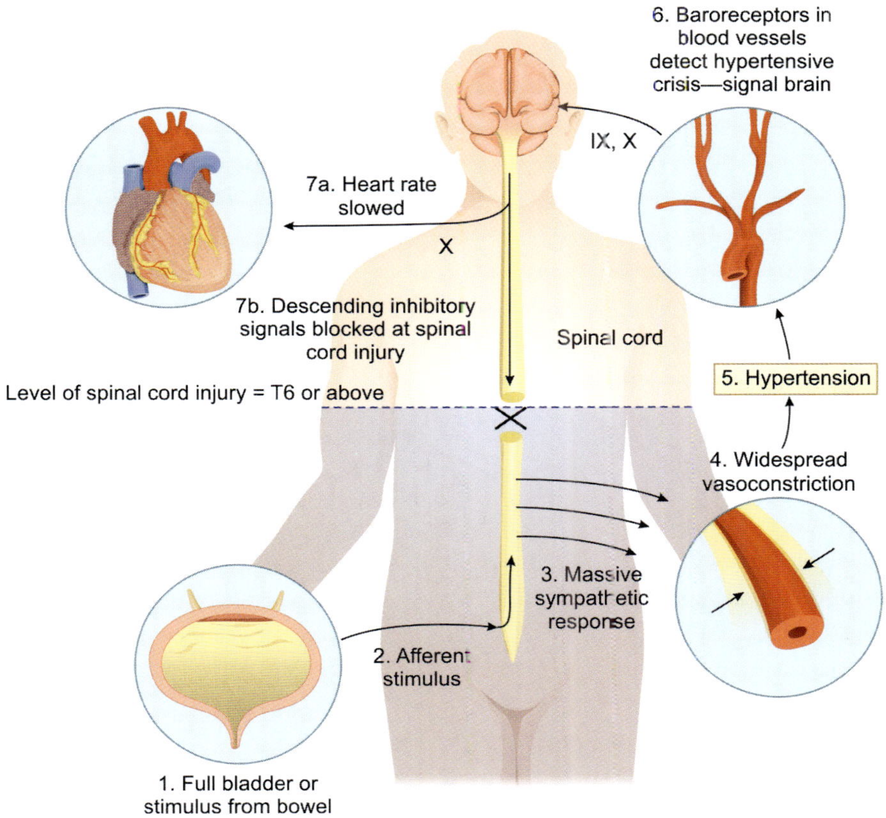

Fig. 4: Diagram illustrating autonomic dysreflexia. The afferent stimulus here is a distended bladder, which triggers a peripheral sympathetic response resulting in vasoconstriction and hypertension. In a person without a SCI, descending inhibitory signal would counteract the rise in blood pressure. Presence of a SCI however blocks these descending signals. Roman numerals refer to cranial nerves.
Source: Adapted from Blackmer 2003.

Dysreflexia

Patients with a spinal cord lesion at T6 and above are at risk of developing autonomic dysreflexia (AD), especially when the lesion is complete. It usually occurs after the resolution of spinal shock, and within the first year post SCI. AD occurs when a spinal reflex mechanism is activated from a noxious stimulus below the level of the lesion which sends afferent impulses to the spinal cord, resulting in a generalized sympathetic response that leads to vasoconstriction below the lesion level.[133] With lesions at or above the T6 level, the splanchnic vascular bed, in addition to the peripheral vasculature, becomes vasoconstricted, causing an elevation of the blood pressure. Central inhibitory pathways that would normally respond to such a rise in blood pressure by modulating the sympathetic response can no longer descend to the sympathetic chain because of the SCI (Fig. 4). Above the level of the lesion, however, the excessive parasympathetic output results in the typical clinical features of AD including peripheral vasodilation, bilateral pounding headache, flushing and sweating in the head and neck region, and the nasal congestion. This contrasts with the lower extremities' piloerection, pallor and cool temperature secondary to the unmodulated sympathetic tone. In addition, an increase in baseline blood pressure by 20–40 mm Hg, or reflex bradycardia from carotid baroreceptor stimulation of the vagus nerve may be signs of AD.[134]

Autonomic dysreflexia must be treated promptly to avoid the potentially serious complications of uncontrolled hypertension. Primary treatment includes sitting the patient upright, removal of any constricting garments to allow the pooling of blood in the lower extremities, and identifying and eliminating the underlying cause. Evaluation of the urinary system with intermittent catheterization or replacement of an indwelling catheter

Table 4: Precipitants of autonomic dysreflexia.[134,135]	
Category	*Noxious stimulus*
Urinary tract	Infection Distension (bladder/urethra) Catheterization or tube kinking Bladder/kidney stones
Anorectal	Bowel obstruction/distension Constipation Colonoscopy Hemorrhoids Anal fissure
Gastrointestinal	Gastroesophageal reflux Ulceration
Dermatologic	Pressure sore Tight clothing Ingrown toenail Blisters
Skeletal	Fracture Joint dislocation
Reproductive	Childbirth Menstruation Testicular torsion Ejaculation Intercourse

is mandatory as the most common cause of AD is an overdistended bladder. Other causes are listed in Table 4 and may guide the physical examination of the patient until the noxious stimuli is found. Medical treatment of hypertension and close monitoring of the patient for persistent hypertension and rebound hypotension is advisable.[131] Given the functional importance of autonomic dysfunction after SCI, subsequent versions of the standard neurologic examination will include some basic assessments of autonomic function.

Psychological Impact

Sustaining a SCI represents a huge traumatic challenge not only physically but psychologically as well. It has been reported that the incidence of anxiety in the spinal cord injured patient population is approximately 25%, and the incidence of clinically significant depression is 27%.[136] Their suicide rate is 2–6 times greater than that for the able-bodied population.[137,138] Physiological counseling for the patient and his/her family should be offered early and pharmacologic interventions should be used. Rehabilitation staff must be active in developing coping strategies with the patient, as well as encouraging peer support and involvement. Substance abuse prevention and treatment programs should be included as well.

PROGNOSIS

Mortality

Early mortality after SCI has been declining over the last 3 decades. The prehospital mortality rate dropped from 38% to 15.8% between the early 1970s to the end of the 21st century.[6,139] This is likely due to the widespread implementation of paramedical services, the formation of regionalized trauma systems, and the dissemination of the ATLS educational course.[140]

Strauss et al.[141] collected data from 30,822 non-ventilator dependent SCI patients between 1972 and 2004. They concluded that of the patients who do reach hospital care within 24 hours of injury, mortality rate in the first 2 years post-injury decreased by 40% over the 30-year study period. They, as well, looked at the two most important prognostic factors for mortality after a SCI: Age and injury severity (level and neurologic grade). Their analysis showed that the odds of dying in the first 2 years post-injury increases steadily with age by 7% per year. With respect to level and grade of injury, they showed that the higher the level of injury in tetraplegia and in complete SCI, the higher the mortality rate; that mortality is higher in patients with tetraplegia compared to paraplegia; and that for a same level of cervical injury, mortality rates are higher in those with AIS grade A (complete) injuries than for those with grade B or C (incomplete) injuries. In patients with paraplegia however, the AIS grade does not affect the mortality rate. Therefore, the AIS grading is an important prognostic factor of mortality for patients with cervical SCI, but not for thoracic or lumbar injuries. Table 5 shows hypothetical life expectancies applicable to a 25-year-old white man victim of a nonviolent SCI and who has survived the first 3 years post-injury period, based on ASIA grade and injury level. Of note, the survival rate during the first 3 years following a SCI is much lower than the ones listed in this. In addition, this entire study excluded ventilator-dependent patients, who generally have a worse survival prognosis. About 7% of SCI patients are discharged from acute hospitalization with continued dependence on the ventilator.[19]

Socioeconomic factors also have a profound effect on mortality. A clear gradation in mortality based on familial income was demonstrated by Krause et al.[142] Those with annual household income of US$25,000 had 2.31 greater odds of mortality and those whose income was between $25,000 and $74,999 had 1.61 greater odds of mortality when compared to those with household incomes of

Table 5: Sample life expectancies for 25-year-old white man: not ventilator dependent, nonviolent etiology and time since injury 3 years, by Injury level and AIS grade.

Group	*Life expectancy (years)*
General population	50.9
C1–3, grade A	25.4
C1–3, grades B and C	32.2
C4, grade A	26.4
C4, grades B and C	34.9
C5, grade A	30.0
C5, grades B and C	35.7
C6–8, grade A	34.7
C6–8, grades B and C	36.7
T1–S5 (paraplegia), grades A, B, and C	37.6
All grade D	44.7

Life expectancy for patients that are < 3 years post- spinal cord injury (SCI) is less than the numbers indicated in this table. Note as well that these numbers do not apply to ventilator-dependent patients or patients whose SCI was of a violent etiology.

Source: Adapted from Strauss 2006 (Adapted with permission on April 14, 2013).

Table 6: Primary and secondary causes of death in patients with chronic spinal cord injury (SCI).

Cause of death	*Underlying cause of death (%)*	*Contributing cause of death (%)*	*Total (%)*
Circulatory system disorder	21.6	18.9	40.5
Nervous system disorder	8.1	27.0	35.1
Neoplasm	24.3	n/a	24.3
Respiratory system disorder	5.4	18.9	24.3
External	13.5	5.5	18.9
Genitourinary system disorder	5.4	10.8	16.2
Endocrine/metabolic disorder	8.1	5.4	13.5
Infectious disease	5.4	8.1	13.5
Gastrointestinal disorder	0.0	13.5	13.5
Musculoskeletal disorder	2.7	0.0	2.7
Congenital disorder	2.7	0.0	2.7
Other/ill-defined conditions	5.4	35.1	37.8

Based on ICD-9 codes, recorded in hospital, of 402 SCI patients enrolled from 994–2000.

Source: Adapted from Garshick 2005 (Adapted with permission on April 14, 2013).

$75,000 or more. Behavioral and psychosocial factors also come into play. Early retrospective studies have shown that alcohol abuse and poor self-care correlate with increased mortality after SCI.[143,144] Later prospective studies demonstrated that being generally more active, being employed, and adapting well after SCI are related to a lower probability of mortality.[145-147]

In patients with chronic SCI, the leading cause of death is neoplasm (24.3%), followed by circulatory system disorders (21.6%). When both underlying and contributing causes of deaths are considered, circulatory system disorder is the leading culprit with 40.5% of patients being affected (Table 6).[148]

Return to Work

Several studies have looked at the rate of employment post SCI. A wide variety of results have been published, likely due to the discrepancies in their definition of employment and the time at data gathering, relative to the time of injury for each patient. Two recent papers reviewed the literature on the subject. Young et al. concluded that approximately 40% of working-age people are employed at 1 year post-injury. This rate increases as the time from injury increases, peaking at 10–12 years post-injury.[149] Ottomanelli et al.[150] drew similar conclusions from the review of 60 articles published from 1978 to 2008; the average rate of any employment after SCI was approximately 35%.[150]

CURRENT TRIALS AND NEW HORIZONS

Intensive scientific research has shed light on the complex pathophysiology of SCI and has led to the development of a number of experimental treatments that are under evaluation in clinical trials. Table 7 lists some of the different pharmacological and biological therapies that are currently being investigated and the rationale for their application. These largely target various aspects of the secondary injury pathophysiology such as disrupted ionic homeostasis, products of lipid peroxidation (oxidative stress), altered neurotransmitter release and receptor function, cellular dysfunction, and inflammatory and immune changes that occur after a SCI.[151] At the time of this writing, these trials are still in relatively early stages and conclusive data demonstrating efficacy is not expected for a number of years.

Table 7: Neuroprotective therapies.

Name of agent	Nature of the agent	MOA in SCI	Animal SCI models	Human research
Minocycline	Tetracycline antibiotic	• Increases IL-10 and decreases TNF-α expression, preventing the exacerbation of the secondary injury in SCI by attenuating neuroinflammation and inhibiting apoptosis.[152,153] • Inhibits excitotoxicity, oxidative stress, apoptotic pathways, and inflammatory mediators released by activated microglia.[153] • Reduces microglial activation.[153]	• Improved neurological and histological outcomes, reduced neuronal and oligodendroglial apoptosis, decreased microglial activation and reduced inflammation[154] • Decreases tissue damage, lesion size, and apoptosis at the site of injury leading to improved functional outcome.[152,155]	A recent phase II placebo-controlled randomized trial of minocycline in acute SCI. Administration of higher doses of this drug to achieve adequate SCF concentration was proven to be safe. Functional outcomes exhibited differences that lacked statistical significance but that may be suggestive of improvement in patients receiving minocycline. Multicenter phase III trial required to hopefully show a statistical significance.[156]
Erythropoietin (EPO)	Glycoprotein hormone (hematopoietic GF)	• Upregulates red blood cell production and mediates tissue protection in response to hypoxia.[157] • Shown to have anti-inflammatory, antioxidant, and antiapoptotic properties.[157]	• EPO IV and subcutaneous promotes tissue protection and improves locomotor performance when compared to control.[158-162] • Single dose of EPO immediately after SCI improved motor function recovery, decreased lesion severity, and increased neuronal regeneration in a rat contusion model of SCI.[163]	An Italian multicenter comparative study of EPO versus methylprednisolone in patients with ASIA A or B traumatic SCI began in 2008. Primary outcome consisted of AIS improvement by at least 1 grade. Recruitment of subjects for this study was aborted at time of this writing.[164]
Riluzole	Benzothiazole anticonvulsant (sodium channel blocker currently approved by the FDA for ALS)	Attenuates secondary damage by decreasing intracellular sodium[165] and inhibiting presynaptic calcium-dependent glutamate release.[166]	Has been shown to increase spared white and gray matter[165] and improve locomotor function[167] in animal models of SCI.	A safety and pharmacokinetic study of Riluzole treatment in patients with traumatic acute SCI is currently underway.[168]
Magnesium	NMDA receptor antagonist	Attenuates excitotoxicity by limiting free radical production and glutamate release, and reduces apoptosis.[169]	High-dose magnesium administration after SCI resulted in significant improvement in functional recovery, apoptosis, and lipid peroxidation.[170]	A combination of magnesium and polyethylene glycol has been developed for administration to humans with SCI, allowing lower doses to be administered.[171] Phase 1 study of healthy human volunteers completed. Phase II study in cervical SCI patients to be initiated in 2013
Anti-Nogo antibodies	Antibody directed against molecules that inhibit neurite growth.[171]	Inhibit the activity of Nogo-A, an inhibitory constituent within CNS myelin that impedes axonal regeneration and/or sprouting		Nonrandomized, multicenter clinical trial in patients with ASIA A thoracic and cervical SCI. Treatment initiated 7–14 days post-injury. Antibody administered via intrathecal infusion over weeks, or via repeated bolus intrathecal injection. Study began in 2006 and was complete in 2011. No results published at time of this writing.[172]

(ALS: amyotrophic lateral sclerosis; GF: growth factor; IV: intravenous; MOA: mechanism of action; MS: multiple sclerosis; NMDA: N-Methyl-D-aspartate; SC: subcutaneous)

Cell transplantation into the injured spinal cord is another area of significant research interest.[173,174] Cells transplanted into the spinal cord may play a number of potential neuroreparative roles. For example, they may secrete neurotrophic factors and provide a permissive environment for axonal sprouting/regeneration by "bridging" the injury site or they may remyelinate demyelinated (but otherwise intact) axons to improve signal transduction across the injury. The use of stem cell technology has created much excitement within the SCI field as the ability to differentiate them into many different cell types raises the potential for them to even replace lost neurons and regenerate axons that might act as "relays" across the injury site.[175]

A large variety of cell substrates have shown promise in preclinical models of SCI including Schwann cells, olfactory ensheathing cells, mesenchymal stem cells, neural stem cells, and embryonic stem cells.[176] A clinical trial of oligodendrocyte progenitor cells derived from human embryonic stem cells was initiated in October 2010 by Geron Corporation (Menlo Park, CA) but was halted just over a year later due to financial considerations after enrolling 5 patients. A clinical trial of neural stem cells was initiated in Zurich, Switzerland, sponsored by Stem Cells Inc., and at the time of this writing has enrolled four patients. A clinical trial of Schwann cells has recently been initiated by the Miami Project to Cure Paralysis. Like the pharmacologic treatments, it will still take many years before evidence of efficacy will be established in such clinical trials of cell transplantation therapies.

REFERENCES

1. Krueger H, Noonan VK, Trenaman LM, et al. The economic burden of traumatic spinal cord injury in Canada. Chronic Dis Inj Can. 2013;33(3):113-22.
2. DeVivo MJ. Causes and cost of spinal cord injury in the United States. Spinal Cord. 1997;35(12):809-13.
3. Sadowsky CL, Margherita A. The cost of spinal cord injury care. Spine. 1999;13(3):593-606.
4. Lenehan B, Street B, Kwon BK, et al. The epidemiology of traumatic spinal cord injury in British Columbia, Canada. Spine (Phila Pa 1976). 2012;37(4):321-9.
5. Couris CM, Guilcher SJ, Munce SE, et al. Characteristics of adults with incident traumatic spinal cord injury in Ontario, Canada. Spinal Cord. 2010;48(1):39-44.
6. Dryden DM, Saunders LD, Rowe BH, et al. The epidemiology of traumatic spinal cord injury in Alberta, Canada. Can J Neurol Sci. 2003;30(2):113-21.
7. Pickett W, Simpson K, Walker J, et al. Traumatic spinal cord injury in Ontario, Canada. J Trauma. 2003;55(6):1070-6.
8. Burke DA, Linden RD, Zhang YP, et al. Incidence rates and populations at risk for spinal cord injury: a regional study. Spinal Cord. 2001;39(5):274-8.
9. Hu R, Mustard CA, Burns C. Epidemiology of incident spinal fracture in a complete population. Spine. 1996;21(4):492-9.
10. Price C, Makintubee S, Herndon W, et al. Epidemiology of traumatic spinal cord injury and acute hospitalization and rehabilitation charges for spinal cord injuries in Oklahoma, 1988–1990. Am J Epidemiol. 1994;139(1):37-47.
11. Van Asbeck FW, Post MW, Pangalila RF. An epidemiological description of spinal cord injuries in The Netherlands in 1994. Spinal Cord. 2000;38(7):420-4.
12. Martins F, Freitas F, Martins L, et al. Spinal cord injuries-epidemiology in Portugal's central region. Spinal Cord. 1998;36(8):574-8.
13. van den Berg MEL, Castellote JM, Mahillo-Fernandez I, et al. Incidence of spinal cord injury worldwide: a systematic review. Neurosurgery. 2010;34(3):184-92.
14. Pickett GE, Campos-Benitez M, Keller JL, et al. Epidemiology of traumatic spinal cord injury in Canada. Spine (Phila Pa 1976). 2006;31(7):799-805.
15. National Spinal Cord Injury Statistical Center. 2012. Spinal cord injury facts and figures at a glance. [online] Available from https://www.nscisc.uab.edu/PublicDocuments/fact_figures_docs/Facts%202012%20Feb%20Final.pdf. [Last accessed July 2019].
16. Statistics Canada. Census snapshot of Canada—Population (age and sex). [online] Available from http://www.statcan.gc.ca/pub/11-008-x/2007006/article/10379-eng.pdf. [Last accessed July 2019].
17. O'Connor PJ. Trends in spinal cord injury. Accid Anal Prev. 2006;38(1):71-7.
18. Pirouzmand F. Epidemiological trends of spine and spinal cord injuries in the largest Canadian adult trauma center from 1986 to 2006. J Neurosurg Spine. 2010;12(2):131-40.
19. Jackson AB, Dijkers M, Devivo MJ, et al. A demographic profile of new traumatic spinal cord injuries: change and stability over 30 years. Arch Phys Med Rehabil. 2004;85(11):1740-8.
20. Sekhon LH, Fehlings MG. Epidemiology, demographics, and pathophysiology of acute spinal cord injury. Spine. 2001;26(24 Suppl): S2-12.
21. Bracken MB, Freeman DH Jr, Hellenbrand K. Incidence of acute traumatic hospitalized spinal cord injury in the United States, 1970–1977. Am J Epidemiol. 1981;113(6):615-22.
22. Kannus P, Niemi S, Palvanen M, et al. Continuously increasing number and incidence of fall-induced, fracture-associated, spinal cord injuries in elderly persons. Arch Intern Med. 2000;160(14):2145-9.
23. Fisher CG, Noonan VK, Dvorak MF. Changing face of spine trauma care in North America. Spine (Phila Pa 1976). 2006;31(11 Suppl):S2-8.
24. Tarazi F, Dvorak MF, Wing PC. Spinal injuries in skiers and snowboarders. Am J Sports Med. 1999;27(2):177-80.

CHAPTER 6

25. Dodwell ER, Kwon BK, Hughes B, et al. Spinal column and spinal cord injuries in mountain bikers: a 13-year review. Am J Sports Med. 2010;38(8):1647-52.
26. Tator CH, Duncan EG, Edmonds VE, et al. Changes in epidemiology of acute spinal cord injury from 1947 to 1981. Surg Neurol.1993;40(3):207-15.
27. Tator CH, Edmonds VE, New ML. Diving: a frequent and potentially preventable cause of spinal cord injury. Can Med Assoc J. 1981;124(10):1323-4.
28. DeVivo MJ, Sekar P. Prevention of spinal cord injuries that occur in swimming pools. Spinal Cord. 1997;35(8):509-15.
29. Tator CH, Provvidenza CF, Lapczak L, et al. Spinal injuries in canadian ice hockey: documentation of injuries sustained from 1943-1999. Can J Neurol Sci. 2004;31(4):461-6.
30. Tator CH, Provvidenza C, Cassidy JD. Spinal injuries in Canadian ice hockey: an update to 2005. Clin J Sport Med. 2009;19(6):451-6.
31. Irwin ZN, Arthur M, Mullins RJ, et al. Variations in injury patterns, treatment, and outcome for spinal fracture and paralysis in adult versus geriatric patients. Spine (Phila Pa 1976). 2004;29(7):796-802.
32. Holly LT, Kelly DF, Counelis GJ, et al. Cervical spine trauma associated with moderate and severe head injury: incidence, risk factors, and injury characteristics. J Neurosurg. 2002;96(3 Suppl):285-91.
33. Mulligan RP, Friedman JA, Mahabir RC. A nationwide review of the associations among cervical spine injuries, head injuries, and facial fractures. J Trauma. 2010;68(3):587-92.
34. Levi AD, Hurlbert J, Anderson PA, et al. Neurologic deterioration secondary to unrecognized spinal instability following trauma: a multicenter study. Spine (Phila Pa 1976). 2006;31(4):451-8.
35. Miller CP, Brubacher JW, Biswas D, et al. The incidence of noncontiguous spinal fractures and other traumatic injuries associated with cervical spine fractures: a ten year experience at an academic medical center. Spine (Phila Pa 1976). 2011;36(19):1532-40.
36. O'Malley KF, Ross SE. The incidence of injury to the cervical spine in patients with craniocerebral injury. J Trauma. 1988;28(10):1476-8.
37. Toscano J. Prevention of neurological deterioration before admission to a spinal cord injury unit. Paraplegia. 1988; 26(3):143-50.
38. Tan HB, Sloan JP, Barlow IF. Improvement in initial survival of spinal injuries: a 10-year audit. Injury. 2005;36(8):941-5.
39. Hachen HJ. Idealized care of the acutely injured spinal cord in Switzerland. J Trauma. 1977;17(12):931-6.
40. Armitage JM, Pyne A, Williams SJ, et al. Respiratory problems of air travel in patients with spinal cord injuries. BMJ. 1990;300(6738):1498-9.
41. Burney RE, Waggoner, R, Maynard FM. Stabilization of spinal injury for early transfer. J Trauma. 1989;29(11):1497-9.
42. Flabouris A. Clinical features, patterns of referral and out of hospital transport events for patients with suspected isolated spinal injury. Injury. 2001;32(7):569-75.
43. Davies G, Deakin C, Wilson A. The effect of a rigid collar on intracranial pressure. Injury. 1996;27(9):647-9.
44. Hunt K, Hallworth S, Smith M. The effects of rigid collar placement on intracranial and cerebral perfusion pressures. Anaesthesia. 2001;56(6):511-3.
45. Kolb JC, Summers RL, Galli RL. Cervical collar-induced changes in intracranial pressure. Am J Emerg Med. 1999;17(2):135-7.
46. Raphael JH, Chotai R. Effects of the cervical collar on cerebrospinal fluid pressure. Anaesthesia. 1994;49(5):437-9.
47. Stambolis V, Brady S, Klos D, et al. The effects of cervical bracing upon swallowing in young, normal, healthy volunteers. Dysphagia. 2003;18(1):39-45.
48. Butman AM, Schelble DT, Vomacka RW. The relevance of the occult cervical spine controversy and mechanism of injury to prehospital protocols: a review of the issues and literature. Prehosp Disaster Med. 1996;11(3):228-33.
49. Plaisier B, Gabram SG, Schwartz RJ, et al. Prospective evaluation of craniofacial pressure in four different cervical orthoses. J Trauma. 1994;37(5):714-20.
50. Powers J. A multidisciplinary approach to occipital pressure ulcers related to cervical collars. J Nurs Care Qual. 1997;12(1):46-52.
51. Bauer D, Kowalski R. Effect of spinal immobilization devices on pulmonary function in the healthy, nonsmoking man. Ann Emerg Med. 1988;17(9):915-8.
52. Totten VY, Sugarman DB. Respiratory effects of spinal immobilization. Prehosp Emerg Care. 1999;3(4):347-52.
53. Chan D, Goldberg RM, Mason J, et al. Backboard versus mattress splint immobilization: a comparison of symptoms generated. J Emerg Med. 1996;14(3):293-8.
54. Hauswald M, Hsu M, Stockoff C. Maximizing comfort and minimizing ischemia: a comparison of four methods of spinal immobilization. Prehosp Emerg Care. 2000;4(3):2502.
55. Sheerin F, de Frein R. The occipital and sacral pressures experienced by healthy volunteers under spinal immobilization: a trial of three surfaces. J Emerg Nurs. 2007;33(5):447-50.
56. American College of Surgeons Trauma Committee: Advanced Trauma Life Support for Doctors: ATLS Student Course Manual, 8th edition. Chicago: American College of Surgeons; 2008.
57. Manoach S, Paladino L. Manual in-line stabilization for acute airway management of suspected cervical spine injury: historical review and current questions. Ann Emerg Med. 2007;50(3):236-45.
58. Ollerton JE, Parr MJ, Harrison K, et al. Potential cervical spine injury and difficult airway management for emergency intubation of trauma adults in the emergency department: a systematic review. Emerg Med J. 2006;23(1):3-11.
59. Mansel JK, Norman JR. Respiratory complications and management of spinal cord injuries. Chest. 1990;97(6):1446-52.
60. Lu K, Lee T, Liang C, et al. Delayed apnea in patients with mid- to lower cervical spinal cord injury. Spine (Phila Pa 1976). 2000;25(11):1332-8.
61. Velmahos GC, Toutouzas K, Chan L, et al. Intubation after cervical spinal cord injury: to be done selectively or routinely? Am Surg. 2003;69(10):891-4.
62. Hassid VJ, Schinco MA, Tepas JJ, et al. Definitive establishment of airway control is critical for optimal outcome in lower cervical spinal cord injury. J Trauma. 2008;65(6):1328-32.

63. Como JJ, Sutton ER, McCunn M, et al. Characterizing the need for mechanical ventilation following cervical spinal cord injury with neurologic deficit. J Trauma. 2005;59(4):912-6.
64. Guly HR, Bouamra O, Lecky FE. Trauma Audit and Research Network: The incidence of neurogenic shock in patients with isolated spinal cord injury in the emergency department. Resuscitation. 2008;76(1):57-62.
65. Mallek JT, Inaba K, Branco BC, et al. The incidence of neurogenic shock after spinal cord injury in patients admitted to a high-volume level I trauma center. Am Surg. 2012;78(5):623-6.
66. Bilello JF, Davis JW, Cunningham MA, et al. Cervical spinal cord injury and the need for cardiovascular intervention. Arch Surg. 2003;138(10):1127-9.
67. Harris MB, Sethi RK. The initial assessment and management of the multiple-trauma patient with an associated spine injury. Spine (Phila Pa 1976). 2006;31(11):S9-15.
68. Markandaya M, Stein DM, Menaker J. Acute treatment options for spinal cord injury. Curr Treat Options Neurol. 2012;14:175-87.
69. Casha S, Christie S. A systematic review of intensive cardiopulmonary management after spinal cord injury. J Neurotrauma. 2011;28(8):1479-95.
70. Levi L, Wolf A, Belzberg H. Hemodynamic parameters in patients with acute cervical cord trauma: description, intervention, and prediction of outcome. Neurosurgery. 1993;33(6):1007-16.
71. Vaccaro AR, Lehman RA Jr, Hurlbert RJ et al. A new classification of thoracolumbar injuries: the importance of injury morphology, the integrity of the posterior ligamentous complex, and neurologic status. Spine (Phila Pa 1976). 2005;30(20):2325-33.
72. McKinley W, Santos K, Meade M, et al. Incidence and outcomes of spinal cord injury clinical syndromes. J Spinal Cord Med. 2007;30(3):215-24.
73. Hayes KC, Hsieh JT, Wolfe DL, et al. Classifying incomplete spinal cord injury syndromes: algorithms based on the International Standards for Neurological and Functional Classification of Spinal Cord Injury Patients. Arch Phys Med Rehabil. 2000;81(5): 644-52.
74. Schneider RC, Cherry G, Pantek H. The syndrome of acute central cervical spinal cord injury. J Neurosurg. 1954;13:546-77.
75. Aarabi BB, Koltz MM, Ibrahimi DD. Hyperextension cervical spine injuries and traumatic central cord syndrome. Neurosurg Focus. 2008;25(5):E9.
76. Pappas CT, Gibson AR, Sonntag VK. Decussation of hind-limb and forelimb fibers in the monkey corticospinal tract: relevance to cruciate paralysis. J Neurosurg. 1991;75(6):935-40.
77. Nathan PW. Effects on movement of surgical incisions into the human spinal cord. Brain. 1994;117(Pt 2):337-46.
78. Levi AD, Tator CH, Bunge RP. Clinical syndromes associated with disproportionate weakness of the upper versus lower extremities after cervical spinal cord injury. J Neurosurg. 1996;38:179-85.
79. Collignon F, Martin D, Lenelle J, et al. Acute traumatic central cord syndrome: magnetic resonance imaging and clinical observations. J Neurosurg. 2002;96(1 Suppl):29-33.
80. Bucy PC, Ladpli R, Ehrlich A. Destruction of the pyramidal tract in the monkey: the effects of bilateral section of the cerebral peduncles. J Neurosurg. 1966;25(1):1-33.
81. Bosch A, Stauffer ES, Nickel VL. Incomplete traumatic quadriplegia: a ten-year review. JAMA. 1971;216(3):473-8.
82. Waters RL, Adkins RH, Sie IH, et al. Motor recovery following spinal cord injury associated with cervical spondylosis: a collaborative study. Spinal Cord. 1996;34:711-5.
83. Ishida Y, Tominaga T. Predictors of neurologic recovery in acute central cervical cord injury with only upper extremity impairment. Spine (Phila Pa 1976). 2002;27(15):1652-7.
84. Penrod LE, Hegde SK, Ditunno JF Jr. Age effect on prognosis for functional recovery in acute, traumatic central cord syndrome. Arch Phys Med Rehab. 1990;71(12):963-8.
85. Roth EJ, Lawler MH, Yarkony GM. Traumatic central cord syndrome: clinical features and functional outcomes. Arch Phys Med Rehab. 1990;71(1):18-23.
86. Lenehan B, Fisher CG, Vaccaro A, et al. The urgency of surgical decompression in acute central cord injuries with spondylosis and without instability. Spine (Phila Pa 1976). 2010;35((21 Suppl)):S180-6.
87. Dvorak MF, Fisher CG, Hoekema J, et al. Factors predicting motor recovery and functional outcome after traumatic centra cord syndrome. Spine (Phila Pa 1976). 2005;30(20):2303-11.
88. Miranda P, Gomez P, Alday R, et al. Brown-Sequard syndrome after blunt cervical spine trauma: clinical and radiological correlations. Eur Spine J. 2007;16(8):1165-70.
89. Roth EJ, Park T, Pang T, et al. Traumatic cervical Brown-Sequard and Brown-Sequard-plus syndromes: the spectrum of presentations and outcomes. Spinal Cord. 1991;29(9):582-9.
90. Pouw MH, van de Meent H, van Middendorp JJ, et al. Relevance of the diagnosis traumatic cervical Brown-Séquard-plus syndrome: an analysis based on the neurological and functional recovery in a prospective cohort of 148 patients. Spinal Cord. 2010;48(8):614-8.
91. Preobrasheski PA. Syphilitic paraplegia with dissociated disturbance of sensation. J Neuropathol Psychiatry. 1904;4:394-433.
92. Cheshire WP, Santos CC, Massey EW, et al. Spinal cord infarction: etiology and outcome. Neurology. 1996;47(2):321-30.
93. Bauer RD, Errico TJ. Cervical spine injuries. In: Errico TJ, Bauer RD, Waugh T (Eds). Spinal Trauma. Philadelphia: JB Lippincott; 1991. pp. 71-121.
94. Suzuki T, Kawaguchi S, Takebayashi T, et al. Vertebral body ischemia in the posterior spinal artery syndrome: case report and review of the literature. Spine (Phila Pa 1976). 2003;28(13):E260-4.
95. Radcliff KE, Kepler CK, Delasotta LA, et al. Current management review of thoracolumbar cord syndromes. Spine J. 2011;11(9):884-92.
96. Harrop JS, Hunt GE, Vaccaro AR. Conus medullaris and cauda equina syndrome as a result of traumatic injuries: management principles. Neurosurg Focus. 2004;16(6):e4.
97. Rahimi-Movaghar V, Vaccaro AR, Mohammadi M. Efficacy of surgical decompression in regard to motor recovery in the stetting of conus medullaris injury. J Spinal Cord Med. 2006;29(1):32-8.

CHAPTER 6

98. Shapiro S. Medical realities of cauda equina syndrome secondary to lumbar disk herniation. Spine. 2000;25(3):348-51.
99. Spector LR, Madigan L, Rhyne A, et al. Cauda equina syndrome. J Am Acad Orthop Surg. 2008;16(8):471-9.
100. Kostuik JP, Harrington I, Alexander D, et al. Cauda equina syndrome and lumbar disc herniation. J Bone Joint Surg Am. 1986;68(3):386-91.
101. Todd NV. Cauda equina syndrome: the timing of surgery probably does influence outcome. Br J Neurosurg. 2005; 19(4):301-6.
102. Delong WB, Polissar N, Neradilek B. Timing of surgery in cauda equina syndrome with urinary retention: meta-analysis of observational studies. J Neurosurg Spine. 2008;8(4):305-20.
103. Amar AP, Levy ML. Pathogenesis and pharmacological strategies for mitigating secondary damage in acute spinal cord injury. Neurosurgery. 1999;44(5):1027-40.
104. Gupta R, Bathen ME, Smith JS, et al. Advances in the management of spinal cord injury. J Am Acad Orthop Surg. 2010;18(4):210-22.
105. Gleave JR, Macfarlane R. Prognosis for recovery of bladder function following lumbar central disc prolapse. Br J Neurosurg. 1990;4(3):205-9.
106. Tator CH. Experimental and clinical studies of the pathophysiology and management of acute spinal cord injury. J Spinal Cord Med. 1996;19(4):206-14.
107. Tator CH. Biology of neurological recovery and functional restoration after spinal cord injury. Neurosurgery. 1998;42(4):696-708.
108. Young W, Bracken MB. The second national acute spinal cord injury study. J Neurotrauma. 1992;9(S1):S397-405.
109. Hall ED. The neuroprotective pharmacology of methylprednisolone. J Neurosurg. 1992;76(1):13-22.
110. Zeidman SM, Ling GS, Ducker TB, et al. Clinical applications of pharmacologic therapies for spinal cord injury. J Spinal Disord. 1996;9(5):367-80.
111. Bracken MB, Collins WF, Freeman DF, et al. Efficacy of methylprednisolone in acute spinal cord injury. JAMA. 1984;251(1):45-52.
112. Bracken MB, Shepard MJ, Collins WF, et al. A randomized, controlled trial of methylprednisolone or naloxone in the treatment of acute spinal-cord injury. Results of the second national acute spinal cord injury study. N Engl J Med. 1990;322(20):1405-11.
113. Bracken MB, Shepard MJ, Holford TR, et al. Administration of methylprednisolone for 24 or 48 hours or tirilazad mesylate for 48 hours in the treatment of acute spinal cord injury. Results of the third national acute spinal cord injury randomized controlled trial: national acute spinal cord injury study. JAMA. 1997;277(20):1597-604.
114. Coleman WP, Benzel E, Cahill DW, et al. A critical appraisal of the reporting of the National Acute Spinal Cord Injury Studies (II and III) of methylprednisolone in acute spinal cord injury. J Spinal Disord. 2000;13(3):185-99.
115. Nesathurai S. Steroids and spinal cord injury: revisiting the NASCIS 2 and NASCIS 3 trials. J Trauma. 1998;45(6):1088-93.
116. Short D. Is the role of steroids in acute spinal cord injury now resolved? Curr Opin Neurol. 2001;14(6):759-63.
117. Sayer FT, Kronvall E, Nilsson OG. Methylprednisolone treatment in acute spinal cord injury: the myth challenged through a structured analysis of published literature. Spine J. 2006;6(3):335-43.
118. Hugenholtz H, Cass DE, Dvorak MF, et al. High-dose methylprednisolone for acute closed spinal cord injury: only a treatment option. Can J Neurol Sci. 2002;29(3):227-35.
119. Hadley MN, Walters BC, Grabb PA, et al. Pharmacological therapy after acute spinal cord injury. Neurosurgery. 2002;50(3 Suppl):S63-72.
120. Bledsoe BE, Wesley AK, Salomone JP. High-dose steroids for acute spinal cord injury in emergency medical services. Prehosp Emerg Care. 2004;8(3):313-16.
121. Eck JC, Nachtigall D, Humphreys SC, et al. Questionnaire survey of spine surgeons on the use of methylprednisolone for acute spinal cord injury. Spine (Phila Pa 1976). 2006;31(9):E250-3.
122. Dimar JR, Glassman SD, Raque GH, et al. The influence of spinal canal narrowing and timing of decompression on neurologic recovery after spinal cord contusion in a rat model. Spine (Phila Pa 1976). 1999;24(16):1623-33.
123. Delamarter RB, Sherman J, Carr JB. Pathophysiology of spinal cord injury. Recovery after immediate and delayed decompression. J Bone Joint Surg Am. 1995;77(7):1042-9.
124. Nystrom B, Berglund JE. Spinal cord restitution following compression injuries in rats. Acta Neurol Scand. 1988;78:467-72.
125. Guha A, Tator C, Endrenyi L. Decompression of the spinal cord improves recovery after acute experimental spinal cord compression injury. Paraplegia. 1987;25(4):324-39.
126. Carlson GD, Minato Y, Okada A, et al. Early time-dependent decompression for spinal cord injury: vascular mechanisms of recovery. J Neurotrauma. 1997;14(12): 951-62.
127. Fehlings MG, Rabin D, Sears W, et al. Current practice in the timing of surgical intervention in spinal cord injury. Spine (Phila Pa 1976). 2010;35:166-73.
128. Fehlings MG, Vaccaro A, Wilson JR, et al. Early versus delayed decompression for traumatic cervical spinal cord injury: results of the Surgical Timing in Acute Spinal Cord Injury Study (STASCIS). PLoS One. 2012;7(2):e32037.
129. Scivoletto G, Morganti B, Molinari M. Early versus delayed inpatient spinal cord injury rehabilitation: an Italian study. Arch Phys Med Rehabil. 2005;86(3):512-6.
130. Sumida M, Fujimoto M, Tokuhiro A, et al. Early rehabilitation effect for traumatic spinal cord injury. Arch Phys Med Rehabil. 2001;82(3):391-5.
131. Kirshblum SC, Priebe MM, Ho CH, et al. Spinal cord injury medicine: 3. Rehabilitation phase after acute spinal cord injury. Arch Phys Med Rehabil. 2007;88(3 Suppl 1):S62-70.
132. Oleson CV, Burns AS, Ditunno JF, et al. Prognostic value of pinprick preservation in motor complete, sensory incomplete spinal cord injury. Arch Phys Med Rehabil. 2005;86(5):988-92.
133. Karlsson AK, Friberg P, Lonnroth P, et al. Regional sympathetic function in high spinal cord injury during mental stress and autonomic dysreflexia. Brain. 1998;121:1711-9.
134. Blackmer J. Rehabilitation medicine: 1. Autonomic dysreflexia. CMAJ. 2003;169(9):931-5.

135. Milligan J, Lee J, McMillan C, et al. Autonomic dysreflexia: recognizing a common serious condition in patients with spinal cord injury. Can Fam Physician. 2012;58(8):831-5.
136. North NT. The psychological effects of spinal cord injury: a review. Spinal Cord. 1999;37(10):671-79.
137. Beedie A, Kennedy P. Quality of social support predicts hopelessness and depression post spinal cord injury. J Clin Psychol Med Settings. 2002;9(3):227-34.
138. Fichtenbaum J, Kirshblum S. Psychologic Adaptation to Spinal Cord Injury. In: Kirshblum S, Campagnola DI, DeLisa JA (Eds). Spinal Cord Medicine. Philadelphia: Lippencott, Williams and Wilkins.
139. Kraus JF, Franti CE, Riggins RS, et al. Incidence of traumatic spinal cord lesions. J Chronic Dis. 1975;28(9):471-92.
140. Kelly DF, Becker DP. Advances in management of neurosurgical trauma: USA and Canada. World J Surg. 2001;25(9):1179-85.
141. Strauss DJ, DeVivo MJ, Paculdo DR, et al. Trends in life expectancy after spinal cord injury. Arch Phys Med Rehabil. 2006;87(8):1079-85.
142. Krause JS, Saunders LL, DeVivo MJ. Income and risk of mortality after spinal cord injury. Arch Phys Med Rehabil. 2011;92(3):339-45.
143. Nehemkis A, Groot H. Indirect self-destructive behavior in spinal cord injury. In: Farberow N (Ed). The many faces of suicide. New York: McGraw Hill; 1980. pp. 99-115.
144. Price M. Causes of death in 11 of 227 patients with traumatic spinal cord injury over a period of nine years. Paraplegia. 1973;11:217-20.
145. Krause JS. Survival following spinal cord injury: a fifteen-year prospective study. Rehabil Psychol. 1991;36(2):89-98.
146. Krause JS, Kjorsvig JM. Mortality after spinal cord injury: a four-year prospective study. Arch Phys Med Rehabil. 1992;73(6):558-63.
147. Krause JS, Sternberg M, Maides J, et al. Mortality after spinal cord injury: an 11-year prospective study. Arch Phys Med Rehabil. 1997;78(8):815-21.
148. Garshick E, KelleyA, Cohen SA. A prospective assessment of mortality in chronic spinal cord injury. Spinal Cord. 2005;43(7):408-16.
149. Young AE, Murphy GC. Employment status after spinal cord injury (1992–2005): a review with implications for interpretation, evaluation, further research, and clinical practice. Int J Rehabil Res. 2009;32(1):1-11.
150. Ottomanelli L, Lind L. Review of critical factors related to employment after spinal cord injury: implications for research and vocational services. J Spinal Cord Med. 2009;32(5):503-31.
151. Gris D, Hamilton EF, Weaver LC. The systemic inflammatory response after spinal cord injury damages lungs and kidneys. Exp Neurol. 2008;211(1):259-70.
152. Stirling DP, Khodarahmi K, Liu J, et al. Minocycline treatment reduces delayed oligodendrocyte death, attenuates axonal dieback, and improves functional outcome after spinal cord injury. J Neurosci. 2004;24(9):2182-90.
153. Stirling DP, Koochesfahani KM, Steeves JD, et al. Minocycline as a neuroprotective agent. Neuroscientist. 2005;11:308-22.
154. Yong VW, Wells J, Giuliani F, et al. The promise of minocycline in neurology. Lancet Neurol. 2004;3(12):744-51.
155. Wells JE, Hurlbert RJ, Fehlings MG, et al. Neuroprotection by minocycline facilitates significant recovery from spinal cord injury in mice. Brain. 2003;126(Pt 7):1628-37.
156. Casha S, Zygun D, McGowan MD, et al. Results of a phase II placebo-controlled randomized trial of minocycline in acute spinal cord injury. Brain. 2012;135(Pt 4):1224-36.
157. Brines M, Cerami A. Emerging biological roles for erythropoietin in the nervous system. Nat Rev Neurosci. 2005;6(6):484-94.
158. Gorio A, Gokmen N, Erbayraktar S, et al. Recombinant human erythropoietin counteracts secondary injury and markedly enhances neurological recovery from experimental spinal cord trauma. Proc Natl Acad Sci. 2002;99(14):9450-5.
159. Gorio A, Madaschi L, Di SB, et al. Methylprednisolone neutralizes the beneficial effects of erythropoietin in experimental spinal cord injury. Proc Natl Acad Sci. 2005; 102(45):16379-84.
160. Kontogeorgakos VA, Voulgaris S, Korompilias AV, et al. The efficacy of erythropoietin on acute spinal cord injury. An experimental study on a rat model. Arch Orthop Trauma Surg. 2009;129(2):189-94.
161. Matis GK, Birbilis TA. Erythropoietin in spinal cord injury. Eur Spine J. 2009;18(3):314-23.
162. Vitellaro-Zuccarello L, Mazzetti S, Madaschi L, et al. Erythropoietin-mediated preservation of the white matter in rat spinal cord injury. Neuroscience. 2007;144(3):865-77.
163. Huang H, Fan S, Ji X, et al. Recombinant human erythropoietin protects against experimental spinal cord trauma injury by regulating expression of the proteins MKP-1 and p-ERK. J Int Med Res. 2009;37(2):511-9.
164. Clinicaltrail.gov. Evaluation of Tolerability and Efficacy of Erythropoietin (EPO) Treatment in Spinal Shock: Comparative Study versus Methylprednisolone (MP). [online] Available from http://www.clinicaltrials.gov/ct2/show/study/NCT00561067. [Last accessed July, 2019]
165. Schwartz G, Fehlings MG. Evaluation of the neuroprotective effects of sodium channel blockers after spinal cord injury: improved behavioral and neuroanatomical recovery with riluzole. J Neurosurg. 2001;94(2 Suppl):245-56.
166. Wang SJ, Wang KY, Wang WC. Mechanisms underlying the riluzole inhibition of glutamate release from rat cerebral cortex nerve terminals (synaptosomes). Neuroscience. 2004;125(1):191-201.
167. Stutzmann JM, Pratt J, Boraud T, et al. The effect of riluzole on post-traumatic spinal cord injury in the rat. Neuroreport. 1996;7(2):387-92.
168. Clinicaltrail.gov. Safety of Riluzole in Patients with Acute Spinal Cord Injury. [online] Available from http://www.clinicaltrials.gov/ct2/show/record/NCT00876889.[Last accessed July, 2019]
169. Lee JS, Han YM, Yoo DS, et al. A molecular basis for the efficacy of magnesium treatment following traumatic brain injury in rats. J Neurotrauma. 2004;21(5):549-61.
170. Suzer T, Coskun E, Islekel H, et al. Neuroprotective effect of magnesium on lipid peroxidation and axonal function after experimental spinal cord injury. Spinal Cord. 1999; 37(7):480-4

CHAPTER 6

171. Caroni P, Schwab ME. Two membrane protein fractions from rat central myelin with inhibitory properties for neurite growth and fibroblast spreading. J Cell Biol. 1988;106(4):1281-8.
172. Clinicaltrail.gov. Acute Safety, Tolerability, Feasibility and Pharmacokinetics of Intrath. Administered ATI355 in Patients with Acute SCI. [online] Available from http://clinicaltrials.gov/ct2/show/record/NCT00406016. [Last accessed July, 2019]
173. Ruff CA, Wilcox JT, Fehlings MG. Cell-based transplantation strategies to promote plasticity following spinal cord injury. Resuscitation. 2012;235(1):78-90.
174. Clinicaltrail.gov. [online] Available from http://www.clinicaltrials.gov/ct2/ results?term= stem+cell+spinal+cord+injury&Search= Search&view=record. [Last accessed July, 2019].
175. Lu P, Wang Y, Graham L, et al. Long-distance growth and connectivity of neural stem cells after severe spinal cord injury. Cell. 2012;150(6):1264-73.
176. Tetzlaff W, Okon EB, Karimi-Abdolrezaee S, et al. A systematic review of cellular transplantation therapies for spinal cord injury. J Neurotrauma. 2011;28(8):1611-82.

CHAPTER 7 Principles of Spine Fusion

S Tim Yoon, Colin G Crosby

INTRODUCTION

The ability to achieve successful fusion or arthrodesis is a critical goal in many spinal surgeries. Spinal fusion is a complex biological process that interacts with anatomic and biomechanical variables. The goal of the surgeon is to optimize biology and biomechanical stability in order to offer the highest chance at successful fusion. An intimate knowledge of the variables and factors associated with spinal fusion is important for surgical planning. In simple terms, spinal fusion is defined as bridging bony union between two and more spinal levels. The technique of spinal fusion is an integral aspect of spinal surgery, and is utilized in a variety of conditions including deformity, fracture, trauma, instability and degenerative process. Since the first reported spinal fusion surgery for the treatment of Pott's disease in 1911 by Albee and for the treatment of deformity by Hibbs, significant advances have been made with the use of internal fixation, surgical techniques, osteobiologics, and other technologies.[1,2] There has been a significant increase in the frequency of spinal fusion surgery throughout the world to treat instability and as a part of deformity correction surgery. Because of the relative difficulty in attaining a high rate of fusion, there have been many new surgical techniques and osteobiologics developed to improve fusion rate. However, there is a proliferation of osteobiologics without high level of evidence of efficacy. This has created great confusion among surgeons. Because there are too many products and techniques currently in use and there are more new products coming to market every year, it is impossible to review all of them. Therefore, it is more important for surgeons to have an understanding of the principles involved in spine fusion and have a guideline to measure the level of evidence of a particular product. The following chapter will discuss the fundamental concepts and principles related to fusion surgery in the spine.

SPINE FUSION TYPES

Generally spinal fusions can be categorized as anterior or posterior fusion. Although they are both designed to create a bony union across two or more vertebra, their geometry, biology, and biomechanics are quite different. Anterior fusions are typically interbody fusions. In this situation, the graft beds are quite close to each other (fusion distance) and the fusion bed area are relatively large. The geometry is such that the ratio between the fusion distance and fusion area is very favorable. The placement of a bone graft between the two fusion beds results in a biological situation that allows more direct bone formation and bypasses endochondral bone formation process. The biomechanics are more advantageous as well because the graft is placed in compression across the fusion bed.

Posterior fusion is quite different. The geometry of intertransverse fusion results in a much longer distance between graft beds. The decorticated fusion bed is often significantly smaller than the interbody fusion bed. This results in a poor fusion distance to fusion area ratio. Furthermore, the bone graft is not protected inside a cavity as in the interbody situation but instead exists in a soft-tissue envelope that can easily disrupt the contiguity of the graft material. Interposed muscle or even the presence of large numbers of fibroblasts can inhibit fusion rates. Because the muscle in the posterior area can exert significant compressive forces, the volume of bone graft must have some compressive resistance and ability to maintain a contiguous scaffold. Primate studies with a soft easily-compressed material (absorbable collagen sponge) resulted in poor results, but after combining a compressive resistant material with the absorbable collagen sponge results were improved. Given that fusion occurs last at the mid-zone between the transverse processes, it is important to maintain a good osteoconductive scaffold throughout the whole fusion process.

The biomechanics of the posterior fusion is also different from the interbody fusion process. In the posterior aspect of the spine there exists a tensile load between the transverse processes compared to the compression force across an anterior fusion. This is exaggerated in the scoliotic spine and often results in a smaller fusion mass in the convexity and a more robust fusion mass on the concavity of the curve. The situation is also aggravated in the patients with a positive sagittal balance, which tends to put more tension across the posterior graft area.

FUSION TECHNIQUES

General principles of good fusion technique include excellent graft bed preparation, good bone grafting, and stabilization. These principles hold for both anterior and posterior spinal fusion. The specific methods are described below.

Anterior cervical discectomy and fusion (ACDF) is a good prototype to discuss anterior fusion. Good technique begins with good exposure. For ACDF, the exposure has to show not only the mid annulus but should be sufficient to clearly visualize the uncovertebral joints bilaterally. Not only does this allow better decompression of the foramen, better exposure allows disk removal from uncus to uncus to provide maximal fusion bed. Sometimes, the less experienced surgeon will not expose laterally enough to allow good preparation of the uncovertebral area. The fusion bed (endplates) must be lightly decorticated. While aggressive decortication provides better marrow and vascular exposure, the interbody fusion bed must have enough mechanical integrity to support the graft and resist subsidence of the graft into the vertebra. The senior author's preferred method is to lightly decorticate the contact areas with the graft but to create deeper decorticated areas lateral to the structural graft and at the center noncontact area. The contact areas of the endplates have been shaped to fit precisely with the graft and avoid any gaps that can form between graft and endplate with poor "carpentry". A good fit between the endplate and graft reduces the osteoblast jumping distance and facilitates ingrowth of bone into the graft.

Fusion rates decline with the number of levels fused especially for ACDFs. This has often been explained as the increasing statistical difficulty in achieving fusion with each bone graft to endplate interface. In a one level fusion, there are two interfaces: one on the superior graft-endplate and another at the inferior graft-endplate interfaces. Given that there is a finite probability of each one of these interfaces not fusing successfully, then there is an ever-increasing rate of nonunion with increasing number of levels to be fused. Indeed the empiric results indicate that fusion rates are the highest with one level fusion and lower with multilevel fusion. Furthermore, empiric observation indicates that lowest levels of the ACDF have the highest likelihood of developing a nonunion.

Anterior fixation does improve stability, decreases subsidence, and increases fusion rate.[3] There are many different types of plate and screw constructs, ranging from very stiff round hole plates to relatively mobile slotted-hole plates. There is some debate about what type of plate screw construct is the best, but the slotted plates are associated with excessive subsidence and are not popular for most situations. It is the opinion of the authors that a relatively stiff construct is superior.

Surgeons can decrease the likelihood of nonunion with multilevel anterior surgery, by several different methods. ACDFs can be converted into corpectomy type constructs. For example, a two level ACDF could be converted into a one level corpectomy.[4] This decreases the number of interfaces that need to heal by two compared to the number of interfaces in a two level ACDF. In another example, a three level ACDF could be converted into a one level corpectomy and a one level ACDF (hybrid construct). Anterior instrumentation with the hybrid type construct, where the points of fixation do not exceed a one level corpectomy, results in a stable biomechanical construct and good clinical success. In contrast, if two contiguous corpectomies are performed (a three level ACDF converted to a two level corpectomy), the biomechanical situation is worsened and leads to a high rate of graft pistoning, subsidence, kyphosis, and possible nonunion. With disk level pathology, a corpectomy can be performed at the top levels, a vertebra is left intact, then another corpectomy can be performed at the lower two levels (Fig. 1). This results in a construct with the same number of fusion interfaces as a two level ACDF. At times, however, multilevel contiguous corpectomies are necessary. In this situation, many

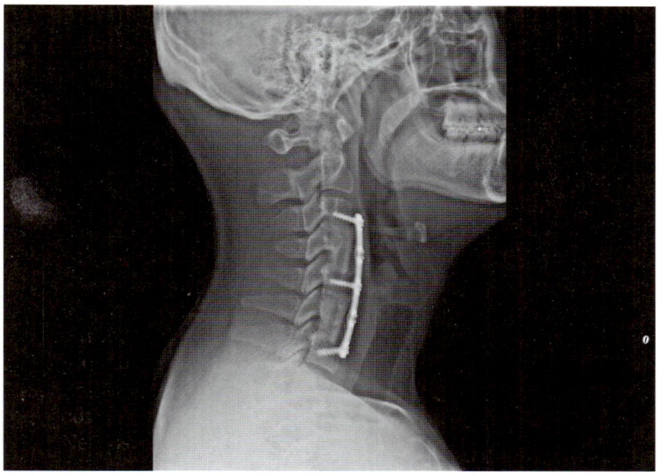

Fig. 1: Hybrid construct of two noncontiguous corpectomies separated by an intact vertebra. This results in a construct with same number of bone to graft interfaces as a two level anterior cervical discectomy and fusion.

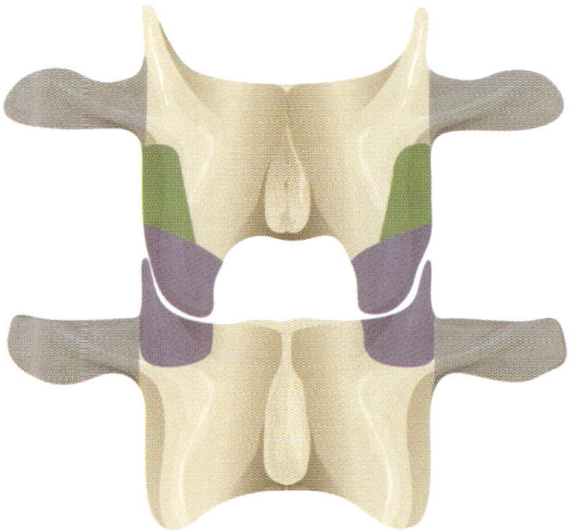

Fig. 2: This schematic diagram represents the anatomic areas of the lumbar spine that can be used for posterolateral bone grafting techniques. Intertransverse fusion bed is colored by gray shade, facet fusion bed is colored blue, and pars fusion bed is colored green.

surgeons prefer to add a posterior instrumented fusion to the treatment plan.

Besides surgical technique as described above, surgeon can choose osteobiologics to improve chances of fusion success. While single level ACDFs have a high fusion rate even with relatively lower-level grafts such as allograft cortical bone, in challenging situations such as multilevel anterior cervical fusion, a high-level graft material may make a significant difference. High-level grafts such as autologous iliac crest or bone morphogenetic proteins (BMPs) increase fusion rates, but have certain disadvantages such as donor site morbidity, increased operative time, cost, or postoperative swelling. It is up to the surgeon to weigh all the pros and cons of each situation to determine the combination of surgical technique and graft material that is appropriate for each situation.

The posterior fusion technique is the most commonly used fusion type in spine surgery. This technique involves fusing the transverse process, the lamina (if available), and often facet joints.[5] This technique is often used in conjunction with lumbar decompression. Because posterior lumbar fusion is such a commonly used technique, surgeons are very familiar with the anatomy and surgical methods. However, it is by no means an easy operation to do well. In fact, even in the best of hands, the fusion rate is often quite far from optimal. As with anterior exposure, good technique starts with excellent exposure. The typical situation involves a laminectomy for neurological decompression. Thus, interlaminar fusion is not available. Therefore, the facet joints and the transverse processes must be exposed for bone grafting. In order to facilitate intertransverse process bone graft, a postero-lateral gutter must be created that will accommodate the graft material without soft-tissue interrupting the graft volume and contiguity. When preparing the graft bed with decortication, one must have an eye to decompressing more than just the transverse processes. The goal is to have as much bone graft material in contact with decorticated bone and to reduce the distance by which new bone needs to form. Therefore, the lateral facet and pars region should be decorticated as well (Fig. 2). The bone graft material should have sufficient volume such that it is in contact with the transverse processes and the decorticated pars and lateral facet joint. As much of the graft should be placed next to the pars and superior articular process of the facet joint as possible as these areas are closer together than between the transverse processes. When the laminectomies are not performed, then the lamina should be decorticated and bone grafted as well. The principle is to decorticate and graft every available surface.

Sometimes graft volume is not sufficient. Several different strategies can be used to deal with this situation. Bone graft extenders are additional material that can be used to add volume when mixed with the autologous bone graft. Allograft bone, synthetics, and demineralized bone matrices (DBMs) have been used for this purpose.

However, there are limits to this technique. If autograft volume is not sufficient to allow good grafting of bilateral intertransverse processes, some surgeons have chosen to graft unilaterally with an adequate amount rather than splitting the graft into two inadequate amounts. For multilevel fusions, this technique seems to be successful.

Facet fusions in posterior fusion are often performed in conjunction with intertransverse process fusion. The rationale for this is to have yet another possible site for fusion to occur and thus increase the overall fusion rate. The facet joints are rather close together and require very little graft material to fill the decorticated graft bed. It takes little additional time and there is no additional exposure that is necessary. However, some surgeons choose not to perform facet fusions. Their rationale is that decorticating the facet joints destabilizes the segment and creates a problem if a nonunion occurs. It is the opinion of the authors that facet fusion should be performed along with intertransverse process fusion on a routine basis when pedicle screw instrumentation is used.

Another important technical point is that the pedicle screw tracks should be created before decortication, and screws should be placed after decortication and bone grafting. Placing the screws first interferes significantly with decortication and grafting. The pedicle screw tracks are created first, but the pedicle screws should be placed after the bone graft is placed. While this leads to minor increase in difficulty placing the pedicle screws, the graft bed preparation and bone grafting can be performed in a much more consistent and successful fashion.

Bone Graft Properties

In many respects, when surgeons are attempting to create a spine fusion, the surgeon is a tissue engineer attempting to engineer bony tissue across two vertebrae. In tissue engineering, three different tissue parts are necessary to optimize for success—scaffold, cells, and factors. The scaffold is necessary to guide the development of new tissue. For bone graft, this is typically a matrix composed of tissue that is favorable to bone cells, has porosity that allows cellular ingrowth, and can be remodeled by bone tissue. This type of matrix (or scaffold) is considered osteoconductive. Cells are absolutely necessary for bone growth and can come from the graft itself or from cells that migrate to the graft from the surrounding tissue. Bone grafts that contain cells that form bone are described as being osteogenic. Factors (small molecules, that are often growth factors) induce cells to migrate into the scaffold, cause cells to differentiate into bone forming cells, and coordinate the bone formation process. Factors that can induce the formation of bone in an ectopic location are defined to be osteoinductive (Table 1).

There are many factors that are involved in bone formation, however, the few factors that have the ability to induce bone formation without other exogenous factors are the truly osteoinductive factors. Naturally occurring osteoinductive factors are confined to molecules in the transforming growth factor-beta (TGF-β) superfamily. The most osteoinductive of these factors are BMP-9, -6, and -2. Of note, not all BMPs and TGF-β family molecules are osteoinductive. Some are more chondrogenic or fibrogenic and at high doses may interfere with bone formation. Osteoinductive BMPs are naturally found in bone. They are thought to be in higher concentrations in cortical bone as compared to cancellous bone. The osteoinductive factors are imbedded in bone tissue and are not active until they are acid treated. Dr Marshall Urist discovered that by acid treating bone, one could identify the osteoinductive components which he called BMP. The initial BMPs extracted from bone were a mixture of many different proteins. However, with the advances in biology,

Table 1: Key properties of various different type of bone graft materials.

Material	*Osteogenic*	*Osteoinductive*	*Osteoconductive*	*Structural support*
Autogenous cancellous bone	+	–	+	–
Autogenous cortical bone	+	–	+/–	+
Allograft cortical bone	–	–	+/–	+
Allograft cancellous bone	–		+	–
Demineralized bone matrix	–	+	+	–
Ceramic	–	–	+	+/–
Bone morphogenetic protein	–	+	–	–

specific BMPs were identified and characterized. BMPs are dimeric molecules that are glycoproteins, which are secreted by cells into the extracellular domain. The BMP dimers can be homodimers (e.g. two BMP-2 molecules) or heterodimers (e.g. one BMP-2 molecule and one BMP-7 molecule). Interestingly, heterodimers of BMP-2 and BMP-7 are thought to be an order of magnitude more potent in bone formation than homodimers of BMP-2 or homodimers of BMP-7. Currently the only commercially available osteoinductive molecule is a recombinant human bone morphogenetic protein-2 (rhBMP-2) homodimer.

SPINE FUSION BIOLOGY

Spinal fusion results in the bony union between two vertebra. This is a cellular process and preparation of the fusion site and soft tissue handling are of utmost importance. Successful fusion requires a population of osteogenic stem cells, adequate vascular supply, a healthy host inflammatory process, and a biologic milieu suitable for bone formation. Meticulous surgical technique must be employed to ensure excellent fusion bed preparation to allow good marrow and blood exposure to the graft material.

Three distinct phases of bone fusion have been described—(1) The inflammatory phase, (2) The reparative phase, and (3) The remodeling phase.[6] The inflammatory phase (weeks 1–3) begins with surgical exposure and decortication. This leads to hematoma formation. A postoperative hematoma is rich with platelets and growth factors including vascular endothelial growth factor (VEGF), platelet-derived growth factor (PDGF), epidermal growth factor (EFG), fibroblast growth factor (FGF), TGF-β, BMP-2, -4, -7, and others.[7]

Adequate blood supply ensures oxygen, nutrients, hormones, and all the necessary ingredients for successful bone fusion to occur. The vascular supply to the fusion site ushers inflammatory cells and allows osteoblastic differentiation through paracrine mechanisms.[8,9] These inflammatory cells including polymorphonuclear cells, lymphocytes, monocytes, and macrophages are thought to be involved in the healing process as they remove necrotic tissues and are part of the initial scaffold of the healing hematoma.[10,11]

The reparative phase (weeks 4–5) begins with this further vascularization of the fusion bed and differentiation of pluripotential mesenchymal cells into chondroblasts and osteoblasts. It is during the later reparative phase that calcification of cartilaginous tissue into immature, woven bone occurs. During this period, 50% of fusion is thought to have occurred.

The final phase is the remodeling phase (weeks 6–12+) during which immature woven bone is systematically remodeled into mature lamellar bone with cortical and cancellous components. This process can continue for many years, however, the majority of remodeling is complete by the 12-week period. This phase model of bone healing was determined using a rabbit model, and thus it can be inferred that the timing of the phases in a human are significantly longer with most estimates ranging from 6 months to 18 months for completion of the remodeling phase.

In this model, mechanically solid fusions occurred during the fourth postoperative week and vascular studies demonstrated that the primary blood supply to the fusion mass originated from the decorticated transverse processes and not the surrounding soft tissues.[12,13] The rabbit model has also shown that bone formation occurs initially from the transverse processes and grows toward each other to join in the intermediate zone between the transverse processes later.

The authors also noted that fusion rates were directly related to the size of the decorticated host site.

BONE GRAFT TYPES

Autologous Cancellous Bone

Autologous cancellous bone is the gold standard of bone graft options. It is a time honored bone graft with a proven track record that offers all three principles of bone graft functionality with its osteogenic, osteoinductive, and osteoconductive properties. Despite the benefits associated with autologous bone grafting, the disadvantages occur with the harvesting of the graft. Autograft harvesting adds time, blood loss, pain, infection risks, cutaneous nerve injury, and iatrogenic fracture risk. The incidence of iliac crest bone graft major complications has been reported between 5% and 10%.[14-16] Sasso and colleagues in a prospective patient satisfaction study of 208 patients demonstrated that 31% of patients after iliac crest harvest have persistent pain at 24 months postoperatively.[17]

The main source of autologous cancellous graft is the iliac crest, which offers a limited supply of bone graft which can be problematic in long fusions, in children, and in the revision setting. Additionally, cancellous autograft offers little mechanical strength and this must be considered in surgical use of this type of graft.

Interestingly, even though autologous cancellous bone is the most abundant source of osteoblastic stem cells, only 1 in 20,000 cells are stem cells capable of bone formation.[18] There is a rich complement of background and stromal cells that are highly metabolically active and are separated from their native blood supply. This creates a relative hypoxic state for the graft cells that cannot be sustained by passive diffusion. Therefore, only cells that are 1–2 mm from the surface of the autograft are able to survive.[19] This limited metabolic state leads to the formation of necrotic debris that must be removed before new bone formation can occur.

Autologous Cortical Bone

Autologous cortical bone offers superior mechanical strength compared to cancellous autograft, yet is less biologically active. Cortical bone contains fewer osteoinductive abilities as the cells are tightly bound within the osteons of cortical bone. Cortical bone lacks the non-osteogenic marrow cells and endothelial cells that are present in cancellous bone. In addition, cortical bone has a lower surface area that reduces the potential for new bone formation. The lower porosity of cortical bone also is a barrier to vascular ingrowth.

The main advantage of cortical autograft over cancellous autograft is the superior mechanical strength that is afforded by the mechanical architecture of the cortical bone. This fact allows immediate mechanical strength at the time of surgery. Once implanted, cortical autograft undergoes creeping substitution that results in decreasing mechanical strength.[19] The process of remodeling and new bone formation can take up to 24 months and is associated with an increased risk of graft failure and collapse.[18] In clinical use, iliac cortical autograft frequently has a component of cancellous autograft that grants both mechanical and biologic properties making it an ideal graft choice for many surgical situations necessitating fusion.

Allograft

The use of allograft bone has been increasing in frequency in structural uses as well as a bone graft extender. The main advantages of allograft use are the elimination of the risks and morbidity of harvesting autograft bone and its availability in large quantities. Structural allografts can be fashioned into numerous functional shapes that allow for precise use by the treating surgeon including blocks, rings, wedges, chips, fibers, dowels, and powder. These surgical time-saving qualities of allograft make it an attractive option to the treating surgeon.

Obviously, allograft is not without its limitations. The process of sterilization and preparation of the graft tissue results in significantly decreased osteoconductive, osteoinductive, and mechanical properties compared to autografts.[20-23] The processing of grafts is in order to remove as many cells as possible to reduce the immunogenic material and allow for successful use in the host. The process of freezing helps to further decrease the immunogenicity; however, this reduces the mechanical strength of the allograft by 50%.[23,24] The modern practices of processing of allograft have resulted in a very low risk of overt immunologic reactions against the donor material. However, on the microscopic level, nearly all allografts result in a histologic subclinical inflammatory reaction.[24] Several animal models have indicated that antigen matching between the host and donor could lead to improved graft assimilation.[22,25,26] However, due to high clinical success rates and the prohibitive costs associated, antigen matching is unfeasible and unwarranted.[27]

In addition to the immunogenicity concerns, the risk of disease transmission is a frequently questioned topic. The risk of disease transmission from allograft that has undergone modern processing and sterilization is approximately 1 in 1,667,000.[28] There have been no reports of bacterial disease transmission and one report of HIV transmission in spinal surgery using allograft.[29] This relatively low risk has been achieved through expedient postmortem harvesting with sterile technique and monitoring of surface cultures and polymerase chain reaction screening for bacterial and viral genomes.[18] Secondary processes such as ethylene oxide sterilization, autoclaving, and high dose irradiation have been employed in the past but have been linked to suboptimal effects on the graft by reducing the biologic and mechanical properties.[24]

Clinical studies comparing allograft to autograft in spinal fusion have been varied in their findings. Some studies have touted the superiority of autograft whereas others have reported similar outcomes. In a prospective randomized controlled trial, Gibson and coauthors showed similar postoperative outcomes in instrumented lumbar fusion patients who received autograft compared to those who received fresh frozen allografts with a follow-up of 6 years.[30]

In a retrospective comparison of 35 patients with allograft to 45 patients with autograft in multilevel anterior cervical discectomy and fusion, Samartzis demonstrated a high fusion rate of 97.5% with either autograft or allograft.[31] The same author demonstrated similar results with single level anterior cervical discectomy and fusion with 35 patients receiving allograft versus 31 patients receiving autograft with 100% and 90.3% fusion rates, respectively.[29] The literature proposes that allograft is particularly valuable in settings that require the graft to serve a significant mechanical or strut function.[32-34]

Demineralized Allograft Bone Matrix

Demineralization of allograft bone by acid extraction is a process that enhances the osteoinductive activity by making growth factors embedded in the allograft more available for bone formation at the expense of decreasing some of the mechanical properties. What remains after the acid extraction is noncollagenous proteins, collagen fibers, and BMPs that are then combined with a carrier material (often sodium hyaluronate) that offers a degree of osteoconductive potential. Bone matrix has also been shown to have a variety of other growth factors including mitogenic factors to promote cell proliferation and angiogenic factors to promote revascularization of the bone graft.[35] In addition, DBM is associated with similar risk of disease transmission as standard allograft preparations.

In rat femur model, Sato and Urist showed that DBM was osteoinductive and synergistic with bone marrow-derived cells in the femoral defect healing.[36] Using a rat model, Peterson and coauthors compared several DBM formulations including Grafton (Osteotech), DBX putty (Synthes), and Allomatrix putty (Wright Medical Technology) with a control model of decortication and were able to demonstrate that spines in the Grafton group had a statistically significant higher rate of fusion compared to control and Allomatrix ($p < 0.05$).[37] In a similar study, Wang and coinvestigators showed that Osteofil and Grafton (Medtronic Sofamor Danek) achieved the highest fusion rate and Dynagraft (Integra Life Sciences) resulting in no fusions.[38] These studies demonstrate a clinical concern regarding the variety of preparations of DBM, which is in part due to the variation of bone quality of the individual donor. However, there is no regulation regarding the process of DBM manufacturing, and thus, the biologic efficacy of DBM can vary significantly as evident by the above rat spinal fusion models. In a study of concentrations of BMP-2 and BMP-7 in commercially available DBM products, Bae and colleagues were able to show marked variability in concentrations of BMPs across the different products and even variability between different batches of the same product.[39]

Use of DBM in human studies has been shown in craniofacial defects, long bone defects, and in spine fusion. In a recent randomized prospective study with 30 patients receiving Grafton DBM with local bone and 16 patients utilizing autologous iliac crest, Kang and colleagues demonstrated 86% fusion rate with Grafton compared to 92% fusion rate with iliac crest.[40] In addition, they showed a statistically significant greater mean intraoperative blood loss in the autologous iliac crest bone graft group compared to the Grafton group ($p < 0.0031$).

Ceramics

Ceramics are a group of synthetic bone grafts consisting of calcium phosphate biomaterials fused into a polycrystalline structure by high temperatures. The majority of calcium phosphate ceramics have a high degree of biocompatibility, but each differs slightly in its bioresorbability characteristics.[41] The two most commonly studied ceramics are composed of either hydroxyapatite (HA) or tricalcium phosphate (TCP). The major role of ceramics is osteoconduction. To facilitate the osteoconductive properties of ceramics, they usually have porous structure that is within range (100–500 um) needed for effective bone ingrowth.[42] In the late stages of bone formation, a ceramic may exert some osteoinductive properties through its affinity to bind osteoinductive proteins such as BMPs, TGF-β, and insulin-like growth factor-binding protein-5 (IGFBP-5) onto a stable surface.[43] The presence of these proteins along with the osteoconductive structure creates an environment that is capable of recruiting local osteoblastic progenitors and inducing bone formation. However, ceramics, as stand-alone substances, are not considered truly osteoinductive.

A mechanical disadvantage of these implants is that they are brittle, having low impact, and fracture resistance.[44] Several studies have shown that ceramic HA does not exhibit extensive bioresorption, and is essentially inert while there is strong evidence that ceramic TCP undergoes biodegradation.[41,45] Furthermore, highly crystalline HA ceramics with limited solubility and remodeling may comprise the late mechanical properties of the bone formed at a fusion site.[41] This concern of reduced mechanical properties was decreased by the work of Muschler and associates who in a series of spinal fusion experiments evaluating a composite of collagen and ceramic (60% HA, 40% TCP) showed that the mechanical properties of successful fusion masses were similar to ones derived from autogenous bone graft despite the presence of unresorbed granules in the fusion mass.[46,47] Importantly, these investigators did note a significantly higher nonunion rate in the ceramic group compared to the autograft group.

Ceramic blocks have been evaluated in goat anterior cervical fusion model with fusion rates ranging from 50% to 70% and single surgeon series of ACDFs with ceramics have been published, but in general the effectiveness of ceramics alone without other graft material for ACDF has not been established.[48,49] Various ceramics have been studied in lumbar spinal fusions with mixed results.[50,51] Ceramics, however, may play a better role as an adjuvant graft when used in conjunction with autograft as a graft extender. It may be useful to fill in voids or gaps left after anterior cervical grafting or other fusion areas to provide additional osteoconductive matrix in a fusion bed that is not fully covered with other bone graft.

Bone Morphogenetic Proteins

As of 2013, two BMPs have undergone pivotal clinical trials for spine fusion indication (rhBMP-2 and rhBMP-7). Recombinant human BMP-7 is also known as OP-1 did not gain full FDA clearance for use in the spine, but has a humanitarian exemption for use in less than 4,000 cases per year under restricted conditions. rhBMP-2 gained FDA approval for use in the lumbar spine in anterior lumbar interbody fusion indication when used in conjunction with an absorbable collagen sponge and a cage. However, surgeons have reported multiple off-label uses of rhBMP-2 in the cervical, thoracic, and lumbar fusion surgery. The literature indicates that in certain situations, fusion rates are increased with the use of rhBMP-2; the appropriate situations for use on these myriad different situations remain to be further delineated. While it is beyond the scope of this chapter to review all the different possible best uses of rhBMP-2 in spinal fusion, it is important for surgeons to understand that the dose and carrier of rhBMP-2 is different for each different fusion surgery type and the possible complications may be different for each of these indications.

REFERENCES

1. Albee FH. Transplantation of a portion of the tibia into the spine for Pott's disease: a preliminary report 1911. Clin Orthop Relat Res. 2007;460:14-6.
2. Hibbs RA. An operation for progressive spinal deformities: a preliminary report of three cases from the service of the orthopaedic hospital. 1911. Clin Orthop Relat Res. 2007; 460:17-20.
3. Wang JC, McDonough PW, Endow KK, et al. Increased fusion rates with cervical plating for two-level anterior cervical discectomy and fusion. Spine (Phila Pa 1976). 2000;25(1):41-5.
4. Wang JC, McDonough PW, Endow KK, et al. A comparison of fusion rates between single-level cervical corpectomy and two-level discectomy and fusion. J Spinal Disord. 2001;14(3):222-5.
5. Wilkins W. Posterolateral fusion of the lumbar and lumbosacral spine. J Bone Joint Surg. 1953;35:1014-8.
6. Boden SD, Schimandle JH, Hutton WC, et al. 1995 Volvo Award in basic sciences. The use of an osteoinductive growth factor for lumbar spinal fusion. Part I: Biology of spinal fusion. Spine (Phila Pa 1976). 1995;20(24):2626-32.
7. Gronthos S, Simmons PJ. The biology and application of human bone marrow stromal cell precursors. J Hematother. 1996;5(1):15-23.
8. Villanueva JE, Nimni ME. Promotion of calvarial cell osteogenesis by endothelial cells. J Bone Miner Res. 1990; 5(7):733-9.
9. Brighton CT, Lorich DG, Kupcha R, et al. The pericyte as a possible osteoblast progenitor cell. Clin Orthop Relat Res. 1992;(275):287-99.
10. Simmons DJ. Fracture healing perspectives. Clin Orthop Relat Res. 1985;(200):100-13.
11. Prolo DJ, Rodrigo JJ. Contemporary bone graft physiology and surgery. Clin Orthop Relat Res. 1985;(200):322-42.
12. Boden SD. Overview of the biology of lumbar spine fusion and principles for selecting a bone graft substitute. Spine (Phila Pa 1976). 2002;27(16 Suppl 1):S26-31.
13. Boden SD. The biology of posterolateral lumbar spinal fusion. Orthop Clin North Am. 1998;29(4):603-19.
14. Younger EM, Chapman MW. Morbidity at bone graft donor sites. J Orthop Trauma. 1989;3(3):192-5.
15. Hu RW, Bohlman HH. Fracture at the iliac bone graft harvest site after fusion of the spine. Clin Orthop Relat Res. 1994;(309):208-13.
16. Ackerman SJ, Mafilios MS, Polly DW Jr. Economic evaluation of bone morphogenetic protein versus autogenous iliac crest bone graft in single-level anterior lumbar fusion: an

evidence-based modeling approach. Spine (Phila Pa 1976). 2002;27(16 Suppl 1):S94-9.
17. Sasso RC, LeHuec JC, Shaffrey C. Iliac crest bone graft donor site pain after anterior lumbar interbody fusion: a prospective patient satisfaction outcome assessment. J Spinal Disord Tech. 2005;18 Suppl:S77-81.
18. Herkowitz H, Garfin S, Eismont F, et al. The Spine, 6th edition. Philadelphia: Saunders-Elsevier; 2006.
19. Muschler GF, Nakamoto C, Griffith LG. Engineering principles of clinical cell-based tissue engineering. J Bone Joint Surg Am. 2004;86-A(7):1541-58.
20. Tomford WW, Starkweather RJ, Goldman MH. A study of the clinical incidence of infection in the use of banked allograft bone. J Bone Joint Surg Am. 1981;63(2):244-8.
21. Tomford WW, Thongphasuk J, Mankin HJ, et al. Frozen musculoskeletal allografts. A study of the clinical incidence and causes of infection associated with their use. J Bone Joint Surg Am. 1990;72(8):1137-43.
22. Stevenson S. The immune response to osteochondral allografts in dogs. J Bone Joint Surg Am. 1987;69(4):573-82.
23. Bauer TW, Muschler GF. Bone graft materials. An overview of the basic science. Clin Orthop Relat Res. 2000;(371):10-27.
24. Pelker RR, McKay J, Troiano N, et al. Allograft incorporation: a biomechanical evaluation in a rat model. J Orthop Res. 1989;7(4):585-9.
25. Stevenson S, Hohn RB, Templeton JW. Effects of tissue antigen matching on the healing of fresh cancellous bone allografts in dogs. Am J Vet Res. 1983;44(2):201-6.
26. Bos GD GV, Powell AE, et al. The effect of histocompatibility matching on canine frozen bone allografts. J Bone Joint Surg. 1983;65:89-96.
27. Muscolo DL, Caletti E, Schajowicz F, et al. Tissue-typing in human massive allografts of frozen bone. J Bone Joint Surg Am. 1987;69(4):583-95.
28. Swenson CL, Arnoczky SP. Demineralization for inactivation of infectious retrovirus in systemically infected cortical bone: in vitro and in vivo experimental studies. J Bone Joint Surg Am. 2003;85-A(2):323-32.
29. Samartzis D, Shen FH, Goldberg EJ, et al. Is autograft the gold standard in achieving radiographic fusion in one-level anterior cervical discectomy and fusion with rigid anterior plate fixation? Spine (Phila Pa 1976). 2005;30(15):1756-61.
30. Gibson S, McLeod I, Wardlaw D, et al. Allograft versus autograft in instrumented posterolateral lumbar spinal fusion: a randomized control trial. Spine (Phila Pa 1976). 2002;27(15):1599-603.
31. Samartzis D, Shen FH, Matthews DK, et al. Comparison of allograft to autograft in multilevel anterior cervical discectomy and fusion with rigid plate fixation. Spine J. 2003;3(6):451-9.
32. Kleinstueck FS, Hu SS, Bradford DS. Use of allograft femoral rings for spinal deformity in adults. Clin Orthop Relat Res. 2002;(394):84-91.
33. Cohen DB, Chotivichit A, Fujita T, et al. Pseudarthrosis repair. Autogenous iliac crest versus femoral ring allograft. Clin Orthop Relat Res. 2000;(371):46-55.
34. Siff TE, Kamaric E, Noble PC, et al. Femoral ring versus fibular strut allografts in anterior lumbar interbody arthrodesis. A biomechanical analysis. Spine (Phila Pa 1976). 1999;24(7):659-65.
35. Linkhart TA, Mohan S, Baylink DJ. Growth factors for bone growth and repair: IGF, TGF beta and BMP. Bone. 1996;19(1 Suppl):1S-12S.
36. Sato K, Urist MR. Induced regeneration of calvaria by bone morphogenetic protein (BMP) in dogs. Clin Orthop Relat Res. 1985;(197):301-11.
37. Peterson B, Whang PG, Iglesias R, et al. Osteoinductivity of commercially available demineralized bone matrix. Preparations in a spine fusion model. J Bone Joint Surg Am. 2004;86-A(10):2243-50.
38. Wang JC, Alanay A, Mark D, et al. A comparison of commercially available demineralized bone matrix for spinal fusion. Eur Spine J. 2007;16(8):1233-40.
39. Bae HW, Zhao L, Kanim LE, et al. Intervariability and intravariability of bone morphogenetic proteins in commercially available demineralized bone matrix products. Spine (Phila Pa 1976). 2006;31(12):1299-306; discussion 307-8.
40. Kang J, An H, Hilibrand A, et al. Grafton and local bone have comparable outcomes to iliac crest bone in instrumented single-level lumbar fusions. Spine (Phila Pa 1976). 2012; 37(12):1083-91.
41. Jarcho M. Calcium phosphate ceramics as hard tissue prosthetics. Clin Orthop Relat Res. 1981;(157):259-78.
42. Klawitter JJ HS. Application of porous ceramics for the attachment of load bearing orthopaedic applications. J Biomed Mater Res A. 1971;2:161.
43. Tan Y, Wang G, Fan H, et al. Expression of core binding factor 1 and osteoblastic markers in C2C12 cells induced by calcium phosphate ceramics in vitro. J Biomed Mater Res A. 2007;82(1):152-9.
44. Bhaskar SN, Brady JM, Getter L, et al. Biodegradable ceramic implants in bone. Electron and light microscopic analysis. Oral Surg Oral Med Oral Pathol. 1971;32(2):336-46.
45. Hoogendoorn HA, Renooij W, Akkermans LM, et al. Long-term study of large ceramic implants (porous hydroxyapatite) in dog femora. Clin Orthop Relat Res. 1984;(187):281-8.
46. Muschler GF, Negami S, Hyodo A, et al. Evaluation of collagen ceramic composite graft materials in a spinal fusion model. Clin Orthop Relat Res. 1996;(328):250-60.
47. Muschler GF, Huber B, Ullman T, et al. Evaluation of bone-grafting materials in a new canine segmental spinal fusion model. J Orthop Res. 1993;11(4):514-24.
48. Pintar FA, Maiman DJ, Hollowell JP, et al. Fusion rate and biomechanical stiffness of hydroxylapatite versus autogenous bone grafts for anterior discectomy. An in vivo animal study. Spine (Phila Pa 1976). 1994;19(22):2524-8.
49. Zdeblick TA, Cooke ME, Kunz DN, et al. Anterior cervical discectomy and fusion using a porous hydroxyapatite bone graft substitute. Spine (Phila Pa 1976). 1994;19(20):2348-57.
50. Epstein NE. A preliminary study of the efficacy of Beta Tricalcium Phosphate as a bone expander for instrumented posterolateral lumbar fusions. J Spinal Disord Tech. 2006; 19(6):424-9.
51. Lerner T, Bullmann V, Schulte TL, et al. A level-1 pilot study to evaluate of ultraporous beta-tricalcium phosphate as a graft extender in the posterior correction of adolescent idiopathic scoliosis. Eur Spine J. 2009;18(2):170-9.

CHAPTER 8

Spinal Infections

Scott D Daffner, Vincent J Miele

INTRODUCTION

Although spinal infections have been reported and treated for centuries, the importance of our understanding of this malady has never been as great as it is today. This is mainly for two reasons. First, we now possess a large armamentarium of medications and surgical interventions with which we can successfully treat this constellation of disease if applied appropriately and in a timely fashion. Second, it appears that the problem is becoming more frequent and destructive which is likely due to the increase in antibiotic-resistant organisms as well as the immunocompromised population. The latter factor is not only a result of the larger surviving human immunodeficiency virus (HIV) population, but increasing prevalence of other immunocompromising disease states such as diabetes mellitus as well as the continuing issues of intravenous (IV) drug abuse.

Spinal infections are a significant source of morbidity and mortality. Complications include instability and deformity, chronic pain, paraparesis, and paraplegia. It is important to recognize that when paresis or plegia does occur, the prognosis for recovery of function is poor.[1] Mortality occurs from the spread of infection, either through the nervous system or through other organs and has a reported overall rate of 5–15%.[2-6] Greater mortality is associated with increasing age (> 60 years), hemodialysis use, diabetes, liver cirrhosis, malignancy, and infective endocarditis.

The term "Spinal Infection" comprises a group of conditions that lie on a spectrum from discitis to vertebral osteomyelitis to abscess. The condition has specific causes as well as characteristic presentations and natural histories and can generally be divided into three categories—pyogenic, granulomatous, and parasitic. Pyogenic are the result of bacterial infection and are the most commonly encountered; the main focus of this chapter will be on this category of disease. Granulomatous pathology results from tuberculosis or fungal infection of the spine. Parasitic spinal infection is the result of organisms that live inside humans or other organisms that act as hosts and are dependent on their hosts because they are unable to produce food or energy for themselves.

PYOGENIC SPINAL INFECTION

Pyogenic infections of the spine are the result of bacterial infection and are the most commonly encountered. They can be broken down into two categories: secondary infections that occur following an invasive spinal procedure and primary infections. This chapter will focus on primary infections. The vast majority of these infections (up to 95%) is structurally identified as involving the disk and surrounding bone and is commonly referred to as pyogenic spondylodiscitis/osteodiscitis. Infections involving just the bone or disk space are referred to as pyogenic spondylitis or discitis, respectively. As would be expected, it is fairly uncommon for the infection to be respectful of the boundary between disk and adjacent vertebral body endplate.

Pyogenic infection is most commonly the result of hematogenous spread of bacteria due to transient (or longer lasting) bacteremia from skin wounds, the urogenital system, the respiratory tract, the gastrointestinal tract, or the oral cavity.[7] Introduction of bacteria into the system can also be the result of IV drug abuse. Several medical conditions and treatments can increase an individual's susceptibility to introduced bacteria. These include chronic steroid use, diabetes mellitus, chronic renal insufficiency, rheumatoid arthritis, and immunocompromise either as a result of chronic disease or iatrogenic as in the case of organ transplant recipients. While patients may have some predisposing factor or clear source of infection such as a urinary tract infection (UTI) or an infected IV line, many patients present with no obvious cause.

Infections typically arise around the vertebral endplates or disk spaces which are likely due to the vascular anatomy of the area. Blood vessels end in a blind loop at the edge of the endplate within the vertebral body. This anatomy creates relatively sluggish blood flow through these high-capacity terminal vessels. While beneficial in allowing nutrients to diffuse through the vessels and endplates into the disk, it also creates an environment in which bacteria can accumulate and flourish in the avascular nucleus pulposus. In addition, the vascular anatomy is such that one segmental artery provides blood flow to the inferior portion of one vertebra and the superior portion of the subjacent vertebra; this explains the tendency for pyogenic vertebral infections to include two adjacent vertebrae and the disk between them.[7] The valveless plexiform venous system of the spine, known as Batson's plexus, also possesses the characteristic of sluggish but large volume flow that predisposes it to the transfer of bacteria via retrograde flow.[8]

Epidemiology

The incidence of osteodiscitis in the general population ranges from 1 in 100,000 to 1 in 250,000 and nearly two cases per 10,000 hospital admissions.[9] A bimodal distribution of ages occurs with discitis, with a peak at the age of 7 years and again at 50 years. The condition is more predominant in males, especially in the older population. Pyogenic spinal infections most frequently involve the lumbar spinal segments (45–50%), followed by the thoracic segments (35%), and the cervical segments (20%).[7,10,11] This is fortunate since, as would be expected, the severe complications of paresis and paralysis more commonly occur with thoracic and cervical region involvement.

Microbiology

Staphylococcus aureus (SA) is the most common organism leading to pyogenic vertebral osteomyelitis. In patients that have a history of frequent hospitalizations or rehabilitation placements, the methicillin resistant form of this organism (MRSA) is more of a concern. Antibiotic resistance has increased in recent years and continues to create challenges in treatment. Other common organisms include *Streptococcus* species, *Escherichia coli*, *Enterococcus*, and *Proteus*. Elderly patients with recurrent UTIs have an increased risk of gram-negative bacilli involvement and in general, *Escherichia coli* and *Proteus* species are more common in patients with UTIs. *Pseudomonas aeruginosa* and *Klebsiella* species are other gram-negative organisms often observed in IV drug users, although they are not seen as commonly as *Staphylococcus aureus*. Mycobacterial species and fungal infections should be considered in immunocompromised patients.

Presentation

Symptoms of spinal infection typically present insidiously and the severity is often dependent on the acuity of the infection. Most patients present with complaints of back or neck pain with localized tenderness. This presentation is often associated with paraspinal muscle spasm. Movement exacerbates these symptoms, which worsen despite normal conservative treatments. Because these symptoms are nonspecific (and common complaints in the general population), the diagnosis is frequently delayed for 2–12 weeks from onset, occasionally extending greater than 3 months.[7,12,13] This delay in initiation of treatment can affect patient outcome and infection recurrence rate.[14] Constitutional symptoms such as fever, chills, weight loss, and symptoms of systemic disease may be present, but are much less common. One study found that while nearly 98% of patients presented with back or neck pain, only 12.5% of patients demonstrated a fever.[12] Neurologic symptoms may be present in up to a third of patients, most frequently radicular in nature.[12,13] As would be expected, cervical and thoracic involvement is more likely to be associated with neurological deficit.

Of note, the condition has a more acute course in children, leading some to speculate that childhood discitis is a separate disease entity and should be considered as such. A sudden onset of back pain, refusal to walk, and irritability are the most common symptoms. Fever is often present, accompanied by local tenderness and limited back motion.

Diagnostic Evaluation

Laboratory Testing

Baseline laboratory studies in any patient suspected of having a spinal infection should include white blood cell count (WBC), erythrocyte sedimentation rate (ESR), and C-reactive protein (CRP) as well as blood cultures. Notably, WBC may be normal in over half of patients[12,13] which is especially true if the infection is not acute. More commonly, ESR is elevated. Similarly, CRP (which is a more specific marker for infection) has demonstrated elevation in over 90% of patients with spinal infections.[7] Because CRP normalizes faster than ESR, it is commonly utilized in following a patient's response to treatment. Positive blood cultures may identify the causative organism in 25–60% of patients, but they may also be negative in up to 75% of patients.[3,11,13] Other laboratory testing may be performed to assess potential causes of infection (e.g. urinalysis and urine culture), or factors that may affect treatment (e.g. nutrition, renal function). Echocardiography is often obtained to evaluate the patient for bacterial endocarditis, which is a common source of discitis and embolic infection throughout the body. Sputum may be used to identify respiratory sources of infection.

Imaging

Plain radiographs often tend to lag behind clinical symptoms by 2–8 weeks and, if obtained early in the infection's course, may appear essentially normal. Patients with discitis and osteomyelitis will typically demonstrate narrowing of the disk space, endplate irregularities, and sclerosis, which may eventually progress to frank bony destruction or instability (coronal or sagittal malalignment). Upright radiographs allow assessment of instability. Frank bony destruction may take 8–12 weeks to become evident (Figs. 1A and B). Also, evident on plain radiographs would be soft tissue evidence of abscess. In the cervical spine, this would be demonstrated by a widened retropharyngeal space. If it occurred in the thoracic spine, a widened paravertebral space would be identified and in the lumbar spine, changes in the psoas shadow could be seen. Computed tomography (CT) may better delineate bony changes and may also provide evidence of associated soft tissue abscess.

Radionuclide studies are helpful in diagnosis of patients with suspected spinal infections. A three-phase technetium Tc-99 study has high sensitivity (approximately 90%) but low specificity (78%) in this setting. When performed in conjunction with a gallium Ga-67 citrate scan, the sensitivity is 90%, specificity is 100%, and diagnostic accuracy is 94%[15] (Table 1).

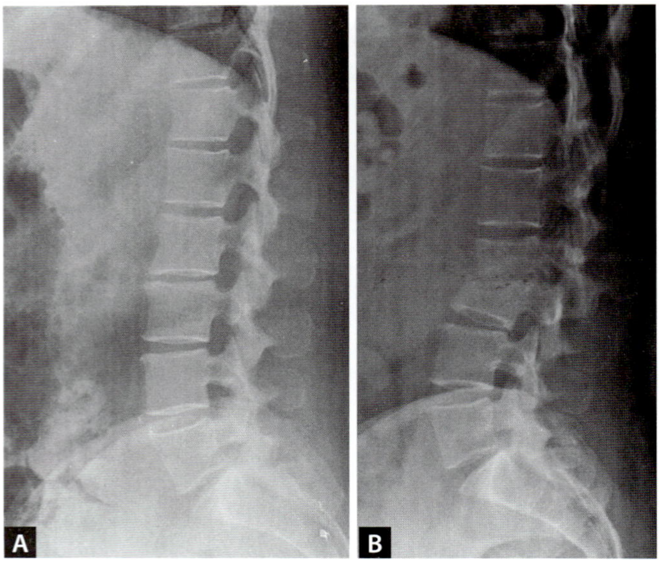

Figs. 1A and B: (A) Lateral radiograph of a 38-year-old woman who presented to her primary care provider with 6 weeks of nonspecific back pain. There is subtle narrowing of the L2–L3 disk space; (B) Lateral radiograph obtained 3 months later after persistent and worsening symptoms showing bony destruction of the L2 and L3 endplates with associated kyphotic deformity.

Table 1: Relative sensitivity, specificity, accuracy of imaging techniques for infection.[15]

Modality	*Sensitivity*	*Specificity*	*Accuracy*
Plain radiography	82	57	73
Bone scan	90	78	86
Bone scan + Gallium scan	90	100	94
MRI	96	92	94

The accuracy of magnetic resonance imaging (MRI) in diagnosing vertebral osteomyelitis has been reported to be 94% with high sensitivity and specificity.[15] MRI has become the imaging modality of choice for patients with suspected vertebral osteomyelitis or discitis. When performed with gadolinium, it has a sensitivity of 96% and specificity of 92%.[16] MRI will show decreased signal on T1-weighted images and increased signal on T2-weighted images (Figs. 2A to D). MRI can also provide evidence that can be used to help differentiate pyogenic osteodiscitis from neoplasm and granulomatous osteodiscitis. Although neoplastic

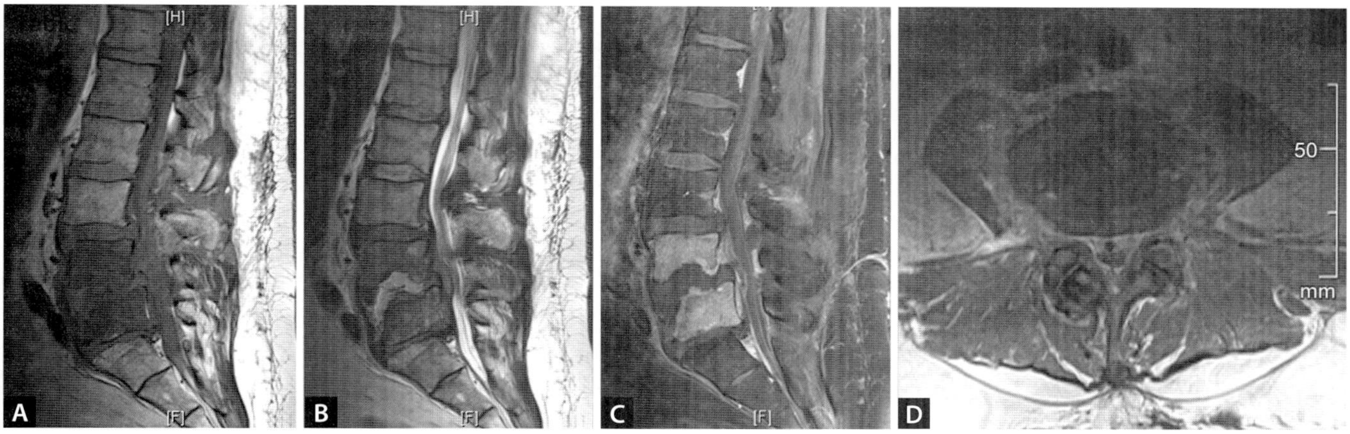

Figs. 2A to D: MRI findings of discitis-osteomyelitis: (A) Sagittal T1-weighted imaging demonstrates decreased signal intensity; (B) Sagittal T2-weighted imaging shows high signal intensity in the disk space and vertebral bodies; (C) Sagittal T1-weighted postcontrast (gadolinium) imaging demonstrates significant enhancement in the bone and epidural space; (D) Axial T1-weighted postcontrast image demonstrating enhancement in the epidural space as well as in the adjacent psoas muscle, suggestive of abscess.

processes may have similar findings, tumors tend to spare the disk space, whereas involvement of the disk space highly favors infection. Granulomatous infections such as tuberculosis have a characteristic finding of involvement of the vertebral bodies with extension under the anterior longitudinal ligament between bodies, but tend to spare the disk space.

Spinal infections are initially identified with imaging changes of osteomyelitis close to the endplates, then progress to involve the disk space. Despite its good sensitivity and specificity, MRI may be unremarkable, or could demonstrate changes attributable to degenerative disease when performed early after onset of symptoms; repeat MRI within 3 weeks, however, can show typical changes associated with infection.[17] The use of MRI to follow resolution of infection after treatment is not recommended, as imaging changes persist (and often appear worse early in the course of treatment) despite improvement in laboratory and clinical findings.[18,19]

Medical Management

While there are no prospective, randomized trials comparing conservative versus surgical management, in the absence of severe or progressive neurologic deficit, structural instability, or systemic sepsis, the initial treatment of vertebral osteomyelitis is nonoperative. Although a presumptive diagnosis can be made in patients with positive blood cultures, and appropriate clinical, laboratory, and imaging findings, definitive diagnosis of vertebral osteomyelitis or discitis requires a tissue biopsy for microbiology. Biopsy should be obtained prior to initiation of antibiotic therapy. The biopsy should be sent for gram stain, aerobic, anaerobic, fungal, and acid fast bacilli (AFB) cultures. In addition, material should be sent for pathology to evaluate for potential neoplastic process. This biopsy can be obtained by interventional radiology with either CT or fluoroscopic guidance, and core biopsy is preferable to fine needle aspirate. Percutaneous biopsy is reported to be positive in approximately 70% of cases.[20] If an initial biopsy is negative, a second attempt should be made; if the second attempt fails to produce a positive culture, an open biopsy may be performed.[3]

If available, an infectious disease consultant should be utilized to recommend, manage, and follow antimicrobial therapy in patients with spinal infections. While the optimal duration and route of antibiotic therapy has yet to be defined, there is a high failure rate if the treatment is performed for less than 4 weeks. Most authors advocate 6–8 weeks of IV treatment. Some stop treatment after this period if the patient has responded appropriately while others then recommend an additional 2 or more months of oral antibiotic therapy. There is no strong evidence that continued oral therapy following parenteral antibiotic treatment has a significant effect on outcome. The efficacy of nonoperative treatment of spinal infections is determined by improvement or resolution of clinical symptoms in conjunction with normalization of ESR and CRP. Generally, before parenteral therapy is discontinued, the ESR should have dropped by one-half to one-third, the patient should have minimal pain on ambulation, and there should be no neurologic deficits.[21,22] If no reduction in ESR or CRP is demonstrated, consideration should be given to repeat biopsy.

The selection and duration of antimicrobial regimen depends on the organism being treated as well as host factors such as nutrition, medical comorbidities, and presence of spinal instrumentation. It has also been suggested that the time from symptom onset to initiation of antibiotic therapy be taken into account. It has been demonstrated that when treatment is delayed for 6–7 weeks after onset of symptoms, antibiotic treatment of only 4–8 weeks is associated with an increased recurrence rate as compared to treatment of 12 weeks and over.[14] Consultation with a clinical nutritionist should be considered to optimize the patient's nutrition.

In addition to antibiotic therapy, conservative treatment consists of immobilization of the affected spinal levels. The goals are to decrease pain, facilitate ambulation, prevent kyphotic deformity, and allow the area to fuse in an anatomically aligned position. Immobilization is accomplished via a well-molded external brace that may be utilized for 3–6 months following initiation of treatment. Follow-up radiographs will show spontaneous fusion of vertebral segments in many cases (Figs. 3A to F). Nonoperative treatment is successful in 75–85% of patients.[7,13]

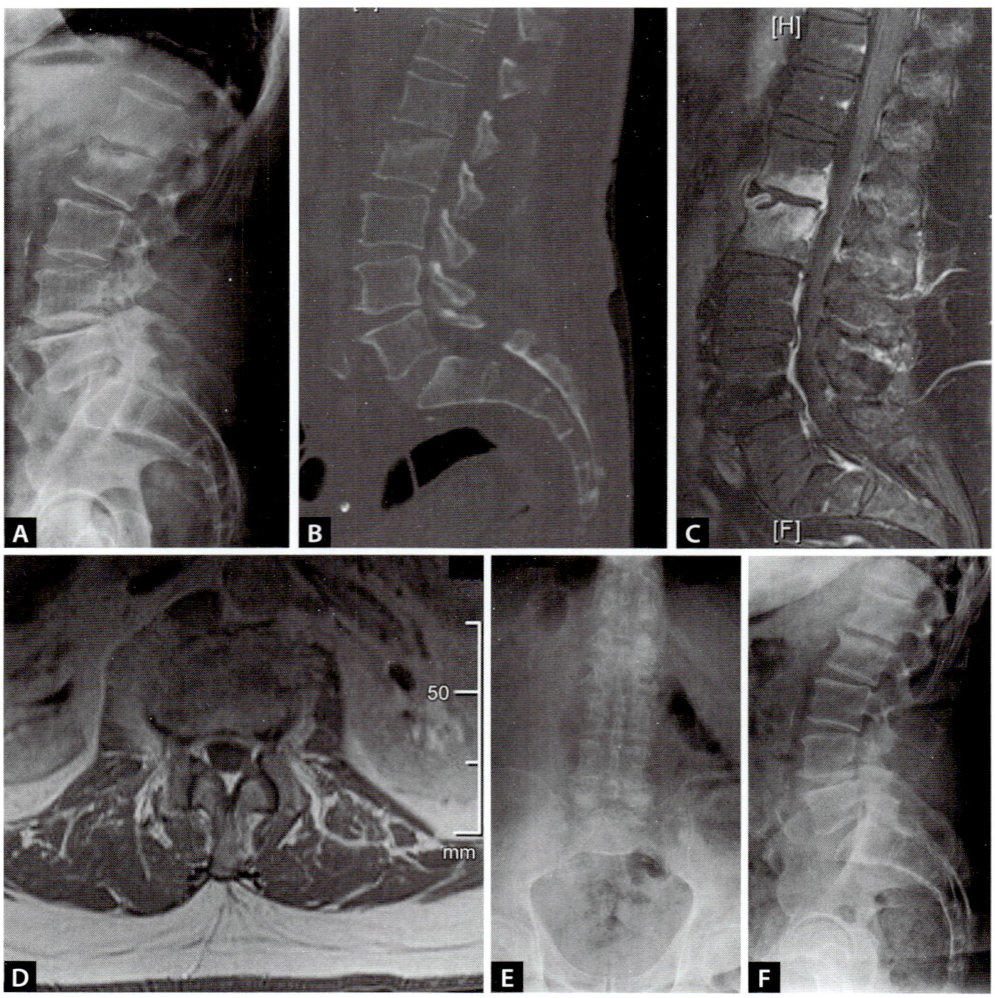

Figs. 3A to F: (A) Lateral radiograph; (B) Sagittal CT; (C) Sagittal T1-weighted postcontrast MRI of a 62-year-old man who presented with 4 months of back pain; (D) Axial T1-weighted postcontrast MRI shows no epidural abscess and minimal enhancement of the adjacent psoas muscle. He had no neurologic deficit, minimal deformity, and well-maintained bony integrity. He was treated with parenteral antibiotics and bracing for 6 weeks; (E) AP; (F) Lateral radiographs obtained 6 months after initiation of treatment demonstrate well-preserved coronal and sagittal alignment with some evidence of autofusion of L1 and L2.

Surgical Indications and Treatment

Indications for surgical intervention for spinal infections include the presence (or progression) of a neurologic deficit due to compression (e.g. abscess), loss or impending loss of structural stability, local kyphosis, need to drain an abscess which is causing systemic sepsis, failure of improvement (improved pain, normalized CRP and ESR) following an appropriate trial of nonoperative treatment, recurrence of infection, and the need to obtain a tissue diagnosis if percutaneous samples are inconclusive (or inaccessible). Generally, only 10–25% of patients require surgical treatment.

Intractable pain should be considered when determining if treatment should be medical versus surgical. While both generally improve pain, surgical treatment tends to improve severe intractable pain more and at a faster rate.[23-25] The improvement in pain from treatment is thought to be secondary to decreased inflammation as well as stabilization of the affected spinal segment. Whether the former or the latter is primarily responsible for pain likely varies between patients. One study demonstrated that while only 26% of patients treated surgically complained of persistent axial mechanical back pain, the conservatively treated group's rate was much higher at 64%.[1] This finding would tend to support the idea that internal stabilization is an important factor in pain control. While bracing is utilized during conservative management of this population to provide stability and spontaneous fusion often occurs, it can take up to 2 years to occur and has been reported to occur in less than half of the treated patients.[26]

The goals of surgical intervention are decompression of neural tissue, specimen collection, removal of all infected and devitalized tissue, evacuation of any abscesses, correction of deformity, and stabilization. With these goals in mind, the surgeon must decide which approach would be most appropriate. Since spinal infections typically involve the vertebral body and disk space, an anterior surgical approach is often recommended. While this approach lends itself well to direct debridement and reconstruction of the infected area, it does have some drawbacks. In the thoracic and lumbar spine, the anterior approach can be more extensive than posterior surgery. Vessels and viscera may be invested in inflammatory tissue, increasing the likelihood of injury as well as operative time that the moribund patient may not tolerate well. Additionally, infection often leads to osteoporosis of surrounding bone which can result in a tenuous foundation for anterior instrumentation.[27] Anterior fusion alone may allow adequate stabilization, particularly if the infection involves a single disk space and has minimal involvement of the adjacent vertebral bodies (Figs. 4A to D). Occasionally, a posterolateral extracavitary approach (e.g. costotransversectomy in the thoracic spine) may be chosen. Such an approach may allow a surgeon to address anterior pathology from a more familiar posterior approach and, in the thoracic spine, may obviate the need for placement of a chest tube.

With multilevel infections or in patients requiring extensive debridement, patients with significant kyphotic or scoliotic deformity, patients with osteoporosis, or in those where surgical approach or body habitus might not allow bracing following an anterior only approach, a combined anterior-posterior approach may be chosen (Figs. 5A to E). The posterior fusion can be safely performed at the same time as the anterior procedure or it may be staged. Combined anterior/posterior approaches for this condition are becoming more common and seem to give better results in terms of decreased postoperative complications and maintenance of deformity correction.[28] Likely due to the more thorough debridement of all necrotic or infected bone and soft tissue, the incidence of infection recurrence has also been demonstrated to decrease with a combined approach.[23,29]

Decompressive laminectomy alone has limited usefulness in spinal infections. It can be utilized for primary epidural abscesses (those that do not involve the vertebral body or disk space). These often present with worsening neurological deficit and the primary goal of surgical intervention is urgent decompression of the neural elements to prevent permanent loss of function. Notably, decompressive laminectomy alone is relatively contraindicated for secondary epidural abscesses (those that arise from infection in the vertebral body or disk space). The reason is mainly because the laminectomy combined with destruction of the anterior supporting structures of the spine from infection will likely result in gross instability.

Following debridement, reconstruction of the anterior column must commonly be performed. Structural autograft, structural allograft, and titanium mesh cages (filled with autograft) have all been used for structural

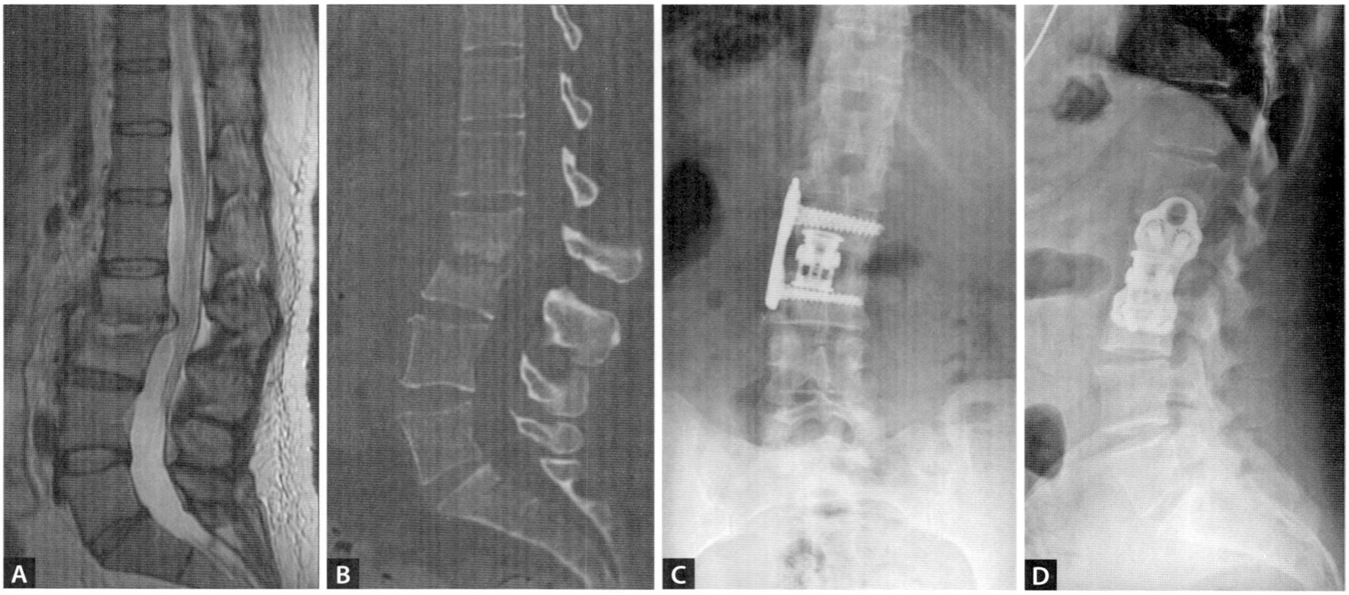

Figs. 4A to D: (A) Sagittal MRI and (B) CT of the patient in Figure 1. Despite the kyphosis, the infection was largely contained in the disk space, allowing preservation of significant bone of the L2 and L3 vertebral bodies, which permitted a stand-alone anterior reconstruction; (C) Anteroposterior; (D) Lateral radiographs obtained 9 months postoperatively.

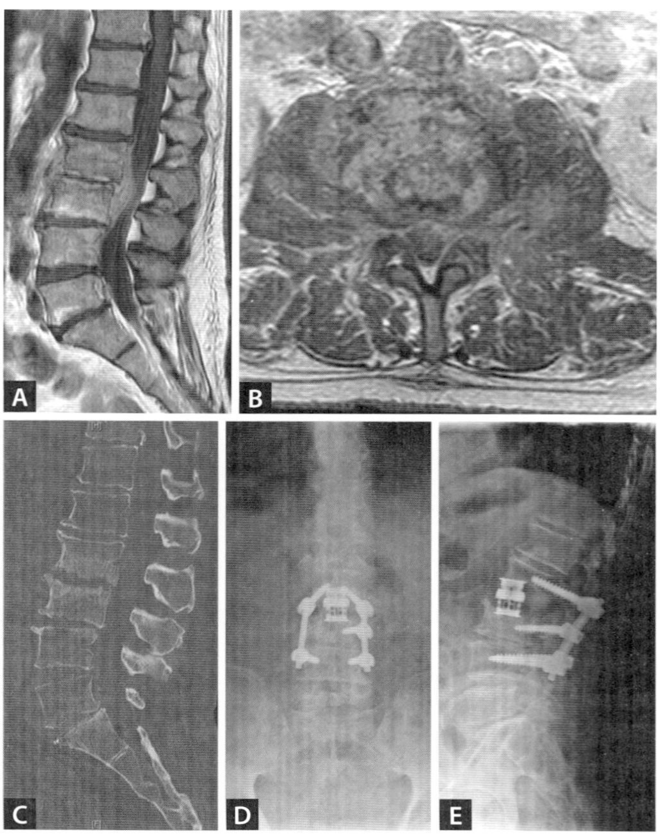

Figs. 5A to E: (A) Sagittal and; (B) Axial T1-weighted postcontrast MRI of a 52-year-old man presenting with 2 months of back pain and 2 months of worsening leg pain and difficulty ambulating, demonstrating discitis-osteomyelitis with a large epidural abscess and; (C) Sagittal CT suggests significant involvement of the L3 vertebral body; (D and E) The patient underwent combined anterior-posterior decompression and reconstruction.

support following anterior debridement. All appear safe and effective, so long as the debridement is complete.[30-33] While tricortical iliac autograft has traditionally been considered the gold standard for strut graft, its use has decreased significantly in favor of cortical bone ring allograft. These grafts have demonstrated excellent rates of fusion and elimination of infection, and eliminate the morbidity associated with autograft donor harvest sites.[32-34] In fact, it has been demonstrated that allograft incorporates at a rate comparable with autograft for spinal osteomyelitis when combined with appropriate medical management.[35] Despite concerns about development of a glycocalyx on spinal implants, which allows bacteria to be more adherent to instrumentation, several studies have found that placement of instrumentation is safe in the setting of infection.[32,33,36,37]

There has been interest in the use of recombinant human bone morphogenetic protein-2 (rhBMP-2) in the spinal infection patient population. Aside from its obvious primary use of increasing the speed and frequency of fusion, its inherent inflammatory properties led to the theory that it could help eradicate the infection locally. While its use is quite controversial, it has been demonstrated that rhBMP-2 in combination with antibiotic therapy as well as a circumferential fusion, can be performed safely and effectively in treatment for the medically nonresponsive patient.[38,39] Importantly, this is an off-label application of rhBMP-2 and it is not FDA approved for use in this setting.

Infection Recurrence

Recurrence of infection may occur after successful initial treatment of spinal infections in 2–8% of patients. Ensuring that the primary source of the infection and its cause are eradicated can minimize the recurrence rate. Modifying medical conditions and behaviors that increase the patient's risk can also reduce recurrence rates. Examples of such interventions include tight control of blood glucose in the diabetic patient, improving nutritional status, and drug and alcohol counseling. As mentioned previously, the time from symptom onset to initiation of antibiotic therapy has been shown to affect recurrence rate of infection. When treatment is delayed for 6–7 weeks after onset of symptoms, antibiotic treatment of only 4–8 weeks is associated with an increased recurrence rate as compared to treatment of 12 weeks and over.[14] Evidence of recurrence would be return of pain or an increase in ESR and CRP. Importantly, while serial radiographic examination is a necessity during treatment, it is performed to detect bony collapse or deformity, not to monitor for recurrence of infection.

Spinal Abscess

Spinal abscesses can be extradural, intradural, or intramedullary and are often the result of untreated or unsuccessfully treated infections. Fortunately, intradural and intramedullary abscesses are rare, with only 100 cases of the latter being reported since the lesion's original description in 1830.[40] Epidural spinal abscesses are the most commonly occurring in this group and have been reported to be present in 2% of spinal infections.[41] If the epidural abscess results from direct seeding of bacteria into the epidural space, it is known as a primary epidural abscess. Extension of infection from the disk space or adjacent bone is much more common and is defined as a secondary epidural abscess.[1,42,43]

On presentation, patients with epidural abscesses are generally more systemically ill than the osteodiscitis patient. The abscesses most commonly cover 3–4 spinal segments and are dorsal to the thecal sac approximately 75% of the time. Symptoms usually evolve from localized pain to radicular pain. If untreated, it is often followed by paresis and plegia. Generally, treatment of these lesions is surgical decompression followed by antibiotic therapy.[44]

Consideration could be given to medical management alone if the patient has had a complete neurological deficit for over 72 hours, is a poor surgical candidate, has no neurological deficit, or has significant multiregional spinal canal involvement.[45] With an epidural abscess, the surgical approach depends on the location of the lesion. A posterior laminectomy can be performed if there is no associated vertebral body abscess. A combined anterior/posterior approach may be required if the lesion is anterior in the thoracic spine or if the abscess is secondary to vertebral osteomyelitis or discitis.[46]

GRANULOMATOUS SPINAL INFECTION

The first description of the natural history of tubercular spondylitis was given by Percival Potts in 1779, and Pott's disease remains the classic example of granulomatous spinal infection.[47] This type of infection occurs when the immune system attempts to wall off substances using macrophages that it perceives as foreign but is unable to eliminate with inflammatory cells such as neutrophils and eosinophils. Granulomatous spondylitis has numerous etiologies and in the developing world and in patients who are immunocompromised. Mycobacteria, fungi, and spirochetes are common pathogens. It is usually the result of hematogenous spread from established foci of disease either in the pulmonary or genitourinary system. It can also be the result of direct extension from a visceral lesion as well as from lymphatic or venous routes.

Granulomatous spinal infections have several key differences from their pyogenic counterparts. Granulomatous pathologic changes usually take longer to develop since there is less of an inflammatory reaction. In addition, the disks are relatively resistant to the infection and may in fact be preserved despite extensive bone loss. Granulomatous spinal infections are more commonly associated with large paraspinal abscesses and frequently result in greater spinal deformity. Treatment consists of prolonged medical treatment of the source of infection. Surgery is often required to correct deformity. Other reasons to perform surgery are similar to those of pyogenic spinal infections such as neurological deficit and instability.

PARASITIC SPINAL INFECTION

Although fairly rare in industrialized nations, a large percentage of the world's population has some form of parasitic infection. Those parasites that invade the nervous system have high morbidity and mortality. Two examples of parasite infections that can involve the spine are schistosomiasis and echinococcosis.

A schistosome is a small flat worm called a fluke that is carried in approximately one in 30 people globally. Humans acquire the fluke by contact with freshwater containing its larvae, which penetrate the skin and migrate into the blood vessels. The parasite uses the patient's blood vessels to travel throughout the body, where they can live for up to 30 years. While they most commonly cause abdominal problems, the fluke can migrate to the spinal cord resulting in myelopathy and paralysis, which is often permanent. Praziquantel is the treatment of choice, but steroids are often given if the patient has spinal cord involvement in an effort to decrease the inflammatory response.[48,49]

Echinococcus is a tapeworm that is common in Africa, Central Asia, southern South America, the Mediterranean, and the Middle East. Infection can result in cyst formation that normally occurs in the liver and lungs. These cysts can, however, develop in the spinal cord resulting in cord compression and paralysis. Treatment consists of albendazole or praziquantel as well as possible surgical removal of the cyst, if accessible.[50,51]

CONCLUSION

Spinal infection remains an important cause of morbidity and mortality. While currently available diagnostic tests and imaging combined with modern antibiotics give the physician powerful tools to improve patient outcome, new challenges such as a growing immunocompromised population and an increasing number of antibiotic-resistant organisms will continue to confront the medical practitioner. Early diagnosis and initiation of culture-specific antibiotic therapy is important in minimizing the adverse sequelae associated with spinal infections, most of which will not require surgical intervention. In those cases that do, current surgical strategies are effective for rapidly decompressing neurological tissue, relieving severe pain, improving deformity, and stabilizing the spine.

REFERENCES

1. Hadjipavlou AG, Mader JT, Necessary JT, et al. Hematogenous pyogenic spinal infections and their surgical management. Spine (Phila Pa 1976). 2000;25(13):1668-79.
2. Akiyama T, Chikuda H, Yasunaga H, et al. Incidence and risk factors for mortality of vertebral osteomyelitis: a retrospective analysis using the Japanese diagnosis procedure combination database. BMJ open. 2013;3(3).
3. Tay BK, Deckey J, Hu SS. Spinal infections. J Am Acad Orthop Surg. 2002;10(3):188-97.
4. Krogsgaard MR, Wagn P, Bengtsson J. Epidemiology of acute vertebral osteomyelitis in Denmark: 137 cases in Denmark 1978-1982, compared to cases reported to the National Patient Register 1991-1993. Acta Orthop Scand. 1998;69(5):513-7.
5. Weinstein MA, Eismont FJ. Infections of the spine in patients with human immunodeficiency virus. J Bone Joint Surg Am. 2005;87(3):604-9.
6. Eismont FJ, Bohlman HH, Soni PL, et al. Pyogenic and fungal vertebral osteomyelitis with paralysis. J Bone Joint Surg Am. 1983;65(1):19-29.
7. Cheung WY, Luk KD. Pyogenic spondylitis. Int Orthop. 2012;36(2):397-404.
8. Batson OV. The vertebral system of veins as a means for cancer dissemination. Prog Clin Cancer. 1967;3:1-18.
9. Frisbie JH, Gore RL, Strymish JM, et al. Vertebral osteomyelitis in paraplegia: incidence, risk factors, clinical picture. J Spinal Cord Med. 2000;23(1):15-22.
10. Hadjipavlou AG, Korovessis PG, Kakavelakis KN. Spine Infections:Medical versus Surgical Treatment Options. In:

Vaccaro AR, Eck JC (Eds). Controversies in Spine Surgery. New York: Thieme; 2010.

11. Jaramillo-de la Torre JJ, Bohinski RJ, Kuntz C 4th. Vertebral osteomyelitis. Neurosurg Clin N Am. 2006;17(3):339-51, vii.
12. Butler JS, Shelly MJ, Timlin M, et al. Nontuberculous pyogenic spinal infection in adults: a 12-year experience from a tertiary referral center. Spine (Phila Pa 1976). 2006;31(23):2695-700.
13. Bettini N, Girardo M, Dema E, et al. Evaluation of conservative treatment of non specific spondylodiscitis. Eur Spine J. 2009;18 Suppl 1:143-50.
14. Grados F, Lescure FX, Senneville E, et al. Suggestions for managing pyogenic (non-tuberculous) discitis in adults. Joint Bone Spine. 2007;74(2):133-9.
15. Modic MT, Feiglin DH, Piraino DW, et al. Vertebral osteomyelitis: assessment using MR. Radiology. 1985;157(1):157-66.
16. An HS, Seldomridge JA. Spinal infections: diagnostic tests and imaging studies. Clin Orthop Relat Res. 2006;444:27-33.
17. Dunbar JA, Sandoe JA, Rao AS, et al. The MRI appearances of early vertebral osteomyelitis and discitis. Clin Radiol. 2010;65(12):974-81.
18. Kowalski TJ, Layton KF, Berbari EF, et al. Follow-up MR imaging in patients with pyogenic spine infections: lack of correlation with clinical features. Am J Neuroradiol. 2007;28(4):693-9.
19. Zarrouk V, Feydy A, Salles F, et al. Imaging does not predict the clinical outcome of bacterial vertebral osteomyelitis. Rheumatology (Oxford). 2007;46(2):292-5.
20. Kornblum MB, Wesolowski DP, Fischgrund JS, et al. Computed tomography-guided biopsy of the spine. A review of 103 patients. Spine (Phila Pa 1976). 1998;23(1):81-5.
21. Conaughty JM, Chen J, Martinez OV, et al. Efficacy of linezolid versus vancomycin in the treatment of methicillin-resistant Staphylococcus aureus discitis: a controlled animal model. Spine (Phila Pa 1976). 2006;31(22):E830-2.
22. Walters R, Rahmat R, Fraser R, et al. Preventing and treating discitis: cephazolin penetration in ovine lumbar intervertebral disc. Eur Spine J. 2006;15(9):1397-403.
23. Kuklo TR, Potter BK, Bell RS, et al. Single-stage treatment of pyogenic spinal infection with titanium mesh cages. J Spinal Disord Tech. 2006;19(5):376-82.
24. Ruf M, Stoltze D, Merk HR, et al. Treatment of vertebral osteomyelitis by radical debridement and stabilization using titanium mesh cages. Spine (Phila Pa 1976). 2007;32(9):E275-80.
25. Emery SE, Chan DP, Woodward HR. Treatment of hematogenous pyogenic vertebral osteomyelitis with anterior debridement and primary bone grafting. Spine (Phila Pa 1976).1989;14(3):284-91.
26. Collert S. Osteomylelitis of the spine. Acta orthopaedica Scandinavica. 1977;48:283-90.
27. Krodel A, Kruger A, Lohscheidt K, et al. Anterior debridement, fusion, and extrafocal stabilization in the treatment of osteomyelitis of the spine. J Spinal Disord. 1999;12(1):17-26.
28. Hee HT, Majd ME, Holt RT, et al. Better treatment of vertebral osteomyelitis using posterior stabilization and titanium mesh cages. J Spinal Disord Tech. 2002;15(2):149-56; discussion 56.
29. Fukuta S, Miyamoto K, Masuda T, et al. Two-stage (posterior and anterior) surgical treatment using posterior spinal instrumentation for pyogenic and tuberculotic spondylitis. Spine (Phila Pa 1976). 2003;28:E302-8.
30. Dimar JR, Carreon LY, Glassman SD, et al. Treatment of pyogenic vertebral osteomyelitis with anterior debridement and fusion followed by delayed posterior spinal fusion. Spine (Phila Pa 1976). 2004;29(3):326-32; discussion 32.
31. McGuire RA, Eismont FJ. The fate of autogenous bone graft in surgically treated pyogenic vertebral osteomyelitis. J Spinal Disord. 1994;7:206-15.
32. Nakase H, Tamaki R, Matsuda R, et al. Delayed reconstruction by titanium mesh-bone graft composite in pyogenic spinal infection: a long-term follow-up study. J Spinal Disord Tech. 2006;19(1):48-54.
33. Fayazi AH, Ludwig SC, Dabbah M, et al. Preliminary results of staged anterior debridement and reconstruction using titanium mesh cages in the treatment of thoracolumbar vertebral osteomyelitis. Spine J. 2004;4(4):388-95.
34. Swanson AN, Pappou IP, Cammisa FP, et al. Chronic infections of the spine: surgical indications and treatments. Clin Orthop Relat Res. 2006;444:100-6.
35. Schuster JM, Avellino AM, Mann FA, et al. Use of structural allografts in spinal osteomyelitis: a review of 47 cases. J Neurosurg. 2000;93(1 Suppl):8-14.
36. Korovessis P, Petsinis G, Koureas G, et al. One-stage combined surgery with mesh cages for treatment of septic spondylitis. Clin Orthop Relat Res.2006;444:51-9.
37. Robertson PA, Rawlinson HJ, Hadlow AT. Radiologic stability of titanium mesh cages for anterior spinal reconstruction following thoracolumbar corpectomy. J Spinal Disord Tech. 2004;17(1):44-52.
38. Chen X, Kidder LS, Lew WD. Osteogenic protein-1 induced bone formation in an infected segmental defect in the rat femur. J Orthop Res. 2002;20(1):142-50.
39. Chen X, Schmidt AH, Tsukayama DT, et al. Recombinant human osteogenic protein-1 induces bone formation in a chronically infected, internally stabilized segmental defect in the rat femur. J Bone Joint Surg Am. 2006;88(7):1510-23.
40. Hart J. Case of Encysted Abscess in the Centre of the Spinal Cord. Dublin Hosp Rep. 1830;5:522-4.
41. Calderone RR, Thomas JC Jr., Haye W, et al. Outcome assessment in spinal infections. Orthop Clin North Am. 1996;27(1):201-5.
42. Khan SH, Hussain MS, Griebel RW, et al. Title comparison of primary and secondary spinal epidural abscesses: a retrospective analysis of 29 cases. Surg Neurol. 2003;59(1):28-33; discussion 33.
43. Kuker W, Mull M, Mayfrank L, et al. Epidural spinal infection. Variability of clinical and magnetic resonance imaging findings. Spine (Phila Pa 1976). 1997;22(5):544-50; discussion 51.
44. Karikari IO, Powers CJ, Reynolds RM, et al. Management of a spontaneous spinal epidural abscess: a single-center 10-year experience. Neurosurgery. 2009;65(5):919-23; discussion 23-4.

45. Sorensen P. Spinal epidural abscesses: conservative treatment for selected subgroups of patients. Br J Neurosurg. 2003;17(6):513-8.
46. Lohr M, Reithmeier T, Ernestus RI, et al. Spinal epidural abscess: prognostic factors and comparison of different surgical treatment strategies. Acta Neurochir (Wien). 2005;147(2):159-66; discussion 166.
47. Pott P. Remarks on that kind of palsy of the lower limbs with is frequently found to accompany a curvature of the spine. London: Printed for J. Johnson; 1779.
48. Ferrari TC. Involvement of central nervous system in the schistosomiasis. Mem Inst Oswaldo Cruz. 2004;99(5 Suppl 1):59-62.
49. Arnon R. Life span of parasite in schistosomiasis patients. Isr J Med Sci. 1990;26(7):404-5.
50. Bahloul K, Ghorbel M, Boudouara MZ, et al. Primary vertebral echinococcosis: four cases reports and review of literature. Br J Neurosurg. 2006;20(5):320-3.
51. Keutgens A, Simoni P, Detrembleur N, et al. Fatal alveolar echinococcosis of the lumbar spine. J Clin Microbiol. 2013;51(2):688-91.

CHAPTER 9 Intradural Spinal Tumors

Yonatan G Keschner, Daniel Lubelski, Gregory R Trost, Edward C Benzel

INTRODUCTION

Intradural spinal tumors are uncommon lesions, representing about 10–15% of neoplasms affecting the central nervous systems.[1] They are classified as either intramedullary or intradural extramedullary based on their relationship to the dura mater and spinal cord parenchyma. Whereas intramedullary tumors are located within the spinal cord parenchyma, intradural extramedullary tumors are located outside the parenchyma.[2] The majority of these tumors are benign low-grade lesions. Intramedullary spinal cord tumors are the less common subtype, accounting for only 5–10% of spinal tumors,[3,4] whereas intradural extramedullary tumors are more common, accounting for 30–40% of all spinal tumors.[3] The remaining 55–60% of spinal tumors are extradural.[2,3] Generally, intramedullary tumors are more common in children and extramedullary tumors are more common in adults.[4] The most frequently encountered intramedullary tumors are ependymomas, astrocytomas, and hemangioblastomas, whereas the most frequently encountered intradural extramedullary tumors are meningiomas, nerve sheath tumors, and paragangliomas. Accurate identification of the specific tumor through clinical symptoms and signs, laboratory findings, and imaging, enable optimal management. Advancements in microsurgical techniques and intraoperative neurophysiological monitoring have revolutionized spinal surgery for such tumors and have improved patient outcomes and survival. In this chapter, the epidemiology, workup, and treatment of the most common intradural tumors is reviewed.

INTRAMEDULLARY TUMORS

Ependymoma

Epidemiology and Natural History

Ependymomas include a range of glial tumors that all share a common origin of ependymal cells that line both the ventricles as well as the spinal central canal.[5] They account for 60% of intramedullary tumors in adults, as opposed to only 12% of intramedullary tumors in children.[2,6,7] Ependymomas tend to occur more commonly in males than females,[3,8] and have a peak incidence in the fourth and fifth decades[6] with a median age of 35 years. The long-term outcomes of low-grade spinal ependymomas following surgical resection tend to be favorable, with 5-year survival rates between 83% and 100%.[2]

Ependymoma refers to a variety of tumor types and are typically categorized by their World Health Organization (WHO) grade: Subependymoma (WHO Grade I), myxopapillary ependymoma (WHO Grade I), benign or "classic" ependymoma (WHO Grade II), and anaplastic ependymoma (WHO Grade III).[8]

Subependymomas are slow growing, benign neoplasms with a good prognosis. They account for about 8% of the ependymal tumors of the spinal cord[9] and are most commonly found in the cervical and cervicothoracic regions.[10] Males are more commonly affected than females.[10]

Myxopapillary ependymomas are almost always benign and associated with a good short-term prognosis. They, however, often recur. They account for nearly 30% of intradural ependymomas,[11] and present in the filum terminale and conus medullaris.[3,4] They are relatively uncommon in pediatric patients with a peak incidence in the fourth decade, and predominantly found in males.[12]

Benign ependymomas are the most common ependymal subtype.[7,13] Their peak incidence is in the fourth decade, with a slight male predominance.[7] They are most commonly found in the cervical spine and are associated with a good prognosis after surgical treatment.[7]

Anaplastic ependymomas are much less common, accounting for only 7% of all ependymal subtypes.[14] They are believed to arise from a malignant transformation of lower grade tumors. They are invasive, poorly differentiated, and generally run a more rapid clinical course, with a substantially worse 10-year survival rate than the other ependymal subtypes.[15] Ependymomas rarely metastasize outside the central nervous system.[16] Patients with neurofibromatosis type II (NF-2) are predisposed to the development of ependymomas and other intradural neoplasms because of a mutation of a tumor suppressor gene located on chromosome 22.[17]

Workup

Symptoms and signs: The diagnosis of intramedullary ependymomas can be delayed by several years due to indolent tumor growth and variable clinical features that may only present in the later stages of the disease.[3,18] Symptoms usually present gradually and are often nonspecific. The majority of patients present with back pain, usually localized at the level of the tumor.[18] Patients may also present with sensory changes, motor deficits, and weakness in specific regions determined by the location of the tumor. Tumors found in the cervical spine may present with upper extremity symptoms, such as atrophy of the upper extremity musculature.[7,18] Tumors found in the thoracic spine may cause spasticity and sensory changes in the lower extremities such as numbness and temperature insensitivity.[18] Tumors found in the lumbar spine often present with leg pain and gait ataxia. Myxopapillary ependymomas, which are most frequently found in the filum terminale and conus medullaris, usually present with local back, leg, or sacral pain. Bladder and sphincter dysfunction may also occur.[3,8,18] Motor impairment and weakness usually occurs late in the disease progression as the surrounding spinal cord is thinned by the growing tumor. These symptoms may present asymmetrically.[19] Malignant lesions and astrocytomas usually cause a more rapid onset of clinical symptoms than benign ependymomas.[19] However, a sudden development of symptoms may occur by hemorrhage of a benign neoplasm.[7]

Laboratory findings/pathology: Ependymomas are classified as five histological subtypes—cellular, myxopapillary, papillary, epithelial, or tancytcic.[11] Mixed cell types are also seen.[4,5] The typical gross appearance of ependymomas is a soft gray to reddish tan color tumor, with a well-circumscribed cleavage plane.[4] Calcifications are rarely observed.[3] Histologically, these tumors usually appear benign. However, the rare anaplastic variant demonstrates clear evidence of malignancy with poorly differentiated cells, increased cellularity, and increased mitotic activity. Cellular ependymomas are the most common subtype. They appear highly cellular, composed of mainly cuboidal and low columnar cells.[11] Perivascular pseudorosettes are a hallmark feature of ependymomas, displayed by clear tumor cells aligning themselves around blood vessels. This helps distinguish them from intramedullary astrocytomas.[4,11] The myxopapillary ependymoma subtype is found almost exclusively in the conus medullaris and filum terminale.[5] They are composed of elongated ependymal cells with spindle-shaped nuclei, and may be found surrounding a blood vessel in a mucoid microcystic matrix.[20] While cystic formation and hemorrhagic regions along the tumor margins can be found in most subtypes, they are most frequently encountered with myxopapillary ependymomas.[3,11] Papillary subtypes are rarely encountered and appear histologically similar to choroid plexus papillomas.[11] The epithelial subtype is characterized by cells arranged in either a linear or glandular formation. In contrast with the perivascular pseudorosettes found in the cellular subtype, epithelial ependymomas usually contain true ependymal rosettes.[11] Tanycytic ependymomas have a similar appearance to astrocytomas, and may contain only subtle perivascular pseudorosettes.[11,21] They contain highly fibrillary and elongated cells.[11]

Imaging: Intramedullary ependymomas commonly present on MRI as focal enlargements of the cervical and upper thoracic regions of the spinal cord. They are well-circumscribed masses that usually contain a well-defined cleavage plain. The majority are located symmetrically in the center of the spinal cord.[5] Ependymomas usually present with uniform contrast enhancement. They are commonly hypointense or isointense on T1-weighted images and hyperintense on T2-weighted images.[3] Polar cysts are commonly found in the cervical and thoracic spinal cord regions.[4] Marked heterogeneous enhancement from intratumoral cysts or hemorrhage can also be seen, whereas calcification is rare. Delineation of intratumoral cysts is more readily seen with gadolinium enhancement.[8] Syrinx formation is a characteristic finding of ependymomas. This is most commonly found in the cervical region, which distinguishes ependymomas from other types of spinal cord tumors.[5] Myxopapillary ependymomas contain unique characteristics, compared to nonmyxopapillary ependymomas and are almost exclusively found in the conus medullaris and filum terminale.[11] They vary in size and may be identified by local bone changes including scalloping of the vertebral bodies and enlargement of the neural foramina. They present as a hyperintense mass on T2-weighted images. However, they may present as hyper-isointense on T1-weighted images with heterogeneous enhancement due to hemorrhagic or cystic formations.[3,8] This contrasts with nonmyxopapillary ependymoma subtypes that usually appear hypointense or isointense on T1-weighted images.[11]

Treatment

Spinal cord ependymomas are slow growing lesions that are best treated with meticulous microsurgical techniques.[22] The goal of surgery is gross total resection and preservation of neurological function.[22,23] They are usually well-circumscribed and are easy to distinguish from the surrounding spinal cord, making them amenable to complete removal.[11] In the majority of cases, gross total resection is sufficient in achieving disease free long-term survival.[14,23,24] It is important to obtain a tissue diagnosis during early phases of the operation in order to determine the nature and grade of the lesion. In the rare case in which the intraoperative tissue biopsy shows a malignant tumor, surgical treatment should be restricted to debulking, since there is little surgical benefit for malignant intramedullary neoplasms.[23] Preoperative neurological status is one of the best predictors of postoperative functional outcomes.[22,23] Therefore, early removal of spinal cord ependymomas often optimizes the chance for preservation of neurological function, though will rarely restore lost function.[20,23] Treatment should not be delayed until development of significant and progressive clinical symptomatology or enlargement of the tumor.[20,23-26]

A dorsal approach is recommended for complete resection. The interface can be visualized through a myelotomy that extends from the rostral to the caudal extent of the tumor.[23] Spinal ependymomas usually appear reddish-gray with a glistening surface, which facilitates the demarcation from the surrounding spinal cord tissue.[4,23] The cleavage plane guides the removal of the tumor from the surrounding spinal cord.[4,27] Larger tumors may require internal decompression with an ultrasonic aspirator.[4,23] The tumor margins are then developed and feeding-arteries are easily identified and cauterized.[4] Detaching the tumor from its ventral cord, where it is supplied by the anterior spinal artery is usually the riskiest part of the procedure.[27] Although, the majority of ependymomas are clearly demarcated from healthy spinal cord tissue, the imperceptible blending with spinal cord tissue is not uncommon. Surgical removal of such indiscernible lesions can be difficult and dangerous.[7,23] Surgical removal of ependymomas poses significant potential risk of postoperative neurological worsening including motor weakness, sensory loss, and loss of autonomic function.[24] Some patients may experience sensory loss in the early period following surgery, which usually resolves within 3 months.[23]

Tumor resection may be performed with intraoperative spinal cord monitoring.[24,26] A change in either motor evoked potentials (MEPs) or somatosensory evoked potentials (SSEPs) signals suggest that the surgery should be suspended for several minutes. If the signal returns to baseline and it is determined that the change in signal was caused by hypotension, anesthesia or temperature changes, surgery may continue while closely monitoring changes in MEPs and SSEPs. However, if after several minutes the MEPs or SSEPs signals do not improve or are lost, one might consider aborting the surgical procedure and accept a subtotal resection.[24,26] Alternatively, a return to surgery as a second stage may be considered in a week or more.

In cases where only a subtotal resection is performed, patients may benefit from postoperative radiation therapy. But in cases of total resection, it is not recommended to treat patients with radiation therapy since the recurrence rate in such patients is very low and because of the negative health risks associated with radiation.[23,24,28,29] The extent of surgical resection is a significant predictor of recurrence-free survival. Gross total resection provides the best long-term survival and preservation of neurological function when compared to subtotal resection and radiation therapy.[14,20,23]

Astrocytoma

Epidemiology and Natural History

Intramedullary spinal cord astrocytomas represent 6–8% of spinal cord tumors.[30] They are the most common pediatric intramedullary spinal cord tumors,[4] comprising 90% of intramedullary tumors in children less than 10 years of age and 60% of adolescent intramedullary tumors.[4,31] These tumors occur equally in males and females and have an average age of presentation of 30 years.[3] The majority of astrocytomas are found in the cervical and thoracic spinal regions.[3,4,8] Pediatric astrocytomas are usually benign, and are most commonly classified as either pilocytic astrocytoma (WHO Grade I) or diffuse (well-differentiated fibrillary) astrocytoma (WHO Grade II). Pilocytic astrocytomas are rare neoplasms and can also be found in young adult patients. Diffuse astrocytomas are the most commonly encountered intramedullary astrocytoma subtype[32] found in both pediatric and adult patients.[4,8,30] Both subtypes are slow-growing neoplasms that usually present with an indolent natural history.[4,34] They are generally associated with long-term survival but are often accompanied by a significant degree of neurological dysfunction because of their infiltrative nature.[31] The preoperative functional scale is the most important prognostic factor in determining the outcome in low-grade astrocytomas.[30] Therefore, patients with less severe or fewer symptoms who are treated early will have the best prognosis. Low-grade astrocytomas have a median survival of about 15 years, with a 70–100% survival at 5 years[2,30] and 50% survival at 10 years.[30] High-grade astrocytomas, such as anaplastic astrocytoma (WHO Grade III) and glioblastoma (WHO Grade IV), account for 10% of intramedullary spinal astrocytomas.[4,30] Glioblastoma is typically seen in only 1.5% of all spinal cord astrocytomas.[3] These tumors are characterized by a rapidly progressing clinical course and poor survival.[9,30] They tend to be associated with severe neurological dysfunction at the time of presentation,[30] and are associated with a high incidence of cerebrospinal fluid tumor dissemination, which can lead to syringomyelia.[4,30] High-grade intramedullary astrocytomas are associated with a median survival of 6–15 months.[2,30] Patients' neurological status and survival is generally unchanged after operation.[30]

Workup

Symptoms and signs: Low-grade spinal astrocytomas present with an indolent course that evolves over a period of months to years before a diagnosis is made.[33] High-grade astrocytomas have a mean duration of symptoms of 6 weeks prior to presentation and significant disability develops on average of 3–5 months[33] after symptom onset. Symptoms are generally nonspecific, most commonly including localized or radiating pain and sensory changes, with motor weakness, gait disturbance, spasticity, and bowel and bladder sphincter dysfunction evolving in the later stages.[3,33] Weakness typically presents in the upper extremities prior to the lower extremities as these tumors most commonly present in the cervical spine.[33] Pediatric patients often present with nonspecific generalized symptoms, in which pain is often the initial complaint, though they may also present later with gait deterioration, motor weakness, torticollis, and kyphoscoliosis.[33] In patients with malignant tumors, pain is followed by a rapid progression of clinical symptoms leading to significant disability.[35] Most patients with high-grade lesions are unable to walk at the time of presentation.[30]

Laboratory findings/pathology: Pathologically, spinal cord astrocytomas are categorized as either low-grade or high-grade tumors. The margins of both low- and high-grade astrocytomas are poorly defined and diffuse.[2] Astrocytomas may progress over several spinal cord segments and can produce a fusiform enlargement of the spinal cord. Many cases develop benign fluid-filled syrinxes, and tumor cysts may be seen in 30% of astrocytomas. Calcification of the tumor is rare.[3] Low-grade tumors include pilocytic (Grade I) and well-differentiated fibrillary astrocytoma or diffuse astrocytoma (Grade II). Grossly, their core appears gray and may resemble normal parenchyma.[36] Microscopically, they are characterized by a diffuse infiltrate of cells that resembles fibrillary cells. They show a low degree of cellularity and mitotic activity, and an absence of necrosis and endothelial microvascular proliferation. Rosenthal fibers and granular eosinophilic bodies may be indicative of a pilocytic astrocytoma.[2] High-grade neoplasms, such as the anaplastic astrocytoma (grade III) and glioblastoma (grade IV), are a lot rarer than the lower-grade neoplasms. Grossly, their core is gray and often surrounded by a reddish cast due to hypercellularity and vascularity.[36] Microscopically, higher-grade astrocytomas have increased cellularity, mitotic activity, and microvascular proliferation. Glioblastomas are destructive and leave very little parenchyma intact in the tumor's core. Necrosis is commonly found.[2]

Imaging: Astrocytomas present as focal enlargements with fusiform expansions, usually in the cervical or thoracic spinal cord. They are not well-circumscribed and have irregular tumor margins. Cystic components, syrinx, and associated edema may also be found.[3] Astrocytomas are usually asymmetrical and located off-center in the spinal cord. They typically affect 1–4 segments of the cord. However, larger, multisegmental tumors can occur, especially with pilocytic astrocytomas.[3,8] Astrocytomas appear hypointense or isointense on T1-weighted images and hyperintense on T2-weighted images. Contrast administration will cause variable enhancement, from uniform to patchy, to no enhancement at all. High-grade astrocytomas tend to contain patchy enhancements with heterogeneous components due to intratumoral cysts or necrosis.[4] Differentiating between tumor cysts and syrinxes is critical. Tumor cysts are generally surrounded by enhancement, while the lining of a syrinx does not show contrast uptake. Delineation of tumor margins from edema, cysts, and syrinxes is facilitated by gadolinium enhanced MRI imaging.[3]

Treatment

Surgery is the primary treatment modality for spinal astrocytomas. The goal of surgery is to obtain a tissue diagnosis of the lesion and to improve neurologic function.[37] Astrocytomas are generally infiltrative and do not have a clear plane of demarcation from normal spinal cord. Thus, it is important for the surgeon to consider the benefit of total or subtotal resection against the risk of neurologic impairment and other morbidity.[37,38] Subtotal resection may be used to reduce the tumor mass in preparation for adjuvant therapy.[33] Fibrillary/diffuse astrocytomas are most common in adults and are usually infiltrating tumors. Their gross appearance is often indistinguishable from the surrounding spinal cord. Hence, total removal is generally not possible. Neurologic deficit and morbidity may occur, even with careful gross total removal of the tumor mass since healthy axons are often trapped within the tumor.[33,38] Pilocytic astrocytomas are commonly found in children and are less infiltrative than the fibrillary subtype. They may displace rather than infiltrate the spinal cord. Thus, pilocytic astrocytomas may be distinguishable from healthy spinal cord tissue and be completely resected without neurological deterioration.[37] If a tissue sample obtained during surgery returns as a high-grade, surgical intervention is usually curtailed. This is due to the highly infiltrative and aggressive nature of malignant astrocytomas for which surgical debulking provides limited benefit.[37,38] In cases of inoperable tumors, radiotherapy may be the best course of treatment.[2,39] Surgical strategy for both infiltrative and noninfiltrative astrocytomas is radical resection of the lesion to the utmost extent while avoiding neurologic impairment and morbidity. This is somewhat facilitated via intraoperative neurophysiological monitoring with SSEPs and MEPs. Intraoperative SSEPs and MEPs are used to guide the surgeon during removal of the lesion by monitoring the functional integrity of the spinal tracts. A deterioration of evoked potentials can be used to help guide the extent of tumor resection. If the evoked potentials remain present during surgical resection, the surgery may continue and resection may be possible.[4,37,39] Ideal surgical candidates are those with either little or no neurological symptoms and in whom independence may be maintained by forestalling the development of severe motor deficits. Surgery may still be beneficial for cases where patients have significant neurological deficits as long as sphincter control or the ability to reposition in bed is maintained.[33] Preoperative clinical status is the best predictor of postoperative outcome.[33,37] Low-grade tumors have a recurrence rate of approximately 25%, whereas high-grade astrocytomas have a much higher recurrence rate at nearly 100%.[2] The postoperative survival of patients with low-grade astrocytomas is generally much greater than patients with high-grade astrocytomas (5-year survival rate of 70–100% versus 6–15 months).[2,30,39]

Hemangioblastoma

Epidemiology and Natural History

Hemangioblastomas are benign (WHO Grade I) tumors of vascular origin that are well-circumscribed but not encapsulated.[4,8] These tumors account for only 1–5% of all spinal cord tumors[40] and 3–8% of all intramedullary tumors.[4] The peak incidence is in the fourth decade[8,41] and the median age at presentation is 35 years.[3] They are predominately found in males.[41] The tumor most frequently affects the thoracic spinal cord but may also develop in the cervical spine.[41] Development of hemangioblastomas in the lower spinal region, such as the cauda equina, conus medullaris, and filum terminale, is uncommon.[40] The majority of hemangioblastomas (60–75%)[40,42] are of intramedullary origin, found specifically in a dorsal or dorsolateral location with subpial attachments.[4,8,40,41] The tumor is usually fed and drained by either the anterior or posterior spinal artery and vein.[40,42] Hemangioblastomas may occur either sporadically or as a result of von Hippel-Lindau (VHL) syndrome. Approximately, 75% of hemangioblastomas are sporadic and the remaining cases are related to VHL syndrome.[43] Patients with VHL syndrome tend to be symptomatic at an earlier age.[4,44] In one series, the average age at presentation was 1–2 decades earlier in patients with VHL syndrome.[43] Also, patients with VHL usually present with multiple tumors, while sporadic hemangioblastomas are usually solitary.[4,44] Patients who undergo uneventful complete removal of the tumor are expected to have good functional outcomes with a significant reduction in morbidity and mortality.[40,41]

Workup

Symptoms and signs: Patients with spinal hemangioblastomas generally complain of pain, weakness, and sensory changes such as impairment of proprioception associated with the typically dorsal spinal cord location of the tumor.[41,42] The tumor's indolent growth pattern causes a slow clinical progression, with a mean duration of 30 months between initial symptoms and admission to the hospital.[41] Isolated cases of catastrophic intramedullary hemorrhage causing radiculopathy and acute paraplegia have been reported,[44] but this is not common. Clinical symptoms in cases with small tumors are thought to be caused by the associated syrinx and not by the tumor itself. However, clinical symptoms in larger tumors are caused by both the syrinx and the tumor mass.[42] There is no difference in clinical symptoms in sporadic versus VHL hemangioblastomas.[42]

Laboratory findings/pathology: Hemangioblastomas are benign, slow growing neoplasms (WHO Grade I). Grossly, they appear highly vascular, fed by small arteries and drained by large prominent veins.[3] These tumors are usually expansive, showing a well-defined border with the spinal cord. The cut surfaces may be bright yellow or bloody. Microscopically, they consist of endothelial cells and large pale stromal cells. The endothelial cells are not atypical as in other spinal tumors and form masses, cords, and thin-walled blood vessels.[45] Stromal cells are usually found between the endothelial cells and have abundant cytoplasm filled with lipid vacuoles and hemosiderin.[45] Hemangioblastomas commonly have cysts lined by fibrillary cells or syrinxes.[45]

Imaging: Hemangioblastomas present as a focal spinal cord mass. Small hemangioblastomas (10 mm or less) appear isointense on T1-weighted images and hyperintense on T2-weighted images. These tumors generally demonstrate intense homogeneous contrast enhancement.[41] Small hemangioblastomas are usually located superficially on the dorsal surface of the spinal cord.[41] Larger hemangioblastomas (10 mm or more) appear hypo- or isointense on T1-weighted images and heterogeneous on T2-weighted images. These tumors generally demonstrate heterogeneous contrast enhancement.[8,41] Vascular flow voids may be seen on noncontrast images caused by the distension and dilation of feeding-arteries and draining veins.[4,42] Syrinx and edema may be present due to venous congestion or arteriovenous shunting. Peritumoral edema results in a low signal on T1-weighted images and a high signal on T2-weighted images. Symptomatic small hemangioblastomas may have relatively large associated syrinxes, whereas asymptomatic ones do not.[41] Gadolinium enhancement is helpful in delineating the nidus of the tumor from the surrounding edema and cysts.[3,46]

Treatment

Gross total resection is the optimal treatment of spinal cord hemangioblastomas. Complete surgical removal is associated with improved functional outcomes and is even indicated for asymptomatic lesions.[41,47] Hemangioblastomas generally have a sharp plane of demarcation with the spinal cord allowing the tumor to be removed in a single piece by following visualization of the tumor margin. Most spinal hemangioblastomas are located dorsally in the spinal cord and may be removed by a dorsal approach, with circumferential dissection of the tumor-pial interface.[4,41,48] A dorsal or dorsolateral approach is also recommended for visualization and resection of lateral tumors.[48] A lesion located in the ventral aspect of the spinal cord may be accessed via a corpectomy. This method provides a more direct route for the removal of the tumor while lowering the risk of perilesional spinal cord injury.[48] Exposure and closure are, however, significantly compromised by this approach. A longitudinal myelotomy is recommended for large tumors in order to gain better access and visualization of the tumor.[4] When vascular flow voids are present in a large spinal tumor on preoperative MRI, angiography is recommended prior to treatment to further evaluate the relationship of the tumor feeding-arteries.[8,41] Excessive intraoperative bleeding interferes with tumor resection and can result in incomplete tumor removal.[41] Therefore, preoperative embolization is very important as it can minimize blood loss during surgery and facilitate the view of the operative bed.[4,41] Although syrinxes are commonly associated with tumors of all sizes, they do not correlate with a positive or negative postoperative outcome.[48] Total removal of the tumor is often associated with syrinx resolution, without the need for additional drainage or for a shunt procedure.[42] Radical excision of spinal hemangioblastomas can be achieved with low morbidity and mortality.[42] Complete removal of the tumor is strongly associated with improved functional outcomes, whereas incomplete removal of the tumor may result in significant morbidity and mortality.[41]

INTRADURAL EXTRAMEDULLARY TUMORS

Meningioma

Epidemiology and Natural History

Spinal meningiomas represent approximately 25% of all primary spinal cord tumors.[49] The majority (greater than 95%) of spinal meningiomas are slow growing benign tumors, corresponding to WHO grade I.[8] They are associated with low rates of recurrence, morbidity and mortality after surgical treatment, and have a good functional outcome.[50] The peak incidence for meningiomas is in the fifth and sixth decades.[8,50] Meningiomas in younger patients are of a different histological subtype and are typically associated with a more aggressive clinical course and a worse prognosis.[8,50] Meningiomas are significantly more common in females than males, with 75–90% of cases affecting females.[4,8,49] Spinal meningiomas originate from arachnoidal cap cells adjacent to the dura near the nerve root sleeve. Less commonly, these tumors may arise from fibroblasts in the dural or pial layers.[4] Approximately, 80% of spinal meningiomas occur in the thoracic spine, 15% in the cervical spine, and 5% in the lumbosacral spine.[3,8] Thoracic meningiomas are usually located dorsolaterally, but are located ventrally in the cervical region.[8] The majority of spinal meningiomas are solitary tumors, with only 1–2% of patients having multiple lesions.[4,8,51] Multiples meningiomas are most often associated with patients who have NF-2.[8,51]

Workup

Symptoms and signs: Meningiomas are slow progressing tumors that are associated with a wide variety of non-specific symptoms. Back pain is the most common initiating symptom found in approximately 50% of patients.[49] Patients may also experience progressive radicular pain, motor weakness, gait instability, and sensory changes.[49] Bladder and bowel dysfunction are less commonly observed in these patients.[3] In advanced stages, tumor growth may lead to the Brown-Séquard syndrome.[49,50] Patients with arachnoid scarring from recurrent tumors tend to present with more severe sensory disturbances, dysesthesia, and pain than those with primary meningiomas.[52]

Laboratory findings/pathology: Meningiomas are tumors that are composed of arachnoid cells. Nearly all meningiomas are solid, well-circumscribed smooth round tumors that grow along the dura mater.[8,49] They are commonly attached to nerve roots, spinal cord, and dura mater.[49] Grossly, the cut surfaces vary from grayish-pink to tan and frequently have calcifications. Microscopically, several histological subtypes exist, including meningothelial, psammomatous, transitional, angiomatous, and fibrous.[3,50] The majority of spinal meningiomas are either meningothelial (29–59%) or psammomatous (21–57%),[50] which histologically exhibit features of whorls and psammoma bodies.[53] The psammomatous subtype is associated with a less favorable neurological outcome postoperatively than the other histological subtypes.[49] This is due to the fact that psammomatous meningiomas are the least cellular of all the subtypes, and the blood vessels and spinal cord roots are more adherent to this histological subtype.[49]

Imaging: Spinal meningiomas are seen on MRI as well-circumscribed tumors with broad dural attachments, usually found in the dorsolateral thoracic region.[3] They tend to be iso- to hypointense on T1-weighted images and slightly hyperintense on T2-weighted images. Except in the calcified areas, meningiomas demonstrate homogenous enhancement after gadolinium administration.[3,8] A distinguishing feature of meningiomas is marginal dural thickening, known as the "dural tail" sign[54] (Fig. 1).

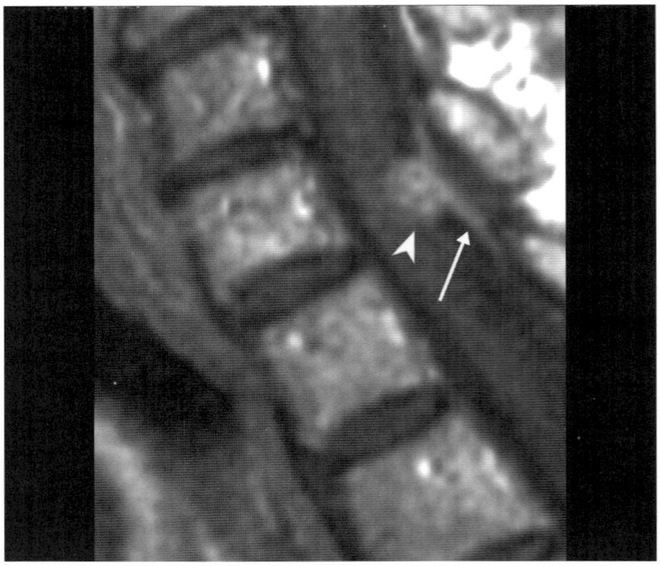

Fig. 1: Meningioma: Sagittal T1-weighted MRI of the upper thoracic spine demonstrating a spinal meningioma (arrowhead) with the associated dural tail (arrow).
Source: Reproduced from Wallace EW. The dural tail sign. Radiology. 2004;233(1):56-7.

Treatment

Complete resection of a spinal cord meningioma is the best modality of treatment for long-term success.[52,55,56] Gross total removal can be achieved in the majority of cases mainly because these tumors tend not to invade the spinal cord or the adjacent bone. Even patients with high-grade preoperative neurological deficits can achieve favorable outcomes.[52] During surgery, it is important to minimize displacement of the spinal cord by undertaking an appropriately wide exposure in order to properly resect the entire tumor.[55,57] Ultrasonography may be used to provide a detailed map of the tumor's location in order to avoid an unnecessarily large dural opening.[57] A variety of strategies can be utilized for removal of spinal meningiomas depending on its location. Dorsal or dorsolateral tumors are best approached through a posterior laminectomy in order to provide adequate exposure and prevent spinal instability.[4,55] In cases in which the tumor is located ventrally or ventrolaterally, a laminectomy or hemilaminectomy at one or two levels with a facetectomy may be sufficient to provide exposure and prevent spinal cord displacement.[55,57] Ventral tumors should be debulked before dissection and the plane between the tumor and the spinal cord should be well exposed before removal.[55] For ventral thoracic tumors, a costotransversectomy or a lateral extracavitary approach may be utilized.[4] In the majority of patients, it is possible to safely resect even large tumors by using a dorsal or dorsolateral laminectomy approach. This approach may even be satisfactory for large ventral meningiomas.[4,55] The operative procedure for tumors with calcifications is more complex because adhesions to the spinal cord must be considered in the surgical strategy. A partial vertebrectomy or costotransversectomy approach is appropriate in patients with calcified ventral or ventrolateral tumors. In rare cases of heavily calcified meningiomas with a ventral or ventrolateral location where internal tumor debulking is not possible, it may be safer to perform a partial or complete vertebrectomy for tumor resection.[55,58] This fortunately is rarely necessary.

En plaque and infiltrative meningiomas are rare subtypes of meningiomas. They are a surgical challenge because they are not associated with a clear tissue demarcation from healthy spinal cord tissue and have a more extensive tumor matrix. En plaque tumors may also invade surrounding tissue structures such as nearby bone, and occasionally show ossifications.[52,57] Like the more common encapsulated meningiomas, the long-term outcome of patients with en plaque or infiltrative meningiomas is related to the extent of resection.[52] While the vast majority of encapsulated tumors can be completely resected, only about half of en plaque tumors can be totally removed.[57]

Total resection of recurrent meningiomas with arachnoid scarring can also be challenging due to the adhesions that can cause spinal cord tethering. The adhesions may make it difficult to distinguish between scar, meningioma, and spinal cord.[52,57] In addition to the complications from tethering, scarring also can cause progressive neurological symptoms from interference with spinal cord blood flow and obstruction of cerebrospinal fluid flow.[52] Surgery for arachnoid scarring is problematic because each attempt at resection can cause more scar to form. Accordingly, it is important to limit arachnoid dissection as much as possible, with the scar tissue dissected sharply and with meticulous hemostasis. Placing a dural graft may provide protection against postoperative retethering and cerebrospinal fluid flow obstruction or leak.[52,57]

Neurophysiological monitoring of both MEPs and SSEPs should be performed in order to guide the surgeon in resecting only neoplastic tissue, while preserving healthy spinal cord tissue. Careful monitoring reduces the likelihood of postoperative neurological deficits.[55,57] Although the most favorable treatment for meningiomas is total resection, adjunctive radiotherapy may be beneficial in cases of subtotal resection and recurrent meningiomas.[55,57,58] Patients with severe preoperative neurological deficits may experience full neurologic recovery after a complete resection.[52,57] Some patients may experience transient neurological worsening after surgery, which usually resolves within 6 months.[52] Tumor recurrence rates are low in Grade I meningiomas, ranging from 0% to 14.7%.[50,55-57] Significantly higher recurrence rates were found in young patients, subtotal resection, en plaque, and infiltrative tumors.[57] One study found that there is a 20% recurrence rate in patients with spinal meningiomas younger than age 21 years.[50]

Schwannoma

Epidemiology and Natural History

Schwannomas, also known as neurilemomas, neurinomas, or neuromas, are derived from neoplastic Schwann cells that arise from dorsal nerve roots in the cervical or lumbar spine. They rarely occur in the thoracic region. Schwannomas are considered benign tumors and are classified as WHO Grade I.[8] They are associated with a favorable prognosis and a life expectancy that is comparable to the general population.[59,60] They are the most common intradural extramedullary spinal tumor, compromising approximately 65% of intradural nerve sheath tumors.[61] They occur in men and women equally[3,4,59] and with a peak incidence between the fourth and sixth decades.[3,4,59] Schwannomas most commonly present as solitary tumors, however, multiple lesions can occur in patients with NF-2.[3,8] Although schwannomas occur most often in adults, they may present in children with NF-2.[8] Schwannomas secondary to NF-2 are associated with a less favorable prognosis and outcome because of their higher recurrence rates and rate of neurological deficits, as well as their greater risk for malignant transformation.[8,60,62] Malignant nerve sheath tumors (MNST), which include malignant schwannomas, are rare, constituting only 0.8–6% of nerve sheath tumors.[60,61] They are associated with a poor prognosis.[60] The survival rate of MNST is variable, with a 5-year survival rate of 10–47%.[60]

Workup

Symptoms and signs: The main presenting symptom in patients with schwannomas is local or radicular pain.[60,61] Motor symptoms, including progressive limb weakness and stiffness, are the second most common presenting signs, followed by sensory changes.[61] Neurological symptoms are caused by their frequent location on the nerve roots. Many patients may only be symptomatic upon palpation of the mass.[60] Schwannomas associated with NF-2 tend to present sooner with more severe neurological deficits. This is due to their faster and more infiltrative growth pattern on nerve roots.[62] Slow growing benign schwannomas have a mean duration of symptoms prior to diagnosis of approximately 30 months.[60,61] However, for faster growing MNST, the mean duration of symptoms prior to diagnosis is approximately 8 months.[60]

Laboratory findings/pathology: Schwannomas are composed of schwann cells associated with fibrous material.[3] They typically arise from a single nerve fascicle and develop asymmetrically. Unlike neurofibromas that encase nerve roots, schwannomas do not contain nerve fibers running through them but rather displace the nerve root.[3] Grossly they appear tan to yellow colored and are well-circumscribed, without significant vascularity. Cellular schwannomas are a benign histological subtype. They are characterized by hypercellularity, moderate mitotic activity, and moderate nuclear atypia. Despite their appearance of a more aggressive tumor, they behave in a benign fashion and carry the same prognosis as the other benign schwannomas.[60] On the other hand, MNST are associated with a poor prognosis. They are characterized by high cellularity with spindle-shaped or polygonal cells, nuclear pleomorphism, and high mitotic activity. MNST also substantially infiltrate surrounding tissue.[60]

Imaging: Spinal schwannomas present with well-defined tumor margins on MRI. Solitary tumors are usually located in the dorsal sensory roots of the cervical or lumbar regions of the spinal cord. Multiple tumors may be present in cases of NF-2. The tumor's growth pattern usually displaces the spinal cord to the contralateral side. This distinguishes them from neurofibromas, which typically encase the nerve.[3] On T1-weighted images, schwannomas appear isointense, and on T2-weighted images they appear markedly hyperintense. Hyperintense signaling on T1-weighted imaging corresponds to hemorrhage. A large schwannoma may protrude out of the neural foramina and

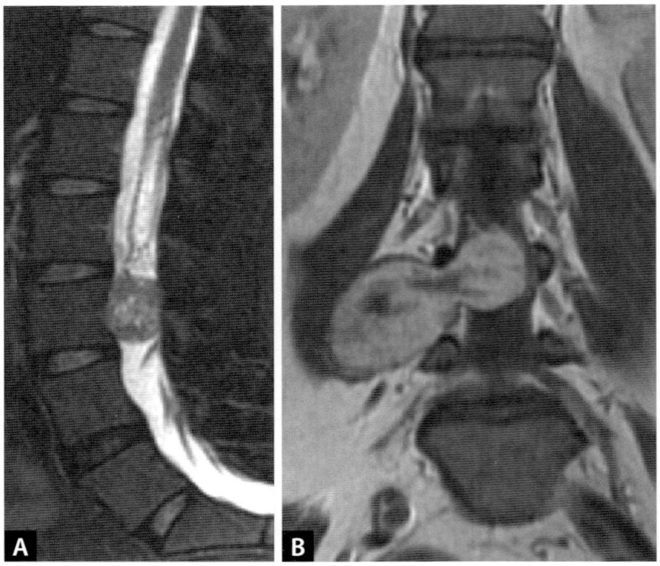

Figs. 2A and B: Schwannoma: (A) Sagittal T2-weighted MR image showing hyperintense intradural extramedullary tumor at the L3–L4 level; (B) Axial T1-weighted MR image showing a dumbbell-shaped mass.[8]

form a dumbbell-shaped mass (Figs. 2A and B). Malignant tumors tend to be associated with irregular margins, compared to benign tumors. However, heterogeneity can be observed in both benign and malignant tumors. This results in a heterogeneous MRI signal resulting from cystic and necrotic regions. Calcification is uncommon in schwannomas. It is possible to differentiate schwannomas from meningiomas by identifying either cystic changes, lack of dural enhancement, or increased peripheral enhancement[3,8,63] that is found in schwannomas.

Treatment

The treatment goal in patients with spinal schwannomas is gross total resection.[64] The majority (90%) of benign schwannomas in patients without NF-2 are amenable to complete resection.[62] The surgical approach depends on the location and anatomy of the lesion. Typically, small and strictly intradural lesions can be removed entirely via laminectomy.[4,62,65,66] Tumor decompression may be required before dissecting and removing large tumors.[62] With large tumors, a more extensive dorsolateral bony removal may be required, followed by spinal stabilization and fusion to avoid instability.[64,66] Ventrally located tumors may require transthoracic or lateral approaches.[4,66] Such approaches should be rarely required if one employs appropriate surgical trajectories and meticulous surgical dissection strategies. After the tumor is exposed, a plane of dissection must be identified on the tumor's surface. Dissection of the tumor requires identification and division of the proximal and distal nerve root tumor attachments.[4] Separating the involved fascicle from the rest of the nerve root can minimize the risk of neurological deterioration.[4,59,64] For tumors arising from the dorsal root, it may be possible to preserve the ventral root by dissecting it off the ventral surface of the tumor.[4] A schwannoma with a dumbbell extension through the nerve root sleeve will usually require a total nerve root resection.[4] In many cases the spinal roots giving rise to schwannomas are nonfunctional at the time of surgery, and therefore, there is little risk of causing further neurological harm by resecting these roots.[64] However, if a total removal will endanger the integrity of vital neural structures, a less radical resection may be considered, since schwannomas are generally slow growing tumors with low recurrence rates.[62,67] In order to minimize and prevent neurological complications, tumor resection may be performed with intraoperative spinal cord monitoring using both SSEPs and MEPs.[26] Direct stimulation of an exposed nerve root can assist the surgeon in differentiating functional roots from nonfunctional roots, thereby reducing postoperative morbidity.[64]

Patients with sporadic schwannomas who have total tumor resection generally remain disease free, with a low risk of recurrence. They do not have a decreased life expectancy compared with the general population. However, patients who have subtotal removal, especially those with NF-2, have a worse prognosis since there is a high incidence of new tumor formation with additional morbidity.[62] Good surgical outcomes are associated with young age, no postoperative spinal cord tethering, first tumor resection operation, and patients without NF-2.[62] Patients without NF-2 and with subtotal removal have an overall recurrence rate of 10% after 5 years.[62,64] However, NF-2 patients have an overall recurrence rate of 40% after 5 years.[62] Thus, it is important to schedule routine clinical and radiological follow-up examinations for patients with subtotal resections or who have NF-2.[62,64]

Radiotherapy is not indicated for benign lesions, but may be beneficial in cases of subtotal resection. MNST carry a very poor prognosis, even after surgery and radiotherapy. Therefore, it is important to consider whether surgery and radiation are appropriate for these patients.[60] The severity of preoperative symptoms is predictive of post-treatment recovery.[59] Patients with preoperative autonomic deficits do not recover significantly, and may still have remaining bladder and bowel deficits. Therefore, it is recommended to intervene early with surgical treatment in order to prevent increased morbidity and autonomic dysfunction in patients.[62,64,67]

Neurofibroma

Epidemiology and Natural History

Neurofibromas are rare, benign nerve sheath tumors that are WHO Grade I.[8] They compromise 3% of all primary spinal tumors,[67] and account for approximately 15–26% of spinal nerve sheath tumors.[61,68] They occur primarily in the ventral nerve roots, and typically surround or engulf the nerve root, in contrast to schwannomas, which commonly displace the nerve root. They are composed of Schwann cells, fibroblasts, and perineurial-like cells embedded in a collagenous matrix.[8] Neurofibromas are commonly solitary tumors, except in patients with neurofibromatosis type I (NF-1). Although most neurofibromas are entirely intradural and extramedullary, about 10–15% are considered both intradural and extradural. This is due to the dumbbell-like growth that extends through the dural nerve root sleeve. Fewer than 1% of neurofibromas are considered intramedullary. These are believed to have arisen from the perivascular nerve sheaths that accompany penetrating spinal cord vessels. Plexiform neurofibromas, commonly found in patients with NF-1, contain subpial extensions and are thus classified as both intramedullary and extramedullary. They are usually associated with proximal nerves.[4] Neurofibromas are distributed relatively evenly throughout the spinal cord. Both men and women are equally affected with the peak incidence occurring between the fourth and sixth decades.[3] Although neurofibromas are commonly benign, plexiform neurofibromas may progress to MNST. MNST usually carry a poor prognosis and are particularly common in patients with NF-1. A better prognosis can be achieved if the tumors are diagnosed at an early stage.[69]

Workup

Symptoms and signs: Patients may present with radicular pain since the majority of neurofibromas originate in spinal roots. Motor deficiency, paresthesia, and numbness may also be seen due to nerve root compression. Patients with sacral lesions most often complain of localized pain in the lower back. Due to the slow indolent growth of benign neurofibromas, neurologic symptoms may be delayed for several years.[3,70,71]

Laboratory findings/pathology: Neurofibromas are composed of Schwann cells, fibroblasts, and pericytes. Grossly they may appear tan to white with an apparent glistening cut surface. Neurofibromas grow as either well-demarcated intraneural tumors or diffusely infiltrate soft tissue at extraneural sites with functioning nerve fascicles traversing through the body of the tumor. In contrast to schwannomas, neurofibromas are more elongated and lobulated masses, that are well-circumscribed but not encapsulated.[72] The architectural growth pattern may be localized, diffuse or plexiform. Microscopically, neurofibroma cells appear twisted or curvilinear spindle-shaped with elongated nuclei present in a myxoid stromal background. Scattered mast cells, lymphocytes, pericytes, and fibroblasts may also be present, with spotted S100-positive pseudomeissnerian corpuscles. Most neurofibromas occur sporadically, although approximately 10% are associated with NF-1. Plexiform neurofibromas are usually diagnostic of NF-1 and are characterized by the intertwining involvement of multiple nerve trunks.[72]

Imaging: Spinal neurofibromas tend to be relatively small and scattered, usually encasing rather than displacing the nerve roots. They are typically rounded or fusiform tumors that are isointense on T1-weighted images and markedly hyperintense on T2-weighted images. Tumor enhancement varies from intense and homogeneous in some lesions to only peripheral enhancement in others. However, after injection of gadolinium, intense homogeneous enhancement is seen. A "target sign" appearance may be present on T2-weighted images, with a centrally decreased signal (Fig. 3). This is usually diagnostic of a benign neurofibroma. Malignant lesions tend to have more irregular margins when compared to benign lesions. Multiple plexiform neurofibromas are often seen in patients with NF-1.[3,8,73]

Treatment

The treatment goal in patients with neurofibromas is gross total resection using careful microsurgical techniques and intraoperative electrophysiologic monitoring when deemed appropriate.[74,75] Neurofibromas are more

CHAPTER 9

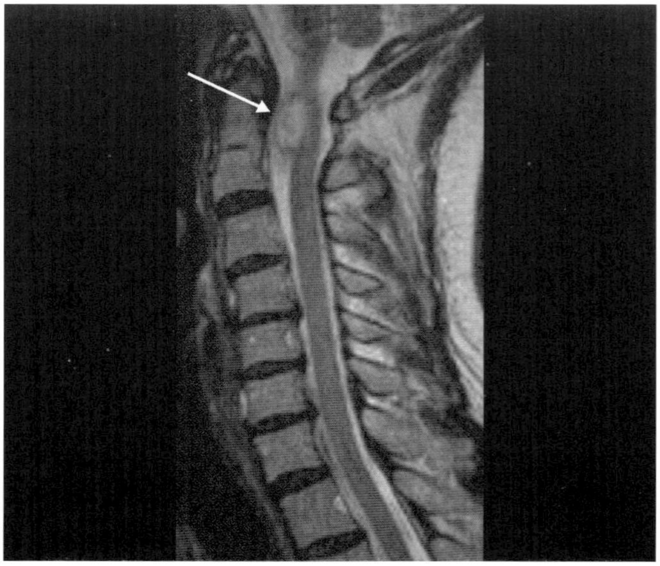

Fig. 3: Nerve sheath tumor: Sagittal T2-weighted MR image demonstrating an intradural extramedullary mass anterolateral to the cervical spinal cord (arrow). The mass demonstrates the familiar "target" sign appearance with central signal intensity that is characteristic of nerve sheath tumors.
Source: Beall DP, Googe DJ, Emery RL, et al. Extramedullary intradural spinal tumors: a pictorial review. Curr Probl Diagn Radiol. 2007;36(5):185-98.

difficult to treat and resect than schwannomas because of the presence of nerve fibers intermingled in the tumor parenchyma.[76] Gross findings will usually show fascicles entering and exiting the tumor at its poles. However, the majority of these nerve fascicles do not yield a nerve action potential and are safe to excise.[68,74,75] It is suggested that the denervation pattern is a result of complete damage to the involved nerve, and that the function of that root is replaced by adjacent segments.[76] Sectioning of the nerve root during the procedure only leads to a neurological deficit in a small fraction of cases.[67,68] In some cases, functioning nerve fascicles are displaced peripherally onto the surface of the tumor or splayed circumferentially around the center of the mass. By using microsurgical techniques, these fascicles may be preserved by dissecting them away from the tumor in the extracapsular plane.[68,74]

Excision of intradural neurofibromas is usually possible via a standard posterior laminectomy approach, since the majority of these tumors are situated dorsally.[4,68] Ventrally located tumors may require transthoracic or lateral approaches. A midline durotomy should be performed to expose the intradural portion of the tumor.[77] After the tumor is exposed, a plane of dissection must be identified on the tumor's surface.[4] Benign nerve sheath tumors are usually well encapsulated.[68,74] The capsule of the tumor should be incised and the mass debulked using an ultrasonic aspirator to allow visualization of the nerve roots entering from the spinal cord.[4,77] Excising the nerve roots is usually necessary for the complete removal of the tumor and rarely leads to a loss of neurological function postoperatively.[74] Intraoperative neurophysiologic monitoring using SSEPs and MEPs can discern functioning nerve fascicles from nonfunctioning nerve fascicles, and may assist in preventing neurologic injury during tumor resection.[78]

Although patients with a solitary neurofibroma usually achieve good outcomes postoperatively with minimal morbidity, plexiform neurofibromas are more difficult to treat and are a significant cause of morbidity and mortality in patients with NF-1.[79] The complexity and limitation in treating plexiform neurofibromas is due to their infiltrative nature, large size, extensive paraspinal spread, and high rate of recurrence.[74,77,79] They do not have a capsule and usually involve multiple adjacent spinal levels leading to myelopathy or multisegmental radiculopathy. Also, because the function of the involved nerve roots is often partially preserved and critical extraspinal structures are generally involved, these lesions are rarely amenable to complete resection without substantial morbidity.[74,77] However, the resection of plexiform neurofibromas can be achieved with acceptable results by utilizing skilled microsurgical techniques and intraoperative neurophysiological monitoring in order to preserve uninvolved rootlets. This should minimize neurologic morbidity and re-establish or maintain neurological function. The treatment must also take into account the systemic nature of NF-1 in order to ensure positive long-term functional outcomes.[77] Preoperative electromyography (EMG) may be useful in predicting the outcome of surgery. If the EMG shows absence of denervation then the risk of postoperative dysfunction is usually low.[76]

Patients with a solitary spinal neurofibromas generally carry an excellent prognosis after complete surgical removal.[62] The recurrence rate is estimated to be 12% and complete relief of pain is expected in over 85% of patients.[67,75] Functional improvements may take several months after surgery to allow neighboring roots that were compressed by the tumor to heal.[67] While functional risk

SECTION 1

of resection is greater in patients with NF-1 disease, tumor removal is still warranted because of the severity of presenting symptoms and the 15% risk of malignant degeneration. Patients that develop malignant tumor degeneration may benefit from high dose radiation.[74] It has been noted that patients treated for plexiform neurofibromas are at a high risk for developing progressive kyphotic spinal deformity after receiving a standard laminectomy procedure. This often necessitates postoperative spinal fusion. However, anatomic reapproximation of the dorsal elements and soft tissues seems to diminish the incidence of postoperative kyphosis.[77]

Paraganglioma

Epidemiology and Natural History

Spinal paragangliomas are rare, slow growing tumors derived from paraganglion cells of neural crest origin. They are typically nonfunctional sympathetic nervous system tumors that are found in the lumbar spine region as well as the conus medullaris, cauda equina or filum terminale.[2,80] In rare cases, they may be functional and secrete catecholamines. They occur most commonly in adults, with only rare cases in children. There is a slight male predominance and the mean age at presentation is in the fourth to fifth decade.[2] These tumors are typically benign (WHO Grade I) but some may be more aggressive and give rise to metastatic spread.[3,8,80-82]

Workup

Symptoms and signs: Patients typically present with clinical signs and symptoms similar to those associated with myxopapillary ependymomas. Symptoms include lower lumbar pain, sensory or motor loss to lower extremities, and bowel and bladder dysfunction. Patients may also complain of pain and discomfort associated with recumbency.[81]

Laboratory findings/pathology: Paragangliomas are solid, highly vascularized growths with thin fibrous capsules. They are well demarcated from adjacent nerve roots with no dural attachments. Grossly they appear reddish-gray due to vascularization.[2] Cystic components may be found.[81] The primary histological feature of paragangliomas is their "zellballen" pattern, which is made up of nests of small, round to polyhedral, cuboidal or columnar cells separated by a fine vascular network. This hallmark feature helps to differentiate from a histologically similar tumor, myxopapillary ependymomas, which have perivascular pseudorosettes.[2,80,83] The predominant cell-type of paragangliomas is the chief cell, which has a characteristic round to oval nucleus containing spotted chromatin. Cellular atypia is rare. Positive immunohistochemical staining for synaptophysin and chromogranin A are specific for diagnosis of a paraganglioma, whereas a negative stain for glial fibrillary acidic protein excludes an ependymoma. Sustentacular cells reactive for S-100 stains are commonly observed with small oval nuclei.[2,80,82]

Imaging: MR imaging of paragangliomas is generally nonspecific, but can typically help narrow the differential diagnosis. The tumor is hypointense to isointense on T1-weighted images and hyperintense on T2-weighted images with hypointense margins due to being well encapsulated. Occasionally, serpiginous flow voids can be seen on T2-weighted images caused by compression of the tumor vessels by the mass or by other adjacent blood vessels; visualization of this characteristic image can be diagnostic for paragangliomas (Figs. 4A to C). The heterogeneous "salt and pepper" appearance produced by gadolinium contrast on T2-weighted images is also characteristic of paragangliomas.[2,8,80-82,84,85]

Treatment

Gross total resection is the best modality of treatment for benign spinal paragangliomas. Although paragangliomas are most commonly nonfunctional secreting tumors, it is important to screen preoperatively for a catecholamine-secreting tumor in order to prevent a hypertensive crisis during excision of the tumor.[2] Surgical treatment is usually curative, with a recurrence rate of less than 5% after total or subtotal removal. Adjuvant radiotherapy does not affect the recurrence rate and is therefore not recommended.[2] The severity of preoperative symptoms is predictive of post-treatment recovery.[82]

CONCLUSION

Intradural spinal cord tumors comprise 10–15% of all central nervous system tumors.[1] These tumors are categorized by location as either intramedullary or intradural extramedullary, and account for 5–10% and 30–40% of all spinal tumors respectively.[3,4] Intramedullary tumors include the ependymomas, astrocytomas, and hemangioblastomas, whereas the intradural

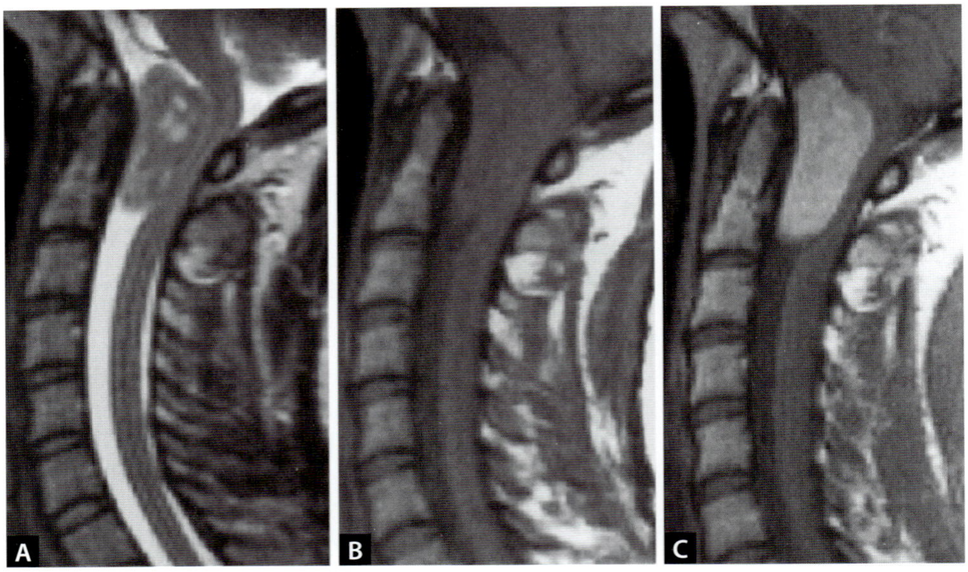

Figs. 4A to C: Paraganglioma: (A) Sagittal T2-weighted MR image showing a well-circumscribed heterogeneous intradural extramedullary tumor in the upper cervical spine; (B) T1-weighted isointense MRI, and (C) T1-weighted MRI showing an intense homogeneous display after injection of gadolinium. The tumor demonstrates flow-voids that are characteristic of hemorrhage and intratumoral vessels in paragangliomas.[80]

extramedullary tumors include the meningiomas, nerve sheath tumors, and paragangliomas; all of these tumors are usually amenable to surgical resection. These tumors typically present with a wide array of nonspecific symptoms and clinical features that includes pain, motor disturbance, sensory loss, and less commonly sphincter disturbance. MRI is the best imaging technique in the evaluation of spinal cord tumors. The tumors' location and relationship to the spinal cord is the most important feature in establishing a diagnosis. A histological workup should be done to confirm the tumor type and grade, which will then guide the treatment plan and prognosis. Tumor type and grade, as well as preoperative functional status, are the common predictors of postoperative outcomes. Improvements in diagnostic capabilities and advancements in microsurgical techniques have created better treatment plans that have led to a minimization of postoperative morbidity and mortality for patients with intradural spinal cord tumors.

REFERENCES

1. Rhines LD, Groves MD. Tumors of the Brain and Spine. New York: Springer US; 2007. pp. 295-328.
2. Traul DE, Shaffrey ME, Schiff D. Part I: Spinal-cord neoplasms—intradural neoplasms. Lancet Oncol. 2007;8(1):35-45.
3. Van Goethem, JWM, van den Hauwe L, Özsarlak Ö, De Schepper AM, , Parizel P. Spinal tumors. Eur J Radiol. 2004;50(2):159-76.
4. Parsa AT, Lee J, Parney IF, et al. Spinal cord and intradural-extraparenchymal spinal tumors: current best care practices and strategies. J Neurooncol. 2004;69(1-3):291-318.
5. Sun B, Wang C, Wang J. MRI features of intramedullary spinal cord ependymomas. J Neuroimaging. 2003;13(4):346-51.
6. Yoshii S, Shimizu K, Ido K, et al. Ependymoma of the spinal cord and the cauda equina region. J Spinal Disord. 1999;12(2):157-61.
7. McCormick PC, Torres R, Post KD, et al. Intramedullary ependymoma of the spinal cord. J. Neurosurg. 1990; 72(4): 523-32.
8. Abul-Kasim K, Thurnher MM, McKeever P, et al. Intradural spinal tumors: current classification and MRI features. Neuroradiology. 2008;50 (4):301-14.
9. Jallo GI, Zagzag D, Epstein F. Intramedullary subependymoma of the spinal cord. Neurosurgery. 1996;38(2):251-7.
10. Dario A, Fachinetti P, Cerati M, et al. Subependymoma of the spinal cord: case report and review of the literature. J Clin Neurosci. 2001;8(1):48-50.
11. Kahan H, Sklar EM, Post MJ, et al. MR characteristics of histopathologic subtypes of spinal ependymoma. Am J Neuroradiol. 1996;17(1):143-50.
12. Celli P, Cervoni L, Cantore G. Ependymoma of the filum terminale: treatment and prognostic factors in a series of 28 cases. Acta Neurochir (Wien). 1993;124(2-4):99-103.
13. Chamberlain MC, Tredway TL. Adult primary intradural spinal cord tumors: a review. Curr Neurol Neurosci Rep. 2011; 11(3):320-8.

14. Waldron JN, Laperriere NJ, Jaakkimainen L, et al. Spinal cord ependymomas: a retrospective analysis of 59 cases. Int J Radiat Oncol Biol Phys. 1993;27(2):223-9.
15. Tominaga T, Kayama T, Kumabe T, et al. Anaplastic ependymomas: clinical features and tumour suppressor gene p53 analysis. Acta Neurochir (Wien). 1995;135(3-4):163-70.
16. Newton HB, Henson J, Walker RW. Extraneural metastases in ependymoma. J Neurooncol. 1992;14(2):135-42.
17. Ueki K, Sasaki T, Ishida T, et al. Spinal tanycytic ependymoma associated with neurofibromatosis type 2—case report. Neurol Med Chir (Tokyo), 2001;41(10):513-6.
18. Schwartz TH, McCormick PC. Intramedullary ependymomas: clinical presentation, surgical treatment strategies and prognosis. J Neurooncol. 2000;47(3):211-8.
19. Epstein FJ, Farmer JP, Freed D. Adult intramedullary spinal cord ependymomas: the result of surgery in 38 patients. J Neurosurg. 1993;79(2):204-9.
20. Boström A, von Lehe M, Hartmann W, et al. Surgery for spinal cord ependymomas: outcome and prognostic factors. Neurosurgery. 2011;68(2):302-8; discussion 309.
21. Goh KY, Velasquez L, Epstein FJ. Pediatric intramedullary spinal cord tumors: is surgery alone enough? Pediatr Neurosurg. 1997;27:34-9.
22. Joaquim AF, Santos MJ, Tedeschi H. Surgical management of intramedullary spinal ependymomas. Arq Neuropsiquiatr. 2009;67(2A):284-9.
23. Lee J, Parsa AT, Ames CP, et al. Clinical management of intramedullary spinal ependymomas in adults. Neurosurg Clin N Am. 2006;17(1):21-7.
24. Manzano G, Green BA, Vanni S, et al. Contemporary management of adult intramedullary spinal tumors-pathology and neurological outcomes related to surgical resection. Spinal Cord. 2008;46(8):540-6.
25. Eroes CA, Zausinger S, Kreth F-W, et al. Intramedullary low grade astrocytoma and ependymoma. Surgical results and predicting factors for clinical outcome. Acta Neurochir (Wien). 2010;152(4):611-8.
26. Matsuyama Y, Sakai Y, Katayama Y, et al. Surgical results of intramedullary spinal cord tumor with spinal cord monitoring to guide extent of resection. J Neurosurg Spine. 2009;10(5):404-13.
27. Sala F, Palandri G, Basso E, et al. Motor evoked potential monitoring improves outcome after surgery for intramedullary spinal cord tumors: a historical control study. Neurosurgery. 2006;58(6):1129-43; discussion 1129-43.
28. Linstadt DE, Wara WM, Leibel SA, et al. Postoperative radiotherapy of primary spinal cord tumors. Int J Radiat Oncol Biol Phys. 1989;16(6):1397-1403.
29. Garcia DM. Primary spinal cord tumors treated with surgery and postoperative irradiation. Int J Radiat Oncol Biol Phys. 1985;11(11):1933-9.
30. Kim MS, Chung CK, Choe G, et al. Intramedullary Spinal Cord Astrocytoma in Adults: Postoperative Outcome. J Neurooncol. 2001;52(1):85-94.
31. Innocenzi G, Raco A, Cantore G, et al. Intramedullary astrocytomas and ependymomas in the pediatric age group: a retrospective study. Childs Nerv Syst. 1996;12(12):776-80.
32. Miller DC. Surgical Pathology of Intramedullary Spinal Cord Neoplasms. J Neurooncol. 2000;47(3):189-94.
33. Houten JK, Cooper PR. Spinal cord astrocytomas: presentation, management and outcome. J Neurooncol. 2000;47(3):219-24.
34. Epstein FJ, Farmer JP, Freed D. Adult intramedullary astrocytomas of the spinal cord. Journal of Neurosurgery. 1992;77(3):355-9.
35. Choi GH, Oh JK, Kim TY, et al. The clinical features and surgical outcomes of pediatric patients with primary spinal cord tumor. Childs Nerv Syst. 2012;28(6):897-904.
36. Dickman CA, Fehlings MG, Gokaslan ZL. Spinal Cord and Spinal Column Tumors: Principles and Practices. New York: Thieme; 2006.
37. Roonprapunt C, Houten JK. Spinal cord astrocytomas: presentation, management, and outcome. Neurosurg Clin N Am. 2006;17(1):29-36.
38. Cristante L, Herrmann HD. Surgical management of intramedullary spinal cord tumors: functional outcome and sources of morbidity. Neurosurgery. 1994;35(1):69-74; discussion 74-6.
39. Jallo GI, Danish S, Velasquez L, et al. Intramedullary low-grade astrocytomas: long-term outcome following radical surgery. J Neurooncol. 2001;53(1):61-6.
40. Biondi A, Ricciardi GK, Faillot T, et al. Hemangioblastomas of the Lower Spinal Region: Report of Four Cases with Preoperative Embolization and Review of the Literature. Am J Neuroradiol. 2005;26(4):936-45.
41. Lee DK, Choe WJ, Chung CK, et al. Spinal cord hemangioblastoma: surgical strategy and clinical outcome. J Neurooncol. 2003;61(1):27-34.
42. Chu BC, Terae S, Hida K, et al. MR findings in spinal hemangioblastoma: correlation with symptoms and with angiographic and surgical findings. Am J Neuroradiol. 2001;22(1):206-17.
43. Neumann HP, Eggert HR, Weigel K, et al. Hemangioblastomas of the central nervous system. A 10-year study with special reference to von Hippel-Lindau syndrome. J Neurosurg. 1989;70(1):24-30.
44. Wanebo JE Lonser RR, Glenn GM, et al. The natural history of hemangioblastomas of the central nervous system in patients with von Hippel-Lindau disease. J Neurosurg. 2003;98(1):82-94.
45. Browne TR, Adams RD, Roberson GH. Hemangioblastoma of the spinal cord: Review and report of five cases. Arch Neurol. 1976;33(6):435-41.
46. Imagama S, Ito Z, Wakao N, et al. Differentiation of localization of spinal hemangioblastomas based on imaging and pathological findings. Eur Spine J. 2011;20(8):1377-84.
47. Pietilä TA, Stendel R, Schilling A, et al. Surgical treatment of spinal hemangioblastomas. Acta Neurochir (Wien). 2000;142(8):879-86.
48. Mandigo CE, Ogden AT, Angevine PD, et al. Operative management of spinal hemangioblastoma. Neurosurgery. 2009;65(6):1166-77.
49. Schaller B. Spinal meningioma: relationship between histological subtypes and surgical outcome? J Neurooncol. 2005;75(2):157-61.

50. Cohen-Gadol AA, Zikel OM, Koch CA, et al. Spinal meningiomas in patients younger than 50 years of age: a 21-year experience. J Neurosurg. 2003;98(3 Suppl):258-63.
51. Chaparro MJ, Young RF, Smith M, et al. Multiple spinal meningiomas: a case of 47 distinct lesions in the absence of neurofibromatosis or identified chromosomal abnormality. Neurosurgery. 1993;32(2):298-301; discussion 301-2.
52. Klekamp J, Samii M. Surgical results for spinal meningiomas. Surg Neurol. 1999;52(6):552-62.
53. Riemenschneider MJ, Perry A, Reifenberger G. Histological classification and molecular genetics of meningiomas. Lancet Neurol. 2006;5(12):1045-54.
54. Alorainy IA. Dural tail sign in spinal meningiomas. Eur J Radiol. 2006;60(3):387-91.
55. Setzer M, Vatter H, Marquardt G, et al. Management of spinal meningiomas: surgical results and a review of the literature. Neurosurg Focus. 2007;23(4):E14.
56. King AT, Sharr MM, Gullan RW, et al. Spinal meningiomas: a 20-year review. Br J Neurosurg. 1998;12(6):521-6.
57. Gottfried ON, Gluf W, Quinones-Hinojosa A, et al. Spinal meningiomas: surgical management and outcome. Neurosurg Focus. 2003;14(6):e2.
58. Roux FX, et al. Intraspinal meningiomas: review of 54 cases with discussion of poor prognosis factors and modern therapeutic management. Surg Neurol. 1996;46(5):458-63; discussion 463-4.
59. Seppälä MT, Haltia MJ, Sankila RJ, et al. Long-term outcome after removal of spinal schwannoma: a clinicopathological study of 187 cases. J Neurosurg. 1995;83(4):621-6.
60. Seppälä MT, Haltia MJ. Spinal malignant nerve-sheath tumor or cellular schwannoma? A striking difference in prognosis. J Neurosurg. 1993;79(4):528-32.
61. el-Mahdy W, Kane PJ, Powell MP, et al. Spinal intradural tumours: Part I—Extramedullary. Br J Neurosurg. 1999; 13(6):550-7.
62. Klekamp J, Samii M. Surgery of spinal nerve sheath tumors with special reference to neurofibromatosis. Neurosurgery. 1998;42(2):279-89; discussion 289-90.
63. Demachi H, Takashima T, Kadoya M, et al. MR imaging of spinal neurinomas with pathological correlation. J Comput Assist Tomogr. 1990;14(2):250-4.
64. Safavi-Abbasi S, Senoglu M, Theodore N, et al. Microsurgical management of spinal schwannomas: evaluation of 128 cases. J Neurosurg Spine. 2008;9(1):40-7.
65. Abernathey CD, Onofrio BM, Scheithauer B, et al. Surgical management of giant sacral schwannomas. J Neurosurg. 1986;65(3):286-95.
66. O'Toole JE, McCormick PC. Midline ventral intradural schwannoma of the cervical spinal cord resected via anterior corpectomy with reconstruction: technical case report and review of the literature. Neurosurgery. 2003;52(6):1482-5; discussion 1485-6.
67. Seppälä MT, Haltia MJ, Sankila RJ, et al. Long-term outcome after removal of spinal neurofibroma. J Neurosurg. 1995;82(4):572-7.
68. McCormick PC. Surgical management of dumbbell tumors of the cervical spine.Neurosurgery. 1996;38(2):294-300.
69. Friedrich RE, Kluwe L, Fünsterer C, et al. Malignant peripheral nerve sheath tumors (MPNST) in neurofibromatosis type 1 (NF1): diagnostic findings on magnetic resonance images and mutation analysis of the NF1 gene. Anticancer Res. 2005;25(3A): 1699-702.
70. Thakkar SD, Feigen U, et al. Spinal tumours in neurofibromatosis type 1: an MRI study of frequency, multiplicity and variety. Neuroradiology. 1999;41(9):625-9.
71. Sanguinetti C, Specchia N, Gigante A, et al. Clinical and pathological aspects of solitary spinal neurofibroma. J Bone Joint Surg Br. 1993;75(1):141-7.
72. Rodriguez FJ, Folpe AL, Giannini C, et al. Pathology of peripheral nerve sheath tumors: diagnostic overview and update on selected diagnostic problems. Acta Neuropathol. 2012;123(3):295-319.
73. Arazi-Kleinmann T, Mor Y, Brand N, et al. Neurofibromatosis diagnosed on CT with MR correlation. Eur J Radiol. 2002; 42(1):69-73.
74. Donner TR, Voorhies RM, Kline DG. Neural sheath tumors of major nerves. J Neurosurg. 1994;81(3):362-73.
75. Levy WJ, Latchaw J, Hahn JF et al. Spinal neurofibromas: a report of 66 cases and a comparison with meningiomas. Neurosurgery. 1986;18(3):331-4.
76. Kim P, Ebersold MJ, Onofrio BM, et al. Surgery of spinal nerve schwannoma. Risk of neurological deficit after resection of involved root. J Neurosurg. 1989;71(6):810-4.
77. Pollack IF, et al. Surgical management of spinal cord compression from plexiform neurofibromas in patients with neurofibromatosis 1. Neurosurgery. 1998;43(2):248-55; discussion 255-6.
78. Nuwer MR. Electrophysiologic evaluation and monitoring of spinal cord and root function. Neurosurg Clin N Am. 1990;1(3):533-49.
79. Needle MN,, Cnaan A, Dattilo J, et al. Prognostic signs in the surgical management of plexiform neurofibroma: the Children's Hospital of Philadelphia experience, 1974-1994. J Pediatr. 1997;131(5):678-82.
80. Sundgren P, Annertz M, Englund E, et al. Paragangliomas of the spinal canal. Neuroradiology. 1999;41(10):788-94.
81. Faro SH, Turtz AR, Koenigsberg RA, et al. Paraganglioma of the cauda equina with associated intramedullary cyst: MR findings. Am J Neuroradiol. 1997;18(8):1588-90.
82. Miliaras GC, Kyritsis AP, Polyzoidis KS. Cauda equina paraganglioma: a review. J Neurooncol. 2003;65(2):177-90.
83. Anderson JR, Gullan RW. Paraganglioma of the cauda equina: a case report. J Neurol Neurosurg Psychiatr. 1987;50(1):100-3.
84. Hsieh CT, Tsai WC, Tang CT, et al. Paraganglioma of the cauda equina. Neurol India. 2009;57(6):833-4.
85. Yang SY, Jin YJ, Park SH, et al. Paragangliomas in the cauda equina region: clinicopathoradiologic findings in four cases. J Neurooncol. 2005;72(1):49-55.

SECTION 2

Pediatric Spine

CHAPTER 10

Evaluation of Back Pain in Children

Hillard T Spencer, Anthony A Scaduto

INTRODUCTION

While transient back pain is a common complaint in children, persistent symptoms warrant a careful evaluation and judicious use of diagnostic testing to evaluate for any specific pathology. This chapter will focus on persistent back pain exclusive of transient symptoms and muscle strains or acute traumatic injuries. To our knowledge, there is no discrete interval that determines "persistence" of symptoms. This judgment must be made by the physician evaluating the patient based on a careful evaluation of the characteristics of the patient's complaint.[1,2]

EPIDEMIOLOGY AND NATURAL HISTORY

A variety of studies have been performed to estimate the prevalence of back pain in the pediatric population. The traditional teaching that back pain in children is a rare entity and usually indicates a pathologic cause has been questioned in prospective studies.[3] It is currently felt that there is in fact a high prevalence of back pain in children with typically benign course in most cases.[4] The change in teaching over the last few decades likely has several explanations, which may include differences in study methodology (medical record retrospective review of patients at large medical centers versus population-based surveys of normal children), definitions of terminology (all back pain, history of back pain, or current persistent back pain), and even perhaps a sociological shift towards a greater awareness of back pain, an increased desire of parents for medical evaluation when a child complains of pain, or changing referral patterns and an increase in specialist care for pediatric back pain. In addition, certain populations such as adolescent high-level athletes may differ from the general population of children and have a high rate of specific injuries leading to back pain.[5] However, in a cross-sectional study performed in Denmark, there was no association between the level of back pain in children and their level of physical activity.[6] The natural history of nonspecific back pain in children has not been clearly defined and it is not clear how childhood episodes of back pain without a discernible etiology relate to complaints later in life. However, there is evidence that family attitudes and experiences with back pain, as well as psychological factors, affect the reporting of back pain in children and adolescents.[7]

WORK-UP (CLINICAL FINDINGS)

Symptoms and Signs

History

Obtaining a complete history is the first step in evaluation of the patient with back pain. The physician should seek to fully characterize the pain, in terms of its location, duration, quality, temporal characteristics (continuous versus intermittent), radiation, exacerbating and relieving factors, and associated symptoms. A history of local symptoms including swelling, tenderness, or a mass should be specifically sought. In addition, careful inquiry about systemic symptoms such as fevers, weight loss, recent infectious processes or any neurologic changes such as headaches, incontinence, or dyscoordination provides important clues for diagnosis of an underlying cause for the back pain. Discitis (infection of the disk space) can occur in children because of the arterial channels around the open apophyses of the vertebral column.[8] Sports participation, e.g. gymnastics, may predispose the patient to a very specific set of injuries such as to the vertebral ring apophysis or the pars interarticularis.[9,10]

Medical history can play a role in the evaluation of a child's back pain and chronic conditions such as cerebral palsy, major medical illnesses, malabsorption syndromes, and certainly any history of malignancy should be explored further. Review of the family medical history can be helpful not only to understand how the child or parent may perceive back pain based on the experience of other family members with back pain, but also to evaluate for the presence of rheumatologic conditions that may be linked to a family history. The social history in some cases can shed light on other reasons for back pain such as substance abuse, psychosocial stress, or abuse at home in cases where no medical reason for back pain can be identified.

Physical Examination

The physical examination of the child with back pain involves certain key elements (Box 1). Visual clues such as alterations in sagittal profile, e.g. hyperlordosis or excessive kyphosis may help to direct the examination to the relevant region. A rigid or structural kyphosis will be notable for failure to reverse with prone hyperextension testing. Scoliosis is often associated with diminished spinal flexibility and the manual examination can help to differentiate between pain due to paraspinal muscle spasms and symptoms localizing to the vertebral column. Provocative testing including lumbar hyperextension tests can help to increase sensitivity for pathology of the pars interarticularis, which occupies a continuum from pars stress to spondylolisthesis.[10] This continuum often coexists with tightness of the hamstrings and lumbar hyperlordosis. If these tests do not yield positive findings, supine flexion, abduction, external rotation stress (FABER) of the hip aids in localizing symptoms derived from sacroiliac joint pathology such as inflammatory arthritides or infections. Finally, a careful neurologic exam, including evaluation of gait, is paramount in identifying disorders of the central or peripheral nervous system.

Box 1: Physical examination.

- General appearance
  - Body habitus—obesity or cachexia
- Spine
  - Inspection
    - Alignment, sagittal profile, shoulder heights, iliac crests
  - Palpation
    - Midline elements, paraspinal muscles
  - Range of motion
    - Forward bending, back/side bending/rotation, prone hyperextension (reversibility of thoracic kyphosis)
  - Provocative testing
    - Stork test
    - Straight leg raise—radicular symptoms versus tight hamstrings (popliteal angle)
    - FABER test—SI joint
- Neurologic
  - Strength
  - Sensation
  - Reflexes—DTR's and long-tract signs, abdominal reflexes
  - Coordination
- Gait
  - Stance—heel-toe pattern, ankle stability, toe-off
  - Swing-foot drop
  - Stride length and symmetry
  - Trendelenburg lurch

The neurologic examination should be tailored to the age of the patient. While an older child may be able to follow commands for manual motor testing and may give accurate responses to sensory testing, the physician must use other clues with the younger child who cannot participate to the same extent. Clues such as asymmetric movement of limbs, a difference in muscle tone, or hyperreflexia may help to localize neurologic deficits. For the child who can participate in the examination, the neurologic exam should include evaluation of strength and muscle tone, sensation, reflexes, coordination and gait. When assessing strength, manual motor testing is generally reliable but the physician must be careful to distinguish between true weakness and hesitancy to produce maximal effort due to pain or fear. It may be useful to involve the parent in coaxing the younger child to perform motor tasks if fear of the examiner is evident. Evaluation of muscle tone may help to distinguish between upper motor neuron lesions with hypertonia and lower motor neuron lesions with diminished muscle tone. Sensory testing in general helps to screen for dermatomal deficits associated with nerve root compression; however, if there is suspicion for an intramedullary spinal cord process or if there is known spinal cord injury, differentiation of mechanosensory information carried through the dorsal column-medial lemniscal tracts and noxious stimuli carried in the spinothalamic tracts becomes paramount. The young patient is likely to cooperate more willingly with testing of temperature sensation, which also follows the spinothalamic pathways, than with testing of nociceptive stimuli. The reflex examination is best performed with a relaxed child. Patellar and Achilles reflexes are easiest to elicit if the patient is sitting with the legs over the edge of the examination table and is distracted by conversation or another task. The Babinski reflex test may be difficult to perform in children depending on age. Asymmetric reflexes are a red flag and require further investigation if the examiner is convinced the finding is not artifactual. Finally, evaluation of coordination and gait provides basic information about cerebellar function. Abnormalities of cerebellar function in a child with back pain should raise suspicion for Chiari malformation, tethered cord syndrome, or syringomyelia and warrant further investigation with cranial-to-caudal neural axis MRI and neurosurgical consultation.[11]

Imaging

Initial Imaging

An algorithmic approach to imaging in pediatric back pain may be useful.[3,12] In general, by the time the patient has been referred for orthopedic evaluation, we consider it prudent to obtain screening radiographs of the affected area of the spine. Ideally, these are limited to the relevant area detected by physical examination in order to keep the effective radiation dose as low as reasonably achievable; however, for young children in particular, back pain is often poorly localized and may in fact present as a limp, necessitating radiographs not only of the spine but also often of the pelvis, hips, and lower limbs. Radiographs provide an excellent initial screening modality for many types of pathology including congenital deformity, many lytic or blastic neoplasms, postinfectious changes, pars injuries, or fractures. Frequently, radiographs will guide the choice of further imaging. Of note, the "winking owl" sign, or lytic destruction of a pedicle leading to absence of the pedicle outline on the posteroanterior spinal radiograph, may help to identify lesions that are otherwise overlooked.

Magnetic Resonance Imaging

The use of magnetic resonance imaging (MRI) has changed the evaluation of numerous disorders of the spine. In diskitis, MRI allows earlier and more accurate detection of the lesion and can be used to evaluate for reconstitution of the disk.[13] It can also aid in distinguishing discitis from osteomyelitis, although these disorders may be part of the same continuum.[8,14]

The presence of neurologic signs should prompt the physician to order MRI with the goal of identifying entities such as compression of nerve roots, spinal cord, or the conus; tethering of the spinal cord; or the rare case of primary spinal cord neoplasia, the most common being astrocytoma.[15] Disk herniation in children, although considered to be fairly uncommon, nonetheless does occur and typically presents with back pain. Perhaps because of its relatively low incidence, the diagnosis is often delayed.[16] It should be suspected in any child with persistent radicular symptoms and should be presumed until proven absent in a child with recent trauma, negative radiographs, and radiculopathy. If there is no focal neurologic deficit, initial nonsurgical management is appropriate, but many patients continue to have pain and receive excellent pain relief with surgical decompression. In particular, disk herniations that are associated with fractures of the vertebral ring apophysis are more likely to require surgery for symptomatic relief.[17] In addition, the presence of a high grade spondylolisthesis, even in the absence of neurologic findings, may warrant obtaining MRI to characterize the position of the intervertebral disk with respect to the slip and to detect disk protrusions that would create risk of neural compression during surgical reduction.

For the patient with extension-based pain and examination suspicious for spondylolysis, but with negative radiographs, MRI can be used to further define early stress changes of the pars interarticularis before radiographic changes are evident.[18] High signal changes on axial T2-weighted MRI in the pars interarticularis as well as in the adjacent pedicle may aid in the early diagnosis of spondylolysis in children, and have been shown to be predictive of healing in patients with pars interarticularis defects proven by CT scan.[19,20] Furthermore, MRI is sensitive to sacroiliitis in many cases when radiographs are negative.[21]

Skeletal Scintigraphy

A nuclear medicine bone scan using Technetium 99, either planar (2-D) or with SPECT, can be a vital tool in localizing pathology and assessing for osteoblastic activity and is particularly useful in young children who have trouble localizing pain or participating with physical examination. Skeletal scintigraphy may also play a role in identification of stress responses in the pars interarticularis, with increased isotope uptake on bone scan correlating with bone marrow edema on MRI.[10] The decision between MRI and bone scan depends on several factors. For one,

CHAPTER 10

the radiation dose associated with SPECT in particular is considerable (estimates: from 2.9 mSv for an average-sized 5-year-old to 4.2 mSv for a 15-year-old child).[22] However, in young children, MRI frequently requires sedation with its attendant risks.[23] In particular, there is a growing body of evidence for long-term neurocognitive effects of general anesthesia in young children.[24] Availability of each modality and consideration of the clinically suspected pathology also weigh into deciding which test is most likely to be diagnostic. It is important to remember that bone scan may be negative with certain tumors and negative scintigraphy does not preclude a pathologic diagnosis.[25]

Computed Tomography

Computed tomography is the study of choice for certain osseous pathologies. In particular, osteoid osteoma and osteoblastoma demonstrate a characteristic nidus on CT scan that aids in distinguishing them from other diagnoses. These pathologies may be clinically suspected if a patient's complaints are not activity related but are relieved by anti-inflammatory medications, and the size of the nidus is the key distinguishing factor between these entities, classically greater than 1.5 or 2 cm for osteoblastoma and smaller for osteoid osteoma. Aneurysmal bone cysts are found in the posterior elements throughout the spine and the extent of involvement can best be delineated with CT scan to aid in planning resection and instrumentation.[26] Malignant tumors, more often localized to the anterior elements (vertebral body), include neuroblastoma and Ewing sarcoma, and are often invasive by the time they are discovered and a CT of the chest to evaluate for pulmonary metastasis is often required. Hematologic malignancy may also involve the spine, and back pain and vertebral body collapse may be the initial presenting complaint in some cases of childhood leukemia.[27]

Laboratory Evaluation

A laboratory workup is useful in certain settings, especially the young child with poorly localized back pain or limp, as well as patients for whom clinical history or examination suggests an inflammatory process and those with systemic complaints. A complete blood count with differential, as well as the erythrocyte sedimentation rate and the C-reactive protein level, help to identify inflammatory or infectious etiologies. If further laboratory workup such as antinuclear antibody, rheumatoid factor, or human leukocyte antigen (HLA) typing is felt to be necessary, we prefer to refer the patient for rheumatologic consultation to ensure continuity of diagnostic and therapeutic decision making.

MEDICAL MANAGEMENT

Initial nonoperative management is possible in many cases of nonspecific childhood back pain. Once a careful evaluation of the patient is complete, and no specific diagnosis is found, it is reasonable to prescribe physical therapy, anti-inflammatory medications and a brief period of activity modification. It is important to remind the patient and parents that the goal is functional rehabilitation and the expected course is a return to normal activities. A conversation with the family often reveals underlying concerns, perhaps due to family perceptions of pain, parents' worries that the child has a malignant process, or to fears that the back pain will interfere with the child's athletic ambitions. It may also reveal that the parents' athletic ambitions for the child are not shared by the patient and the complaint of back pain may be a manifestation of the wish to cease participation in a sport.

Prior to concluding that there is no pathophysiologic cause of the patient's complaint, it is incumbent on the physician to systematically consider the entire differential diagnosis in order to avoid delaying a diagnosis and missing a therapeutic window in some cases. The differential roughly falls into the major categories of developmental, traumatic, infectious, inflammatory, degenerative, and neoplastic diagnoses (Box 2). Developmental causes encompass structural abnormalities of the spine, such as scoliosis, either congenital (due to bony malformation) or idiopathic, kyphosis (e.g., Scheuermann disease), hyperlordosis, some of the subtypes of spondylolysis, congenital stenosis, and transitional vertebrae or Bertolotti's syndrome.[28] Although adolescent idiopathic scoliosis often presents with back pain, there has been some debate in the medical literature regarding the question of whether patients with idiopathic scoliosis actually have a higher lifetime risk of disabling back pain than the general population. In a 50-year follow-up study of 117 patients with idiopathic scoliosis who ended up not undergoing surgical treatment, it was noted that 61% of patients with scoliosis stated they had chronic back pain, significantly more than the 35% rate in the control group, but the authors noted that of the patients who

Box 2: Differential diagnosis of pediatric back pain.

- *Developmental* causes encompass structural abnormalities of the spine, such as scoliosis, either congenital (due to bony malformation) or idiopathic, kyphosis (e.g. Scheuermann disease), hyperlordosis, some of the subtypes of spondylolysis, congenital stenosis, and transitional vertebrae or Bertolotti's syndrome.
- *Traumatic* etiologies of back pain encompass acute injuries (outside the scope of this chapter—refer to chapter on spine fractures) and repetitive strain injuries, commonly in the adolescent athlete. These repetitive strain injuries may include some cases of spondylolysis, disk disease, and zygapophyseal joint sprains, as well as apophyseal ring injuries, ALL/PLL strain, and muscular strain.
- *Infectious* causes of back pain include osteomyelitis (typically hematogenous), discitis, paraspinal abscess (e.g. psoas abscess), meningitis, or epidural abscess.
- *Inflammatory* etiologies, such as juvenile arthritis, ankylosing spondylitis or other seronegative spondyloarthropathies, are often revealed when inflammatory markers prove to be elevated or sacroiliac pain is present.
- *Degenerative* causes of back pain, such as intervertebral disk herniation, disk space narrowing, or desiccation, although considered most common in the adult population, may be found in children as well, particularly adolescents.
- *Neoplastic* causes are many, including benign tumors such as osteoid osteoma, osteoblastoma (classically in the posterior elements), intermediate tumors such as eosinophilic granuloma, aneurysmal bone cyst, and chordoma, as well as malignant causes such as Ewing sarcoma, lymphoma, or rhabdomyosarcoma; not to mention both benign and malignant tumors of the neural axis such as schwannoma, neurofibroma, and neurofibrosarcoma.

(ALL/PLL: anterior longitudinal ligament/posterior longitudinal ligament))

reported pain, over two-thirds said that they experienced only low or moderate levels of pain and the authors concluded that even untreated scoliosis causes little functional impairment over a lifetime.[29] The question arises, however, whether patients who were not included in the analysis may have differed in characteristics or level of pain than the other patients. Certainly, for children who present with scoliosis and back pain, the physician should diligently seek any other cause for the pain such as osteoid osteoma, spondylolysis or spondylolisthesis, sacroiliitis, or neurologic abnormalities including tethering of the spinal cord or tonsillar herniation.

Scheuermann kyphosis commonly presents in the adolescent with parents noting "poor posture" and the patient complaining of back pain. While the exact etiology is poorly understood, it is often grouped with other osteochondroses of childhood.[30] The cause of pain in Scheuermann disease may be inflammation of the vertebral apophysis, leading to growth abnormalities and anterior wedging of the vertebral body. Scheuermann disease is diagnosed in a patient with end plate changes (Schmorl's nodes) and anterior wedging of 5° or more in three contiguous vertebral bodies, classically in the thoracic region. In the Danish Twin Registry, which includes all twin births in Denmark in the last 130 years (73,000 pairs), there is a 3.6% incidence of Scheuermann disease in males and 2.1% incidence in females and a significantly higher disease concordance in monozygotic than in dizygotic twins, suggesting a strong genetic component to the disease.[31] There is sparse long-term data on the natural history of untreated Scheuermann disease or on the results of surgical intervention.[32] One natural history study with an average of 32 years of follow-up on 67 patients with Scheuermann kyphosis (mean kyphosis angle of 71°) suggested that patients with Scheuermann kyphosis had a higher intensity of back pain than age and sex-matched controls, and jobs with a lower level of physical activity, but no difference in work days missed due to back pain or presence of back pain that interfered with daily activities, or in educational level achieved.[33] In general, moderate kyphosis with some reversibility on prone hyperextension testing can be managed with observation or bracing, and surgery should be reserved for severe deformity or deformity that progresses after skeletal maturity, as the surgical procedure carries a not insignificant risk of complications (14%) including acute neurologic injury (1.9%), according to an analysis based on surgeon-entered data (2001–2004) from the SRS database.[34] Thoracic disk herniation may occur in some patients with Scheuermann kyphosis, most often at the apex of the deformity, and can necessitate surgical treatment to prevent permanent neurologic injury.[35]

Hyperlordosis of the lumbar spine is often seen in patients who present with back pain, and could be a factor in the development of spondylolysis due to increased load on the posterior spinal elements. A study of 29 patients with bilateral L5 pars interarticularis fractures and matched controls showed a higher mean angle of lordosis and angle of sacral inclination in the patients with spondylolysis than in the control group.[36] However, even in the absence of injury to the pars interarticularis, hyperlordosis can be associated with zygapophyseal inflammation or facet syndrome or paraspinal muscle spasms as well as with hamstring tightness and many children with this constellation of findings will benefit from a physical therapy referral for a home exercise program of hamstring stretches, core stability, and antilordosis postural re-education. If imaging studies reveal injury to the pars interarticularis, initial nonoperative management is appropriate with a 15° antilordotic lumbosacral orthosis combined with the physical therapy program. In a study of 104 athletes with back pain and spondylolysis, there were 40 individuals who had to stop sports participation due to severity of back pain and 35 of those patients were able to resume their original sport at an average of 5.4 months after initiation of treatment with antilordotic bracing.[37]

Spinal stenosis is rare in average-height children but can be symptomatic in children with achondroplasia. Patients may present with back pain or neurologic symptoms. There is little role for nonoperative management if the patient is experiencing neurologic changes. Compression of neural structures can best be detected by MRI. A study comparing patients with achondroplasia below age 18 who were treated with decompression and instrumentation versus decompression without instrumentation showed that the patients who underwent instrumented fusion at the time of decompression had a lower risk of requiring revision surgery and a greater improvement in symptoms than the other patients.[38]

Discitis, or inflammation of the intervertebral disk space, is generally considered to be caused by infection although an offending pathogen frequently cannot be isolated. There is often elevation of erythrocyte sedimentation rate and C-reactive protein, with a variable white blood cell count. The yield of cultures from biopsy of the affected disk space has been reported to be as low as 0% in some series although others report better yields.[14,39] As a result of these low yields on culture, biopsy is generally only performed for patients who fail to show improvement after initiation of rest and antibiotic therapy. The onset is often insidious and diagnosis may be delayed as there are often no early radiographic findings. Loss of lumbar lordosis may be the earliest radiographic finding. However, with clinical suspicion for spinal infection in children, MRI is now considered the most sensitive method of early detection and differentiation between discitis and osteomyelitis.[8] Treatment generally consists of rest and antibiotic therapy directed toward *Staphylococcus aureus* which has been described as the most common pathogen in some series.[40] In a series of cases of children between the ages of 1 to 3 years at the Hospital for Children, London, 63% presented with refusal to walk, 50% presented with inability to flex the lumbar spine, 40% with loss of lumbar lordosis, and 27% with a complaint of back pain.[13] MRI was obtained in select cases for clinical follow-up to demonstrate resolution and recovery of the disk, although the time required was significant in some cases, over 2 years, and radiographs showed persistent loss of disk or vertebral height in many patients in that series.

SURGICAL INDICATIONS AND TREATMENT

Other than scoliosis, the two conditions mentioned above that are most likely to be seen by the pediatric orthopedic spinal surgeon and progress to require surgical treatment, are spondylolisthesis and Scheuermann kyphosis. These two topics will be touched on here with further details of the surgical techniques covered elsewhere in this book.

Spondylolysis/Spondylolisthesis

Surgical treatment is considered in cases of spondylolisthesis that have failed conservative management with brace immobilization, physical therapy, and symptomatic treatment, continuing to show instability on flexion/extension views, progression of the slip beyond Meyerding Grade 2, or in some instances, pain refractory to a thorough course of nonoperative management. In carefully selected cases, with slips less than 25%, a repair of the pars interarticularis may be attempted, provided there is no significant intervertebral disk disease on MRI that is a better explanation for the patient's symptoms. Several techniques for pars repair are available, including Buck's translaminar screw repair for compression of the defect, or bone grafting with a variety of internal fixation methods such as a rod-screw construct, a screw-cable construct, or a pedicle screw-laminar hook construct, with all reporting reasonable rates of pars union and pain relief when patients are selected appropriately.[41-44] Dysplastic spondylolisthesis is more likely to progress and is not amenable to a pars repair, thus requiring an instrumented posterior fusion. For higher-grade spondylolisthesis that fails conservative management either due to continued progression beyond grade 2 or unrelenting pain, instrumented fusion is the procedure of choice, with combined posterior pedicle screw fixation and anterior intervertebral support now the widely accepted standard.[45] A reduction or partial reduction of the slip may be necessary to achieve satisfactory anterior intervertebral support in the highest grades, with wide decompression mandatory to lower the risk of neurologic injury during reduction.[46]

Scheuermann Kyphosis

The fact that disagreement exists regarding the origin, treatment, and prognosis of Scheuermann's disease, creates difficulty in determining clear operative indications.[32] Long-term follow-up studies of both nonoperatively and operatively treated patients have failed to show a relationship between radiographic outcomes and clinical outcomes.[47,48] However, in general, for patients who have progressive curves beyond 75° of kyphosis with persistent severe pain despite compliance with brace treatment, surgical treatment may be considered, with the goal of obtaining moderate curve reduction and spinal fusion.[49] Because of significant concern for obtaining fusion and maintaining correction, the prior standard of care was a combined anterior and posterior fusion.[50] However, due to advances in technology and surgical technique, it is now considered the norm to use an all-posterior approach; anterior release or interbody fusion is not thought to be necessary when utilizing modern posterior pedicle-screw instrumentation systems combined with Ponte osteotomies at the apical levels.[51]

COMPLICATIONS

Spondylolisthesis

In a report of the morbidity and mortality index of the Scoliosis Research Society, 605 pediatric patients were identified who underwent surgical treatment for isthmic or dysplastic spondylolisthesis from 2004 to 2007. The authors reported an overall complication rate of 10.4%, with the most frequent being postoperative neurologic deficit (5%), wound infection (2%), and dural tear (1.3%).[52] It is interesting to note a parallel paper from the same database and time period regarding surgery in adults for isthmic and degenerative spondylolisthesis, with a much larger cohort of patients (10,242 patients) and a similar total complication rate of 9.2%.[53] Thus, regardless of patient age, it is clear that complications from these surgical procedures are very common.

Scheuermann Kyphosis

Even in experienced hands, surgical treatment of Scheuermann kyphosis is associated with a significant risk of complications (14% overall), according to an analysis based on surgeon-entered data (2001–2004) from the SRS database.[34] In that analysis, wound infection was the most common complication (3.9%) and acute neurologic injury was also documented (1.9%), with overall complications being more common in adult patients (22%) than in pediatric patients (12%). In this data, the rate of complications was not significantly different when comparing all-posterior spinal fusion procedures to those with a same-day combined anterior and posterior surgical procedure. Discussing these risks with the patient and family members prior to surgery is therefore of paramount importance. Finally, curve decompensation with either proximal or distal junctional kyphosis can occur, and has been associated with failure to fuse to the appropriate level and disruption of junctional ligamentum flavum.[54]

PROGNOSIS

There is little prospective clinical outcome data for surgical treatment of spondylolisthesis. However, three retrospective outcome studies from Finland with long-term follow-up are available. A retrospective analysis of 108 pediatric patients with low-grade slips treated by posterior or posterolateral fusion, that obtained 83% follow-up at a mean of 20.8 years, suggested that overall results were satisfactory as measured by the Oswestry Disability Index and the Scoliosis Research Society questionnaire. However, there was significant variation in these outcomes and 14% of patients reported back pain often or very often at rest.[55] In a separate retrospective analysis of 70 pediatric patients with high grade slips treated with posterolateral, anterior, or circumferential fusion in situ, that achieved 84% follow-up after a mean of 17.2 years, these authors found again a significant variation in outcomes measured by the same measures, but concluded that circumferential fusion was superior to either the posterolateral or anterior techniques.[56] This group of surgeons also looked at 22 patients between 1983 and 1991 to compare 11 who had reduction for high-grade slips to 11 who had in-situ fusion for high-grade slips, and concluded that the Oswestry Disability Index and the Scoliosis Research Society questionnaire results were superior for the in-situ fusion group, although the in-situ group had a higher rate of nerve root impingement at the L5–S1 level on MRI, which the authors reported was asymptomatic.[57] The limitation may be the older techniques utilized during that study period. One other retrospective study of 49 children with high-grade spondylolisthesis comparing outcomes among cohorts treated with and without surgery showed that higher slip angle was associated with a poorer outcome score, and concluded that "operative intervention for the symptomatic patient achieves similar long-term results compared with patients whose minimal symptoms do not warrant surgery."[58]

Outcome data for surgical treatment of Scheuermann kyphosis is similarly sparse. One retrospective study has shown higher scores on the Scoliosis Research Society questionnaire in a cohort of patients treated with all-posterior technique than in a similar cohort of patients treated with combined anterior-posterior spinal fusion.[59] Another retrospective study has shown a lower rate of complications in patients treated with posterior techniques alone, compared to patients treated with combined anterior-posterior approaches, but outcome scores on the Scoliosis Research Society questionnaire were not significantly different.[60] A retrospective analysis of 63 patients treated with either exercise, bracing, or surgical fusion found at 10–28-year follow-up that patients treated by bracing or surgery had improved self-image, and patients with kyphosis over 70° at follow-up had an inferior functional result, but the final degree of kyphosis was not different between treatment groups, a finding that suggests to us these results may not be applicable to currently practiced surgical techniques.[61] To our knowledge, however, there is no randomized study comparing outcome scores between operative and nonoperative management of patients with Scheuermann kyphosis, so the choice of intervention remains dictated largely by the patient's level of symptoms. In summary, data on surgical outcomes lags behind current surgical techniques due to rapid advances in the field of pediatric spinal surgery in the past few decades, and this information deficit will require further research to aid in defining surgical indications for these conditions.

REFERENCES

1. Afshani E, Kuhn JP. Common causes of low back pain in children. Radiographics. 1991;11(2):269-91.
2. Rodriguez DP, Poussaint TY. Imaging of back pain in children. Am J Neuroradiol. 2010;31(5):787-802.
3. Bhatia NN, Chow G, Timon SJ, et al. Diagnostic modalities for the evaluation of pediatric back pain: a prospective study. J Pediatr Orthop. 2008;28(2):230-3.
4. Feldman DS, Hedden DM, Wright JG. The use of bone scan to investigate back pain in children and adolescents. J Pediatr Orthop. 2000;20(6):790-5.
5. Curtis C, d'Hemecourt P. Diagnosis and management of back pain in adolescents. Adolesc Med State Art Rev. 2007;18(1): 140-64, x.
6. Wedderkopp N, Leboeuf-Yde C, Bo Andersen L, et al. Back pain in children: no association with objectively measured level of physical activity. Spine (Phila Pa 1976). 2003;28(17):2019-24; discussion 2024.
7. Balagué F, Skovron ML, Nordin M, et al. Low back pain in school children. A study of familial and psychological factors. Spine (Phila Pa 1976). 1995;20(11):1265-70.
8. Early SD, Kay RM, Tolo VT. Childhood diskitis. J Am Acad Orthop Surg. 2003;11(6):413-20.
9. Katz DA, Scerpella TA. Anterior and middle column thoracolumbar spine injuries in young female gymnasts. Report of seven cases and review of the literature. Am J Sports Med. 2003;31(4):611-6.
10. Spencer HT, Sokol LO, Glotzbecker MP, et al. Detection of pars injury by SPECT in patients younger than age 10 with low back pain. J Pediatr Orthop. 2013;33(4):383-8.
11. Inoue M, Minami S, Nakata Y, et al. Preoperative MRI analysis of patients with idiopathic scoliosis: a prospective study. Spine (Phila Pa 1976). 2005;30(1):108-14.
12. Feldman DS, Straight JJ, Badra MI, et al. Evaluation of an algorithmic approach to pediatric back pain. J Pediatr Orthop.2006;26(3):353-7.
13. Brown R, Hussain M, McHugh K, et al. Discitis in young children. J Bone Joint Surg Br. 2001;83(1):106-11.
14. Wenger DR, Bobechko WP, Gilday DL. The spectrum of intervertebral disc-space infection in children. J Bone Joint Surg Am. 1978;60(1):100-8.
15. Huisman TA. Pediatric tumors of the spine. Cancer Imaging. 2009;9(Special issue A):S45-48.
16. Haidar R, Ghanem I, Saad S, et al. Lumbar disc herniation in young children. Acta Paediatr. 2010;99(1):19-23.
17. Lavelle WF, Bianco A, Mason R, et al. Pediatric disk herniation. J Am Acad Orthop Surg. 2011;19(11):649-56.
18. Yamane T, Yoshida T, Mimatsu K. Early diagnosis of lumbar spondylolysis by MRI. J Bone Joint Surg Br. 1993;75(5):764-8.
19. Sairyo K, Katoh S, Takata Y, et al. MRI signal changes of the pedicle as an indicator for early diagnosis of spondylolysis in children and adolescents: a clinical and biomechanical study. Spine (Phila Pa 1976). 2006;31(2):206-11.
20. Sakai T, Sairyo K, Mima S, et al. Significance of magnetic resonance imaging signal change in the pedicle in the management of pediatric lumbar spondylolysis. Spine (Phila Pa 1976). 2010;35(14):E641-5.
21. Pagnini I, Savelli S, Matucci-Cerinic M, et al. Early predictors of juvenile sacroiliitis in enthesitis-related arthritis. J Rheumatol. 2010;37(11):2395-401.
22. Fahey FH, Treves ST, Adelstein SJ. Minimizing and communicating radiation risk in pediatric nuclear medicine. J Nucl Med. 2011;52(8):1240-51.

23. Auerbach JD, Ahn J, Zgonis MH, et al. Streamlining the evaluation of low back pain in children. Clin Orthop Relat Res. 2008;466(8):1971-7.
24. McCann ME, Soriano SG. General anesthetics in pediatric anesthesia: influences on the developing brain. Curr Drug Targets. 2012;13(7):944-51.
25. Sanpera I, Jr., Beguiristain-Gurpide JL. Bone scan as a screening tool in children and adolescents with back pain. J Pediatr Orthop. 2006;26(2):221-5.
26. Zenonos G, Jamil O, Governale LS, et al. Surgical treatment for primary spinal aneurysmal bone cysts: experience from Children's Hospital Boston. J Neurosurg Pediatr. 2012;9(3):305-15.
27. Santangelo JR, Thomson JD. Childhood leukemia presenting with back pain and vertebral compression fractures. Am J Orthop (Belle Mead NJ). 1999;28(4):257-60.
28. Quinlan JF, Duke D, Eustace S. Bertolotti's syndrome. A cause of back pain in young people. J Bone Joint Surg Br. 2006;88(9):1183-6.
29. Weinstein SL, Dolan LA, Spratt KF, et al. Health and function of patients with untreated idiopathic scoliosis: a 50-year natural history study. JAMA. 2003;289(5):559-67.
30. Atanda A Jr, Shah SA, O'Brien K. Osteochondrosis: common causes of pain in growing bones. Am Fam Physician. 2011;83(3):285-91.
31. Damborg F, Engell V, Andersen M, et al. Prevalence, concordance, and heritability of Scheuermann kyphosis based on a study of twins. J Bone Joint Surg Am. 2006;88(10):2133-6.
32. Tsirikos AI, Jain AK. Scheuermann's kyphosis; current controversies. J Bone Joint Surg Br. 2011;93(7):857-64.
33. Murray PM, Weinstein SL, Spratt KF. The natural history and long-term follow-up of Scheuermann kyphosis. J Bone Joint Surg Am. 1993;75(2):236-48.
34. Coe JD, Smith JS, Berven S, et al. Complications of spinal fusion for Scheuermann kyphosis: a report of the Scoliosis Research Society morbidity and mortality committee. Spine (Phila Pa 1976). 2010;35(1):99-103.
35. Kapetanos GA, Hantzidis PT, Anagnostidis KS, et al. Thoracic cord compression caused by disk herniation in Scheuermann's disease: a case report and review of the literature. Eur Spine J. 2006;15(Suppl 5):553-8.
36. Bugg WG, Lewis M, Juette A, et al. Lumbar lordosis and pars interarticularis fractures: a case-control study. Skeletal Radiol. 2012;41(7):817-22.
37. Iwamoto J, Takeda T, Wakano K. Returning athletes with severe low back pain and spondylolysis to original sporting activities with conservative treatment. Scand J Med Sci Sports. 2004;14(6):346-51.
38. Baca KE, Abdullah MA, Ting BL, et al. Surgical decompression for lumbar stenosis in pediatric achondroplasia. J Pediatr Orthop.2010;30(5):449-54.
39. Ryoppy S, Jaaskelainen J, Rapola J, et al. Nonspecific diskitis in children. A nonmicrobial disease? Clin Orthop Relat Res. 1993(297):95-9.
40. Chandrasenan J, Klezl Z, Bommireddy R, et al. Spondylodiscitis in children: a retrospective series. J Bone Joint Surg Br. 93(8):1122-5.
41. Buck JE. Direct repair of the defect in spondylolisthesis. Preliminary report. J Bone Joint Surg Br. 1970;52(3):432-7.
42. Gillet P, Petit M. Direct repair of spondylolysis without spondylolisthesis, using a rod-screw construct and bone grafting of the pars defect. Spine (Phila Pa 1976). 1999;24(12):1252-6.
43. Kakiuchi M. Repair of the defect in spondylolysis. Durable fixation with pedicle screws and laminar hooks. J Bone Joint Surg Am. 1997;79(6):818-25.
44. Songer MN, Rovin R. Repair of the pars interarticularis defect with a cable-screw construct. A preliminary report. Spine (Phila Pa 1976). 1998;23(2):263-69.
45. Molinari RW, Bridwell KH, Lenke LG, et al. Anterior column support in surgery for high-grade, isthmic spondylolisthesis. Clin Orthop Relat Res. 2002(394):109-120.
46. Molinari RW, Bridwell KH, Lenke LG, et al. Complications in the surgical treatment of pediatric high-grade, isthmic dysplastic spondylolisthesis. A comparison of three surgical approaches. Spine (Phila Pa 1976). 1999;24(16):1701-11.
47. Poolman RW, Been HD, Ubags LH. Clinical outcome and radiographic results after operative treatment of Scheuermann's disease. Eur Spine J. 2002;11(6):561-9.
48. Ristolainen L, Kettunen JA, Heliovaara M, et al. Untreated Scheuermann's disease: a 37-year follow-up study. Eur Spine J. 2012;21(5):819-24.
49. Lowe TG. Scheuermann's disease. Orthop Clin North Am. 1999;30(3):475-87, ix.
50. Herndon WA, Emans JB, Micheli LJ, et al. Combined anterior and posterior fusion for Scheuermann's kyphosis. Spine (Phila Pa 1976). 1981;6(2):125-30.
51. Tsutsui S, Pawelek JB, Bastrom TP, et al. Do discs "open" anteriorly with posterior-only correction of Scheuermann's kyphosis? Spine (Phila Pa 1976). 2011;36(16):E1086-92.
52. Fu KM, Smith JS, Polly DW Jr., et al. Morbidity and mortality in the surgical treatment of six hundred five pediatric patients with isthmic or dysplastic spondylolisthesis. Spine (Phila Pa 1976). 2011;36(4):308-12.
53. Sansur CA, Reames DL, Smith JS, et al. Morbidity and mortality in the surgical treatment of 10,242 adults with spondylolisthesis. J Neurosurg Spine. 2010;13(5):589-93.
54. Denis F, Sun EC, Winter RB. Incidence and risk factors for proximal and distal junctional kyphosis following surgical treatment for Scheuermann kyphosis: minimum five-year follow-up. Spine (Phila Pa 1976). 2009;34(20):E729-34.
55. Helenius I, Lamberg T, Osterman K, et al. Scoliosis research society outcome instrument in evaluation of long-term surgical results in spondylolysis and low-grade isthmic spondylolisthesis in young patients. Spine (Phila Pa 1976). 2005;30(3):336-41.
56. Helenius I, Lamberg T, Osterman K, et al. Posterolateral, anterior, or circumferential fusion in situ for high-grade spondylolisthesis in young patients: a long-term evaluation using the Scoliosis Research Society questionnaire. Spine (Phila Pa 1976). 2006;31(2):190-6.

CHAPTER 10

57. Poussa M, Remes V, Lamberg T, et al. Treatment of severe spondylolisthesis in adolescence with reduction or fusion in situ: long-term clinical, radiologic, and functional outcome. Spine (Phila Pa 1976). 2006;31(5):583-90; discussion 591-2.
58. Lundine KM, Lewis SJ, Al-Aubaidi Z, et al. Patient outcomes in the operative and nonoperative management of high-grade spondylolisthesis in children. J Pediatr Orthop. 2014;34(5):483-9.
59. Koptan WM, Elmiligui YH, Elsebaie HB. All pedicle screw instrumentation for Scheuermann's kyphosis correction: is it worth it? Spine J. 2009;9(4):296-302.
60. Lee SS, Lenke LG, Kuklo TR, et al. Comparison of Scheuermann kyphosis correction by posterior-only thoracic pedicle screw fixation versus combined anterior/posterior fusion. Spine (Phila Pa 1976). 2006;31(20):2316-21.
61. Soo CL, Noble PC, Esses SI. Scheuermann kyphosis: long-term follow-up. Spine J. 2002;2(1):49-56.

CHAPTER 11 Congenital Scoliosis

Kaine C Onwuzulike

INTRODUCTION AND BACKGROUND

Scoliosis, a three-dimensional rotational deformity of the spine, is one of the oldest diseases known to mankind. It is a complex group of disorders, which can begin embryologically in congenital forms; however, it is most common during late childhood and adolescence, particularly in girls. The classification of scoliosis is divided into four major categories: (1) idiopathic (unknown causation, subclassified as infantile, juvenile, and adolescent); (2) congenital [failure or formation (hemivertebrae), failure of segmentation (unilateral bars), or mixed]; (3) neuromuscular (myopathic and neurogenic disorders); and (4) syndromic (associated with a syndrome). We will focus most of our attention in this chapter on the congenital subtype.

Congenital scoliosis is defined as spinal deformity resulting from the presence of ≥1 vertebral malformations. It is a direct result of failure of vertebral formation, segmentation, or combination of the two arising from abnormal vertebral development. These malformations occur during embryogenesis (weeks 4–6 of gestation) when other vital organ systems in particular the genitourinary, musculoskeletal, and cardiovascular are forming as well. During embryogenesis, the axial skeleton forms via somitogenesis resulting in transient segments of tissue called somites. Perturbations during this process can give way to vertebral malformations, including uneven segments (hemivertebrae and wedge vertebrae), fused segments (block vertebrae), and alterations in midline fusion (butterfly vertebrae).[1] The malformations are always present at birth and can occur in any part of the spinal column; however, the development of the scoliosis may occur over time. The results of these combined malformations result in a three-dimensional asymmetric growth of the spine resulting in varying degrees of spinal and axial skeletal deformity.[2] The high incidence of associated abnormalities in other organ systems can lead to significant adverse health issues in affected individuals in addition to imposing significant financial constraints on families and the medical system.

The true prevalence of congenital scoliosis is unknown; however, we estimate the overall incidence to be ~1 in every 1,000 live births. Although there is currently no known cause for its development, it appears to be influenced by various external factors such as maternal carbon monoxide exposure, gestational diabetes, and various medications, most notably certain antiepileptic drugs. Besides the 5–10% risk of congenital scoliosis for future siblings of patients with multiple vertebral anomalies, true Mendelian genetic underpinnings remain elusive.[3]

CLASSIFICATION

Congenital scoliosis results from a failure of segmentation, formation, or mixed form (Fig. 1). The classification scheme proposed by Winter and Moe remains one of the most useful and predictive schematics.[2] The vast majority (80%) of anomalies may be classified as either failures of segmentation or formation with the remaining being of mixed form. Defects of formation result in either wedge vertebrae or hemivertebrae. A wedge vertebra results from partial failure of vertebral body formation on one side but maintains bilateral pedicles. Hemivertebrae on the other hand are due to a complete failure of the formation of half of the vertebrae. Hemivertebrae can occur at ipsilateral adjacent levels of the spine producing significantly asymmetrical spine development, or it may occur in

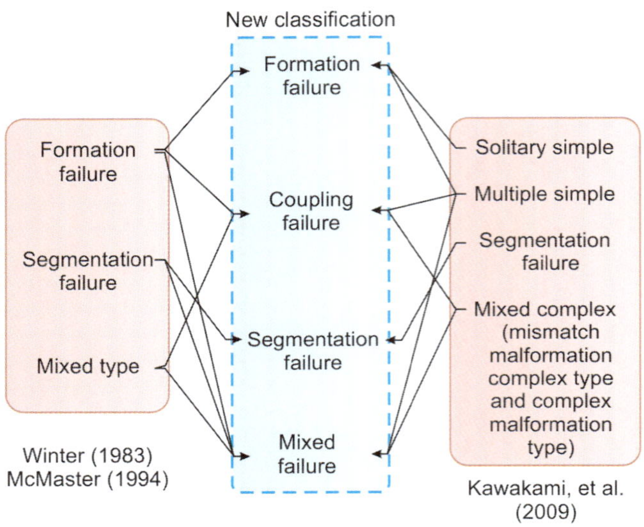

Fig. 1: Classification of congenital scoliosis.

conjunction with hemivertebrae on the contralateral side of the spine separated by one or more healthy vertebrae. There are three main subtypes:

1. *Fully segmented (65%)*: It contains a normal disk both above and below the anomaly.
2. *Partially segmented (22%)*: It is fused to the neighboring vertebrae ipsilaterally with an open disk space on the contralateral side.
3. *Nonsegmented (12%)*: It contains no intervening disk space between the adjacent vertebrae.

Defects of segmentation are characterized by abnormal bony connections between adjacent vertebrae. These can be bilateral and symmetrical resulting in block vertebrae. They are caused by unilateral bony fusions, bars, and act as a unilateral growth tether. In some instances, a segmentation defect crosses an ipsilateral formation defect resulting in a unilateral bar and contralateral hemivertebrae. Mixed defects although common are notoriously hard to characterize given their abnormal anatomy and resulting severe deformity. Scoliosis caused in this manner results in multiple vertebral anomalies with associated rib and thoracic cage developmental abnormalities as well. Risk of progression with each of these subtypes cannot be accurately predicted by the anticipated potential for either unbalance growth due to failures of formation or growth retardation due to tethering created by failures of segmentation.[4,5] The highest risk occurs in situations where there is unbalanced growth opposite the asymmetric tether as in unilateral unsegmented bar with contralateral hemivertebrae. The rate of progression is highly variable but is known to be around 5–10° per year with the most rapid course within the first 5 years of life and from ages 10 years to 14 years. Invariably, those who show deformities within the 1st year of life have the worst overall prognosis.

There have been other proposed classification schemes for congenital scoliosis included by Kawakami et al. by using a three-dimensional classification system, which categorizes congenital scoliosis into 4 types: solitary simple, multiple simple, complex, and segmentation failure. A more recent classification system by Kawakami et al. introduces the concept of coupling failure, which is defined as vertebral anomalies with either anterior or posterior discordancy, or both (anterior, posterior, and anteroposterior type) (Fig. 2).

ASSOCIATED CONDITIONS

Greater than half of individuals with congenital scoliosis, in which progression of curvature often leads to secondary organ involvement, have other associated malformations. Neurologic abnormalities are common and can occur in up to 40% of individuals. Most of these are intraspinal anomalies with diastematomyelia being the most common. Others include intradural lipoma, syringomyelia, Chiari malformation, and tethered cord. Patients with congenital cardiac abnormalities have also been found to have a higher association of scoliosis. The cardiac defects range from atrial and ventricular septal defects, which are the most common abnormalities, to complex congenital heart defects, such as tetralogy of Fallot and transposition of the great vessels. A renal ultrasound remains the mainstay for the identification of these features. The incidence of renal anomalies and congenital scoliosis has been reported to range from 25% to 35%. Common findings include unilateral renal agenesis, renal duplication, ectopic kidney, reflux, and horseshoe kidney. Musculoskeletal anomalies occur frequently and include disorders such as clubfeet, Sprengel deformity, Klippel-Feil deformity, and developmental dysplasia of the hip. A relatively well-known morbidity associated with large progressive curves is the development of restrictive lung disease, which is believed to be a function of both altered lung function and constriction of the chest wall.[6]

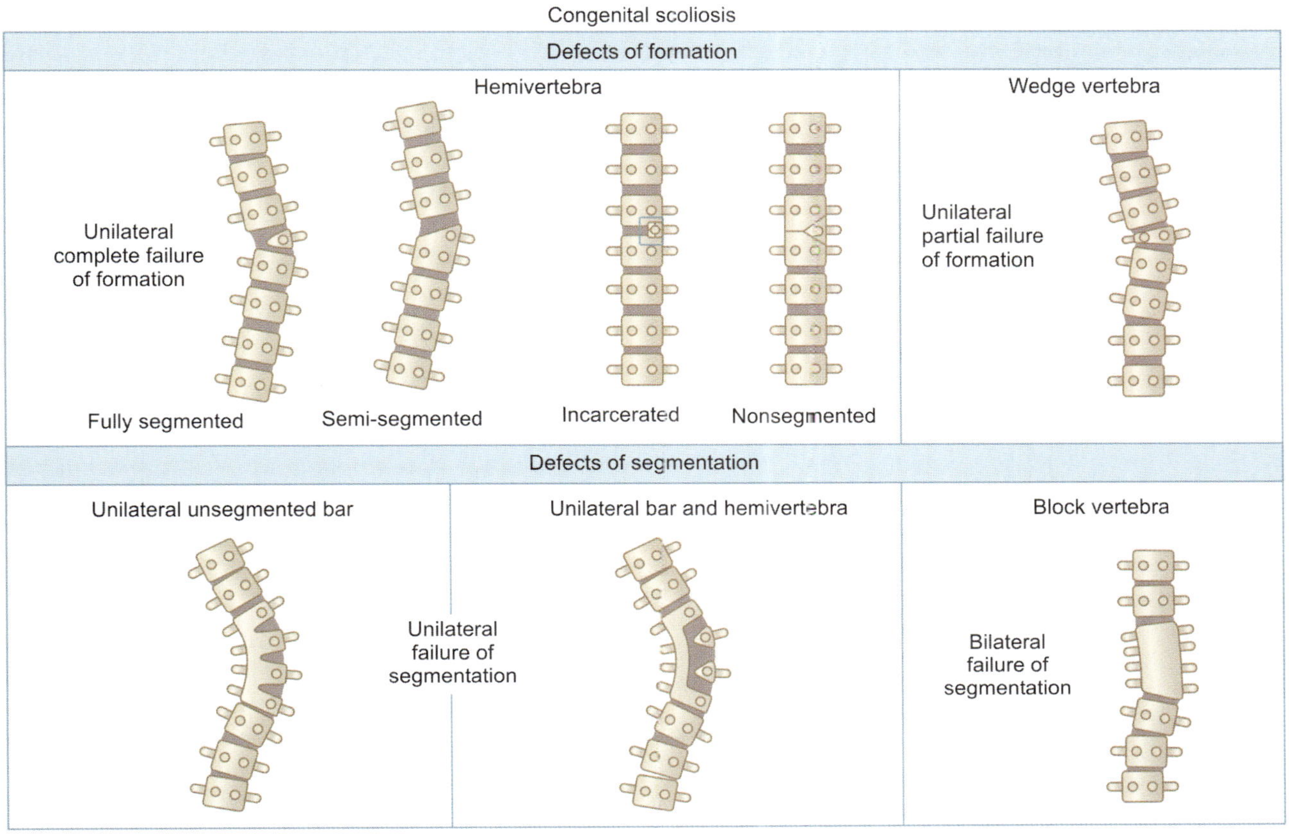

Fig. 2: Schematic representation of defects of formation and segmentation.

PHYSICAL EXAMINATION

Clinical evaluation of patients with congenital scoliosis should begin with a comprehensive medical history including prenatal and birth history, previous medical conditions, and a detailed review of systems. It should be inclusive of the patient's height and weight given the effect of (remaining) growth in curve progression. Of vital importance is documentation of when deformity was first noted. The skin and extremities should be inspected for cutaneous stigmata of spinal dysraphism. These include but are not limited to abnormal pigmentation, hairy patches, or skin tags over the cutaneous region of the spine. Additional physical findings can include: uneven or elevated musculature on one side of the spine; a rib prominence or a prominent shoulder blade (rib hump), caused by rotation of the ribs in thoracic scoliosis; and the appearance of lower extremity length inequality (lumbar curve). Musculoskeletal anomalies such as clubfoot, Sprengel and Klippel-Feil deformities, and developmental dysplasia should prompt investigation of scoliosis in all adolescent patients.

Due to the high incidence of associated renal anomalies, renal ultrasound has become part of the mainstay and evaluating individuals with known scoliosis. In this same manner, cardiac screening by way of echocardiogram is also recommended for patients known to have congenital scoliosis. Given the association of curve progression with pulmonary disease, there should be specific attention paid to children who exhibit hypercarbia or hypoxemia. The most common mechanism for evaluation in this setting is via capillary blood gas and serum hemoglobin analysis.

Symptoms of scoliosis are initially subtle to mild; however, they may become progressive in severe cases and lead to several complications. Detailed evaluation and workup of these patients for associated visceral and neuraxis abnormalities are crucial prior to any surgical intervention. Although consistent criteria for timing of surgical intervention have not been readily established, the rapid progression of deformity at a prepubertal age carries a morbid prognosis and surgical intervention is most often required. Although imaging algorithms across centers vary substantially, three-dimensional radiographic imaging is becoming a mainstay in the management and surgical planning of these patients.

MANAGEMENT

Children with congenital scoliosis require very close observation during growth and in particular until skeletal maturity has been reached. As mentioned previously, although the underlying abnormalities are present at birth, the phenotypically manifestations may not fully manifest until later in development. This underscores the importance of appropriate classification along with the predicted natural history in disease treatment. Even in cases of initial observation, the patient should be monitored with radiographs, initially in 3-month intervals and subsequently in 6–12-month intervals depending on the type of malformation and risk of future progression. For more complex lesions or those associated with an underlying syndrome, more detailed imaging of the soft tissues and neuraxis may entail imaging via CT and MRI as well.

Noninvasive Treatment

There are several noninvasive treatment modalities for congenital scoliosis including bracing, casting, and traction. Little evidence exists in support of bracing alone in congenital scoliosis. It is rarely indicated as these curves are exceptionally rigid and unresponsive to such measures. It may, however, be used as a time-buying maneuver or in combination with other treatments. Bracing is typically reserved for relatively mature patients with documented nonprogression and balanced spinal curves. There are, however, a few exceptions in which it may be considered: compensatory curve above or below the congenital segment, long sweeping congenital curves with a known flexible component, and in the maintenance of truncal and spinal balance during growth. Bracing is absolutely contraindicated in scoliosis types with known poor prognosis such as that with a unilateral bar and contralateral hemivertebrae.[7,8]

Serial derotational casting (Figs. 3A to C) has recently come into favor as a potential "time-buying strategy" for congenital scoliosis. It emphasizes extension, derotation, and flexion of the spine and relies on casting forces to correct spinal deformity during periods of rapid growth. This is mainly to hinder the development of the crankshaft

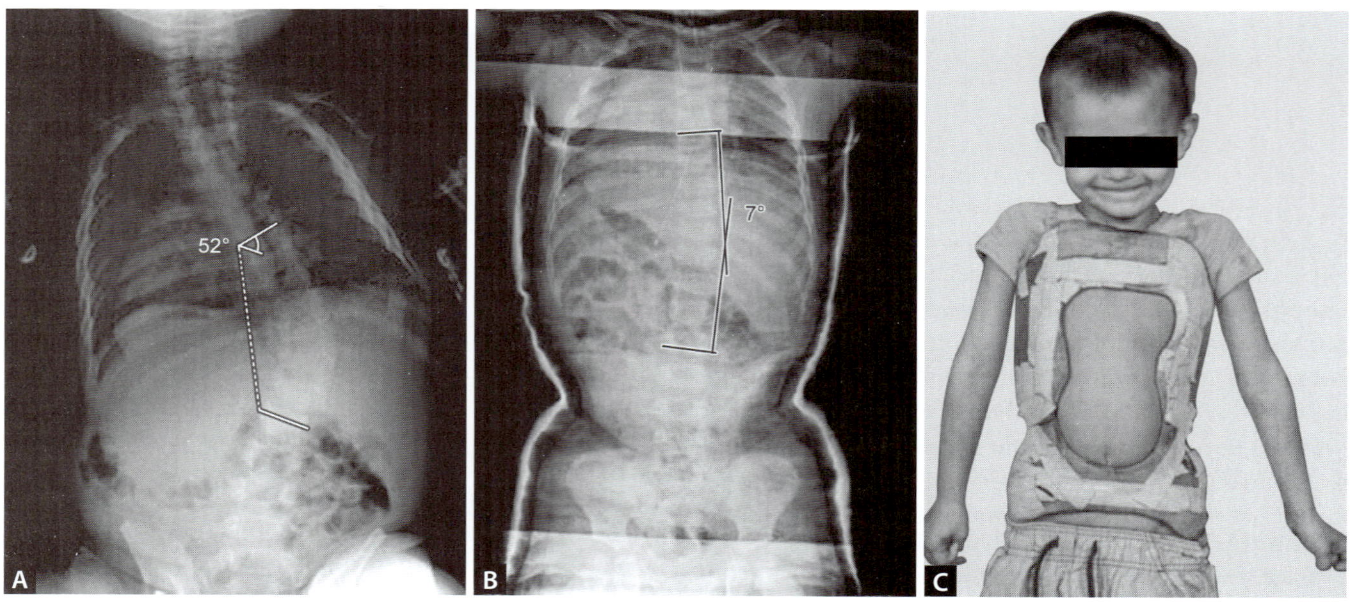

Figs. 3A to C: (A) Posteroanterior radiograph of a 3-year-old boy with idiopathic early onset scoliosis with a progressive curve measuring >50°. (B) Posteroanterior radiograph of the same patient 6 months later after the derotational cast has been applied. (C) Frontal photograph of the same patient showing the cutouts and molding of the cast.

phenomenon and associated impaired respiratory function that can be seen with early long posterior fusions. These time-buying strategies are often useful given the high complication rate seen with prolonged invasive growing rod treatment. Bess et al. reported that the complication rate in such techniques increases by 24% with each lengthening procedure and decreases by 13% for every year of increase in the patient's age at the time of index surgery. Key factors to consider when deciding to employ serial derotational casting include age, etiology, major curve angle, presence of kyphosis, and progression rate.[9]

Halo traction provides another means of nonoperative management and is often used as a viable adjunct in the treatment of severe scoliosis, and has a relatively safe profile. Caution must be exercised in patients with sharp, short, or highly angulated deformities, and is contraindicated in kyphoscoliosis. Its most common application is preoperatively prior to posterior fusion. Its efficacy is derived by maximizing correction of stiff deformities in preparation for surgery. It can be remarkably well tolerated as patients are allowed to be mobile during this treatment. Its added advantage belies its ability to allow patients to maximize nutrition and improved pulmonary function and bone density prior to undergoing definitive treatment. Length of traction is generally between 2 weeks and 12 weeks during which up to 44% of deformity correction can be achieved. In general, between 30% and 50% of total body weight can be tolerated by the patient provided routine neuro checks are obtained. Complications associated with halo gravity traction include pin site infection and loosening.

Early Surgical Treatment

The history of surgical intervention is quite storied and almost unprecedented, with the first attempt being centuries ago. Before we discuss modern surgical treatment, we will first divulge into the history and evolution of its practice. The first recorded attempt of correction of spinal deformity was documented in *Srimad Bhagavata Maha Purana*, an Indian religious mythological book written circa 3500 BC and 1800 BC, where Lord Krishna (a Hindu deity) cured a female devotee with scoliosis by exerting pressure on her back with upward traction on her chin. There have been myriad attempts in the presurgical era to address scoliosis. Hippocrates (460–370 BC) devised

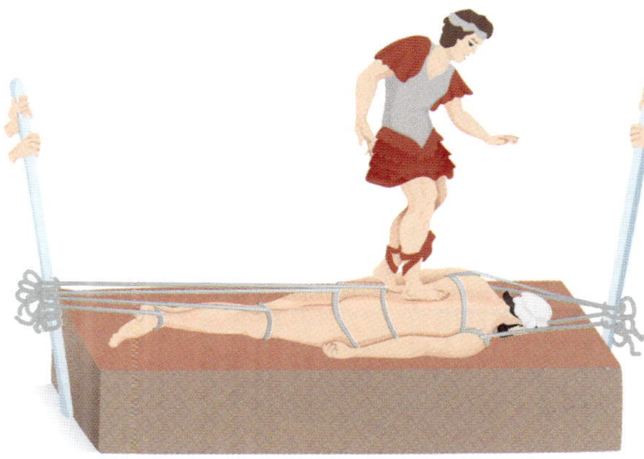

Fig. 4: Hippocrates relied on certain devices for spinal manipulation and traction.

and relied on certain devices for spinal manipulation and traction (Fig. 4). He advocated the use of scamnum and succession (shaking) methodologies for patients with such deformities. Galen, who is credited for the description and use of the terms scoliosis, kyphosis, and lordosis, used a combination of axial traction and direct pressure to treat spinal deformities.

Prior to the Medical Renaissance, all attempts at the correction of scoliosis were without an intimate knowledge of the anatomy and biomechanical properties of the spine. Leonardo da Vinci (1452–1519) first meticulously described the anatomy and biomechanics of the spine, and in doing so described the intimate relationship of the various curvatures and articulations between the spinal vertebrae, sectioning them into the three parts as we know today, i.e. cervical, thoracic, and lumbar along with their associated lordotic and kyphotic curvatures, respectively. Giovanni Alfonso Borelli (1608–1679), widely considered the father of spinal biomechanics, wrote the first text on biomechanics entitled *De Motu Animalium* (Fig. 5). He theorized that scoliosis is derived from an imbalance of the vertebral muscles, and his illustration of a crooked tree strapped to a straight stake remains the symbol of orthopedic surgery today.

The aforementioned pioneers soon thrust the medical consortium into the surgical era, replete with equally progressive pioneers and modern contemporaries. The first surgical expose to treat scoliosis was reported in the mid-19th century. Jules Rene Guerin (1801–1886), a French orthopedist, initiated the operative management for scoliosis via a series of percutaneous myotomies of the

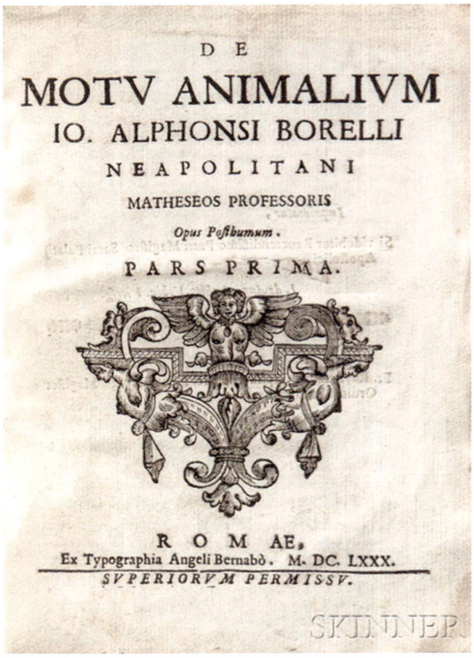

DE
MOTV ANIMALIVM
IO. ALPHONSI BORELLI
NEAPOLITANI
MATHESEOS PROFESSORIS
Opus Posthumum.
PARS PRIMA.
ROMAE,
Ex Typographia Angeli Bernabò. M. DC. LXXX.
SVPERIORVM PERMISSV.

Fig. 5: Hippocrates' wrote over 50 medical books, many of which are included in the *Hippocratic Collection* (*Corpus Hippocraticum*).

vertebral musculature. His postoperative management consisted of bracing, which is still used in the perioperative period in modern day.

A revolution occurred in the surgical management with the discovery and use of X-rays. This allowed for the visualization of pre- and postoperative subjects and their respective curvatures. A seminal event occurred in the early 20th century with the establishment of fusion techniques by Dr Russell Hibbs (1869–1933). His partner Joseph Risser is credited for the development of the "Risser Sign", a radiological feature characterized in the anteroposterior orientation classifies the ossification of the iliac epiphysis and is beneficial in delineating cessation of skeletal growth in conjunction with the ideal timing for surgical intervention. Another widely used and monumentally important radiographic measure, the Cobb angle, was introduced by its namesake, John Cobb, and is considered the gold standard with respect to objective descriptions of scoliosis measurements.[10,11]

Modern Surgical Treatment

Current guidelines regarding surgical intervention for congenital scoliosis suggest intervention for deformities that are increasing in severity or anomalies that are predicted to have a high risk of future progression. Historically, it has been noted to be easier to prevent a deformity rather than correct one, which belies the importance in keen observation and knowledge of the natural history and type of anomaly. Goals of surgery are to arrest further progression of curvature and to improve global balance while maximizing unobstructed future growth without disturbing neurological function. This requires knowledge of a wide array of techniques to be included in the surgical armamentarium. Surgical treatment of such patients carries a risk of neurological injury greater than that of patients with idiopathic spinal deformities. Often neurosurgical treatment for comorbidities such as tethered and split cord malformation can occur simultaneously or prior to definitive curvature correction. These dual surgeries depend greatly on the complexity of procedure, and require definitive input from the neurosurgeon.[12] Prior to initiation of surgery, a comprehensive medical evaluation detailing the spinal anomalies, pulmonary function, and nutritional status of the patient is required. Treatment is generally categorized into procedures that will prevent or control versus those which correct the deformity in question.[13,14]

In Situ Fusion

It is relatively safe procedure and is typically employed in cases where the curve is predicted to worsen or there has been known progression. In situ fusion can halt progression and is ideal for a small curve. It is most frequently used in cases of a unilateral bar or a unilateral bar with contralateral hemivertebrae. Fusion levels should encompass the vertebrae of the measured Cobb angle and should extend to a level above and below the anomalous segment(s). In situ arthrodesis over a short segment is associated with minimal limited loss in spinal height and has durable long-term results. Its success is based on complete facet resection, decortication, and use of abundant auto- or allograft material. A side effect of such posterior fusion in the face of open anterior growth plates with normal disk spaces is the development of the crankshaft phenomenon, which is thought to occur secondary to continued growth of the anterior elements of the spine after solid posterior spinal fusion causing vertebral bodies and disks to bulge laterally toward the convexity and to pivot on the posterior fusion, causing loss of correction, increase in vertebral rotation, and recurrence of the rib hump.[15]

Convex Hemiepiphysiodesis

This is a partial growth arrest procedure particularly effective when there is little to no concave growth potential as in unilateral failure of formation resulting in hemivertebrae. While most correction is obtained initially in the postoperative cast, some correction can be achieved over time depending on age and growth potential of the child. These procedures are typically performed anteriorly with extirpation of the disk and growth plates, along with anterior spinal fusion plus a posterior spinal hemiarthrodesis (on the convexity side). They are typically reserved for patients younger than 5 years with only modest deformity. Both, convex hemiepiphysiodesis and in situ fusion, are generally low risk; however, they offer limited correction.

Hemivertebrae Excision

Hemivertebrae excision, described initially by Bradford and then subsequently by Klemme et al., is traditionally a sequential anterior excision followed by posterior excision, which results in a circumferential exposure of the affected spine allowing removal of the disks above and below the hemivertebra in addition to the bone itself. The associated lamina and pedicle are removed and the convexity of the curve is compressed posteriorly allowing for instrumented fusion. The excision of hemivertebrae provides an immediate correction of the congenital deformity and restoration of global balance. It is a safe and effective tool for treating isolated hemivertebrae. The optimal indication for hemivertebrae resection is similar to those of convex hemiepiphysiodesis and in situ fusion, that being the patient less than 5 years of age with a radical lumbar or lumbosacral hemivertebrae and corresponding truncal imbalance. Differences in technique include combined anterior/posterior and posterior only hemivertebrae excision, which itself is a labor intensive procedure best performed at high-volume institutions with an experienced caregivers.[4]

Distraction-based Techniques

Nonfusion instrumentation techniques aim to moderate progressive spinal deformity while allowing for spinal growth via serial lengthening procedures, until the child reaches an appropriate size and maturity prior to undergoing definitive fusion. These techniques apply longitudinal forces, which bypass the apex of the curve. This allows fusing only short segment at the end of the construct and allows for relatively unobstructed chest wall development. Instrumentation in these cases is attached to the spine ribs and/or pelvis. They are considered growth friendly and include traditional growing rods, magnetically controlled growth rods, and vertical expandable prosthetic titanium rib (VEPTR) constructs. Preserving growth with control of spinal deformity in young children is an attractive and formidable concept. This is especially applicable when the deformity is recognized early in its evolution.

Vertical Expandable Prosthetic Titanium Ribs

Traditional surgical management, including fusion in situ and hemiepiphysiodesis, has not been effective in addressing the multithoracic deformity and insufficiency in patients with multiple congenital abnormalities of the developing spine. Furthermore, arthrodesis frequently limits the growth of the thoracic spine and lungs resulting in constriction and poor pulmonary performance. Drs Robert Campbell and Melvin Smith developed VEPTR in an ongoing effort to treat thoracic insufficiency syndrome (TIS) in which the function of the thorax is insufficient to support the normal growth and development of the spinal column. VEPTR is most commonly used for congenital scoliosis with fused ribs, in which the device is implanted to maximize thoracic volume and symmetry via the distraction and lengthening of the constricted hemithorax via a transverse opening-wedge thoracostomy of the concave side, typically through osteotomy of fused ribs or intercostal muscle lysis (Fig. 6). Scoliosis is initially corrected by the thoracostomy, and the thoracic reconstruction is further stabilized by the addition of a rib to spine or rib to pelvis VEPTR construct. Bracing is not required postoperatively and VEPTRs are subsequently lengthened every 4–6 months with final fusion being performed once skeletal maturity is attained. Complications related to the use of VEPTR have paralleled that of other growth preservation systems. The most common entities being anchor migration, implant failure, wound infection, and loss of control of the deformity.[16]

Growing Rods

Harrington initially described the technique of fusionless spine surgery in children younger than 10 years of age with the use of a single subperiosteal distraction rod. His

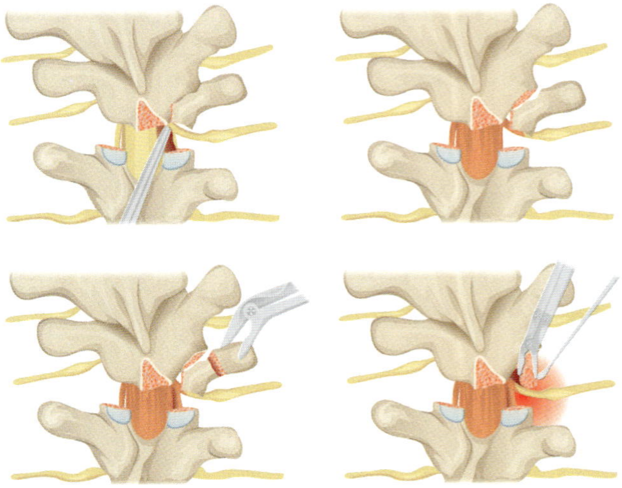

Fig. 6: Hemivertebrae excision.

initial description has been subsequently modified with numerous variations existing on the technique. Progressive deformities in patients without rib anomalies and a physiologically segmented spine are classic indications for submuscular rod construct(s) with solid fixation of 1 motion segment at both ends and scheduled lengthenings to facilitate growth.[17] They can be implanted as a single rod or dual rod constructs, which themselves seem to confer a select advantage with respect to complication rates, reoperations, gain in length, and control of deformity. More progressive options include magnetically controlled growing rods, which allow lengthening procedures without the need of anesthesia or surgical intervention (Figs. 7A and B).

Spinal Instrumentation

As discussed previously, the history of operative intervention for scoliosis spans well over a century and encompasses both instrumented and noninstrumented fusion, growth-friendly and magnetically controlled implants. Indications for instrumentation and fusion of pediatric deformity cases vary with the age, diagnosis, and severity. Congenital scoliosis presents one of the most challenging aspects of deformity correction surgery. Performing an instrumented fusion in a young child impedes growth of the thorax and soft tissues and organs within it and may result in the crankshaft phenomenon. Although anterior arthrodesis may combine with posterior

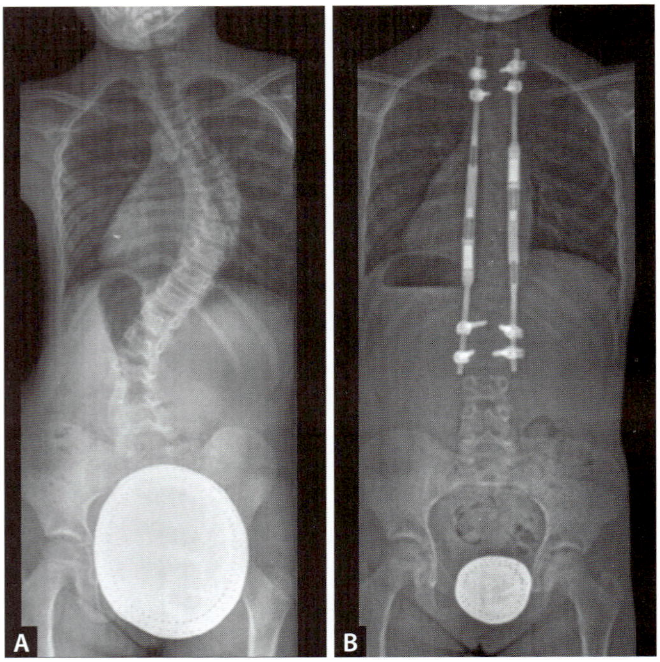

Figs. 7A and B: (A) PA radiograph of a 7-year-old patient with early onset idiopathic scoliosis. (B) Two years postoperative PA radiograph after 6 lengthenings with magnetically controlled growing rods.

spinal fusion to prevent the crankshaft phenomenon, this can result in significant loss of trunk height. When surgery is indicated, surgical implants that allow for some spinal growth are preferable. Such growth friendly implants have been classified into three distinct categories, each defined by the innate correction strategy. These include—distraction, compression, and guided growth systems. While the various detailed surgical procedures and nuances for each type of deformity correction are beyond the scope of this chapter, we will address general surgical tenets with respect to deformity correction.

After comprehensive analysis of the deformity, the natural history, and documentation of progression, surgery is usually indicated. A multimodality evaluation of the patient is necessary to assess and manage any associated anomalies, cardiopulmonary function, and nutritional status. The surgeon should have access to a versatile system with the robust inventory of various size implants for each patient. Facetectomies, ligamentum flavum resection, posterior osteotomies, and anterior discectomies are often employed when treating long severe and rigid curves. Vertebral column resection is a technically demanding procedure for use in the most rigid, deformed, fused, and unsegmented areas when there are no further options for correction. Surgical treatment carries a slight-to-moderate risk of neurological injury; however, the primary goal of treatment, irrespective of etiology, is preventing further progression of the curve magnitude. The use of neuromonitoring is a must. Over the past century, substantial understanding and improvement in the surgical correction of scoliosis have been made. The array of surgical options should be inclusive of techniques encompassing the array of encountered pathologies. The explicit goals of management of patients with congenital scoliosis are appropriate spinal alignment with balanced spine, maximized cardiopulmonary function, optimized spinal height, and maintenance of neurological function.[18]

Segmental instrumentation enables application of corrective forces, including cantilevering, rotation, transverse traction, distraction, and compression, resulting in kyphosis or lordosis, respectively. The use of pedicle screws for posterior instrumented spinal fusion is the preferred and most widely used modality for deformity correction in skeletally mature individuals. They have been shown to be both safe and reliable.

Advantages

Major advantages of the definitive surgical procedures are that they prevent further curve progression and in some cases help to restore spinal alignment prior to final fusion. Above all, they help to allow for further spine and truncal growth, which enhances the space available for the lungs and stabilizes pulmonary functions. This is critically important in the developing child and is a major goal of this type of treatment in very young children.

OPERATIVE DETAIL AND PREPARATION

Operative preparation begins with an experienced team. During preadmission testing, appropriate nasal cultures are obtained for possible methicillin-resistant *Staphylococcus aureus*.

Standard blood work is also performed. Prior to surgery, PA and lateral standing as well as anteroposterior (AP) supine maximum bending radiographs are obtained. Appropriate measurements are made to determine flexibility, which will be an aid in determining the proximal and distal end vertebrae of the fusion. At the time of surgery, intravenous and intra-arterial lines are inserted. Most patients will receive intrathecal morphine as an adjuvant to postoperative pain management. The spinal cord monitoring lines are inserted at this time. The patient is then positioned in the prone position on a Jackson table. This allows for proper truncal and extremity support and avoidance of pressure on the abdomen that will increase venous pressure and postoperative bleeding. Patients receive intraoperative antibiotics as well as an antifibrinolytic to help minimize blood loss. It is important that fluoroscopy or an intraoperative computed tomography (CT) scanner be available to assist during the procedure. Bipolar sealer device has recently been shown to be very effective to further decrease intraoperative blood loss.

Following appropriate prepping and draping, the skin is marked for the incision. A Bovie cord is used as a guide to create a straight line incision. The subcutaneous tissues are infiltrated with a 1 to 500,000 saline and epinephrine solution. This helps to constrict the superficial vessels and minimize blood loss. The fascia is exposed and split over the spinous processes of the vertebrae to be instrumented. Further infusion of the saline and epinephrine solution is performed down to the lamina. Subperiosteal dissection is then carried out. Intraoperative radiography or fluoroscopy is used to identify the planned end vertebrae for instrumentation. The spine has been completely cleared of muscle and soft tissues. Facetectomies are performed and the underlying cartilage is removed. This will enhance fusion. Once the facetectomies have been completed, instrumentation can be performed. There are a variety of instrumentation techniques. These include all-pedicle screw constructs, hybrid constructs with thoracic hooks and lumbar pedicle screws, and all-hook constructs. The two former techniques are the most widely used today. When pedicle screws are used, the posterior entrance to the pedicle is exposed by removing all overlying cortical bone. The pedicle is then probed and the site felt with the ball-tipped probe. Preoperative radiographs are utilized to determine the approximate diameter of the screws. This is also helpful in determining the length of the screws. The site is then tapped, if nontapping screws are to be used. If self-tapping screws are utilized, then tapping is not necessary. Once the desired pattern of implants on both the right and left sides of the spine has been performed, fluoroscopy is used to check the screws alignment, particularly their direction and length. If acceptable, then electromyographic (EMG) stimulation of all pedicle screws is performed. There is typically stimulation up to

30 milliamperes (mA). Transmission of signals of less than 10 mA is of concern for a medial breach of the pedicle. Higher amplitude usually is not significant. The concavity rod is inserted first. This can be a 5.0, 5.5, or 6.35 titanium or cobalt chrome rod depending on the size of the patient. Stainless steel can also be considered but is less common due to the associated nickel allergy. Once it is properly aligned, the rod is then rotated away from the concavity until it appears entirely straight when viewed from a posterior aspect. Beginning with a proximal or distal approach, the first set screw is tightened and compression or distraction is applied between the screws. The convex of the rod is inserted next and the opposite compression–distraction mode is performed. The spine will typically look completely straight at the end of the procedures. A final check with either fluoroscopy or CT is then performed. If the alignment is satisfactory and spinal cord monitoring normal, the wound is irrigated. The exposed bone is then decorticated and this bone plus an additional 90–120 mm from homologous cancelous bone cubes are applied throughout the spine. The wound is closed in layers. This usually consists of the fascia and subcutaneous tissues. A single drain is placed on the top fascia and brought out over one of the iliac crests. This helps to remove any postoperative blood. The skin is closed with a running subcuticular closure. Steri-Strips (3M Healthcare Products, St Paul, MN) and sterile dressings are then applied. The patient is then returned to bed and final radiographs are obtained. Particular attention is paid to the chest to be certain that a pneumothorax has not occurred. If the final radiographs are satisfactory, the patient is awakened, the neurological status is checked, and the patient is sent to the postanesthesia care unit (PACU).

Newer less invasive surgical treatments are emerging, which include minimally invasive spinal deformity correction. There is a steep learning curve associated with these techniques; however, they offer significantly less blood loss, less muscle disruption, decreased length of stay, and less cosmetic scarring. They also seem to offer the same degree of correction in comparison to more traditional open methods.

OPERATIVE PLANNING AND SPECIAL EQUIPMENT

Preoperative planning begins when the patient has met the appropriate criteria for surgical intervention. This is based on the measurements on the preoperative PA standing radiograph of the entire spine. Once this decision has been made, then additional studies are necessary. The flexibility of the spine is assessed by preoperative AP supine maximum right- and left-bending radiographs of the entire spine. These angles are measured using the same levels as were obtained from the standing radiographs. Flexibility helps to determine the upper and lower vertebrae to be instrumented. The final flexibility assessment is made intraoperatively with a traction radiograph. In this technique, the anesthesiologist applies traction to the patient's head and a resident, fellow, or clinical nurse applies traction to the feet. Gentle but maximum traction is applied and a repeat AP radiograph of the entire spine is obtained. Again, the same measurement levels are utilized. The end vertebrae are determined by the most horizontal vertebrae from proximal and distal aspects and by using the center sacral line. This line should pass between the pedicles and be relatively centered. Bending radiographs are also useful because they demonstrate the motion in the disk space. The disk space that reverses its alignment on the side-bending films is usually quite flexible and can also be utilized to help determine the end vertebrae.[19,20]

A considerable amount of special equipment is necessary in performing spinal deformity surgery in addition to the appropriate implants. This includes the use of intraoperative fluoroscopy and/or CT scanner. Intrathecal morphine and antifibrinolytic are administered to help in management of pain postoperatively and perioperative blood loss. A bipolar sealing device will be very effective in further decreasing intraoperative blood loss. Of course, all patients require antibiotics to minimize the risk for postoperative infection—one of the more serious complications of this type of surgery.

KEY STEPS OF THE PROCEDURE/OPERATIVE NUANCES

All the steps in the procedure of spinal deformity correction are critically important. The reader can probably tell by now that there are several key points. These include antibiotic administration to decrease the risk of an acute postoperative infection; the administration of intrathecal morphine to aid in postoperative pain management; the use of antifibrinolytic medications, such as tranexamic acid and epsilon aminocaproic acid, to decrease intraoperative blood loss; the use of a bipolar sealing device to further enhance the control of intraoperative spinal cord monitoring, including transcranial motor and somatosensory evoked potentials; and a detailed knowledge of spinal anatomy. Decreasing blood loss results in better exposure of the spine intraoperatively, has less of a physiological impact postoperatively, helps speed overall recovery, and lower costs. Intrathecal morphine will result in decreased pain and fewer pain related complications and helps to speed the patient's overall recovery.[21]

Perhaps the most important operative nuance is understanding the spinal anatomy, particularly that of the pedicles. They become more oblique in the upper thoracic spine and more vertical in the lumbar spine. Awareness of this anatomical change allows more accurate probing and insertion of pedicle screws. This results in fewer medial breaches and reduces the possibility of neurological injury.

HAZARDS/RISKS/AVOIDANCE OF PITFALLS

The greatest risk in pediatric spinal deformity surgery occurs intraoperatively, when nerve root and spinal cord injury are most likely to occur. This is usually an iatrogenic complication. A thorough knowledge of anatomy as well as experience performing this type of surgery is critically important to help minimize complications. The highest risk for neurological injury occurs in children who have congenital scoliosis. Given the rigid, inflexible curves, multiple types of procedures including osteotomies and hemivertebrae excision may need to be incorporated at the time of correction. These are intense and technically demanding procedures. Knowledge of spinal anatomy and experience will help the surgeon to minimize the risk. Many times, these complications can be minimized or prevented entirely by intraoperative spinal cord monitoring. An experienced monitoring technician is mandatory in this type of surgery.[22]

Other risk factors include hypotension, which can affect blood flow to the spinal cord and results in neurological injury. It is essential that hypotensive anesthesia, commonly performed in this type of surgery, be maintained with a pressure of approximately 70 mm Hg. If neurological changes are seen, raising the blood pressure is the first and many times the most crucial step in reversing any potential monitoring changes.

SALVAGE AND RESCUE

This section deals primarily with the onset of intraoperative spinal cord monitoring changes. This is very critical change and one that must be managed appropriately to prevent any impending spinal cord or neurological problem. The first steps when intraoperative spinal cord monitoring changes have occurred are to stop the procedure, raise the blood pressure back physiological levels, and be certain the patient is hemodynamically stable by giving blood replacement, if necessary. If these actions do not result in improvement in spinal cord monitoring over a 5–10-minute interval, then a wake-up test must be performed. This consists of reversing the anesthesia and having somebody at the patient's feet to assess for movement when the patient is asked to move the feet by the anesthesiologist. The surgeon's role is to be certain the patient does not shift on the Jackson table because there is a potential for a fall. If the spinal cord monitoring changes reverse and the patient's wake-up test shows voluntary motion in the feet, anesthesia is reintroduced even though the mean arterial blood pressure may be higher. The procedure can then resume. However, if there are recurrent spinal cord monitoring changes, it is best to abort the procedure, close the wound, and come back in 1–2 weeks to complete the process. The patient then undergoes an urgent evaluation to be certain that there are no other abnormalities, such as an extradural or intradural hematoma, that may be applying pressure on the spinal cord or nerve roots. This is best assessed by postoperative MRI.

OUTCOMES AND POSTOPERATIVE COURSE

The authors assess outcomes of pediatric spinal deformity surgery on several factors. First and foremost are the avoidance of complications, safe deformity correction, restoration of physiological frontal and sagittal plane alignment and balance, and no need for further surgery. These are achieved by detailed preoperative assessment of the patient, appropriate determination of the end vertebrae, and meticulous surgical procedure and appropriate postoperative management.[7]

POSTOPERATIVE CONSIDERATIONS

The postoperative management of patients following spinal deformity surgery is vital. There are significant variations across centers; however, certain mandates remain paramount for optimal care. Generally, children and adolescents with idiopathic scoliosis do not want to wear orthosis. However, it may be necessary for some patients with neuromuscular and congenital scoliosis to use an orthosis, because it will help their sitting alignment and function. Children are placed on protected activities for 5 months postoperatively. This means no organized sports or gym. Nevertheless, they are allowed to engage in individual activities, such as swimming, jogging, or bicycle riding. They are more than capable of doing routine household chores. The main goal is to avoid activities in which the patient is subject to falls or injuries until the spine has had adequate time for initial healing. Patients with neuromuscular scoliosis may return to physical therapy when they are comfortable. The therapist should avoid any truncal activities. Patients with syndromic scoliosis are more variable, depending on their preoperative functional level.

COMPLICATIONS

Complications in spinal deformity surgery in children and adolescents are relatively uncommon but are higher than of adolescent idiopathic types due to the repetitive nature of the lengthening procedures, increased instrumentation along with their inherent stresses on the mobile developing spine. The risks for neurological injury, which is the most severe complication of this type of surgery, can vary significantly. Postoperative infection occurs in 2–8% of patients and increases with frequency and proximity of interventions. The risk for bone implant and metal failure in the immediate postoperative period is rare. Late pseudarthrosis is also uncommon and is usually manifested by a broken rod. Late infection is more likely, especially an acute postoperative infection. Younger children, neuromuscular and syndromic children, and higher curve magnitude as well as rigid immobile spines are associated with higher complication rates.

CONCLUSION

The history of spinal deformity spans centuries, with early pioneers utilizing novel inventions and various forms of treatments including observation, traction, bracing, and casting to address this relative unknown. With the advent of novel techniques and practices, surgical intervention has become the mainstay with minimal morbidity and relatively no mortality. This has resulted in the achievement of spinal arthrodesis with arrest of curve progression, allowing those affected to live normal lives, and in many cases pursue activities previously relegated to those without such ailments such as contact sports. Recent advances in operative and nonoperative techniques and understanding regarding the importance of preserving the thoracic space have improved the morbidity and mortality of children with progressive congenital scoliosis. Better outcomes favor simple procedures with a low complication profile. VEPTR may be beneficial for select patients with congenital scoliosis and fused ribs with TIS. In situ fusion or hemiepiphysiodesis are viable options when there is little deformity present; however, further progression is likely to occur. More severe deformities will require instrumentation and arthrodesis, which should be done after reaching skeletal maturity. For severe and rigid deformities, osteotomies and resections to balance the spine may be required.

With renewed focus on global craniocervical alignment, we are now more than anytime previously, appropriately, and sufficiently armed with knowledge and techniques to positively impact those affected with congenital scoliosis and offer them optimal interventions, improvement in global alignment, and hastened recovery.

REFERENCES

1. Shah SA, Song K. Congenital Scoliosis. Chapter 18.
2. Erol B, Tracy MR, Dormans JP, et al. Congenital scoliosis and vertebral malformations: characterization of segmental defects for genetic analysis. J Pediatr Orthop. 2004;24(6):674-82.
3. Heary RF, Madhavan K. Genetics of scoliosis. Neurosurgery. 2008;63(Suppl 3):222-7.
4. Hedequist D, Emans J. Congenital scoliosis: a review and update. J Pediatr Orthop. 2007;27(1):106-16.
5. Lopez-Sosa F, Guille JT, Bowen JR. Rotation of the spine in congenital scoliosis. J Pediatr Orthop. 1995;15(4):528-34.
6. McPhail GL, Howells SA, Boesch RP, et al. Obstructive lung disease is common in children with syndromic and congenital scoliosis: a preliminary study. J Pediatr Orthop. 2013;33(8):781-5.
7. Heary RF, Bono CM, Kumar S. Bracing for scoliosis. Neurosurgery. 2008;63(Suppl 3):125-30.
8. Kawakami N, Koumoto I, Dogaki Y, et al. Clinical impact of corrective cast treatment for early onset scoliosis: is it a worthwhile treatment option to suppress scoliosis progression before surgical intervention? J Pediatr Orthop. 2018;38(10):e556-61.
9. Hasler CC. Early-onset scoliosis: contemporary decision-making and treatment options. J Pediatr Orthop. 2018;38(Suppl 1):S13-20.
10. Heary RF, Madhavan K. The history of spinal deformity. Neurosurgery. 2008;63(Suppl 3):5-15.
11. Pahys JM, Guille JT. What's new in congenital scoliosis? J Pediatr Orthop. 2018;38(3):e172-9.

12. Sansone JM, Mann D, Noonan K, et al. Rapid progression of scoliosis following insertion of intrathecal baclofen pump. J Pediatr Orthop. 2006;26(1):125-8.
13. Beauchamp EC, Anderson RCE, Vitale MG. Modern surgical management of early onset and adolescent idiopathic scoliosis. Neurosurgery. 2019;184(2):291-304.
14. McGirt MJ, Mehta V, Garces-Ambrossi G, et al. Pediatric tethered cord syndrome: response of scoliosis to untethering procedures. J Neurosurg Pediatr. 2009;4(3):270-4.
15. Terek RM, Wehner J, Lubicky JP. Crankshaft phenomenon in congenital scoliosis: a preliminary report. J Pediatr Orthop. 1991;11(4):527-32.
16. Flynn JM, Emans JB, Smith JT, et al. VEPTR to treat nonsyndromic congenital scoliosis: a multicenter, mid-term follow-up study. J Pediatr Orthop. 2013;33(7):679-84.
17. Elsebai HB, Yazici M, Thompson GH, et al. Safety and efficacy of growing rod technique for pediatric congenital spinal deformities. J Pediatr Orthop. 2011;31(1):1-5.
18. Tis JE, Karlin LI, Akbarnia BA, et al. Growing Spine Committee of the Scoliosis Research Society. Early onset scoliosis: modern treatment and results. J Pediatr Orthop. 2012;32(7):647-57.
19. Iorio J, Orlando G, Diefenbach C, et al. Serial casting for infantile idiopathic scoliosis: radiographic outcomes and factors associated with response to treatment. J Pediatr Orthop. 2017;37(5):311-6.
20. Larson N, Polly DW Jr, Guidera KJ, et al. The accuracy of navigation and 3D image-guided placement for the placement of pedicle screws in congenital spine deformity. J Pediatr Orthop. 2012;32(6):e23-9.
21. Smith JS, Abel MF, Shaffrey CI, et al. Decision-making in pediatric spinal deformity. Neurosurgery. 2008;63(Suppl 3):54-68.
22. Fletcher ND, Larson AN, Richards BS, et al. Current treatment preferences for early onset scoliosis: a survey of POSNA members. J Pediatr Orthop. 2011;31(3):326-30.

CHAPTER 12

Idiopathic Scoliosis

Richard E Bowen, Natalie L Leong

EPIDEMIOLOGY AND NATURAL HISTORY

Definitions

Scoliosis is a musculoskeletal condition in which there is deviation of the spinal cord by at least 10° in the coronal plane; curvature of the spine that measures less than 10° is called spinal asymmetry. This chapter will focus on idiopathic scoliosis, which has no well-established etiology, as opposed to congenital, syndrome-associated, or neuromuscular scoliosis. Idiopathic scoliosis is classified by age of onset. Infantile idiopathic scoliosis is characterized by an onset at age 0 to 3 years, juvenile idiopathic scoliosis has an onset from 4 years to 10 years, and adolescent idiopathic scoliosis has an onset from 11 years to 17 years, while adult idiopathic scoliosis is defined as cases with onset past 17 years of age.[1] Additionally, curves are described based on the location of the apex, or most laterally deviated and most horizontal vertebra at the center of the curve (Table 1).[1] The location of a curve has implications on the likelihood of progression and thus the treatment of the curve. In some cases, there is an apical disk but not a single apex vertebra, and thus two apex vertebrae are defined. The end vertebrae define the outer limits of the curve, and are the most angulated from the horizontal. The central sacral vertical line (CSVL), a vertical line that bisects the sacrum, is used for assessing the balance of the spine in relation to the pelvis. The stable vertebra is the most cephalad vertebra distal to the curve that is bisected by the CSVL. The neutral vertebra is the most cephalad vertebra that remains without transverse plane rotation.[1]

Table 1: Classification of curves by location.

Curve type	*Location of apex*
Cervical	C2–C6
Cervicothoracic	C7–T1
Thoracic	T2–T11
Thoracolumbar	T11–L4
Lumbar	L2–L4
Lumbosacral	L5 or below

Epidemiology

Infantile idiopathic scoliosis is rare, accounting for only 1% of the cases of pediatric idiopathic scoliosis, and 60% of patients with this diagnosis are males.[2] Juvenile idiopathic scoliosis accounts for 10–15% of idiopathic scoliosis, and tends toward boys with left sided curves at the lower end of the age spectrum of 4 to 10 years, while girls with right thoracic curves are more common at the upper end of the age spectrum.[3] Adolescent idiopathic scoliosis is the most common form of idiopathic scoliosis and is estimated to have a prevalence of 2–4%, with a prevalence of curves greater than 30° estimated at 0.2% and curves greater than 40° at 0.1%.[4,5] Adolescent idiopathic scoliosis is 2 to 10 times more prevalent in females than males, with approximately equal prevalence in 10° curves and a progressive increase in female predominance with higher degree curves.[4]

Etiology

Even after decades of research, there is no single universally accepted theory regarding the etiology and pathogenesis of scoliosis. While a specific gene or set of genes has not been identified as the cause of idiopathic scoliosis, the observation of increased prevalence of scoliosis among relatives of individuals with scoliosis supports the presence of genetic factors. It is estimated that approximately 11% of first-degree relatives of individuals with scoliosis also have scoliosis.[6] When both parents have scoliosis, the chance of an affected child is 50 times greater than the general population.[7] Furthermore, in monozygotic twins with at least one affected individual, the rate of concordance is 73–92%, as compared to dizygotic twins, in which the rate is lower, at 36–63%.[8,9] Also, the rate of curve progression is nearly identical in affected twins. Recently, Kruse et al. performed a study of 140 families in which more than one member was affected by scoliosis.[10] It was found that 36% of sons with affected mothers had scoliosis, while 85% of daughters of affected fathers had scoliosis. Furthermore, affected males were more likely to transmit scoliosis to offspring of either sex (80%) as compared to affected females (56%), and siblings of males with scoliosis were more likely to be affected than siblings of females with scoliosis.[10] This data is explained by the Carter effect, in which the less commonly affected sex carries a higher load of deleterious genes and is thus more likely to transmit the condition to offspring. Overall, this data supports a polygenic inheritance in adolescent idiopathic scoliosis, in which males have a higher threshold for scoliosis-related genes before scoliosis is observed. A myriad of candidate genes that affect the extracellular matrix, such as, those coding for collagen, fibrillin, and elastin, have been proposed.[11,12] However, to date, there is no single gene that has been found to be responsible for idiopathic scoliosis.

With recent advances in the field of biology, there has been increasing interest in finding epigenetic explanations for scoliosis. Epigenetics is the study of heritable traits that are not encoded in the sequence of DNA base pairs, and three major modes of epigenetic inheritance are DNA methylation, histone modifications, and noncoding RNAs that modify gene expression.[13] It is thought that environmental factors are able to influence the expression of genes through epigenetics. For example, it was found that biomechanical stress and estradiol can affect the gene expression of cultured osteoblasts, with significantly higher levels of nitrous oxide and COX-2 expressed in cells from patients with adolescent idiopathic scoliosis (AIS) as compared to cells from healthy controls.[14] Also, maternal age has been studied as an environmental factor that affects the risk of scoliosis through epigenetics; an association was found between younger mothers and males with truncal asymmetry.[15] Also, it has been proposed that infant exposure to neurotoxins in heated swimming pools increases the likelihood of AIS, but this has yet to be proven.[16,17]

Alternatively, it has been proposed that deficiencies in bone, ligament, muscles, or central nervous system are related to the pathogenesis of idiopathic scoliosis. Because it has been found that bone density was lower in patients with AIS than in age-matched controls both in the spine and in the femur, it was proposed that osteopenia may somehow be part of the etiology of scoliosis rather than a consequence.[18,19] Also, histologic analysis of the multifidus muscle at the musculotendinous junction revealed discontinuities in sarcolemmal membranes, and associated structural disorganization of the tendons, suggesting a primary muscle etiology for AIS.[20] Differences in collagen cross-linking have also been found in the intervertebral disks between patients with scoliosis and controls,[21] with more cross-links on the convex side of the curve than the concave side. However, abnormalities in cross-linking have not been confirmed in the collagen of spinal ligaments.[22,23] Because soft tissue conditions such as Marfan's and Ehlers-Danlos are associated with scoliosis, it is reasonable that subtle defects in any of the tissues of the spine may be responsible for idiopathic scoliosis. Likewise, conditions of the central nervous system such as cerebral palsy are associated with scoliosis, so it is plausible that deficiencies in the nervous system can also cause idiopathic scoliosis. Using dichotic listening tests, it was determined that children with scoliosis had more left-right asymmetry in cortical organization.[24] Interestingly, it has also been found that idiopathic scoliosis has a much lower incidence (1.2%) in hearing impaired children than the national incidence across all children (4-10%).[25] It has been suggested that equilibrial dysfunction is associated with scoliosis,[26] however, in a more recent study of labyrinthine function through caloric testing for nystagmus in patients with idiopathic scoliosis, no differences were observed between AIS patients and controls.[27] Based on the high rates of scoliosis in chickens after pinealectomy, it has been hypothesized that the melatonin deficiency seen post-pinealectomy can cause scoliosis, as melatonin receptors are found in areas of the spinal cord associated with postural control.[28] It has been found in small series that some girls with AIS have minimal expression of the melatonin receptor MT2.[29,30] However, studies of melatonin levels in patients with scoliosis have been inconclusive.[31-34]

Abnormalities in spinal growth have also been suggested as a cause of scoliosis, as scoliosis tends to progress and develop at times of rapid spinal growth. It has been theorized that scoliosis can be due to relative anterior spine overgrowth.[35] It was found that peak height velocity was greater and the period of peak growth was shorter in girls with AIS as compared to healthy controls.[36] Additionally, it has been proposed that inheritance of a sagittal profile that is less resistant to rotatory forces can predispose to scoliosis; it was found that fathers but not mothers of girls with severe progressive AIS had significantly flatter sagittal spine profiles.[37]

Risk Factors for Progression

Naturally, the ability to predict risk of curve progression is instrumental in guiding treatment of idiopathic scoliosis. Scoliosis progresses most rapidly during periods of peak skeletal growth, which are observed in infancy and during puberty. Mehta identified two radiographic risk factors for progression of infantile idiopathic scoliosis—rib vertebral angle difference (RVAD) and phase of the rib head.[38] In his report of 135 patients with infantile idiopathic scoliosis, 80% of patients with RVAD <20° spontaneously resolved, while 83% of patients with RVAD >20° progressed. Juvenile idiopathic scoliosis is often characterized by curve progression with potential for serious sequelae such as cardiopulmonary compromise. In AIS, it is well established that curve progression is associated with peak growth velocity.[39] However, the challenge is that there is no way to directly and accurately measure growth velocity. Instead, surrogates such as patient age, bone age,[40] menarche, Risser sign,[41] and closure of the triradiate cartilage[42] are used to predict remaining growth and likelihood of progression. Curves with an apex above T12 were more likely to progress than lumbar curves.[43] Recently it has been suggested that three-dimensional morphologic parameters of the spine such as 3D wedging of apical disks, lower junctional vertebral axial rotation, torsion, height/width ration of T6, and whole spine height/width ratio, are more predictive of curve progression in AIS than traditional two-dimensional parameters such as Cobb angle.[44] The magnitude of the curve can be used to predict curve progression at skeletal maturity. Thoracic curves of less than 30° tended not to progress, while progression tended to occur at approximately 1° per year in curves that were between 50° and 75°. Lumbar curves generally progressed if they were greater than 30° at skeletal maturity.[45,46]

Adult Natural History

More than two-thirds of patients with scoliosis continue to have curve progression past skeletal maturity.[45] Aside from the most severe thoracic curves of greater than 90°, which are associated with increased mortality from heart failure and cor pulmonale, there does not appear to be an increase in mortality in AIS.[46] Adults with scoliosis have higher rates of back pain than non-affected counterparts,46 and possibly higher rates of disability.[47,48] 65% of adults with scoliosis reported chronic back pain as compared to 35% of controls in long-term follow-up;[49] even adults with mild curves had an increased prevalence of fatigue-like back pain. As one might expect, patients with curves greater than 80° were found to be more likely to experience shortness of breath.[49] Also, there are psychosocial effects associated with having a physical deformity. It has been found that women with scoliosis are less likely to get married than women without scoliosis,[50] although this effect is more pronounced in nonidiopathic scoliosis.[51]

CLINICAL WORK-UP

School Screening

In many cases, idiopathic scoliosis is asymptomatic and first detected through routine school screening, which has been widely instituted in the United States, most commonly in the fifth and sixth grades. The goal behind school screening is to diagnose scoliosis at an age when bracing is still an option. However, school screening for idiopathic scoliosis is controversial given the low prevalence of clinically significant curves that are not already apparent, the cost of school screening, and the rate of false positives.[52-54] In 1996, the United States Preventative Services Task Force (USPSTF) published guidelines regarding school screening of scoliosis, concluding that there was sufficient evidence to recommend for or against school screening.[55] However, in 2004, the USPSTF guidelines were revised, stating that the harms of school screening, such as unnecessary follow-ups and false positives, may outweigh the benefits.[56] Currently, the American Association of Orthopaedic Surgeons (AAOS) and the Scoliosis Research Society (SRS) do continue to recommend school screening,[57] and school screening continues to be fairly common. In an attempt to improve the over-referral and false-positive rates in school screening, suggestions have been made to further select the population that is screened.[58] However, it has been shown that restricting screening may miss significant curves.[59] In addition, early efforts are underway to investigate the feasibility of remote school screening, by acquiring three-dimensional images of students' backs.[60]

History

In evaluating a new patient for scoliosis, a thorough history and physical examination must be performed. A focused history can provide much information that can assist in diagnosis and treatment. The patient should be asked whether he or she has pain, although back pain is a common complaint that is not necessarily due to scoliosis. The patient and parent's perception of whether the curve is progressing should also be ascertained. The patient's overall rate of growth and any pubertal changes, particularly the timing of menarche in females, should be determined. Any limitations in the patient's functional status should be elicited, with attention to any bowel or bladder dysfunction. A family history focusing on any history of scoliosis or other neuromuscular conditions in family members should be obtained. Also, the reason for seeking care should be elicited.

Physical Examination

The overall symmetry of the patient should be assessed with the patient standing, with attention to the levels of the shoulders, waist, and pelvis as viewed from both anteriorly and posteriorly. Lateral translation of the head with respect to the gluteal cleft can be assessed by dropping a plumb line from C7. Any leg length discrepancy should be measured, as this can cause pelvic obliquity and thus a functional scoliosis, which should be differentiated from idiopathic scoliosis. The Adams forward bend test (Fig. 1) is a preliminary screening test for scoliosis, and is performed by having the patient bend at the waist with knees straight and palms together. Any asymmetry observed should be measured using a scoliometer to determine the angle of trunk rotation (ATR). An ATR of 5–7° corresponds to a Cobb angle of 15–20°. The correlation coefficient between ATR and Cobb angle has been found to be good at 0.7.[61] In recent years, iPhone applications have been used in place of traditional scoliometers, and have been shown to be at least as good at measuring ATR.[62,63] Three-dimensional surface topography has been proposed to measure trunk rotation in place of a scoliometer, but has proved to have inferior sensitivity and specificity.[64]

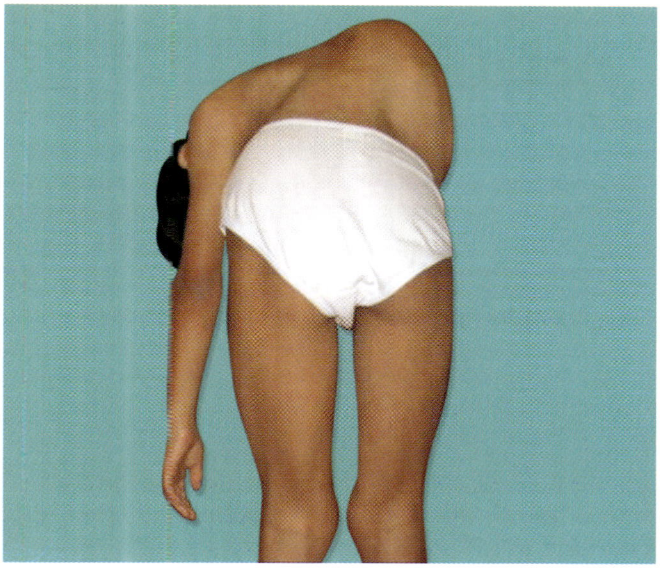

Fig. 1: The Adams forward bend test, which in this case shows a large right-sided rib prominence due to vertebral rotation at the apex of the curve. The direction of rotation (posterior elements toward the midline) is constant in idiopathic scoliosis.

A full neurologic examination should be performed, with attention to any muscle weakness, sensory deficits, or abnormal reflexes. In particular, absence or abnormality of the superficial abdominal reflex is associated with syringomyelia and myogenic scoliosis.[65] The skin should be examined, and any café-au-lait spots or axillary freckling, as seen in neurofibromatosis, or hairy spots, associated with spinal dysraphism, should be noted. Attention should be paid to abnormal laxity, as seen in Marfan's or Ehlers-Danlos and other connective tissue disorders. In the presence of any of these abnormal findings, a high index of suspicion should be maintained for nonidiopathic scoliosis.

Imaging

Scoliosis Plain Films

The Cobb angle has been used to quantify the severity of scoliotic curves in the coronal plane (Figs. 2A to C). On a posteroanterior (PA) radiograph, the cranial and caudal end vertebrae of the curve are identified as the most tilted vertebrae. Then, lines are drawn at the superior end plate of the cranial end vertebrae and at the inferior end plate of the caudal end vertebrae. Next, lines are drawn perpendicular to each of these, and the angle at which these lines cross

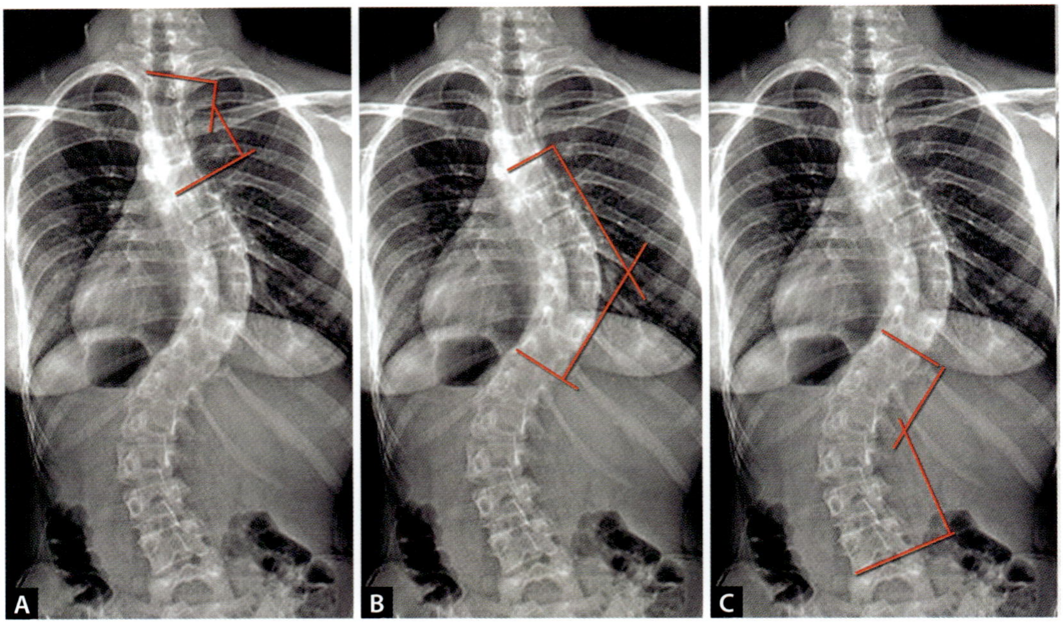

Figs. 2A to C: The Cobb angle is the angle measured between the upper endplate of the upper end vertebrae and lower end plate of the lower end vertebrae for each curve.

is measured as the Cobb angle. When multiple curves are present, a separate Cobb angle should be measured for each curve. The intra- and inter-observer error has traditionally been estimated to be approximately 5°; this should be considered before determining whether a curve has progressed.[66] Of note, it has been found that intra- and inter-observer reliability of Cobb angle measurements is lower in juvenile idiopathic scoliosis (JIS) than in AIS, possibly due to ill-defined endplates in the JIS patients.[67]

Recently, the digital methods of Cobb measurement have shown promise in improving the accuracy of measurement. Using a digital measurement system with pre-selected end vertebrae, the 95% confidence intervals for intra- and inter-observer reliability were found to be +1.30° and +1.26°, respectively.[68] Mok et al. compared manual and computer-based Cobb angle measurements, and found inter-observer reliability to be high except when digital images were printed onto two unstitched films.[69] Additionally, smartphone applications have been developed to measure Cobb angles, and have been found to be at least equivalent to conventional methods.[70,71]

Lateral radiographs are used to quantify thoracic kyphosis (T2–T12, normal 20–50°) and lumbar lordosis (L1–S1, normal 31–79). In patients with main thoracic curves, T5–T12 kyphosis is generally measured, and normal is between 10° and 40°. For proximal thoracic curves, T2–T5 kyphosis is also important, and in patients with thoracolumbar curves, T10–L2 kyphosis (normal = 0) is measured as well. Pelvic incidence, which is a constant variable for any particular patient quantifying sacral tilt relative to the pelvis, can also be measured. Increased pelvic incidence values are associated with increased thoracic kyphosis and lumbar lordosis, and differences in pelvic incidence may explain the wide range of normal values for thoracic kyphosis and lumbar lordosis. The technique of lateral radiographs influences overall sagittal balance, with the patient's hands resting in the supraclavicular fossa most reflective of normal posture while allowing for adequate visualization of the thoracic vertebrae.

Several different methods of stress radiographs quantify curve flexibility and disk mobility at the limits of the end vertebrae, including supine bending radiographs, traction radiographs, and push prone radiographs. Of the three modalities, supine bending radiographs are dependent on patient effort and may not reflect the true amount of flexibility of the various curves but are used most often (Figs. 3A to D). Push prone and traction radiographs require two assistants to perform. Compared to bending radiographs, push prone radiographs most

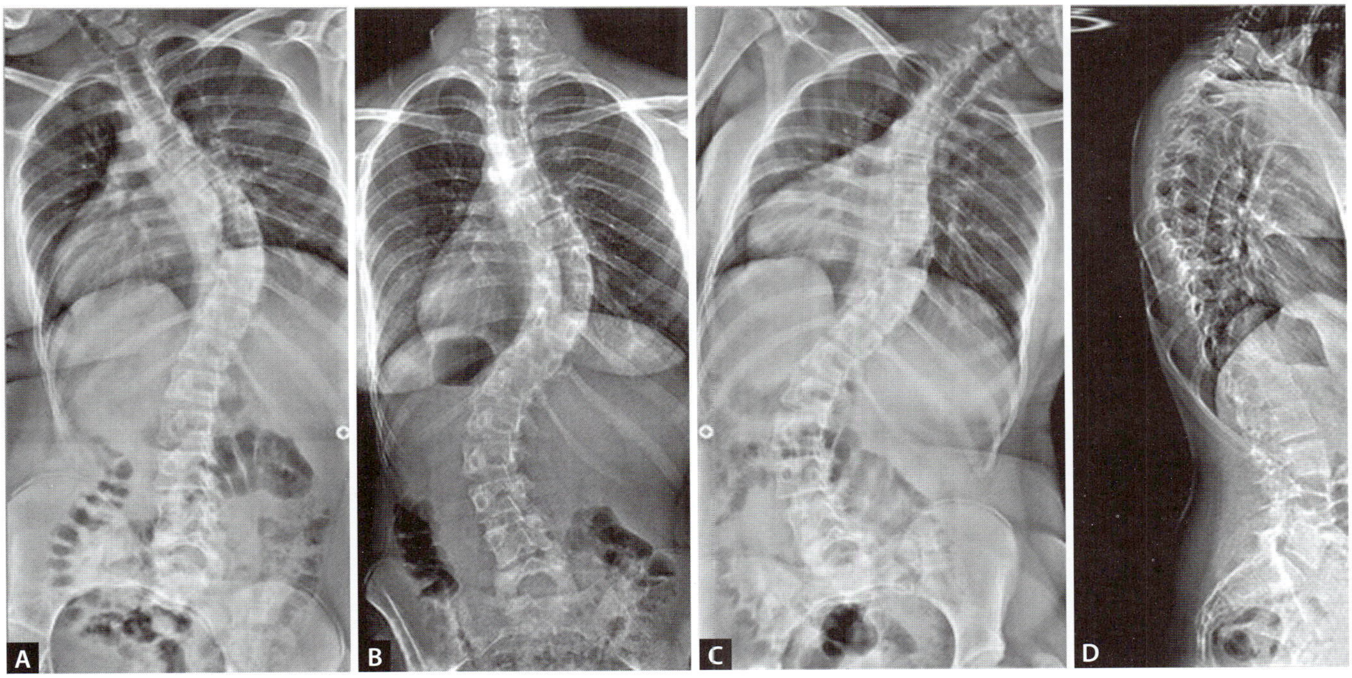

Figs. 3A to D: A complete set of preoperative radiographs includes upright anteroposterior (AP) or posteroanterior (PA), lateral, and flexibility films. In this case, left (A) and right (C) supine bending radiographs were used to assess curve flexibility and rotational correction, which is helpful in determining which curves are structural.

accurately reflect the residual lumbar curve in selective thoracic fusions.

Magnetic Resonance Imaging

In patients with idiopathic scoliosis, advanced imaging modalities such as magnetic resonance imaging (MRI) are generally not required. However, if there is a suspicion that a curve may indeed not be idiopathic, an MRI can be useful to help rule out other pathologies. In addition, patients with a hyperkyphotic sagittal profile in the thoracic spine are at increased risk of syringomyelia[72] and should have an MRI. Additionally, MRI may be indicated in left thoracic curves, male patients, rapidly progressive curves, infantile or juvenile patients, and in patients with abnormal neurologic examination (including asymmetric abdominal reflexes). The MRI should be of the entire spine, and rule out any tumors, syringomyelia, spinal dysraphism, or tethered cord.

CLASSIFICATION

Multiple classification systems have been developed to describe scoliotic curves, in order to facilitate communication, research, and guide treatment. The King-Moe classification consists of five types of curves: (1) thoracic and lumbar curve with larger lumbar curve, (2) thoracic and lumbar curve with larger thoracic curve, (3) single thoracic curve, (4) long lumbar curve with L4 tilted into the curve, and (5) double thoracic curve.[73] While this classification system is relatively simple and can guide surgical treatment, it is not comprehensive.

Based on standard preoperative radiographs (standing PA and lateral, and supine bending), Lenke et al. developed a classification system which describes most curve patterns. The classification was developed in part to improve intra- and inter-observer reliability as compared to the King-Moe classification, as well as to include lumbar curve types.[74] The system combines data from three categories to determine overall curve type. The first value considers the three main locations of coronal spinal deformity (main thoracic, proximal thoracic, thoracolumbar/lumbar). Using the common curve locations, patients are classified into one of six curve types (main thoracic, double thoracic, double major, triple major, thoracolumbar/lumbar, and thoracolumbar/

lumbar—main thoracic). Bending radiographs help determine if a particular curve is structural (corrects to <25°) or not for purposes of assigning curve type. Next, the lumbar curve apical translation is classified into either group A, B, or C depending on if the CSVL falls between, on, or outside of the apical vertebrae pedicles on an upright radiograph. Lastly, in the sagittal plane, patients are ordinally classified into decreased, normal, or increased T5-T12 kyphosis (–, N, or +). Despite studies questioning the inter-observer reliability of the system, the significance of a structural proximal thoracic curve, and the importance of the lumbar modifier,[75-78] the system is the most widely used in America currently (Table 2).

Table 2: Lenke scoliosis curve classification.

Curve type	*L-spine modifier*	*Sagittal thoracic profile*
1. Main thoracic	A. CSVL between pedicles	–: <10°
2. Double thoracic	B. CVSL touches apical body	N: 10–40°
3. Double major	C. CVSL medial to pedicles	+: >40°
4. Triple major		
5. Thoracolumbar/ Lumbar		
6. Thoracolumbar/ Lumbar-main thoracic		

(CSVL: central sacral vertical line)

The Risser scale is the most commonly used, although not necessarily reliable, radiographic marker of skeletal maturity. As seen on the anteroposterior (AP) radiographs of the iliac crest, the Risser scale is a system for classifying the ossification of the iliac apophysis as it progresses from lateral to medial, and ranging from 0 (no ossification) to V (fully ossified) (Figs. 4A to F). The entire process of

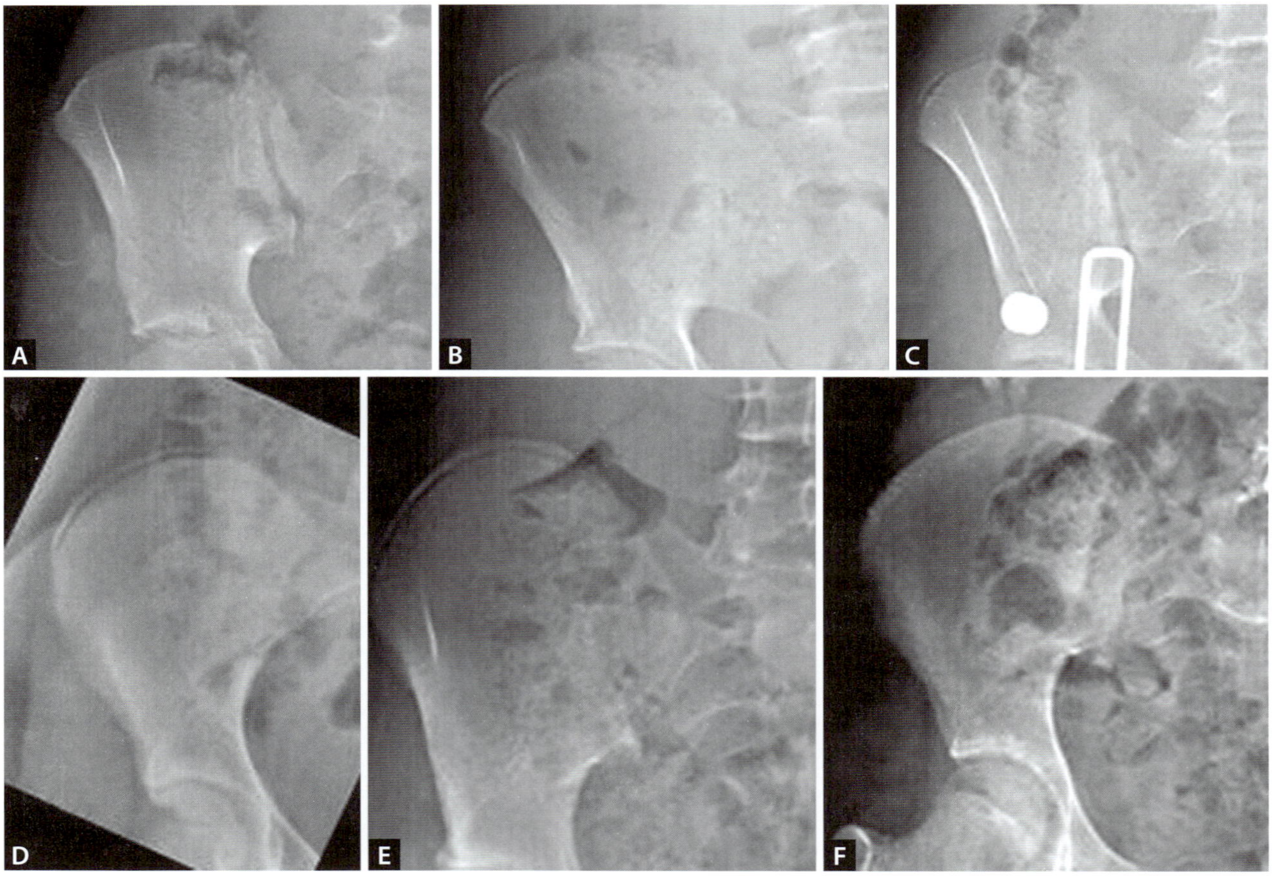

Figs. 4A to F: The Risser sign (progressive ossification of the iliac apophysis) is one measure of skeletal maturity. (A) Risser 0; (B) Risser 1; (C) Risser 2; (D) Risser 3; (E) Risser 4; (F) Risser 5. Note that the patient in "A" also has an open triradiate cartilage, further signifying the patient has not yet achieved peak height velocity.

ossification takes place over 1.5 to 2 years. However, it has been suggested that the Risser sign is of limited utility given that the calcification of the iliac apophysis occurs after peak growth velocity.[79] In fact, the Risser sign was found to most accurately predict whether a person has reached age 14, at stage IV.[80,81] Still, the Risser sign is often used due to the convenience of being able to see the iliac crest on scoliosis films without obtaining additional films.

Another method of assessing skeletal maturity is by taking hand radiographs and referencing to the standardized images in the book of Greulich and Pyle,[82] but the accuracy of this method is not optimal in the juvenile age group. More recently, a modified version of the Tanner-Whitehouse-III score, which is based on the radiographic appearance of the epiphyses of the distal part of the radius, the distal part of the ulna, and small bones of the hand, was found to correlate more strongly with scoliotic progression than Risser or Greulich and Pyle-based predictions.[83] Additionally, the status of the triradiate cartilage can be used, as it closes before the iliac apophysis appears, during Risser 0, better correlating with maximal spinal growth.[84] However, this would require obtaining a separate pelvis film.

MEDICAL MANAGEMENT

In many cases of patients referred for orthopedic spine evaluation, conservative management is appropriate. In small curves, minimally progressive curves, and patients at or nearing skeletal maturity, reassurance, and observation is often all that is required.

Historically, electrical stimulation has been used to treat scoliosis, as applied through surface-stimulation on the convex portion of the deformity. However, this method is less popular given a lack of evidence supporting its effectiveness.[43] In a large meta-analysis, the weighted mean proportion of success for lateral electric stimulation was 0.39, as compared to 0.49 for observation alone.[85]

In patients with significant skeletal growth remaining, a brace, or spinal orthosis, can be considered. While a brace is unlikely to permanently correct a curve, it can help prevent further progression. Generally, this is indicated when a curve progresses past 25°.[86] In a prospective study of brace efficacy in preventing curve progression, it was found that at least 2 years after brace weaning, 68/284 of compliant patients and 46/71 of noncompliant patients experienced curve progression of at least 6°, with compliance defined as at least 20 hours of brace wear daily.[87] It has been suggested that bracing is not as effective in males because their spines are stiffer,[88] however, more recent analysis has demonstrated that the reason for more curve progression in males is poor brace compliance.[89] Many different types of braces are available, as outlined here.

The Milwaukee brace, or cervico-thoraco-lumbo-sacral orthosis (CTLSO), was a traditional brace that provides longitudinal traction between the neck and pelvic girdle with lateral translation forces applied to the curve apex as directed between the pads and the chest wall. The mechanism of correction is thought to be a combination of passive pressure applied by the pad on the apex and active avoidance of the pads by the thoracic musculature. The brace was originally prescribed to be worn 23 hours daily with an accompanying exercise program. As an early spinal orthosis used to treat scoliosis, the Milwaukee brace had several notable drawbacks, namely limited patient and parent acceptance and compliance due to the visible nature of the neckpiece and uprights. Additionally, it has been demonstrated through a case series by Olin and Ponseti that the use of a Milwaukee brace without an intraoral device can lead to maxillofacial deformities due to the pressure applied by the most cephalad portion of the orthosis.[90]

Underarm braces, also known as thoraco-lumbo-sacral orthoses (TLSOs), have become more popular because they are not as externally apparent. The Boston brace (Fig. 5) is widely studied, which is fitted by modifying an

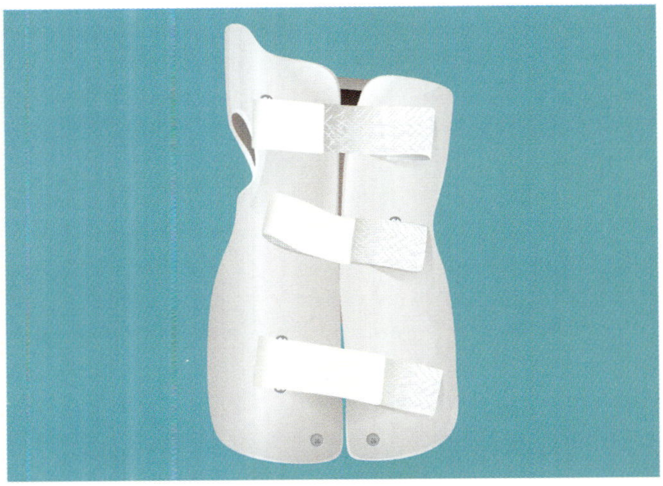

Fig. 5: The Boston thoraco-lumbo-sacral orthosis (TLSO), from behind demonstrating the Velcro straps.

CHAPTER 12

"off-the-shelf" module based on patient measurements. In long-term follow-up of patients treated with the Boston brace, 9% had surgery, 13% had curve progression to greater than 45°, and 69% had curve progression less than 6°.[91] However, as in all other braces, efficacy is highly dependent on patient acceptance of the brace. Other TLSO braces include the Wilmington brace, which is made of a circumferential thermoplastic material that is less rigid than the Boston brace. The SpineCor brace is a flexible derotational brace that works through dynamic derotation. In a prospective randomized controlled trial, it was found that the SpineCor brace was less effective and did not have any higher compliance than a rigid orthosis.[92] To date, the highest level of evidence for use of a TLSO has been demonstrated by the BrAIST trial,[93] in which 242 patients across 25 sites in North America were randomized to watchful waiting versus TLSO bracing until they reached skeletal maturity or their curves progressed to greater than 50°. It was found that bracing was associated with 72% rate of treatment success, as compared to 48% in the observation group, with the dramatic difference in efficacy leading to early cessation of the study.[94]

Because bracing is often associated with a psychological burden and poor compliance, part-time or nighttime braces are alternate options. They generally work by hyper-correcting the deformity.[95] The Charleston nighttime bending brace is designed to produce a trunk bend that is so severe that it can prevent walking. In a prospective study of the Charleston brace, it was found that in a cohort of patients with previously untreated AIS and curves of 25–40°, the brace was 78% successful overall, with higher success rates in thoracolumbar and lumbar curves.[96] Another popular nighttime brace is the Providence brace, which is molded using computer-assisted design and works through the application of controlled, direct, lateral, and rotational opposing forces on the trunk to push the curve apex toward midline or past it.[96] In a prospective study of 102 girls who wore the Providence brace, 76% did not experience curve progression; as with the Charleston brace, the highest rates of success were observed with thoracolumbar and lumbar curves.[97] In a direct comparison of lumbar curves, patients using the Providence brace had 92% correction of their primary curves and a 27% rate of progression, while wearers of the Boston brace had 50% correction and 22% progression.[98] Currently, a prospective randomized controlled trial, CONTRAIS, is underway to compare the use of nighttime bracing versus a physical activity prescription in adolescents with idiopathic curves between 25° and 40°;[99] the results of this study may provide more definitive evidence on the use of night bracing.

Efforts have been made to better understand the effects of bracing in idiopathic scoliosis. Mahaudens et al. studied the effects of short-term brace wear, finding that while there was correction of the primary curve, a brace alters gait by reducing pelvis, hip, and shoulder motion.[100] Additionally, bracing of AIS patients caused a decrease in duration of gluteus medius activity as measured by electromyography (EMG) but no significant effect on EMG activity of lumbopelvic muscles, muscular mechanical work, and energy consumption during gait.[100] In order to better understand the morphological changes of the spine with a brace in place, 3D reconstructions of biplanar stereoradiography have been used; such imaging demonstrates wide variability in the effect of brace treatment in almost every parameter.[101]

SURGICAL INDICATIONS AND TREATMENT

Surgical indications for idiopathic scoliosis depend on patient age (or more precisely, patient skeletal age), curve location, curve flexibility, and curve magnitude.

Infantile and Juvenile Idiopathic Scoliosis (Age <10)

In young patients, treatment strategies are different than in the adolescent because of the significant growth remaining (both vertebral and chest wall) and continued lung development. The definition of "young" is not absolute, with some authors using age 5 (when thoracolumbar spine growth is >2 cm/year), 2–8 (when pulmonary alveolar duplication, or "alveolarization", may be complete), or age 10 years (when achieved thoracic cavity volume is 50%) as a cut-off.[102-105] Achieving control of spinal curvature while preserving spinal growth (particularly thoracic spinal growth) and maintaining chest wall compliance is the main treatment principle in these patients.

Serial Casting (Mehta, Risser)

The authors consider serial body casting as a surgical procedure, as it is performed in an operating room under anesthetic. Historically, spinal casting was described in the mid-20th century, and recently there has been renewed interest in the technique. There are two different types of serial spinal casting described: Mehta (derotational) and Risser (translational).[106-108] Both require special tables

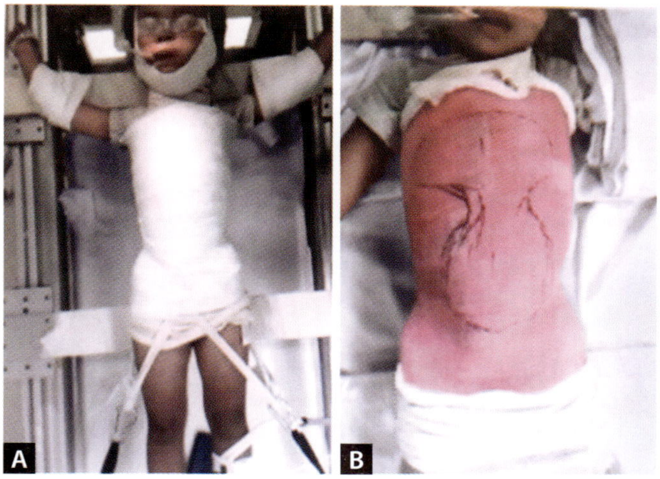

Figs. 6A and B: A patient with infantile idiopathic scoliosis on the Mehta casting table before (A) and after (B) application of a Mehta scoliosis cast.

and general anesthesia to perform. Patients with infantile idiopathic scoliosis, and occasionally juvenile idiopathic scoliosis, are candidates for serial casting. In the infantile population, indications include a progressive curve greater than 20° or a rib vertebral angle difference (RVAD) of >20° upon presentation.[109] There is no lower age limit to spinal casting, although it is rare to initiate casting before age 1, and most patients who undergo casting start approximately at age of 18 months. Mehta casting is more successful when initiated in the young with smaller, progressive curves, and complete curve resolution is possible in these patients (Figs. 6A and B). The upper age limit for casting becomes a practical one, as it is difficult for an older, larger patient to function in society in a body cast. Casts are generally changed every 3–6 months. If spinal curvature decreases to 10°, then the patient can be transitioned into a TLSO for 18–24 hours of daily wear. If there is complete resolution of curvature, observation is warranted. It is assumed that if there is complete resolution of deformity, outcomes in these patients will approach that of the normal population. If there is progression of curvature despite casting, an alternate method of treatment is instituted, which depends on the patient age.

Fletcher et al. described initiation of casting in idiopathic patients at up to 6.1 years of age. The upper curve magnitude limit for casting is up to 80°,[110] although most authors use 60° as an upper limit. Fletcher et al. and Sanders et al. found that although older patients with larger curves do not have complete resolution of their curves with serial casting, they do derive benefits through a delay in curve progression and surgical intervention, with potential avoidance of growth stunting surgery. Sanders et al. showed no significant curve progression in 49/55 patients casted for infantile idiopathic scoliosis with casting initiated at an average age of 2.2 years and an average Cobb angle of 52° at 1 year minimum follow-up.[109]

Posterior Growth Friendly Surgery (Growing Rods, Shilla, VEPTR)

Growth friendly surgeries include posterior-based instrumentation systems, such as growing rods and, more recently, the Shilla technique and the vertical expandable prosthetic titanium rib (VEPTR). Posterior growing rods and the Shilla technique both are not FDA approved in the United States for use in children, and their application is an off-label indication. With the VEPTR system, FDA approval is under a Humanitarian Device Exemption. The concept with all of these systems is surgical control of spinal curvature with limited or no spinal fusion to allow for continued growth. Typically, growing rods are implanted with local fusion around proximal and distal anchors, and a proximal and distal rod (or rods) connected within a distraction sleeve or by tandem rod connectors. The intervening vertebrae are not exposed surgically, and the rods lie in an intramuscular (or subcutaneous) location. Either single or dual rods can be implanted, and they can be used with or without an apical fusion (Fig. 7). Akbarnia et al. found that dual rods without an apical fusion resulted in the most preservation of spinal growth and curve control.[111] Rods are most often surgically lengthened every 6–12 months, until the curve progresses beyond a threshold value (100–120°), until no further length is gained, if severe kyphosis develops, or if the patient is skeletally mature.[112,113] At skeletal maturity, a definitive spinal fusion is often performed. Recently, a magnetic growing rod system (not currently available for use in the United States), which achieves rod lengthening without surgery through an externally applied magnet, has been developed with encouraging early results.[114]

The VEPTR device was initially devised for use in patients with congenital thoracic scoliosis and fused ribs, it also can be used in patients with early-onset idiopathic scoliosis and thoracic insufficiency syndrome.[115,116] Smith et al. treated patients with progressive curvature beyond 50–60° refractory to casting and bracing initially with a

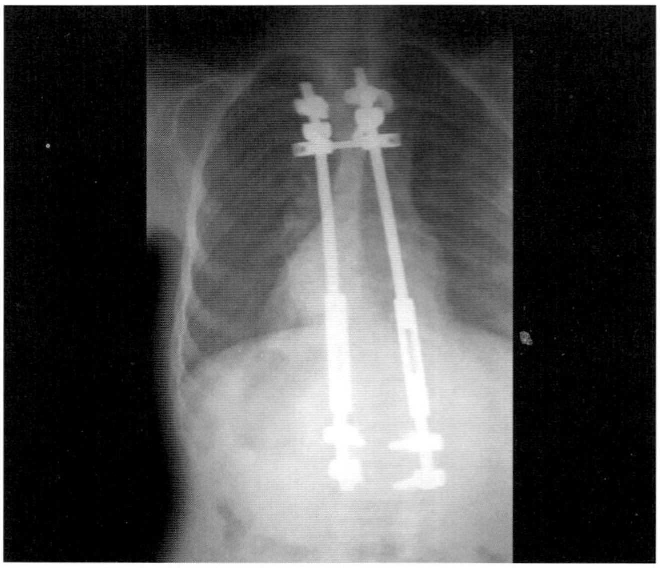

Fig. 7: An example of a growing rod construct in a patient with juvenile idiopathic scoliosis who had curve progression despite thoraco-lumbo-sacral orthosis (TLSO) bracing.

bilateral rib to pelvis VEPTR devices and serial distraction surgeries. They found that, although curve control and spinal growth were maintained, 39% of ambulatory patients developed a clinically significant crouch gait due to positive sagittal balance with this strategy. Revision of the VEPTR devices to include distal vertebral (instead of pelvic) anchors alleviated this problem,[115] which is now his recommended strategy.

The Shilla procedure is a posterior spine-guided growth system. It involves performing an apical fusion with pedicle screws and inserting proximal and distal anchors with a specially designed screw that allows the spinal rods to slide within the screw head. The rods are left purposefully long either proximally or distally (or both). With growth, the proximal and distal anchors grow toward the ends of the rods. Short-term follow-up in a small group of patients <10 years of age, with curves >50°, showed good curve correction with a minor complication rate of approximately 50%, which is similar to complication rates with other growth friendly spine implants. The Shilla system has the added benefit of eliminating lengthening surgeries.[117]

The indications for spinal derotational casting versus growth friendly spine surgery are unclear. Many authors apply growth friendly spine surgery in patients with progressive curves above 50–60° less than 10 years old. Some authors will choose posterior growth friendly surgery only after curve progression despite serial casting or bracing regardless of curve size (in patients of appropriate age and curve magnitude for serial casting). At this time, there are no direct comparison studies between growth friendly surgery and serial spinal casting. It seems prudent to treat progressive curvature in the young patient with casting or bracing, and to reserve surgical intervention for young patients with curve progression despite casting or bracing.

Outcomes of treatment for growing rods, Shilla, or VEPTR in idiopathic scoliosis are difficult to ascertain because most reports in the literature include evaluation of patient populations with mixed diagnoses (neuromuscular, congenital, etc.). However, studies show modest growth of the thoracolumbar spine during treatment, and complication rates in upward of 50% of patients over time. Most complications are either infectious or implant-related (proximal or distal anchor failure, rod breakage).[116,118] Nevertheless, growing rod, Shilla, or VEPTR treatment in these patients may delay final fusion and allow for spinal growth in the childhood years.

Anterior Vertebral Body Growth Modulation (Vertebral Tethering, Vertebral Body Stapling)

Anterior growth modulation surgery is another type of growth friendly spine surgery whereby there is anterior-based compression of the convexity of a curvature. According to the Heuter-Volkmann principle, decreased convex growth in the face of continued concave vertebral body growth can lead to improving curvature with subsequent growth. The most commonly applied techniques for growth modulation currently are vertebral body stapling and vertebral body tethering. Both have similarities in that they are anterior-based instrumentation systems that can be inserted via thoracoscopy or a limited thoracotomy in a child in a time window with sufficient growth remaining to have corrective potential, but not so much growth remaining that there could be curve over-correction.

Vertebral body stapling (VBS) typically uses shape-memory alloy staples which are implanted across the disk space and vertebral end plate on the convexity of the curvature. Because of the unique metallurgical properties of the staple, the tines of the staple change from a straight

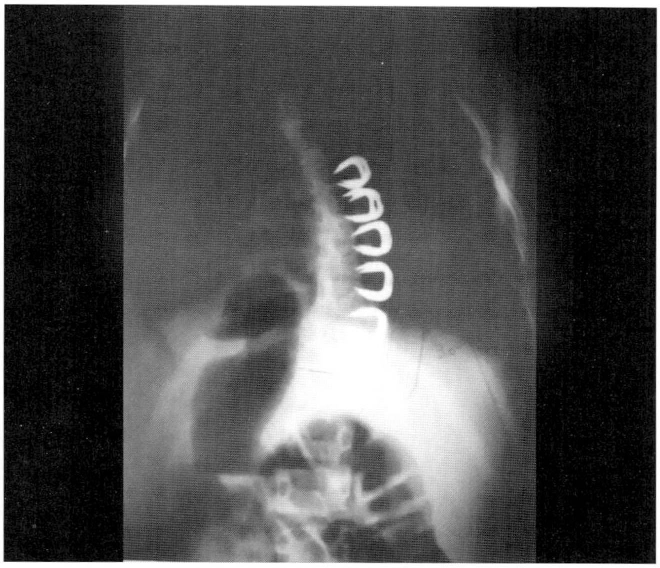

Fig. 8: A patient with late juvenile idiopathic scoliosis who underwent anterior vertebral body stapling for a progressive thoracic curve.

position at cool temperatures to an inward-curved position at body temperature. This results in "compression" across the disk and vertebral apophysis, where vertical vertebral growth occurs (Fig. 8). Indications for VBS as described by both Betz et al. and Lavelle et al. include patients between 8 and 13 (girls) or 15 (boys) with significant growth remaining (generally Risser 0 or 1 and/or 1 year of growth remaining according to bone age) and curves less than 45°.[119,120] Thoracic hyperkyphosis beyond 40° is also a relative contraindication, and allergy to nickel (the staples are an alloy that includes nickel) is an absolute contraindication. As there is limited data regarding this technique, the surgical indications are not universally accepted. Also, there is much overlap between the inclusion criteria for vertebral body stapling and bracing, which has limited the widespread use of vertebral body stapling.

More recently, vertebral body tethers, which have been studied in several animal models, have been used clinically.[121] In this case report, an 8 + 6-year-old male with a progressive thoracic curve despite bracing underwent surgical placement of anterior body screws with a flexible polypropylene tether tensioned on the convex curve side. With 4 years of growth, the curve corrected from 40° to 8°, with no significant increase in thoracic kyphosis. Anterior vertebral body growth modulation devices are currently not FDA approved for use in children. Although the results are encouraging, much more clinical data need to be shown before this can be recommended as a widespread treatment.

Adolescent Idiopathic Scoliosis (>11 years)

By age 11, much of the thoracic spinal height (>75%) and volume (>50%) has been achieved, and lung alveolar cell duplication has slowed. Treatment strategies during adolescence focus on preventing further curve progression while preserving as many spinal motion segments as possible, maintaining or achieving global spinal balance, and decreasing spinal curvature. As mentioned previously, this may be accomplished by bracing in moderate sized curves in skeletally immature patients, or with spinal fusion if curvature (particularly thoracic curvature) progresses beyond 50°.

Surgical goals can be looked at from the point of view of the surgeon or patient. A survey of spinal deformity surgeons revealed the surgeon's primary surgical goals in performing a spinal fusion are achievement of a solid spinal fusion to prevent curve progression into adult life, maintenance of global coronal and sagittal spinal balance, and maintenance of lumbar lordosis. Secondary surgical goals include maximizing spinal mobility, Cobb angle correction, and rotational deformity correction. There was wide variability from surgeon to surgeon on which goals (other than coronal and sagittal balance) were most important.[122] Thus, there is often variability on how each surgeon approaches spinal deformity surgically. With respect to patient's expectations of surgery, the majority focuses on the absence of pain as well as postoperative appearance (specifically shoulder symmetry, back appearance, and their surgical scar).[123] Thus, the primary goals of the patient are not often in line with the primary goals of the surgeon.

Surgical Approach

Spinal fusion can be undertaken via a posterior, anterior, or combined anterior and posterior surgical approach. The most common approach for all curve types is a posterior one, and this trend has increased over the last decade. An anterior diskectomy and fusion may be added to a posterior fusion in patients at risk of continued significant anterior growth, which in the face of a posterior fusion could result in twisting of the anterior column around the fixed posterior fusion mass ("crankshaft" phenomenon).[124]

Crankshaft is specifically defined radiographically as curve progression of >10° or an increase in RVAD of >10° within an instrumented fusion. Patients at greatest risk for crankshaft have not yet achieved their peak height velocity (Risser 0, triradiate cartilage open).[42] There is some evidence that use of pedicle screws (which extend to the anterior column) may decrease the risk of crankshaft, although it may also be that increased curve correction with pedicle screws makes it more difficult to detect significant crankshaft.[125]

Anterior diskectomy (or posterior-based osteotomies) combined with posterior instrumented fusion can be performed to increase curve flexibility in large, stiff curves. Dobbs et al. showed equal curve correction in stiff idiopathic curves >90° with combined anterior release/posterior instrumented fusions versus posterior instrumented fusions with pedicle screw fixation and selective use of posterior column shortening osteotomies.[126] Anterior release surgery tends to increase kyphosis and decrease postoperative pulmonary function, while posterior osteotomies tend to create lordosis and increase surgical blood loss. For thoracic curves, in either setting (risk of crankshaft or large, stiff curves), the anterior fusion can be performed thoracoscopically to decrease surgical morbidity in a modified prone position.[127] If the curve extends into the lumbar spine, minimally invasive, transpsoas muscle approaches can be used to gain access to the intervertebral disks. Both techniques increase surgical time to posterior instrumented spinal fusion surgery, and multiple authors have shown no benefit to using either technique in moderate sized, flexible curves.[128,129] The surgeon should consider these issues when deciding between techniques.

In North America, anterior instrumented fusions are uncommonly performed. The most common setting is in the patient with a thoracolumbar scoliosis without structural associated curves (Figs. 9A to C). Anterior diskectomy renders the spine more flexible, and anterior compression/derotation anterior instrumentation (either single or dual rod) gives the surgeon powerful deformity correction tools which often allow the surgeon to choose a lowest instrumented vertebra (LIV) one level proximal as compared to a posterior approach (i.e. LIV of L3 versus L4).[130] The use of posterior Ponte osteotomies has increased the posterior instrumented corrective power[131,132] and decreased the number of anterior instrumented fusions for thoracolumbar scoliosis. In a comparison of techniques, the short segment anterior instrumented fusions result in more saved motion segments distally, more LIV translation postoperatively, increased thoracolumbar kyphosis, and similar clinical outcomes.[131]

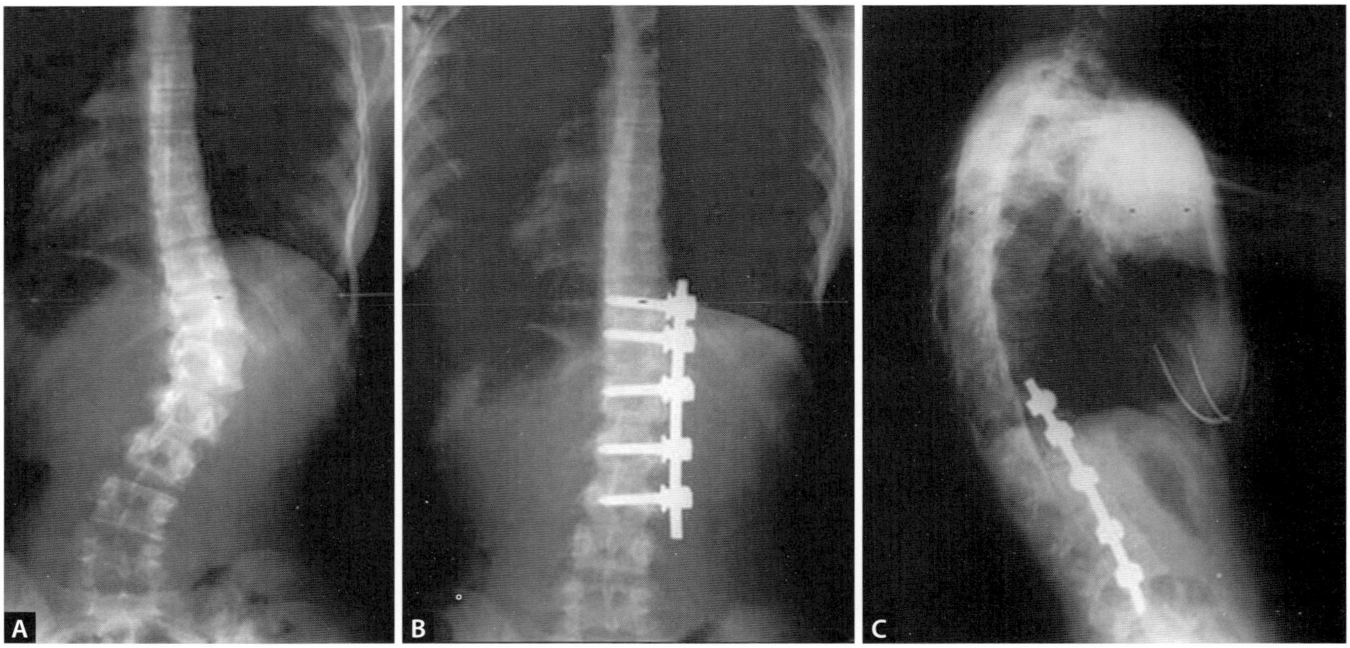

Figs. 9A to C: An example of an anterior instrumented spinal fusion for an apex thoracolumbar scoliosis.

The second setting where anterior instrumented fusion occurs is for right main thoracic curves (most often thoracoscopically). Thoracoscopic anterior instrumented thoracic fusion is performed in select centers. Early problems with pseudoarthrosis and rod failure have largely been circumvented with increased diameter rods made of stiffer materials and greater attention to bone grafting the intervertebral disk spaces. One advantage of anterior instrumented fusion for main thoracic scoliosis is improved restoration of normal thoracic kyphosis (and therefore lumbar lordosis) as compared to a posterior approach.[133] When comparing posterior to anterior thoracoscopic fusions in these patients, surgical times are shorter for posterior fusions, more levels are fused with posterior approaches, and clinical outcomes are similar.[134] Anterior thoracic open fusions result in a permanent decrease in pulmonary function as measured by pulmonary function testing but are an option depending on surgeon experience. Thoracoscopic techniques and anterior open thoracolumbar techniques result in mild, temporary decreases in pulmonary function. Anterior instrumented fusions still play an important role in the treatment of main thoracic and thoracolumbar curve patterns.

Choice of Fusion Levels

The Lenke curve classification aids the surgeon in selective fusion levels by defining which curves are structural versus nonstructural. In general, all structural curves should be included in the fusion mass. Also, fusions should not end at the apex of a deformity (in the coronal, sagittal, or transverse plane). While there is wide agreement on these principles, there is great variability in the specific choice of proximal and distal fusion levels from surgeon to surgeon when considering any curve type.[135] This variability relates to surgeon experience, surgical objectives, surgical approach, and anticipated correction. To discuss the choice of fusion levels, the concepts of the neutral vertebrae (NV), stable vertebrae (SV), upper and lower end vertebrae (UEV and LEV), and upper and lower instrumented vertebrae (UIV and LIV) should be reviewed. Choosing a LIV too proximal risks postoperative adding-on, while choosing a LIV too distal unnecessarily sacrifices motion segments and might lead to future adjacent-segment degenerative disk disease. This issue is particularly relevant when choosing distal fusion levels in thoracolumbar and lumbar curves, where limited motion segments below the fusion are available.

Nevertheless, the literature has tried to refine selection of distal fusion levels and indications for selective thoracic fusion for Lenke 1 and 3 type curves. Suk et al. have suggested that, if there is no more than a 2-level difference between the neutral vertebrae and the end vertebrae, then fusion should extend to the neutral vertebrae.[136] Cao et al. suggested the LIV should be no more than 1 cm deviated from the CSVL on preoperative radiographs.[137] In practice, most selective thoracic fusions end distally at SV-1 or SV-2, and most fusions including a lumbar curve end at L3 (or less commonly L4). Proximally, most fusions involving the thoracic spine end at T2 (if there is a proximal thoracic curve), T3, or T4. In the case of an isolated thoracolumbar curve being treated by posterior fusion, the proximal fusion level is usually the upper end vertebrae (if this is not the apex of a deformity in the sagittal or transverse planes). The articles by both Cho et al. and Erikson et al. summarize the topic well,[138,139] as does a recent review article by Trobisch et al.[140] Fusion levels in anterior instrumented fusions are selected differently. Most often, using the end vertebrae as the upper and lower instrumented vertebrae is performed, unless the short segment fusion technique is used for a thoracolumbar curve. In that situation, a 3-level (if the apex is a vertebrae) or 4-level (if the apex is a disk) instrumented fusion with overcorrection is performed.[141]

Choice of Implants

Implant choice involves implant material, type, and density. Available implant rod materials include stainless steel, titanium alloys, and cobalt-chrome alloys. When choosing a material, two material properties are most important: stiffness (proportional to Young's modulus of elasticity) and yield stress. Stiffness of a rod is also impacted by rod diameter, with stiffness increasing to the 4th power of the diameter. Stiffness is reflected by the rod's ability to hold and achieve correction. In general, titanium alloys have a Young's modulus of between 55 Gpa and 110 Gpa, while stainless steel and cobalt-chrome alloys have a Young's modulus of 210–240 Gpa.[142] Thus, choice of a stiffer material allows for use of smaller diameter rods to achieve the same rod stiffness. Titanium alloys in general have a higher yield stress than stainless steel, which means they are less brittle or likely to catastrophically fail ("break") in the face of cyclic micromotion (but are more sensitive to surface irregularities, or "notches"). Other factors important in choosing implant material are MRI-compatibility and impact on infection risk. Di Silvestre et al. showed a higher late infection rate in idiopathic scoliosis patients treated with a posterior instrumented spinal fusion with stainless steel versus titanium implants.[143]

Anchor types include spinous process wires, sublaminar wires or polymers, pedicle hooks, laminar hooks (lumbar or thoracic), transverse process hooks, and pedicle screws. While a full discussion of anchor types is beyond the scope of this chapter, most recent studies in idiopathic scoliosis have concentrated on the relative ratio of hooks to pedicle screws utilized in posterior fusion constructs, and to a lesser extent the density of anchors per levels fused. So-called second generation spine implants (Cotrel-Dubousset) allowed for segmental spinal fixation with hooks. With the appearance of pedicle screw fixation came "hybrid" (hook and screw) constructs, typically with pedicle screws serving as the lower rod anchors and hooks in the thoracic spine. With either hook or hybrid constructs, there was more emphasis placed on distraction and compression forces to achieve curve correction. Anchor placement was selected to distract in the concavity of curvature, level the lowest instrumented vertebrae, and compress across the thoracolumbar junction and the convexity of the curvature. Distraction forces tended to increase kyphosis (not undesirable in the thoracic spine). With increasing use of pedicle screws in the thoracic spine, "all pedicle screw" constructs are more common, and the concept of distraction and compression as corrective forces has decreased in importance. The concepts of anchor density (number of anchors used per vertebral level) and pedicle screw density (number of pedicle screws used per vertebral level) have been examined as they relate to surgical outcome. Studies have not shown consistently improved patient outcomes with higher density pedicle screw constructs in moderate sized main thoracic curves, although there is good evidence that radiographic measures are improved with higher density pedicle screw constructs.[144-146] As higher density pedicle screw constructs are more costly than lower density hybrid constructs, cost is an issue. For moderate sized, flexible curves, both strategies can lead to good results (Figs. 10A and B). Perhaps the most incremental benefit from use of higher density pedicle screw constructs in idiopathic scoliosis will be realized in patients with severe, stiff curves, in patients with osteopenic bone, and/or in patients with increased risk of pseudoarthrosis.

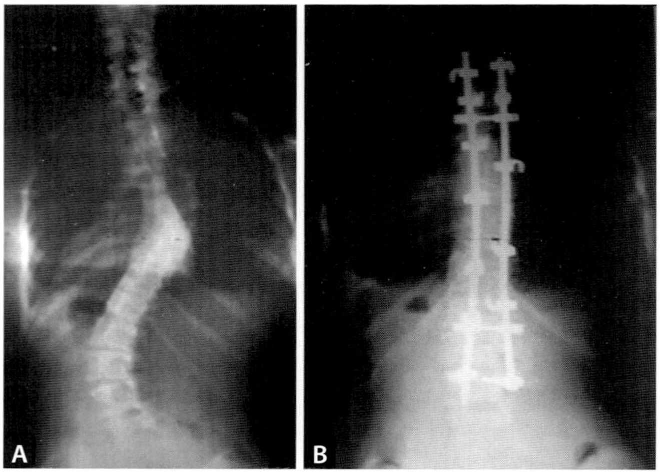

Figs. 10A and B: An example of a posterior instrumented spinal fusion using a hybrid construct in a moderate sized, flexible double major curve.

Modes of Correction

Safe correction of global and local spinal deformity during spinal fusion is one of the major goals of surgery. Multiple corrective maneuvers are available to the surgeon depending on each patient's curve pattern and personality. Multiple corrective maneuvers are often used in the same patient. Correction may be acute or gradual. In large stiff curves, it may be safer to perform correction gradually. Halo-gravity or halo-femoral traction are possible. Halo-gravity traction is done preoperatively over several weeks. Specially modified wheelchairs and walkers allow for the patient to be mobile during the process. Halo-femoral traction is usually performed intraoperatively at the start of surgery and may be adjusted gradually during surgery. More recently, the concept of internal distraction was introduced by Buchowski et al.[147] This involves placing temporary anchors proximal and distal to the curve (attached to the spine, ribs, and/or pelvis) at the start of spinal exposure and distracting gradually during surgical exposure and implant placement.

Acute modes of corrections aim to improve coronal curvature, sagittal profile, and vertebral rotation. Rod derotation involves contouring a spinal rod into normal sagittal shape, placing it within spinal anchors 90° from its desired position, and rotating the rod into the correct plane. This has the effect of correcting both coronal and sagittal parameters. It can only be done in curves whose coronal apices are located near the normal sagittal apices (T8 and L5). It is less useful in thoracolumbar curves. Other modes of correction in the coronal and sagittal plane are cantilever bending, apical translation, in-situ rod contouring, and end vertebrae compression/distraction to "level" the LIV. Direct vertebral rotation is an important corrective maneuver which addresses the transverse plane deformity of scoliosis, which involves applying a force couple (most effectively through bilateral pedicle screws) to an individual vertebra to rotate it about its center point, correcting the rotational deformity.

Thoracoplasty

If direct vertebral rotation cannot correct the rib prominence associated with large thoracic curves, a thoracoplasty may be performed (either at the same time as posterior instrumented spinal fusion or at a separate surgical setting). This involves resecting portions of the apical ribs on the convex side of the curvature. Typically, no more than five consecutive ribs are partially resected, and no more than 4 cm of each rib is removed. If too many ribs or too much length are removed, a flail chest may result. Also, a mild but permanent decrease in pulmonary function is associated with thoracoplasty. Newton et al. found modest decrease in forced vital capacity age percentile (FVC%) after posterior instrumented spinal fusion (PISF) plus thoracoplasty (in the neighborhood of 5%) versus a 1% increase with PSF without thoracoplasty.[148] Lonner found that, for mild preoperative ATR (<9%), using direct vertebral rotation (DVR) versus thoracoplasty versus both led to similar clinical measures of postoperative ATR, but for large preoperative ATR, doing both a DVR and a thoracoplasty led to better clinical outcome.[149] Although improved curve correction with modern implants has greatly decreased the rotational deformity that thoracoplasty surgery addresses, it still is a surgical procedure that may be used in patients with residual, cosmetically-unacceptable rib prominence after (or in conjunction with) posterior instrumented spinal fusion. A discussion of the respiratory consequences associated with thoracoplasty should be thoroughly discussed with the patient before undertaking this procedure.

PROGNOSIS AFTER SURGERY

Outcomes

Outcomes after spinal fusion for idiopathic scoliosis can be measured radiographically or clinically. Radiographic measures include amount of deformity correction in all planes. Clinical outcomes take the form of patient- or patient proxy-based outcomes questionnaires like the SRS-30 and the Spinal Appearance Questionnaire (among others). Neither modality alone paints a comprehensive picture of the "true" outcome after spinal fusion for scoliosis. However, use of a combination of radiographic and clinical outcome measures represents a "best effort" at understanding true treatment outcomes. Also, scoliosis is a disease with far reaching consequences. The outcome of interest is not only the outcome in the short- (2 year) or medium- (5–10 year) term, but the health status far into adult life. Studies with long-term follow-up have particular value in this situation, and ideally would compare surgically treated to nonoperatively treated patients. With this being said there are no such studies currently.

The goal of treatment in progressive infantile or juvenile scoliosis patients is to preserve spinal growth while controlling spinal deformity until the patient attains an age at which spinal fusion can be feasibly performed. Since there are no good long-term follow-up studies of operatively treated patients with infantile or juvenile idiopathic scoliosis, outcomes must be extrapolated from existing studies in adolescent patients. At first glance, outcome after spinal fusion in young idiopathic patients might be thought to be similar. However, young idiopathic patients often are treated with growth sparing surgery, and they tend to have stiffer curves at time of final fusion, longer fusions, and require more spinal osteotomies.[150] Therefore, it can be safely assumed that they likely have more surgical complications and are more at risk for adjacent segment disease than in adolescent idiopathic scoliosis in general. However, it must be remembered that the natural history of these patients without surgery is poorer than in adolescent idiopathic scoliosis, with higher mortality (respiratory and /or cardiopulmonary failure) than matched controls in the general population.[151]

When comparing radiographic outcomes between anterior and posterior instrumented fusions, correction rates are similar in the coronal plane. In a study by Newton et al. which compared anterior to posterior instrumented thoracic fusions, similar curve correction (57%) was obtained, with higher blood loss with posterior approaches and higher operative time with anterior approaches. Anterior instrumented fusions resulted in over 2 times more patients having normal 15–40° thoracic kyphosis (43% vs. 18%). Anterior open (versus thoracoscopic) instrumented fusions resulted in a significant decrease in pulmonary function at 2-year post-surgery and offered no clear benefit to the patient as compared to posterior or thoracoscopic instrumented fusion.[134]

In most published studies, radiographic deformity correction in the coronal plane is superior with posterior pedicle screw constructs as compared to hook or hybrid constructs. Yilmaz et al. showed coronal Cobb correction percent with hook, hybrid, and pedicle screw constructs to be approximately 50, 60, and 70%.[152] They also found a trend toward postoperative worsening of thoracic kyphosis (average 10° loss of kyphosis, with an average of 11° post-surgery) with pedicle screw constructs versus hook and hybrid constructs (2° increase, with an average of >20° of kyphosis). Despite these differences, there were no differences in global SRS-22 outcomes scores, although there were higher patient satisfaction scores in the pedicle screw group. Lowenstein et al. showed similar findings, with improved coronal but worsening sagittal measures in the thoracic spine with pedicle screw versus hybrid constructs (72% vs. 60% coronal correction; 10° average loss of kyphosis with an average of <20° post-surgery).[153] Also, increased implant density (number of anchors per level fused) has little effect on 3-plane correction in moderate (50–60°) thoracic scoliosis, with approximately 65% coronal curve correction and 5° loss of thoracic kyphosis in high and low density pedicle screw constructs (> or <1.3 TPS per level).[144] Other authors have demonstrated similar findings in a similar group of patients.[154] It is possible that increased thoracic pedicle screw density may have a more pronounced corrective effect in larger, stiffer curves. Luhmann et al. showed that, in patients with curves between 70° and 100°, pedicle screw constructs gave similar correction percentages (48%) to combined anterior release and posterior instrumented fusion (48%) which was superior to hook and hybrid constructs (38% and 34%).[129] Watanabe et al. showed similar results in a group of patients with different diagnosis (many idiopathic) with coronal curvature above 100°.[155] Clinically, pedicle screw constructs may have improved transverse plane correction (decrease in rib prominence) as compared to hybrid constructs due to the possibility of direct vertebral rotation of the apical vertebrae. However, it is difficult to find definitive evidence of this in the literature. Arlet and Ouellet et al. showed similar transverse plane correction clinically with pedicle screw versus hybrid constructs.[156] Fu and Kawakami showed that, for patients with flexible thoracic scoliosis, pedicle screw use and direct vertebral rotation gave similar rotational correction as anterior instrumented fusion, and superior correction to hook or wire constructs.[157] Patients with rib prominence correction using direct vertebral rotation may avoid thoracoplasty and the associated negative impact on long-term pulmonary function. To summarize radiographic outcomes, good (>50%) coronal curve correction is achievable with a variety of posterior constructs as well as anterior instrumented constructs. Improved coronal correction can be expected with pedicle screws and increased implant density constructs. Pedicle screws constructs consistently show worsening of thoracic hypokyphosis when compared to hook or hybrid constructs and with anterior instrumentation (Figs. 11A to D). Rotational correction is perhaps superior using pedicle screws and a direct vertebral body rotation maneuver in flexible thoracic curves.

Clinically, there is minimal to mild correlation between coronal and transverse deformity correction and patient or physician perceived improvement in appearance.[152,156,158] Smucny et al. showed a mild increase (positive assessment) of appearance in patients treated with pedicle screw versus hybrid posterior constructs.[158] However, the difference in curve correction was only 7%, and only coronal measurements were listed. Arlet et al. studied the clinical appearance as judged by patients, non-physicians, and spine surgeons blinded to the type of instrumentation in operatively treated patients (either pedicle screw or hybrid posterior constructs) with main thoracic curves between 40° and 70°. They found no relationship among patient outcome, appearance scores, and instrumentation type (although there was over 70% curve correction in both groups).

Clinically, in the short term, there is post-surgical pain in the months following surgery. By 6 months post-surgery, approximately 80–93% of patients have low levels of pain nearing their baseline status. Patients with increased pain beyond 6 months (in the absence of surgical complications) were more likely to have preoperative negative emotions related to their back and more anxiety.[159-161] Mid-term (5–15 year)

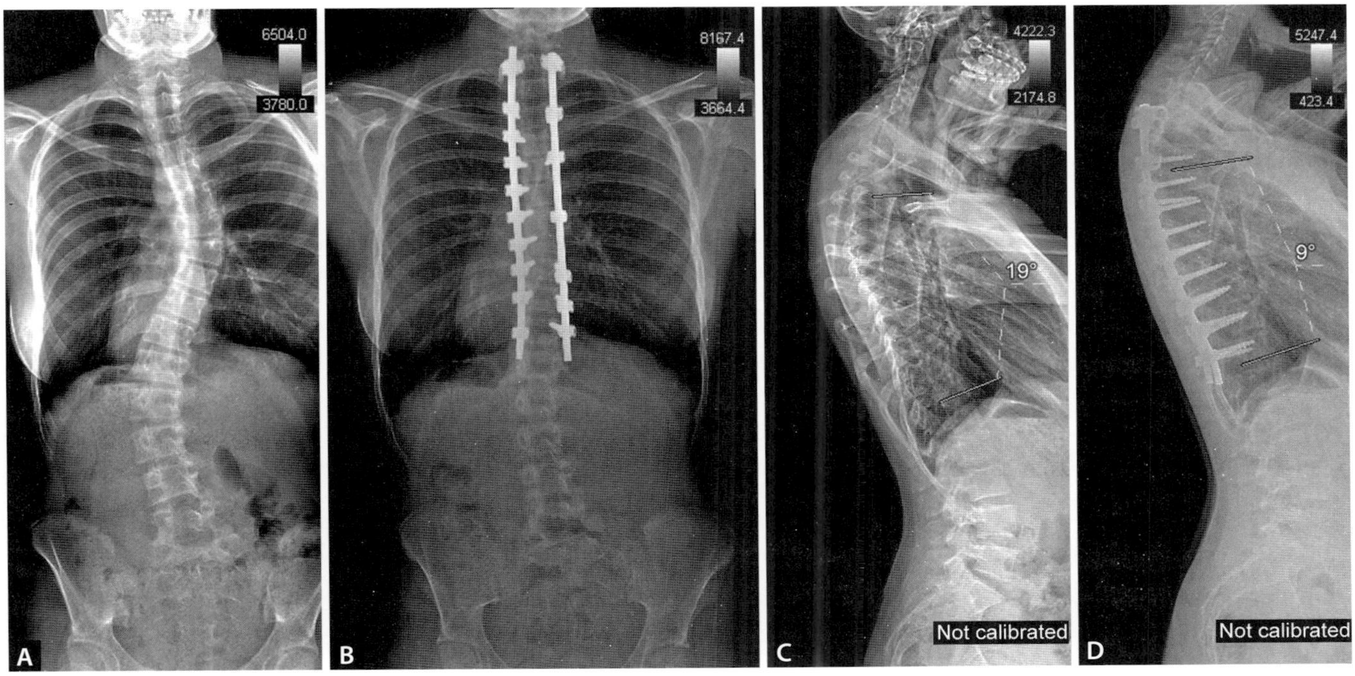

Figs. 11A to D: A patient with a main thoracic scoliosis treated with a high density pedicle screw construct. There has been good correction of the coronal (A and B) and transverse components of the deformity, but there has been worsening of the thoracic hypokyphosis (C and D), which is seen more often with high density pedicle screw constructs.

outcomes demonstrate generally low levels of pain (<30% of respondents with significant pain) and high levels of societal function (>70% without self-reported employment restrictions).[162] Akazawa et al. studied patient-based outcomes in AIS patients treated with spinal fusion to age- and sex-matched control patients at 21–41 years post-surgery. As compared to normal controls, patients with adolescent idiopathic scoliosis after spinal fusion had similar amounts of back pain and mental health status, but decreased reported physical function and body self-image using SRS-22 and Roland-Morris Disability Questionnaire outcomes measures.[163] Other authors have found similar rates of pain as compared to the general population.[164] Kepler provides a good review of the topic.[165]

Adjacent Segment Disease

By performing an appropriate selective fusion, mobile adjacent spinal segments remain. If only a few mobile segments remain, they are subjected to increased stresses, and there is the potential risk of developing future degenerative disk disease at these levels. This has been examined in the literature for thoracolumbar fusions extending to the low lumbar spine, and has not been studied proximal to the fusion mass. This was reported initially with first-generation posterior implant systems (Harrington rods) primarily in the setting of long fusions ending at L4 or L5. In addition to adjacent segment disease, these patients also had loss of sagittal contours ("flat back" syndrome). Cochran et al. showed significant low back pain in 24% of patients fused with Harrington rod instrumentation on average 16 years after surgery, 71% of whom were fused to either L4 or L5.[166] Helenius found a 20 + % rate of degenerative disks in the unfused lumbar spine of thoracic-fused AIS patients with Harrington rods, but this did not correlate to back pain as compared to controls.[167] Perez-Grueso found degenerative disk disease below thoracic fusions in patients fused using second-generation implant systems, despite improved sagittal contour as compared to Harrington rod fusions.[168] However, the degeneration was not at the adjacent segment but rather most commonly at L5S1, at a rate similar to normal controls in other studies, and patients did not have increased rates of back pain. Although a more distal lumbar fusion results in radiographic disk degeneration, low back pain does not always correlate to the radiographic findings. Moreover,

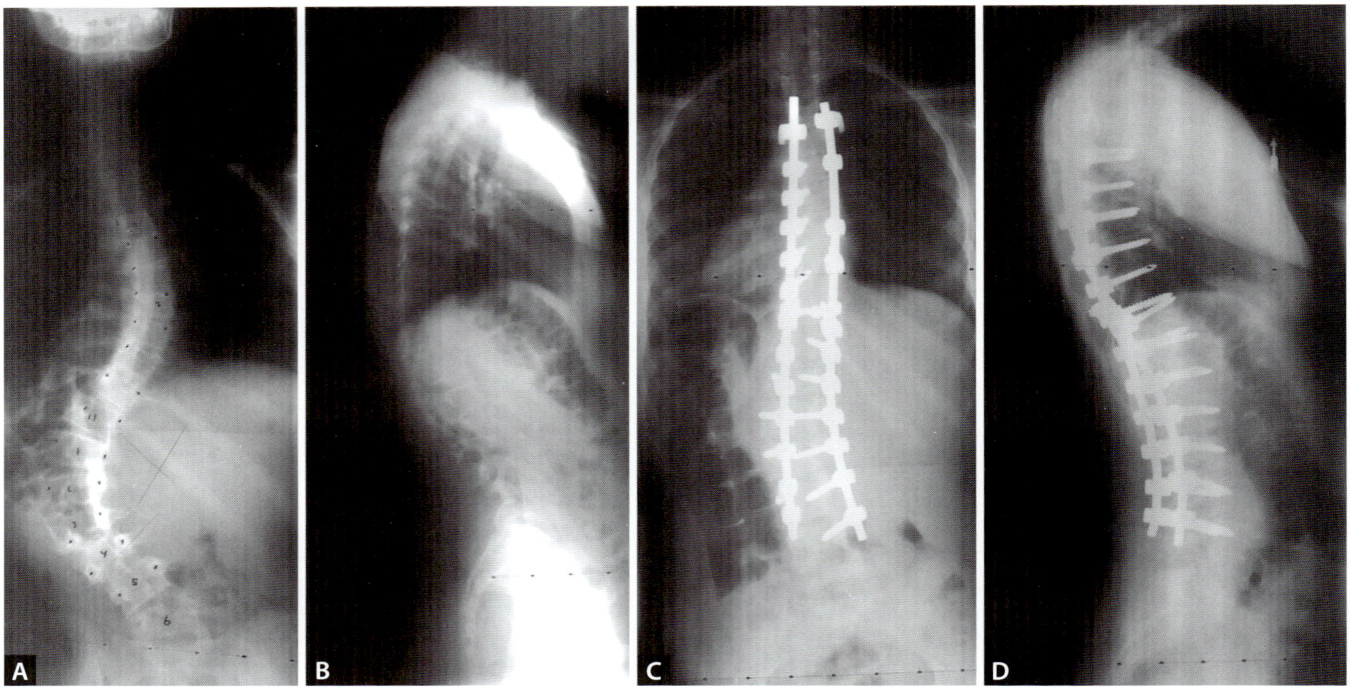

Figs. 12A to D: A patient with a severe thoracolumbar/main thoracic scoliosis with a significantly translated lower end vertebrae treated with posterior instrumented spinal fusion. Although there has been good curve correction, because there are only two mobile disk segments below this fusion, there is concern for future development of adjacent segment disease.

in patients with low back pain and radiographic disk degeneration, it is unclear if it is the degeneration or the abnormal postoperative sagittal contour (or both) that are the primary cause of low back pain in these patients (Figs. 12A to D).

COMPLICATIONS

Complications often result in reoperations, either in the early postoperative period or several months to years later. Overall, reoperation rates range from 4% to 20%.[78,169] Most revisions are performed for dislodged implants, pseudarthroses, implant prominence, or infection.

Neurologic Complications

Neurologic complications are a rare but potentially devastating complication after spinal surgery. Multi-modality spinal cord monitoring is recommended to detect spinal cord injuries intraoperatively. This includes use of somatosensory evoked potentials (SSEP), in which a distal nerve stimulus, which primarily ascends through the dorsal columns of the spinal cord, causes a measurable effect over the proximal somatosensory cortex; and motor evoked potentials (MEP), in which a proximal motor cortical stimulus, which descends through the ventral columns of the spinal cord, causes muscle activity distally. The article by Schwartz et al. gives a comprehensive review of use of SSEP and MEP in scoliosis surgery. Another modality includes the monitoring of triggered electromyographic (t-EMG) activity over the thoracic nerve root innervated abdominal wall muscles.[170] If there is EMG activity below a threshold electrical impulse intensity to a stimulus transmitted through a pedicle screw, this can signify a medial or inferior pedicle breach. However, the sensitivity of threshold stimulation of pedicle screws is poor, varies with the spinal; level being tested, and differs on the concave versus convex side of the spine, making this modality of questionable benefit.[171,172]

Recognition of an intraoperative spinal cord monitoring change requires immediate attention. Steps to reverse any potential injury after ruling out technical causes of a monitoring change include removing any surgical implant that may be impinging on neural elements, raising the blood pressure to a mean arterial pressure (MAP) at or above baseline awake levels, ensuring that oxygen saturation levels are 100%, and maintaining a hematocrit above 30%. The order of these steps depends on the exact clinical scenario immediately preceding the change in spinal cord monitoring signals. If there is no improvement of the neural monitoring changes in a short time frame (15–30 minutes), consideration should be given to giving a neuroprotective antioxidant medication, demonstrated to have modest neuroprotective benefit and result in modest recovery from spinal cord injury. The most commonly used agent is high-dose methylprednisolone according to the NASCIS II protocol for spinal cord injury,[173] although its use is controversial due to the medication's side effect profile. If there is no complete resolution of spinal cord monitoring signals after these steps, an intraoperative wake up test should immediately be performed. If the results of the wake up test are abnormal or equivocal, removal of all spinal implants should be considered with abortion of the procedure, and rapid 3-D imaging should be performed. No good literature exists on when to return to the operating room in the face of an iatrogenic spinal cord injury, but most authors wait for weeks to months to witness stabilization of the neurologic deficit. A good review article giving practical treatment algorithms in the setting of iatrogenic spinal cord injury was recently authored by Pahys et al.[174]

Neurologic complications can involve the peripheral or central nervous system. Peripheral nerve injuries are often the result of arm patient positioning or pressure on the lateral femoral cutaneous nerve and most often represent temporary neurapraxia.[175,176] Spinal cord injury can be caused by direct injury with a surgical instrument or implant, vascular insult by ligation of segmental vessels supplying the anterior spinal cord or by ischemia caused by stretch of the anterior spinal artery, compression by bone graft or hemostatic material.[170,177,178] Coe et al. summarized data on AIS patients from the SRS database in the years 2001–2003 and found a spinal cord injury rate of 0.26, 0.32, and 1.75% for anterior, posterior, and combined surgeries.[169] Of these, over 60% had complete recovery of the injury. The article by Mooney et al. gives a good summary of recognition and management of spinal cord injury.[179]

Infection

There are two types of postoperative infections: acute and chronic. Acute as defined by Clark et al., occurs within the first year after surgery.[180] Treatment of acute infections includes surgical irrigation and debridement, retention of implants for spinal stability, long-term suppressive antibiotics, and possibly application of negative pressure wound therapy devices if there are no exposed neural elements.[181] Late infections are thought to be the result of slow-growing bacteria (often skin flora such as *S. aureus, S. epidermidis, P. acnes*, or *K. kingae*) present at the time of the index procedure that can take years to develop. Hedequist et al. have written an excellent review article on the subject, and emphasize that in addition to a thorough irrigation and debridement, instrumentation removal is essential to complete eradication of the infection (once a solid fusion mass is present).[182]

Some risk factors for infection are modifiable by the surgeon; some are not. There is good evidence that proper use and timing of preoperative prophylactic antibiotics (a first generation cephalosporin if no contraindication exists) decreases surgical site infections.[183] There is some evidence that the type of metal instrumentation used affects infection rates. Both Soultanis et al. and De Silvestre et al. have shown higher late infection rates in posterior instrumented spinal fusions with first generation stainless steel implants as compared to newer titanium alloy implants.[143,184] It is unknown if this is in fact a material or a design issue. Many proposed interventions to decrease surgical site infection extrapolate findings from adult spine fusion patients or nonidiopathic scoliosis patients to the adolescent idiopathic population. These include using a chlorhexidine skin presurgical scrub (both before hospital admission and as a surgical preparation solution), using vancomycin powder placed in the surgical wound before closure, soaking bone graft in gentamicin, and presurgical treatment of nasal colonization by methicillin-resistant *Staphylococcus aureus* (MRSA) with mupirocin ointment. Although the above practices are safe, there is insufficient evidence to determine their efficacy at this time.[185,186]

Adding-on

Adding-on is defined as progression of spinal curvature in the unfused levels just above and/or below a previous spinal fusion. Adding-on may occur in the coronal or

CHAPTER 12

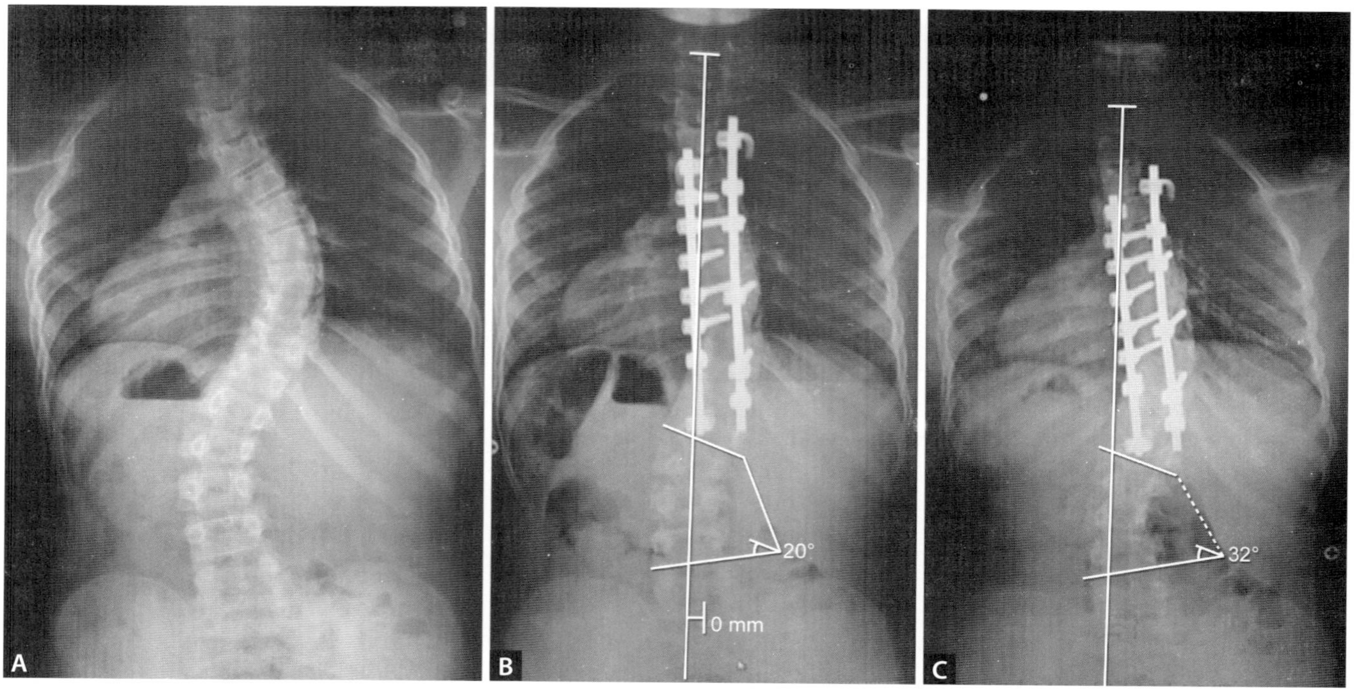

Figs. 13A to C: Early adding-on in a Risser 0 patient who underwent a posterior instrumented spinal fusion for main thoracic scoliosis. There has been small (3°) progression of the lumbar curve associated with 1 additional cm of left lateral translation of the C7 plumb line from the center sacral vertebral line one year after surgery. Close observation in this skeletally immature patient is warranted, as further adding-on may be expected.

sagittal or transverse plane. Coronal adding-on is defined as progression of disk tilt just above or below a fusion. It can be quantified by an increase of translation of the vertebrae just above or below fusion from the CSVL (or C7 plumb). Adding-on is thought to be related to upper and lower instrumented vertebrae (UIV or LIV) selection. In general, choosing an IV that is significantly deviated from the CSVL and/or stops short of the end vertebrae may result in postoperative adding-on. Some authors suggest adding-on is more likely in skeletally immature regardless of IV choice, but this is unclear[187] (Figs. 13A to C).

Sagittal adding-on is also known as progressive junctional kyphosis. It is defined as an increase in sagittal curvature of >10° over preoperative values just above or below an instrumented fusion. Risk factors for junctional kyphosis are choosing an IV with pre-existing segmental kyphosis (an IV selection error), not restoring sagittal alignment within the fusion (failure of correction of hypokyphosis), or perhaps using a construct with pedicle screws at the most proximal aspect of the fusion (implant related).

Decompensation

Spinal decompensation can be defined as a lack of sagittal or coronal balance after an instrumented fusion. Decompensation can be due to improper exclusion of a structural curve from fusion, overcorrection of a curve in a selective fusion, improper selection of fusion levels, or failure to restore proper sagittal balance within a fusion. Decompensation can be stable or progressive after surgery. Examples of stable decompensation can include postoperative proximal or distal junctional kyphosis, or coronal imbalance due to the LIV being significantly translated from the CSVL. Progressive decompensation is a result of adding-on (described above).

Pseudoarthrosis/Implant Failure

The goal of spinal implants in the context of fusion for scoliosis is to rigidly hold the spine in position while spinal fusion takes place. Although there are cases of implant failure due to implant design reasons, most cases of implant failure are due to development of pseudoarthrosis.

Overall, the pseudoarthrosis rate is in the range of 1–3% for idiopathic scoliosis. Published pseudoarthrosis rates are higher with anterior thoracic instrumented fusions than anterior dual-rod instrumented thoracolumbar fusions or posterior instrumented fusions. In separate studies by Yoon and Newton comparing 4.0 mm stainless steel to 4.75 mm titanium alloy rods in anterior instrumented thoracic fusions, there was a nearly 3-fold increase in the pseudoarthrosis rate (21% vs. 8%), and 13% of the patients who had a 4.0 mm stainless steel rod experienced rod breakage.[188,189] This led to the abandonment of 4.0 mm stainless steel rods in this setting. Using meticulous diskectomy and autograft bone, Newton et al. found an 8% rate of unfused disk spaces in anterior instrumented fusions,[189] and the same senior author has reported a 3% rate of disk space nonfusion more recently at 5-year post-surgical follow-up.[190] Posteriorly, there has been a trend of decreasing pseudoarthrosis rates with more rigid posterior constructs. Posterior pedicle screw constructs have led to a decrease in pseudoarthrosis rates on the order of <1% (versus >2% with hybrid constructs). This topic is well discussed by both Kuklo et al. and Ramo et al.[191,192]

Implant-related

First and second generation posterior spinal implant systems were more prominent over the posterior elements ("higher profile"). Occasionally, particularly in thin patients, these prominent posterior implants could be a source of skin irritation and pain. With the advancement of spine implants, the profile of constructs has been decreased. The elements of a construct that are most often prominent are cross-links. Partial implant removal often succeeds at relieving the pain.

Implants can also dislodge or be malpositioned initially. Implants that dislodged were in an appropriate position initially but migrated into a different one. Kuklo et al. discussed dislodgement being more common with hooks because they are not rigid points of fixation.[191] Campos et al. proposed that car accidents can cause hook dislodgement.[193] Malpositioned implants, however, are located in an unintended position immediately after placement. This does not necessarily mean that all postoperative implants in an unintended position are malpositioned. Screws can migrate (or "plow") into an unintended position by placing force upon them during the performance of deformity correction maneuvers. This was demonstrated by Wagner et al., who confirmed appropriately located screws with intraoperative CT scan images before performing corrective maneuvers, only to find with postoperative imaging screws that were abutting the aorta.[194] There are many articles that describe the misplacement of pedicle screws. Screw misplacements can occur in any direction, with most focus in the literature being placed on medial misplacements because of the risk of neurologic impingement. Screws with small (<2 mm) medial pedicular breaches into the canal rarely cause symptoms, whereas large (>4 mm) medial pedicular breaches often cause symptoms. In the best of hands, pedicle screw accuracy rates when considering large medial breaches are 94%.[195,196] Screw misplacement can either be described on a per-screw or per-patient basis. Because most constructs involve multiple screws, the per-patient misplacement rate (approximately 10% in many studies) will be higher than the significant per-screw misplacement rate (approximately 5% in many studies).[197-199] In studies where any detectible pedicle breach was detected on routine postoperative CT scans, approximately 15% of screws are misplaced.[197] What to do with a malpositioned screw is unclear. Revision surgical rates (screw removal) for malpositioned screws are less than 1%, with most screw removals occurring in asymptomatic cases.[200] If an implant is malpositioned or has displaced into a potentially dangerous position, implant removal is a logical solution.

Finally, late operative site pain is the name of focal back in the absence of infection, prominent implants, or pseudoarthrosis. Though unclear, the pain is thought to be caused by aseptic loosening with resultant metal debris formation leading to an inflammatory response. Metal debris could be from corrosion or from micromotion before fusion happens.[201] This is a diagnosis of exclusion. Implant removal (even partial) can be helpful in these situations.

REFERENCES

1. Working Group on 3-D Classification and the Terminology Committee. SRS Terminology Committee and Working Group on Spinal Classification Revised Glossary of Terms. From: scoliosis research society website, accessed 9/16/19 (https://www.srs.org/professionals/online-education-and-resources/glossary/revised-glossary-of-terms).
2. Scoliosis Research Society. (2013). Infantile Scoliosis. From scoliosis research society website, accessed 9/16/19 (https://www.srs.org/professionals/online-education-and-resources/conditions-and-treatments/infantile-scoliosis).

3. Scoliosis Research Society. (2013). Juvenile Scoliosis. From scoliosis research society website, accessed 9/16/19 (https://www.srs.org/professionals/online-education-and-resources/conditions-and-treatments/juvenile-scoliosis).
4. Roach JW. Adolescent idiopathic scoliosis. Orthop Clin North Am. 1999;30(3):353-65, vii-viii.
5. Miller NH. Cause and natural history of adolescent idiopathic scoliosis. Orthop Clin North Am. 1999;30(3):343-52, vii.
6. Riseborough EJ, Wynne-Davies R. A genetic survey of idiopathic scoliosis in Boston, Massachusetts. J Bone Joint Surg Am. 1973;55(5):974-82.
7. MacEwen G, Cowell H. Familial incidence of idiopathic scoliosis. JBJS. 1970;52A:405.
8. Kesling KL, Reinker KA. Scoliosis in twins. A meta-analysis of the literature and report of six cases. Spine (Phila Pa 1976). 1997;22(17):2009-14; discussion 2015.
9. Inoue M, Minami S, Kitahara H, et al. Idiopathic scoliosis in twins studied by DNA fingerprinting: the incidence and type of scoliosis. J Bone Joint Surg Br. 1998;80(2):212-7.
10. Kruse LM, Buchan JG, Gurnett CA, et al. Polygenic threshold model with sex dimorphism in adolescent idiopathic scoliosis: the Carter effect. J Bone Joint Surg Am. 2012;94(16):1485-91.
11. Carr AJ, Ogilvie DJ, Wordsworth BP, et al. Segregation of structural collagen genes in adolescent idiopathic scoliosis. Clin Orthop Relat Res. 1992;274:305-10.
12. Miller NH, Mims B, Child A, et al. Genetic analysis of structural elastic fiber and collagen genes in familial adolescent idiopathic scoliosis. J Orthop Res. 1996;14(6):994-9.
13. Burwell RG, Dangerfield PH, Moulton A, et al. Whither the etiopathogenesis (and scoliogeny) of adolescent idiopathic scoliosis? Incorporating presentations on scoliogeny at the 2012 IRSSD and SRS meetings. Scoliosis. 2013;8(1):4.
14. Moldovan F, Villemure I, Fendri K, et al. Adolescent idiopathic scoliosis (AIS): netabolic factors, biomechanical stress and estrogen impact. Stud Health Technol Inform. 2012;176:452.
15. Grivas TB, Mihas C, Mazioti C, et al. Maternal age at birth: does it dictate the epigenotypic expression of the trunkal asymmetry of a child? Stud Health Technol Inform. 2012;176:36-42.
16. McMaster ME, Lee AJ, Burwell RG. Indoor heated swimming pools: the vulnerability of some infants to develop spinal asymmetries years later. Stud Health Technol Inform. 2006;123:151-5.
17. McMaster ME. Heated indoor swimming pools, infants, and the pathogenesis of adolescent idiopathic scoliosis: a neurogenic hypothesis. Environ Health. 2011;10:86.
18. Cheng JC, Guo X. Osteopenia in adolescent idiopathic scoliosis. A primary problem or secondary to the spinal deformity? Spine (Phila Pa 1976). 1997;22(15):1716-21.
19. Cheng JC, Qin L, Cheung CS, et al. Generalized low areal and volumetric bone mineral density in adolescent idiopathic scoliosis. J Bone Miner Res. 2000;15(8):1587-95.
20. Khosla S, Tredwell SJ, Day B, et al. An ultrastructural study of multifidus muscle in progressive idiopathic scoliosis. Changes resulting from a sarcolemmal defect at the myotendinous junction. J Neurol Sci. 1980;46(1):13-31.
21. Duance VC, Crean JK, Sims TJ, et al. Changes in collagen cross-linking in degenerative disc disease and scoliosis. Spine (Phila Pa 1976). 1998;23(23):2545-51.
22. Ponseti IV. Lesions of the skeleton and of other mesodermal tissues in rats fed sweet-pea (Lathyrus odoratus) seeds. J Bone Joint Surg Am. 1954;36-A(5):1031-58.
23. Venn G, Mehta MH, Mason RM. Characterisation of collagen from normal and scoliotic human spinal ligament. Biochim Biophys Acta. 1983;757(2):259-67.
24. Goldberg CJ, Dowling FE, Fogarty EE, et al. Adolescent idiopathic scoliosis and cerebral asymmetry. An examination of a nonspinal perceptual system. Spine (Phila Pa 1976). 1995;20(15):1685-91.
25. Woods LA, Haller RJ, Hansen PD, et al. Decreased incidence of scoliosis in hearing-impaired children. Implications for a neurologic basis for idiopathic scoliosis. Spine (Phila Pa 1976). 1995;20(7):776-80; discussion 781.
26. O'Beirne J, Goldberg C, Dowling FE, et al. Equilibrial dysfunction in scoliosis: cause or effect? J Spinal Disord. 1989;2(3):184-9.
27. Kapetanos G, Potoupnis M, Dangilas A, et al. Is the labyrinthine dysfunction a causative factor in idiopathic scoliosis? Stud Health Technol Inform. 2002;91:7-9.
28. Kono H, Machida M, Saito M, et al. Mechanism of osteoporosis in adolescent idiopathic scoliosis: experimental scoliosis in pinealectomized chickens. J Pineal Res. 2011;51(4):387-93.
29. Man GC, Wong JH, Wang WW, et al. Abnormal melatonin receptor 1B expression in osteoblasts from girls with adolescent idiopathic scoliosis. J Pineal Res. 2011;50(4):395-402.
30. Man GC, Wang WW, Yeung BH, et al. Abnormal proliferation and differentiation of osteoblasts from girls with adolescent idiopathic scoliosis to melatonin. J Pineal Res. 2010;49(1):69-77.
31. Machida M, Dubousset J, Imamura Y, et al. Melatonin. A possible role in pathogenesis of adolescent idiopathic scoliosis. Spine (Phila Pa 1976). 1996;21(10):1147-52.
32. Hilibrand AS, Blakemore LC, Loder RT, et al. The role of melatonin in the pathogenesis of adolescent idiopathic scoliosis. Spine (Phila Pa 1976). 1996;21(10):1140-6.
33. Bagnall KM, Raso VJ, Hill DL, et al. Melatonin levels in idiopathic scoliosis. Diurnal and nocturnal serum melatonin levels in girls with adolescent idiopathic scoliosis. Spine (Phila Pa 1976). 1996;21(17):1974-8.
34. Fagan AB, Kennaway DJ, Sutherland AD. Total 24-hour melatonin secretion in adolescent idiopathic scoliosis. A case-control study. Spine (Phila Pa 1976). 1998;23(1):41-6.
35. Guo X, Chau WW, Chan YL, et al. Relative anterior spinal overgrowth in adolescent idiopathic scoliosis: result of disproportionate endochondral-membranous bone growth? Summary of an electronic focus group debate of the IBSE. Eur Spine J. 2005;14(9):862-73.
36. Chazono M, Soshi S, Kida Y, et al. Height velocity curves in female patients with idiopathic scoliosis. Stud Health Technol Inform. 2012;176:202-5.
37. Janssen MM, Vincken KL, van Raak SM, et al. Sagittal spinal profile and spinopelvic balance in parents of scoliotic children. Spine J. 2013;13(12):1789-800.

38. Mehta MH. The rib-vertebra angle in the early diagnosis between resolving and progressive infantile scoliosis. J Bone Joint Surg Br. 1972;54(2):230-43.
39. Little DG, Song KM, Katz D, et al. Relationship of peak height velocity to other maturity indicators in idiopathic scoliosis in girls. J Bone Joint Surg Am. 2000;82(5):685-93.
40. Biondi J, Weiner DS, Bethem D, et al. Correlation of Risser sign and bone age determination in adolescent idiopathic scoliosis. J Pediatr Orthop. 1985;5(6):697-701.
41. Risser JC. The Iliac apophysis; an invaluable sign in the management of scoliosis. Clin Orthop. 1958;11:111-9.
42. Sanders JO, Little DG, Richards BS. Prediction of the crankshaft phenomenon by peak height velocity. Spine (Phila Pa 1976). 1997;22(12):1352-6; discussion 1356-7.
43. Peterson LE, Nachemson AL. Prediction of progression of the curve in girls who have adolescent idiopathic scoliosis of moderate severity. Logistic regression analysis based on data from the Brace Study of the Scoliosis Research Society. J Bone Joint Surg Am. 1995;77(6):823-7.
44. Nault ML, Mac-Thiong JM, Roy-Beaudry M, et al. Three-dimensional spine parameters can differentiate between progressive and nonprogressive patients with AIS at the initial visit: a retrospective analysis. J Pediatr Orthop. 2013; 33(6):618-23.
45. Weinstein SL, Ponseti IV. Curve progression in idiopathic scoliosis. J Bone Joint Surg Am. 1983;65(4):447-55.
46. Weinstein SL, Zavala DC, Ponseti IV. Idiopathic scoliosis: long-term follow-up and prognosis in untreated patients. J Bone Joint Surg Am. 1981;63(5):702-12.
47. Nilsonne U, Lundgren KD. Long-term prognosis in idiopathic scoliosis. Acta Orthop Scand. 1968;39(4):456-65.
48. Mayo NE, Goldberg MS, Poitras B, et al. The Ste-Justine Adolescent Idiopathic Scoliosis Cohort Study. Part III: Back pain. Spine (Phila Pa 1976). 1994;19(14):1573-81.
49. Weinstein SL, Dolan LA, Spratt KF, et al. Health and function of patients with untreated idiopathic scoliosis: a 50-year natural history study. JAMA. 2003;289(5):559-67.
50. Nachemson A. A long-term follow-up study of non-treated scoliosis. Acta Orthop Scand. 1968;39(4):466-76.
51. Akazawa T, Minami S, Kotani T, et al. Health-related quality of life and low back pain of patients surgically treated for scoliosis after 21 years or more of follow-up: comparison among nonidiopathic scoliosis, idiopathic scoliosis, and healthy subjects. Spine (Phila Pa 1976). 2012;37(22):1899-903.
52. Yawn BP, Yawn RA, Hodge D, et al. A population-based study of school scoliosis screening. JAMA. 1999;282(15):1427-32.
53. Yawn BP, Yawn RA. The estimated cost of school scoliosis screening. Spine (Phila Pa 1976). 2000;25(18):2387-91.
54. Lee CF, Fong DY, Cheung KM, et al. Costs of school scoliosis screening: a large, population-based study. Spine (Phila Pa 1976). 2010;35(26):2266-72.
55. Guide to Clinical Preventive Services, 2nd edition. Report of the US Preventive Services Task Force. Baltimore (MD): Williams & Wilkins; 1996.
56. Guide to Clinical Preventive Services, 3rd edition. Periodic Updates US Preventive Services Task Force. Rockville (MD): Agency for Healthcare Research and Quality (US); 2002.
57. Richards BS, Vitale M. AAOS-SRS-POSNA-AAP Position Statement. Screening for Idiopathic Scoliosis in Adolescents 2007.
58. Bunnell WP. Selective screening for scoliosis. Clin Orthop Relat Res. 2005;434:40-5.
59. Lee CF, Fong DY, Cheung KM, et al. Referral criteria for school scoliosis screening: assessment and recommendations based on a large longitudinally followed cohort. Spine (Phila Pa 1976). 2010;35(25):E1492-8.
60. Glinkowski W, Michoński J, Glinkowska B, et al. Telediagnostic 3D school screening of back curvatures and posture using structured light method: pilot study. Stud Health Technol Inform. 2012;176:291-4.
61. Coelho DM, Bonagamba GH, Oliveira AS. Scoliometer measurements of patients with idiopathic scoliosis. Rev Bras Fisioter. 2013;17(2).
62. Izatt MT, Bateman GR, Adam CJ. Evaluation of the iPhone with an acrylic sleeve versus the Scoliometer for rib hump measurement in scoliosis. Scoliosis. 2012;7(1):14.
63. Franko OI, Bray C, Newton PO. Validation of a scoliometer smartphone app to assess scoliosis. J Pediatr Orthop. 2012;32(8):e72-5.
64. Chowanska J, Kotwicki T, Rosadzinski K, et al. School screening for scoliosis: can surface topography replace examination with scoliometer? Scoliosis. 2012;7(1):9.
65. Fujimori T, Iwasaki M, Nagamoto Y, et al. The utility of superficial abdominal reflex in the initial diagnosis of scoliosis: a retrospective review of clinical characteristics of scoliosis with syringomyelia. Scoliosis. 2010;5:17.
66. Carman DL, Browne RH, Birch JG. Measurement of scoliosis and kyphosis radiographs. Intraobserver and interobserver variation. J Bone Joint Surg Am. 1990;72(3):328-33.
67. Modi HN Chen T, Suh SW, et al. Observer reliability between juvenile and adolescent idiopathic scoliosis in measurement of stable Cobb's angle. Eur Spine J. 2009;18(1):52-8.
68. Srinivasalu S, Modi HN, Smehta S, et al. Cobb angle measurement of scoliosis using computer measurement of digitally acquired radiographs-intraobserver and interobserver variability. Asian Spine J. 2008;2(2):90-3.
69. Mok JM, Berven SH, Diab M, et al. Comparison of observer variation in conventional and three digital radiographic methods used in the evaluation of patients with adolescent idiopathic scoliosis. Spine (Phila Pa 1976). 2008;33(6):681-6.
70. Qiao J, Liu Z, Xu L, et al. Reliability analysis of a smartphone-aided measurement method for the Cobb angle of scoliosis. J Spinal Disord Tech. 2012;25(4):E88-92.
71. Jacquot F, Charpentier A, Khelifi S, et al. Measuring the Cobb angle with the iPhone in kyphoses: a reliability study. Int Orthop. 2012;36(8):1655-60.
72. Ouellet JA, LaPlaza J, Erickson MA, et al. Sagittal plane deformity in the thoracic spine: a clue to the presence of syringomyelia as a cause of scoliosis. Spine (Phila Pa 1976). 2003;28(18):2147-51.
73. King HA, Moe JH, Bradford DS, et al. The selection of fusion levels in thoracic idiopathic scoliosis. J Bone Joint Surg Am. 1983;65(9):1302-13.

CHAPTER 12

74. Lenke LG, Betz RR, Harms J, et al. Adolescent idiopathic scoliosis: a new classification to determine extent of spinal arthrodesis. J Bone Joint Surg Am. 2001;83-A(8):1169-81.
75. Richards BS, Hasley BP, Casey VF. Repeat surgical interventions following "definitive" instrumentation and fusion for idiopathic scoliosis. Spine (Phila Pa 1976). 2006;31(26):3018-26.
76. Ilharreborde B, Even J, Lefevre Y, et al. How to determine the upper level of instrumentation in Lenke types 1 and 2 adolescent idiopathic scoliosis: a prospective study of 132 patients. J Pediatr Orthop. 2008;28(7):733-9.
77. Miyanji F, Pawelek JB, Van Valin SE, et al. Is the lumbar modifier useful in surgical decision making?: defining two distinct Lenke 1A curve patterns. Spine (Phila Pa 1976). 2008;33(23):2545-51.
78. Ward WT, Rihn JA, Solic J, et al. A comparison of the lenke and king classification systems in the surgical treatment of idiopathic thoracic scoliosis. Spine (Phila Pa 1976). 2008;33(1):52-60.
79. Little DG, Sussman MD. The Risser sign: a critical analysis. J Pediatr Orthop. 1994;14(5):569-75.
80. Wang W, Zhen X, Sun X, et al. The value of different Risser grading systems in determining growth maturity of girls with adolescent idiopathic scoliosis. Stud Health Technol Inform. 2012;176:183-7.
81. Wittschieber D, Schmeling A, Schmidt S, et al. The Risser sign for forensic age estimation in living individuals: a study of 643 pelvic radiographs. Forensic Sci Med Pathol. 2013;9(1):36-43.
82. Greulich W, Pyle S. Radiographic atlas of skeletal development of the hand and wrist. Stanford, CA: Stanford University Press; 1959.
83. Sanders JO, Khoury JG, Kishan S, et al. Predicting scoliosis progression from skeletal maturity: a simplified classification during adolescence. J Bone Joint Surg Am. 2008;90(3):540-53.
84. Ryan PM, Puttler EG, Stotler WM, et al. Role of the triradiate cartilage in predicting curve progression in adolescent idiopathic scoliosis. J Pediatr Orthop. 2007;27(6):671-6.
85. Rowe DE, Bernstein SM, Riddick MF, et al. A meta-analysis of the efficacy of non-operative treatments for idiopathic scoliosis. J Bone Joint Surg Am. 1997;79(5):664-74.
86. Nachemson AL, Peterson LE. Effectiveness of treatment with a brace in girls who have adolescent idiopathic scoliosis. A prospective, controlled study based on data from the Brace Study of the Scoliosis Research Society. J Bone Joint Surg Am. 1995;77(6):815-22.
87. Brox JI, Lange JE, Gunderson RB, et al. Good brace compliance reduced curve progression and surgical rates in patients with idiopathic scoliosis. Eur Spine J. 2012;21(10):1957-63.
88. Karol LA. Effectiveness of bracing in male patients with idiopathic scoliosis. Spine (Phila Pa 1976). 2001;26(18):2001-5.
89. Yrjönen T, Ylikoski M, Schlenzka D, et al. Results of brace treatment of adolescent idiopathic scoliosis in boys compared with girls: a retrospective study of 102 patients treated with the Boston brace. Eur Spine J. 2007;16(3):393-7.
90. Olin W, Ponseti I. Orthodontic considerations for the patient wearing a Milwaukee Brace. Iowa Orthop J. 2011;31:22-9.
91. Lange JE, Steen H, Gunderson R, et al. Long-term results after Boston brace treatment in late-onset juvenile and adolescent idiopathic scoliosis. Scoliosis. 2011;6:18.
92. Wong MS, Cheng JC, Lam TP, et al. The effect of rigid versus flexible spinal orthosis on the clinical efficacy and acceptance of the patients with adolescent idiopathic scoliosis. Spine (Phila Pa 1976). 2008;33(12):1360-5.
93. Weinstein SL, Dolan LA, Wright JG, et al. Design of the Bracing in Adolescent Idiopathic Scoliosis Trial (BrAIST). Spine (Phila Pa 1976). 2013;38(21):1832-41.
94. Weinstein SL, Dolan LA, Wright JG, et al. Effects of bracing in adolescents with idiopathic scoliosis. N Engl J Med. 2013;369(16):1512-21.
95. Grivas TB, Rodopoulos GI, Bardakos NV. Night-time braces for treatment of adolescent idiopathic scoliosis. Disabil Rehabil Assist Technol. 2008;3(3):120-9.
96. Lee CS, Hwang CJ, Kim DJ, et al. Effectiveness of the Charleston night-time bending brace in the treatment of adolescent idiopathic scoliosis. J Pediatr Orthop. 2012;32(4):368-72.
97. D'Amato CR, Griggs S, McCoy B. Nighttime bracing with the Providence brace in adolescent girls with idiopathic scoliosis. Spine (Phila Pa 1976). 2001;26(18):2006-12.
98. Yrjönen T, Ylikoski M, Schlenzka D, et al. Effectiveness of the Providence nighttime bracing in adolescent idiopathic scoliosis: a comparative study of 36 female patients. Eur Spine J. 2006;15(7):1139-43.
99. Abbott A, Möller H, Gerdhem P. CONTRAIS: CONservative TReatment for Adolescent Idiopathic Scoliosis: a randomised controlled trial protocol. BMC Musculoskelet Disord. 2013;14:261.
100. Mahaudens P, Banse X, Mousny M, et al. Very short-term effect of brace wearing on gait in adolescent idiopathic scoliosis girls. Eur Spine J. 2013;22(11):2399-406.
101. Courvoisier A, Drevelle X, Vialle R, et al. 3D analysis of brace treatment in idiopathic scoliosis. Eur Spine J. 2013; 22(11):2449-55.
102. Canavese F, Dimeglio A. Normal and abnormal spine and thoracic cage development. World J Orthop. 2013;4(4):167-74.
103. DiMeglio A, Dimeglio A, Canavese F, et al. Growth and adolescent idiopathic scoliosis: when and how much? J Pediatr Orthop. 2011;31(1 Suppl):S28-36.
104. Zeltner TB, Burri PH. The postnatal development and growth of the human lung. II. Morphology. Respir Physiol. 1987;67(3):269-82.
105. Dunnill M. Quantitative methods in the study of pulmonary pathology. Thorax. 1962;17:320.
106. Cotrel Y, Morel G. The elongation-derotation-flexion technic in the correction of scoliosis. Rev Chir Orthop Reparatrice Appar Mot. 1964;50:59-75.
107. Mehta MH. Growth as a corrective force in the early treatment of progressive infantile scoliosis. J Bone Joint Surg Br. 2005;87(9):1237-47.
108. Risser JC. Scoliosis treated by cast correction and spine fusion. Clin Orthop Relat Res. 1976;116:86-94.
109. Sanders JO, D'Astous J, Fitzgerald M, et al. Derotational casting for progressive infantile scoliosis. J Pediatr Orthop. 2009;29(6):581-7.
110. Fletcher ND, McClung A, Rathjen KE, et al. Serial casting as a delay tactic in the treatment of moderate-to-severe early-onset scoliosis. J Pediatr Orthop. 2012;32(7):664-71.

111. Akbarnia BA, Cheung K, Noordeen H, et al. Next generation of growth-sparing techniques: preliminary clinical results of a magnetically controlled growing rod in 14 patients with early-onset scoliosis. Spine (Phila Pa 1976). 2013;38(8):665-70.
112. Thompson GH, Akbarnia BA, Kostial P, et al. Comparison of single and dual growing rod techniques followed through definitive surgery: a preliminary study. Spine (Phila Pa 1976). 2005;30(18):2039-44.
113. Schroerlucke SR, Akbarnia BA, Pawelek JB, et al. How does thoracic kyphosis affect patient outcomes in growing rod surgery? Spine (Phila Pa 1976). 2012;37(15):1303-9.
114. Cheung KM, Cheung JP, Samartzis D, et al. Magnetically controlled growing rods for severe spinal curvature in young children: a prospective case series. Lancet. 2012; 379(9830):1967-74.
115. Smith JT. Bilateral rib-to-pelvis technique for managing early-onset scoliosis. Clin Orthop Relat Res. 2011;469(5):1349-55.
116. Schulz JF, Smith J, Cahill PJ, et al. The role of the vertical expandable titanium rib in the treatment of infantile idiopathic scoliosis: early results from a single institution. J Pediatr Orthop. 2010;30(7):659-63.
117. McCarthy RE, Luhmann S, Lenke L, et al. The shilla growth guidance technique for early-onset spinal deformities at 2-year follow-up: a preliminary report. J Pediatr Orthop. 2014;34(1):1-7.
118. Farooq N, Garrido E, Altaf F, et al. Minimizing complications with single submuscular growing rods: a review of technique and results on 88 patients with minimum two-year follow-up. Spine (Phila Pa 1976). 2010;35(25):2252-8.
119. Betz RR, Ranade A, Samdani AF, et al. Vertebral body stapling: a fusionless treatment option for a growing child with moderate idiopathic scoliosis. Spine (Phila Pa 1976). 2010;35(2):169-76.
120. Lavelle WF, Samdani AF, Cahill PJ, et al. Clinical outcomes of nitinol staples for preventing curve progression in idiopathic scoliosis. J Pediatr Orthop. 2011;31(1 Suppl):S107-13.
121. Crawford CH, Lenke LG. Growth modulation by means of anterior tethering resulting in progressive correction of juvenile idiopathic scoliosis: a case report. J Bone Joint Surg Am. 2010;92(1):202-9.
122. Majdouline Y, Aubin CE, Robitaille M, et al. Scoliosis correction objectives in adolescent idiopathic scoliosis. J Pediatr Orthop. 2007;27(7):775-81.
123. Koch KD, Buchanan R, Birch JG, et al. Adolescents undergoing surgery for idiopathic scoliosis: how physical and psychological characteristics relate to patient satisfaction with the cosmetic result. Spine (Phila Pa 1976). 2001;26(19):2119-24.
124. Dubousset J, Herring JA, Shufflebarger H. The crankshaft phenomenon. J Pediatr Orthop. 1989;9(5):541-50.
125. Sarlak AY, Atmaca H, Buluç L, et al. Juvenile idiopathic scoliosis treated with posterior arthrodesis and segmental pedicle screw instrumentation before the age of 9 years: a 5-year follow-up. Scoliosis. 2009;4:1.
126. Dobbs MB, Lenke LG, Kim YJ, et al. Anterior/posterior spinal instrumentation versus posterior instrumentation alone for the treatment of adolescent idiopathic scoliotic curves more than 90 degrees. Spine (Phila Pa 1976). 2006;31(20):2386-91.
127. Sucato DJ, Elerson E. A comparison between the prone and lateral position for performing a thoracoscopic anterior release and fusion for pediatric spinal deformity. Spine (Phila Pa 1976). 2003;28(18):2176-80.
128. Halanski MA, Cassidy JA. Do multilevel Ponte osteotomies in thoracic idiopathic scoliosis surgery improve curve correction and restore thoracic kyphosis? J Spinal Disord Tech. 2013;26(5):252-5.
129. Luhmann SJ, Lenke LG, Kim YJ, et al. Thoracic adolescent idiopathic scoliosis curves between 70 degrees and 100 degrees: is anterior release necessary? Spine (Phila Pa 1976). 2005;30(18):2061-7.
130. Li M, Ni J, Fang X, et al. Comparison of selective anterior versus posterior screw instrumentation in Lenke5C adolescent idiopathic scoliosis. Spine (Phila Pa 1976). 2009;34(11):1162-6.
131. Geck MJ, Macagno A, Ponte A, et al. The Ponte procedure: posterior only treatment of Scheuermann's kyphosis using segmental posterior shortening and pedicle screw instrumentation. J Spinal Disord Tech. 2007;20(8):586-93.
132. Hee HT, Yu ZR, Wong HK. Comparison of segmental pedicle screw instrumentation versus anterior instrumentation in adolescent idiopathic thoracolumbar and lumbar scoliosis. Spine (Phila Pa 1976). 2007;32(14):1533-42.
133. Newton PO, Yaszay B, Upasani VV, et al. Preservation of thoracic kyphosis is critical to maintain lumbar lordosis in the surgical treatment of adolescent idiopathic scoliosis. Spine (Phila Pa 1976). 2010;35(14):1365-70.
134. Newton PO, Marks MC, Bastrom TP, et al. Surgical treatment of Lenke 1 main thoracic idiopathic scoliosis: results of a prospective, multicenter study. Spine (Phila Pa 1976). 2013;38(4):328-38.
135. Lenke LG, Betz RR, Haher TR, et al. Multisurgeon assessment of surgical decision-making in adolescent idiopathic scoliosis: curve classification, operative approach, and fusion levels. Spine (Phila Pa 1976). 2001;26(21):2347-53.
136. Suk SI, Lee SM, Chung ER, et al. Determination of distal fusion level with segmental pedicle screw fixation in single thoracic idiopathic scoliosis. Spine (Phila Pa 1976). 2003;28(5):484-91.
137. Cao K, Watanabe K, Kawakami N, et al. Selection of lower instrumented vertebra in treating Lenke type 2A adolescent idiopathic scoliosis. Spine (Phila Pa 1976). 2014;39(4):E253-61.
138. Cho RH, Yaszay B, Bartley CE, et al. Which Lenke 1A curves are at the greatest risk for adding-on and why? Spine (Phila Pa 1976). 2012;37(16):1384-90.
139. Erickson MA, Baulesh DM. Lowest instrumented vertebra selection in AIS. J Pediatr Orthop. 2011;31(1 Suppl):S69-76.
140. Trobisch PD, Ducoffe AR, Lonner BS, et al. Choosing fusion levels in adolescent idiopathic scoliosis. J Am Acad Orthop Surg. 2013;21(9):519-28.
141. Bernstein RM, Hall JE. Solid rod short segment anterior fusion in thoracolumbar scoliosis. J Pediatr Orthop B. 1998;7(2):124-31.
142. Wedemeyer M, Parent S, Mahar A, et al. Titanium versus stainless steel for anterior spinal fusions: an analysis of rod stress as a predictor of rod breakage during physiologic loading in a bovine model. Spine (Phila Pa 1976). 2007;32(1):42-8.

CHAPTER 12

143. Di Silvestre M, Bakaloudis G, Lolli F, et al. Late-developing infection following posterior fusion for adolescent idiopathic scoliosis. Eur Spine J. 2011;20(Suppl 1):S121-7.
144. Bharucha NJ, Lonner BS, Auerbach JD, et al. Low-density versus high-density thoracic pedicle screw constructs in adolescent idiopathic scoliosis: do more screws lead to a better outcome? Spine J. 2013;13(4):375-81.
145. Howard A, Donaldson S, Hedden D, et al. Improvement in quality of life following surgery for adolescent idiopathic scoliosis. Spine (Phila Pa 1976). 2007;32(24):2715-8.
146. Donaldson S, Hedden D, Stephens D, et al. Surgeon reliability in rating physical deformity in adolescent idiopathic scoliosis. Spine (Phila Pa 1976). 2007;32(3):363-7.
147. Buchowski JM, Bridwell KH, Lenke LG, et al. Epidural spinal cord compression with neurologic deficit associated with intrapedicular application of hemostatic gelatin matrix during pedicle screw insertion. Spine (Phila Pa 1976). 2009;34(13):E473-7.
148. Newton PO, Perry A, Bastrom TP, et al. Predictors of change in postoperative pulmonary function in adolescent idiopathic scoliosis: a prospective study of 254 patients. Spine (Phila Pa 1976). 2007;32(17):1875-82.
149. Lonner BS, Auerbach JD, Estreicher MB, et al. Pulmonary function changes after various anterior approaches in the treatment of adolescent idiopathic scoliosis. J Spinal Disord Tech. 2009;22(8):551-8.
150. Flynn JM, Tomlinson LA, Pawelek J, et al. Growing-rod graduates: lessons learned from ninety-nine patients who completed lengthening. J Bone Joint Surg Am. 2013; 95(19):1745-50.
151. Pehrsson K, Larsson S, Oden A, et al. Long-term follow-up of patients with untreated scoliosis. A study of mortality, causes of death, and symptoms. Spine (Phila Pa 1976). 1992;17(9):1091-6.
152. Yilmaz G, Borkhuu B, Dhawale AA, et al. Comparative analysis of hook, hybrid, and pedicle screw instrumentation in the posterior treatment of adolescent idiopathic scoliosis. J Pediatr Orthop. 2012;32(5):490-9.
153. Lowenstein JE, Matsumoto H, Vitale MG, et al. Coronal and sagittal plane correction in adolescent idiopathic scoliosis: a comparison between all pedicle screw versus hybrid thoracic hook lumbar screw constructs. Spine (Phila Pa 1976). 2007;32(4):448-52.
154. Yang S, Jones-Quaidoo SM, Eager M, et al. Right adolescent idiopathic thoracic curve (Lenke 1 A and B): does cost of instrumentation and implant density improve radiographic and cosmetic parameters? Eur Spine J. 2011;20(7):1039-47.
155. Watanabe K, Lenke LG, Bridwell KH, et al. Efficacy of perioperative halo-gravity traction for treatment of severe scoliosis (≥100°). J Orthop Sci. 2010;15(6):720-30.
156. Arlet V, Ouellet JA, Shilt J, et al. Subjective evaluation of treatment outcomes of instrumentation with pedicle screws or hybrid constructs in Lenke Type 1 and 2 adolescent idiopathic scoliosis: what happens when judges are blinded to the instrumentation? Eur Spine J. 2009;18(12):1927-35.
157. Fu G, Kawakami N, Goto M, et al. Comparison of vertebral rotation corrected by different techniques and anchors in surgical treatment of adolescent thoracic idiopathic scoliosis. J Spinal Disord Tech. 2009;22(3):182-9.
158. Smucny M, Lubicky JP, Sanders JO, et al. Patient self-assessment of appearance is improved more by all pedicle screw than by hybrid constructs in surgical treatment of adolescent idiopathic scoliosis. Spine (Phila Pa 1976). 2011;36(3):248-54.
159. Bastrom TP, Marks MC, Yaszay B, et al. Prevalence of postoperative pain in adolescent idiopathic scoliosis and the association with preoperative pain. Spine (Phila Pa 1976). 2013;38(21):1848-52.
160. Connelly M, Fulmer RD, Prohaska J, et al. Predictors of postoperative pain trajectories in adolescent idiopathic scoliosis. Spine (Phila Pa 1976). 2014;39(3):E174-81.
161. Sanders JO, Carreon LY, Sucato DJ, et al. Preoperative and perioperative factors effect on adolescent idiopathic scoliosis surgical outcomes. Spine (Phila Pa 1976). 2010;35(20):1867-71.
162. Bas T, Franco N, Bas P, et al. Pain and disability following fusion for idiopathic adolescent scoliosis: prevalence and associated factors. Evid Based Spine Care J. 2012;3(2):17-24.
163. Akazawa T, Minami S, Kotani T, et al. Long-term clinical outcomes of surgery for adolescent idiopathic scoliosis 21 to 41 years later. Spine (Phila Pa 1976). 2012;37(5):402-5.
164. Takayama K, Nakamura H, Matsuda H. Low back pain in patients treated surgically for scoliosis: longer than sixteen-year follow-up. Spine (Phila Pa 1976). 2009;34(20):2198-204.
165. Kepler CK, Meredith DS, Green DW, et al. Long-term outcomes after posterior spine fusion for adolescent idiopathic scoliosis. Curr Opin Pediatr. 2012;24(1):68-75.
166. Cochran T, Irstam L, Nachemson A. Long-term anatomic and functional changes in patients with adolescent idiopathic scoliosis treated by Harrington rod fusion. Spine (Phila Pa 1976). 1983;8(6):576-84.
167. Helenius I, Remes V, Yrjönen T, et al. Comparison of long-term functional and radiologic outcomes after Harrington instrumentation and spondylodesis in adolescent idiopathic scoliosis: a review of 78 patients. Spine (Phila Pa 1976). 2002;27(2):176-80.
168. Pérez-Grueso FS, Fernández-Baíllo N, Arauz de Robles S, et al. The low lumbar spine below Cotrel-Dubousset instrumentation: long-term findings. Spine (Phila Pa 1976). 2000;25(18):2333-41.
169. Coe JD, Arlet V, Donaldson W, et al. Complications in spinal fusion for adolescent idiopathic scoliosis in the new millennium. A report of the Scoliosis Research Society Morbidity and Mortality Committee. Spine (Phila Pa 1976). 2006;31(3):345-9.
170. Schwartz DM, Auerbach JD, Dormans JP, et al. Neurophysiological detection of impending spinal cord injury during scoliosis surgery. J Bone Joint Surg Am. 2007;89(11):2440-9.
171. Samdani AF, Hwang SW, Miyanji F, et al. Direct vertebral body derotation, thoracoplasty, or both: which is better with respect to inclinometer and scoliosis research society-22 scores? Spine (Phila Pa 1976). 2012;37(14):E849-53.
172. de Blas G, Burgos J, Regidor I, et al. Recording diffusion responses from contralateral intercostal muscles after stimulus-triggered electromyography: refining a tool for the assessment of thoracic pedicle screw placement in an experimental porcine model. Spine (Phila Pa 1976). 2009;34(11):E391-6.

173. Bracken MB, Shepard MJ, Collins WF, et al. A randomized, controlled trial of methylprednisolone or naloxone in the treatment of acute spinal-cord injury. Results of the Second National Acute Spinal Cord Injury Study. N Engl J Med. 1990;322(20):1405-11.
174. Pahys JM, Guille JT, D'Andrea LP, et al. Neurologic injury in the surgical treatment of idiopathic scoliosis: guidelines for assessment and management. J Am Acad Orthop Surg. 2009;17(7):426-34.
175. Tejwani SG, Scaduto AA, Bowen RE. Transient meralgia paresthetica after pediatric posterior spine fusion. J Pediatr Orthop. 2006;26(4):530-3.
176. Diab M, Smith AR, Kuklo TR, et al. Neural complications in the surgical treatment of adolescent idiopathic scoliosis. Spine (Phila Pa 1976). 2007;32(24):2759-63.
177. Lewis SJ, Gray R, Holmes LM, et al. Neurophysiological changes in deformity correction of adolescent idiopathic scoliosis with intraoperative skull-femoral traction. Spine (Phila Pa 1976). 2011;36(20):1627-38.
178. Buchowski JM, Bhatnagar R, Skaggs DL, et al. Temporary internal distraction as an aid to correction of severe scoliosis. J Bone Joint Surg Am. 2006;88(9):2035-41.
179. Mooney JF, Bernstein R, Hennrikus WL, et al. Neurologic risk management in scoliosis surgery. J Pediatr Orthop. 2002;22(5):683-9.
180. Clark CE, Shufflebarger HL. Late-developing infection in instrumented idiopathic scoliosis. Spine (Phila Pa 1976). 1999;24(18):1909-12.
181. Li Y, Glotzbecker M, Hedequist D. Surgical site infection after pediatric spinal deformity surgery. Curr Rev Musculoskelet Med. 2012.
182. Hedequist D, Haugen A, Hresko T, et al. Failure of attempted implant retention in spinal deformity delayed surgical site infections. Spine (Phila Pa 1976). 2009;34(1):60-4.
183. Milstone AM, Maragakis LL, Townsend T, et al. Timing of preoperative antibiotic prophylaxis: a modifiable risk factor for deep surgical site infections after pediatric spinal fusion. Pediatr Infect Dis J. 2008;27(8):704-8.
184. Soultanis K, Mantelos G, Pagiatakis A, et al. Late infection in patients with scoliosis treated with spinal instrumentation. Clin Orthop Relat Res. 2003;411:116-23.
185. Gans I, Dormans JP, Spiegel DA, et al. Adjunctive vancomycin powder in pediatric spine surgery is safe. Spine (Phila Pa 1976). 2013;38(19):1703-7.
186. Glotzbecker MP, Riedel MD, Vitale MG, et al. What's the evidence? Systematic literature review of risk factors and preventive strategies for surgical site infection following pediatric spine surgery. J Pediatr Orthop. 2013;33(5):479-87.
187. Sponseller PD, Betz R, Newton PO, et al. Differences in curve behavior after fusion in adolescent idiopathic scoliosis patients with open triradiate cartilages. Spine (Phila Pa 1976). 2009;34(8):827-31.
188. Yoon SH, Ugrinow VL, Upasani VV, et al. Comparison between 4.0-mm stainless steel and 4.75-mm titanium alloy single-rod spinal instrumentation for anterior thoracoscopic scoliosis surgery. Spine (Phila Pa 1976). 2008;33(20):2173-8.
189. Newton PO, White KK, Faro F, et al. The success of thoracoscopic anterior fusion in a consecutive series of 112 pediatric spinal deformity cases. Spine (Phila Pa 1976). 2005;30(4):392-8.
190. Newton PO, Upasani VV, Lhamby J, et al. Surgical treatment of main thoracic scoliosis with thoracoscopic anterior instrumentation: a five-year follow-up study. J Bone Joint Surg Am. 2008;90(10):2077-89.
191. Kuklo TR, Potter BK, Lenke LG, et al. Surgical revision rates of hooks versus hybrid versus screws versus combined anteroposterior spinal fusion for adolescent idiopathic scoliosis. Spine (Phila Pa 1976). 2007;32(20):2258-64.
192. Ramo BA, Richards BS. Repeat surgical interventions following "definitive" instrumentation and fusion for idiopathic scoliosis: five-year update on a previously published cohort. Spine (Phila Pa 1976). 2012;37(14):1211-7.
193. Campos M, Dolan L, Weinstein S. Unanticipated revision surgery in adolescent idiopathic scoliosis. Spine (Phila Pa 1976). 2012;37(12):1048-53.
194. Wagner MR, Flores JB, Sanpera I, et al. Aortic abutment after direct vertebral rotation: plowing of pedicle screws. Spine (Phila Pa 1976). 2011;36(3):243-7.
195. Ledonio CG, Polly DW, Vitale MG, et al. Pediatric pedicle screws: comparative effectiveness and safety: a systematic literature review from the Scoliosis Research Society and the Pediatric Orthopaedic Society of North America task force. J Bone Joint Surg Am. 2011;93(13):1227-34.
196. Kuklo TR, Lenke LG, O'Brien MF, et al. Accuracy and efficacy of thoracic pedicle screws in curves more than 90 degrees. Spine (Phila Pa 1976). 2005;30(2):222-6.
197. Smorgick Y, Millgram MA, Anekstein Y, et al. Accuracy and safety of thoracic pedicle screw placement in spinal deformities. J Spinal Disord Tech. 2005;18(6):522-6.
198. Di Silvestre M, Parisini P, Lolli F, et al. Complications of thoracic pedicle screws in scoliosis treatment. Spine (Phila Pa 1976). 2007;32(15):1655-61.
199. Suk SI, Kim WJ, Lee SM, et al. Thoracic pedicle screw fixation in spinal deformities: are they really safe? Spine (Phila Pa 1976). 2001;26(18):2049-57.
200. Hicks JM, Singla A, Shen FH, et al. Complications of pedicle screw fixation in scoliosis surgery: a systematic review. Spine (Phila Pa 1976). 2010;35(11):E465-70.
201. Cook S, Asher M, Lai SM, et al. Reoperation after primary posterior instrumentation and fusion for idiopathic scoliosis. Toward defining late operative site pain of unknown cause. Spine (Phila Pa 1976). 2000;25(4):463-8.

CHAPTER 13

Neuromuscular Scoliosis

David Gurd, Siddharth A Badve

INTRODUCTION

Scoliosis, though commonly believed to be a coronal curvature, is actually a three-dimensional deformity affecting the axial, sagittal, and coronal alignment of the spine. Based on the age of appearance, it has been broadly classified as pediatric and adult scoliosis. Pediatric scoliosis includes a wide variety of conditions which could be either congenital or developmental. On the other hand, scoliosis in the adult population is possibly related to a pre-existing spinal curvature, degenerative process or a combination of both. A clinician often comes across children with spinal deformity or a concern for scoliosis in the practice. The etiology, natural history, and the management protocols of different forms of pediatric scoliosis can vary significantly. For a clinician, understanding these concepts is important, not just from the diagnostic perspective but also for initiating timely therapeutic intervention. Appropriate management of pediatric scoliosis can significantly improve the quality of life (QOL) of these patients and avoid both short, as well as long-term complications.

A working classification of pediatric scoliosis is given below:

- Congenital
- Developmental:
  - *Idiopathic scoliosis*: It is further subclassified as—
    - Adolescent idiopathic scoliosis and
    - Early onset scoliosis (which includes the infantile and the juvenile variants)
    - Neuromuscular (NM) scoliosis.

Based on the primary condition, it is further subclassified by the Scoliosis Research Society as neuropathic and myopathic variety. The details of this classification have been provided in the epidemiology section of this chapter.

Scoliosis is a common manifestation of various NM disorders. Impaired voluntary muscle function and loss of proprioception are the key factors that contribute to the progressive spinal deformity. In spite of the diverse causes, these curves share many common features. The majority of the NM curves are typically long thoracolumbar C-shaped curves. The classical deformity pattern is kyphoscoliosis, but lordoscoliosis could also be present. Involvement of the sacrum causing pelvic obliquity is also a common feature and can lead to difficulties with seating. The severity of the curve tends to increase with worsening NM involvement. The associated systemic manifestations of the primary disorder can be significant and need to be taken into consideration during the evaluation and treatment of these patients.

EPIDEMIOLOGY AND NATURAL HISTORY

The Scoliosis Research Society has classified the NM scoliosis based on the neuropathic and myopathic etiology. The neuropathic causes can be further subclassified into upper and lower motor neuron conditions. The upper motor neuron conditions include the following:

- Cerebral palsy
- Spinocerebellar degeneration:
  - Friedreich's ataxia
  - Charcot-Marie-Tooth disease
  - Roussy-Levy syndrome
- Syringomyelia
- Spinal cord tumor.

The lower motor neuron causes include:

- Poliomyelitis and other viral myelitides
- *Spinal muscular atrophy*: Werdnig-Hoffmann disease, Kugelberg-Welander disease
- *Dysautonomic disorders*: Riley-Day syndrome.

Neuromuscular scoliosis secondary to conditions like myelodysplasia and traumatic spinal cord injuries could result from both upper and lower motor neuron involvement.

The myopathic conditions include:

- Arthrogryposis
- Muscular dystrophies:
  - Duchenne and Becker
  - Limb-girdle
  - Facioscapulohumeral
- Congenital hypotonia
- Myotonia dystrophica.

The degree of the NM involvement significantly influences the presence and severity of the scoliosis. The prevalence of scoliosis could vary from 10 to 100%.[1-4] In static encephalopathy, the incidence in nonambulatory patients is 62% while the incidence in the bedridden population is as high as 100%.[5,6] In patients with myelodysplasia, the prevalence of congenital spinal deformities ranges from 7 to 20% while that of developmental type is 52–89%.[7] Increased awareness of the use of folic acid during pregnancy has decreased the incidence of neural tube defects and the associated spinal deformities. Another author has described the prevalence of spinal deformities in various NM disorders as follows—cerebral palsy (25%), myelodysplasia (60%), spinal muscular atrophy (SMA) (67%), Friedreich ataxia (80%), Duchenne muscular dystrophy (DMD) (90%), and traumatic paralysis in younger children (100%).[4]

Neuromuscular scoliosis develops early in childhood. In contrast to adolescent idiopathic scoliosis (AIS), the NM curves tend to develop earlier and continue to progress even after skeletal maturity. Curve progression is typically gradual but can be rapid with the onset of puberty, deteriorating neurologic function, shunt malfunction, or prolonged time in a wheelchair. The worsening of the deformity could also be attributed to progressive conditions like Duchenne's muscular dystrophy. On the other hand, in static conditions like cerebral palsy, the weakened trunk muscles may not be able to support the growing skeletal and body mass causing the deformity to worsen.

Cerebral Palsy

In cerebral palsy (CP or static encephalopathy), muscular dysfunction in tandem with asymmetric spasticity and the effect of gravity appear to be responsible for the development of spinal deformity. Pelvic obliquity and hip imbalance often coexist with large cerebral palsy curves, indicating a generalized muscular imbalance to be a predisposing factor.[5,6] Saito et al. studied the natural history of scoliosis in cerebral palsy patients and determined the important risk factors for progression. These include spinal curvature greater than 40° before the age of 15 years, having total body involvement, being bedridden, and having a thoracolumbar curve.[5] Thometz and Simon in their study of skeletally mature institutionalized patients with cerebral palsy found the rate of scoliosis progression to be 0.8°/year for curves < 50° and 1.4°/year for curves > 50° (Fig. 1).[3]

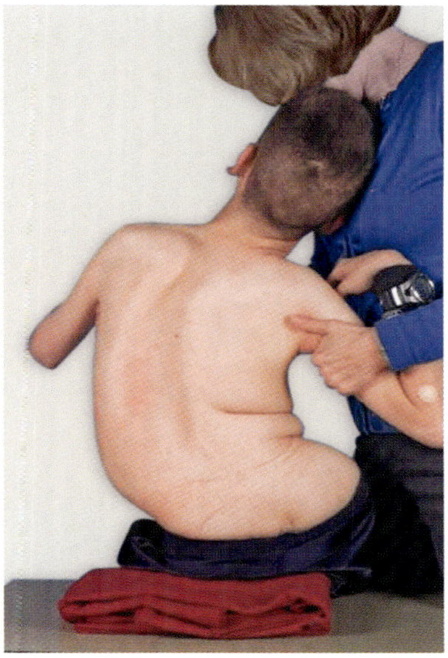

Fig. 1: A clinical illustration of a patient with neuromuscular scoliosis secondary to cerebral palsy. Note the pelvic tilt and costopelvic impingement on the right side.

Myelodysplasia

For the patients with myelodysplasia, the major factors that influence curve progression include the motor level, the ambulatory status, and the last intact laminar arch. The minor factors include hip subluxation and the severity of lower extremity spasticity.[7] The curve generally tends to develop before the age of 15 years, following which appearance of a spinal deformity is not common.[9] Presence of tethered cord could predispose to rapid curve progression[7] (Figs. 2A and B).

CHAPTER 13

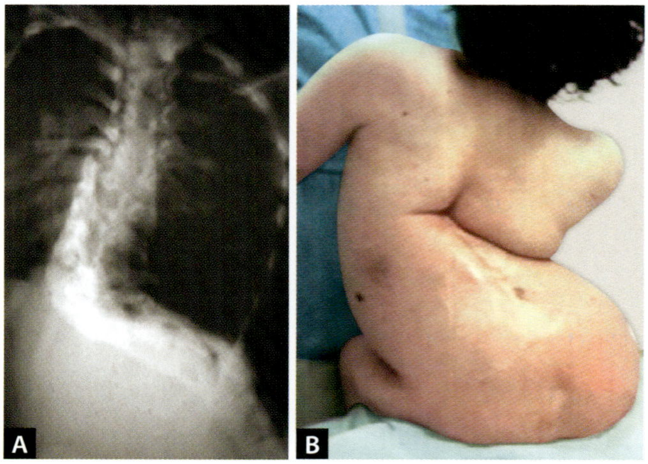

Figs. 2A and B: A posteroanterior radiograph (A) and a clinical illustration (B) of a patient with neuromuscular scoliosis secondary to myelodysplasia. Note the costopelvic impingement on the right side along with the scar of previous surgery.

Spinal Muscular Atrophy

In spinal muscular atrophy, the severe variants tend to develop scoliosis in the first 2 years of life, but the curve may not attain severe magnitude due to a very limited life expectancy. On the other hand, in the milder variants the spinal deformity may appear after the age of 2 years, and tends to progress mostly in the nonambulatory patients.[10-12] Schwentkar and Gibson reported that the ability to walk correlated directly with the severity of scoliosis.[12] In a study by Evans et al., scoliosis developed in all patients who had SMA type 1 or 2 but only developed in approximately half of the patients who had SMA type 3. The age at the time of onset of scoliosis increased in accordance with the severity of the SMA. The natural history of untreated scoliosis includes loss of independent function of the upper extremities secondary to the necessity to support the trunk, ischial bursitis with necrosis, and fairly appreciable back pain.[10] Severe spinal deformities can lead to cardiopulmonary impairment.

Duchenne Muscular Dystrophy

In DMD, the incidence of scoliosis progression is reported to be 95%.[13] Curves can rapidly worsen to a significant severity. Based on the severity of progression, Oda et al. have classified the curves into three categories: Type I has rapid progression of scoliosis with kyphosis, Type II shows transition of kyphosis to lordosis while Type III has a mild deformity.[14] With the progression of the disease, pulmonary function is compromised due to intercostal muscle weakness, increased chest wall stiffness and a weak cough reflex. Worsening of the scoliotic curvature further impairs the lung function. Cardiopulmonary failure is a common cause of death in this patient population.[13,14]

Friedreich's Ataxia

Scoliosis in patients with Friedreich's ataxia is a common feature and can have a variable course. Progression has been associated with the growth spurt and curves that appear early in life, but progression may continue even after skeletal maturity.[15] The muscle function does not appear to influence the rate of progression.[15] The curve pattern appears to behave as an idiopathic scoliosis. Some of the deformities are nonprogressive or progress very slowly. Once the ataxia develops, the disease runs a steady downhill course without remission. The patients usually succumb to primary cardiomyopathy by the third or the fourth decade, many not living long enough to experience scoliosis progression that necessitates any treatment.[15]

Rett Syndrome

Rett syndrome is a neurodevelopmental disorder that predominantly affects young females.[16] Spinal deformity is a common musculoskeletal manifestation and tends to progress with advanced stages of the disease.[16-18] Rapid worsening of the curve has been known to occur.[16] Rate of progression is variable and correlates to the extent of neurologic affection due to the disease.[17,18]

Arthrogryposis

The incidence and the behavior of curves in arthrogryposis are variable. In one of the studies, the incidence has been reported to vary from 30% to 67%.[19] The data about natural history of this condition is scarce. Some of the curves may progress rapidly and end up with a rigid deformity.[19]

In general, the course of the spinal deformity is predominantly influenced by the type of primary condition and its overall severity. Even when the underlying disease is unchanged, with growth, the weak trunk muscles cannot balance the increased body mass. In comparison to idiopathic scoliosis, the curve progression is much more common and can continue even after skeletal maturity. As the scoliosis worsens, the ability to sit erect may also deteriorate, causing severe functional and pulmonary impairment. Loss of the sitting balance can necessitate

SECTION 2

the use of the hands for support rather than being used for other purposeful activities. Unlike AIS, even moderate curves severely impair the pulmonary function, due to the pre-existing respiratory muscle weakness.[4]

CLINICAL FINDINGS AND DIAGNOSTIC WORK-UP

Cerebral Palsy

A multidisciplinary approach is ideal for evaluation of patients with a cerebral palsy curve. The nonspinal manifestations of the condition should be taken into consideration in formulating the management. Birth history, overall development, and milestones along with the extent of neurological involvement should be analyzed in detail. Ambulatory status, use of wheel chair, overall physical and mental function, growth spurt, upper extremity function, feeding problems, respiratory function, and hip involvement are vital factors that should be reviewed.[20] Based on their ambulatory capacity, the patients can be classified as walkers, sitters or bedridden. Use of baclofen, botox, antiepileptics, and other medications should be noted. History should also include the details about the rate of curve progression and its impact on the general health. Family members and care takers could be a useful source of information. It is also equally important to understand the patients, families, and caretakers goals.

The general physical examination should assess for gait, sitting and standing posture, nutritional status, growth and development, signs of puberty, and the degree of spasticity. A detailed evaluation of the respiratory system and the pulmonary function is helpful in formulating the management plan. The musculoskeletal examination should include evaluation of range of motion of the major joints, muscle tone, and motor strength. Tight hamstrings can cause decreased lumbar lordosis; conversely hip flexure contracture can increase the lordosis. Abduction or adduction contracture of the hips may contribute to the lumbar-pelvic[20] malalignment. The presence of a dislocated hip can result in pelvic obliquity which could produce a compensatory scoliosis. Conversely, the scoliotic deformity may lead to pelvic obliquity which may cause a hip deformity.[20]

Spinal examination should focus on the nature and magnitude of decompensation, shoulder balance, and pelvic obliquity.[20] The effect of scoliosis on the sitting and standing balance should be noted. Flexibility of the curve and costopelvic impingement is additional important factor. Presence of skin problems and decubitus ulcers should also be noted.

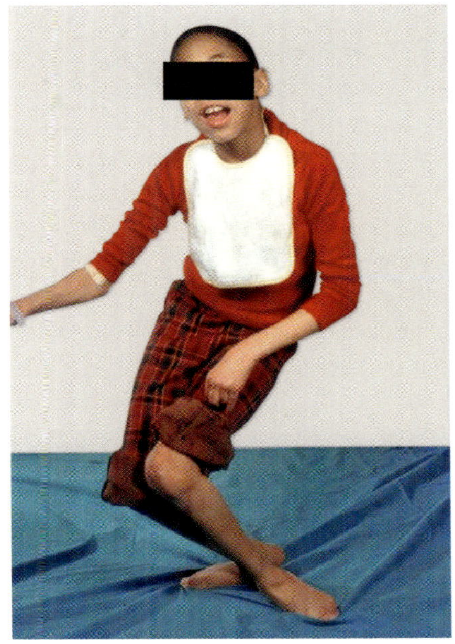

Fig. 3: A clinical illustration of standing posture in patient with cerebral palsy. Note the lower extremity joint contractures.

Additional evaluation by internist, neurologist, pulmonologist, orthotist, and other specialists, when appropriate, is of immense help in planning and coordinating the overall management (Fig. 3).

Myelodysplasia

Developmental curve of greater than 20° magnitude was defined as scoliosis.[7,9] Smaller curves often resolve without intervention.[7,9] Kyphosis is often a component of the deformity and can present early. Myelodysplasia can be associated with other neurological conditions like hydrocephalus, tethered spinal cord, and mental retardation.[7] Rapid curve progression in association with increased muscle tone, bladder dysfunction, limb deformities along with back discomfort is a manifestation of a tethered cord.[21,22] Development of hydrocephalus can complicate the condition in these patients and often needs shunt procedures at an early stage. Renal anomalies, bladder and bowel incontinence, and chronic urinary tract infection are common and require appropriate treatment. In myelodysplasia, due to similar congenital changes vertebral anomalies have been associated with the presence of congenital renal defects.[23] Contractures of the lower extremities and issues related to insensate skin could add to the problems with positioning and infection. Latex allergy is a concern in this patient population and is seen in 9–40% patients. Because this can lead to a life-threatening IgE-mediated hypersensitivity reaction, patients with myelodysplasia should be treated in a latex-free environment.[24]

Periodic patient evaluation is of importance to identify the changes in the spinal balance, neurological, and functional status. The physical examination should be carried on similar lines as cerebral palsy. Evaluation by other specialists including neurosurgeon, pediatrician, neurologist, pulmonologist, occupational, and physical therapist can help with the coordination of management.

Spinal Muscular Atrophy

Spinal muscular atrophy is an autosomal recessive disorder that is characterized by degeneration of the anterior horn cells. It causes generalized paralysis of proximal trunk muscles. Based on the variability of severity, SMA has been classified into three variants. Type I is the most severe with a very limited life expectancy while Type III is least severe with mild functional impairment.[10] Patients with the Type I and II variants tend to develop early scoliosis. The majority of Type II patients are nonambulators and tend to develop rapid scoliosis progression. Type III patients, due to the mild affection in general, have a relatively lower incidence of scoliosis occurrence.[11,12]

Duchenne Muscular Dystrophy

Duchenne muscular dystrophy is a common X-linked recessive disorder affecting male patients. Females generally tend to be carriers. It is caused by deficiency of the muscle protein dystrophin which plays an important role in muscle cellular stability. The disease may present with delay in walking and the symptoms become more pronounced after the 3rd year. The early signs include pseudohypertrophy of calf muscles and proximal muscle weakness. This weakness may be identified as the Gower's sign where the patient gets up by walking their hands up their knees when rising from a seated position. Altered walking, flat feet and contractures of hips, knees and ankles may also be the associated features. Affected children tend to lose the ability to ambulate independently by the end of the first decade of life.[25] At this stage, cardiac and pulmonary involvement is common along with mild mental impairment. During the early second decade, the patients tend to have hyperlordosis which eventually develops in to a progressive kyphoscoliosis with the worsening of the muscular function.[13,14] The progression of the spinal deformity tends to worsen the pulmonary function which limits the survival beyond the second decade.[26] Becker's muscular dystrophy is a milder form of muscular dystrophy with delayed and less severe presentation. This also correlates with a lower incidence and lesser severity of scoliosis.

Friedreich's Ataxia

Friedreich's ataxia is a hereditary and progressive neurodegenerative disorder affecting the spinocerebellar function. The diagnosis is based on a set of primary clinical findings: appearance of the symptoms before the age of 25 years, ataxia and absence of deep tendon reflexes in the lower extremities, positive Babinski sign, impairment of upper extremity motor and sensory function, and dysarthria.[15] Scoliosis is one of the secondary symptoms and needs careful screening.

Rett Syndrome

Rett syndrome is a progressive neurological disorder linked to a gene mutation located on the X chromosome. It almost exclusively affects females. The syndrome presents as a cluster of clinical manifestations in four stages. These include psychomotor regression, autistic behavior, nonpurposeful stereotypical hand movements, ataxia, gait apraxia and microcephaly.[16,17] Scoliosis tends to develop in the late stages, especial stage IV due to muscle insufficiency.[17]

Arthrogryposis

Arthrogryposis is a generic term used to describe more than 150 distinct disorders in children manifesting with multiple congenital contractures. Clinical presentation includes joint contractures affecting both upper and lower extremities. Scoliosis tends to develop in the first few years of life and tends to progress rapidly[19] (Fig. 4).

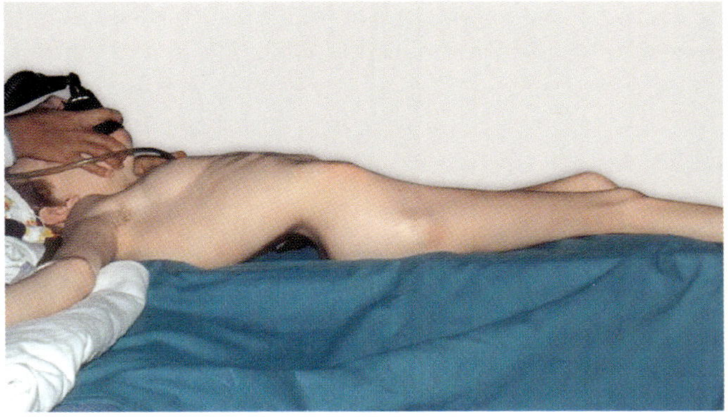

Fig. 4: A clinical illustration demonstrating hyperlordosis as a component of spinal deformity in neuromuscular scoliosis.

DIAGNOSTIC EVALUATION

Radiologic Assessment

Plain radiographs are the cornerstone in the initial evaluation of a NM spinal deformity. Full length radiographs provide vital insight in the nature, magnitude, and flexibility of the curves. There is no consensus about the frequency or technique for the radiographs, though it is reasonable to perform posteroanterior and lateral radiographs every 6 months. Based on the functional ability, the radiographs could be obtained in standing, sitting or supine position and should be performed in the most functional position. When possible, attempt should be made to obtain bending views preferably in standing erect or supine positions preoperatively for surgical planning. If the patient is unable to cooperate enough to actively bend, then traction, push-pull radiographs or fulcrum-bending radiographs are very useful for preoperative assessment and planning. Additional radiographic information can be obtained about the presence of vertebral anomalies, appearance of the rib cage, pelvic obliquity, presence of spondylolisthesis, and hip involvement. In the cerebral palsy variants with the involvement of bilateral lower extremities, the incidence of spondylolisthesis could be as high as 21%.[27] If hip involvement is suspected, detailed radiographic assessment of the hips is helpful.

In the patients with myelodysplasia, preoperative localization of level of dysraphism is important to note. Serial radiographs every 6 months are valuable in documenting curve progression. In a small group of patients, progressive kyphosis with a relatively stable scoliosis can complicate the course of the disease. It affects the sitting posture and can also lead to skin breakdown

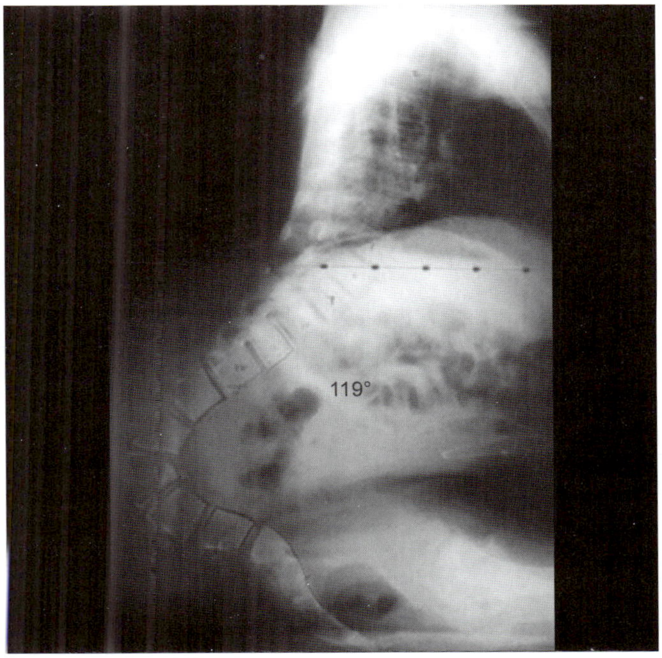

Fig. 5: A lateral radiograph demonstrating lumbar kyphosis as a predominant component of spinal deformity in patient with myelodysplasia.

over the apex of the deformity. Periodic radiographic evaluation can help with early identification of the kyphotic component. Progressive kyphosis in myelodysplasia is resistant to conservative measures and often requires surgical intervention[7] (Fig. 5).

Magnetic Resonance Imaging

The need for magnetic resonance imaging (MRI) is dictated by the etiology of spinal deformity. It is indicated in conditions like myelodysplasia to evaluate the commonly associated conditions like syringomyelia, hydromyelia, and tethered cord. Imaging of the brain is helpful in studying associations like Chiari malformation and hydrocephalus.[7] In patients with myelodysplasia, a MRI of the spine should be done as early as first 2 years of life and repeated when clinically indicated. The indication of MRI in cerebral palsy patients with scoliosis includes sudden progression of the deformity and change in the neurological status.[20]

Computed Tomography

A computed tomography (CT) scan can aid in defining the skeletal details in relation to the spinal deformity. Vertebral anomalies which could be present in conditions like myelodysplasia can be identified in detail.[7] Knowledge of the anatomic details of the vertebrae could help decide the nature and size of the spinal instrumentation to be used. It is also of importance when planning complex deformity correction with the use of procedures like vertebral column resection or a three column osteotomy. Intraoperative CT imaging can also be used in appropriately indicated situations.

Serum Creatine Phosphokinase Levels

Raised creatine phosphokinase is a marker for muscle necrosis and is helpful in the diagnosis of myopathies.[25] In the common variants like Duchenne and Becker muscular dystrophy, the Creatine phosphokinase levels may be elevated up to 100 times the normal.[28]

Electromyography

It is of value in the diagnosis of myopathies, although differentiating the various types may eventually require a muscle biopsy.[28] Conditions like Duchenne and Becker muscular dystrophy show signs of myopathy. The electromyographic findings diagnostic for SMA include denervation induced fibrillation potentials and a regular spontaneous motor unit activity. Muscle tremor defect may be present while the nerve conduction velocity in the motor fibers is usually normal. These findings increase in the frequency and magnitude with the progression of the disease.

Muscle Biopsy

It is indicated when the primary condition is unknown and a myopathic cause is suspected. Histopathological analysis can identify the type of the myopathy and thus help with the prognosis of both the primary condition as well as the spinal deformity. The biopsy is characterized by variations of fiber size in internal nuclei, split fibers, degenerating and regenerating fibers, and fibrofatty tissue deposition.[28] Additional tests on the muscle biopsy specimen include immunohistochemistry and immunoblotting for dystrophin.[25]

MEDICAL MANAGEMENT

Medical treatment of NM scoliosis includes observation, bracing and the use of sitting support systems.[4] Pharmacologic agents like baclofen and botulinum are often used to control spasticity. These modalities are generally suited for smaller and flexible curves and in younger patients.

Observation

It is ideal for very mild curves and as a temporary measure, especially in skeletally immature patients. Moderate stable curves in mature patients can also be observed. It should involve periodic clinical and radiological evaluation. Any signs of curve progression should be carefully watched for, so as to initiate timely intervention measures.[4] It is common for clinicians to employ the criteria of observing curves less than 20–25°, as in the treatment of idiopathic scoliosis.[7,20,29-34] Generally, observation can be continued until the curves begin to cause functional impairment. Close coordination with the caregivers can be valuable in the identification of curve progression or functional impairment due to the spinal deformity.

Bracing

Control of the curve progression by orthotic treatment in NM conditions is difficult. Bracing could have a temporary role by possibly delaying the curve progression especially until the skeletal growth is complete. Earlier studies have concluded that the use of a brace is usually ineffective in halting the progression of the spinal deformity.[29,30] Bracing could specifically be helpful in ambulatory patients with decreased muscle tone and short thoracolumbar curves of moderate severity.[30] The curve magnitude at which bracing can be considered in NM scoliosis is still ill defined, although it is a common practice to brace curves greater than 20–30° range.[7,29-34] Spinal braces can also help support the spine to improve the sitting balance. On the contrary, use of rigid spinal braces negatively impacts the pulmonary function by restricting the chest expansion in the setting of weakened respiratory musculature.[11,31] It could also contribute to skin problems and pressure ulcers. Softer spinal braces can to some extent avoid the pulmonary and skin problems while supporting the trunk.[32,33] A study by Kotwicki et al. concluded that correctly fitted orthosis can improve function, prevent some of the complications, and to some extent delay the need for surgery.[34]

Sitting Support Systems and Other Treatment Modalities

Molded wheel chairs with inserts and other sitting support systems are widely used, but it is unclear if they have any

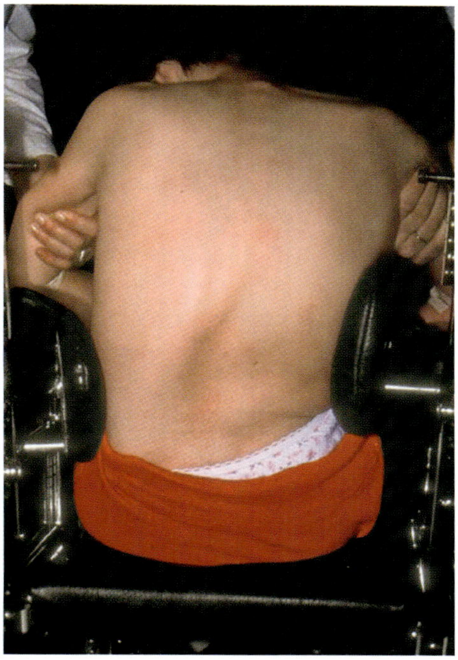

Fig. 6: A clinical illustration demonstrating a sitting support used in the management of neuromuscular scoliosis secondary to cerebral palsy.

effect in slowing or prevention curve progression. They do tend to provide trunk support to maintain the sitting balance and achieve static correction of the deformity.[35] Similarly, physical therapy and electrical stimulation has not shown to be of any value in the treatment of the spinal malalignment. Nuzzo et al. reported the short-term results in a small group of NM scoliosis patients treated with botulinum and they observed either no worsening or some reduction in the curve magnitude[36] (Fig. 6).

Cerebral Palsy

Braces are used for the temporary control of the spinal deformity in these patients. But in the long-term, bracing has not shown to change the course of the scoliosis in view of the long and flexible nature of these curves.[29,30] On the other hand, the ambulatory cerebral palsy population with shorter and structural curves tends to benefit with bracing for curve control.[30] Soft spinal orthosis have been shown to have a favorable profile in term of pulmonary and skin complications.[33] Bracing and sitting supports like a molded wheelchair, in the appropriate groups of patients can improve the quality of care and social interaction by helping the sitting balance.[35,37]

Myelodysplasia

Minor curves could have a self-limiting course and may not need any intervention.[7] Some of the curves may have a neurologic etiology like a tethered cord or syringomyelia and addressing this causative problem may be the only treatment that is required. Curves less than 20° can be observed with periodic radiographs while in curves of greater magnitude, especially in younger children, bracing can be considered.[7,38,39] Bracing does not stop the progression of the curve, but it may delay the progression, so as to allow for trunk growth till the fusion procedure can be considered.[7,30,38] Insensate skin, poor pulmonary function, and obesity could be a few of the factors that can make bracing a challenge in this population.[31-33]

Spinal Muscular Atrophy

The role of bracing is to temporarily support the spine to improve the overall sitting balance.[10,12] It can also help prevent painful costopelvic impingement in adult patients.[10] Bracing could possibly delay the deformity progression in younger patients with larger curves 40° or greater, until spinal fusion is feasible and safe.[10,12,40] It has been found to fairly effective in the Type III variant but ineffective in the Type I variant.[40] Patient compliance could be a major limiting factor in the use of long-term bracing. The effect of bracing on the already compromised lung function in SMA patients can be considered a relative contraindication for brace treatment.[11,31]

Duchenne Muscular Dystrophy

With the disease progression, the spinal curvature as well as the cardiopulmonary function tends to worsen.[13,14,21] Orthotic treatment of scoliosis in Duchenne muscular dystrophy (DMD) has shown to slow down the progression, but is ineffective in halting the process.[13,41,42] With a period of bracing, the window of opportunity for the surgical intervention may be lost as the patient is too debilitated and risk associated with surgery may become unacceptable as the curve becomes too large. Thus, bracing is not an acceptable treatment option during early treatment of scoliosis in DMD.[41-43] Wheel chairs with trunk supports could be helpful to maintain trunk balance in those awaiting spinal fusion.[43]

Friedreich's Ataxia

An attempt at bracing with these patients does not appear to change the natural progression of the spinal curves.[15,44-46]

CHAPTER 13

Braces are very poorly tolerated and could even limit ambulation. Orthotic treatment could have a role in delaying the surgery in skeletally immature patients.[15,44,46] Wheelchairs and other positioning devices could help in improving sitting balance. Physical therapy and other modalities do not appear to influence the outcome of the scoliosis.[15]

Rett Syndrome

As with scoliosis associated with other NM conditions, orthotic treatment appears to have a limited role in the management. Bracing does not affect the progression of the curvature.[18,47-50] It could be of some value in improving the trunk balance and delaying the need for fusion in skeletally immature children.[50]

Arthrogryposis

The role of conservative options in the management of arthrogrypotic spinal deformities appears to be controversial. Sarwak et al. in their study reported partial stretching to be effective in the treatment of trunk muscular contractures.[50,51] Greggi et al. have recommended an attempt at early full time bracing as there is no verified criteria to predict curve progression.[19] On the contrary, other studies have not reported any significant benefit with orthotic treatment in the control of the curve.[19,50,52]

SURGICAL TREATMENT

The goal of surgical treatment in NM scoliosis is to prevent further progression of deformity and to correct the torso to a safe and comfortable position while preserving the pulmonary function, thus facilitating the care and comfort of these patients. This is achieved by correction of the scoliosis and the pelvic tilt with fusion of the spine in a balanced alignment to prevent further progression of the deformity.[7,20,40,45,49,52] The stable realigned spinopelvic relationship helps with the restoration of the sitting balance without hand support, improved ability to use the upper extremities for purposeful activities and an erect posture to facilitate social interaction. Preservation and if possible, improvement of the pulmonary function by preventing the deformity progression is also a vital goal. The ultimate aim is to enhance the QOL for this patient population.

In view of the major medical comorbidities associated with the NM conditions, the role and the timing of the surgical intervention is always a matter of debate.[53] The majority of these patients have an impaired cardiopulmonary function and a very high susceptibility to respiratory infections.[7,20,26,53] Neurological problems could be significant and may include hydrocephalus, CSF shunts, epilepsy, ataxia, poor mentation, baclofen pumps, etc.[7,53] Aspiration and gastrointestinal issues like feeding problems and chronic constipation are extremely common. Anemia and malnourishment are frequently associated.[53] Osteopenia due to lack of activity and the use of antiepileptic medication is another concern in this population.[54,55] All these factors make the patients relatively poor surgical candidates. Scoliosis surgery involves prolonged anesthesia and extensive exposure for long segment fusion that mostly includes the pelvis. These surgeries are associated with significant blood loss and fluid and electrolyte disturbance. The risk of neurological worsening is also a factor to be considered. Postoperative complications both short and long-term are significant, sometimes necessitating a revision surgery. This background makes the decision of surgical intervention in these patients a major endeavor with serious potential risks.

Multiple studies support the role of surgical treatment in the management of NM scoliosis. Bohtz et al. in a retrospective review of 50 consecutive patients with cerebral palsy, evaluated the outcome of surgical scoliosis correction measured by the subjective change in the health-related quality of life (HRQL) and the objective radiologic changes. Their results indicated that life quality improved after surgical scoliosis correction in patients with cerebral palsy. There is a high satisfaction rate of patients and their caregivers. Subjective changes in HRQL after the operation do not correlate with objective radiographic changes brought about by the operation. This indicates that the present operative indications and the obtained correction are adequate to achieve an improvement of the subjective HRQL in this patient group.[56] A study by Watanabe et al. evaluated the clinical outcomes and satisfaction associated with the surgical treatment of NM spinal deformity secondary to cerebral palsy in 84 patients and families. The evaluation included subjective assessment of the expectation, cosmesis, function, patient care, QOL, pulmonary function, pain, health status, self-image, and satisfaction along with objective assessment of the operative complications and radiographs. Both patients as well as parents were satisfied with the surgical outcome of the scoliosis correction, but the functional improvement after the surgery was only marginal.[57] Mercado et al. performed a systemic review of literature pertaining to the effect of spinal fusion on the QOL in NM scoliosis patients. They concluded that studies regarding QOL in NM patients after spinal fusion are of low quality of evidence. Spinal fusion improves the QOL in patients with static encephalopathy and muscular dystrophy, but this improvement was not noted in the patients with spina bifida.[58] A study of spinal surgery in NM scoliosis in 100 consecutive patients by Larsson et al. compared the long-term outcomes to the preoperative status. The assessments comprised sitting, angle of scoliosis, lung function, reaching, pain estimation, activities of daily living (ADL), care given, and time used for resting. Improvement after surgery was shown in the Cobb angle, lung function, seating position, ADL, and the time used for resting. In a comparison between the 1-year follow-up and the long-term follow-up, there were further improvements in sitting, ADL, and care given but an increased Cobb angle. These results were in line with the assessments reported by patients and relatives suggesting a sustained benefit from the surgery.[59] Larsson et al. in another study evaluated the effect of spinal fusion in patients with paralytic scoliosis in relation to function in terms of impairments, activities in terms of disabilities, and dependence in terms of handicaps 1 year postoperatively, with emphasis on subgroups. The patients with paralytic scoliosis maintained or improved their function and level of independence 1 year after surgery. The subjectively assessed results obtained from the patients and relatives also showed a positive outcome of surgery. Weight distribution on a seating surface was improved, but continued to be uneven.[60] A study by Bridwell et al. assessed the patient/parent satisfaction, clinical/functional ways in which spinal fusion affected patients along with the complications and the ultimate radiographic result in 44 patients with DMD and SMA. The evaluation included function, self-image, cosmesis, pain, pulmonary status, patient care, QOL, and satisfaction. The study indicated that spinal fusion benefits most of the patients, even though these diseases have a progressively deteriorating course. Cosmesis, QOL, and overall satisfaction rated the highest.[61] Analysis of spinal fusion in patients with total body involvement in cerebral palsy was done by Comstock et al. They concluded that corrective spinal surgery is indicated and is beneficial for most patients. Additionally, despite the surgical complexity and expected complications, the overall good surgical results and patient and caregiver satisfaction noted at 85%, was high.[62] In another study, Askin et al. performed a prospective, functional assessment based on physical ability and independence in daily activities of patients who had severe physical handicaps and spinal deformities secondary to NM etiologies and were undergoing scoliosis surgery. The level of physical independence was evaluated before surgery, including the ability to sit, ambulate, and complete activities of daily living. Evaluation was done before surgery, 6 months after surgery, and 12 months after surgery. A subjective assessment of cosmesis also was made. They reported deterioration in the initial 6 months after the surgery, followed by improvement to return to the preoperative level of function. No further improvement in the function was noted after 12 months. Cosmetic results were extremely gratifying to the patients and their caregivers. The study concluded that corrective spinal surgery in patients with severe physical handicap should be performed early to preserve function and should not be dictated solely by the severity of the curvature. Improvement in the patient's level of independence may not necessarily occur after truncal stabilization.[63]

Thus, despite the high risks and potential complications associated with the surgical treatment, the benefits are evident. Surgical intervention appears to preserve and, in some cases, improve the function in patients with NM scoliosis, although the level of evidence is still low. The satisfaction rate among the patients, parents and care givers, in terms of QOL for the patients, is high.

Systemic Perioperative Medical Considerations

A thorough preoperative assessment is the key for limiting the complications associated with surgery. Perioperative management by a multispecialist team that includes the anesthesiologist, pediatric internist, pulmonologist, rehabilitation specialist, in addition the operating surgeon is vital for a successful surgical outcome. The following is the list of the important systemic issues that need special attention.

Cardiopulmonary Problems

Patients with DMD are known to have cardiomyopathy and arrhythmias.[25,53,65] Similarly cardiomyopathy, especially left ventricular hypertrophy, is a common association with Friedreich's ataxia.[15,46,64] Restrictive lung disease secondary to severe thoracic spinal deformities may induce

CHAPTER 13

pulmonary hypertension that in turn may result in cor pulmonale.[53] Impaired muscle function can contribute to a weak respiratory effort. Recurrent aspiration of the gastric contents can lead to pulmonary fibrosis.[53] These factors make the patients highly susceptible to frequent respiratory infections and other complications especially in the early postoperative period. A detailed clinical evaluation, radiological and laboratory work-up that includes studies like chest radiograph, echocardiography, and pulmonary function tests can assess the cardiopulmonary function and help initiate the necessary treatment measures. In the group of patients with severe mental impairment, pulmonary function tests may not be a viable option and actions like laughing, coughing, crying, and screaming that involve a ventilator function can provide valuable data.[65]

Hematologic Problems

Scoliosis surgery in patients with NM conditions is associated with significant blood loss.[65] Antiepileptic medications like valproic acid can prolong the bleeding time and increase the surgical blood loss by affecting the platelet function. The routine laboratory tests of complete blood count, prothrombin time, and partial thromboplastin time will not adequately screen for the platelet-mediated effects of valproic acid.[66] In such situations, an effort should be made to wean the patients off valproic acid or replace it with suitable medication. Agents like aminocaproic and aprotinin acid have been used safely in scoliosis surgery in NM patient population and have shown to decrease the blood loss.[67,68] Aminocaproic acid appears to be the more cost effective option.[25] In general, the perioperative support system should be geared up for a significant blood loss with a ready availability of blood products.

Gastrointestinal Problems

Lack of tone and coordination of the muscles of deglutition can contribute to episodes of acute aspiration, especially in the perioperative period.[53] Swallowing evaluation can help address these issues and the appropriate measures like dietary modification, tube feeding or gastrostomy can be initiated. Most of these patients have chronic constipation and impaired bowel motility. Postspinal surgery ileus and use of opioids can further potentiate this problem. An aggressive bowel protocol and optimal hydration can help mitigate the constipation.[53,65] Superior mesenteric artery syndrome was a complication seen in lean patients undergoing acute correction of the spinal deformity due to the obstruction of duodenum. Use of nonsegmental instrumentation and cast immobilization in supine position in the postoperative period were thought to be the causative factors. Advent of segmental instrumentation and early mobilization following the surgery appear to have decreased the incidence of this problem.[53]

Nutritional Status

Chronic malnourishment and poor hydration can predispose these patients to surgical site and systemic infection, impaired wound healing, wound dehiscence, and osseous nonunion. Preoperative albumin levels and total lymphocyte count are good indicators of the nutritional status.[25] In a study by Jevsevar and Karlin, patients with serum albumin levels greater than 3.5g/L and total lymphocyte count greater than 1,500 cells/mm^3 had a significantly lower rate of infection, a shorter period of endotracheal intubation after the operation, and a shorter period of hospitalization.[69]

Operative Indications

A number of factors influence the decision for surgical intervention in NM scoliosis, with the curve magnitude being most important. Generally, curves reaching the magnitude of 40–50° or more are considered appropriate for surgical fusion.[7,15,19,20,26,40,41,43-46,49,50,53,70-73] Attention should also be given to factors like skeletal maturity, medical comorbidities and the care needs of the patient. The influence of the nature and severity of the primary NM condition on the progression of the scoliosis should also be taken into account. Failure of the orthotic treatment in arresting the rapid progression of the curve could be an important factor indicating the need for surgical intervention. On the other hand, some patients with worsening curves may not be suitable for brace treatment due to either obesity or skin problems. Under certain circumstances, the sagittal imbalance may be the predominant component that influences the operative decision. The surgical indications for each NM condition are discussed below.

Cerebral Palsy

The surgical decision making in scoliosis with cerebral palsy is dependent on a number of different factors like the curve progression, mental status, change in the functional status, seating difficulties, and the issues involved in

SECTION 2

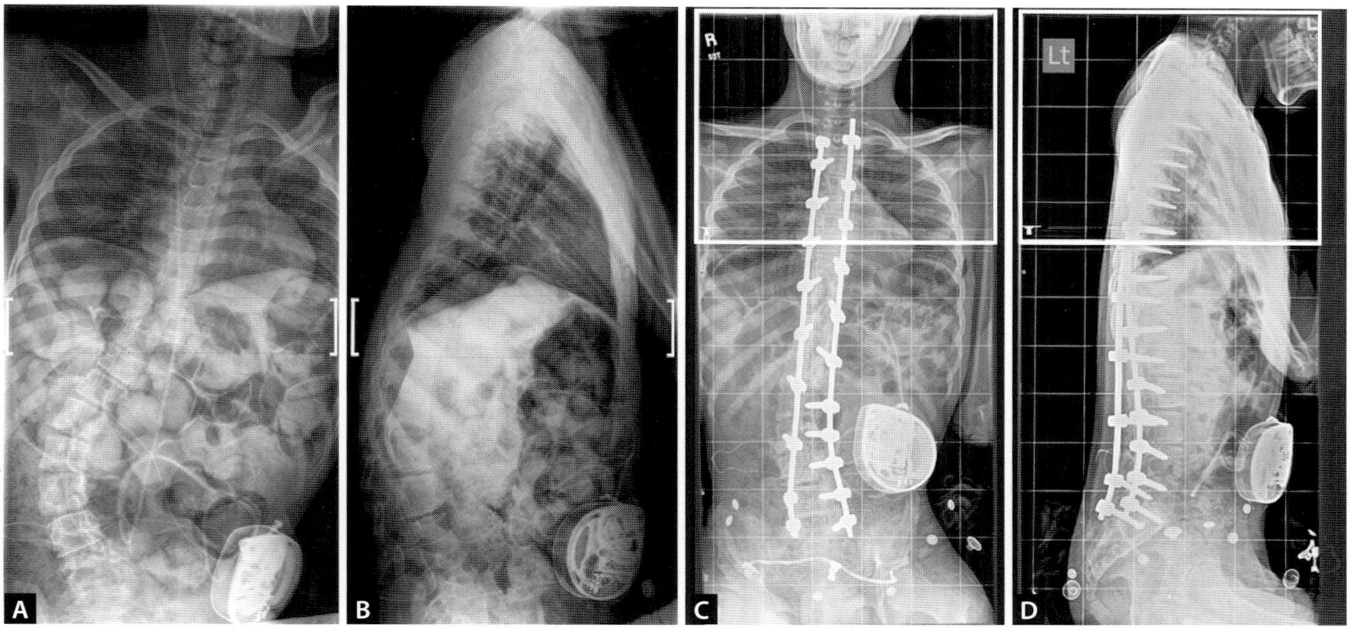

Figs. 7 A to D: Pre- and postoperative posteroanterior (A and C) and lateral (B and D) radiographs of a patient with neuromuscular scoliosis secondary to cerebral palsy treated with posterior spinal fusion to the sacrum.

caring for the patient. Cerebral palsy patients with sound mental functions can be considered for surgery if the curve reaches a magnitude of 50° in a skeletally immature child (>10-years old) or when curve progression (>5°) is noted on serial radiographs.[20,53,70] In patients with mental impairment and significant body involvement, curve progression (>5–10°) on serial radiographs is an indication for surgical intervention even at a lesser magnitude.[70] Additionally, deterioration in the functional status in the form of impairment of sitting balance, increasing difficulty with patient care and maintaining the hygiene, development of pressure sores due to worsening posture and pressure distribution are the other factors that can contribute to the surgical decision making[20,53,70] (Figs. 7A to D).

Myelodysplasia

The majority of the indications for a spinal fusion in myelodysplasia are similar to those in adolescent idiopathic scoliosis.[74] Curves more than 40–50°, progressive curves, significant sitting imbalance, deterioration in the functional status, and issues related to caring and hygiene are the major reasons to consider operative intervention.[7,53,71] Ideally, spinal fusion should be carried out, only after achieving maximal truncal growth (>10 years age). Hip contractures should be addressed prior to attempting scoliosis correction.[53] In a subgroup of patients with myelodysplasia, progressive kyphosis is the major deformity component that can result in problems like skin breakdown on the spinal prominence, postural problems due to trunk shortening and increased pressure over the abdominal viscera. Thus, progressive symptomatic kyphosis is another indication for surgical treatment.[7]

Spinal Muscular Atrophy

The role of surgery is individualized, based on the type of SMA, severity of the curve and the rate of progression. In general, large progressive curves not responding to orthotic treatment that negatively impact the posture and sitting balance, pulmonary status and the functional capacity in patients with a reasonable life expectancy are considered appropriate for operative correction. A curve severity of 50–60° in a child with almost adult truncal growth (>10 years old) is considered appropriate for spinal fusion.[40,72] When indicated, the surgery should be performed before the pulmonary and general health status is too impaired to withstand any intervention.

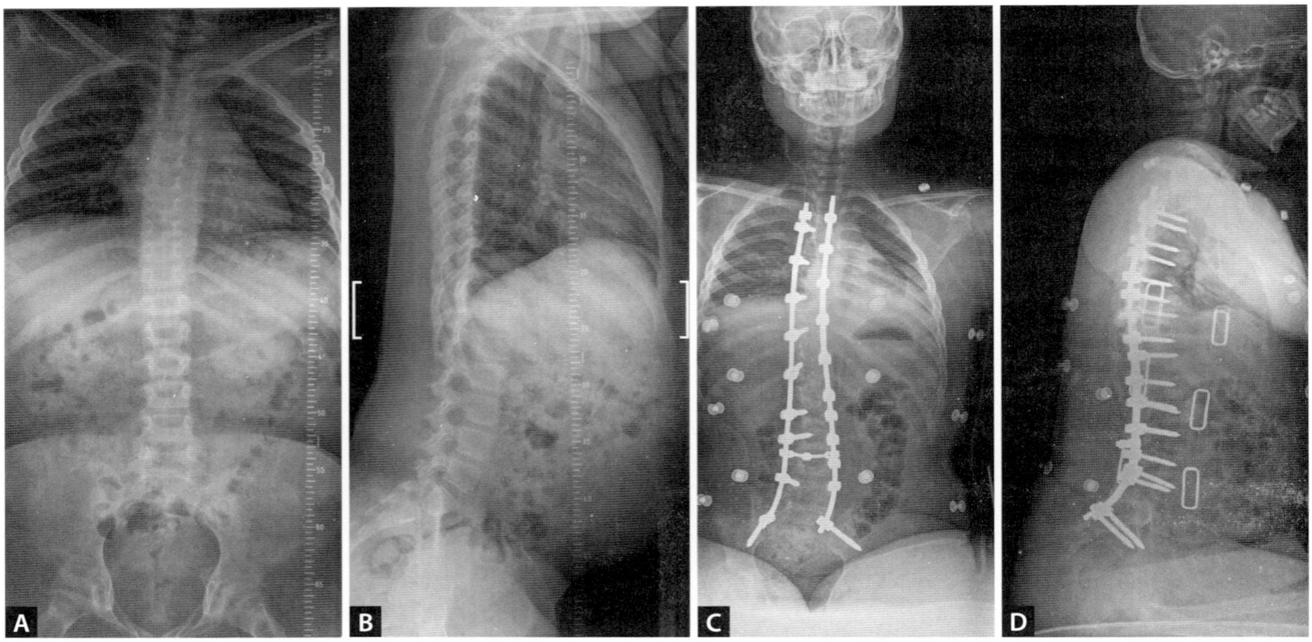

Figs. 8A to D: Pre- and postoperative posteroanterior (A and C) and lateral (B and D) radiographs of a patient with neuromuscular scoliosis secondary to Duchenne muscular dystrophy treated with posterior spinal fusion with extension to the sacrum.

Shapiro et al.concluded that early surgery, when curve magnitude was not so great, would allow for improved outcomes and less complications.[75]

Duchenne Muscular Dystrophy

There is a consensus about the role of early spinal fusion in scoliosis secondary to DMD, particularly before the deterioration of the cardiopulmonary function. A number of authors have recommended operative intervention when the curve reaches 20° and the forced vital capacity is greater than 40%. The incidence of perioperative pulmonary complications significantly increases in patients with vital capacity > 30%[26,41,43,53] (Figs. 8A to D).

Friedreich's Ataxia

Scoliotic deformities in Friedreich's ataxia are managed on the principles similar to those of adolescent idiopathic scoliosis. Curves greater than 40° in the coronal plane with documented progression in a skeletally immature patient are treated with spinal fusion.[15,44-46,73] Stable curves between 40–60° in patient after completion of skeletal maturity can be observed.[15,73]

Rett Syndrome

Due to paucity of studies, the indications of operative treatment in scoliosis secondary to Rett syndrome are not clear.[49,50,53] The surgical indications include rapidly progressive curves with sitting imbalance. Skeletal maturity, severity and stiffness of the spinal curve and the truncal height are some of the factors that need consideration in the decision-making.[50,53]

Arthrogryposis

Again, lack of adequate data prevents defining the accurate role of surgical treatment in arthrogrypotic spinal deformities. These curves tend to progress rapidly and develop into very rigid deformities involving the pelvis. Hence, spinal fusion is indicated early, before progression to a rigid deformity or development of pelvic obliquity.[19,51,52] Greggi et al. recommended early surgery in aggressive curves that exceed 40° with marked thoracic hyperkyphosis, hyperlordosis or pelvic obliquity.[19] Sarwak et al. described a curve magnitude of 50° as an indication for spinal fusion.[51] On the other hand, Daher et al. found the development of thoracic lordosis as an important indicator for surgical intervention.[52]

Spinal Instrumentation

There has been a tremendous evolution in the spinal instrumentation techniques in the past few decades. The purpose of NM scoliosis surgery is the correction of the spinal curvature and the pelvic tilt and fusion of the spine in a balanced alignment, so as to prevent further progression of the deformity and preserve the pulmonary function.[7,20,40,45,49,52] Based on the current standard of treatment, this is typically achieved by performing instrumented spinal fusion.

The early sixties witnessed the introduction of the Harrington compression and distraction system for spinal fusion. Although the Harrington rod was a major improvement in the surgical treatment of spinal deformities, the correction obtained was not optimal and the incidence of pseudoarthrosis was high.[76,77] Moreover, following the surgery, a significant period of bed rest and external immobilization in a cast was mandatory.[76] The development of segmental spinal fixation was a major step in the modern treatment of spinal deformities. The Luque method of segmental sublaminar wire fixation was one of the first such techniques. It provided an improved spinal fixation to the lamina with better stability and correction of the scoliotic curve.[78,79] In contrast to the Harrington rod system the rate of complications, especially pseudoarthrosis, was significantly low.[76,78,79] Long-term postoperative bracing was not mandatory, which was major advantage in the NM population.[76,78,79] A number of modifications of the Luque method are popular in NM scoliosis surgery. The Galveston technique modification facilitated the rods to be fixed to the pelvis so as to address the pelvic obliquity.[80,81] The unit rod technique incorporated the Galveston portion of the pelvic fixation into the Luque system, thus achieving both spinal and pelvic fixation using the same rod.[82,83] Thus the segmental sublaminar wire technique revolutionized the treatment of NM scoliosis. The advantages include ease of use, low cost, low complication rate, and excellent coronal correction. The disadvantages include inadequate sagittal and rotational correction, semirigid correction that can allow settling and some loss of correction and a higher possibility of proximal junctional kyphosis due to the disruption of the interspinous ligaments.[53]

The development of hooks was the next step in the spinal deformity correction. The hooks allowed for the compression and distraction, thus allowing both coronal and sagittal correction. Cotrel-Dubousset and other hook-based systems have been fairly popular for use in spinal deformity surgery.[84]

The development of pedicle screw-based systems is the latest addition to the instrumentation available in NM scoliosis surgery. Pedicle screws achieve a three column fixation into the vertebra, thus providing rigid stabilization. This allow for compression, distraction, rod rotation, in-situ rod bending and when appropriate, direct vertebral derotation maneuvers for correction of even rigid spinal deformities by a posterior only approach. Pedicle screws are reported to be safe and effective in the management of NM scoliosis.[85-87] Based on the study by Whitaker et al., posterior instrumentation and arthrodesis using pedicle screw anchorage can safely end in the lower lumbar region, in a select group of patients. Pedicle screw fixation can be useful in the cerebral palsy patients developing spinal deformity following posterior laminectomy for rhizotomy, where sublaminar wires fixation is not an option.[87,88] In myelodysplasia, where posterior elements may be malformed or absent, pedicle screws can help obtain stable anchorage in the available osseous structure.[7] It is also suitable for use in the presence of a baclofen pump, where the rod can easily be inserted under the shunt, something not possible with a unit rod.[87]

Use of hybrid fixation using the combination of screws, wires, and hooks is indicated in certain situations and may help with good curve correction.[86,89] Hybrid constructs can also help with limiting the implant costs.

Extension of Fixation to the Pelvis

One of the important aspects of surgical management of NM scoliosis involves the decision concerning extension of the fusion to the pelvis. Conventional indications for the inclusion of the pelvis in the spinal fusion include severe pelvic obliquity with sitting imbalance and contractures of lower extremity, especially in the nonambulatory patients.[7,20,53,56,32,83,90-96] The purpose of fusion to the pelvis is the improvement and maintenance of sitting balance by correcting the pelvic obliquity. On the contrary, for patients with a good ambulatory function, stopping the fusion in the lumbar spine appears to be safe and effective. This is especially applicable to patients with mild pelvic obliquity (<15°) and minimal lower extremity contractures[77,86,91,97,98] (Figs. 9A and B).

CHAPTER 13

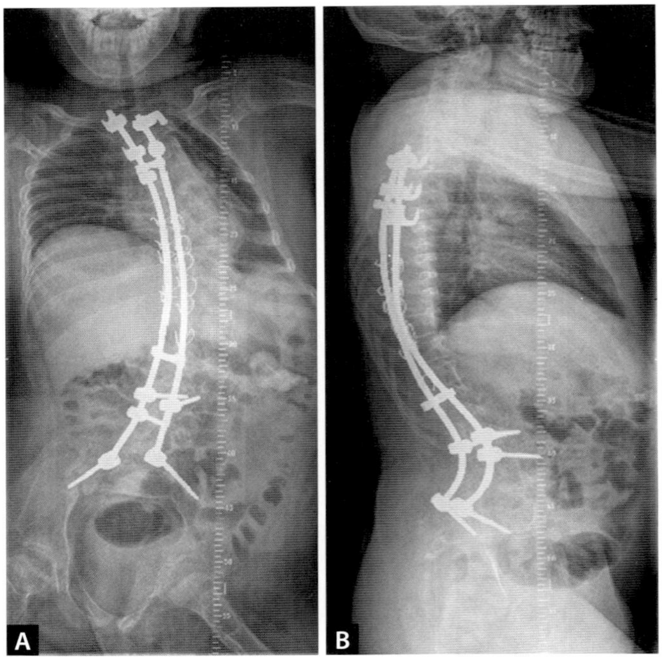

Figs. 9A and B: (A) A posteroanterior; and (B) Lateral radiograph of a patient with neuromuscular scoliosis treated with extension of fusion to the pelvis using iliac screws.

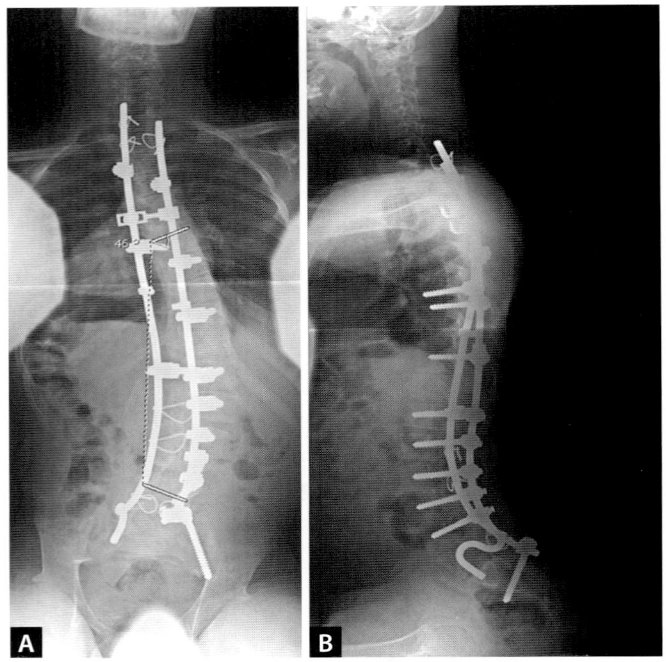

Figs. 10A and B: (A) A posteroanterior; and (B) Lateral radiograph demonstrating neuromuscular scoliosis managed by spinopelvic fixation. Note the type of spinopelvic fixation, Dunn-McCarthy technique on the left side and iliac screw on the right side.

A number of other factors need to be taken into account when considering pelvic fixation. The inclusion of pelvis in the fusion complicates the surgery significantly. It is associated with increased blood loss and longer surgical time.[86,99,100] A number of studies have suggested that extension of fusion to pelvis is suitable only for nonambulatory patients.[86,101] Studies have noted that mobility at the lumbosacral junction provides functional advantages in transferring and performing weight shifts while sitting and ambulating particularly in patients with minimal pelvic obliquity.[91,97] On the other hand, Tsirikos et al. attributed the myth about the impairment of ambulation in cerebral palsy after pelvic fusion to the outcomes from early attempts at instrumenting to the pelvis using straight Harrington rods, which removed all lumbar lordosis and created "lumbar flat back." In addition, many of the instrumentation systems used initially in the surgical management of NM scoliosis were not rigid enough to achieve a solid spine fusion without long periods of bed rest and body casting. These prolonged periods of postoperative immobilization had a detrimental effect on the ambulatory capacity of the patients. In their series of patients with the use of unit rod, patients had a good restoration of the spinal sagittal alignment and were mobilized early. In conclusion, Tsirikos et al. reported no change in the ambulatory status of the patients undergoing successful fusion to the pelvis for scoliosis secondary to spastic cerebral palsy.[102] Thus, there appears to be obvious ambiguity in the literature concerning the inclusion of pelvis in the fusion construct. The decision for pelvic fixation in NM scoliosis should be individualized and be based on the ambulatory status, ability to sit independently, severity of the pelvic obliquity and the lower extremity contractures, affecting overall sitting balance of the patient (Figs. 10A and B).

A wide variety of pelvic fixation techniques have been developed. Some of the commonly used techniques include Galveston, Dunn-McCarthy, Warner-Fackler, McCall, STIF, Iliac screw, Amrita, Colorado II, Four rod technique, etc. The reader is recommended to refer to the appropriate literature for the detailed description of each of these techniques (Figs. 11A and B).

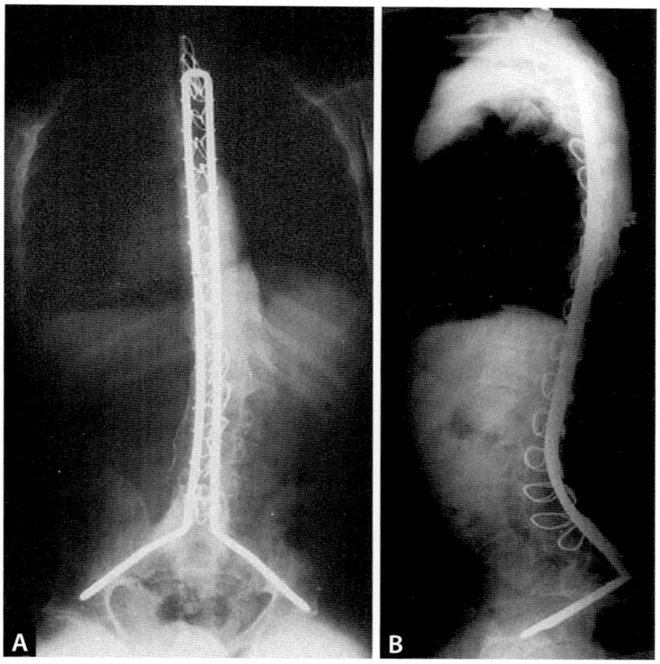

Figs. 11A and B: A posteroanterior (A) and lateral radiograph (B) demonstrating the use of unit rod in the management of neuromuscular scoliosis with spinopelvic fixation.

Surgical Approaches

Role of Anterior Surgery

Anterior release in combination with a posterior instrumented fusion has been well described in the surgical management of NM scoliosis.[7,20,59,77,84,86,94,96] The indication for concomitant anterior surgery is to improve correction in large (>70°) and stiff (<30% correction on lateral bending radiograph) curves with apex rotation of more than 25–30°.[86,96] Anterior surgery helps improve the flexibility of the curve, thus facilitating greater correction.[7,20,77,86,96] It can also decrease the rate of pseudoarthrosis by providing more surface area for fusion.[7,20,59,96] In skeletally immature patients, in combination with posterior fusion, it can help prevent the crankshaft phenomenon.[7,20,59,62] Comstock et al. in the study of skeletally immature patients undergoing surgical correction of NM scoliosis, concluded that the best correction and long-term outcomes were observed in those treated with both anterior and posterior procedure.[62] In spinal deformities secondary to myelodysplasia, where the posterior elements could be deficient, anterior arthrodesis alone or in combination with posterior fusion may be the cornerstone in achieving deformity correction.[7,71,103-108]

Anterior surgery, in spite of all its benefits, could potentially contribute to a higher rate of complications especially in the perioperative period. An anterior procedure can increase the surgical time, blood loss, pulmonary complications, and the overall morbidity related to the surgery.[83,85,90,96,101,109] The long-term compromise in the pulmonary function secondary to a thoracotomy is well known.[90,101,109] This is of immense importance, based on the fact that majority of the NM scoliosis patients have a number of preexisting comorbidities along with an impaired cardiopulmonary function.[7,15,20,25,26,46,53,64,65] Thus, an additional anterior surgery can increase the surgical risk substantially in this fragile patient population. This restricts the role of anterior release surgery mostly for the management of stiffer and larger curves.[96] The various anterior approaches include transthoracic, thoracoabdominal, and lumbar retroperitoneal. The dependence on an access surgeon for an anterior exposure is not infrequent. Video-assisted thoracoscopic surgery (VATS) has been used in the treatment of idiopathic scoliosis and is shown to have a less adverse effect on the pulmonary function. Its role in NM scoliosis as treatment is still unexplored. A steep learning curve and the requirement of appropriate equipment are the other potential factors that may limit its use.[53]

Role of Posterior Surgery

A number of studies have reported excellent curve correction and rate of fusion by posterior surgery without an anterior release.[46,56,85,86,89,96,109] The evolution of segmental instrumentation systems, especially the use of pedicle screws, has made the posterior surgical correction of the spinal deformities very convenient.[85,89,96,109] Pedicle screws by virtue of the control over the three spinal columns help manipulate the curve very effectively.[85,109] The posterior surgical approach is simple and is known universally. In severe and rigid deformities, a variety of osteotomies can be used to achieve the desired result. The advantages of avoiding anterior surgery in the medically fragile NM patient population are numerous and have already been discussed. Posterior spinal fusion has thus evolved into a safe, effective and less morbid option for the surgical treatment of majority of patients with NM scoliosis (Figs. 12A and B).

Postoperative Care

A spinal fusion surgery for NM scoliosis causes a significant physiological insult to medically vulnerable host. A dedicated pediatric intensive care unit provides an optimal setting for the immediate postoperative management. Frequently, these children are kept intubated and on a ventilatory support for 24–48 hours, but early weaning should be attempted when possible. Aggressive resuscitative measures can prevent serious postoperative complications in this fragile patient population.

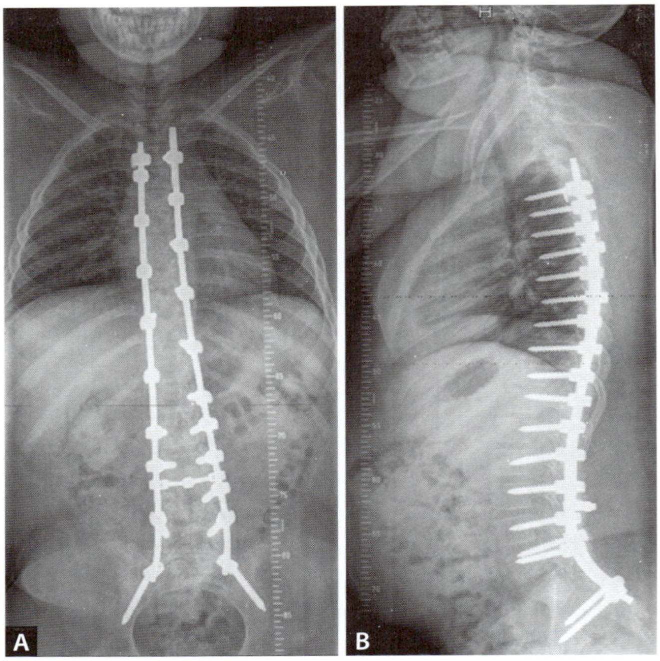

Figs. 12A and B: (A) A posterior-anterior; and (B) Lateral radiograph demonstrating posterior pedicle screw only construct in the management of neuromuscular scoliosis.

Once stabilized, early mobilization out of the bed is immensely helpful in promoting pulmonary toilet and preventing pressure sores. A rehabilitation team accustomed to the care of the NM patient population is vital. Postoperative bracing can be considered to promote early mobilization, especially if there is a concern about the stability provided by the spinal instrumentation and the quality of the bone stock. Pressure sores and effect of the brace on the pulmonary function should be kept in mind when bracing is considered (Figs. 13A to D).

COMPLICATIONS

The common postoperative complications after a major spinal surgery in children tend to occur more frequently and are at times more pronounced in the NM scoliosis patient population. This could be attributed to the multitude of the associated medical problems in this population. A number of studies of the surgical management of NM scoliosis have reported the rate of complications to be

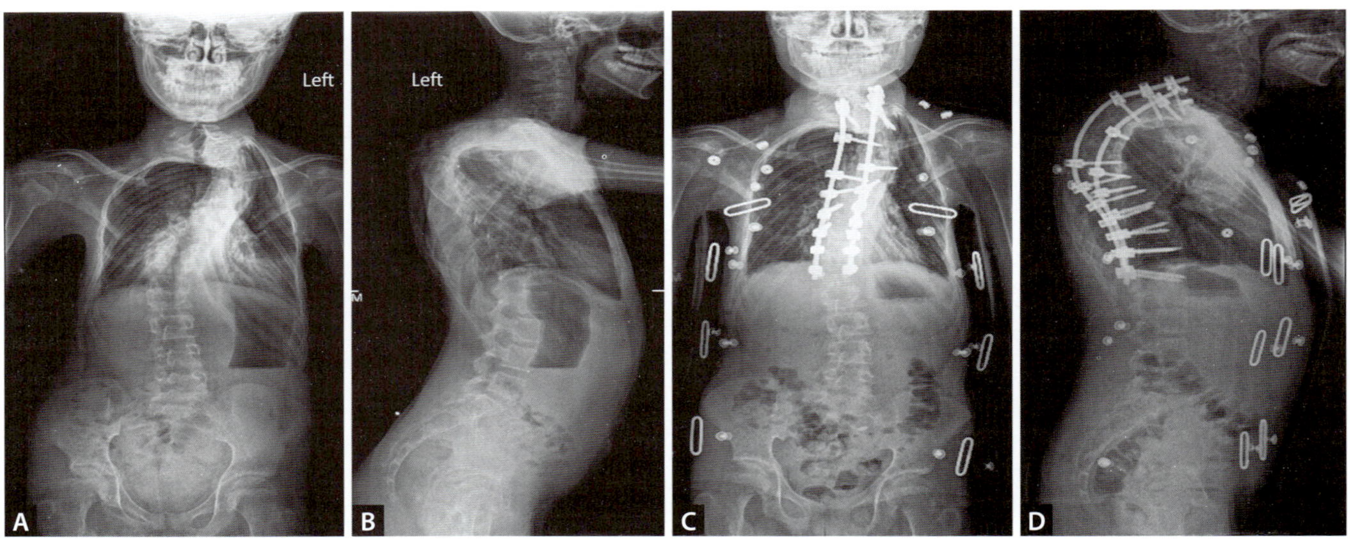

Figs. 13A to D: Pre- and postoperative posteroanterior (A and C) and lateral (B and D) radiographs demonstrating a neuromuscular kyphoscoliotic deformity affecting the thoracic spine which was managed by posterior spinal fusion.

ranging from 24% to 75%.[53,70,90,91,110,111] For convenience, complications occurring before the discharge from the hospital are termed early, while those occurring after the discharge are late.

Early Complications

Pulmonary Complications

Due to the pre-existing pulmonary compromise, these patients are prone to develop atelectasis, pleural effusion, and pneumonia. Prolonged endotracheal intubation and ventilator dependence is the other problem commonly encountered. Involvement of a pulmonologist and respiratory therapist is valuable. Aggressive pulmonary toilet with the help of repeated suctioning, chest physical therapy, positioning and early mobilization is vital in the management of these issues.[53,110-112]

Urinary Complications

The incidence urinary tract infection has been reported to range from 9% to 22%. Prolonged presence of a urinary catheter can be a contributing factor. Urinary retention after the removal of the catheter is another commonly encountered problem. When indicated, early urinary cultures can be obtained for the appropriate management of the infection. The myelodysplasia population often has chronic colonization of the bacteria in their lower urinary tract. Perioperative prophylactic antimicrobial therapy appears to have a role in limiting the infection.[53,110-112]

Cardiovascular Complications

Surgery for NM scoliosis is associated with significant blood loss that can lead to hemodynamic compromise and cardiac stress. Patients often need resuscitation with large volumes of fluids and blood products in the perioperative period. This can contribute to fluid and electrolyte imbalance and deranged coagulation parameters. Hence, every attempt should be made to minimize the blood loss and for recycling of lost blood with the use of a cell saver. Transfusion reactions, although rare, can complicate the surgical course. Therefore, intensive monitoring in the perioperative period and prompt correction of these abnormalities is warranted.[110-112]

Gastrointestinal Complications

Impaired bowel motility is a very common problem in the NM population. Ileus can be precipitated post spinal fusion, especially if a retroperitoneal approach is used. Opioid medications which form the mainstay of the pain management can further worsen the gut mobility. Oral intake may be impaired, resulting in malnutrition. Aggressive bowel protocol and appropriate hydration can help restore the gut mobility. When indicated, parenteral nutrition should be considered till the bowel function is restored.[70,110-112]

Neurological Complications

Neurological compromise, although rare, can still occur during the surgical management the spinal deformity. It could be related to spinal manipulation, instrumentation or hemodynamic factors. Neurological monitoring during the surgery can help avoid this problem.

Late Complications

Infections and Wound Complications

Various studies have reported the infection rate in NM scoliosis surgery in a range of 4–14%.[91,112-114] The potential factors that have been described as a high risk for infection include severe neurologic involvement, myelodysplasia, presence of a ventriculoperitoneal shunt, use of allograft, malnutrition, urinary tract infection, and excessive blood loss with requirement of blood transfusion.[25,69,113,114] A high index of suspicion is necessary to identify especially a low grade or quiescent wound infection. A timely irrigation and debridement can help eradicate early wound infection. Appropriate antibiotics should be selected based on the bacterial cultures obtained from the wound. In case of a deep delayed wound infection with an adequately fused spine, removal of instrumentation may be necessary.

Fusion-related Complications

The management of NM scoliosis involves long segment instrumented fusions extending from the upper thoracic spine to the lower lumbar spine or the sacrum and pelvis when indicated. Inappropriate selection of the fusion level distally can predispose to residual pelvic obliquity and sitting imbalance. On the other hand, proximal junctional kyphosis can result from inappropriate selection of the proximal level of the fusion.[91,98] Pseudoarthrosis and failure of instrumentation are complications seen late during the follow-up. The lumbosacral and the thoracolumbar regions are the most common sites for the nonunion. Frequently, this problem is asymptomatic and may not be progressive. A group of patients may present with pain, loss of correction, and displaced implant, which requires revision surgery.[77,82,83,90,91,98,109,111] Bell et al. have reported the rate

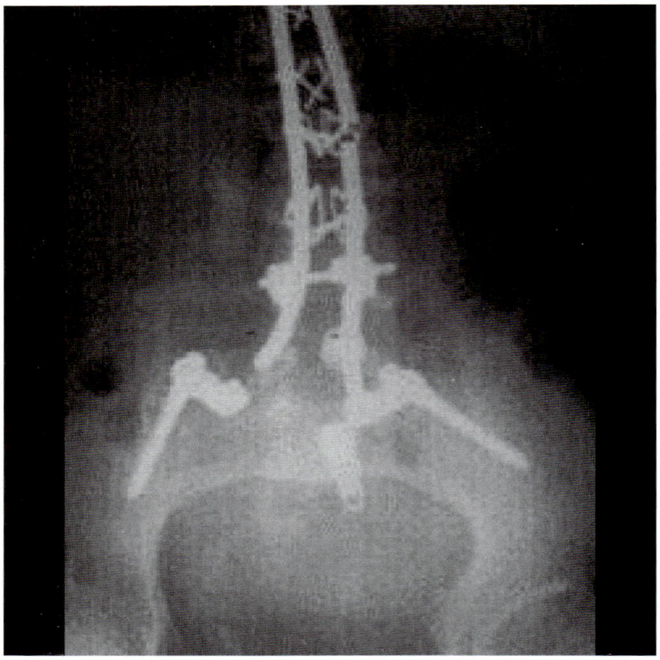

Fig. 14: A posteroanterior radiograph demonstrating failure of fixation secondary to pseudoarthrosis in the lumbosacral region.

of pseudoarthrosis to be 7.5% at an average of 30 month follow-up.[82] While Boachie-Adjei et al. have reported the rate of pseudoarthrosis at 6.5% and that of instrumentation failure at 15%.[90] Crankshaft phenomenon is a concern in skeletally immature children undergoing posterior spinal fusion, especially with the use of earlier nonsegmental instrumentation systems. It could lead to some loss of the deformity correction. Use of segmental instrumentation, pedicle screws in particular, due to the virtue of three column control, appears to limit this problem[83,98,109] (Fig. 14).

PROGNOSIS

The natural history of untreated NM scoliosis has been discussed earlier part of this chapter. In majority of the patients, progression of the spinal deformity is predominantly influenced by the type of primary condition and its severity.[5,7-9,11-19] The worsening spinal deformity has an adverse impact on the sitting balance, pulmonary function, and the overall QOL for these patients. Spinal fusion appears to preserve, and in select situations, improve some of these parameters.[56-63] It does not change the course of the primary NM condition. Most of these children have significant multiple systemic comorbidities that tend to influence their general well-being and survival. In general, the prognosis of the patient is dictated by the type and severity of the primary neurological or myopathic disease (Table 1).[53,70]

Table 1: Evidence-based table.

Author, journal, year	*Design*	*LoE*	*Topic*	*F/U (m)*	*Measures*	*Main results*
Saito, Lancet, 1998[5]	R	IV	Natural history of scoliosis in cerebral palsy	207	Cobb angle	Risk factors for progression, > 40°, < 15 years, total body involvement, being bedridden, thoracolumbar curve
Thomez, JBJS Am, 1988[8]	R	IV	Curve progression	195	Cobb angle	Risk factors for progression, large curves at skeletal maturity, spastic quadriplegia, thoracolumbar or lumbar curve, bedridden
Trivedi, JBJS Am, 2002[9]	R	IV	Clinical and radiologic predictors for development of scoliosis in myelomeningocele	112.8	Cobb angle	Factors include clinical motor level, ambulatory status, and last intact laminar arch
Oda, J Pedatr Orthop,1998[14]	R	IV	Natural course of spinal deformity	48	Cobb angle, spinal alignment, vital capacity	Surgery if curve > 30° and vital capacity > 35%

Contd...

Contd...

Author, journal, year	*Design*	*LoE*	*Topic*	*F/U (m)*	*Measures*	*Main results*
Potaczek, Chir Narzadow Ruchu Ortop Pol, 2010[16]	R	IV	Rett syndrome curve progression preoperatively, course of surgery and finally radiological and subjective results of treatment	37	Cobb angle, blood loss, caregiver satisfaction	Surgery for curves 40–50° is safe. Nonambulatory patients fused to pelvis.
Greggi, Scoliosis, 2010[19]	R	IV	Role of surgical treatment	50	Clinical, radiological—Cobb angle, fusion	Brace for curves< 40°, surgery for larger curves.
Pierz, J Peadatr Orthop, 2000[21]	R	IV	Effects of detethering on scoliosis in myelomeningocele	60	Cobb angle	Detethering improves curves < 40°
Emans, JBJS Am, 1992[24]	R	IV	Allergy to latex in myelodysplasia			
Kennedy, Thorax, 1995[26]	R	III	Effect of surgery on lung function in DMD	84	Cobb angle, % forced vital capacity	Spinal surgery in DMD does not alter lung function nor does it affect survival
Hennrikus, J Pediatr Orthop, 1993[27]	P	II	Incidence of spondylolisthesis in ambulatory CP patients		Clinical, radiographic	Incidence same as in general population, not related to hip flexion contracture
Miller, J Pediatr Orthop, 1996[29]	P	II	Impact of orthosis on scoliosis progression in CP	67	Cobb angle	Orthosis had no effect on curve progression. Apical vertebral rotation is an indicator for progression
Olafsson, J Pediatr Orthop, 1999[30]	R	IV	Brace treatment in NM	37	Cobb angle, compliance	Brace treatment effective in hypotonia and short thoracolumbar curves < 40° and spastic short lumbar curves
Morillon, Ann Readapt Med Phys, 2007[31]	R	III	Impact of spinal bracing on lung function		Spirometry	Spinal bracing in NM disease leads to significant respiratory impairment
Kotwici, Disabil Rehabil Assist Technol, 2008[34]	P	II	Technical particularities of construction and application of trunk orthosis in nonambulatory patients		Clinical, subjective	Correctly orthosis can improve the function, prevent complications and postpone the surgical treatment
Homes KJ, Clin Biomech (Bristol, Avon), 2003[35]	P	II	Effects of special seating on lateral spinal curvature in CP with scoliosis		Cobb angle	Significant scoliosis correction can be obtained in CP with special seating
Terjesen, Dev Med Child Neurol, 2000[37]	R	IV	Evaluate clinical results of treatment and factors influencing rate of scoliosis progression	24	Cobb angle	Age and initial correction in orthosis were the only variables significantly influencing the rate of progression
Marchesi, Acta Orthop Belg, 1991[39]	R	IV	Clinical and radiological evolution of scoliosis treated conservatively in myelomeningocele	120	Clinical, Cobb angle	Conservative treatment for curves less than 50° and spinal stabilization in curvatures over 50

Contd...

Contd...

Author, journal, year	*Design*	*LoE*	*Topic*	*F/U (m)*	*Measures*	*Main results*
Milbrandt, J Pediatr Orthop, 2008[46]	R	IV	Evaluate the demographics, progression, nonoperative and operative treatment of spinal deformities in patients with Friedreich's ataxia	45	Cobb angle	Patients with Friedreich's ataxia need to be screened for scoliosis and counseled about the high rate of surgical fusion
Farhat, Neurology, 2002[54]	C	II	Determine the effect of antiepileptics on vitamin D levels and bone density		Bone mineral density and serum 25 hydroxy-vitamin D	Epilepsy and its therapy, are risk factors for low bone density, irrespective of vitamin D levels
Joyce NC, Phys Med Rehabil Clin N Am, 2012[55]	SR	III	Reviews of literature regarding bone health in neuromuscular disease			Therapeutic effect of available osteoporosis treatments
Bohtz, J Pediatr Orthop, 2011[56]	R	IV	Evaluate outcome of surgical scoliosis correction measured by the subjective change in the HRQL and the objective radiologic changes	24	HRQL, radiological, Cobb angle	Life quality improved after surgical scoliosis correction in patients with CP, but does not correlate with radiological changes
Watanabe, Spine (Phila Pa 1976), 2009[57]	R	IV	Evaluate the clinical outcomes and satisfaction associated with the surgical treatment of neuromuscular spinal deformity due to CP	74	Patient expectation, cosmesis, function, patient care, quality of life, pulmonary function, pain, health status, self-image, and satisfaction, complications, and radiographic data	CP patient/parents were satisfied with the results of the spinal deformity surgery
Mercado, Spine (Phila Pa 1976), 2007[58]	SR	IV	To determine if QOL is improved by scoliosis surgery in neuromuscular patients.			Grade C recommendation: Spinal fusion improves QOL in CP and muscular dystrophy. Spinal fusion does not improve QOL in spina bifida.
Larsson, Spine (Phila Pa 1976), 2005[59]	P	II	Long-term follow-up of functioning in patients with NM scoliosis after surgery	84.5	Sitting, angle of scoliosis, lung function, reaching, pain, activities of daily living, care given and time for resting	Comparison of the preoperative and long-term follow-ups showed that patients were mostly improved
Bridwell, Spine (Phila Pa 1976), 1999[61]	R	IV	To assess patient/parent satisfaction and clinical/functional ways in which spinal fusion affected patients	93.6	Evaluate function, self-image, cosmesis, pain, pulmonary status, patient care, quality of life, and satisfaction	Spinal fusion with segmental spinal instrumentation benefits most patients

Contd...

Contd...

Author, journal, year	*Design*	*LoE*	*Topic*	*F/U (m)*	*Measures*	*Main results*
Comstock, Spine (Phila Pa 1976), 1998[62]	R	IV	Analyze the results of spinal fusion in patients with total-body-involvement CP		Physical examination and a personal interview conducted with the patient, parents, and primary caregiver.	High patient and caregiver satisfaction confirm that corrective spinal surgery is indicated and is beneficial for most patients with total-body-involvement CP and scoliosis
Askin, Spine (Phila Pa 1976), 1997[63]	P	II	Whether improving spinal alignment and truncal balance improved the functional abilities of handicapped patients	12	Ability to sit, ambulate, and complete activities of daily living	Spinal surgery in patients with severe physical handicap should be performed early to preserve function and should not be dictated solely by the severity of the curvature
Chambers, J Pediatr Orthop, 1999[66]	R	III	Evaluate the effect of valproic acid on blood loss during spine surgery		Bleeding time, blood loss	Potential association between VPA use and increased blood loss
Thompson, Spine (Phila Pa 1976), 2008[67]	R	III	Evaluate the effectiveness of Amicar in decreasing perioperative blood loss in patients with NM scoliosis surgery		Perioperative blood loss	Amicar was effective in decreasing perioperative blood loss and transfusion requirements in patients with NM scoliosis
Kasimian, Eur Spine J, 2008[68]	R	III	Evaluate the safety and efficacy of aprotinin in pediatric NM scoliosis patients undergoing spinal fusion		Perioperative blood loss	Aprotinin resulted in decreased blood loss and a decreased rate of transfusions in children with NM scoliosis
Dias, J Pediatr Orthop, 1996[83]	R	IV	Surgical correction of spinal deformity using a unit rod in children with CP	33.6	Clinical, Cobb angle	Objective of improving the child's ability to sit more comfortably was accomplished with spinal fusion
Piazolla, Eur Spine J, 2011[84]	R	IV	Cotrel-Dubousset instrumentation in NM	142	Clinical, blood loss, Cobb angle	CD technique provides lasting correction of spinal deformity in patients with NM scoliosis
Modi, Spine (Phila Pa 1976), 2009[85]	R	IV	Effectiveness and amount of correction using posterior-only pedicle screw construct	36	Clinical, modified Rancho Los Amigos Hospital system criteria, Cobb angle	Satisfactory coronal and sagittal correction with posterior-only pedicle screw fixation without higher complication rate in CP patients
Whitaker, Spine (Phila Pa 1976), 2000[86]	R	IV	Safety and efficacy of stopping posterior instrumentation constructs in the lumbar spine with pedicle screw anchorage	62	Clinical, radiological, Cobb angle	Posterior instrumentation and arthrodesis using lumbar lower instrumented vertebra pedicle screw anchorage can be performed safely and effectively, in selected patients with scoliosis and minimal pelvic obliquity
Li, Microsurgery, 2008[88]	R	IV	Deformity of lumbar spine after selective dorsal rhizotomy for spastic cerebral palsy	75	Clinical, radiological	Cerebral palsy patients may develop spinal deformity after selective dorsal rhizotomy

Contd...

Contd...

Author, journal, year	*Design*	*LoE*	*Topic*	*F/U (m)*	*Measures*	*Main results*
La Rosa, Eur Spine J, 2011[89]	R	IV	To verify the validity of this spinal fixation implant in the surgical treatment of patients affected by NM scoliosis	36	Clinical, radiological, blood loss	Universal clamps technique appeared safe and effective and its mechanical performance is comparable to all-level screws construct
Broom, J Bone Joint Surg Am, 1989[91]	R	IV	Spinal fusion augmented by Luque-rod segmental instrumentation for NM	42	Clinical, radiological, Cobb angle	Luque-rod segmental instrumentation with posterior spinal fusion is an effective treatment for NM scoliosis
Ferguson, Orthop Clin North Am, 1988[92]	EO	V	Considerations in the treatment of CP patients with spinal deformities			Use of L-rod instrumentation to stabilize the spinal deformity in the CP patient
Majd, Spine (Phila Pa 1976), 1997[95]	P	II	The study followed the natural history of untreated scoliosis to determine whether a decline in functional status is related to curve progression		Clinical, radiological, Cobb angle	A definite correlation exists between deformity size and functional decline and decubiti
Auerbach, Spine (Phila Pa 1976), 2009[96]	R	IV	Compare coronal and sagittal plane radiographic outcomes in patients undergoing either a combined anteroposterior spinal fusion or a posterior-only fusion		Clinical, Radiological, Cobb angle	Excellent correction in severe pelvic obliquity can be achieved in smaller, more flexible curves using an all construct and posterior spinal fusion, and in larger, less flexible curves using an anterior release with PSF
Sussman, J Pediatr Orthop, 1996[98]	R	IV	Posterior instrumentation and fusion of the thoracolumbar spine for treatment of NM scoliosis	66	Clinical, Radiological, Cobb angle	Those patients with significant growth remaining, or with severe deformities, may benefit by preliminary anterior release and fusion or inclusion of the pelvis and sacrum
Mubarak, J Pediatr Orthop, 1993[99]	R	IV	Spinal fusion in DMD fixation and fusion to the sacropelvis		Clinical, radiological, forced vital capacity	Recommendation for operation should be made when their curve is > 20° and if their forced vital capacity is > 40%. T2 to L5 fusion adequate
Sengupta, Spine (Phila Pa 1976), 2002[100]	R	IV	To determine whether fixation to the sacropelvis is always necessary for adequate stabilization of scoliosis in DMD	42	Clinical, radiological, Cobb angle	Lumbar fixation to L5 is adequate if the surgery is performed early, soon after becoming wheelchair bound, and with smaller curves and minimal pelvic obliquity. Pelvic fixation may be necessary in older children, who have larger curves and established pelvic obliquity
Tsirikos, Spine (Phila Pa 1976), 2003[102]	R	IV	To evaluate the effect of spinal fusion from T1–T2 to the sacrum with pelvic fixation using unit rod instrumentation on the ambulatory potential of these patients	33	Clinical, radiological, gait analysis	Spine surgery with fusion extending to the pelvis in ambulatory patients with cerebral palsy provided excellent deformity correction and preserved their ambulatory function

Contd...

Contd...

Author, journal, year	*Design*	*LoE*	*Topic*	*F/U (m)*	*Measures*	*Main results*
Banta, Spine (Phila Pa 1976), 1990[103]	R	IV	Combined anterior and posterior fusion for spinal deformity in myelomeningocele	66	Clinical, radiological, Cobb angle	Anterior fusion of the dysraphic spine allows greater correction of both spinal deformity and pelvic obliquity in addition to contributing significant strength to the fusion mass
Sponseller, Clin Orthop Relat Res, 1999[107]	R	IV	Determine whether the infection rate could be decreased, adequate correction and pelvic balance could be provided, and posterior surgery could be avoided in myelomeningocele	24	Clinical, radiological, blood loss	Anterior only fusion and instrumentation may have significant advantages, but only for selected patients with thoracolumbar curves less than 75°, compensatory curves less than 40°, no increased kyphosis, and no syrinx
Stella, Eur J Pediatr Surg, 1998[108]	R	IV	Surgical approach in the treatment of scoliosis associated with myelomeningocele	74	Clinical, radiological	The combined anterior and posterior instrumentation and fusion gave the best correction of deformity and reduced the rate of pseudoarthrosis
Keeler, Spine (Phila Pa 1976), 2010[109]	R	IV	Is anterior releasing necessary when intraoperative halofemoral traction is used?	24	Clinical, radiological, blood loss	When intraoperative halofemoral traction is used, PSF-only surgery for NMS can provide excellent curve correction and spinal balance
Benson, Spine (Phila Pa 1976), 1998[110]	R	IV	To provide current data on the results and complications of patients who have undergone spinal fusion for NM	40	Clinical, radiological, Cobb angle	With current surgical techniques and perioperative management in an experienced center, the results for patients undergoing spinal fusion for NM have been improved, and major complications have been minimized
Lonstein, Spine (Phila Pa 1976), 2012[111]	R	IV	Results and complications after spinal fusion for NM scoliosis in CP and using luque galveston instrumentation	45.6	Clinical, radiological, Cobb angle	Spinal fusion in NM with Luque-Galveston technique is a safe and effective procedure. Pseudarthroses were detected late and were the main reason for additional surgery
Mohamad, J Pediatr Orthop, 2007[112]	R	IV	Perioperative complications after surgical correction in neuromuscular scoliosis		Clinical, radiological	Patients with NM are at high risk of developing perioperative complications after surgical correction of their deformity (overall rate, 33.1%)
Master, Spine (Phila Pa 1976), 2011[114]	R	III	Determine risk factors for postoperative wound infections after surgery for NM as well as the causative organisms and the results of treatment	55.2	Clinical, radiological	The presence of a ventriculoperitoneal shunt is a statistically significant risk factor for wound infection after corrective surgery for NM. Wound infection is associated with pseudarthrosis and prolonged hospitalization

(C: cross sectional; EO: expert opinion; FU: follow up; HRQL: health-related quality of life; LoE: level of evidence; NM: neuromuscular scoliosis; P: prospective; QOL: quality of life; R: retrospective; SR: systemic review)

CHAPTER 13

REFERENCES

1. Bleck EE: Orthopaedic management in cerebral palsy. In: Clinics in developmental medicine. Philadelphia: JB Lippincott; 1987.
2. Balmer GA, MacEwen GD: The incidence and treatment of scoliosis in cerebral palsy. J Bone Joint Surg. 1970;52(1):134-7.
3. Madigan RR, Wallace SL. Scoliosis in the institutionalized cerebral palsy population. Spine (Phila Pa 1976). 1981;6(6):583-90.
4. Lonstein JE: Neuromuscular spinal deformities. In: The pediatric spine principles and practice, 2nd edition. Philadelphia: Lippincott Williams & Wilkins; 2001. pp. 789-96.
5. Saito N, Ebara S, Ohotsuka K, et al. Natural history of scoliosis in spastic cerebral palsy. Lancet. 1998;351(9117):1687-92.
6. Hodgkinson I, Berard C, Chotel F, et al. Pelvic obliquity and scoliosis in non-ambulatory patients with cerebral palsy: A descriptive study of 234 patients over 15 years of age. Rev Chir Orthop Reparatrice Appar Mot 2002;88(4):337-41.
7. Guille JT, Sarwark JF, Sherk HH, et al. Congenital and Developmental Deformities of the Spine in Children With Myelomeningocele. J Am Acad Orthop Surg. 2006;14(5):294-302.
8. Thometz JG, Simon SR. Progression of scoliosis after skeletal maturity in institutionalized adults who have cerebral palsy. J Bone Joint Surg Am. 1988;70(9):1290-6.
9. Trivedi J, Thomson JD, Slakey JB, et al. Clinical and radiographic predictors of scoliosis in patients with myelomeningocele. J Bone Joint Surg Am. 2002;84 (8):1389-94.
10. Evans GA, Drennan JC, Russman BS. Functional classification and orthopedic management of spinal muscular atrophy. J Bone Joint Surg Br. 1981;63B(4):516-22.
11. Tangsrud SE, Carlson KC, Lund-Peterson I, et al. Lung function measurements in young children with spinal muscular atrophy: a cross-sectional survey on the effect of position and bracing. Arch Dis Child. 2001;84(6):521-4.
12. Schwentker EP, Gibson DA. The orthopedic aspects of spinal muscular atrophy. J Bone Joint Surg Am. 1976;58(1):32-8.
13. Cambridge W, Drennan JC. Scoliosis associated with Duchenne muscular dystrophy. J Pediatr Orthop. 1987;7(4):436-40.
14. Oda T, Shimizu N, Yonenobu K, et al. Longitudinal study of spinal deformity in spinal deformity in Duchenne muscular dystrophy. J Pedatr Orthop. 1993;13(4):478-88.
15. Labelle H. Spinal deformities in Friedreich's Ataxia. In: The Pediatric Spine Principles and Practice, 2nd edition. Philadelphia: Lippincott Williams & Wilkins; 2001. pp. 809-18.
16. Potaczek T, Jasiewicz B, Tesiorowski M, et al. Scoliosis in Rett syndrome-own experience. Chir Narzadow Ruchu Ortop Pol. 2010;75(1):17-23.
17. Lidstrom J, Stokland E Hagberg B. Scoliosis in Rett syndrome: Clinical and biologic aspects. Spine (Phila Pa 1976). 1994;19(14):1632-5.
18. Holm VA, King HA. Scoliosis in the Rett syndrome. Brain Dev. 1990;12:151-3.
19. Greggi T, Martikos K, Pipitone E, et al. Surgical treatment of scoliosis in a rare disease: arthrogryposis. Scoliosis. 2010;9;5:24.
20. McCarthy JJ, D'Andrea LP, Betz RR. Scoliosis in the child with cerebral palsy. J Am Acad Orthop Surg. 2006;14(6):367-75.
21. Pierz K, Banta J, Thomson J, et al. The effect of tethered cord release on scoliosis in myelomeningocele. J Pediatr Orthop. 2000;20(3):362-5.
22. Sarwark JF, Weber DT, Gabrieli AP, et al. Tethered cord syndrome in low motor level children with myelomeningocele. Pediatr Neurosurg. 1996;25(6):295-301.
23. Tori JA, Dickson JH. Association of congenital anomalies of the spine and kidneys. Clin Orthop Relat Res. 1980;148:259-62.
24. Emans JB. Current concepts review: Allergy to latex in patients who have myelodysplasia. J Bone Joint Surg Am. 1992;74:1103-9.
25. Bushby K, Finkel R, Birnkrant DJ, et al. Diagnosis and management of Duchenne muscular dystrophy, part 1: diagnosis, and pharmacological and psychosocial management. Lancet Neurol. 2010;9(1):77-93.
26. Kennedy JD, Staples AJ, Brook PD, et al. Effect of spinal surgery on lung function in Duchenne muscular dystrophy. Thorax. 1995;50(11):1173-8.
27. Hennrikus WL, Rosenthal RK, Kasser JR. Incidence of spondylolisthesis in ambulatory cerebral palsy patients. J Pediatr Orthop. 1993;13(1):37-40.
28. Hoffman EP, Fischbeck KH, Brown RH, et al. Characterization of dystrophin in muscle biopsy specimens from patients with Duchenne's or Becker's muscular dystrophy. N Engl J Med. 1988;318(21):1363-8.
29. Miller A, Temple T, Miller F. Impact of orthosis on the rate on the rate of scoliosis progression in children with cerebral palsy. J Pediatr Orthop. 1996;16(3):332-5.
30. Olafsson Y, Saraste H, Al-Dabbagh Z. Brace treatment in neuromuscular spine deformity. J Pediatr Orthop. 1999;19(3):376-9.
31. Morillon S, Thumerelle C, Cuisset JM, et al. Effect of thoracic bracing on lung function in children with neuromuscular disease. Ann Readapt Med Phys. 2007;50(8):645-50.
32. Letts M, Rathbone D, Yamashita T, et al. Soft Boston orthosis in the management of neuromuscular scoliosis: A preliminary report. J Pediatr Ortho. 1992;12(4):470-4.
33. Leopando MT, Moussavi Z, Holbrow J, et al. Effect of soft Boston orthosis on pulmonary mechanics in cerebral palsy. Pediatr Pulmonol. 1999;28(1):53-8.
34. Kotwicki T, Durmala J, Czubak J. Bracing for neuromuscular scoliosis: orthosis construction to improve the patient's function. Disabil Rehabil Assist Technol. 2008;3(3):161-9.
35. Homes KJ, Michael SM, Thorpe SL, et al. Management of scoliosis with special seating for nonambulatory spastic cerebral palsy population—A biomechanical study. Clin Biomech. 2003;18(6):480-7.
36. Nuzzo RM, Walsh S, Boucherit T, et al. Counterparalysis for treatment of paralytic scoliosis with botulinum toxin type A. Am J Orthop (Belle Mead NJ). 1997;26(3):201-7.

37. Terjesen T, Lange JE, Steen H. Treatment of scoliosis with spinal bracing in quadriplegic cerebral palsy. Dev Med Child Neurol. 2000;42(7):448-54.
38. Müller EB, Nordwall A, Oden A. Progression of scoliosis in children with myelomeningocele. Spine (Phila Pa 1976). 1994;19(2):147-50.
39. Marchesi D, Rudeberg A, Aebi M. Development in conservatively treated scoliosis in patients with myelomeningocele (patients of the years 1964-1977). Acta Orthop Belg. 1991;57(4):390-8.
40. Sucato DJ. Spine deformity in spinal muscular atrophy. J Bone Joint Surg Am. 2007;89(Suppl 1):148-54.
41. Sussman MD. Advantage of early spinal stabilization and fusion in patients with Duchenne muscular dystrophy. J Pediatr Orthop. 1984;4(5):532-7.
42. Weimann RI, Gibson DA, Moseley CF, et al. Surgical stabilization of spine in Duchenne muscular dystrophy. Spine. 1983;8(7):776-80.
43. Hann G, Mubarak S. Muscular dystrophy. In: The Pediatric Spine Principles and Practice, 2nd edition. Philadelphia: Lippincott Williams & Wilkins. 2001. pp. 819-32.
44. Cady RB, Bobechko WP. Incidence, natural history, and treatment of scoliosis in Friedreich's ataxia. J Pediatr Orthop. 1984;4(6):673-6.
45. Daher YH, Lonstein JE, Winter RB, et al. Spinal deformities in patients with Friedrich's ataxia: a review of 19 patients. J Pediatr Orthop. 1985;5(5):553-7.
46. Milbrandt TA, Kunes JR, Karol LA. Friedreich's ataxia and scoliosis: the experience at two institutions. J Pediatr Orthop. 2008;28(2):234-8.
47. Harrison DJ, Webb PJ. Scoliosis in Rett syndrome: Natural history and treatment. Brain Dev. 1990;12(1):154-6.
48. Huang TJ, Lubickey JP, Hammerberg KW. Scoliosis in Rett syndrome. Orthop Rev 1994;23(12):931-7.
49. Keret D, Basset GS, Bunnell WP, et al. Scoliosis in Rett syndrome. J Pediatr Orthop 1988;8(2):138-42.
50. Barnes MJ. Other Neuromuscular deformities. In: The Pediatric Spine Principles and Practice, 2nd edition. Philadelphia: Lippincott Williams & Wilkins; 2001. pp. 881-91.
51. Sarwark JF, MacEwen GD, Scott CL. A multidisciplinary approach to amyoplasia congenita ("classic arthrogryposis"). Orthop Trans. 1986;10:130. [Google Scholar].
52. Daher YH, Lonstein JE, Winter RB, et al. Spinal deformities in patients with arthrogryposis. A review of 16 patients. Spine (Phila Pa 1976). 1985;10(7):609-13.
53. Newton PO, Frances F, Wenger D, et al. Neuromuscular scoliosis. In: Rothman-Simone The Spine, 5th edition. Philadelphia : Saunders Elsevier; 2006. pp. 535-64.
54. Farhat G, Yamout B, Mikati MA, et al. Effect of antiepileptic drugs on bone density in ambulatory patients. Neurology. 2002;58(9):1348-53.
55. Joyce NC, Hache LP, Clemens PR. Bone health and associated metabolic complications in neuromuscular diseases. Phys Med Rehabil Clin N Am. 2012;23(4):773-99.
56. Bohtz C, Meyer-Heim A, Min K. Changes in health-related quality of life after spinal fusion and scoliosis correction in patients with cerebral palsy. J Pediatr Orthop. 2011;31(6):668-73.
57. Watanabe K, Lenke LG, Daubs MD, el al. Is spine deformity surgery in patients with spastic cerebral palsy truly beneficial? a patient/parent evaluation. Spine (Phila Pa 1976). 2009;34(20):2222-32.
58. Mercado E, Alman B, Wright JG. Does spinal fusion influence quality of life in neuromuscular scoliosis? Spine (Phila Pa 1976). 2007;32(19 Suppl):S120-5.
59. Larsson EL, Aaro SI, Normelli HC, et al. Long-term follow-up of functioning after spinal surgery in patients with neuromuscular scoliosis. Spine (Phila Pa 1976). 2005;30(19):2145-52.
60. Larsson EL, Aaro S, Oberg B. Activities and functional assessment 1 year after spinal fusion for paralytic scoliosis. Eur Spine J. 1999;8(2):100-9.
61. Bridwell KH, Baldus C, Iffrig TM, et al. Process measures and patient/parent evaluation of surgical management of spinal deformities in patients with progressive flaccid neuromuscular scoliosis (Duchenne's muscular dystrophy and spinal muscular atrophy). Spine (Phila Pa 1976). 1999;24(13):1300-9.
62. Comstock CP, Leach J, Wenger DR. Scoliosis in total-body-involvement cerebral palsy. Analysis of surgical treatment and patient and caregiver satisfaction. Spine (Phila Pa 1976). 1998;23(12):1412-24.
63. Askin GN, Hallett R, Hare N, et al. The outcome of scoliosis surgery in the severely physically handicapped child. An objective and subjective assessment. Spine (Phila Pa 1976). 1997;22(1):44-50.
64. Tsirikos AI, Smith G. Scoliosis in patients with Friedreich's ataxia. J Bone Joint Surg Br. 2012;94(5):684-9.
65. Pruijs JE, van Tol MJ, van KesterenRG, et al. Neuromuscular scoliosis: Clinical evaluation pre- and postoperative. J Pediatr Orthop B. 2000;9(4):217-20.
66. Chambers HG, Weinstein CH, Mubarak SJ, et al. The effect of valproic acid on blood loss in patients with cerebral palsy. J Pediatr Orthop. 1999;19(6):792-5.
67. Thompson GH, Florentino-Pineda I, Poe-Kochert C, et al. Role of Amicar in surgery for neuromuscular scoliosis. Spine (Phila Pa 1976). 2008;33(24):2623-9.
68. Kasimian S, Skaggs DL, Sankar WN, et al. Aprotinin in pediatric neuromuscular scoliosis surgery. Eur Spine J. 2008;17(12):1671-5.
69. Jevsevar DS, Karlin LI. The relationship between preoperative nutritional status and complications after an operation for scoliosis in patients who have cerebral palsy. J Bone Joint Surg Am. 1993;75(6):880-4.
70. Lonstein JE. Spinal deformities due to cerebral palsy. In: The Pediatric Spine Principles and Practice, 2nd edition. Philadelphia: Lippincott Williams & Wilkins; 2001. pp. 797-807.
71. McMaster MJ. Anterior and posterior instrumentation and fusion of thoracolumbar scoliosis due to myelomeningocele. J Bone Joint Surg Br. 1987;69(1):20-5.
72. Daher YH, Lonstein JE, Winter RB, et al. Spinal surgery in spinal muscular atrophy. J Pediatr Orthop. 1985;5(4):391-5.

CHAPTER 13

73. Labelle H, Tohmé S, Duhaime M, et al. Natural history of scoliosis in Friedreich's ataxia. J Bone Joint Surg Am. 1986;68(4):564-72.
74. Lindseth RE. Myelomeningocele spine. In: The Pediatric Spine Principles and Practice, 2nd edition. Philadelphia: Lippincott Williams & Wilkins; 2001. pp. 845-68.
75. Shapiro F, Bresnan MJ. Orthopaedic management of childhood neuromuscular disease. Part I: spinal muscular atrophy. J Bone Joint Surg Am. 1982;64(5):785-9.
76. Sullivan JA, Conner SB. Comparison of Harrington instrumentation and segmental spinal instrumentation in the management of neuromuscular spinal deformity. Spine (Phila Pa 1976). 1982;7(3):299-304.
77. Lonstein JE, Akbarnia A. Operative treatment of spinal deformities in patients with cerebral palsy or mental retardation. An analysis of one hundred and seven cases. J Bone Joint Surg Am. 1983;65(1):43-55.
78. Luque ER. Segmental spinal instrumentation for correction of scoliosis. Clin Orthop Relat Res. 1982;(163):192-8.
79. Taddonio RF. Segmental spinal instrumentation in the management of neuromuscular spinal deformity. Spine (Phila Pa 1976). 1982;7(3):305-11.
80. Allen BL Jr, Ferguson RL. The Galveston technique for L rod instrumentation of the scoliotic spine. Spine (Phila Pa 1976). 1982;7(3):276-84.
81. Allen BL Jr, Ferguson RL. L-rod instrumentation for scoliosis in cerebral palsy. J Pediatr Orthop. 1982;2(1):87-96.
82. Bell DF, Moseley CF, Koreska J. Unit rod segmental spinal instrumentation in the management of patients with progressive neuromuscular spinal deformity. Spine (Phila Pa 1976). 1989;14(12):1301-7.
83. Dias RC, Miller F, Dabney K, et al. Surgical correction of spinal deformity using a unit rod in children with cerebral palsy. J Pediatr Orthop. 1996;16(6):734-40.
84. Piazzolla A, Solarino G, De Giorgi S, et al. Cotrel-Dubousset instrumentation in neuromuscular scoliosis. Eur Spine J. 2011;20 Suppl 1:S75-84.
85. Modi HN, Hong JY, Mehta SS, et al. Surgical correction and fusion using posterior-only pedicle screw construct for neuropathic scoliosis in patients with cerebral palsy: a three-year follow-up study. Spine (Phila Pa 1976). 2009;34(11):1167-75.
86. Whitaker C, Burton DC, Asher M. Treatment of selected neuromuscular patients with posterior instrumentation and arthrodesis ending with lumbar pedicle screw anchorage. Spine (Phila Pa 1976). 2000;25(18):2312-8.
87. Jones-Quaidoo SM, Yang S, Arlet V. Surgical management of spinal deformities in cerebral palsy. A review. J Neurosurg Spine. 2010;13(6):672-85.
88. Li Z, Zhu J, Liu X. Deformity of lumbar spine after selective dorsal rhizotomy for spastic cerebral palsy. Microsurgery. 2008;v28(1):10-2.
89. La Rosa G, Giglio G, Oggiano L. Surgical treatment of neurological scoliosis using hybrid construct (lumbar transpedicular screws plus thoracic sublaminar acrylic loops). Eur Spine J. 2011;20(Suppl 1):S90-4.
90. Boachie-Adjei O, Lonstein JE, Winter RB, et al. Management of neuromuscular spinal deformities with Luque segmental instrumentation. J Bone Joint Surg Am. 1989;71(4):548-62.
91. Broom MJ, Banta JV, Renshaw TS. Spinal fusion augmented by Luque-rod segmental instrumentation for neuromuscular scoliosis. J Bone Joint Surg Am. 1989;71(1):32-44.
92. Ferguson R, Allen B Jr. Considerations in the treatment of cerebral palsy patients with spinal deformities. Orthop Clinics North Am. 1988;19(2):419-25.
93. Lonstein JE. The Galveston technique using Luque or Cotrel-Dubousset rods. Orthop Clin North Am. 1994;25 (2):311-20.
94. Maloney W, Rinsky LA, Gamble JG. Simultaneous correction of pelvic obliquity, frontal plane, and sagittal plane deformities in neuromuscular scoliosis using a unit rod with segmental sublaminar wires. J Pediatr Orthop. 1990;10(6):742-9.
95. Majd ME, Muldowny DS, Holt RT. Natural history of scoliosis in the institutionalized adult cerebral palsy population. Spine (Phila Pa 1976). 1997;22(13):1461-6.
96. Auerbach JD, Spiegel DA, Zgonis MH, et al. The correction of pelvic obliquity in patients with cerebral palsy and neuromuscular scoliosis: is there a benefit of anterior release prior to posterior spinal arthrodesis? Spine (Phila Pa 1976). 2009;34(21):E766-74.
97. Sussman M. Is fusion to the sacrum necessary in patients with progressive flaccid neuromuscular disease? Orthop Trans. 1987;11:123-4.
98. Sussman MD, Little D, Alley RM, et al. Posterior instrumentation and fusion of the thoracolumbar spine for treatment of neuromuscular scoliosis. J Pediatr Orthop. 1996;16(3):304-13.
99. Mubarak SJ, Morin WD, Leach J. Spinal fusion in Duchenne muscular dystrophy: fixation and fusion to the sacropelvis? J Pediatr Orthop. 1993;13(6):752-7.
100. Sengupta DK, Mehdian SH, McConnell JR, et al. Pelvic or lumbar fixation for the surgical management of scoliosis in Duchenne muscular dystrophy. Spine (Phila Pa 1976). 2002;27(18):2072-9.
101. Swank SM, Cohen DS, Brown JC. Spine fusion in cerebral palsy with L-rod segmental spinal instrumentation. A comparison of single and two-stage combined approach with Zielke instrumentation. Spine (Phila Pa 1976). 1989;14(7):750-9.
102. Tsirikos AI, Chang WN, Shah SA, et al. Preserving ambulatory potential in pediatric patients with cerebral palsy who undergo spinal fusion using unit rod instrumentation. Spine (Phila Pa 1976). 2003;28(5):480-3.
103. Banta JV. Combined anterior and posterior fusion for spinal deformity in myelomeningocele. Spine 1990;15(9):946-52.
104. Ward WT, Wenger DR, Roach JW. Surgical correction of Myelomeningocele scoliosis: A critical appraisal of various spinal instrumentation systems. J Pediatr Orthop. 1989;9(3):262-8.

105. Parsch D, Geiger F, Brocai DR, et al. Surgical management of paralytic scoliosis in myelomeningocele. J Pediatr Orthop B. 2001;10(1):10-7.

106. Banit DM, Iwinski HJ, Talwalkar V, et al. Posterior spinal fusion in paralytic scoliosis and myelomeningocele. J Pediatr Orthop. 2001;21(1):117-25.

107. Sponseller PD, Young AT, Sarwark JF, et al. Anterior only fusion for scoliosis in patients with myelomeningocele. Clin Orthop Relat Res. 1999;(364):117-24.

108. Stella G, Ascani E, Cervellati S, et al. Surgical treatment of scoliosis associated with myelomeningocele. Eur J Pediatr Surg. 1998;8(Suppl 1):22-5.

109. Keeler KA, Lenke LG, Good CR, et al. Spinal fusion for spastic neuromuscular scoliosis: is anterior releasing necessary when intraoperative halo-femoral traction is used? Spine (Phila Pa 1976). 2010;35(10):E427-33.

110. Benson ER, Thomson JD, Smith BG, et al. Results and morbidity in a consecutive series of patients undergoing spinal fusion for neuromuscular scoliosis. Spine (Phila Pa 1976). 1998;23(21):2308-17.

111. Lonstein JE, Koop SE, Novachek TF, et al. Results and complications after spinal fusion for neuromuscular scoliosis in cerebral palsy and static encephalopathy using luque galveston instrumentation: experience in 93 patients. Spine (Phila Pa 1976). 2012;37(7):583-91.

112. Mohamad F, Parent S, Pawelek J, et al. Perioperative complications after surgical correction in neuromuscular scoliosis. J Pediatr Orthop. 2007;27(4):392-7.

113. Szöke G, Lipton G, Miller F, et al. Wound infection after spinal fusion in children with cerebral palsy. J Pediatr Orthop. 1998;18(6):727-33.

114. Master DL, Connie PK, Son-Hing J, et al. Wound infections after surgery for neuromuscular scoliosis: risk factors and treatment outcomes. Spine (Phila Pa 1976). 2011;36(3):E179-85.

CHAPTER 14

Juvenile Kyphosis (Scheuermann's Disease)

Luiz Roberto Vialle, Emiliano Vialle, Orlando Colina

DEFINITION AND HISTORICAL BACKGROUND

Scheuermann's disease (SD) is a thoracic or thoracolumbar hyperkyphosis secondary to wedging of the vertebral body during growth. Its true incidence is unknown, ranging from 1% to 8% of the population and being more common in males (ratio varies up to 7/1). One-third of the patients may also present with a mild scoliosis.[1,2]

Although previous descriptions of thoracic and thoracolumbar kyphosis are known, credit is given to Holger Werfel Scheuermann, a Danish physician who in 1920 differentiated the rigid juvenile kyphosis from the flexible postural kyphosis, and identified the wedging of the vertebrae as the cause of deformity. He was the first to describe such radiographic characteristics, naming it "*osteochondritis deformans juvenilis dorsi*", in an attempt to associate it with the femoral head osteochondritis described by Calvé and Perthes.[3]

ETIOLOGY

Scheuermann's classic description of the deformity suggested an avascular necrosis of the vertebral endplates leading to vertebral wedging. The exact etiology is unknown, and most authors agree that it is probably multifactorial.

A genetic autosomal dominant pattern of inheritance has been described by some authors. Halal described five families in which the disease seems to follow an autosomal dominant pattern of inheritance. Findlay reported a family in which Scheuermann's juvenile kyphosis was present in three successive generations with male-to-male transmission.[4,5] Recently, Damborg reported the heritability of SD to be 0.74, in a study using the Danish Twin Registry.[6] This study emphasizes the importance of genetics over environmental factors on SD.

An error in collagen aggregation has also been described by Aufdermaur, leading to changes on the ossification process of the endplates.[7] Other authors have detailed the histologic changes of both cartilage and vertebral endplates as mosaic-like, with reduced amount of collagen and increased proteoglycan content. This would then lead to an early growth arrest in affected areas, and acceleration in the normal ones, resulting in the wedge-shaped vertebrae and increased kyphosis.[8] Box 1 summarizes the most common theories on the etiology of SD.

The source of pain, during such process, would be secondary to postural changes and insufficient musculature to compensate for the increasing kyphosis. Cervical and lumbar regions would tend to extend in an effort to compensate the posture, also causing pain. In adults, this can lead to disk degeneration and facet arthritis, both in the kyphotic segment and in the compensating regions.

DIAGNOSIS AND CLASSIFICATION OF SCHEUERMANN'S DISEASE

The definition of normal thoracic kyphosis varies in the literature from 10° to 50°, being more prominent in males,

Box 1: List of most common etiologies for Scheuermann's disease.

- Osteochondritis, epiphysitis
- Genetic autosomic trait
- Collagen defect
- Defective endplates
- Juvenile osteoporosis
- Hormonal abnormality (growth hormone)
- Strenuous manual labor
- Vitamin A deficiency
- Poliomyelitis
- Prolonged sitting

and increasing from adolescence until adulthood, where a natural progression of kyphosis is seen due to degenerative changes. Due to the wide range on the definition of thoracic kyphosis, it should always be evaluated with the entire spine for a valid comprehension of the sagittal alignment. The thoracolumbar junction (from T10 to L2), another area of interest of SD, can measure from 3° of lordosis to 20° of kyphosis.[9] The two most used definitions of SD were established by Sorensen[10] (1964) and by Bradford[11] (1977). Sorensen's criteria for diagnosis of SD are wedging of more than 5° in three consecutive vertebrae, with typical endplate irregularities on a lateral radiograph.

Bradford's criteria include:

- Irregular vertebral endplates
- Narrowing of the intervertebral disk space
- Wedging of 5° or more in one or more vertebrae
- An increase of normal kyphosis beyond 40°.

Many have criticized both criteria for being too arbitrary. For example, by Sorensen's criteria any kyphosis with less than three deformed vertebrae would be excluded, and by Bradford criteria, the threshold for kyphosis (40°) is not supported by sound data, having in mind the great variability of thoracic kyphosis in the general population. Schlenzka and Arlet tried to be more inclusive with the following diagnostic criteria for thoracic juvenile kyphosis (or Type I kyphosis):[12]

- Wedging of more than 5° in one or more vertebrae in the thoracic or thoracolumbar region
- Endplate irregularities
- Disk space narrowing
- Increased thoracic or thoracolumbar kyphosis.

Although SD is typically a thoracic problem, several authors have reported on a lumbar presentation of adolescent kyphosis, starting with Lindemann,[13] and followed by Edgren and Vaino,[14] who have defined the characteristics of endplate changes during the growth period as well as its appearance after the end of growth. The lumbar, or type II kyphosis, would then be defined by three obligatory criteria, and three facultative criteria:

Obligatory criteria:

1. Endplate irregularities in one or more vertebral bodies of the thoracolumbar or lumbar segment
2. Increased sagittal diameter of vertebral bodies
3. Disk space narrowing.

Facultative criteria:

1. Apophyseal separation
2. Loss of lumbar lordosis or lumbar kyphosis
3. Schmorl's nodes.

Other authors, such as Blumenthal,[15] Wenger,[1] and Murray,[16] have tried to further divide and differentiate thoracic and lumbar kyphosis, with small variations on the description mentioned above:

- Blumenthal subdivided the lumbar form in type I (three or more wedged vertebrae); type IIa (atypical form, with endplate irregularities, Schmorl's nodes and disk space narrowing); and type IIb (acute traumatic intraosseous disk herniation).
- Wenger divided SD in type I (thoracic) and type II (thoracolumbar), where the second type would develop at a later age and be more painful, due to mechanical overloading.
- Murray classified SD according to their apex, with a cephalic type (apex from T1–T8) and caudal type (apex at T9–T12).

One must assume that these are variations on the same subject, and that such distinct determinations do not change the principles of management of SD.

CLINICAL FINDINGS AND DIFFERENTIAL DIAGNOSIS

The clinical presentation of SD is secondary to back pain and cosmetic disturbance. In the adolescence, it is usually noticed by a relative or caretaker, as an abnormal posture during exercise or sitting. In the adult, pain becomes the chief complaint, followed by cosmesis.

Although more frequent in the lumbar form of SD, pain seems to be more intense and limit daily activities in curve with a more proximal apex and a more severe angulation.[16] There is also some suggestion that patients with lumbar SD have a tendency to develop lumbar stenosis.[17]

Physical examination is typical, with hyperkyphosis and compensatory hyperlordosis of the cervical and lumbar spine. There is usually nice coronal balance, and a negative sagittal balance. Such negative balance has a tendency not to change over time, even after treatment.[18]

The examination allows the physician to evaluate the rigidity of the curve, both by forward bending, or by having the patient prone and asking him to lift his head and extend the spine. This allows for differential diagnosis with postural kyphosis, where the curve is harmonic during

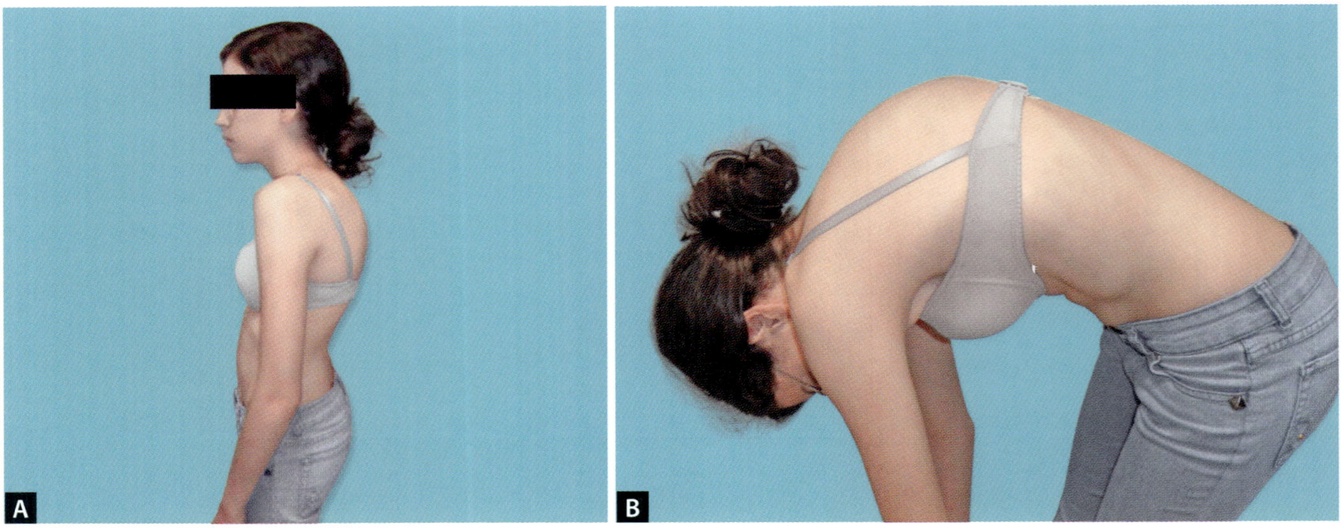

Figs. 1A and B: (A) Lateral aspect of a Scheuermann's patient with an 80° curve; (B) Angular kyphosis during forward bending.

forward bending, and correct with extension in prone position[19] (Figs. 1A and B).

If the patient complains of low back pain, investigation should also be directed toward the lumbosacral junction, as there is an increased incidence of spondylolysis and spondylolisthesis, with some studies showing lysis in up to 50% of SD cases. The hypothesis for that is the increased stress on the pars interarticularis secondary to compensatory hyperlordosis.[20]

Muscle examination might reveal tenderness above and below the deformity, and hamstring and pectoral tightness being common findings. Although most patients will have no neurology, this step of the examination is crucial for the differential diagnosis of SD with other, less frequent, forms of kyphosis (Table 1). Spinal cord compression has been described in SD in curves with severe angulation, due to herniated disks and dural cysts.[21-23]

IMAGING

Conventional radiographs give enough information for confirming the diagnosis and planning patient's treatment. MRI helps in differential diagnosis, and can also show the endplate and disk abnormalities in a detailed manner (Figs. 2A and B)

Plain lateral panoramic radiographs of the entire spine allow measurements of both the thoracic kyphosis and the compensatory lordosis (Fig. 3A).

Table 1: Main differential diagnosis of Scheuermann's disease.

Idiopathic thoracic hyperkyphosis	
Neuromuscular	Skeletal dysplasia
Spinal cord tumor	Infection
Postlaminectomy kyphosis	Tumor
Post-traumatic kyphosis	
Connective tissue disorders	
Congenital kyphosis	

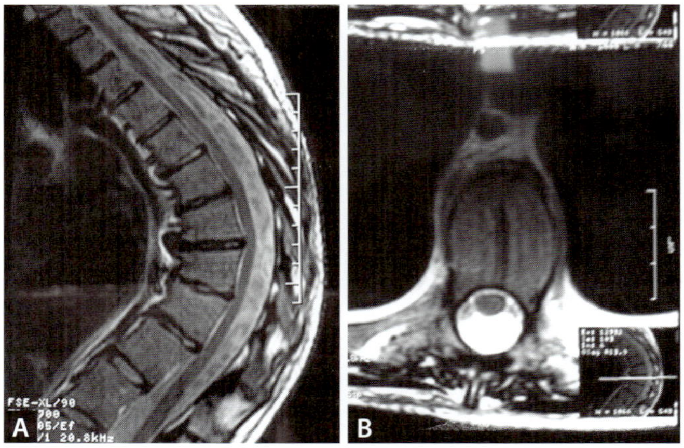

Figs. 2A and B: MR imaging characteristics of Scheuermann's disease.

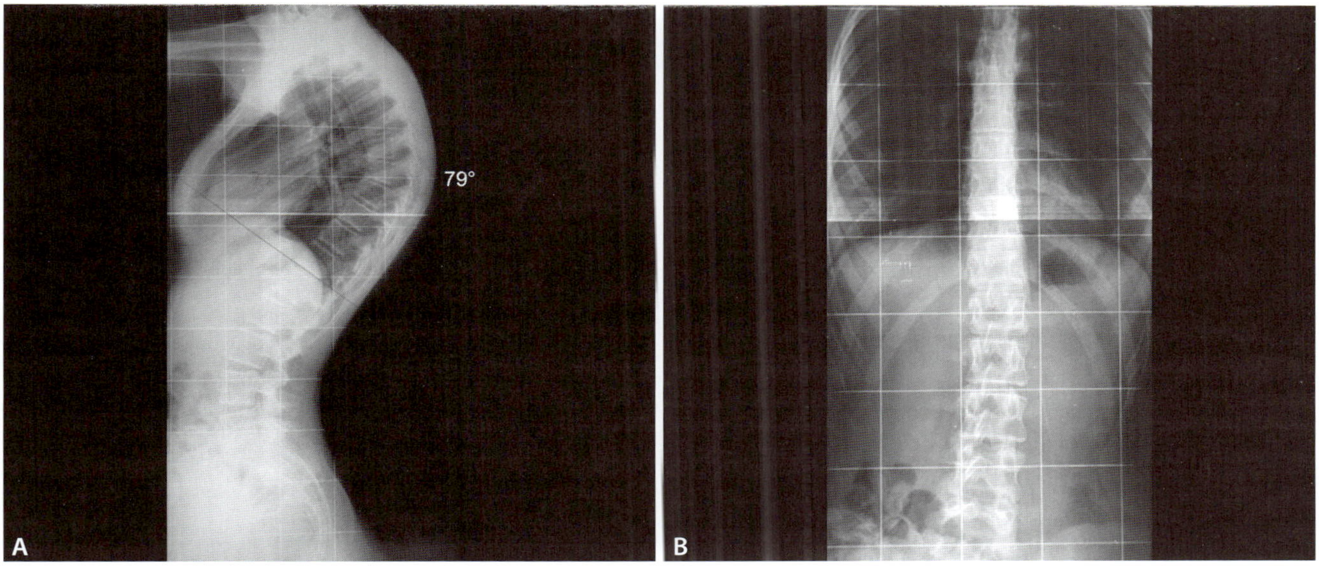

Figs. 3A and B: (A) Typical appearance of Scheuermann's thoracic kyphosis with a compensatory hyperlordosis; (B) Anteroposterior imaging showing secondary scoliosis, commonly associated with Scheuermann's disease.

Anteroposterior radiographs allow for evaluation of secondary scoliosis (Fig. 3B), and an extension film with the patient on supine position with a sandbag under the apex of the deformity evaluates the flexibility of the curve.

Measurement of the deformity is performed using the Cobb method, usually from T5 to T12, and must include lumbar lordosis and transitional curves (upper thoracic and thoracolumbar zones), all fundamental on treatment planning.

Although MRI has no diagnostic purpose, and the possibility to have a better view of the endplate and disk changes, its main use is to determine spinal cord compression at the apex of the deformity in severe curves and in patients with neurologic symptoms. The authors do not use MRI routinely for patients with normal neurologic examination and during conservative treatment, but due to the magnitude of the correction achieved with modern instrumentation, preoperative MRI has become part of the preoperative routine.

TREATMENT

Although the natural history of SD is benign, with nonlimiting pain and normal cardiopulmonary function on those cases that do not exceed 100° of kyphosis, it can bring significant back pain, physical embarrassment, and interference with social activities.[16]

It has been shown that curves above 45° progress during growth, and continue to increase through adulthood.[24]

In cases above 70°, the cosmetic impairment becomes significant, as well as the clinical symptoms, and although there is no significant data on the progression of the deformity, some worsening is expected during adulthood, partially because of natural history of thoracic kyphosis, partially due to progressive loss of compensation mechanisms for the sagittal imbalance (meaning lumbar lordosis and pelvic tilt).

Such natural history seems to be less favorable in the lumbar type of SD, where more pain and progression might be expected with follow-up.[25]

The general objectives of treatment include:
- Prevention of progression
- Pain relief
- Deformity correction
- Cosmetic improvement.

The choice of treatment varies according to patient's age, severity of the kyphosis, and patient's symptoms and expectations.

Conservative Treatment

The initial option for most patients is nonoperative treatment, which includes physical therapy and the use of orthesis. Some authors advocate conservative management of the curves, with satisfactory results, in patients with confirmed radiologic diagnosis of SD, flexible curves, and remaining growth potential.

The authors usually offer a program of back exercises and muscle contractures stretching for adolescents with curves below 60° and adults with mild symptoms. For those skeletally immature, and with curves above 60°, bracing is considered. The authors use a lateral hyperextension X-ray to access the flexibility of the curve, and if it is rigid and no correction is seen, then bracing is unlikely to be effective. Some authors have stated that a 40% correction is needed for bracing to be effective.[26] Contrary to scoliosis bracing, in SD the goal is to obtain correction through reduction of vertebral wedging by means of bone remodeling. As the apex of the kyphosis is usually cranial to T8, the Milwaukee brace is preferred over a thoracolumbosacral orthosis (TLSO).

Bradford has reported on the factors that influenced negatively the correction of SD:

- Kyphosis greater than 65°
- Skeletal maturity
- Vertebral wedging above 10°.[27,28]

After longer follow-up, the same group of authors has shown that bracing can be effective in curves up to 74°. Results have shown a 50% correction of the deformity during the bracing, with some loss of correction over time.[28] Other studies have compared the Milwaukee to the Boston brace, showing better correction with the Milwaukee, but a significant lower compliance with brace wearing with its use. Gutowski has also shown that the use of brace for 16 hours had the same results to 23 hours of use, and the Boston brace provided adequate correction for curves up to 70°, and reserved the Milwaukee brace for curves of larger magnitude.[29]

Duration of treatment has various ranges, but the authors follow and adapt the rule of the "four 6's" described by Crawford.[26] They advocated 6 weeks of hyperextension cast, Milwaukee brace for 6 months, gradual removal of the brace for 6 weeks, and finally sleeping in the brace for 6 months. The authors have removed the hyperextension cast on their protocol, and emphasized physical therapy and extension exercises in their treatment plan, without significant loss of correction on their patients.

Surgical Treatment

The benign natural history of SD, the importance of cosmesis and functional impairment must be weighed against the risks and magnitude of surgical management, and be individualized to each patient's needs and expectations.

General surgical indications would include:

- Progressive thoracic kyphosis greater than 75° in the skeletally immature
- Thoracolumbar kyphosis above 50°, usually associated with pain despite conservative management
- Failure of conservative treatment to arrest deformity progression
- Cosmetic deformity that is unacceptable to the patient and his family
- Sharp and angular deformity
- Pulmonary compromise (rare, unless curve greater than 100°)
- Neurologic deficit (usually due to associated conditions, such as a disk herniation or dural cysts).

Before surgery, preoperative assessment of the patient should include a thorough neurological examination, MR imaging, lung functional tests (for curves above 90°) and an evaluation of muscle tightness, especially the hamstrings. Hosman has shown that patients with tight hamstrings had little lumbar adaptation capacity, leading to significant worsening of the negative sagittal balance and increased risk of junctional kyphosis after surgery.[30]

Surgery for SD can be performed by means of posterior, anterior, or combined approaches.

The early results of surgical treatment by means of posterior approach only, using Harington instrumentation, yielded a high rate of nonunion, hardware complications and loss of correction, and led to the addition of anterior release followed by posterior fusion as the standard of care for many years.[18,31-33]

The anterior release can be performed by means of open or thoracoscopic procedures. Although the authors have experience with the thoracoscopic release, their current preference is to use a minimally invasive, open procedure, releasing from 6 to 8 disks adjacent to the apex of the deformity. The anterior longitudinal ligament and the disk are completely removed, and the disk space is packed with bone auto or allograft. Although allowing for better correction, anterior approach is not without consequences, and its limitations involve the extra time and cost of an additional procedure, a potential reduction in pulmonary capacity, hemothorax, pneumothorax, and pulmonary embolism.

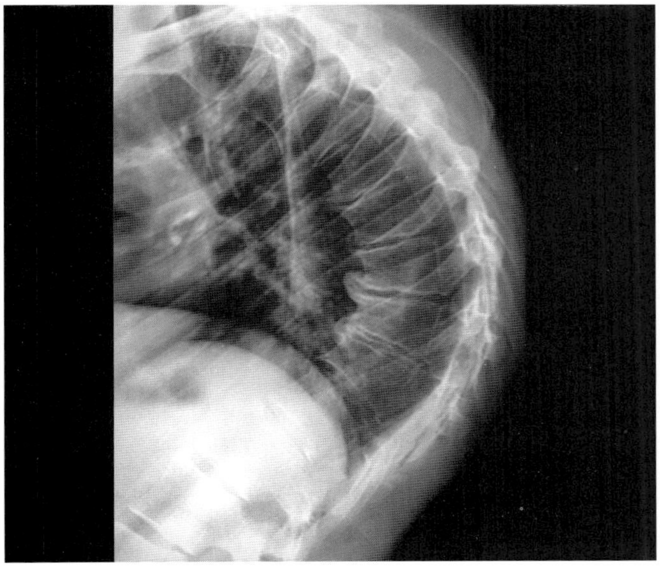

Fig. 4: Osteophytes at the apex of the deformity may limit the correction of posterior only surgery.

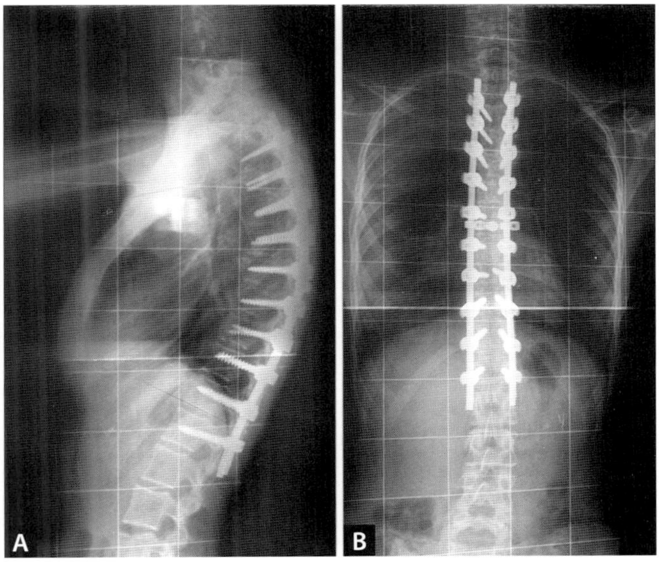

Figs. 5A and B: Multilevel pedicle screw instrumentation for posterior only correction of Scheuermann's disease. (A) Lateral image; (B) Anteroposterior image.

Our current indications for anterior release include curves above 90° and the presence of osteophytes at the apex, in which a posterior approach with pedicle screw instrumentation and osteotomies would not achieve sufficient correction (Fig. 4).

The advent of multilevel pedicle screw instrumentation and multilevel posterior column shortening osteotomies (known as Ponte osteotomies) has largely increased the capabilities of posterior correction, obviating the need for anterior approach, even in severe and rigid deformities (Figs. 5A and B).[34-36]

Surgical Strategy

Surgical correction must be carefully planned in order to avoid overcorrection, neurological complications, and junctional (both proximal and distal) kyphosis. Correction should aim the upper normal range of kyphosis, between 40° and 50°. With modern instrumentation, some curves can easily be overcorrected, increasing the risks of the abovementioned complications.[18]

The proximal extent of fusion has been subject of debate, with some advocating the end vertebra of the deformity, and others suggesting the inclusion of the first lordotic vertebra above the deformity, for reducing the risks of junctional kyphosis. This would require imaging of the cervicothoracic junction for a better understanding of the compensation mechanisms. Winter has advocated that besides level selection, preserving the cranial ligament structure and facets is critical for avoiding postoperative decompensation and the postoperative "goose neck" posture. He also postulated that some deformities extend further up and some patients might need fixation up to C7 or T1 for avoiding decompensation.[37]

The distal point of fixation has traditionally been the vertebra below the first lordotic disk in the lumbar area, usually L1 or L2.[18,38] This has clearly not solved the problem of distal junctional kyphosis, leading to the suggestion that two lordotic disks should be included in the fusion area.[39] Lenke et al. have brought some light to the subject as they have coined the sagittal stable vertebra concept, in which the last vertebra of the fixation should be the most proximal vertebra touched by a line drawn vertically from the posterior superior corner of the sacrum on the lateral radiographs. They have shown that this method significantly reduced the distal complications, in comparison to the traditional inclusion of the first lordotic disk.[40]

The author's strategy follows the outlined steps:

1. Curve correction planning, to 40–50°, or 50% correction for curves above 90°
2. Definition of the need for an anterior release, in curves above 90° and with osteophytes at the apex of deformity. If necessary, the authors perform complete disk removal and anterior longitudinal

ligament release at four to six levels at the apex of the deformity, using a minimally invasive open left-sided approach
3. Defining the upper instrumented level to the first vertebra above the end vertebra
4. Defining the caudal instrumented level using the sagittal stable vertebra
5. *Pedicle screw planning*: Bilateral pedicle screws at the three cranial and caudal vertebrae, followed by unilateral pedicle screws on the remaining vertebrae, switching sides at each level (Figs. 6A and B)
6. Three levels of Ponte osteotomies above and below the apex of the curve (a total of six osteotomies)
7. Patient positioning in an extension frame
8. Normovolemic hemodilution, immediately prior to the procedure, usually not needing additional blood transfusion or the use of a cell saver
9. Neurophysiologic monitoring
10. Gradual correction with previously bent rods to the desired residual kyphosis
11. Decortication, auto/allograft of the instrumented area
12. Vancomycin powder (1 g) over the surgically exposed area
13. Closure by layers with subfascial drainage for 24 hours.

Complication Avoidance and Management

The most feared complication is neurologic deficit. The Scoliosis Research Society has determined the risk of neurologic injury during SD surgery to be 1 per 700 cases.[41] Causes include direct trauma during surgery, stretch to the spinal cord during correction, and vascular injury, either by disruption of blood supply or due to hypotension. Abnormalities of the spinal canal can also be involved, and preoperative MRI should rule out spinal canal stenosis, dural cysts and syringomyelia, especially in severe curves. The best way to prevent neurologic injury is to be aware of such risks, using careful surgical technique, adequate control of blood pressure, and moderate correction of the curve under neurophysiological monitoring.

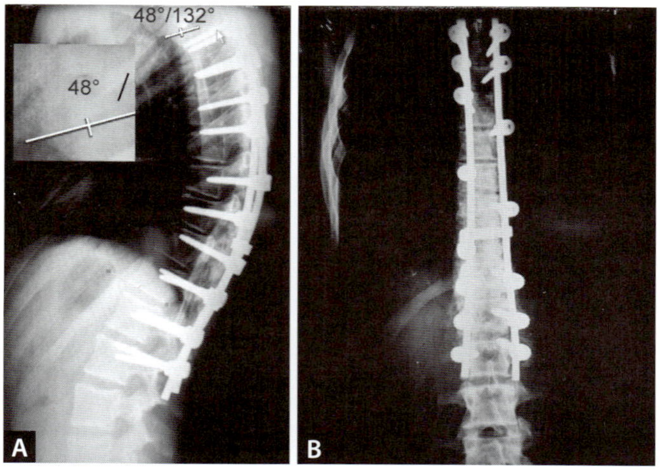

Figs. 6A and B: Representation of the author's surgical strategy for Scheuermann's disease.

Junctional kyphosis has been defined as a kyphosis above 10° between the first uninstrumented vertebra and the last instrumented vertebra, both cranially and caudally. As some cases might be asymptomatic, radiographic awareness during follow-up is required for early identification and management. Management, with extension of the instrumented area, is usually only needed if the patient is symptomatic or cosmesis is severely affected, Lonner has found this problem to be clinically relevant in about 5% of the patients operated for SD. In the same study, the authors pointed out that the main cause of junctional kyphosis was either over-correction, or inadequate (short) determination of the fusion levels.[42]

Nonunion may also be a problem, as in any long fusion. The authors attribute the reduction of their nonunion rate on SD to not using instrumentation at all levels, thus allowing more area for the graft and fusion mass.

CONCLUSION AND FINAL REMARKS

- Although the natural history of SD is benign, untreated patients suffer from significant back pain and cosmetic issues through their lives.
- Conservative treatment yields good results for patients with flexible curves and growth potential.
- Surgical treatment should be carefully discussed with the patient and his family, and surgical planning is the key for a successful outcome.
- A summary of the current literature is presented on Table 2.

TOP 6 ARTICLES

1. *Hosman et al. Spine; 2003*: In this retrospective case series, the authors emphasized the importance of identifying patients with tight hamstrings (popliteal

Table 2: Level-of-evidence summary table for Scheuermann's kyphosis.

Author, journal, year	*Design*	*LoE*	*Topic*	*F/U*	*Measures*	*Main results*
Blumenthal, Spine, 1987	R	IV	Lumbar Scheuermann's kyphosis	N/A	Radiographic characteristics	One of the few studies to address lumbar variant of SK, proposal for a classification
Murray, JBJS-A, 1993	R	IV	Natural history of SK	32 years	Quality of life, pulmonary function	Few differences in quality of life Pulmonary function reduced in curves >100°
Lowe, Spine, 1994	R	IV	Spinal balance and reasons for postoperative decompensation	2 years	Radiographic measurements	Overcorrection was the main cause of junctional kyphosis proximally, and instrumentation above the first lordotic vertebrae distally
Bradford, JBJS-A, 1974	R	IV	Brace treatment for SK		Radiographic measurements	Determined the ideal indications for brace treatment for SK
Sachs, JBJS-A, 1987	R	IV	Brace treatment for SK	5 years	Radiographic measurements	Longest follow-up on conservative treatment of SK
Hosman, Spine, 2003	R	III	Influence of tight hamstrings of the management of SK		Radiographic measurements	Patients with tight hamstrings are prone to overcorrection and decompensation
Geck, JSDT, 2007	R	IV	Surgical treatment of SK		Radiographic measurements	Describes in detail the advantages of the posterior procedure known as the Ponte osteotomy
Lee, Spine, 2006	R	III	Comparison of posterior only versus circumferential surgery			Showed the superiority of posterior only surgery for SK
Hosman, Spine, 2002	R	IV	Comparison of posterior only versus circumferential surgery	4.5 years	Radiographic measures Oswestry scores Satisfaction rates	Minimizes the need for anterior release in SK
Denis, Spine, 2009	R	IV	Identification of risk factors for junctional kyphosis	Minimum 5 years	Clinical and radiographic data	Defines the causes of junctional kyphosis and gives surgical recommendations
Poolman, ESJ, 2002	PC	III	Prospective evaluation of surgical treatment for SK	75 months	Clinical and radiographic data	No correlation between clinical and radiographic data
Cho, Spine, 2009	R	IV	Distal fusion level for SK	2 years	Radiographic data	Defines the sagittal stable vertebra concept
Lonner, Spine, 2007	R	IV	Identification of risk factors for junctional kyphosis	2 years	Radiographic data	Defines risk factors for proximal junctional kyphosis

(F/U: follow-up; LoE: level of evidence; PC: prospective cohort; RCT: randomized controlled trial; R: retrospective; SK: Scheuermann's kyphosis)

CHAPTER 14

angle >30°). Patients with tight hamstrings were considered as lumbar compensators, and were prone to overcorrection and postsurgical imbalance.

2. *Hosman et al. Spine; 2002*: A cohort of 33 patients was reviewed for comparing anteroposterior (n = 17) and posterior (n = 16) techniques, showing no difference after 4.5 years follow-up. The authors also recommend limiting correction to the upper limits of normal kyphosis (40–50°), minimizing the need for anterior release.
3. *Murray et al. JBJS-Am; 1993*: This study on the natural history of SD with 32 years of follow-up showed worse quality of life and more physical limitation, in comparison with a control group matched for age and sex.
4. *Poolman et al. Eur Spine J; 2002*: One of the few prospective studies on the surgical treatment of SD questioned the indications of surgical treatment on curves below 75°, due to late loss of correction at the final follow-up. Patients who had loss of correction did not seem to have worse clinical outcome.
5. *Cho et al. Spine; 1999*: The authors define the concept of sagittal stable vertebra, changing the concept of distal instrumentation for SD.
6. *Geck et al. JSDT; 2007*: This paper describes the posterior shortening osteotomy for the thoracic spine, known as the Ponte procedure, which has expanded the corrective possibilities of the posterior approach for SD.

REFERENCES

1. Wenger DR, Frick SL. Scheuermann kyphosis. Spine. 1999;24(24):2630-9.
2. Scholes P, Latimer B, Diglovanni B, et al. Vertebral alterations in Scheuermann's kyphosis. Spine. 1991;16(5):509-15.
3. Scheuermann HW. The classic: kyphosis dorsalis juvenilis. Clin Orthop Relat Res. 1977;(128):5-7.
4. Halal F, Gledhill RB, Fraser C. Dominant inheritance of Scheuermann's juvenile kyphosis. Am J Dis Child. 1978; 132(11):1105-7.
5. Findlay A, Conner AN, Connor JM. Dominant inheritance of Scheuermann's juvenile kyphosis. J Med Genet. 1989; 26(6):400-3.
6. Damborg F, Engell V, Nielsen J, et al. Genetic epidemiology of Scheuermann's disease. Acta Orthop. 2011;82(5):602-5.
7. Aufdermaur M, Spycher M. Pathogenesis of osteochondrosis juvenilis Scheuermann. J Orthop Res. 1986;4(4):452-7.
8. Ippolito E, Ponseti IV. Juvenile kyphosis: histological and histochemical studies. J Bone Joint Surg Am. 1981;63(2):175-82.
9. Vialle E, Vialle LR. Postura e equlíbrio sagital do adolescente. Clínica Ortopédica. 2005;6(1):45-8.
10. Sorensen K. Scheuermann's Juvenile Kyphosis: Clinical Appearances, Radiography, Aetiology, and Prognosis. Copenhagen: Enjar Munksgaard Forlag; 1964.
11. Bradford DS. Juvenile kyphosis. Clin Orthop Relat Res. 1977; 128:45-55.
12. Arlet V, Schlenzka D. Juvenile Kyphosis (Scheuermann's Disease). In: Aebi M, Boos N (Eds). Spinal Disorders. Berlin Heidelberg: Springer-Verlag; 2008. pp. 765-96.
13. Lindemann K. Die Lumbale Kyphose im Adoleszentenalter. Z Orthop. 1933;58:54-65.
14. Edgren W, Vainio S. Osteochondrosis juvenilis lumbalis. Acta Chir Scand Suppl. 1957;227:3-47.
15. Blumenthal S, Roach J, Herring J. Lumbar Scheuermann's. A clinical series and classification. Spine. 1987;9:929-32.
16. Murray PM, Weinstein SL, Spratt KF. The natural history and long-term follow-up of Scheuermann kyphosis. J Bone Joint Surg Am. 1993;75(2):236-48.
17. Tallroth K, Schlenzka D. Spinal stenosis subsequent to juvenile lumbar osteochondrosis. Skeletal Radiol. 1990;19:203-5.
18. Lowe TG, Kasten MD. An analysis of sagittal curves and balance after Cotrel-Dubousset instrumentation for kyphosis secondary to Scheuermann's disease. A review of 32 patients. Spine. 1994;19(15):1680-5.
19. Vialle LR. Coluna Torácica. In: de Barros Filho TEP, Lech O (Eds). Exame Físico em Ortopedia. São Paulo: Sarvier; 2001. pp. 20-36.
20. Ogilvie J, Sherman J. Spondylolysis in Scheuermann's disease. Spine. 1987;12:251-3.
21. Bhojraj SY, Dandawate AV. Progressive cord compression secondary to thoracic disc lesions in Scheuermann's kyphosis managed by posterolateral decompression, interbody fusion and pedicular fixation. A new approach to management of a rare clinical entity. Eur Spine J. 1994;3(2):66-9.
22. Klein DM, Weiss RL, Allen JE. Scheuermann's dorsal kyphosis and spinal cord compression: case report. Neurosurgery. 1986;18(5):628-31.
23. Yablon JS, Kasdon DL, Levine H. Thoracic cord compression in Scheuermann's disease. Spine. 1988;13(8):896-8.
24. Ponte A, Gebbia F, Eliseo F. Non-operative treatment of adolescent hyperkyphosis. Orthop Trans. 1985;9:108.
25. Lowe TG. Kyphosis of the thoracic and thoracolumbar spine in the pediatric patient: surgical treatment. Instr Course Lect. 2004;53:493-500. Review.
26. Agabegi S, Kazemi N, Crawford A. Pediatric Kyphosis: Scheuermann Disease and Congenital Deformity. In: Herkowitz H, Garfin S, Eismont F, Bell G, Balderston R (Eds). Rothman Simeone The Spine, 6th edition. Philadelphia: Saunders; 2011.

27. Bradford DS, Moe JH, Montalvo FJ, et al. Scheuermann's kyphosis and roundback deformity. Results of Milwaukee brace treatment. J Bone Joint Surg Am. 1974;56(4):740-58.
28. Sachs B, Bradford D, Winter R, et al. Scheuermann kyphosis. follow-up of Milwaukee-brace treatment. J Bone Joint Surg Am. 1987;69(1):50-7.
29. Gutowski WT, Renshaw TS. Orthotic results in adolescent kyphosis. Spine. 1988;13(5):485-9.
30. Hosman AJ, de Kleuver M, Anderson PG, et al. Scheuermann Kyphosis: the importance of tight hamstrings in the surgical correction. Spine. 2003;19:2252-9.
31. Bradford DS, Moe JH, Montalvo FJ, et al. Scheuermann's kyphosis. Results of surgical treatment by posterior spine arthrodesis in twenty-two patients. J Bone Joint Surg. 1975;57A:439-48.
32. Herndon W, Emans B, Micheli L, et al. Combined anterior and posterior fusion for Scheuermann's kyphosis. Spine. 1981;6:125-30.
33. Lim M, Green D, Billinghurst J. Scheuermann kyphosis: safe and effective surgical treatment using multisegmental instrumentation. Spine. 2004;29:1789-94.
34. Geck MJ, Macagno A, Ponte A, et al. The Ponte procedure: posterior only treatment of Scheuermann's kyphosis using segmental posterior shortening and pedicle screw instrumentation. J Spinal Disord Tech. 2007;20(8):586-93.
35. Lee S, Lenke L, Kuklo T. Comparison of Scheuermann kyphosis correction by posterior-only thoracic pedicle screw fixation versus combined anterior/posterior fusion. Spine. 2006;21:2316-21.
36. Hosman A, de Kleuver M, Anderson P. Analysis of the sagittal plane after surgical management for Scheuermann's disease: a view on overcorrection and the use of anterior release. Spine. 2002;27:167-75.
37. Denis F, Sun EC, Winter RB. Incidence and risk factors for proximal and distal junctional kyphosis following surgical treatment for Scheuermann kyphosis: minimum five-year follow-up. Spine. 2009;34(20):E729-34.
38. Sturm F. Dobson J, Armstrong G. The surgical management of Scheuermann's disease. Spine. 1993;18:685-91.
39. Poolman R, Bee H, Ubags L. Clinical outcome and radiographic results after operative treatment of Scheuermann disease. Eur Spine J. 2002;11:561-9.
40. Cho KJ, Lenke LG, Bridwell KH, et al. Selection of the optimal distal fusion level in posterior instrumentation and fusion for thoracic hyperkyphosis: the sagittal stable vertebra concept. Spine. 2009;34(8):765-70.
41. Cheh G, Lenke LG, Padberg AM, et al. Loss of spinal cord monitoring signals in children during thoracic kyphosis correction with spinal osteotomy: why does it occur and what should you do? Spine. 2008;33(10):1093-9.
42. Lonner BS, Newton P, Betz R, et al. Operative management of Scheuermann's kyphosis in 78 patients: radiographic outcomes, complications, and technique. Spine. 2007;32(24):2644-55.

CHAPTER 15 Pediatric Trauma

Theodore J Choma, Daniel G Hoernschemeyer, Sumit K Gupta

EPIDEMIOLOGY AND NATURAL HISTORY

Pediatric spinal trauma is not entirely different from adult spinal trauma; there are still primary issues of neurological function and mechanical stability that need to be addressed with each patient. But, given the differences in morphology and biomechanics between the growing spines of children and adults, it makes some sense to explore pediatric spinal trauma as a separate topic in this chapter.

Spine trauma in children is less common than in adults, and represents between 2.7% and 9% of all spinal trauma.[1-3] The most common mechanisms of injury include motor vehicle accidents, pedestrians struck by a moving vehicle, falls from height, athletic injuries, nonaccidental injury, and birth related trauma. Cervical level injuries account for a larger proportion of injuries in children than in adults.[4-7] The patterns of injury are different in children due to unique anatomic features of the immature spine, including unossified growth centers, unfused synchondroses, ligamentous laxity, different orientation of facet joints, and relatively larger head size.

Spinal Cord Injury

If the osseoligamentous injury to the pediatric spine exceeds certain limits, the energy imparted on the spinal cord may cause acute injury. This basic fact pertains to children as well as adults. There are, however, distinct patterns of mechanical failure in the pediatric spine that may cause injury and we will explore them. In general though, traumatic spinal cord injury (SCI) involves acute deformation (strain) of the neural parenchyma. This is responsible for the initial neurological deficit, but tissue damage may continue in the hours following the acute traumatic event, as a result of cord swelling, ischemia, and programmed cell death resulting in the totality of the neurological deficit.

Fortunately, pediatric SCI seems to be a relatively rare event, occurring with incidence of 1–27 children/million/year in European countries.[8] It had been estimated that of the approximately 250,000 patients living in the United States, some 37,500 of them were under age 15 in 2005. In 2011, 10% of patient who sustained new SCI were of age 17 or younger.[9] The chief causes for pediatric SCI remain motor vehicle accidents (37.4%), violence (22.8%), and sports (23.9%).[9] Children between the ages of 4 to 8 years old with SCI due to motor vehicle accidents were most likely to be suboptimally restrained; children with abdominal wall ecchymosis had associated vertebral fractures and SCI in 11% of cases.[10]

Cervical Injury

Cervical spine injuries represent about 1–2% of all pediatric trauma.[4,11,12] 60–80% of spine trauma includes the cervical region in children, compared to 30–40% in adults.[5-7,13] Children younger than 8 years of age usually have upper cervical spine injuries, and those over 8 have a higher incidence of lower cervical spine injuries similar to adults.[4-7,11-15] This predilection of younger children for upper cervical spine injuries can be attributed to biomechanical and physiological features of the immature spine. These include incomplete ossification, anterior vertebral wedging, and horizontal orientation of facet joints, ligamentous laxity, underdeveloped neck musculature, and larger relative head size. The larger head/body ratio causes an increased torque and acceleration stress on the upper cervical spine such that the fulcrum of rotation in the immature spine is much higher (around C2–C3) compared to adolescents and adults (C4–C5).

Thoracolumbar Injury

Pediatric thoracolumbar spine injuries are relatively uncommon injuries, comprising 7% of presenting pediatric trauma patients in one recent series.[16] These injuries are more likely to occur as a result of a motor vehicle accident, but can also occur from falls or child abuse.[17,18] Spine fractures in the thoracic and lumbar areas occur most commonly in the adolescent population as a result of a high energy injury from axial loading, flexion, distraction or shear forces to the spine.[19] Multiple studies have shown nontrivial rates of noncontiguous thoracolumbar spinal injury. As such, it is prudent to obtain imaging of the entire spine once a single traumatic injury is identified.[17]

EVALUATION AND IMAGING

It may be difficult to obtain an accurate history from a child at the initial evaluation, so it is necessary to have a high level of suspicion for spine injuries with particular mechanisms of injury. When assessing the child who has been involved in a high-energy injury mechanism, the team should maintain a high index of suspicion for spinal trauma until proven otherwise. The most common causes of cervical spine injury in children are motor vehicle accidents, sports injuries, or pedestrian-struck injuries, so they should elicit caution in the physician. Infants are more prone to child abuse and injuries from fall. The incidence of sport-related and motor vehicle-related injury increases with age. The common presenting symptoms for cervical injury include neck pain and unwillingness or inability to move the neck. Patients may additionally complain of headaches or neurological symptoms. Infants may present with fussiness, unexplained weakness, hypotonia, weakness, bowel or bladder dysfunction, or respiratory depression. Any evidence of head or facial trauma, altered sensorium, or loss of consciousness should alert the examiner to the possibility of cervical spine trauma. Localized pain or tenderness are the most common signs of thoracolumbar trauma, although these are not particularly sensitive nor specific.[16]

Examination for neurological function can be difficult in the very young or uncooperative patient. The child may be in pain, or anxious due to unfamiliar surroundings. It is often easier to examine babies and infants while they are held in their caregivers arms, rather than placing them on an examining table, if possible. Effort should be made to allow a parent to be present during the examination. Physical examination includes inspection and palpation of the entire back followed by a detailed neurological examination. Complete sensory and motor examination should be performed and documented on every child who is able to understand and cooperate with the examination. If the child's age or mental status does not allow a complete examination, Babinski, abdominal, bulbocavernosus, and deep tendon reflexes should still be assessed.

Any child with a suspected cervical spine injury should be immobilized using a well-fitting cervical spine collar, and on a spine board. It is important to immobilize the entire spine, since there is a 6–12% incidence of a noncontiguous injury being present.[20-22] If appropriately sized collars are not available, the neck may be immobilized by placing rolled up towels on either side of the head to prevent rotation. The use of standard adult spine boards in a child can cause undesirable flexion of the neck, due to the larger head size (Fig. 1).[23] If boards with an appropriate head cut out are not available, the torso should be placed on blankets for elevation. While it is prudent to consider these precautions in children, studies have failed to correlate poor alignment with adverse neurological outcome.[24]

Imaging

Unlike in adults, there are no established guidelines to aid the physician in clearing the pediatric cervical spine.[25] The National Emergency X-radiography Utilization Study (NEXUS) outlined criteria for clinical clearance in adults

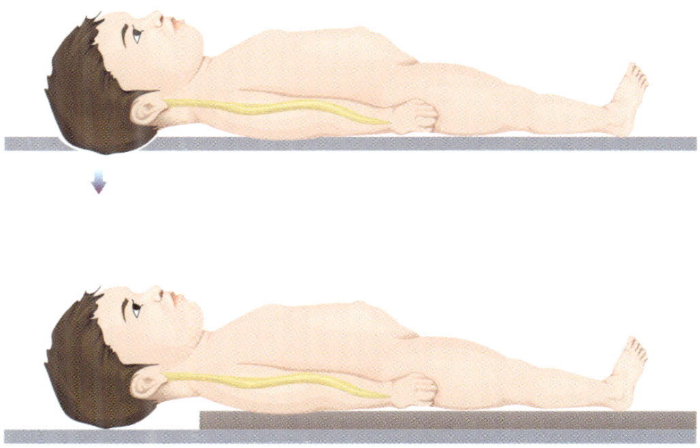

Fig. 1: The large head of children is accommodated on a spinal board by either having an occipital recess in the board, or elevating the torso with 25 mm of padding.
Source: Green NE, Swintkowski MF (Eds). Skeletal Trauma in Children, 4th edition. Philadelphia: Elsevier.

which included absence of midline neck pain, focal neurological deficits, intoxication, distracting injuries or altered mental status. The validity of this rule in children has been studied by Viccellio et al.[26] They retrospectively looked at 3065 patients under the age of 18, assessed for trauma and found that no injuries would have been missed when applying the NEXUS criteria. However, their study only included 88 children under the age of 2 years, and none had cervical spine injuries. They concluded that NEXUS criteria may decrease pediatric cervical spine imaging by 20% but should not be used for infants or toddlers. A recent case report described an odontoid fracture in a 3-year-old girl after a motor vehicle collision, who did not fulfill the NEXUS criteria.[27] The authors stressed that cervical spine imaging should be considered in any patient with a high-risk mechanism of injury.

Initial radiographs include a cross table lateral, anteroposterior (AP), and open-mouth odontoid views. Oblique radiographs may be more effective in showing details of the pedicle and facet joints. CT scans are the best test to evaluate for bony injury and are highly sensitive and specific for detecting instability.[28] Flexion-extension views can further aid in diagnosing instability in an awake and cooperative child. MRI is the study of choice to evaluate SCI and other soft tissues including ligaments and intervertebral disks.

Normal Spinal Development

The spine undergoes a process of maturation from birth until it reaches the final adult morphology. It is important for the clinician treating spine injuries in children to understand the differences in anatomy when compared to adults in order to correctly identify injuries. The atlas and axis have unique characteristics, whereas the subaxial vertebrae from C3 to L5 follow a common developmental pathway.

Atlas: Three ossification centers are present in the atlas (Figs. 2A and B). The ventral arch ossification center is usually not visible at birth. In 33% of children it is visible after 3 months, and in 81% after 1 year, and 100% by age 3.[29] The two dorsal neural arches start to ossify at 7 weeks gestation and are visible at birth.[30] The dorsal synchondrosis fuses by age 3 years and the ventral synchondroses (neurocentral synchondroses) close by age 7.[30,31]

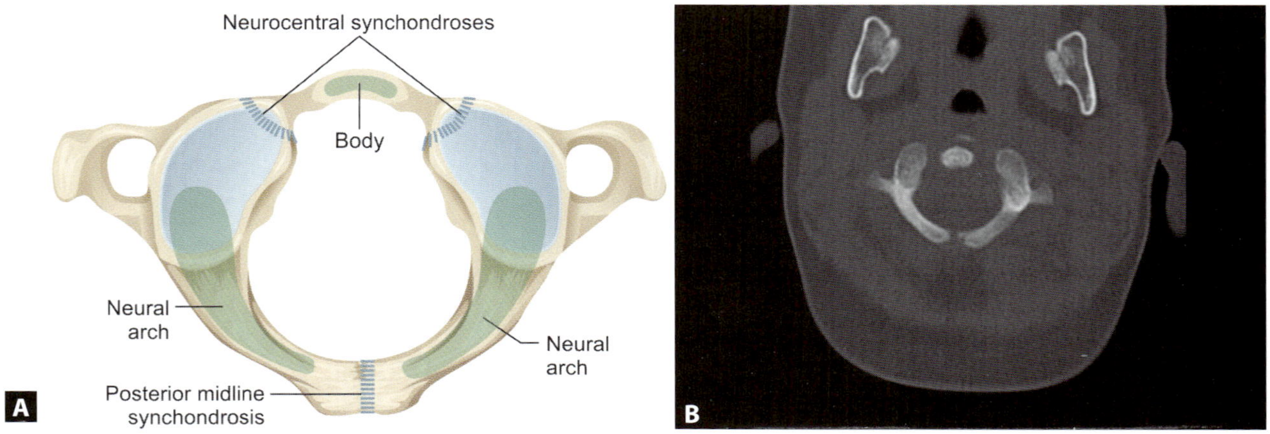

Figs. 2A and B: (A) The ossification centers and synchondroses of the atlas. The neural arch ossification centers form during the seventh gestational week, whereas the ossification center within the body of C1 becomes visible during the first year of life. The posterior midline synchondrosis fuses at about the third year of life. The neurocentral synchondroses about the atlas body fuse around the age of 7 years. (B) Correlative axial CT scan of C1 in a 10-month old.

Source: Figure A from Gore PA, Chang S, Theodore N. Cervical spine injuries in children: attention to radiographic differences and stability compared to those in the adult patient. Semin Pediatr Neurol. 2009;16(1):42-58.

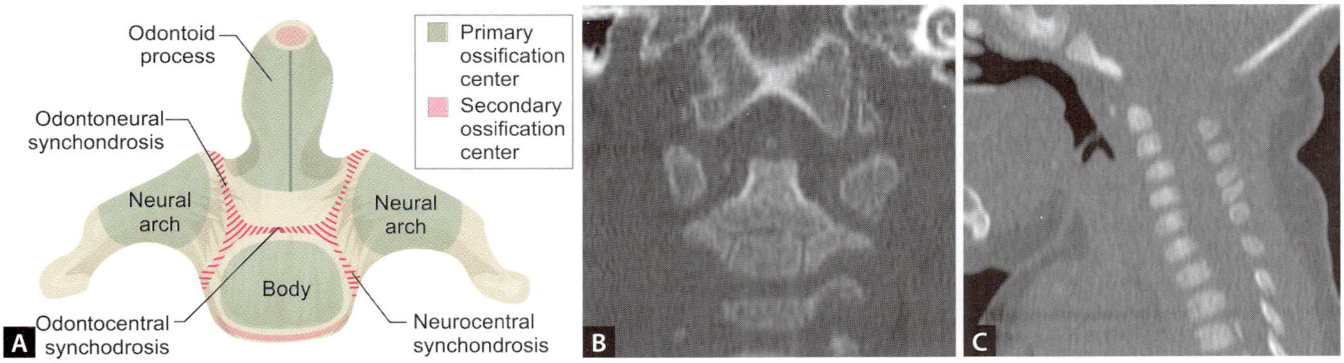

Figs. 3A to C: (A) The ossification centers and synchondroses of the axis. Two ossification centers fuse in the midline to form the odontoid process by the seventh gestational month. The body of C2 fuses to the odontoid between ages 3 and 6 years. The neurocentral synchondroses about the body also fuse between ages 3 and 6 years. The secondary ossification center at the apex of the odontoid appears between ages 6 and 8 years and fuses with the dens around the age of 12 years. (B) Correlative coronal CT from a 5-month-old child shows the synchondrosis between the odontoid and body of C2, and the neurocentral synchondroses. (C) Correlative sagittal CT of the same child shows the synchondrosis between the odontoid and body of C2.

Source: Fig. A from Gore PA, Chang S, Theodore N. Cervical spine injuries in children: attention to radiographic differences and stability compared to those in the adult patient. Semin Pediatr Neurol. 2009;16(1):42-58.

Axis: The axis has four ossification centers—one each for the posterior neural arches, one for the body, and one for the odontoid (Figs. 3A to C). The ossification center of the odontoid comprises of two distinct ossific nuclei which fuse in utero at 7 months gestation. By age 3–6 years, the body fuses with the dens. However, this fusion line, the subdental synchondrosis, can be seen until age 11 and may be mistaken for a fracture.[30] The tip of the dens has its own ossification center that appears at age 6 and fuses to the body of the dens by age 12. The posterior arches fuse at an age of 3 years and fuse to the body of C2 by age 6.

Subaxial (C3-C7), thoracic and lumbar vertebrae: The subaxial cervical spine, thoracic, and lumbar spine develop in a similar manner. Each vertebral level is composed of three ossification centers—one anteriorly for the body, and one for each posterior neural arch (Figs. 4A and B). The neural arches fuse posteriorly by age 3 and with the neurocentral synchondroses fusing at age 3–6. Secondary ossification centers develop at the tips of the transverse processes, spinous process, facets, and at the superior and inferior apophyseal rings. These ossification centers persist until the third decade of life.[30]

The height of the vertebral body at birth is similar to or slightly smaller than the intervertebral disk when seen on plain radiographs. This is not a true measurement of vertebral body height, as the endplates have not ossified, thus falsely portraying the bodies as smaller and corresponding disks bigger than they truly are. A cleft exists in the anterior wall of the mid-portion of the vertebral bodies. This represents a nutrient artery and is usually visible on plain radiographs until age 3–6.[32] A similar posterior cleft is also visible (containing the basivertebral vein and nutrient artery) but this persists into adulthood.

The facet joint orientation changes with age. It is initially more horizontal and gradually becomes more vertical. Due to this, there is initially less resistance to anterior motion. Along with increased elasticity of interspinous ligaments, joint capsules and cartilaginous end plates, this may be an explanation for pseudosubluxation that is often seen in the pediatric cervical spine.

The anatomy of the immature cervical spine creates several unusual features on radiographs and these must not be confused with traumatic injury. Compared to adults, children under the age of 8 have relatively horizontal facet joint orientation, and increased ligamentous laxity, leading to increased vertebral movement.[33] Pseudosubluxation is seen most often at C2–C3 and is also seen at C3–C4. Swischuk described the spinolaminar line (Figs. 5A and B) to differentiate between pseudosubluxation and pathologic subluxation.[34]

The atlanto-dens interval (ADI) in children younger than 8 can be between 3 mm and 5 mm. In adults this distance should be 3 mm or less. Anterior wedging on the bodies of cervical vertebra does not imply a fracture. Anterior wedging of less than 3 mm is within normal

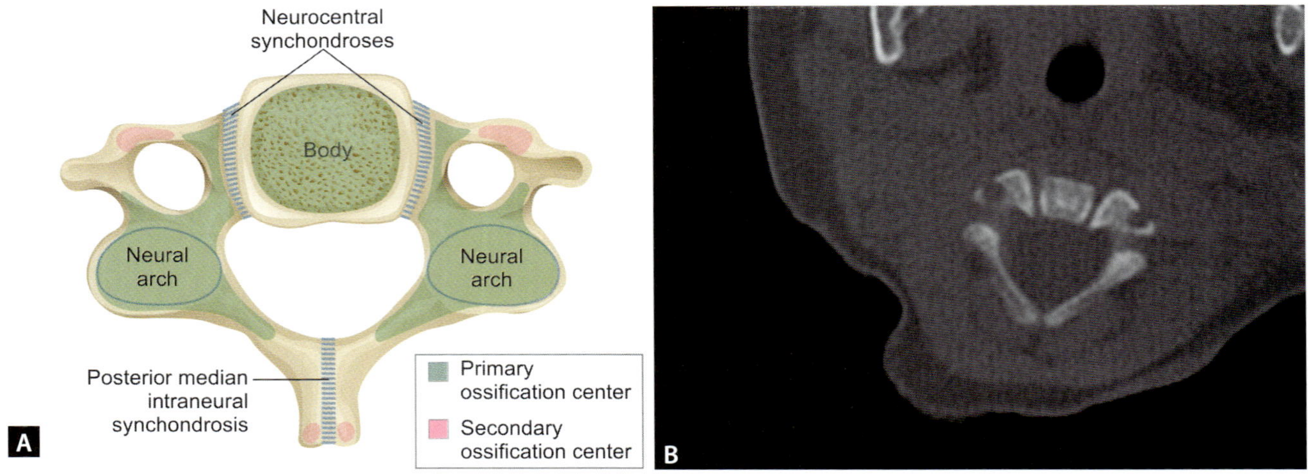

Figs. 4A and B: (A) The ossification centers and synchondroses of a subaxial vertebra. The development of the subaxial cervical spine is highly conserved from C3 through C7. Ossification of the centrum is present by the fifth gestational month. The arches fuse in the midline by the age of 2–3 years. The neurocentral synchondroses fuse between the ages of 3–6 years. (B) Correlative sagittal CT from a 15 week-old infant.
Source: Figure A from Gore PA, Chang S, Theodore N. Cervical spine injuries in children: attention to radiographic differences and stability compared to those in the adult patient. Semin Pediatr Neurol. 2009;16(1):42-58.

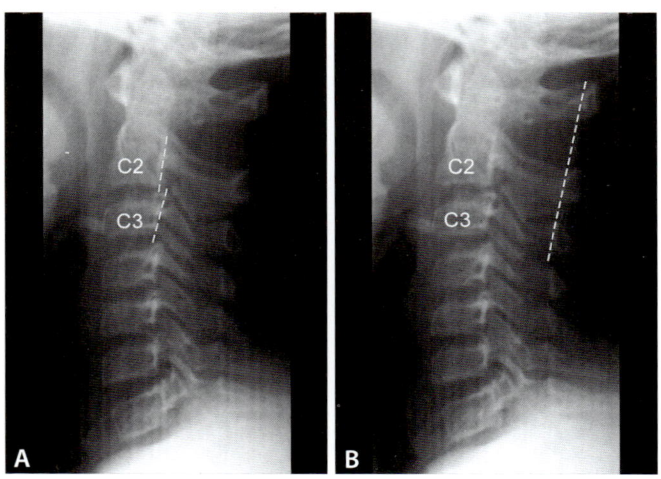

Figs. 5A and B: (A) Forward displacement of C2–C3 seen on lateral C-spine radiograph when placing posterior vertebral body lines. (B) The diagnosis of pseudosubluxation is made after drawing the spinolaminar line.
Source: Shaw M, Burnett H, Wilson A, et al. Pseudosubluxation of C2 on C3 in polytraumatized children: prevalence and significance. Clin Radiol. 1999;54(6):377-80.

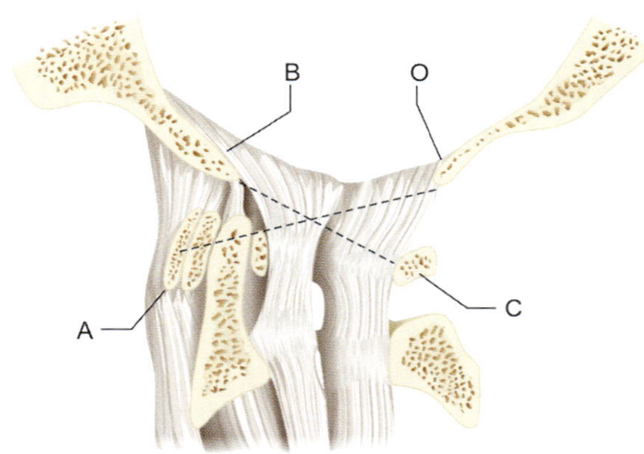

Fig. 6: Power's ratio measurement, ratio is BC/OA; A value greater than 1 indicates anterior displacement of the occiput on C1 and less than 0.55 indicates posterior displacement. (A: anterior arch of C1; B: basion; C: posterior arch of C1; O: opisthion).
Source: Spiteri V, Kotnis R, Singh P, et al. Cervical dynamic screening in spinal clearance: now redundant. J Trauma. 2006;61(5):1171-7; discussion 1177.

limits. Loss of cervical lordosis is common with flexion and is restored in extension radiographs. Secondary ossification centers, unfused synchondroses, and unfused ring apophysis can be mistaken for fractures.

Evaluation of alignment at the craniocervical junction on lateral cervical spine radiographs can be evaluated in several ways.[35,36] Powers et al. described a ratio calculated by dividing the distance from the basion to the posterior arch of the atlas by the distance between the opisthion to the anterior arch of the atlas (Fig. 6).[37] A ratio of greater than 1 or less than 0.55 represents anterior or posterior displacement of the atlanto-occipital joint. Kaufman et al.

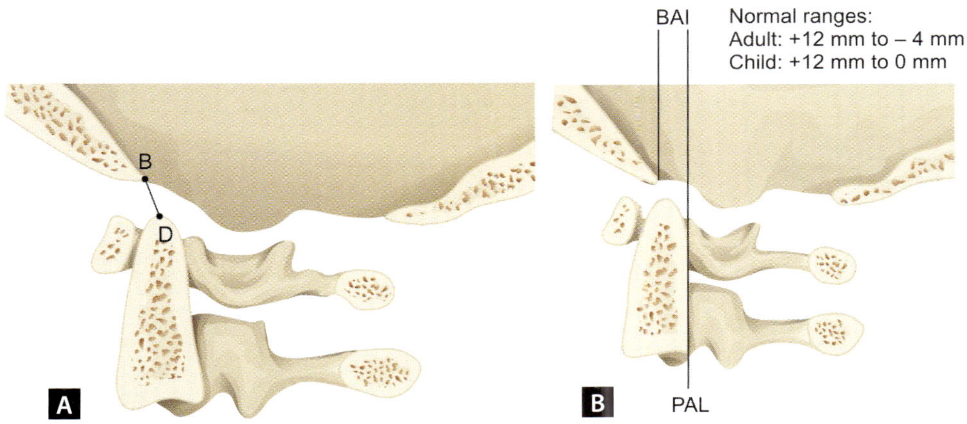

Figs. 7A and B: (A) Basion dens interval and, (B) Basion axial interval should be less than 12 mm. A value > 12 mm suggests atlanto-occipital dissociation.

Source: Pang D, Nemzek WR, Zovickian J. Atlanto-occipital dislocation—part 2: the clinical use of (occipital) condyle-C1 interval, comparison with other diagnostic methods, and the manifestation, management, and outcome of atlanto-occipital dislocation in children. Neurosurgery. 2007;61(5):995-1015; discussion 1015.

looked at the distance between the occipital condyle and the superior facet of C1 on lateral radiographs and found that this distance should never exceed 5 mm.[38] Harris et al. described the "rule of 12" which evaluates the distance between the basion and the rostral tip of the odontoid process, as well as the basion and the rostral extension of the posterior cortical margin of the axis (Figs. 7A and B).[39] These measures are called the basion dens interval (BDI) and basion axial interval (BAI) respectively. In patients over the age of 13, both these distances measure less than 12 mm. In children less than 12 years of age, the BDI is less reliable due to the variable ossification of the den. However, the BAI should remain less than 12 at all ages.

COMMON PATTERNS OF INJURY IN THE GROWING SPINE TREATMENT AND PROGNOSIS

Sciwora

Since Pang and Wilberger described the phenomenon of SCI without radiographic abnormality (SCIWORA) in 1982, treating physicians have gained MRI as a common imaging option.[40] This has improved our understanding of the processes of SCIWORA. In some cases, ligaments and/or disks are completely ruptured, despite the lack of injury to the bony structures. In other SCIWORA cases, it appears the restraining soft tissues are significantly more com-pliant in the young child (< 8 years old) than in the older child or adult.[41,42] This may allow the spine to momentarily deform enough to cause spinal cord injury, but spontaneously reduce so as to appear normal on routine imaging. Some combination of these mechanisms may be at play in 30–40% of children who sustain traumatic myelopathy,[43] and multiple series have demonstrated the predilection for SCIWORA in younger children (< 10 years) than older children.[44,45] Furthermore, these children tend to sustain more severe SCI patterns.

It should be remembered that not all SCIWORA injuries affect the cervical spinal cord. 13% of SCIWORA injuries can occur to the thoracic cord, usually as a result of motor vehicle injury.[43] Unfortunately, it must also be remembered that occult instability in children's spines may put them at risk for delayed neurological compromise as SCIWORA has been described in children up to 4 days following traumatic injury.[40] Treatment of SCIWORA has been supportive of fluid status and blood pressure for cord perfusion. Operative stabilization can be considered when obviously unstable injuries are demonstrated, or brace immobilization for 3 months in cases of true SCIWORA, and no MRI abnormality of the supporting structures. Assessment of spinal stability with flexion-extension radiographs is recommended in the acute setting and at late follow-up, even when the MRI is negative for extraneural injury, but neither spinal angiography nor myelography are recommended in these patients.[46] The main predictor of outcomes in children with SCIWORA appears to be neurological status at presentation, with more severe lesions having a worse prognosis.[43] There is some evidence that those patients with normal

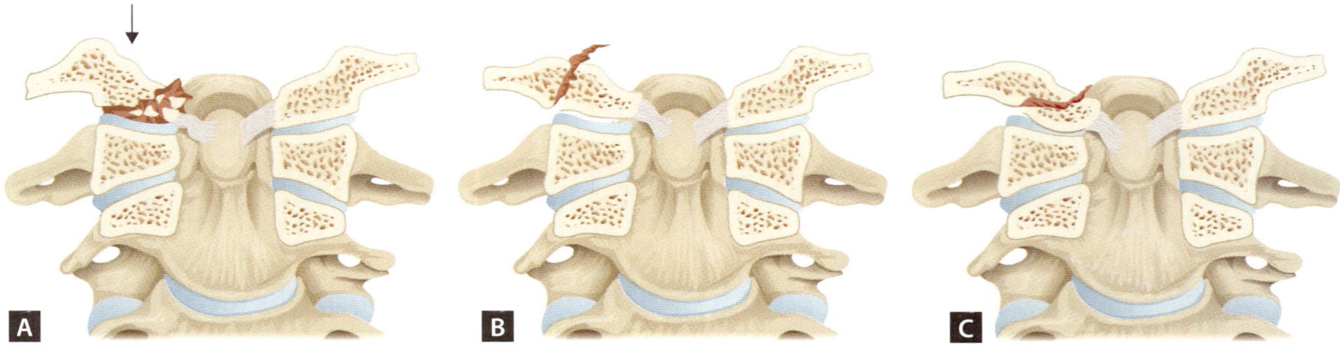

Figs. 8A to C: Anderson and Montesano classification of occipital condyle fractures. (A) Type I injuries are comminuted, impaction fractures caused by axial loading. (B) Type II injuries are impaction or shear fractures extending into the base of the skull. (C) Type III injuries are alar ligament avulsion fractures.

Source: Maddox JJ, Rodriguez-Feo JA 3rd, Maddox GE, et al. Nonoperative treatment of occipital condyle fractures: an outcomes review of 32 fractures. Spine (Phila Pa 1976). 2012;37(16):E964-8.

MRI's at presentation have better prognosis, and those demonstrating cord transection or cord hemorrhage have a far worse prognosis for neurological return.[47]

Occipital Condyle Fractures

The inability to diagnose occipital condyle fractures (OCFs) on plain radiographs has resulted in this injury being historically under-reported.[48] Widespread use of CT and MR imaging has led to an increased awareness of this entity.

Occipital condyle fractures in children are usually associated with motor vehicle or sporting accidents, head injury and loss of consciousness.[49] Injury to cranial nerves, brain stem or high spinal cord is frequently present.

Anderson and Montesano's classification is most widely used.[50] They describe three types of injuries—Type 1 is an impacted fracture of the occipital condyle, Type II is a basilar skull fracture which extends into the occipital condyle and Type III is an avulsion fracture of the condylar fragment (Figs. 8A to C). Some Type IIs and all Type IIIs are considered to be unstable. Tuli et al. proposed a different classification system based on the degree of ligamentous injury reflected by the presence of a displaced OCF observed on CT and determination of occipito-C1–C2 instability on X-ray, CT and MRI. They described three types—Type 1 is a nondisplaced fracture, Type 2A is a displaced stable fracture, and Type 2B is a displaced unstable fracture.[51]

Treatment of unstable injuries is generally nonsurgical, with a rigid collar or halo vest for 8 weeks. The osseous injury heals predictably well-including restoration of mobility and eradication of pain. However, neurological deficits may not resolve completely. Early diagnosis and management is essential to prevent secondary displacement of fragments resulting in delayed cranial nerve injury or compression of brain stem.[49]

Atlanto-Occipital Dissociation

Atlanto-occipital dislocation (AOD) is a rare injury and is associated with a high mortality rate. Improved prehospital care, a high index of suspicion, early recognition with better imaging techniques, and rapid stabilization and treatment has led to improved survival rates.[36] Children appear to be at a higher risk for this injury due to larger relative head size, horizontal atlanto-occipital joints, and smaller occipital condyles.[52]

The most common cause of AOD is motor vehicle crashes, although direct traumas, deployment of airbags, and forceps delivery have been described.[53-55] The mechanism is believed to be a hyperextension, resulting in traumatic rupture of the alar and apical ligaments, and the tectorial membrane, allowing the cranium to move with respect to the cervical spine. Traynelis et al. described a classification system in adults based on the direction of displacement of the cranium—Type I is anterior, Type II is primarily longitudinal distraction, and Type III is posterior.[56] Harris et al. also described a fourth type which is combined anterior translation and distraction.[57]

The clinical presentation can be variable. Neurological signs can vary from absence of neurological deficit to complete quadriplegia with respiratory failure.[52,36] Coexisting intracranial injuries are common and may obscure the findings of the clinical examination. The diagnosis should be suspected in any patient with major trauma who demonstrates agonal respirations, irregular heart rate, lower cranial nerve abnormalities or asymmetric motor deficits.[36]

The diagnosis can often be made with careful scrutiny of plain radiographs. Several methods have been described to detect instability in the atlanto-occipital joint. The Power's ratio, Harris et al.'s "rule of 12," and Kaufmann's method have been described earlier in the chapter. CT and MRI are useful adjuncts to confirm the diagnosis and evaluate the osseous and soft tissue structures.

Initial management includes stabilizing the injury, which is best accomplished initially with a halo vest. However, external immobilization alone is unpredictable in restoring ligamentous stability, and these injuries usually require surgical stabilization through occipitocervical fusion once the patient is clinically stable enough for surgery. Isolated occiput (C0) to C1 fusion can be done in cases where there is no C1–C2 instability[58] and preserves C1–C2 rotational motion. Fixation may be achieved with either transarticular C0–C1 screws, or occipital keel (midline)—C1 lateral mass screws and rods (Figs. 9A and B). The transarticular screw construct is biomechanically more stable. Structural bone graft is used to help achieve fusion. Rib and iliac crest grafts have both been used successfully.[36] In most cases, the fusion will extend down to C2. The construct can include C1 lateral mass screws with C2 pars or pedicle screws, or a transarticular screw at C1–C2; with midline occipital screws. Postoperative protocol usually involves immobilization with a halo vest for 6 weeks.

Atlanto-occipital dislocation remains a very severe injury with a high mortality rate. Higher mortality rates are associated with complete neurological injury, severe distraction (Basion-Dens Interval > 16 mm), and high Injury Severity Score.[59] However, with early identification and prompt management, outcomes may be more favorable than previously thought.

Atlas Fractures

Fractures of the ring of C1 (Jefferson fractures) are rare in children.[60-62] The usual mechanism is an axial load on the top of the head. The patient will usually present with pain and torticollis. Neurological deficit is uncommon. The forces are distributed from the occipital condyles to the atlantal lateral masses, pushing them centrifugally, causing the C1 ring to fail in tension. The fracture may go through bone, or unossified synchondroses, and these can be difficult to identify. The extent of separation of the lateral masses of C1 depends on the velocity of injury and ultimately the integrity of the trtansverse atlantal ligament (TAL). Lateral mass displacement totaling more than 6.9 mm is usually associated with TAL disruption and instability.[61]

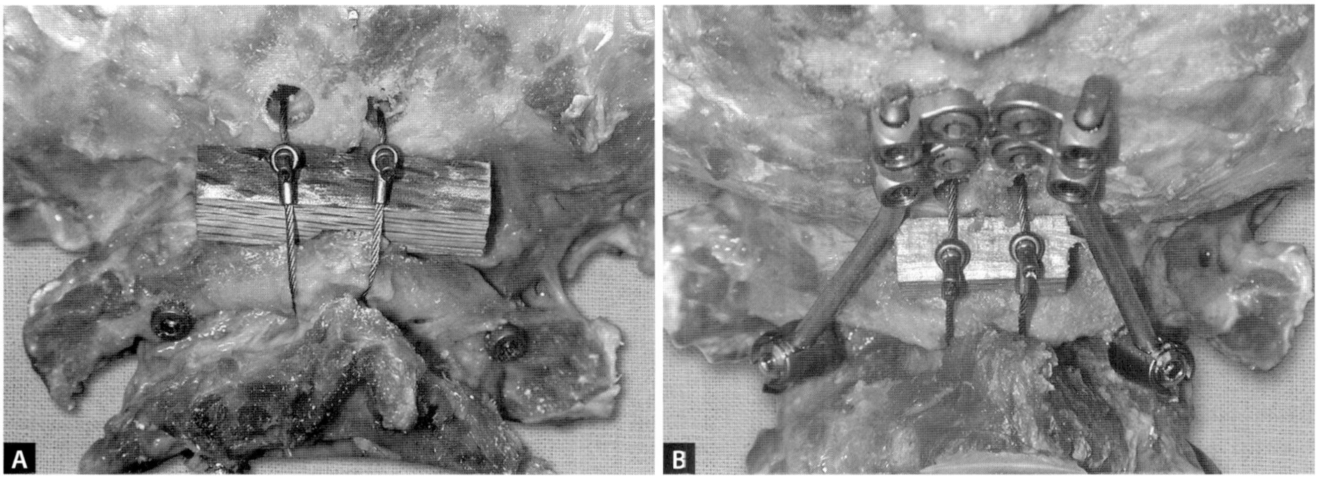

Figs. 9A and B: Fixation of occiput to C1. (A) Transarticular screw and structural bone graft. (B) Occipital keel screw and C1 lateral mass screws.[58]

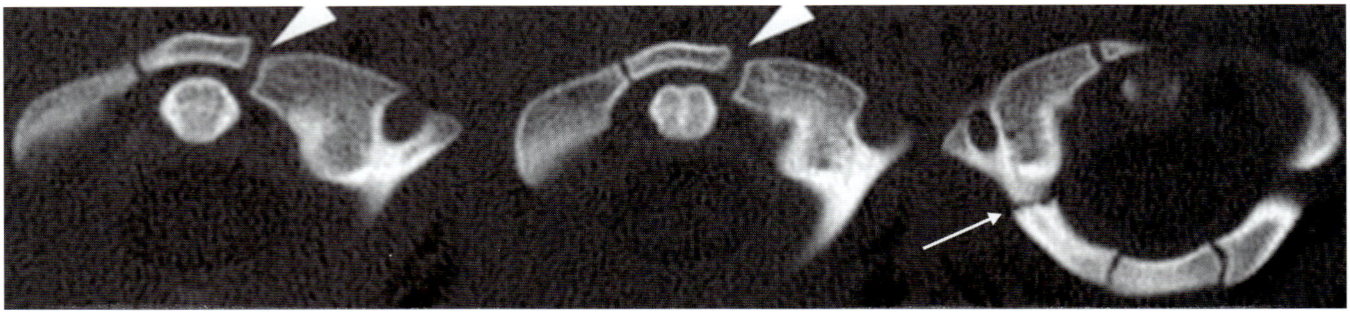

Fig. 10: Jefferson fracture. Axial CT scans showing a disruption of the synchondrosis at the left side of the anterior arch (arrowheads) and a fracture on the right side of the posterior arch (arrow). Note that this child has two posterior arch synchondroses which is a variant of normal.[61]

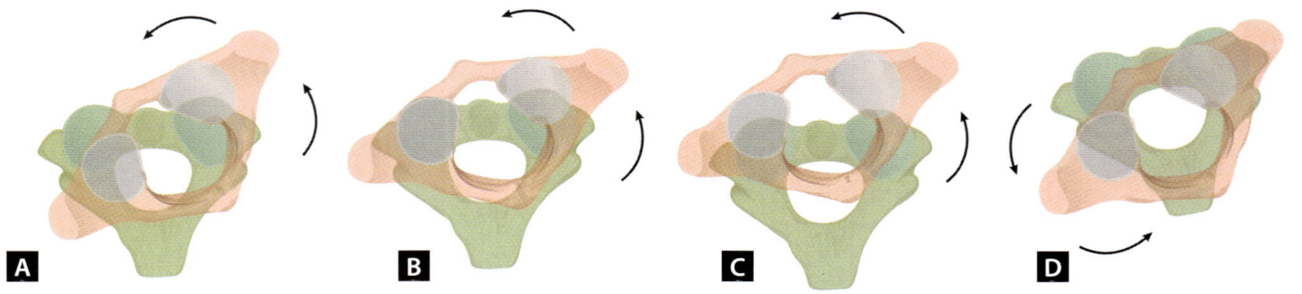

Figs. 11A to D: The four types of rotatory fixation. (A) Type I—rotatory fixation with no anterior displacement and the odontoid acting as the pivot; (B) Type II—rotatory fixation with anterior displacement of 3–5 mm, one lateral articular process acting as the pivot; (C) Type III—rotatory fixation with anterior displacement of more than 5 mm; and (D) Type IV—rotatory fixation with posterior displacement.[66]

CT scan is the study of choice for detecting these injuries (Fig. 10). MRI images will show high signal intensity in synchondroses, consistent with acute injury, and can verify the integrity of the TAL.

Treatment of these injuries in children is generally nonsurgical. Halo vest or other rigid immobilization is applied for a period 3 weeks up to 3 months.[63,61] There is little indication in the literature of the need for surgical intervention in children with this injury.

Atlantoaxial Rotatory Subluxation

Atlantoaxial rotatory subluxation (AARS) is a rotational deformity of C1 on C2 associated with significant loss of motion. The etiology is usually traumatic or associated with upper respiratory infection (Grisel's syndrome) or inflammation. AARS is more common in children due to the unique anatomy of the upper cervical spine. The dens-facet angle in the axis is steeper in children than in adults.[64] Meniscus-like synovial folds are found in the occiput-C1 and C1-C2 facet joints in the immature spine which may invaginate and block spontaneous reduction.[64] Infection or inflammation in the neck may cause hyperemia in the atlantoaxial region as there is a direct connection between the pharyngovertebral veins and the periodontoidal venous plexus and suboccipital venous sinuses.[65]

Fielding et al. classified AARS into four subtypes (Figs. 11A to D).[66] Type 1 is rotatory displacement without anterior translation. The odontoid acts as a pivot and the transverse and alar ligaments are intact. This is the most common type.[65] Type 2 involves rotatory fixation with anterior displacement of less than 5 mm. This signifies transverse ligament deficiency and is the second most common type. Type 3 is a rotatory fixation with greater than 5 mm of anterior displacement, and indicates transverse and alar ligament deficiency. Type 4 involves posterior translation of C1 on C2. This type is rare and occurs with a deficient odontoid process.

Children usually present with torticollis with the head held in a "cock-robin" position. The neck is tilted to one side, but the head is rotated to face the other side

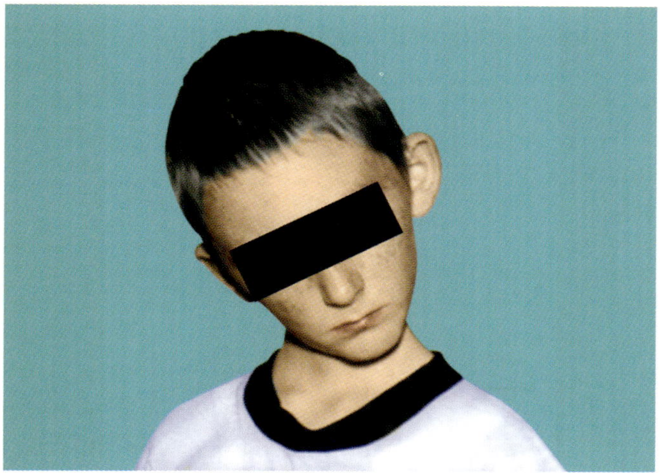

Fig. 12: Cock-robin position in a child with AARS. The neck is tilted to the right and the head is rotated to the left.[65]

(Fig. 12). The deformity is rigid and usually only partially correctable actively and passively. There is often pain and muscle spasm. Neurological compromise is rare in Type 1 and atraumatic cases, but may be present in traumatic Type 2–4 injuries.

Diagnosis is made by demonstrating fixed rotation of C1 on C2 with a dynamic test. Plain radiographs are difficult to interpret due to the overlap of the skull on the occipito-atlanto-axial complex (Figs. 13A to D). The open mouth odontoid view shows asymmetry of the lateral masses with the anterior mass appearing wider and closer to midline. The test of choice for the diagnosis is a CT scan (Figs. 13A to D). Axial cuts can adequately show the rotation of the atlas on the axis. When there is anterior or posterior displacement, a static CT will make the diagnosis. In type 1 torticollis, the static CT appearance is identical to that in a normal subject who holds his head in a rotated and tilted position. Patients are therefore initially scanned in the Cock-Robin position, and then scanned again while holding their head in the maximum corrected position. In AARS, C1 will not rotate over C2 as in normal individuals.

Early diagnosis and treatment generally results in favorable outcomes without surgical intervention.[65,67] In patients presenting acutely with less than 1 week of symptoms, often a soft collar with appropriate analgesics is sufficient. If the deformity persists, or in patients presenting with symptoms greater than 1 week old, halter traction should be first attempted. If this is unsuccessful, skeletal traction with a halo ring can be used to apply higher weights. In patients who do not respond to traction, surgical correction involves C1–C2 or C0–C2 fusion.

Odontoid Fractures

Odontoid fractures are one of the most common fractures of the cervical spine in children. Unlike those seen in adults, odontoid fractures in young children do not occur through bone at the base of the dens but at a lower level within the body of C2 as a separation through the unossified dentocentral synchondrosis.[68] The most common mechanism of injury is forced flexion in motor vehicle accidents, occurring in children in forward facing car seats.[69]

Spinal cord injury is uncommon with this fracture, though transient paresthesia and weakness has been reported.[68] Most fractures of the odontoid are displaced anteriorly and the diagnosis can be made on lateral radiographs, unless there has been spontaneous reduction of the fracture. An MRI scan is helpful in these cases.

Odontoid fractures in children generally heal well. The fracture is reduced by extension of the head to achieve at least 50% apposition. If adequate reduction is not achieved by simple extension, halter traction or skeletal traction with a halo ring is usually effective. Immobilization with a Minerva or halo brace for 6–12 weeks is usually sufficient for fracture healing.

Acute injuries must be differentiated from os odontoideum This is an anatomical abnormality in which the tip of the odontoid process lacks continuity with the body of C2 (Fig. 14).[70] Os odontoideum may be discovered incidentally or on evaluation for neck pain or neurological symptoms after trauma. The etiology is widely debated in the literature. Some authors believe that it is a developmental lesion resulting from a failure of fusion of two ossific nuclei, while others believe it is a post-traumatic pseudarthrosis.[70-72] There is an increased incidence of os odontoideum in patients with Klippel-Feil syndrome, Down's syndrome, multiple epiphyseal dysplasia, or other skeletal dysplasias as compared to the general population.[71]

Os odontoideum can present as an incidental finding in an asymptomatic patient, or can cause symptoms such as neck pain, torticollis, headache, or myelopathy. The diagnosis can often be made on plain radiographs. Lateral flexion-extension radiographs should be obtained to assess for instability. The os moves with the anterior arch of C1, so the radiograph should be assessed for displacement

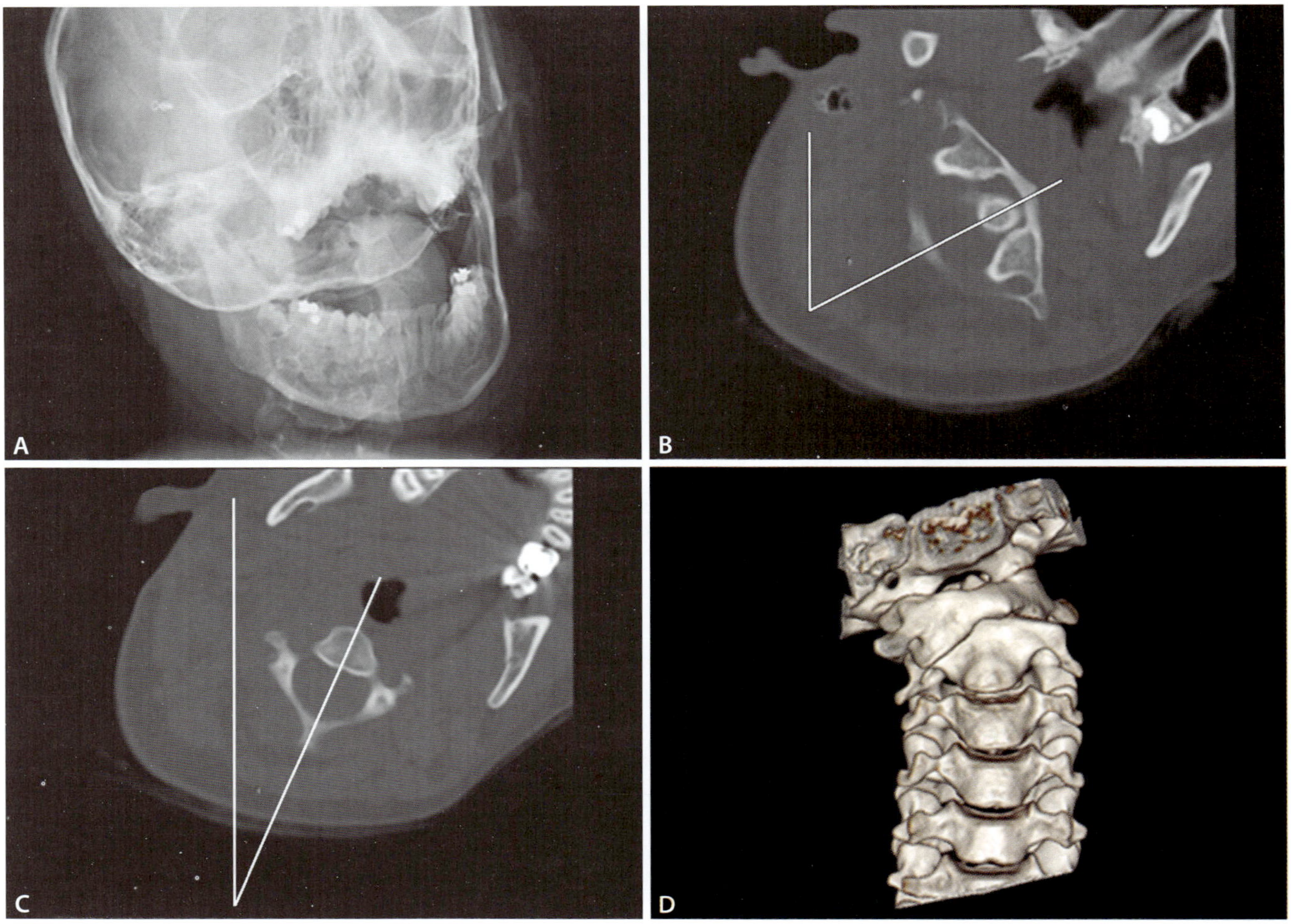

Figs. 13A to D: Atlantoaxial rotatory subluxation. (A) Plain radiographs are often hard to interpret. The lateral masses are difficult to view on this open mouth odontoid view due to superimposition of the skull. CT scans show that the C1 (B) is rotationally misaligned on C2 (C). (D) 3D reconstruction of CT images shows a Type 2 AARS.

between the bodies of C1 and C2, and the space available for the cord.

Treatment of asymptomatic os odontoideum is controversial. Several authors have recommended to simply observe these patients, as the risk of sudden neurological injury is low.[70,73-75] However, others have suggested that even asymptomatic patients should be offered surgical stabilization, as there are no guidelines to predict which ones will progress to neurological injury.[75,76] Most authors do agree that symptomatology or radiographic evidence of instability are indications for surgical stabilization.

C1–C2 stabilization is most often achieved with transarticular screws or fixation with lateral mass, pedicle or laminar screws or hooks. These techniques generally confer greater stability and have largely replaced older graft/wiring techniques such as the Gallie and Brooks procedures.[70]

Hangman's Fractures

Traumatic spondylolisthesis of C2 or Hangman's fracture can occur in children. The mechanism of injury is forced hyperextension. This fracture is rarely associated with neurological injury as the space available for the cord actually increases due to a break in the ring of C2. The diagnosis can be made on plain radiographs; however, it must not be confused with a persistent synchondrosis of the axis which is a normal variant. Treatment usually consists of immobilization in a hard collar, Minerva cast or halo vest. If the fracture does not heal, posterior or anterior fusion can be performed.

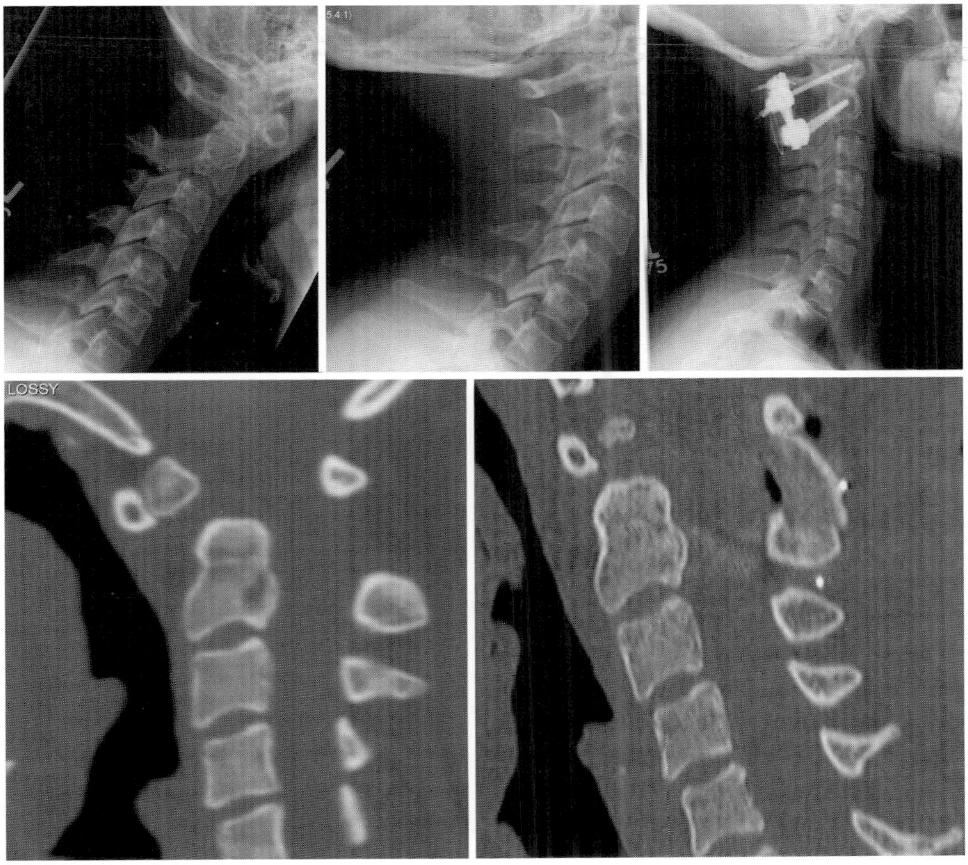

Fig. 14: CT scan showing os odontoideum.[75]

Subaxial Injuries

Subaxial spine injuries are more commonly seen in older children and adolescents. Injuries can include bony or cartilaginous (end plate) fractures, facet dislocations, fracture dislocations, or ligamentous injury. Most of these injuries occur between C5 and C7, reflecting a distal shift in the fulcrum of cervical motion.[7] Most of these injuries can be treated with external immobilization, but some may require surgical stabilization if they do not heal with immobilization alone.[7] The most grossly unstable will require primary surgical fusion as in adults.

Thoracolumbar Apophyseal Ring Injuries

Apophyseal ring injuries typically occurs in the adolescent years, but have been reported in the young adult population.[77] The vertebral ring apophysis begins to ossify at 6 years of age and fuses around age 17. Tensile stresses in flexion are thought contribute to the apophyseal ring avulsion fracture.[78] The apophysis is tightly bound to the annulus of the disk resulting in an associated avulsion fracture identified in 28% of adolescent disk herniations.[79] Most of these fractures occur in the lumbar region but they have also been identified at the level of the spinal cord. The size and location of the apophyseal ring fracture are best identified on CT myelogram which can also better identify any bony fragment in the canal.[80] An MRI can be used to visualize any protrusion of the disk into the spinal canal but it may make it difficult to see the fracture, thus leading to a delay with the correct diagnosis.

Adolescents with apophyseal ring injuries can have a wide variation in their presenting symptoms depending on the size and displacement of the fracture. Patients with large, centrally displaced apophyseal fragments will often present with more severe back pain and neurological symptoms than that seen with an isolated lumbar disk herniation.[79]

Various treatment options have been reported throughout the literature ranging from an anterior decompression and fusion to microdiscectomy with bilateral hemilaminectomies to remove the large bony fragment. A 2012 literature review of 19 articles found the posterior discectomy with excision of the apophyseal fracture without spine fusion to be the preferred treatment of choice.[81]

Thoracolumbar Burst Fractures

Pediatric burst fractures are relatively rare due to greater flexibility of the pediatric spine and thicker annular fibers in the disk.[82] Occurring as the result of a primarily axial compressive load to the spine, these fractures result in disruption of the anterior and middle columns, potentially leading to retropulsion of fracture fragments into the spinal canal.[83] Neurologic injury in pediatric burst fractures is correlated more strongly with the level of fracture, with thoracic fractures having higher risk, than with the percentage of canal compromise seen on CT scan.[82]

While the initial evaluation begins with plain X-rays of the spine, the CT scan is much more valuable in assessing the extent of the injury. Assessment of kyphosis, canal compromise, and loss of vertebral height at the injury sight are best determined on the CT scan. An MRI can be helpful in further evaluating the posterior ligamentous structures of the pediatric spine, helping to differentiate between stable and unstable burst fractures.

While a stable burst fracture can be treated nonoperatively in a hyperextension cast or brace, an unstable burst fracture is best treated surgically. The assessment of stability, already somewhat controversial, is more difficult in the pediatric thoracolumbar spine given the lack of clinical evidence upon which to base criteria. The goals of operative intervention are to correct any excessive kyphotic deformity, protect the spinal cord from injury, stabilize the fracture, and allow for early mobilization. In one study looking at pediatric burst fractures, operatively treated injuries had a decreased length of stay in the hospital and there is no progression of their sagittal plane deformity compared to the burst fractures treated nonoperatively.[84]

Treatment options for pediatric burst fractures consist of a posterior only instrumented fusion or an anterior fusion with corpectomy and strut grafting combined with a posterior spine fusion. Efforts are made in the pediatric spine to save levels posteriorly, especially in the lumbar region. Recent literature has reported the use of short-segment hybrid constructs using universal clamps in combination with pedicle screws to limit the number of fusion levels.[85]

Chance Fracture

A Chance fracture is the result of a flexion-distraction injury to the pediatric spine which can occur from an improperly worn seat belt. At injury, the instantaneous center of rotation is at a point ventral to the vertebral body and the posterior elements fail in tension. Commonly referred to as "seat belt syndrome," 40–50% of these pediatric spine fractures will have associated intra-abdominal injuries requiring further evaluation. A high index of suspension should be raised when bruising and discoloration are seen across a child's abdomen. An abdominal CT scan can identify life-threatening injuries.[86]

Plain radiograph, CT scan, and an MRI of the spine can help to determine if the injury is purely ligamentous or it also involves disruption of the bone. In a study looking at MRI evaluation of pediatric Chance fractures, one-third of patients were found to have bony involvement through the pedicle and vertebral body while the other two-thirds were found to have fractures through the superior or inferior physeal endplates. No disk injuries were identified.[87]

Nonoperative treatment using a hyperextension brace or cast may be considered when there is a bony injury with no intra-abdominal injuries. A posterior spine fusion with instrumentation is the gold standard when ligamentous disruption is seen on the MRI. Looking at outcome of these injuries, one study reported 6 year follow-up on pediatric Chance fractures demonstrating more pain and disability when treated nonoperatively.[88]

Compression Fractures

In a review of all pediatric spine fractures, compression fractures were found to be the most common, accounting for 42% of all spine fractures in children.[89] By definition, a compression fracture only involves the anterior column of the spine, leaving the middle column intact. Therefore, these fractures are felt to be quite stable and SCI is extremely rare. When these fractures occur, failure of the superior and inferior endplates may be seen, causing more pain for the child. Anterior wedging and loss of height can be identified on plain radiographs of the spine, but long cassette radiographs of the spine case will best assess any kyphotic deformity and overall sagittal alignment. While most of these injuries occur as the result of trauma, compression fractures have been reported in patients with acute lymphoblastic leukemia (ALL) after chemotherapy.[90]

Compression fractures are best treated nonoperatively. Less than 20% loss of vertebral height should be monitored for pain control with mobilization as tolerated. When pain is poorly controlled and loss of vertebral height exceeds 20%, a TLSO may be considered. Spontaneous remodeling after loss of vertebral height can occur in children under 10 years of age.[91]

Fracture Dislocations

Fracture dislocation injuries of the pediatric spine are relatively rare injuries that involve all three columns of the spine. As a result, these are highly unstable and usually associated with neurologic injury. Surgery is required to stabilize the spine and protect the cord from further injury. Fracture dislocations in the pediatric spine occur most commonly at the thoracolumbar junction. While the vast majority of these injuries happen as a result of high energy accidents, traumatic thoracolumbar spine fracture dislocations have been reports as a result of child abuse.[18]

Treatment of these pediatric spine fractures may need to be delayed if more life-threatening injuries have occurred and the patients are hemodynamically unstable. Due to these associated injuries, the mortality rate for these high-energy injuries is quite high. Reduction and stabilization of these fractures can often be accomplished through a posterior approach with transpedicular fixation. A level-of-evidence (Table 1) is attached at the end of the chapter.

Table 1: Level-of-evidence for C-spine.

Author, journal, year	*Design*	*LoE*	*Topic*	*F/U (m)*	*Measures*	*Main results*
Anderson, Spine, 1988	Case Series	IV	Occipital condyle fractures	12		Description of classification
Beier, J Neurosurg Peds, 2012	R	IV	AARS	Na		Acute patients can be managed in a collar, subacute and late presenters may need surgery
Brockmeyer, Childs Nerv Syst, 2012	PC	II	Pediatric C-spine clearance	3	Flex-Ex radiographs	Initial use of CT and plain radiographs, recommend flexex radiographs over MRI for ligamentous injury
Chaput, J Trauma, 2011	R	IV	AOD	6	Survival, Neurologic status, ISS	High ISS, BDI or complete neurological deficit associated with mortality
Firth, Spine, 2012	R	IV	Spine trauma—noncontiguous spine injuries (NCSI)	56	Incidence of NCSI after trauma	11.7% NCSI. 16% initially missed. 24% of NCSI patients had neurological injury
Garrett, Neurosurgery, 2010	Rev		AOD			Review article
Hofbauer, J Tr Acute Care Surg, 2012	R	IV	Spine injury in pediatric polytrauma	20	Location and incidence of neurological injury	Most common injury is thoracic spine followed by TBI. Younger children more commonly have upper spine injury
Hosalkar, JBJSAm, 2005	R	IV	AOD outcomes in children	50	Neurological outcome after AOD	69% mortality. 1/5 surviving patients were neurologically normal
Klimo, J Neurogurg Spine	R	IV	Os odontoideum outcomes after surgical fixation	14	Neurological function	90% improvement of symptoms
Mortazavi, Childs Nerv Syst, 2011	R	IV	NCSI	7.5	Neurologic outcome	73% normal neurologic function, 4% incomplete SCI, 8% complete SCI
Parent, J Neurotrauma, 2011	Sys Rev	IV	Pediatric SCI	Na	Various outcomes after SCI	Pediatric patients have better neurological recovery. Preadolescent have high chance of scoliosis
Viccellio, Pediatrics, 2001	PC	III	Cervical spine injury in children	Na	NEXUS	NEXUS performed well in children

(AARS: atlanto-axial rotatory subluxation; AOD: atlanto-occipital dissociation; BDI: basion dens interval; Childs Nerv Syst: child's nervous system; ISS: injury severity score; J Tr Acute Care Surg: Journal of Trauma and Acute Care Surgery; JBJSAm: Journal of Bone and Joint Surgery, American; J Neuro Trauma: Journal of Neurotrauma; J Trauma: Journal of Trauma; J Neurosurg Peds: Journal of Neurosurgery, Pediatrics; J Neurosurg Spine: Journal of Neurosurgery, Spine; LoE: level-of-evidence; Na: not applicable/not reported; NEXUS: National Radiographic X-radiographic Utilization Study; PC: prospective cohort; R: retrospective; Rev: review; SCI: spinal cord injury; Sys Rev: systematic review; TBI: traumatic brain injury)

REFERENCES

1. Ruge JR, Sinson GP, McLone DG, et al. Pediatric spinal injury: the very young. J Neurosurg. 1988;68(1):25-30.
2. Osenbach RK, Menezes AH. Pediatric spinal cord and vertebral column injury. Neurosurgery. 1992;30(3):385-90.
3. Hamilton MG, Myles ST. Pediatric spinal injury: review of 174 hospital admissions. J Neurosurg. 1992;77(5):700-4.
4. Kokoska ER, Keller MS, Rallo MC, et al. Characteristics of pediatric cervical spine injuries. J Pediatr Surg. 2001;36(1):100-5.
5. McCall T, Fassett D, Brockmeyer D. Cervical spine trauma in children: a review. Neurosurg Focus. 2006;20(2):E5.
6. Tilt L, Babineau J, Fenster D, et al. Blunt cervical spine injury in children. Curr Opin Pediatr. 2012;24(3):301-6.
7. Jones TM, Anderson PA, Noonan KJ. Pediatric cervical spine trauma. J Am Acad Orthop Surg. 2011;19(10):600-11.
8. Augutis M, Abel R, Levi R. Pediatric spinal cord injury in a subset of European countries. Spinal Cord. 2006;44(2):106-12.
9. National Spinal Cord Injury Statistical Center. (2011). NSCISC: The 2011 Annual Statistical Report for the Spinal Cord Injury Model Systems. [online] Available from https://www.nscisc.uab.edu/Public/2011%20Annual%20Report%20-%20Complete%20Public%20Version.pdf. [Last accessed July, 2019].
10. Achildi O, Betz RR, Grewal H. Lapbelt injuries and the seatbelt syndrome in pediatric spinal cord injury. J Spinal Cord Med. 2007;30(Suppl 1):S21-4.
11. Platzer P, Jaindl M, Thalhammer G, et al. Cervical spine injuries in pediatric patients. J Trauma. 2007;62(2):389-96; discussion 394-6.
12. Hofbauer M, Jaindl M, Hochtl LL, et al. Spine injuries in polytraumatized pediatric patients: characteristics and experience from a Level I trauma center over two decades. J Trauma Acute Care Surg. 2012;73(1):156-61.
13. Ramrattan NN, Oner FC, Boszczyk BM, et al. Cervical spine injury in the young child. Eur Spine J. 2012;21(11):2205-11.
14. Eleraky MA, Theodore N, Adams M, et al. Pediatric cervical spine injuries: report of 102 cases and review of the literature. J Neurosurg. 2000;92(1 Suppl):12-7.
15. Basu S. Spinal injuries in children. Front Neurol. 2012;3:96.
16. Junkins EP Jr, Stotts A, Santiago R, et al. The clinical presentation of pediatric thoracolumbar fractures: a prospective study. J Trauma. 2008;65(5):1066-71.
17. Dogan S, Safavi-Abbasi S, Theodore N, et al. Thoracolumbar and sacral spinal injuries in children and adolescents: a review of 89 cases. J Neurosurg. 2007;106(6 Suppl):426-33.
18. Bode KS, Newton PO. Pediatric nonaccidental trauma thoracolumbar fracture-dislocation: posterior spinal fusion with pedicle screw fixation in an 8-month-old boy. Spine (Phila Pa 1976). 2007;32(14):E388-93.
19. Santiago R, Guenther E, Carroll K, et al. The clinical presentation of pediatric thoracolumbar fractures. J Trauma. 2006;60(1):187-92.
20. Firth GB, Kingwell SP, Moroz PJ. Pediatric noncontiguous spinal injuries: the 15-year experience at 1 pediatric trauma center. Spine (Phila Pa 1976). 2012;37(10):E599-608.
21. Mahan ST, Mooney DP, Karlin LI, et al. Multiple level injuries in pediatric spinal trauma. J Trauma. 2009;67(3):537-42.
22. Mortazavi MM, Dogan S, Civelek E, et al. Pediatric multilevel spine injuries: an institutional experience. Childs Nerv Syst. 2011;27(7):1095-100.
23. Herzenberg JE, Hensinger RN, Dedrick DK, et al. Emergency transport and positioning of young children who have an injury of the cervical spine. The standard backboard may be hazardous. J Bone Joint Surg Am. 1989;71(1):15-22.
24. Curran C, Dietrich AM, Bowman MJ, et al. Pediatric cervical-spine immobilization: achieving neutral position? J Trauma. 1995;39(4):729-32.
25. Burns EC, Yanchar NL. Using cervical spine clearance guidelines in a pediatric population: a survey of physician practices and opinions. CJEM. 2011;13(1):1-6.
26. Viccellio P, Simon H, Pressman BD, et al. A prospective multicenter study of cervical spine injury in children. Pediatrics. 2001;108(2):E20.
27. Maxwell MJ, Jardine AD. Paediatric cervical spine injury but NEXUS negative. Emerg Med J. 2007;24(9):676.
28. Brockmeyer DL, Ragel BT, Kestle JR. The pediatric cervical spine instability study. A pilot study assessing the prognostic value of four imaging modalities in clearing the cervical spine for children with severe traumatic injuries. Childs Nerv Syst. 2012;28:699-705.
29. Wang JC, Nuccion SL, Feighan JE, et al. Growth and development of the pediatric cervical spine documented radiographically. J Bone Joint Surg Am. 2001;83(8):1212-8.
30. Lustrin ES, Karakas SP, Ortiz AO, et al. Pediatric cervical spine: normal anatomy, variants, and trauma. Radiographics. 2003;23(3):539-60.
31. Gore PA, Chang S, Theodore N. Cervical spine injuries in children: attention to radiographic differences and stability compared to those in the adult patient. Semin Pediatr Neurol. 2009;16(1):42-58.
32. Byrd SE, Comiskey EM. Postnatal maturation and radiology of the growing spine. Neurosurg Clin N Am. 2007;18(3):431-61.
33. Copley LA, Dormans JP. Cervical spine disorders in infants and children. J Am Acad Orthop Surg. 1998;6(4):204-14.
34. Swischuk LE. Anterior displacement of C2 in children: physiologic or pathologic. Radiology. 1977;122(3):759-63.
35. Eubanks JD, Gilmore A, Bess S, et al. Clearing the pediatric cervical spine following injury. J Am Acad Orthop Surg. 2006;14(9):552-64.
36. Hosalkar HS, Cain EL, Horn D, et al. Traumatic atlanto-occipital dislocation in children. J Bone Joint Surg Am. 2005;87(11):2480-8.
37. Powers B, Miller MD, Kramer RS, et al. Traumatic anterior atlanto-occipital dislocation. Neurosurgery. 1979;4(1):12-7.
38. Kaufman RA, Carroll CD, Buncher CR. Atlanto-occipital junction: standards for measurement in normal children. Am J Neuroradiol. 1987;8(6):995-9.
39. Harris JH Jr, Carson GC, Wagner LK. Radiologic diagnosis of traumatic occipitovertebral dissociation: 1. Normal occipitovertebral relationships on lateral radiographs of supine subjects. Am J Roentgenol. 1994;162(4):881-6.

40. Pang D, Wilberger JE Jr. Spinal cord injury without radiographic abnormalities in children. J Neurosurg. 1982;57(1):114-29.
41. Sullivan CR, Bruwer AJ, Harris LE. Hypermobility of the cervical spine in children; a pitfall in the diagnosis of cervical dislocation. Am J Surg. 1958;95(4):636-40.
42. Taylor AR. The mechanism of injury to the spinal cord in the neck without damage to vertebral column. J Bone Joint Surg Br. 1951;33-B(4):543-7.
43. Pang D. Spinal cord injury without radiographic abnormality in children, 2 decades later. Neurosurgery. 2004;55(6):1325-42; discussion 1342-23.
44. Yngve DA, Harris WP, Herndon WA, et al. Spinal cord injury without osseous spine fracture. J Pediatr Orthop. 1988;8(2):153-9.
45. Osenbach RK, Menezes AH. Spinal cord injury without radiographic abnormality in children. Pediatr Neurosci. 1989;15(4):168-74; discussion 175.
46. Rozzelle CJ, Aarabi B, Dhall SS, et al. Spinal cord injury without radiographic abnormality (SCIWORA). Neurosurgery. 2013;72 (Suppl 2):227-33.
47. Dare AO, Dias MS, Li V. Magnetic resonance imaging correlation in pediatric spinal cord injury without radiographic abnormality. J Neurosurg. 2002;97(1 Suppl):33-9.
48. Neeman Z, Bloom AI. Occipital condyle fractures in the pediatric population. Radiographics. 2003;23(6):1699-701; author reply 1699-701.
49. Momjian S, Dehdashti AR, Kehrli P, et al. Occipital condyle fractures in children. Case report and review of the literature. Pediatr Neurosurg. 2003;38(5):265-70.
50. Anderson PA, Montesano PX. Morphology and treatment of occipital condyle fractures. Spine (Phila Pa 1976). 1988;13(7):731-6.
51. Tuli S, Tator CH, Fehlings MG, et al. Occipital condyle fractures. Neurosurgery. 1997;41(2):368-76.
52. Ehlinger M, Charles YP, Adam P, et al. Survivor of a traumatic atlanto-occipital dislocation. Orthop Traumatol Surg Res. 2011;97(3):335-40.
53. McKenna DA, Roche CJ, Lee WK, et al. Atlanto-occipital dislocation: case report and discussion. CJEM. 2006;8(4):50-3.
54. Angel CA, Ehlers RA. Images in clinical medicine. Atloido-occipital dislocation in a small child after air-bag deployment. N Engl J Med. 2001;345(17):1256.
55. Saveika JA, Thorogood C. Airbag-mediated pediatric atlanto-occipital dislocation. Am J Phys Med Rehabil. 2006;85(12):1007-10.
56. Traynelis VC, Marano GD, Dunker RO, et al. Traumatic atlanto-occipital dislocation: a case report. J Neurosurg. 1986;65(6):863-70.
57. Harris JH Jr, Carson GC, Wagner LK, et al. Radiologic diagnosis of traumatic occipitovertebral dissociation: 2. Comparison of three methods of detecting occipitovertebral relationships on lateral radiographs of supine subjects. Am J Roentgenol. 1994;162(4):887-92.
58. Garrett M, Consiglieri G, Kakarla UK, et al. Occipitoatlantal dislocation. Neurosurgery. 2010;66(3 Suppl):48-55.
59. Chaput CD, Torres E, Davis M, et al. Survival of atlanto-occipital dissociation correlates with atlanto-occipital distraction, injury severity score, and neurologic status. J Trauma. 2011;71(2):393-5.
60. Vilela MD, Peterson EC. Atlantal fracture with transverse ligament disruption in a child: a case report. J Neurosurg Pediatr. 2009;4(3):196-8.
61. AuYong N, Piatt J Jr. Jefferson fractures of the immature spine. Report of 3 cases. J Neurosurg Pediatr. 2009;3(1):15-9.
62. Korinth MC, Kapser A, Weinzierl MR. Jefferson fracture in a child—illustrative case report. Pediatr Neurosurg. 2007; 43(6):526-30.
63. Judd DB, Liem LK, Petermann G. Pediatric atlas fracture: a case of fracture through a synchondrosis and review of the literature. Neurosurgery. 2000;46(4):991-4; discussion 994-5.
64. Kawabe N, Hirotani H, Tanaka O. Pathomechanism of atlantoaxial rotatory fixation in children. J Pediatr Orthop. 1989;9(5) 569-74.
65. Roche CJ, O'Malley M, Dorgan JC, et al. A pictorial review of atlanto-axial rotatory fixation: key points for the radiologist. Clin Radiol. 2001;56(12):947-58.
66. Fielding JW, Hawkins RJ. Atlanto-axial rotatory fixation (fixed rotatory subluxation of the atlanto-axial joint). J Bone Joint Surg Am. 1977;59(1):37-44.
67. Beier AD, Vachhrajani S, Bayerl SH, et al. Rotatory subluxation: experience from the Hospital for Sick Children. J Neurosurg Pediatr. 2012;9(2):144-8.
68. Hosalkar HS, Greenbaum JN, Flynn JM, et al. Fractures of the odontoid in children with an open basilar synchondrosis. J Bone Joint Surg Br. 2009;91(6):789-96.
69. Odent T, Langlais J, Glorion C, et al. Fractures of the odontoid process: a report of 15 cases in children younger than 6 years. J Pediatr Orthop. 1999;19(1):51-4.
70. Klimo P Jr, Coon V, Brockmeyer D. Incidental os odontoideum: current management strategies. Neurosurg Focus. 2011; 31(6):E10.
71. Bach CM, Arbab D, Thaler M. Treatment strategies for severe C1C2 luxation due to congenital os odontoideum causing tetraplegia. Eur Spine J. 2013;22(1):29-35.
72. McHugh BJ, Grant RA, Zupon AB, et al. Congenital os odontoideum arising from the secondary ossification center without prior fracture. J Neurosurg Spine. 2012;17(6):594-7.
73. Spierings EL, Braakman R. The management of os odontoideum. Analysis of 37 cases. J Bone Joint Surg Br. 1982;64(4):422-8.
74. Fielding JW, Hensinger RN, Hawkins RJ. Os Odontoideum. J Bone Joint Surg Am 1980;62(3):376-83.
75. Arvin B, Fournier-Gosselin MP, Fehlings MG. Os odontoideum: etiology and surgical management. Neurosurgery. 2010;66(3 Suppl):22-31.
76. Klimo P Jr, Kan P, Rao G, et al. Os odontoideum: presentation, diagnosis, and treatment in a series of 78 patients. J Neurosurg Spine. 2008;9(4):332-42.
77. Yang IK, Bahk YW, Choi KH, et al. Posterior lumbar apophyseal ring fractures: a report of 20 cases. Neuroradiology. 1994;36(6):453-5.
78. Sairyo K, Goel VK, Masuda A, et al. Three-dimensional finite element analysis of the pediatric lumbar spine. Part I:

CHAPTER 15

pathomechanism of apophyseal bony ring fracture. Eur Spine J. 2006;15(6):923-9.

79. Chang CH, Lee ZL, Chen WJ, et al. Clinical significance of ring apophysis fracture in adolescent lumbar disc herniation. Spine (Phila Pa 1976). 2008;33(16):1750-4.
80. Dake MD, Jacobs RP, Margolin FR. Computed tomography of posterior lumbar apophyseal ring fractures. J Comput Assist Tomogr. 1985;9(4):730-2.
81. Wu X, Ma W, Du H, et al. A review of current treatment of lumbar posterior ring apophysis fracture with lumbar disc herniation. Eur Spine J. 2013;22(3):475-88.
82. Vander Have KL, Caird MS, Gross S, et al. Burst fractures of the thoracic and lumbar spine in children and adolescents. J Pediatr Orthop. 2009;29(7):713-9.
83. Denis F. The three column spine and its significance in the classification of acute thoracolumbar spinal injuries. Spine (Phila Pa 1976). 1983;8(8):817-31.
84. Lalonde F, Letts M, Yang JP, et al. An analysis of burst fractures of the spine in adolescents. Am J Orthop (Belle Mead NJ). 2001;30(2):115-20.
85. Ilharreborde B, Hirsch C, Presedo A, et al. Circumferential fusion with anterior strut grafting and short-segment multipoint posterior fixation for burst fractures in skeletally immature patients: a preliminary report. J Pediatr Orthop. 2012;32(5):440-4.
86. Choit RL, Tredwell SJ, Leblanc JG, et al. Abdominal aortic injuries associated with chance fractures in pediatric patients. J Pediatr Surg. 2006;41(5):1184-90.
87. de Gauzy JS, Jouve JL, Violas P, et al. Classification of chance fracture in children using magnetic resonance imaging. Spine (Phila Pa 1976). 2007;32(2):E89-92.
88. Mulpuri K, Jawadi A, Perdios A, et al. Outcome analysis of chance fractures of the skeletally immature spine. Spine (Phila Pa 1976). 2007;32(24):E702-7.
89. Carreon LY, Glassman SD, Campbell MJ. Pediatric spine fractures: a review of 137 hospital admissions. J Spinal Disord Tech. 2004;17(6):477-82.
90. Kakihara T, Watanabe A, Imai C, et al. Chemotherapy-induced multiple vertebral compression fractures in a boy with acute lymphoblastic leukemia. Pediatr Int. 2002;44(6):683-5.
91. Hasler C, Jeanneret B. Pediatric spinal injuries. Orthopade. 2002;31(1):65-73.

CHAPTER 16 Pediatric Spinal Column: Congenital Anomalies

Juliann Kwak Lee, Mauricio Silva

SPINAL COLUMN

Basilar Impression

The encroachment of the foramen magnum secondary to the superior migration of the odontoid process is known as basilar impression. The congenital form of basilar impression is often associated with other abnormalities of the upper cervical spine, including hypoplasia of the occipital condyles or the atlas, odontoid abnormalities, atlanto-occipital synostosis, or abnormalities of the ring of the atlas leading to lateral displacement of the lateral masses. Basilar impression is commonly seen in patients with achondroplasia and Klippel-Feil syndrome.[1]

It has been postulated that the underdevelopment of the occipital somites as a result of insufficient paraxial mesoderm, with an associated shortening of the clivus and anteroposterior enlargement of the foramen magnum, is responsible for the development of the congenital form of basilar impression.[2]

With proximal migration of the dens, the lower portion of the brain stem can be impacted. Children with basilar impression often demonstrate a short, stiff neck, but can be asymptomatic until the second or third decade of life.[3] At times, symptoms are elicited by minor trauma. Clinically, patients present with neck pain, muscle weakness, posterior column and spinothalamic tract dysfunction, a low hairline, a webbed, short and stiff neck, and localized torticollis.[3]

Diagnosis of basilar impression is usually made on plain lateral radiographs of the cervical spine. Several lines have been described to diagnose basilar impression, including the lines of Chamberlain, McGregor, McRae, and Wackenheim.[1] While the definition of each line is different, they all assess the amount of proximal migration of the dens. A migration of the dens above the level of the opening of the foramen magnum is likely to result in neurologic deficits.[1] While screening can be effectively performed with plain radiographs, the assessment of the potential impingement of neural structures is better accomplished with the use of magnetic resonance imaging (MRI).

The use of traction with the aim of reducing the compression of neural structures by the dens is usually considered as the first line of treatment for patients with basilar impression. If successful, a posterior stabilization and fusion can be used to maintain the reduction. If reduction is not achieved by traction, a transoral decompression, followed by posterior stabilization and fusion, might be required.[3]

Atlantoaxial Instability and Down Syndrome

Down syndrome (trisomy 21) is probably the most common human malformation pattern, affecting about 1:660 live births.[4] In addition to cardiac, ophthalmologic, gastrointestinal, infectious and endocrine disorders,[5-7] multiple musculoskeletal issues have been recognized in patients with Down syndrome. These include cervical instability, hip abnormalities, patellofemoral instability, and foot deformities. Laxity of ligamentous structures, commonly seen in patients with Down syndrome, is thought to be associated with the origin of these musculoskeletal issues.[8]

Cervical instability can be observed both at the occipitocervical junction and at the atlantoaxial junction. Of the two, atlantoaxial instability has been more commonly described in this population.[4,8-19] The integrity of the odontoid process (dens of C2) and the transverse ligament, which holds the dens of C2 against the atlas, have been described as the two major structures supplying stability of the atlantoaxial joint.[20] Laxity of the transverse ligament in patients with Down syndrome is thought to be associated with an increased mobility at the C1–C2 level,[8] with a resultant increase in the distance between the posterior surface of the anterior arch of C1 and the anterior surface of the dens of C2 (atlantodens interval, or ADI). As the ADI increases, the space available for the cord (SAC) decreases. Therefore, determination of the ADI provides valuable information to assess the risk of cord compression. It has been reported that between 10% and 30% of patients with Down syndrome have an ADI of more than 4–5 mm.[6,8,9,21-24] In general, an ADI of >10 mm can lead to a significantly decreased SAC, eventually resulting in the development of myelopathy. While radiographic evaluation of the ADI provides indirect information regarding the SAC, MRI evaluation of the spinal canal with supervised flexion/extension[4] has gained popularity as an effective tool to qualitatively assess the spinal cord and SAC.[6]

It has been suggested that, in patients with Down syndrome, abnormal radiographic findings (represented by an increased ADI) do not directly correlate with neurologic abnormalities.[25] Therefore, the assessment of the Down syndrome patient must include a complete history of the type and amount of physical activity performed by the patient, a careful physical and neurological examination, and a radiographic evaluation of the cervical spine. Cervical stenosis secondary to instability can manifest by a history of diminished physical activity, gait disturbance, hyperreflexia, the presence of primitive reflexes, and loss of bladder control.[4,6]

Pizutillo and Herman proposed an algorithm for the management of patients with Down syndrome that takes into account both, clinical and radiological findings.[6] According to this algorithm—(1) patients who are asymptomatic and have an ADI of less than 4.5 mm can continue performing full, unrestricted activities; (2) those who are asymptomatic and have a normal neurological examination, but in whom the ADI is between 4.5 mm and 10 mm, are considered at risk; therefore, they must avoid high contact activities such as boxing, diving, football, gymnastics, ice hockey, rugby, soccer, and wrestling; (3) those who are symptomatic and demonstrate neurological abnormalities, in whom the ADI is between 4.5 mm and 10 mm, but have a normal MRI evaluation of the spinal cord, should be managed with close clinical observation and activity restriction; (4) symptomatic patients in whom the MRI evaluation of the spinal cord is abnormal and those with an ADI greater than 10 mm should undergo surgical stabilization.

If surgical management is chosen, a thorough medical evaluation and preoperative planning should be performed. It has been noted that patients with Down syndrome have an increased risk of postoperative complications, including wound dehiscence, infection, loss of reduction, nonunion, junctional instability, and neurological deterioration.[26] The risks and benefits of the operation should be clearly discussed with the patient's family.

Dens Anomalies

Odontoid hypoplasia, aplasia, and os odontoideum have been described in multiple congenital syndromes including 22q11.2 deletion syndrome, Down syndrome, Dyggve-Melchior-Clausen syndrome, Goldenhar syndrome, Hurler syndrome, Kozlowski spondylometaphyseal dysplasia, Maroteaux-Lamy mucopolysaccharidosis syndrome, metatropic dysplasia, Morquio syndrome, mucopolysaccharidoses, multiple epiphyseal dysplasia, pseudoachondroplasia, and spondyloepimetaphyseal dysplasia, among others.[4]

An intact, normal sized, odontoid is a critical component of the C1–C2 stability mechanism. Odontoid congenital malformations, including hypoplasia, aplasia and os odontoideum, that result in an incompetent odontoid process, usually lead to instability and compression of the spinal cord, both in flexion and extension.[27] In patients with pseudoachondroplasia, the instability due to the presence of os odontoideum seems to increase with age;[28] therefore, continued surveillance is of critical importance. As is the case with other entities associated with C1–C2 instability, congenital abnormalities of the dens can present with a broad range of clinical findings, from mild local symptoms (neck pain, headaches) to severe myelopathy.[29] A complete history, a careful physical and neurological examination, and a thorough radiographic evaluation of the cervical spine is required. As it is with patients with Down syndrome, it is critical to obtain a complete history of the type and amount of physical activity performed by the patient with congenital anomalies of the odontoid. While everyday physiological loads might be tolerated in the presence of congenital anomalies of the odontoid, minor trauma can lead to neurological injury in such cases. In general, plain odontoideum. Based on the radiographic position of the tip of the dens, the os odontoideum can be orthotopic (in its anatomic position) or dystopic (in any other position). Dynamic lateral radiographs are useful to determine the presence of instability. If surgery is planned, a high-resolution, multiplanar computed tomography (CT) scan should be obtained to assess the anatomy of the os odontoideum and any other associated cervical or skull base anomalies.

In general, patients with neurological symptoms or with significant neck pain should be considered for surgical stabilization.[27] C1–C2 fusion with either semi-rigid (wires or cable constructs) or rigid fixation (trans-articular screws and plate, or rod and screw constructs) can be achieved.[4] Rigid fixation may be difficult and risky in the small bones of infants and young children.

Atlanto-occipital Fusion (Assimilation of the Atlas, Occipitocervical Synostosis)

The fusion of the occiput to the atlas, a failure of segmentation between the 4th occipital and 1st cervical sclerotomes, occurs in about 25% of the population,[30] can be partial or complete, and can be bony or fibrous.[31] This congenital anomaly rarely presents as an isolated deformity; it usually presents in conjunction with basilar invagination, Chiari malformation, Klippel-Feil syndrome or fusion of the second and third cervical vertebrae.[15,32]

The presence of an atlanto-occipital fusion results in heavy mechanical demands at the atlantoaxial segment which, associated with an often weakened or absent transverse atlantal ligament,[33] can result in instability.[1] As the instability progresses, basilar invagination can ensue.[1] Patients with an atlanto-occipital fusion usually become symptomatic due to the instability at the extremities, weakness, numbness, hyperreflexia, spasticity, a short neck, limited neck mobility, and a low hair line.[1,32] Unilateral atlanto-occipital fusion can present as a torticollis in a young child. Once suspected, adequate imaging modalities, including plain radiographs, CT scan, and MRI should be obtained.

An atlanto-occipital fusion, especially in the presence of atlantoaxial instability, constitutes a serious risk to severe neurological impairment and death. Modification of activities, bracing, and traction, can be used for patients without evidence of segmental instability or neurological compromise. Once neurological signs and symptoms develop, consideration should be given to surgical management. In the presence of an anterior arch of C1 fused to the occiput without associated atlantoaxial instability, the resection of the posterior elements of the atlas can be considered.[1] In the presence of instability, decompression and fusion should be included in the surgical plan.[1]

Klippel-Feil Syndrome

While a congenital segmentation defect of some or all cervical vertebrae is the common denominator of this syndrome,[34-36] a wide spectrum of anomalies that include congenital scoliosis, rib abnormalities, deafness, Sprengel's deformity, synkinesia, cervical ribs, and genitourinary and cardiovascular abnormalities have been associated with it.[36] A triad of short neck, low posterior hairline, and severe restrictions of cervical motion was originally described with this syndrome;[37] however, it is now apparent that, of all patients with congenital defects of the cervical spine, fewer than 50% have all three signs present.[34,36] Some estimation would suggest that Klippel-Feil syndrome occurs in approximately 1:40,000 births, with a slight female predilection.[38] It appears to have a multifactorial etiology.[34]

Earlier classification schemes of Klippel-Feil syndrome were based on the anatomic distribution of the fused segments. With recent advances in genetic mapping, the mode of inheritance, in combination with the location of the most rostral synostosis, has been used as the base for a new classification system.[39] Klippel-Feil 1 (KF1), with an autosomal recessive inheritance, demonstrates fusions at C1 with or without more caudal fusions; Klippel-Feil 2 (KF2), with an autosomal dominant inheritance, has the most rostral fusion at C2–C3; Klippel-Feil 3 (KF3), with either autosomal dominant or recessive inheritance, demonstrates isolated fusions of the cervical spine caudal to C1 and C2–C3; and Klippel-Feil 4 (KF4), with an X-linked dominant inheritance pattern, is associated with congenital cervical synostosis, congenital hearing loss, and the Duane anomaly (Wildervanck syndrome).[39]

In general, the type and severity of the cervical fusions and associated anomalies can influence the evaluation, natural history, and treatment of the disease. While an asymptomatic cervical synostosis is occasionally found incidentally on radiographs made for a different purpose, patients with Klippel-Feil syndrome are usually diagnosed after complaints of pain, neurologic symptoms, and/or decreased mobility of the cervical spine.[36] Once a synostosis of the cervical spine has been found, it is imperative to obtain high quality radiographs of the entire cervical, thoracic, and lumbar spine to assess the magnitude of the fusion, to evaluate for other abnormalities, and to monitor for the development of scoliosis.[36,40] If instability or stenosis is suspected, magnetic resonance imaging should be obtained to determine the space available for the cord, to assess the presence and severity of spinal stenosis caused by the synostosis, and to rule-out the presence of other abnormalities, including syringomyelia, diastomyelia, or tethered cord.[36] Given the wide spectrum of anomalies that can be associated with Klippel-Feil syndrome, a comprehensive assessment that includes neurologic, cardiovascular, renal, audiologic, gastrointestinal, respiratory and dermatologic evaluation should be considered.[40]

Clinically, the presentation of Klippel-Feil syndrome patients is quite variable; they can be asymptomatic and have a synostosis incidentally found on a radiograph, have decreased range of motion of the neck due to cervical spinal abnormalities, present with cervical or radicular pain from degenerative changes, or complain of symptoms related to abnormalities in organ systems that undergo embryological development at the same time as the cervical spine.[36,40] While the presentation might be variable, it is key to recognize the presence of syndrome in order to address possible issues regarding cervical instability, hypermobility, stenosis and degeneration.[34,36,41] Symptomatic instability has been specifically associated with three fusion patterns: (1) fusion at C2–C3 in the presence of occipitocervical synostosis; (2) multilevel fusion in the presence of an abnormal occipitocervical junction; (3) two fused segment separated by an open interspace.[42]

Most patients with stable fusion patterns will be asymptomatic.[35] Symptomatic treatment, including modification of activities, bracing, and traction, can be used for patients without evidence of segmental instability or neurological compromise.[40,42] However, it is important to recognize that minor traumatic events have resulted in catastrophic spinal cord injuries.[1,43-49] In the presence of symptomatic segmental instability or neurologic compromise, surgical stabilization of the abnormal region of the cervical spine should be considered.[36]

Muscular Torticollis

Torticollis, defined as a head tilted and abnormally rotated, can be a primary deformity due to typical congenital muscular shortening or secondary to osseous malformations, inflammation, or neurogenic disorders. Up to 82% of all torticollis appear to be of congenital origin;[50] Klippel-Feil syndrome and its associated osseous malformations, ocular disorders, brachial plexus palsy, and lesions involving the central nervous system (including posterior fossa and cervical tumors, syringomyelia, and Arnold-Chiari malformations) account for the majority of the remaining cases.[50] Basilar impression, atlanto-occipital anomalies, unilateral absence of C1, familial cervical dysplasia, and atlantoaxial rotatory displacement are among the osseous abnormalities that can result in torticollis.

With congenital muscular torticollis, a painless contracture of the sternocleidomastoid muscle leads to an ipsilateral head tilt and a contralateral head rotation. This deformity, which is typically noted in the first 2 months of life, has been associated with hip dysplasia,[51,52] metatarsus adductus, and clubfoot.[53] Although the etiology of congenital muscular torticollis remains unclear, fibrosis of the sternocleidomastoid muscle due to an intramuscular bleed or a compartment syndrome,[54] primary myopathy[55] or intrauterine crowding have been proposed as possible causes.

SPINAL CORD

Myelomeningocele

Neural tube defects are the most common severely disabling birth defects of the central nervous system, including the spinal cord and brain.[56] The main types of neural tube defects are anencephaly, encephalocele, and spina bifida. In particular, spina bifida includes meningocele and myelomeningocele. Meningocele is characterized by a posterior vertebral defect that allows for a protrusion of a cystic sac containing meninges but no spinal cord. There can be minimal disability. More commonly, myelomeningocele is a herniation of a cystic sac containing meninges and spinal cord through the posterior vertebral defect. Invariably, there is associated neurologic deficit, which results with disabling handicaps. In myelomeningocele, this protrusion of the neural contents can occur anywhere along the spinal column

SECTION 2

but is most common in the lumbar region. The degree of disability depends on the level of the lesion.

The nervous system develops by the formation of a tubular structure or neurulation, and this closure is completed by 24 to 26 days of gestation. The myelomeningocele is thought to form when the neural folds fail to fuse or when a rupture of a previously closed neural tube occurs. Thus the myelomeningocele is formed by the protrusion of spinal cord and meninges within a cyst-like sac through the defect in the posterior vertebral arches. Often times, there is no skin covering this protrusion. Other concomitant abnormalities of the spinal cord are split cord malformation, diastematomyelia, and vertebral bony anomalies that may cause congenital scoliosis and kyphosis.

The incidence of myelomeningocele is less than 1 in 1,000 births in the United States. At birth, defects are noted more common in females than males, with a ratio of 1.2:1.0. The precise cause of neural tube defects is not exactly known but possible predisposing factors are diabetes mellitus, family history, exposure to anticonvulsants or nutritional, and dietary deficiencies.[57] In particular, research data has shown that maternal vitamin deficiencies, especially of folate, play a role in the pathogenesis of neural tube defects, suggesting that supplementation may be preventative.[58-60] Currently, the Food and Drug Administration recommends that women of childbearing age who are planning to become pregnant take 0.4 mg of folic acid before conception and during early pregnancy. The Centers for Disease Control and Prevention also recommend that high-risk women receive 4 mg of folate per day. Advanced technologies have allowed more sensitive means for prenatal diagnosis by serum markers as well as by more sophisticated ultrasound and imaging modalities.

The diagnosis of myelomeningocele is determined in utero. The serum marker for alpha-fetoprotein is a standard part of the maternal screening tests and is elevated with fetal neural tube defects. If an elevated maternal alpha-fetoprotein level is detected, amniocentesis is performed to check the amniotic fluid for alpha-fetoprotein. In addition, ultrasound evaluation of the fetus is used to confirm the diagnosis and evaluate the fetus for additional anomalies.

Over 90% of children with myelomeningocele also have hydrocephalus, which is an imbalance between the production and absorption of cerebrospinal fluid (CSF). This incidence is related to the neurological level of the lesion; the higher level of the lesion, the greater incidence. Cerebrospinal shunting usually alleviates hydrocephalus. Children who do not require shunting have a better prognosis for upper extremity function, trunk balance, and gait.[61]

The neurosurgical approach for newborns with myelomeningocele is sac closure within 48 hours of birth, with subsequent ventriculoperitoneal shunting for hydrocephalus. Timely surgical closure of the exposed neural elements prevents spinal infection and improves patient survival. Recently a prospective study has shown that in utero closure of the defect may allow future better motor function and decrease need for ventriculoperitoneal shunting, however without beneficial consequence for urologic function.[62] This study did also note that in utero sac closure can lead to higher morbidity/mortality for the mother and fetus. In addition, the neurosurgeon will be actively assessing for shunt malfunction, brainstem compromise by the Arnold-Chiari II malformation, the development of syringomyelia, and symptoms consistent with a tethered cord.[63,64]

Shunt malfunction or infection can result in further neurological deterioration, such signs of shunt failure include nausea, vomiting, and severe headaches. Hydrocephalus can also result in syringomyelia, which is an accumulation of fluid in the enlarged central canal of the spinal cord. Syringomyelia can cause problems in patients with myelomeningocele including an increasing level of paralysis of the lower extremities, progressive scoliosis, and weakness of the upper extremities. Brainstem abnormalities, as in Arnold Chiari malformation, can coexist with hydrocephalus. The type II Chiari malformation is most often seen with children with myelomeningocele and is characterized by caudal displacement of the medulla oblongata into the cervical neural canal through the foramen magnum. This displacement causes dysfunction of the lower cranial nerves. Symptoms can include nystagmus, stridor, difficulty in swallowing, and depressed cough reflex. Tethered cord is also a consistent finding in children with myelomeningocele. Clinical signs of cord tethering are loss of motor function, development of spasticity in the lower extremities such as in the medial hamstrings and ankle dorsiflexors and evertors, development of scoliosis before age 6 years, increase lumbar lordosis, and changes in urologic function.

Urologic evaluation begins with postnatal urodynamic evaluation of bladder function. The goals for urologic treatment include maintaining continence, preserving renal function, and minimizing the frequency of urinary tract infections.

Patients with myelomeningocele have latex hypersensitivity, presumably acquired from repeated exposure starting early in life. This allergy is type I, IgE-mediated, and can cause anaphylaxis and death.

Classification for myelomeningocele is based on three neurological regions of the lesion. Group I patients have a thoracic or high lumbar lesion typically without quadriceps function. These patients are unlikely to become community ambulators. Group II patients have a low lumbar lesion and can demonstrate good quadriceps and medial hamstring function with poor gluteus medius strength. These patients are likely able to ambulate though require AFOs and assistive devices for stability. Group III patients have lower level lesion at the sacrum with minimal disability and can ambulate without external support and may not require any orthoses. The distinction for independent ambulation is seen in children with lesions between L4 and L3, where the walking child demonstrates knee extension power. Prerequisites for walking include a spinal sagittal and coronal balance, absence of hip and knee contractures, and plantigrade supple or braceable feet.

Tethered Cord and Occult Spinal Dysraphism

Tethered Cord Syndrome

Tethered cord syndrome describes a pathologic fixation or traction of the spinal cord from an abnormally low position such that the spinal cord undergoes mechanical stretch, distortion, and possible ischemia.[65] Many conditions, including myelomeningocele and occult spinal dysraphisms, can be the cause of cord tethering.

Problems of tethered cord arise in areas involving sensorimotor, urologic, and orthopedic issues. Sensorimotor symptoms present as pain, delayed walking, sensory loss, and motor weakness.[66] Urologic dysfunction begins to manifest with persistent urinary tract infections due to incomplete emptying, urinary incontinence or impotence, and hydronephrosis secondary to reflux. Orthopedic changes from tethered cord appear in gait disturbances, progressive foot deformities, and scoliosis.[67,68] The radio imaging of choice is MRI. It is important to obtain a complete evaluation of the spinal cord to rule out adjacent anomalies such as syrinx or Chiari malformation.

The treatment for tethered cord is surgical release from a posterior approach.[69] Many advocate surgical release even if the patient is asymptomatic, in order to prevent future neurologic deterioration. Good prognosis of surgical untethering is correlated to a shorter duration of symptoms.[65]

Occult Spinal Dysraphism

Occult spinal dysraphism (OSD) refers to a spectrum of congenital anomalies characterized by an incomplete fusion of midline mesenchymal, bony, or neural elements of the spine. This collection of malformations is thought to arise from incomplete formation of the dorsal midline structures during early embryogenesis. Occult spinal dysraphism is characterized by skin-covered lesions without exposed neural tissue such as focal hairy patches, caudal appendage or hemangioma.[70,71] These pathologic entities may be found in isolation or in various combinations and are often associated with midline cutaneous changes typically over the lumbosacral area as described above. Specific pathologies that makeup the constellation of OSD include split cord malformation, filum terminale syndrome, lipomyelomeningocele, dermal sinus tracts, neurenteric cyst, and anterior sacral meningocele. The true incidence of OSD is not known, and unlike myelomeningocele, OSD is usually diagnosed only in patients with cutaneous stigmata or symptoms or is found incidentally after investigation for unrelated problems.[72]

Split Cord Malformation

Split cord malformation is a form of closed neural tube defect in which the spinal cord is longitudinally split by a fibrous band or bone spicule. There are two types of split cord phenomenon, as described by Pang and coworkers in 1992.[73,74] The embryonic mechanisms are common between the two types; there the defect in the midline ectoendodermal adhesion tract during gastrulation determines the classification between the two types of split cord malformations. Type I, previously termed diastematomyelia, consists of two hemicords contained within separate dural tubes, separated by an osteocartilaginous septum that extends from the vertebral body to the neural arches. This septum is rigid and entirely extradural. Type II consists of the hemicords residing within a common dural tube, without the rigid bisecting septum.

Split cord malformations are typically seen in females, where they may initially present with spinal cord dysfunction or scoliosis, often times from congenital vertebral anomalies and hemivertebrae and block vertebrae.[75,76] About 50–80% of patients with split cord malformations may demonstrate cutaneous findings, which do not necessarily locate the level of the pathology. The cord above and below the split cord is generally normal and symmetrical, with 10% of malformations demonstrating asymmetry.

Neurologic symptoms may not arise until adulthood, when traction of the spinal cord against the restricting septum/bony spur which prohibits the ascent of the cord. The average age of presentation can manifest as early as 5 years old, demonstrating gait disturbances. If an adult is presenting for the first time, the common complaints are low back pain or shooting pain down the leg. Traction or tethered cord symptoms also include sensory changes, urologic dysfunction, abnormal spine curvature, typically kyphoscoliosis.

Radiography of choice is MRI, where the coronal and axial views will delineate the split cord malformation clearly. The entire spine should be evaluated to detect any other secondary occult spinal dysraphisms such as associated tight filum terminale, a lipoma, a dermoid cyst or a second spur.

Indications for surgery include progressive neurologic deficit and prophylactically resection of the spur or release of any tethering prior to scoliosis surgery. The surgical goal is to release the traction from the fibrous, bony septum in order to relieve symptoms, preserve function, and reverse neurologic deficits.[77] Complications include persistent CSF leakage and less likely, epidural hemorrhage. Long-standing deformities and scoliosis are unlikely to improve, but studies have shown that bowel and bladder dysfunction can improve up to 40%, neurologic sensorimotor may return approximately 5–10%, and reliably, pain can improve.[77]

Dermal Sinus Tract

Dermal sinus tracts are remnants of the incomplete neural tube closure that consist of epithelial-lined tract extending from the skin surface to the spinal fascia, dura mater or spinal cord. They result from abnormal ectodermal adhesion of the neural tube to the dermis. These lesions can be found anywhere along the dorsal midline of the neural axis, but are more common in the lumbosacral region.[78] Lumbosacral tracts ascend the midline to their destination, whereas cranial dermal sinuses descend from their origin. A dermal sinus may occur as a solitary lesion or in combination with other spinal dysraphism such as split cord malformation and midline bony anomalies.[78,79]

The small dimpling or opening may be overlooked in the physical examination and the dermal sinus may not be discovered until there are signs of cord tethering or persistent infections. Chronic bouts of meningitis,[80] especially by unusual organisms, and epidural and subdural abscesses have been reported,[81] and can often be the first indication for a dermal sinus. Dermal sinus tracts may be associated with spinal fluid drainage, intradural dermoid or epidermoid cysts and spinal cord tethering. Common cutaneous finding associated with dermal sinus tracts include a pit, flat capillary hemangiomas, hypertrichosis, subcutaneous lipomas, drainage of debris or fluid from the pit and signs of local infection. In addition to symptoms consistent with tethered cord, a common neurological finding is spinal cord compression secondary to the mass effect of intradural dermoid cyst growth.

Clinical identification of the dermal sinus may be enough for diagnosis, but MRI studies are necessary to determine the extent of the sinus tract involvement as well as any associated spinal pathology.[78,82] Treatment in the past has consisted of either superficial resection or intradural surgical exploration.[79] However, currently it is recommended that the tract be traced surgically to its termination and resected with any terminal dermoids.[83,84]

Lipomeningocele

Lipomeningocele may resemble a closed myelomeningocele, however the neural elements remain inside and only the lipoma mass protrudes through the spina bifida defect. Typically, this can present in a newborn as a subcutaneous mass in the midline dorsal lumbosacral region. There can be associated cutaneous manifestations as well as anorectal and urogenital anomalies.[85] Children, who are older than 1-year-old, may develop progressive symptoms consistent with tethered cord syndrome.

The presence of lipomeningocele can be detected, as early as in utero, however with ultrasound techniques,[86] it is still difficult to exclude myelomeningocele. The imaging modality of choice is MRI, where fatty tumors are clearly visualized on T1-weighted images. The typical MRI of a lipomeningocele shows a low-lying conus with the fatty mass located dorsally or caudally.

The treatment for lipomeningocele is recommended surgical resection and untethering. The preferred timing for the lipoma resection is during infancy, thus becoming prophylactic surgery to prevent the onset of neuromotor deterioration and urologic dysfunction.[87,88] Early surgery has shown to be effective and safe, as well as maximizing functional outcome. Orthopedic evaluation is also warranted because of the associated deformities observed in this condition, most commonly cavovarus or equinovarus foot deformities.[89]

Filum Terminale Syndrome

The filum terminale is a viscoelastic band that stabilizes the distal end of the cord and decreases its movement within the spinal canal. However certain pathologies such as abnormal thickening or fatty infiltration can cause tension or traction of the cord, thereby causing a tethered cord syndrome.[90] A hypertrophied filum terminale can allow the conus medullaris to be bound in a low position, preventing natural ascension of the cord with development. The conus typically sits at the L1–L2 interspace, however it is abnormal if it sits below L2 at age 5 years or older. Though there may be visible cutaneous manifestations of an abnormal filum terminale, the first presenting symptoms may be progressive urologic dysfunction[91] and uncoordinated bladder activity, consistent with signs of tethered cord. Orthopedic issues involve progressive scoliosis,[92] leg/foot atrophy, lower extremity weakness or spasticity.[93]

Magnetic resonance imaging is the best modality to evaluate filum terminale pathology. The MRI will clearly show the location of the caudally displaced filum and stretched out conus, the fatty infiltration in the T1-weighted scans or the thickening of the filum.[94] Once identified, the symptomatic patient is recommended to undergo surgical untethering or sectioning of the filum to relieve the traction effect on the cord. Many surgeons may also advocate prophylactic untethering or sectioning in the asymptomatic patient with a low-lying conus to prevent future neuromotor deterioration.[95]

Neurenteric Cysts

Spinal neurenteric cysts, also known as enterogenous cysts, are infrequent congenital abnormalities believed to be derived from an abnormal connection between the primitive endoderm and ectoderm during the 3rd week of embryogenesis. This abnormal connection results in lesions within the spinal axis that are heterotopic mucus-secreting epithelium reminiscent of the gastrointestinal tract.[96] These cysts are not necessarily confined to the spinal column, but can be found within the brain, mediastinum, abdomen, pelvis or in a subcutaneous region. Most neurenteric cysts are located in the intradural/extramedullary compartment, while less than 10% of lesions are divided between an intradural/intramedullary or extradural location. Neurenteric cysts are classically described as solitary lesions in the cervical region, located anterior or anterolateral to the cord.[96] If bone abnormalities are present, they are likely to involve the anterior column. However other studies have shown that these cysts also arise dorsal to the cord in the thoracolumbar region. Often, the presence of the cyst can be associated with another forms of occult spinal dysraphism, scoliosis, and spina bifida.[97] In addition, neurenteric cysts can coexist with visceral abnormalities of the gastrointestinal, renal, and cardiac systems.

Adult patients may present with focal back pain, myelopathic changes or radicular symptoms. The pediatric population exhibits a more variable clinical picture, including meningitis, incontinence, and paraplegia. As with the previously discussed spinal lesions, MRI can clearly elucidate location of the neurenteric cyst, especially in the T2-weighted images, as well as reveal other associated anomalies. Surgical excision is the preferred treatment with goal of complete resection without neural compromise. Most cysts are located intramedullary and extradural, which allows a more straightforward dissection plane and successful complete resection. Resolution of neuromotor deficits from the cyst is essentially achieved with complete surgical excision.[98] However the cysts that are located intradural may contain adhesions and allow for only a partial resection, which then increases the risk of recurrence of cyst formation and of neuromotor changes.

Anterior Sacral Meningocele

Anterior sacral meningocele is a rare spinal dysraphism, where there is a herniation of dural sac through a defect in the anterior surface of the spine, typically in the sacrum. The sac is typically composed of the outer dural membrane and inner arachnoid membrane, and contains cerebrospinal fluid and variable neural elements. Anterior sacral meningocele may have concomitant genitourinary malformations. However, unlike the typical myelomeningocele, there is no hydrocephalus or Chiari malformation.

This entity usually presents in adulthood as a pelvic mass, where patients complain of pressure on their pelvic structures.[99] When symptoms arise in infants and children, their main complaints are chronic constipation or urinary difficulties.[100] Anteroposterior radiographs may show a lucent defect or complete absence of the sacrum. Abdominal ultrasound can help diagnose anterior sacral meningocele and distinguish it from a cystic pelvic mass. But MRI is the best imaging modality to delineate the communication between the spinal canal and the anterior portion of the vertebral column.[100]

There have been reports of morbidity of pelvic obstruction with labor[101] or rectum erosion and fistula formation[102,103] followed by infection such as meningitis.[104] Therefore, it is recommended that patients with anterior sacral meningocele undergo surgical closure of the communication between the meningocele and subarachnoid space and meningocele excision to decompress the pelvic structures.[105,106] Also, if necessary, cord detethering should be performed.

Sacral Agenesis

Sacral agenesis is an uncommon congenital disorder that denotes absence of part or all of lower sacral and coccygeal vertebral segments.[107,108] Typically, this vertebral column disorder is accompanied by a wide range of abnormalities,[109] especially involving the gastrointestinal system and genitourinary tract.[110,111] Children will typically present with persistent urinary tract infections, bladder dysfunction, and constipation. Classic clinical findings include the "Buddha" sitting position with the arms resting on the hips to provide sitting support to the upper spine. Often times, knee flexion contractures and clubfeet are present. Treatment is based on individual's orthopaedic needs.[112] Lower extremity contractures and deformities can be released and corrected. Lumbosacral stabilization to the pelvis may be warranted for patients who have sitting imbalance or discomfort.

REFERENCES

1. Klimo P, Rao G, Brockmeyer D. Congenital anomalies of the cervical spine. Neurosurg Clin N Am. 2007;18:463-78.
2. Marin-Padilla M. Cephalic axial skeletal-neural dysraphic disorders: embryology and pathology. Can J Neurol Sci. 1991;18:153-69.
3. Goel A, Bhatjiwale M, Desai K. Basilar invagination: a study based on 190 surgically treated patients. J Neurosurg. 1998;88:962-8.
4. McKay SD, Al-Omari A, Tomlinson LA, et al. Review of cervical spine anomalies in genetic syndromes. Spine (Phila Pa 1976). 2012;37:E269-77.
5. Mik G, Gholve PA, Scher DM, et al. Down syndrome: orthopedic issues. Curr Opin Pediatr. 2008;20:30-6.
6. Pizzutillo PD, Herman MJ. Cervical spine issues in Down syndrome. J Pediatr Orthop. 2005;25:253-9.
7. van Allen MI, Fung J, Jurenka SB. Health care concerns and guidelines for adults with Down syndrome. Am J Med Genet. 1999;89:100-10.
8. Caird MS, Wills BP, Dormans JP. Down syndrome in children: the role of the orthopaedic surgeon. J Am Acad Orthop Surg. 2006;14:610-9.
9. Brockmeyer D. Down syndrome and craniovertebral instability. Topic review and treatment recommendations. Pediatr Neurosurg. 1999;31:71-7.
10. Burke SW, French HG, Roberts JM, et al. Chronic atlanto-axial instability in Down syndrome. J Bone Joint Surg Am. 1985;67:1356-60.
11. Davidson RG. Atlantoaxial instability in individuals with Down syndrome: a fresh look at the evidence. Pediatrics. 1988;81:857-65.
12. Hankinson TC, Anderson RC. Craniovertebral junction abnormalities in Down syndrome. Neurosurgery. 2010;66:32-8.
13. Martel W, Tishler JM. Observations on the spine in mongoloidism. Am J Roentgenol Radium Ther Nucl Med. 1966;97:630-8.
14. Martel W, Uyham R, Stimson CW. Subluxation of the atlas causing spinal cord compression in a case of Down's syndrome with a "manifestation of an occipital vertebra". Radiology. 1969;93:839-40.
15. Menezes AH, Ryken TC. Craniovertebral abnormalities in Down's syndrome. Pediatr Neurosurg. 1992;18:24-33.
16. Morton RE, Khan MA, Murray-Leslie C, et al. Atlantoaxial instability in Down's syndrome: a five year follow up study. Arch Dis Child. 1995;72:115-8.
17. Nader-Sepahi A, Casey AT, Hayward R, et al. Symptomatic atlantoaxial instability in Down syndrome. J Neurosurg. 2005;103:231-7.
18. Pueschel SM, Scola FH. Atlantoaxial instability in individuals with Down syndrome: epidemiologic, radiographic, and clinical studies. Pediatrics. 1987;80:555-60.
19. Pueschel SM, Scola FH, Pezzullo JC. A longitudinal study of atlanto-dens relationships in asymptomatic individuals with Down syndrome. Pediatrics. 1992;89:1194-8.
20. White AA, Panjabi MM. The clinical biomechanics of the occipitoatlantoaxial complex. Orthop Clin North Am. 1978;9:867-78.
21. Doyle JS, Lauerman WC, Wood KB, et al. Complications and long-term outcome of upper cervical spine arthrodesis in patients with Down syndrome. Spine (Phila Pa 1976). 1996;21:1223-31.

CHAPTER 16

22. Ferguson RL, Putney ME, Allen BL. Comparison of neurologic deficits with atlanto-dens intervals in patients with Down syndrome. J Spinal Disord. 1997;10:246-52.
23. Pueschel SM, Scola FH, Tupper TB, et al. Skeletal anomalies of the upper cervical spine in children with Down syndrome. J Pediatr Orthop. 1990;10:607-11.
24. Taggard DA, Menezes AH, Ryken TC. Treatment of Down syndrome-associated craniovertebral junction abnormalities. J Neurosurg. 2000;93:205-13.
25. Roy M, Baxter M, Roy A. Atlantoaxial instability in Down syndrome—guidelines for screening and detection. J R Soc Med. 1990;83:433-5.
26. Crostelli M, Mariani M, Mazza O, et al. Cervical fixation in the pediatric patient: our experience. Eur Spine J. 2009;18(Suppl 1):20-8.
27. Klimo P, Coon V, Brockmeyer D. Incidental os odontoideum: current management strategies. Neurosurg Focus. 2011;31:E10.
28. Shetty GM, Song HR, Unnikrishnan R, et al. Upper cervical spine instability in pseudoachondroplasia. J Pediatr Orthop. 2007;27:782-7.
29. Rowland LP, Shapiro JH, Jacobson HG. Neurological syndromes associated with congenital absence of the odontoid process. AMA Arch Neurol Psychiatry. 1958;80:286-91.
30. McRae DL, Barnum AS. Occipitalization of the atlas. Am J Roentgenol Radium Ther Nucl Med. 1953;70:23-46.
31. Ryken TC, Menezes AH. Cervicomedullary compression by separate atlantal lateral mass. Pediatr Neurosurg. 1993;19:165-8.
32. Hensinger RN. Osseous anomalies of the craniovertebral junction. Spine (Phila Pa 1976). 1986;11:323-33.
33. Wackenheim A. Occipitalization of the ventral part and vertebralization of the dorsal part of the atlas with insufficiency of the transverse ligament. Neuroradiology. 1982;24:45-7.
34. Kaplan KM, Spivak JM, Bendo JA. Embryology of the spine and associated congenital abnormalities. Spine J. 2005;5:564-76.
35. Theiss SM, Smith MD, Winter RB. The long-term follow-up of patients with Klippel-Feil syndrome and congenital scoliosis. Spine (Phila Pa 1976). 1997;22:1219-22.
36. Tracy MR, Dormans JP, Kusumi K. Klippel-Feil syndrome: clinical features and current understanding of etiology. Clin Orthop Relat Res. 2004;424:183-90.
37. Klippel M, Feil A. The classic: a case of absence of cervical vertebrae with the thoracic cage rising to the base of the cranium (cervical thoracic cage). Clin Orthop Relat Res. 1975;109:3-8.
38. Thomsen MN, Schneider U, Weber M, et al. Scoliosis and congenital anomalies associated with Klippel-Feil syndrome types I-III. Spine (Phila Pa 1976). 1997;22:396-401.
39. Clarke RA, Catalan G, Diwan AD, et al. Heterogeneity in Klippel-Feil syndrome: a new classification. Pediatr Radiol. 1998;28:967-74.
40. Herman MJ, Pizzutillo PD. Cervical spine disorders in children. Orthop Clin North Am. 1999;30:457-66, ix.
41. Pizzutillo PD, Woods M, Nicholson L, et al. Risk factors in Klippel-Feil syndrome. Spine (Phila Pa 1976). 1994;19:2110-6.
42. Copley LA, Dormans JP. Cervical spine disorders in infants and children. J Am Acad Orthop Surg. 1998;6:204-14.
43. Ducker TB. Cervical myeloradiculopathy: Klippel-Feil deformity. J Spinal Disord. 1990;3:439-40.
44. Elster AD. Quadriplegia after minor trauma in the Klippel-Feil syndrome. A case report and review of the literature. J Bone Joint Surg Am. 1984;66:1473-4.
45. Epstein NE, Epstein JA, Zilkha A. Traumatic myelopathy in a seventeen-year-old child with cervical spinal stenosis (without fracture or dislocation) and a C2-C3 Klippel-Feil fusion. A case report. Spine (Phila Pa 1976). 1984;9:344-7.
46. Hall JE, Simmons ED, Danylchuk K, et al. Instability of the cervical spine and neurological involvement in Klippel-Feil syndrome. A case report. J Bone Joint Surg Am. 1990;72:460-2.
47. Rouvreau P, Glorion C, Langlais J, et al. Assessment and neurologic involvement of patients with cervical spine congenital synostosis as in Klippel-Feil syndrome: study of 19 cases. J Pediatr Orthop B. 1998;7:179-85.
48. Sherk HH, Dawoud S. Congenital os odontoideum with Klippel-Feil anomaly and fatal atlanto-axial instability. Report of a case. Spine (Phila Pa 1976). 1981;6:42-5.
49. Southwell RB, Reynolds AF, Badger VM, et al. Klippel-Feil syndrome with cervical compression resulting from cervical subluxation in association with an omo-vertebral bone. Spine (Phila Pa 1976). 1980;5:480-2.
50. Ballock RT, Song KM. The prevalence of nonmuscular causes of torticollis in children. J Pediatr Orthop. 1996;16:500-4.
51. Hummer CD, MacEwen GD. The coexistence of torticollis and congenital dysplasia of the hip. J Bone Joint Surg Am. 1972;54:1255-6.
52. von HJ, Green DW, Burke SW, et al. The relationship between developmental dysplasia of the hip and congenital muscular torticollis. J Pediatr Orthop. 2006;26:805-8.
53. Lincoln TL, Suen PW. Common rotational variations in children. J Am Acad Orthop Surg. 2003;11:312-20.
54. Davids JR, Wenger DR, Mubarak SJ. Congenital muscular torticollis: sequela of intrauterine or perinatal compartment syndrome. J Pediatr Orthop. 1993;13:141-7.
55. Tang S, Liu Z, Quan X, et al. Sternocleidomastoid pseudotumor of infants and congenital muscular torticollis: fine-structure research. J Pediatr Orthop. 1998;18:214-8.
56. Northrup H, Volcik KA. Spina bifida and other neural tube defects. Curr Probl Pediatr. 2000;30:313-32.
57. Sandler AD. Children with spina bifida: key clinical issues. Pediatr Clin North Am. 2010;57:879-92.
58. Folic acid for the prevention of neural tube defects. American Academy of Pediatrics. Committee on Genetics. Pediatrics. 1999;104:325-7.
59. Oakley GP. Elimination of folic acid-preventable neural tube defects. Am J Prev Med. 2008;35:606-7.
60. Wolff T, Witkop CT, Miller T, et al. Folic acid supplementation for the prevention of neural tube defects: an update of the evidence for the U.S. Preventive Services Task Force. Ann Intern Med. 2009;150:632-9.
61. Battibugli S, Gryfakis N, Dias L, et al. Functional gait comparison between children with myelomeningocele: shunt versus no shunt. Dev Med Child Neurol. 2007;49:764-9.
62. Adzick NS, Thom EA, Spong CY, et al. A randomized trial of prenatal versus postnatal repair of myelomeningocele. N Engl J Med. 2011;364:993-1004.

63. Ansari S, Nejat F, Yazdani S, et al. Split cord malformation associated with myelomeningocele. J Neurosurg. 2007;107:281-5.
64. Piatt JH, Jr. Syringomyelia complicating myelomeningocele: review of the evidence. J Neurosurg. 2004;100:101-9.
65. Cornette L, Verpoorten C, Lagae L, et al. Tethered cord syndrome in occult spinal dysraphism: timing and outcome of surgical release. Neurology. 1998;50:1761-5.
66. James HE, Walsh JW. Spinal dysraphism. Curr Probl Pediatr. 1981;11:1-25.
67. Archibeck MJ, Smith JT, Carroll KL, et al. Surgical release of tethered spinal cord: survivorship analysis and orthopedic outcome. J Pediatr Orthop. 1997;17:773-6.
68. McGirt MJ, Mehta V, Garces-Ambrossi G, et al. Pediatric tethered cord syndrome: response of scoliosis to untethering procedures. Clinical article. J Neurosurg Pediatr. 2009;4:270-4.
69. Lew SM, Kothbauer KF. Tethered cord syndrome: an updated review. Pediatr Neurosurg. 2007;43:236-48.
70. Singh DK, Kumar B, Sinha VD, et al. The human tail: rare lesion with occult spinal dysraphism—a case report. J Pediatr Surg. 2008;43:e41-3.
71. Tubbs RS, Wellons JC, Iskandar BJ, et al. Isolated flat capillary midline lumbosacral hemangiomas as indicators of occult spinal dysraphism. J Neurosurg. 2004;100:86-9.
72. Guggisberg D, Hadj-Rabia S, Viney C, et al. Skin markers of occult spinal dysraphism in children: a review of 54 cases. Arch Dermatol. 2004;140:1109-15.
73. Pang D. Split cord malformation: Part II: Clinical syndrome. Neurosurgery. 1992;31:481-500.
74. Pang D, Dias MS, Ahab-Barmada M. Split cord malformation: Part I: A unified theory of embryogenesis for double spinal cord malformations. Neurosurgery. 1992;31:451-80.
75. Ersahin Y, Mutluer S, Kocaman S, et al. Split spinal cord malformations in children. J Neurosurg. 1998;88:57-65.
76. Mahapatra AK. Split cord malformation—A study of 300 cases at AIIMS 1990-2006. J Pediatr Neurosci. 2011;6:S41-5.
77. Proctor MR, Scott RM. Long-term outcome for patients with split cord malformation. Neurosurg Focus. 2001;10:e5.
78. Radmanesh F, Nejat F, El KM. Dermal sinus tract of the spine. Childs Nerv Syst. 2010;26:349-57.
79. Ackerman LL, Menezes AH. Spinal congenital dermal sinuses: a 30-year experience. Pediatrics. 2003;112:641-7.
80. Wang YM, Chuang MJ, Cheng MH. Infected spinal dermal sinus tract with meningitis: a case report. Acta Neurol Taiwan. 2011;20:188-91.
81. Chen CY, Lin KL, Wang HS, et al. Dermoid cyst with dermal sinus tract complicated with spinal subdural abscess. Pediatr Neurol. 1999;20:157-60.
82. Barkovich AJ, Edwards MS, Cogen PH. MR evaluation of spinal dermal sinus tracts in children. Am J Neuroradiol. 1991;12:123-9.
83. Ackerman LL, Menezes AH, Follett KA. Cervical and thoracic dermal sinus tracts. A case series and review of the literature. Pediatr Neurosurg. 2002;37:137-47.
84. Coumans JV, Walcott BP, Redjal N, et al. En bloc excision of a dermal sinus tract. J Clin Neurosci. 2011;18:554-8.
85. Rendeli C, Ausili E, Tabacco F, et al. Urodynamic evaluation in children with lipomeningocele: timing for neurosurgery, spinal cord tethering and followup. J Urol. 2007;177:2319-24.
86. Sharony R, Aviram R, Tohar M, et al. Prenatal sonographic detection of a lipomeningocele as a sacral lesion. J Clin Ultrasound. 2000;28:150-2.
87. Macejko AM, Cheng EY, Yerkes EB, et al. Clinical urological outcomes following primary tethered cord release in children younger than 3 years. J Urol. 2007;178:1738-42.
88. Satar N, Bauer SB, Scott RM, et al. Late effects of early surgery on lipoma and lipomeningocele in children less than 1 year old. J Urol. 1997;157:1434-7.
89. Gourineni P, Dias L, Blanco R, et al. Orthopaedic deformities associated with lumbosacral spinal lipomas. J Pediatr Orthop. 2009;29:932-6.
90. Tehli O, Hodaj I, Kural C, et al. A comparative study of histopathological analysis of filum terminale in patients with tethered cord syndrome and in normal human fetuses. Pediatr Neurosurg. 2011;47:412-6.
91. Steinbok P, Kariyattil R, MacNeily AE. Comparison of section of filum terminale and non-neurosurgical management for urinary incontinence in patients with normal conus position and possible occult tethered cord syndrome. Neurosurgery. 2007;61:550-5.
92. Chern JJ, Dauser RC, Whitehead WE, et al. The effect of tethered cord release on coronal spinal balance in tight filum terminale. Spine (Phila Pa 1976). 2011;36:E944-9.
93. Cornips EM, Vereijken IM, Beuls EA, et al. Clinical characteristics and surgical outcome in 25 cases of childhood tight filum syndrome. Eur J Paediatr Neurol. 2012;16:103-17.
94. Fabiano AJ, Khan MF, Rozzelle CJ, et al. Preoperative predictors for improvement after surgical untethering in occult tight filum terminale syndrome. Pediatr Neurosurg. 2009;45:256-61.
95. Wehby MC, O'Hollaren PS, Abtin K, et al. Occult tight filum terminale syndrome: results of surgical untethering. Pediatr Neurosurg. 2004;40:51-7.
96. de Oliveira RS, Cinalli G, Roujeau T, et al. Neurenteric cysts in children: 16 consecutive cases and review of the literature. J Neurosurg. 2005;103:512-23.
97. Rauzzino MJ, Tubbs RS, Alexander E, et al. Spinal neurenteric cysts and their relation to more common aspects of occult spinal dysraphism. Neurosurg Focus. 2001;10:e2.
98. Savage JJ, Casey JN, McNeill IT, et al. Neurenteric cysts of the spine. J Craniovertebr Junction Spine. 2010;1:58-63.
99. Liu L, Li J, Huang S, et al. Adult anterior sacral meningoceles misdiagnosed as pelvic cysts. Br J Neurosurg. 2011;25:532-3.
100. Mohta A, Das S, Jindal R. Anterior sacral meningocele presenting as constipation. J Pediatr Neurosci. 2011;6:40-3.
101. Manson F, Comalli-Dillon K, Moriaux A. Anterior sacral meningocele: management in gynecological practice. Ultrasound Obstet Gynecol. 2007;30:893-6.
102. Fitzpatrick MO, Taylor WA. Anterior sacral meningocele associated with a rectal fistula. Case report and review of the literature. J Neurosurg. 1999;91:124-7.
103. Sanchez AA, Iglesias CD, Lopez CD, et al. Rectothecal fistula secondary to an anterior sacral meningocele. J Neurosurg Spine. 2008;8:487-9.

104. Miletic D, Poljak I, Eskinja N, et al. Giant anterior sacral meningocele presenting as bacterial meningitis in a previously healthy adult. Orthopedics. 2008;31:182.
105. Ashley WW, Wright NM. Resection of a giant anterior sacral meningocele via an anterior approach: case report and review of literature. Surg Neurol. 2006;66:89-93.
106. Jeon BC, Kim DH, Kwon KY. Anterior endoscopic treatment of a huge anterior sacral meningocele: technical case report. Neurosurgery. 2003;52:1231-3.
107. Estin D, Cohen AR. Caudal agenesis and associated caudal spinal cord malformations. Neurosurg Clin N Am. 1995;6:377-91.
108. Pang D. Sacral agenesis and caudal spinal cord malformations. Neurosurgery. 1993;32:755-78.
109. Emami-Naeini P, Rahbar Z, Nejat F, et al. Neurological presentations, imaging, and associated anomalies in 50 patients with sacral agenesis. Neurosurgery. 2010;67:894-900.
110. Emami-Naeini P, Nejat F, Rahbar Z, et al. Urological manifestations of sacral agenesis. J Pediatr Urol. 2012;8:181-6.
111. Levitt MA, Patel M, Rodriguez G, et al. The tethered spinal cord in patients with anorectal malformations. J Pediatr Surg. 1997;32:462-8.
112. Caird MS, Hall JM, Bloom DA, et al. Outcome study of children, adolescents, and adults with sacral agenesis. J Pediatr Orthop. 2007;27:682-5.

CHAPTER 17

Spondylolysis and Spondylolisthesis

Haariss Ilyas, Keith Bachmann, Joel Kolmodin, Siddharth A Badve, Ryan Goodwin

INTRODUCTION

Spondylolysis and spondylolisthesis are common spinal pathologies that a clinician comes across in children and adolescents. The term "spondylolysis" refers to anatomic defect of the pars interarticularis without displacement of that specific vertebral body (Fig. 1). "Spondylolisthesis" refers to a defect of the pars interarticularis resulting in either anterior or posterior displacement of that specific vertebral body in relation to its caudal vertebral segment. Both these conditions could be an incidental radiologic finding and symptomatic. On the contrary, both conditions can symptomatically present with low back, with or without neurological manifestations in the pediatric and adolescent population. A variety of etiologies can result in the development of spondylolysis and spondylolisthesis. Upright posture appears to predispose humans to the development of this pathology.

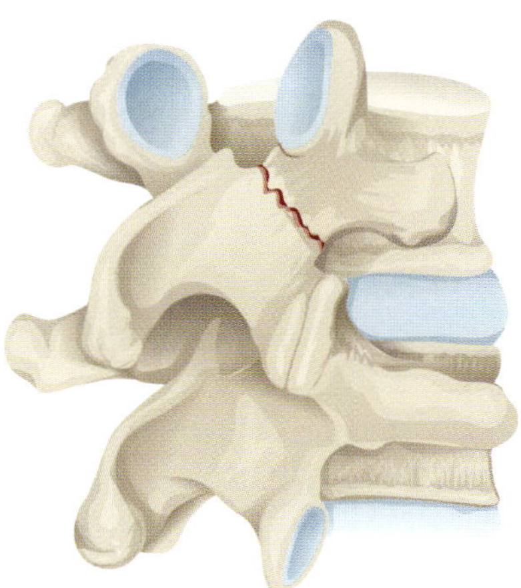

Fig. 1: Spondylolysis.

EPIDEMIOLOGY AND CLASSIFICATION

The current literature reports a 5% incidence of spondylolysis in general population.[1-5] It is found to be much higher in some population subgroups.[4-7] Ambulation in an upright posture transmits significant physiologic stress across the posterior elements of the lumbar spine. This could be a basic predisposing mechanism in the evolution of this pathology in humans. Spondylolysis is almost nonexistent in nonambulatory population.[8] Activities involving repetitive hyperextension and rotational motion in the lumbar spine are a well-known causative factor. Accordingly, spondylolysis is commonly seen in gymnasts, divers, cricket fast bowlers, American football players, and even some dancers. The incidence of spondylolysis in some of high-performance athletes is as high as 47%.[9,10] Genetic factors have also been hypothesized to contribute in the evolution of this condition. A study by Albanese et al. reports high incidence of pars defects and spina bifida occulta in families of patients with spondylolysis.[4,6,7] Spondylolysis typically affects the caudal vertebrae in the lumbar spine, L5 vertebra being most commonly affected. Symptomatic lesions are classically seen at L4 levels. Affection of more cephalad vertebrae in the lumbar spine is less common.[5,11] The pathologic lesion of spondylolysis can vary from a bony stress reaction to a complete structural discontinuity in the pars interarticularis. The bony stress reaction can manifest as either sclerotic changes on radiographs or a CT scan or bone edema on MRI.[5]

Spondylolisthesis is a consequence of structural instability of the lumbar motion segment leading to either anterior or posterior displacement of the affected vertebrae in relation to the vertebrae directly caudal.

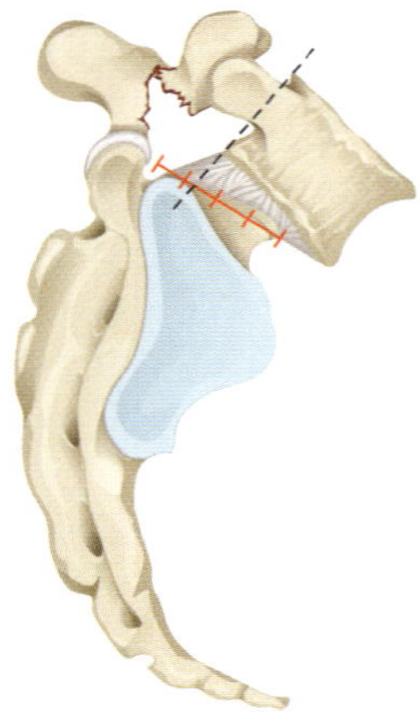

Fig. 2: The Meyerding classification system based on the grade of slip.

The causative factors contributing to this pathology could either be congenital/dysplastic or acquired. Acquired spondylolisthesis can further be classified as lytic, degenerative, traumatic, iatrogenic, or pathologic. Spondylolisthesis, in addition to causing back pain, can also contribute to the compromise of the neurological elements therein causing symptoms. The dysplastic and lytic variants, which are the most common presentations in children, are mostly seen at L5–S1, while the degenerative variant is often seen at the L4–5 level.[5]

Several classification systems for spondylolisthesis have been described in the literature, including the Meyerding classification system (Fig. 2). This anatomic classification describes the different grades of spondylolisthesis based on the severity of the slip. Although very easy to use, it does not address the other factors related to the pathology.[12]

The Wiltse-Newman classification takes into consideration both the etiological and anatomical factors. The comprehensive nature and the ease of application make it one of the most widely used classifications. Based on the pathogenesis, it describes five different variants of spondylolisthesis.[13]

Type I is the dysplastic type, which is a consequence of a developmental anomaly of the L5–S1 facet region. The sacral articulation as well as the pars are hypoplastic and are unable to withstand the sheer stresses across the lumbosacral junction ultimately leading to the slip. A number of studies have described the incidence of the dysplastic variant at 14–21%.[13,14]

Type II is the isthmic variant and is based on the pathologic lesion involving the pars interarticularis. Wiltse attributed the evolution of the type II lesion to the genetic predisposition of the pars to fatigue failure.[15] It is further subclassified into three subvariants. Type IIA, which is the most common variant of spondylolisthesis, is the consequence of a fatigue fracture in the pars. Chronic repetitive stress due to a variety of activities involving the hyperextension of the lumbar spine appears to be the etiology. The fracture defect is obvious due to the lack of healing. Type IIB refers to the presence of an elongated pars interarticularis. This pathology results as a development of chronic, recurrent microfractures that ultimately heal under distraction stress. Type IIC involves an acute disruption of the pars interarticularis.

Type III, the degenerative variant, is due to long-standing intersegmental instability, most commonly seen at the L4–5 level. Type IV is a traumatic variant that develops due to a fracture in the posterior elements, other than the pars. Lastly, type V refers to spondylolisthesis due to pathologic bone disease, such as the presence of tumor.

Another classification system has been descried by Marchetti and Bartolozzi, which broadly categorizes spondylolisthesis in either developmental or acquired types. This classification system has not achieved a very wide acceptance, possibly due to its complex nature and a confusing taxonomy.[5,16]

NATURAL HISTORY

The natural history of both spondylolysis and spondylolisthesis has been reported in the literature (Table 1). These reports are largely based on lower levels of evidence because the majority of the literature is based on retrospective reviews. Additionally, some studies do not differentiate between the isthmic and dysplastic variants. The Wiltse-Newman classification provides a sound background for understanding the etiopathogenesis of both spondylolysis and spondylolisthesis.

Dysplastic spondylolisthesis, often identified in pediatric patients, has an incidence of progression that is much higher than the other variants. The study by McPhee et al. reported the rate at 32% in contrast to the isthmic type, where it is much lower (4%).[17] In the dysplastic type, the posterior elements are intact although hypoplastic, as the slip progresses, there is gradual canal compromise. This contributes to cauda equina (L5 and the sacral roots) compression with neurological dysfunction. Patients tend

Table 1: Outline of literature.

Author, journal, year	*Design*	*LoE*	*Topic*	*F/U (m)*	*Measures*	*Main results*
Fredrickson BE, Baker D, McHolick WJ, et al. J Bone Joint Surg Am, 1984	P	I	The natural history of spondylolysis and spondylolisthesis	300	Clinical and radiological	Defect result of cartilaginous anlage, hereditary predisposition,and association with spina bifida. Progression of a slip was unlikely after adolescence and the slip was never symptomatic in the population that we studied
Turner RH, Bianco AJ, J Bone Joint Surg Am, 1971	P	IV	Spondylolysis and spondylolisthesis in children and teenagers	–	Clinical and radiological	Only symptomatic grades I and II need treatment. Grades III and IV need surgical treatment
Cavalier R, Herman MJ, Cheung EV, et al. J Am Acad Orthop Surg, 2006	Review	IV	Spondylolysis and spondylolisthesis		Review of literature	Diagnosis, natural history, and nonsurgical management
Albanese M, Pizzutillo PD, J Pediatr Orthop, 1982	Cross-sectional	I	Family study of spondylolysis and spondylolisthesis		Interview, clinical and radiological	Hereditary predisposition
Rosenberg NJ, Bargar WL, Friedman B, Spine (Phila Pa 1976), 1981	Cross-sectional	I	The incidence of spondylolysis and spondylolisthesis in nonambulatory patients	–	Radiological	Spondylolysis represents a fatigue fracture resulting from activities associated with ambulation
Congeni J, McCulloch J, Swanson K, Am J Sports Med, 1997	P	III	Lumbar spondylolysis in athletes	–	Clinical and radiological	Computed tomography scans can play a very important role in management
Micheli LJ, Wood R, Arch Pediatr Adolesc Med, 1995	R	II	Back pain in young athletes	–	Clinical and radiological	Significant differences in the major causes of low back pain (LBP) in young athletes compared with general adult population
Saraste H, J Pediatr Orthop, 1987	P	I	Long-term clinical and radiological follow-up of spondylolysis and spondylolisthesis	240	Clinical and radiological	Risk factors for low back symptoms were greater than 25% slipping, low lumbar index in L5 spondylolysis, spondylolysis at the L4 level, and early disk degeneration
Wiltse LL, Newman PH, Macnab I, Clin Orthop Relat Res, 1976	R	II	Classification of spondylolysis and spondylolisthesis	–	Radiological	Etiological and anatomical factors
Boxall D, Bradford DS, Winter RB, et al. J Bone Joint Surg Am, 1979	R	II	Management of severe spondylolisthesis in children and adolescents	–	Clinical and radiological	Arthrodesis relieves symptoms but progression of the slip can continue
McPhee IB, O'Brien JP, McCall IW, et al. Australas Radiol, 1981	R	II	Progression of lumbosacral spondylolisthesis	12	Clinical and radiological	Progression only in adolescents. Dysplastic 32% and isthmic 4%
Sys J, Michielsen J, Bracke P, et al. Eur Spine J, 2001	R	IV	Nonoperative treatment of active spondylolysis in elite athletes	13.2	Clinical and radiological	Healing occurs in unilateral lesions. Stable nonunion does not preclude good clinical outcome
Debnath UK, Freeman BJ, Grevitt MP, et al. Spine (Phila Pa 1976), 2007	P	II	Clinical outcome of symptomatic unilateral stress injuries of the lumbar pars interarticularis	24	Clinical and radiological	Nonoperative treatment gives good results
Beutler WJ, Fredrickson BE, Murtland A, et al. Spine (Phila Pa 1976), 2003	P	II	The natural history of spondylolysis and spondylolisthesis	540	Clinical and radiological	Subjects with pars defects follow a clinical course similar to that of the general population, with a marked slowing of slip progression with each decade

Contd...

Contd...

Author, journal, year	*Design*	*LoE*	*Topic*	*F/U (m)*	*Measures*	*Main results*
Harris IE, Weinstein SL, J Bone Joint Surg Am, 1987	R	III	Long-term follow-up of patients with grade-III and IV spondylolisthesis: treatment with and without posterior fusion	288	Clinical and radiological	Both groups could live an active life. Symptomatic patients did well with in-situ fusion
Ravichandran G, AJR Am J Roentgenol, 1980	C	II	A radiologic sign in spondylolisthesis		Radiological	Isolated lateral deviation and rotation of a spinous process seen in anteroposterior radiographs of the lumbar spine that seems to be associated with pathology in the pars interarticularis
Boden SD, Wiesel SW, Spine (Phila Pa 1976), 1990	C	II	Lumbosacral segmental motion in normal individuals	–	Clinical and radiological	Overlap between symptomatic and asymptomatic patients may be significantly decreased (eightfold) by calculating dynamic motion, rather than static vertebral positions
Dunn AJ, Campbell RS, Mayor PE, Rees D, Skeletal Radiol, 2008	R	IV	Radiological findings and healing patterns of incomplete stress fractures of the pars interarticularis	–	Radiological	Incomplete fracture of the pars interarticularis represents a stage of the evolution of a complete stress fracture. The direction of fracture propagation is consistent, and complete healing can be achieved in most cases with appropriate clinical management
Johnson DW, Farnum GN, Latchaw RE, et al. AJR Am J Roentgenol, 1989	R	IV	MR imaging of the pars interarticularis	–	Radiological	Four situations in which the pars can simulate spondylolysis on sagittal MR images: (1) Sclerosis of the neck of the pars; (2) Partial volume imaging of the degenerative spur of the superior facet slightly lateral to the pars; (3) Partial facetectomy; and (4) Osteoblastic metastatic replacement of the marrow of the pars
Hollenberg GM, Beattie PF, Meyers SP, et al. Spine (Phila Pa 1976), 2002	R	IV	Stress reactions of the lumbar pars interarticularis: the development of a new MRI classification system	–	Radiological	MR findings of stress reactions and spondylolysis of the lumbar pars interarticularis can be reliably classified into five grades by experienced readers
Saifuddin A, Burnett SJ, Clin Radiol, 1997	C	II	The value of lumbar spine MRI in the assessment of the pars interarticularis	–	Clinical and radiological	MRI was found to have a sensitivity of 57–86%, specificity of 81–82%, positive predictive value of 14–18%, and negative predictive value of 97–99% for the diagnosis of a pars defect
Bellah RD, Summerville DA, Treves ST, et al. Radiology, 1991	R	IV	LBP in adolescent athletes: detection of stress injury to the pars interarticularis with single-photon emission computed tomography (SPECT)	–	Radiological	SPECT can be used to detect stress injury not seen with planar bone imaging or radiography and is recommended in evaluation of LBP in young athletes
Sakai T, Sairyo K, Mima S, et al. Spine (Phila Pa 1976), 2010	P	II	Significance of magnetic resonance imaging signal change in the pedicle in the management of pediatric lumbar spondylolysis	–	Radiological	MRI at the 3rd month during follow-up can indicate whether the conservative treatment is being successful or not

Contd...

Contd...

Author, journal, year	*Design*	*LoE*	*Topic*	*F/U (m)*	*Measures*	*Main results*
Fujii K, Katoh S, Sairyo K, et al. J Bone Joint Surg Br, 2004	R	IV	Union of defects in the pars interarticularis: the radiological outcome after conservative treatment	–	Radiological	The site of the defects in the pars, the presence or development of spondylolisthesis, the condition of the contralateral pars, the degree of lumbar lordosis, and the degree of lumbar inclination all significantly affected union
Sairyo K, Sakai T, Yasui N, J Bone Joint Surg Br, 2009	R	IV	Conservative treatment of lumbar spondylolysis: the radiological signs which predict healing		Radiological	Early-stage defect on CT and high-signal change in the adjacent pedicle on a T2-weighted MR scan are useful predictors of bony healing of a pars defect in children after conservative treatment
Sairyo K, Sakai T, Yasui N, et al. J Neurosurg Spine, 2012	R	IV	Brace treatment: determine in what types of spondylolysis bone healing can be achieved and how long it takes	–	Radiological	Patients with early-stage defects are the best candidates for conservative treatment with a hard brace because more than 90% of such cases can be healed in 3 months
Anderson K, Sarwark JF, Conway JJ, et al. J Pediatr Orthop, 2000	R	IV	Quantitative assessment with SPECT imaging of stress injuries of the pars interarticularis and response to bracing	–	Clinical and radiological	The data, which use SPECT scintigraphy, supports prompt treatment with brace immobilization for acute spondylolysis in children and adolescents
Ranawat VS, Dowell JK, Heywood-Waddington MB, Injury, 2003	R	IV	Stress fractures of the lumbar pars interarticularis in athletes	–	Clinical and radiological	Conservative measures are treatment of choice, Buck's repair as the operation of choice if conservative measures fail
Sairyo K, Sakai T, Mase Y, et al. Arch Orthop Trauma Surg, 2011	R	IV	Purpose of this study is to clarify the cause of LBP associated with pars defects in athletes	–	Clinical and radiological	Study showed that inflammation was always present at the pars defects and in some cases at the adjoining facet joints
Pizzutillo PD, Hummer CD, Pizzutillo PD, Hummer CD, 1989	R	IV	Nonoperative treatment for painful adolescent spondylolysis or spondylolisthesis	80	Clinical and radiological	Nonoperative treatment of degrees of spondylolisthesis of less than or equal to grade 2 can reliably relieve pain in two-thirds of patients
Klein G, Mehlman CT, McCarty M, J Pediatr Orthop, 2009	M	IV	Nonoperative treatment of spondylolysis and grade I spondylolisthesis in children and young adults	–	Clinical and radiological	Majority of patients treated nonoperatively will have a successful clinical outcome after at least 1 year. Bracing does not seem to influence this outcome. In contrast to the high rate of success with clinical parameters, most defects did not heal with nonoperative treatment suggesting that a successful clinical outcome does not depend on healing of the lesion. Lesions diagnosed at the acute stage were more likely to heal after nonoperative treatment as were unilateral defects when compared with bilateral defects
O'Sullivan PB, Phyty GD, Twomey LT, et al. Spine (Phila Pa 1976), 1997	P	I	To determine the efficacy of a specific exercise intervention in the treatment of patients with chronic LBP and a radiologic diagnosis of spondylolysis or spondylolisthesis	–	Clinical	A "specific exercise" treatment approach appears more effective than other commonly prescribed conservative treatment programs in patients with chronically symptomatic spondylolysis or spondylolisthesis

Contd...

Contd...

Author, journal, year	*Design*	*LoE*	*Topic*	*F/U (m)*	*Measures*	*Main results*
Helenius I, Lamberg T, Osterman K, et al. Spine (Phila Pa 1976), 2005	R	IV	To evaluate the usefulness of the SRS questionnaire and compare it with ODI and radiographic parameters in patients with isthmic spondylolisthesis	–	–	Long-term clinical and radiographic outcomes after posterolateral fusion of low-grade spondylolisthesis were satisfactory. Inverse correlations between the outcomes and amount of slip at final follow-up observation
Frennered AK, Danielson BI, Nachem-son AL, et al. Spine (Phila Pa 1976), 1991	R	IV	Midterm follow-up of young patients fused in situ for spondylolisthesis	98	Clinical and radiological	Indication for operative treatment in patients with low-grade slip is relative
Ekman P, Möller H, Tullberg T, et al. Spine (Phila Pa 1976), 2007	R	II	To compare the outcome of posterior lumbar interbody fusion (PLIF) and posterolateral fusion (PLF) in adult isthmic spondylolisthesis	24	Clinical and radiological	Type of fusion, PLIF or PLF, does not affect the 2-year outcome of surgical treatment of adult isthmic spondylolisthesis
Sudo H, Oda I, Abumi K, et al. J Neurosurg Spine, 2006	–	I	Biomechanical study on the effect of five different lumbar reconstruction techni-ques on adjacent-level intradiskal pressure and lamina strain	–	Biomechanical	If the number of fused levels can be reduced by using PLIF to correct local kyphosis, then this procedure may be valuable for reducing adjacent-segment degenerative changes
Kakiuchi M, J Bone Joint Surg Am, 1997	R	IV	Repair of the defect in spondylolysis: Durable fixation with pedicle screws and laminar hooks	25	Clinical and radiological	The method used for direct repair of the defect of the pars interarticularis in these patients proved to be simple and effective
Schlenzka D, Remes V, Helenius I, Eur Spine J, 2006	R	IV	The aim of the present study was to assess the long-term clinical, functional, and radiographic outcome of direct repair of the pars using cerclage wire fixation—Scott technique versus posterolateral in-situ fusion in young patients with symptomatic spondylolysis or low-grade isthmic spondylolisthesis	180	Clinical and radiological	After direct repair, the ODI deteriorated with time leading to a clinically moderate but statistically significant difference in favor of segmental fusion. Lumbar spine mobility was decreased after direct repair. The theoretical benefits of direct repair could not be proven
Labelle H, Roussouly P, Berthonnaud E, et al. Spine (Phila Pa 1976), 2004	C	II	Investigate the role of pelvic anatomy and its effect on the global balance of the trunk in developmental spondylolisthesis	–	Clinical and radiological	Study participants with an increased pelvic incidence (PI) appear to be at higher risk of presenting a spondylolisthesis, and an increased PI may be an important factor predisposing to progression in developmental spondylolisthesis
Labelle H, Mac-Thiong JM, Roussouly P, Eur Spine J, 2001	–	III	The purpose of this article is to review the work done within the spinal deformity study group (SDSG) over the past decade, which has led to a classification incorporating this recent knowledge	–	Radiological	L5–S1 spondylolisthesis are a heterogeneous group with various adaptations of their posture. Reduction techniques should preferably be used in subjects with evidence of abnormal posture, in order to restore global spinopelvic balance and improve the biomechanical environment for fusion

Contd...

Contd...

Author, journal, year	*Design*	*LoE*	*Topic*	*F/U (m)*	*Measures*	*Main results*
Lenke LG, Bridwell KH, Bullis D, et al. J Spinal Disord, 1992	R	IV	Results of in-situ fusion for isthmic spondylolisthesis	–	Clinical and radiological	Despite this surprisingly low fusion rate, overall clinical improvement was noted in >80% of patients with preoperative symptoms of back pain, leg pain, or hamstring tightness
Grzegorzewski A, Kumar SJ, J Pediatr Orthop, 2000	R	IV	In-situ posterolateral spine arthrodesis for grades III, IV, and V spondylolisthesis	144	Clinical and radiological	In-situ posterolateral arthrodesis with a large amount of autogenous bone graft followed by immobilization in a pantaloon cast yields a solid arthrodesis and provides satisfactory results
Carragee EJ, J Bone Joint Surg Am, 1997	P	I	Prospective study of single-level posterolateral arthrodesis, with or without posterior decompression, for the treatment of isthmic spondylolisthesis in adults	54	Clinical and radiological	The addition of decompression to arthrodesis, performed with or without instrumentation, for the treatment of low-grade isthmic spondylolisthesis in patients who do not have a serious neurological deficit does not appear to improve the result and may significantly increase the rates of pseudoarthrosis and unsatisfactory results
Smith MD, Bohlman HH, J Bone Joint Surg Am, 1990	R	IV	Spondylolisthesis treated by a single-stage operation combining decompression with in-situ posterolateral and anterior fusion	24–144	Clinical and radiological	A solid fusion was obtained in all patients, and all had major or complete neurological recovery. The results did not deteriorate with time
Poussa M, Schlenzka D, Seitsalo S, et al. Spine (Phila Pa 1976), 1993	R	IV	Surgical treatment of severe isthmic spondylolisthesis in adolescents: Reduction or fusion in situ	56.5 and 59.8	Clinical and radiological	Reduction procedures were associated with a higher number of complications and reoperations. No neurologic complications occurred in the reduction group. Based on this study, in-situ fusions are to be preferred in adolescents with severe spondylolisthesis
Muschik M, Zippel H, Perka C, Spine (Phila Pa 1976), 1997	R	IV	Surgical management of severe spondylolisthesis. Anterior fusion in situ versus anterior spondylodesis with posterior transpedicular instrumentation and reduction	125 and 67	Clinical and radiological	Anterior spondylodesis including posterior instrumentation and reduction was superior to the simple anterior fusion in situ for normalization of the lumbosacral profile and osseous consolidation of the spondylodesis. This result was not reflected in the clinical evaluation
Molinari RW, Bridwell KH, Lenke LG, et al. Spine (Phila Pa 1976), 1999	R	IV	Complications in the surgical treatment of pediatric high-grade, isthmic dysplastic spondylolisthesis. A comparison of three surgical approaches	36	Clinical and radiological	Circumferential procedures result in the highest rate of fusion and are effective in achieving fusion in those patients with established pseudoarthrosis. Outcomes of function, pain, and satisfaction are excellent in those in whom fusion is achieved. The risks in circumferential fusion-reduction procedures are acceptable
Petraco DM, Spivak JM, Cappadona JG, et al. Spine (Phila Pa 1976), 1996	–	II	To quantify the change in length of the L5 nerve root associated with reduction of spondylolisthesis, correction of slip angle, and changing disk height	–	Cadaveric	The findings suggest that the risk of stretch injury to the L5 nerve with reduction of a high-grade spondylolisthesis is not linear; with 71% of the total L5 nerve strain occurring during the second half of reduction, partial reduction may be a significantly safer treatment approach for high-grade spondylolisthesis than complete reduction

Contd...

Contd...

Author, journal, year	*Design*	*LoE*	*Topic*	*F/U (m)*	*Measures*	*Main results*
Dubousset J, 1997	R	IV	Treatment of spondylolysis and spondylolisthesis in children and adolescents	–	Clinical and radiological	When the lumbosacral angle is not improved to 100° or more by hyperextension and traction, an anterior console interbody fusion is added before the posterolateral fusion
Hanson DS, Bridwell KH, Rhee JM, et al. Spine (Phila Pa 1976), 2002	R	IV	To demonstrate the efficacy of partial reduction and fibular dowel graft placement in the treatment of high-grade isthmic spondylolisthesis	240	Clinical and radiological	Fibular strut grafting is a useful surgical adjunct in high-grade spondylolisthesis that is partially reduced. Clinical and radiographic outcomes were satisfactory. Our experience shows that there is no significant difference between allograft and autograft. All struts healed and remodeled by the ultimate follow-up, and there was only one instance of fibula fracture
Lehmer SM, Steffee AD, Gaines RW, Spine (Phila Pa 1976), 1994	R	IV	A study was performed on the two-stage Gaines procedure for the treatment of spondyloptosis, evaluating indications, techniques, results, and patient satisfaction	35	Clinical and radiological	Despite the relatively high complication rate, with appropriate patient selection, planning, and surgical technique, this procedure appears to be a sound method for treating severe cases of spondyloptosis, yielding very high patient satisfaction
Schoenecker PL, Cole HO, Herring JA, et al. J Bone Joint Surg Am, 1990	R	IV	Cauda equina syndrome after in-situ arthrodesis for severe spondylolisthesis at the lumbosacral junction	–	Clinical and radiological	An acute cauda equina syndrome that follows a seemingly uneventful in-situ arthrodesis for spondylolisthesis is best treated by an immediate decompression that includes resection of the posterosuperior rim of the dome of the sacrum and the adjacent intervertebral disk. In addition, posterior insertion of instrumentation and reduction of the lumbosacral spondylolisthesis should be considered
Fantini GA, Pappou IP, Girardi FP, et al. Spine (Phila Pa 1976), 2007	R	IV	Incidence of major vascular injury during anterior lumbar spinal surgery, attempt to identify predisposing risk factors, and management techniques	–	Clinical and radiological	Current or previous osteomyelitis or diskogenic infection, previous anterior spinal surgery, spondylolisthesis, osteophyte formation, transitional lumbosacral vertebra, and anterior migration of interbody device point to an increased risk of vascular injury during anterior lumbar spinal surgery
Newton PO, Johnston CE, J Pediatr Orthop, 1997	R	IV	Analysis and treatment of poor outcomes following in-situ arthrodesis in adolescent spondylolisthesis	56	Clinical and radiological	Patients with the most severe kyphosis (slip angle) had the greatest chance of a poor result

to present with L5 radiculopathy, neurogenic claudication, or even bowel or bladder symptoms. The tendency for slip progression as well as the appearance of early neurological symptoms may encourage the patients to seek early medical attention. This has been corroborated by a number of studies which report a higher incidence of surgical intervention in the dysplastic spondylolisthesis patients.[5,18,19]

The evolution of the isthmic variant could usually be attributed to a phenomenon of chronic overloading of the pars interarticularis, especially in populations predisposed to spondylolysis. Sport and physical activities that involve repetitive hyperextension, rotation, or torsional forces in flexion may be a strong causative factor.[20-22] The lesion tends to start as a stress reaction and may develop into a distinct pars defect if the torsional force persists. Early stress reactions that are unilateral may heal with adequate immobilization that limits the extension and reduces the distorting forces.[20,21]

Based on the study by Wiltse, the association of spina bifida with individuals with pars defect is 13 times more than that in the general population. Additional, near relatives of an individual with spondylolisthesis are five times more likely to have spondylolisthesis themselves.[6] Albanese et al. reported spondylolysis and spondylolisthesis incidence rates of 29% and 21% in nuclear family members, if the index patient has dysplastic or isthmic defects, respectively.[7] Frederickson et al. demonstrate a difference in the incidence of isthmic spondylolysis based on age, reporting 4.4% and 6% at ages 6 years and 18 years, respectively.

The majority of individuals with isthmic spondylolysis are clinically asymptomatic and may never show progression of the slip. The incidence of slip progression is less than 4% and is more likely to occur in females, individuals presenting prior to puberty, and individuals with high-grade slips (>50%).[14,17,20] Beutler et al. additionally have reported that bilateral pars defects, compared to unilateral defects, are also more likely to progress to a slip in adulthood. Nevertheless, low-grade isthmic spondylolisthesis (Meyerding I or II) as a result of bilateral pars defects clinically progressed similar to an unaffected population. Slip progression diminished as each individual aged, and no individual reached a slip of 40% or higher. Additionally, this study did not demonstrate a relationship between development of slip progression and clinical low back pain.[23] Harris and Weinsten evaluated high-grade slips (Meyerding grade III or IV), comparing nonoperative management versus in-situ fusion. In the nonoperative cohort, 36% of patients were asymptomatic, 55% had occasional back pain, and 45% had developed neurologic symptoms. At the final follow-up, with an average of 18 years, all individuals were leading active lives with only minor adjustments in lifestyle.[24]

CLINICAL EVALUATION

Symptoms and Signs

A detailed clinical evaluation is an essential part of the clinical evaluation. This should include a thorough orthopedic examination of the spine, and hips, as well as a neurological examination. It should be noted that a spondylolysis with or without a low-grade spondylolisthesis may be an incidental radiographic finding with the patient being completely asymptomatic.

The usual presentation for spondylolysis with low-grade spondylolisthesis is an adolescent presenting with insidious onset low back pain mostly related to activities. These children are often involved in high impact and physically demanding sports and strongly relate their symptoms to these activities. An episode of acute back injury is not uncommon, although it may have made the underlying symptoms more noticeable. It is always a matter of debate if the injury is the cause of the spondylolysis or just a factor that has irritated a preexisting dormant lesion. Frank neurological symptoms are not a usual feature of a spondylolysis with low-grade spondylolisthesis. The fibrotic tissue in the area of a long-standing pars defect may irritate the existing nerve root to cause radicular symptoms. High-grade spondylolisthesis can contribute to radiculopathy, claudication, and even bladder and bowel symptoms.

Occasionally, the presentation may be with a concern for scoliosis with back discomfort. It is not uncommon for individuals, particularly with high-grade spondylolisthesis to present with a scoliosis either as an idiopathic variety, secondary to chronic muscle spasms, or listhesis of the vertebrae. The scoliosis is secondary to the spondylolisthesis and often disappears once the primary cause is appropriately addressed.

During the clinical evaluation, it is convenient to have the patient dressed in a gown or underwear. The global spinal alignment should be addressed. A high-grade spondylolisthesis is often associated with a loss of lumbar lordosis (LL). A scoliotic curvature can also be noted in the coronal plate secondary to a painful muscle spasm. It may be possible to palpate a step off, or a difference in depth, of the spinous processes at the affected levels. A vertical sacrum secondary to a posterior pelvic tilt (PT) may also be evident. The spinal range of motion may be associated with considerable discomfort, especially with extreme extension. Significant paraspinal muscle spasm is an indicator of a painful lesion.

On examination of the lower extremities, a hamstring spasm or contracture may contribute to the flexed posture of knees and hips. This could force the patient to walk with a shorter stride length. A straight leg test helps gauge the extent of the hamstring spasm by measuring the popliteal angle.

An elaborate neurological examination includes evaluation of both motor and sensory function of the lower extremities, as well as deep tendon reflexes. The indication for a rectal examination includes presence of bladder and other neurological symptoms, especially with a background of a grade III or IV slip.

Radiological Imaging

The purpose of imaging in lumbar spondylolysis is to detect the presence of a defect, delineate acute versus chronic pathologies, identify healed fibrous nonunions, assist with prognosis and treatment, and also provide insight on the native spine's healing potential. In the presence of spondylolisthesis, imaging will also outline the severity of the slip, the extent of neurological compromise, and the presence of any anatomical changes.

Plain Radiography

Plain radiography is the most commonly used screening tool for evaluating the pathology of back pain. In settings of spondylolysis and spondylolisthesis, imaging generally includes an anterior-posterior (AP), lateral, and oblique X-rays, which are taken at a 45° angle. The AP X-ray displays the global coronal alignment, while the lateral demonstrates sagittal alignment and the presence and extent of a slip, as described in Meyerding classification (Figs. 3A to C).[12] Obvious pars defects can sometimes be appreciated on these films; however, the oblique views can be more accurate in detecting this pathology. The "scotty dog sign" has been well-described in the oblique view for detecting slips. The neck of the dog represents the pars interarticularis and can present with a defect in patients with spondylolisthesis. The ear represents the superior articular process and the foreleg is the inferior articular process on one side, while the tail and hind leg mirror this image on the opposite side. The body of the "scotty dog" represents the lamina. Since other anatomical parts of the posterior elements are also visible on this X-ray, a relative comparison of the pars allows for the evaluation of dysplastic or elongated pars. Despite its utility, the oblique X-ray also has limitations in evaluating spondylolysis.

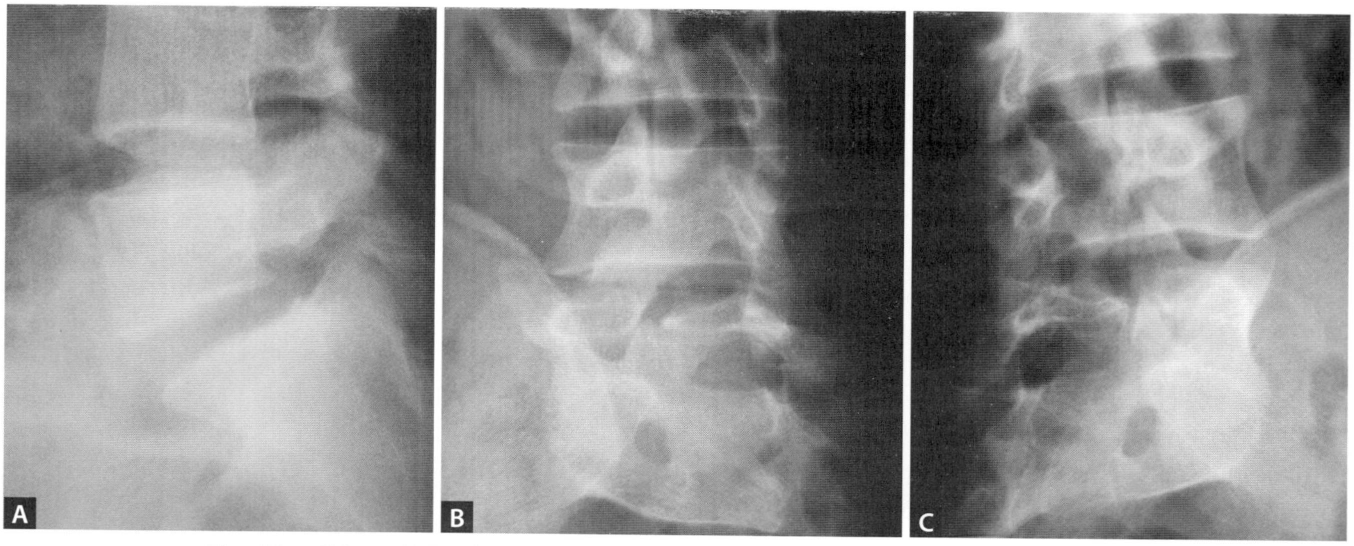

Figs. 3A to C: Lateral (A) and oblique (B and C) of spondylolysis and with Grade 1 spondylolisthesis.

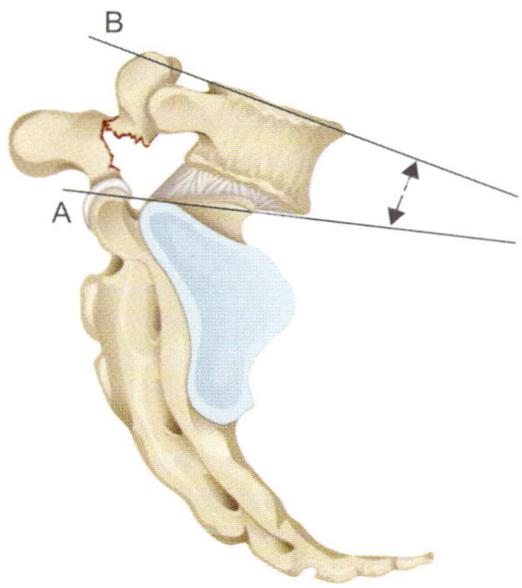

Fig. 4: The concept of slip angle: It is the angle subtended by a line parallel to the superior endplates of L5 and another to that of S1.

Due to the natural morphology of the pars interarticularis involving all three spatial dimensions, it often remains difficult to capture an orthogonal radiograph.[25-27]

The lateral X-ray remains the most insightful in evaluating spondylolisthesis. A vertical line can be drawn along the posterior border of the lumbar vertebral bodies, and any vertebrae discontinuous with this line will be a sign of spondylolisthesis.[28] Additionally, in patients who are symptomatic, lateral flexion-extension radiography reveal the mobility of the slip, and display how much the affected vertebral body moves forward in flexion, and reduces in extension. Traditionally, 4 mm of anterior or posterior translation has been used as a cut-off for instability.[29,30] The lateral X-ray of all slips should also be analyzed for determining the slip angle. The slip angle quantifies the presence of kyphosis at the lumbosacral junction in the setting of spondylolisthesis. This angle is measured by first drawing a line tangential to the posterior border of the sacrum. The slip angle is the angle formed between a line perpendicular to this line and a line drawn tangential to the superior endplate of L5 (Fig. 4). Current literature reports that slip angles greater than 50° are more likely to progress, be unstable, and have higher postoperative complications.[14]

Computed Tomography

CT scans are a powerful tool in evaluating spine pathologies as they allow thinly-sliced images across all three spatial fields. In the presence of a pars fracture, a discontinuity of the neural arch in the axial plane is evidence and correlates with a pars defect (Figs. 5A and B).[5,25,31] Additionally, isthmic spondylolysis in the presence or absence of a slip can result in posterior translation of the posterior elements, and subsequently an increased AP width of the spinal canal in the sagittal plane, which can be distinguished from degenerative spondylolisthesis which would have a shortened diameter.[25,32]

CT scans are also valuable to evaluate the presence of physiologic and pathologic healing, whether complete or incomplete, of a pars defect. In the presence of physiologic stress, the body's natural response is to fill the pars defect with fibrous or fibrocartilaginous tissue. Ossification of the tissue in or adjacent to the pars defect can become pathologic if it results in stenosis of either the exiting or descending nerve root, resulting in symptomatic root compression. These pathologic lesions are referred to as Gill's nodules.[25] Additionally, although not applicable in all patients, CT scans can also provide insight on the acuity of the defect. In chronic pars defects, the bony margins adjacent to the defect are sclerotic as compared to acute defects which present with narrow and noncorticated borders.[25]

In spite of the utility of CT scans in diagnosing and evaluating spondylolysis, including high sensitivity and specificity, the high radiation exposure limits the role of CT as a screening tool. In practice, CT is useful in determine the healing response and also to study the anatomic details of the pars defect when surgery is being contemplated.[5,25]

Magnetic Resonance Imaging

MRI is a commonly used modality in the evaluation and diagnosis of spondylolysis and spondylolisthesis. In additional to providing multiplanar imaging, it provides an evaluation of the neural elements, potential nerve compression, and bone metabolism. The lack of radiation risk, particularly in the pediatric population, is a definitive advantage of using MRI rather than considering a CT scan as a screening tool.[5,25] For completeness purposes, each MRI should include sagittal and reverse angle oblique axial images in both T1-weighted sequences as well as fluid-sensitive protocols [such as short-tau inversion recovery (STIR) or T2-weighted images].[32,33]

T1-weighted sequences are best for evaluating anatomy, and hence, a pars defect is best seen on T1 where there is a discontinuity of bone cortex and marrow in the pars region. T1 sequences are preferred for this finding as

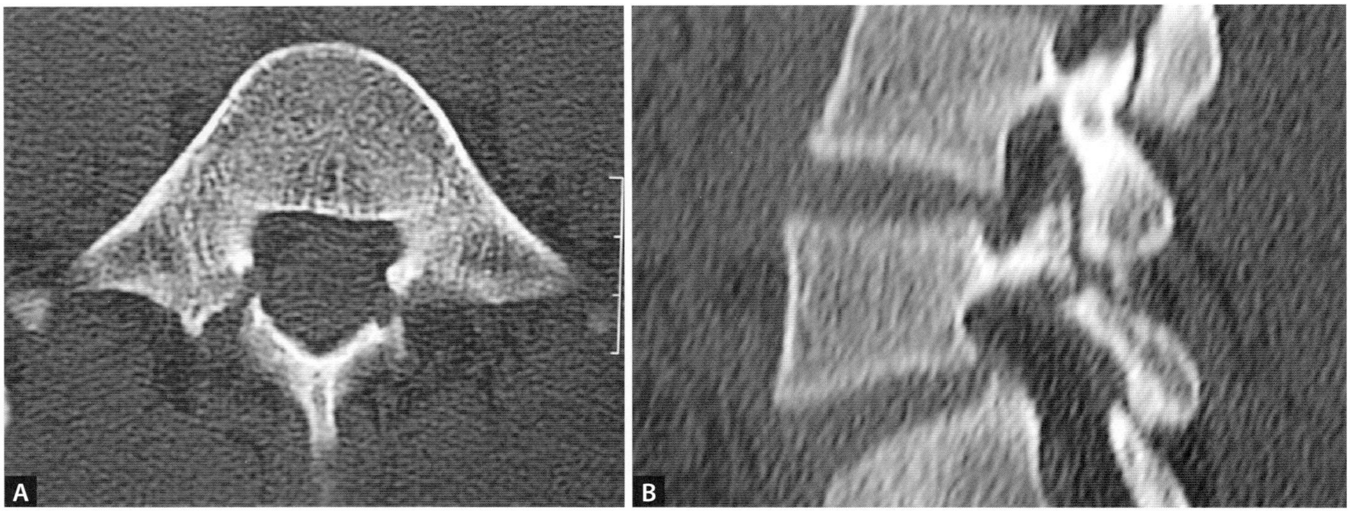

Figs. 5A and B: Axial (A) and sagittal (B) images of a CT scan of isthmic spondylolysis.

bone marrow naturally is hyperintense, and its absence in a defect can be appreciated.[34] In the combined interpretation of multiple sequences of an MRI, further data regarding the acuity, severity, presence of healing, and chronicity of a pars defect can also be evaluated, as outlined by Hollenberg et al. in their proposed classification system:[35]

- *Grade 0 (normal)*: Intact cortical borders and normal marrow signal (T1 sequences).
- *Grade 1 (stress reaction)*: Intact cortical margins of the pars (T1 sequence) in the setting of marrow edema of the pars (fluid-sensitive sequence). This may or may not have signal changes in the adjacent pedicle or facet.
- *Grade 2 (incomplete fracture)*: Bone marrow edema (fluid-sensitive sequence) + incomplete cortical fracture through the pars.
- *Grade 3 (complete active fracture)*: Complete defect (T1) in the setting of bone marrow edema (fluid-sensitive sequence).
- *Grade 4 (nonunion/inactive fracture)*: Complete defect without any bone marrow edema.

As outlined earlier, the presence of bone marrow edema on a fluid-sensitive sequence (STIR or fat-saturated T2) suggests an acute and active pathology, whether it be a stress reaction or fracture. The lack of bone marrow edema suggests a chronic or inactive fracture without active metabolic activity.[35] Despite the vast amount of information that can be extracted from an MRI, their interpretation can still present a challenge. The presence of cortical continuity on T1 sequences may not always be definitive in MRIs in diagnosing spondylolysis, and as a result MRIs may have higher false-positive rates and lower positive predictive values.[5,25,33,36,37] Thus, the role of MRI in diagnosing young patients with stress reactions or symptomatic spondylolytic defects is evolving.

In patients with neurological complaints or deficits on examination, MRI provides exceptional cross-sectional evaluation of the neural elements as well as potential etiology, including Gill's nodules, stenosis, foraminal narrowing, disk herniation, and central stenosis. Specific to spondylolysis and nerve compression, MRI is an exceptional tool to evaluate both lateral recess and foraminal stenosis and narrowing.[5,25] Thus, with the ability to evaluate the neural elements and no radiation risks, despite the limitations, MRI continues to be an advantageous modality for the diagnosis and evaluation of spondylolysis and spondylolisthesis.

Single-photon Emission Computed Tomography

Single-photon emission computed tomography (SPECT) is a fairly sensitive imaging modality in diagnostic evaluation of spondylolysis with a greater capability to localize abnormal bone locations. Due to its high sensitivity, a normal SPECT can practically eliminate spondylolysis as a source of clinical back pain. Additionally, SPECT can potentially identify cases of spondylolysis and pars stress reactions prior to being able to be seen on radiography.

Recent studies evaluated patients who underwent spinal fusion for spondylolysis and found that the cohort with a positive preoperative SPECT had significantly greater improvement than those with a negative preoperative SPECT.[38,39]

Although a negative SPECT can be reliably rule out spondylolysis, the specificity of SPECT is not as impressive. False positives are well-documented, including in asymptomatic patients.[40,41] Additionally, different pathologies may mimic spondylolysis in terms of SPECT findings, including facet degeneration or infection. Furthermore, SPECT cannot be used to reliably differentiate unilateral versus bilateral pars defects. Therefore, despite the high sensitivity of SPECT imaging for spondylolysis, the presence of false positives, lack of pathology specificity, and use of radiation make it a suboptimal screening modality.[42,43]

MEDICAL MANAGEMENT

Stress Reaction and Early Pars Fracture

As outlined earlier, MRI and CT are useful modalities to diagnose spondylolysis and can subsequently stratify the progression and severity of the defect. As described as grade 1 changes, the bony anatomy of the pars can be intact; however, a stress reaction in the marrow of the pars, pedicle, and adjacent facet can form. Current literature reports that the potential for healing for a stress reaction or an early pars fracture is excellent.[5,44-46] Unilateral lesions tend to heal better than the bilateral variants, with current reports success rates of 81% with nonoperative management.[5,20,21] From an imaging standpoint, hyper-intensity on a fluid-sensitive MRI sequence in a pedicle adjacent to the pars defect has also been identified as predictive factor of successful nonoperative management.[46]

The goal of nonsurgical treatment is to achieve relief of symptoms with healing of the lesion. Contrary to almost all other fractures in orthopedics, the treatment goal is resolution of symptoms rather than obtain a bony union, as a fibrous nonunion can alleviate symptoms as well. As discussed earlier, certain hyperextension maneuvers have been identified as inciting spondylolysis, and hence, immobilization in a brace preventing trunk extension and rotation can provide a milieu of tissue healing. Immobilization in a thoracolumbosacral orthosis (TLSO) for a period of 6–12 weeks is indicated for the child or adolescent with a stress reaction of the pars. Immobilization may be discontinued once pain-free lumbar extension and rotation can be demonstrated and follow-up evaluation with repeat CT documents progressive healing.[5] Sairyc et al. prospectively evaluated the effectiveness of TLSO bracing in 63 defects. They divided their patients into four categories: (1) Early (hairline fractures), (2) Progressive (no sclerosis) with bone edema at the adjacent pedicle, (3) Progressive with no bone edema at the adjacent pedicle, and (4) Inactive lesions (sclerotic bone changes). Their study reported healing rates on CT scan of 94%, 64%, 27%, and 0%, respectively. While the vast majority of early and active defects healed nonoperatively, none of the sclerotic/inactive lesions healed with immobilization, highlighting that there is a window of opportunity for nonoperative care.[47]

Following adequate conservative treatment, it is not uncommon to see a group of patients with good pain relief but absence of osseous union. The pars defect is bridged by fibrous tissue to achieve a stable pain-free "fibrous union". This result does not preclude an optimal clinical outcome in the long-term.[5,20,48]

After the discontinuation of the period of rest and immobilization, patients need to undergo a graded rehabilitation protocol. Motions that can contribute to hyperextension and rotational stressors to the pars could potentially aggravate the symptoms and should be avoided. In order to prevent recurrent injuries and symptoms, physical therapy should be incorporated in the treatment protocol, focused on strengthening the patient's core, hip flexor, and hamstring stretching. After an optimal trial of conservative treatment and a skilled sports rehabilitation therapy, it is possible to attain the preinjury level of function and performance in the majority of these patients.[5,20,48,49]

Spondylolysis (Isthmic) with a Chronic Pars Defect

It is a common scenario for children, adolescents, and athletes to present with back pain with the radiological work-up demonstrating a well-defined pars defect. These lesions, when chronic, involve a fibrous union across the site of the defect equivalent to the development of a pseudoarthrosis. This chronic spondylolytic lesion is usually pain free and does not impair the patient's function. A thorough search for other sources of low back should be conducted before focusing on the pars defect as the etiology.

In an active pediatric and adolescent patient population, repetitive, physically demanding sports, and other activities may cause sufficient irritation at the site of the spondylolysis to induce inflammatory changes. This could be a source of chronic back pain causing activity limitations. Sairyo et al. studied the pathophysiology of low back pain in athletes with chronic pars defects. They identified 12 pars defects that were in their terminal stage and had achieved a pseudoarthrosis on CT and subsequently underwent MRI. They noted that fluid-sensitive MRI sequences demonstrated inflammation at the site of the defect in all 12 patients. Interestingly, 58% of the pars defects had inflammation in either the cranial or caudal facet joint on MRI. Subsequently, the authors hypothesize that symptomatic back pain in the setting of chronic pars fracture may originate from adjacent facet joint inflammation.[50]

Once an alternate source of low back pain has been ruled out, the treatment of a symptomatic chronic pars defect involves conservative measures to alleviate pain. A period of rest or activity modification, a short period of nonsteroidal anti-inflammatory drugs (NSAIDs), reassurance to the anxious parents, and physical therapy rehabilitation are the cornerstones of the treatment. A lumbar corset may be helpful in providing comfort and also limiting some of the provocative activities involving extremes of motion.[5,51-54] The physical therapy exercises should involve core strengthening along with stretching of the tight lumbodorsal fascia and hamstring muscles.[5,55]

Low-grade Spondylolisthesis

The incidence of progression and development of neurological complications differs significant in the isthmic and dysplastic variants of spondylolisthesis.[5,17-19] Accordingly, the role of conservative management is determined by the natural history of the two common types of spondylolisthesis.

The natural course of a low-grade (grade I or II) isthmic spondylolisthesis is fairly benign, with a very low risk of progression.[5,17] The likelihood of slip progression gradually decreases with every decade of life.[23] Episodes of back pain in slips that are radiologically stable can be managed in a fashion similar to that described earlier. The mainstay of treatment includes a period of rest and activity modification, physical therapy, and symptomatic measures for pain control. No long-term activity modification is necessary and children and athletes can pursue their activities and sports of choice. Detailed patient and family counseling about the diagnosis and the natural history with a stress on the low incidence of slip progression are often very helpful.[5,53,54,56] The role of bracing is still not clear, but it can help improve comfort and slow down an overtly active patient. Bell et al. in their study of brace treatment of symptomatic spondylolisthesis concluded that progression of spondylolysis to a slip, as well as the progression of spondylolisthesis are not rare events, occurring in 15–40% of reported series. Significant progression, in some cases from grade II to grade IV, has been reported. When a slip progression occurs, it is most likely when the patient is experiencing a period of rapid adolescent growth. Brace treatment relieved symptoms in this entire patient group with grade I and II spondylolisthesis. LL and sacral inclination were decreased during the period of brace treatment. No progression was demonstrated in any patients with grade I or grade II spondylolisthesis, once brace treatment was initiated. The mechanism whereby bracing prevents progression may be through decreasing shear stress as the involved segment by a decrease in lordosis in the brace. Though this series presents a small patient cohort, the fact that no individuals progressed to requiring surgery for intractable pain or for progression of slip warrants consideration of this treatment modality in symptomatic patients with grade I or II spondylolisthesis.[57] Nevertheless, the lack of progression that Bell et al. have attributed to bracing could purely be that low-grade spondylolisthesis has a benign natural clinical course.

Dysplastic spondylolisthesis, in contrast to the isthmic variant, could progress aggressively, especially around the period of adolescent growth spurt. The consequent symptoms could include back pain along with worsening neurological complaints. In the progressive slips, early surgical intervention may become necessary to avoid neurological complications.[5,17-19] Thus, it is mandatory to identify and closely follow the low dysplastic variants, especially during adolescence. Late progression has been reported to be rare.[17]

High-grade Spondylolisthesis

Stable high-grade slips that are asymptomatic can be managed with observation, as the current literature does not endorse prophylactic fusion in grade III and IV slips.[5,24] Harris et al. provided 18-year follow-up in a comparative study and found that the patients treated nonoperatively did not report major limitations in their activity and only reported minor modifications in their lifestyle to cope with their minor symptoms.[24] On the other hand, individuals with high-grade spondylolisthesis with significant symptoms have been documented to respond poorly to conservative measures.[5,53] Pizzutillo et al. reviewed 12 patients with high-grade spondylolisthesis and reported that such patients are more appropriately treated by surgical stabilization.[53]

SURGICAL INDICATIONS AND TREATMENT

Spondylolysis and Low-grade Spondylolisthesis

The mainstay of treatment of pediatric patients with back pain is due to spondylolysis and low-grade spondylolisthesis conservative management. Surgical treatment can be considered when these patients fail a reasonable period (6 months or more) of conservative treatment (Figs. 6A to D). Appearance and progression of neurological symptoms is another indication for considering early operative intervention. Methods for surgical management of spondylolysis are broad, and include both an in-situ repair of the pars defect and segmental fusion.

One of the most common, simple, and widely used technique for managing L5 pars defects and low-grade lytic spondylolisthesis is in-situ posterior-lateral fusion across the L5–S1 segment. The advent of pedicle screws has provided to a powerful tool to obtain rigid fixation, achieve high rates of fusion, minimize complications, and eliminate the need of postoperative bracing. Helenius et al. performed a retrospective study of 108 patients with low-grade spondylolisthesis with an average follow-up time of just over 20 years who were treated with posterior and posterolateral fusion. They reported nonunion rates of 34% and 13%, respectively. They reported that increased anterior residual slip and subsequent lumbosacral kyphosis resulted in a cosmetic deformity, manifested by worse scores for appearance in clothes, attractiveness, and self-image. Nevertheless, the study demonstrated that posterolateral fusion (PLF) is a viable and successful treatment modality for low-grade spondylolisthesis.[58] These findings were further reinforced by Frennered et al. who reported a 67% satisfaction rate with in-situ PLF with a 6% pseudoarthrosis rate.[59]

The role of lumbar interbody fusion in pediatric and adolescent patients with low-grade spondylolisthesis has not been well-delineated in the current literature. Theoretically, interbody fusion has the potential to decrease pseudoarthrosis rates, allows the surgeon to reduce slips without have to rely exclusively on posterolateral fixation as the isolation form of rigid fixation, and corrects and subsequently prevents lumbosacral kyphosis. Additionally, an appropriately-sized interbody device also has the potential to provide indirect decompression of both foraminal and lateral recess stenosis.[60-64] Unfortunately, these advantages have not been unequivocally demonstrated in the literature. Ekman et al. performed a prospective study comparing posterior lumbar interbody fusion (PLIF)

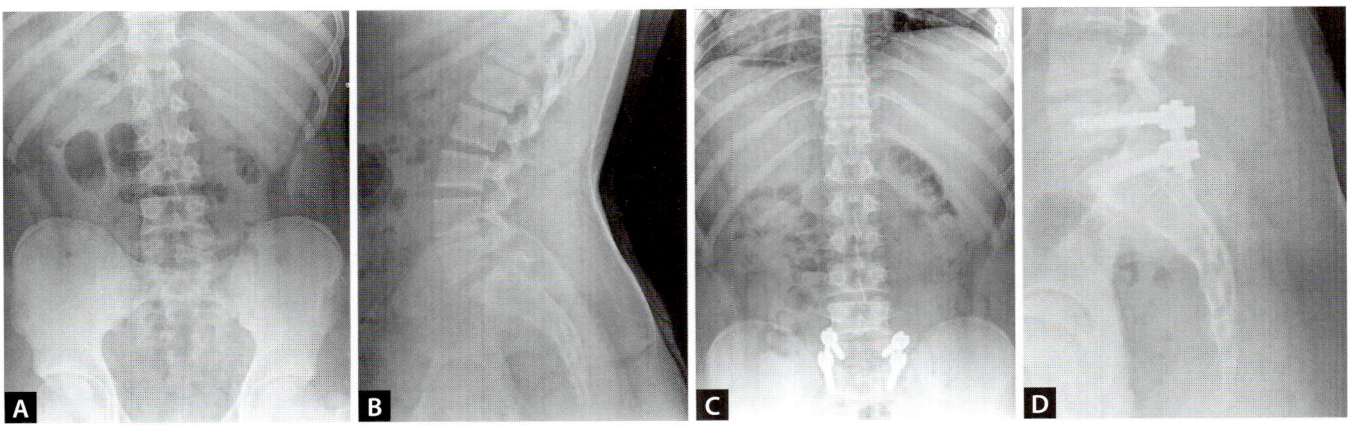

Figs. 6A to D: Preoperative (A and B) and postoperative (C and D) and anteroposterior and lateral radiographs of a 17-year-old male with chronic back pain secondary to spondylolysis and grade I listhesis not responding to conservative treatment. The patient underwent L5–S1 posterior lumbar interbody fusion (PLIF) with a satisfactory result.

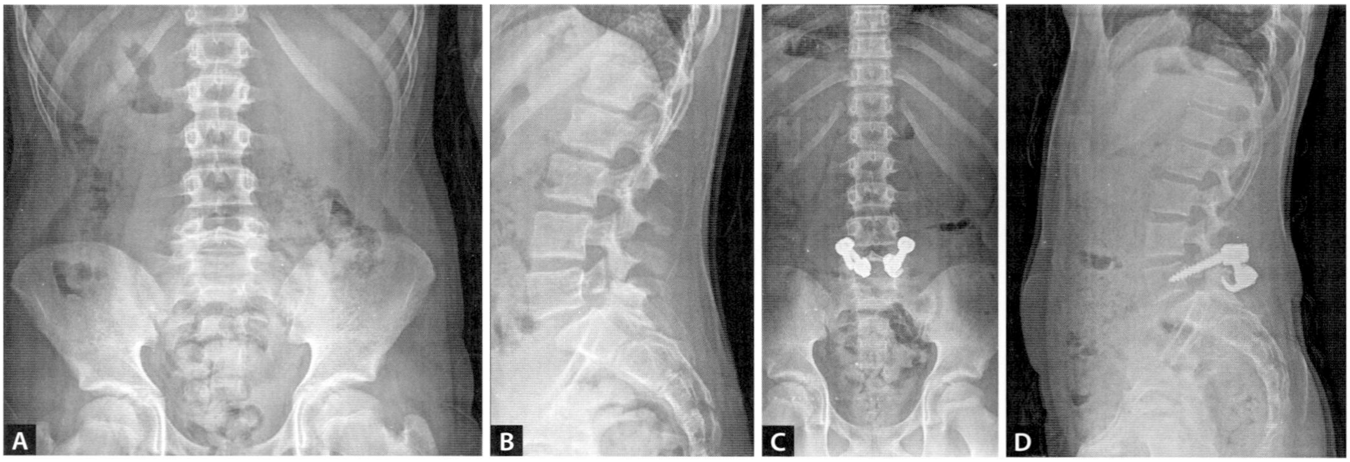

Figs. 7A to D: Preoperative AP (A) and lateral (B) X-rays of spondylolysis with subsequent treatment with pars repair with hook and pedicle screws (C and D).

with PLF in patients with adult isthmic spondylolisthesis and found that there was no significant difference in clinical outcomes between the cohorts.[60] Appropriately designed, matched, and powered studies focused on the pediatric and adolescent population with low-grade lytic spondylolisthesis would be of great utility in further demarcating the role of interbody fusion techniques.

Pars repair is an attractive alternative to fusion because of the sparing spinal motion segments. The initial techniques for pars repair were predominantly successful for defects at L1 through L4 levels possibly due to the nonrigid nature of fixation. Advent of newer fixation devices, such as pedicle screws and hooks, has helped to achieve satisfactory results at all the lumbar segments including L5 (Figs. 7A to D).[65-67] A detailed search for other sources of low back pain, before considering surgery for pars repair, is logical. As discussed, a complete history and examination as well as adequate imaging evaluation should be completed. MRI is a commonly used investigation in the diagnosis of the pars defect as a source of pain.[50] CT and SPECT can also be helpful in the diagnostic work-up, although not used often due to radiation concerns. Temporary relief of back pain after the area of the pars defect has been infiltrated with lidocaine is another helpful diagnostic modality.[67] Individuals with single-level defects, minimal slippage, a normal intervening disk, and no radicular symptoms are the best candidates for pars repair.[65] A number of procedures for the repair of the pars defect have been described. Each of these is technically demanding. Techniques with the more rigid modes of fixation appear to have better healing rates for the pars defect.[66-69] In the direct fixation of pars defects described by Buck, the defect should be exposed, debrided, and decorticated to facilitate bony healing. Then, a neutralization screw is placed across the defect with supplemental bone graft.[68]

The Scott wiring technique has also been described to repair pars defects. This technique involves passing a wire through both transverse processes, looping them through the spinous process in a tension-band like construct to immobilize and compress the pars defect.[69] Kakiuchi described a technique which used a rod to compress across the pars defect by anchoring it to a screw in the cephalad pedicle and a hook under the caudal lamina with bone grafting. He reported that 100% of pars defects united using this method. The rod is first secured to the pedicle screw at the affected level and then to a laminar hook, which is attached to the trailing edge of the lamina. This technique provides more rigid fixation with a pedicle screw and a greater compression force with a laminar hook as well.

The advantage of repairing the pars defect versus short segment fusion in low-grade slips has not been substantiated in the literature. Schlenzka et al. compared pars repair using the Scott wiring techniques versus uninstrumented posterolateral in-situ fusion with approximately 15-year follow-up.[70] The authors reported that the fusion group ultimately yielded superior clinical outcomes over time while there was no significant difference in functional and radiographic outcomes. Of note, the authors did report decreased lumbar mobility of the operative level in the repair group as well, the preservation of which is a goal in direct repair. In the future, it will be helpful to have studies comparing the long-term outcomes of procedures for pars repair and segmental spinal fusion using modern instrumentation techniques.

High-grade Spondylolisthesis

Unlike low-grade spondylolisthesis, high-grade slips are less amenable to conservative modes of treatment. A few studies have demonstrated that nonoperative treatment may be of utility in a small cohort of patients with insignificant symptoms. In terms of surgery, the current literature reports satisfactory long-term outcomes in the treatment of high-grade spondylolisthesis.[14,23,24,59,65]

Operative intervention is often indicated in symptomatic high-grade slips; however, the optimal surgical procedure is often a matter of debate. The most commonly described surgical techniques include posterolateral fusion, with or without postural reduction, instrumented interbody fusion with partial reduction, and combined anterior and posterior fusion with partial excision of the L5 body and possible sacral dome osteotomy. Each of these techniques has associated benefits and risks. The ultimate goal of surgical treatment is to provide definitive symptomatic relief, including back pain and any neurological sequelae, by obtaining adequate fusion and decompression, as indicated. Attempt at restoration of the physiologic lumbopelvic alignment should be considered when safely possible.

The surgical planning should be based on careful analysis of the presenting complaints (back pain, L5 radiculopathy, and bowel and bladder disturbances due to sacral root dysfunction), clinical deformity (altered posture and gait changes due to global sagittal malalignment and hamstring tightness), neurologic function (weakness in the L5 or sacral root distribution, rectal tone), and spinal imaging (hypoplasia of the posterior elements of L5, size of the L5 transverse process, anatomical changes in the sacral dome, foraminal and central stenosis, and segmental mobility). The other critical factors that need consideration include the surgeon's experience and familiarity with a particular technique and availability of resources (intraoperative neuromonitoring, anesthetic and perioperative support). A detailed discussion with both the patient and patient's family should include the risks, benefits, and realistic expectations from surgical intervention.[65]

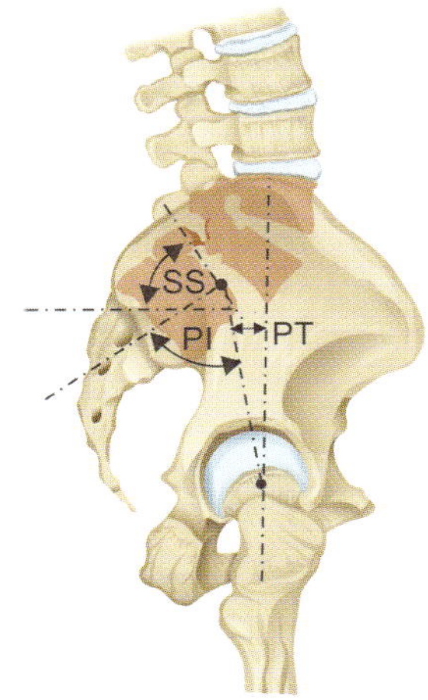

Fig. 8: The important spinopelvic parameters—pelvic tilt, pelvic incidence, and sacral slope.

Spinopelvic Alignment in High-grade Spondylolisthesis

There has been increased focus and evaluation of sagittal alignment in spine surgery recently. Parameters such as pelvic incidence (PI), sacral slope (SS), PT, and LL have all been well-described in the literature (Fig. 8). A retrospective study by Labelle et al. found that these measurements were significantly higher when compared to the general population. Furthermore, the authors concluded that the difference in these parameters also increased with greater severity of spondylolisthesis. Although SS and PT are position dependent, PI is a morphological measurement that is specific to each individual. Individuals are able to clinically retrovert and antevert their pelvis, hence altering their SS and PT; however, PI is a fixed variable that is surrogate for assessing the "verticality" of the fixed sacrum within the pelvis. Hence, when the pelvis changes positions, the sacrum does as well, maintaining a constant PI (Figs. 9A and B). The authors subsequently hypothesize that a higher PI is a risk factor for developing spondylolisthesis.[71] This appears to be an intuitively logical phenomenon as higher PIs result in greater SS, while altered mechanical stress in the posterior elements predisposes the vertebral bodies to be in a position of "shear" rather than "compression".[72]

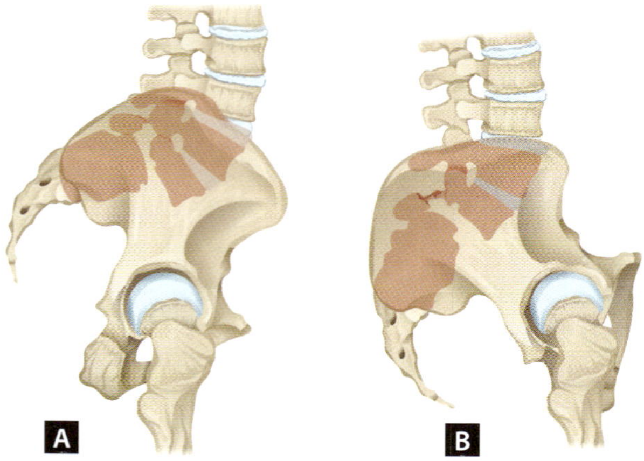

Figs. 9A and B: Balanced (A) and unbalanced pelvis (B).

Mac-Thiong et al. from the Spinal Deformity Study Group created a new classification of spondylolisthesis with inclusion of sagittal parameters and excluding dysplastic characteristics. They proposed five types of slips based on lateral imaging of the spine.[73] The slip is first defined as low grade (<50% of a slip) or high grade (>50% of a slip). Type 1 is a low-grade spondylolisthesis with a PI under 60° and type 2 is a low-grade spondylolisthesis with a PI greater than 60°. In high-grade spondylolisthesis, the SS/PT ratio is evaluated. If balanced, it is categorized as type 3. Types 4 and 5 are for high-grade spondylolisthesis with an unbalanced sacropelvic morphology. In type 5, there is global sagittal imbalance, as measured by the C7 plumb line, comparison to type 4 which maintains global sagittal balance.[74]

Despite the nuances of this classification system, it is critical in highlighting the diversity of anatomy and morphology in patients with spondylolisthesis. Hence, clinicians should be keen on assessing a patient's posture, slip severity, global and focal and sagittal alignment/balance, and clinical examination in the process of determining a treatment course.

SURGICAL TECHNIQUES

In-situ Posterolateral Fusion

In-situ PLF remains one of the most commonly used and simple techniques for surgical treatment of high-grade spondylolisthesis. There is minimal risk of neurological complications. The relief of symptoms is fairly predictable, with the majority of patients reporting improvement in the back pain and neurological complaints (Figs. 10A to C). Successful fusion has been reported in more than 70% of treated patients. Development of radiological pseudoarthrosis may not preclude clinical symptomatic relief. In patients developing radiological pseudoarthrosis, progression of the slip is unusual and even if present, is minor and not clinically significant.[14,65,75] Notably, long-term follow-up of patients undergoing in-situ fusion has not demonstrated an increased incidence of adjacent segment degeneration.[14,24,59,65,75-79]

Technically, this surgery can be done from either a standard midline incision or a bilateral parasagittal Wiltse approach.[65,80] The Wiltse approach permits direct access to the posterolateral portions of the spine, including the transverse processes, facets, and sacral alae, yet avoids destabilization of the posterior elements. If lumbar decompression is indicated, the midline incision should be performed. Nerve root decompression may be necessary in some cases, but bilateral laminectomy and pars debridement (i.e. Gill decompression) are not routinely performed unless the patient presents with neurological symptoms.[65,81] After removal of the facets and decortication of the bony structures, bone graft can be placed along the lateral gutters, promoting a PLF mass.[65,77] The preference of the authors is to perform a midline approach with pedicle screw instrumentation.

Postoperative immobilization by a pantaloon spica casting or bracing with a TLSO is used for 8–12 weeks. Postoperative postural reduction of the slip angle by molding the brace into increased lumbosacral lordosis (hyperextension) is an effective method of improving the slip angle and overall sagittal balance of individuals with severe but partially mobile deformities.[65,82]

The critics of in-situ fusion argue about a number of factors including the lack of cosmetic improvement due to inadequate restoration of the physiologic spinopelvic alignment, a relatively higher incidence of pseudoarthrosis that could potentially contribute to back pain and neurological symptoms. In patients undergoing in-situ PLF with compression of the thecal sac, the Gill fragment with the posterior elements of L5 is completely excised. This significantly reduces the bone surface area available for the posterolateral fusion. The fusion mass incorporating the small L5 transverse processes, especially in the adolescent population, may not be robust enough to withstand the shear forces in an unstable

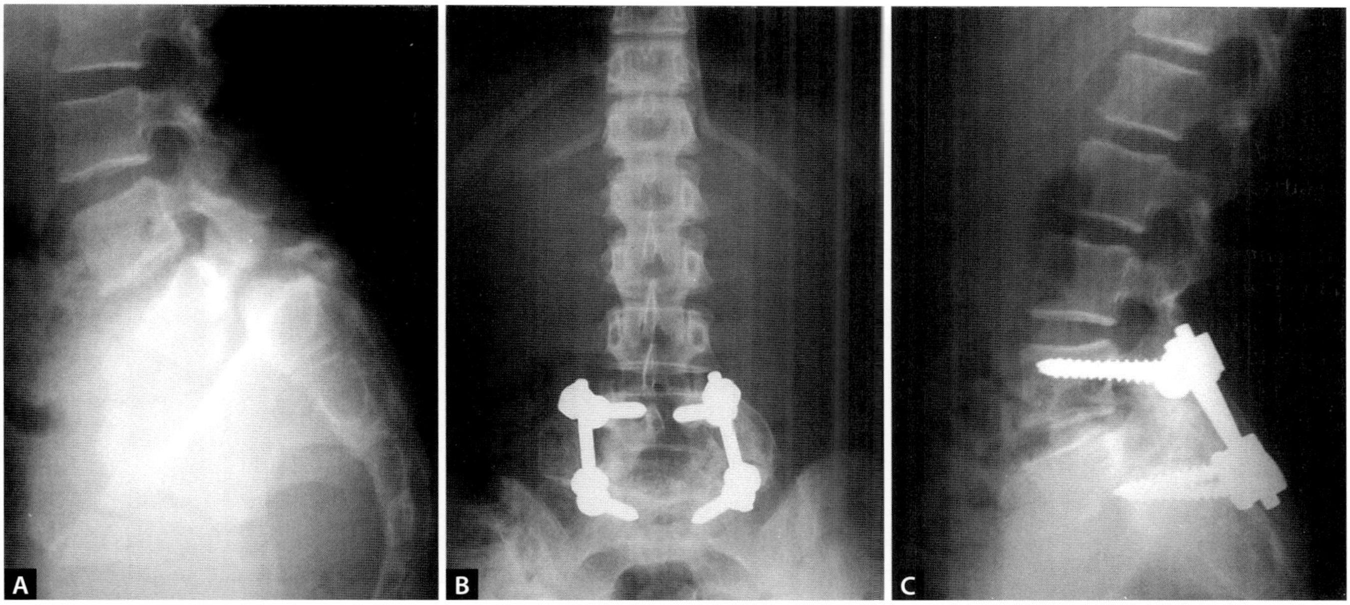

Figs. 10A to C: Preoperative lateral X-ray (A) demonstrating spondyloptosis, subsequently treated with in-situ fusion (B and C).

high-grade slip. Thus, in-situ PLF with decompression may have to be combined with L5–S1 interbody fusion.[83] In high-grade slips, the minimal overlap of the L5 and S1 bodies and altered anterior anatomy and proximity to critical retroperitoneal structures may make anterior interbody fusion fairly difficult in this region. Alternative techniques exist to obtaining interbody fusion, including transforaminal lumbar interbody fusion (TLIF) and PLIF.

There are few studies that have directly compared the in-situ fusion versus fusion with reduction in the surgical treatment of high-grade slips. Poussa et al. performed a retrospective study comparing long-term effects of reduction and fusion and in-situ fusion in high-grade spondylolysis. At an average follow-up of just under 15 years, the authors found that in-situ fusion was associated with both higher clinical outcomes and adjacent segment disease on MRI. Of note, the in-situ fusion group had a large subgroup that included fusion extension to L4 and all had interbody fusion at L5–S1.[84]

Muschik et al. retrospectively compared clinic-radiologic outcomes between isolated anterior in-situ fusion and combined AP fusion with reduction. The authors found that reduction with circumferential fusion resulted in lower rates of pseudoarthrosis, superior slip angle, and lumbosacral alignment without a significant difference in the clinical outcomes.[85]

Molinari et al. compared three surgical techniques for high-grade spondylolisthesis, including posterior fusion from L4 to S1 without decompression, posterior fusion with decompression, and reduction and circumferential fusion. They reported pseudoarthrosis to be 45%, 29%, and 0%, respectively without any significant difference in clinical outcomes among patients who did achieve bony fusion among the three groups. Given the high pseudoarthrosis rates in isolated posterior fusion, the authors highlight the clinical effectiveness of circumferential fusion.

High-grade Slip Reduction with Fusion

The advent of versatile posterior spinal instrumentation systems and availability of modern neurological monitoring have made intraoperative reduction of high-grade slips surgically safe and possible. Postural reduction with a cast has historically been an option, but has nearly been eliminated in the present era. Nevertheless, surgical reduction of high-grade slips remains technically demanding and should be carried out only in appropriately indicated cases. The major disadvantage of in-situ fusion involves the high incidence of pseudoarthrosis and the inability in restoring the normal pelvic balance. The risk factors for pseudoarthrosis include excessive mobility

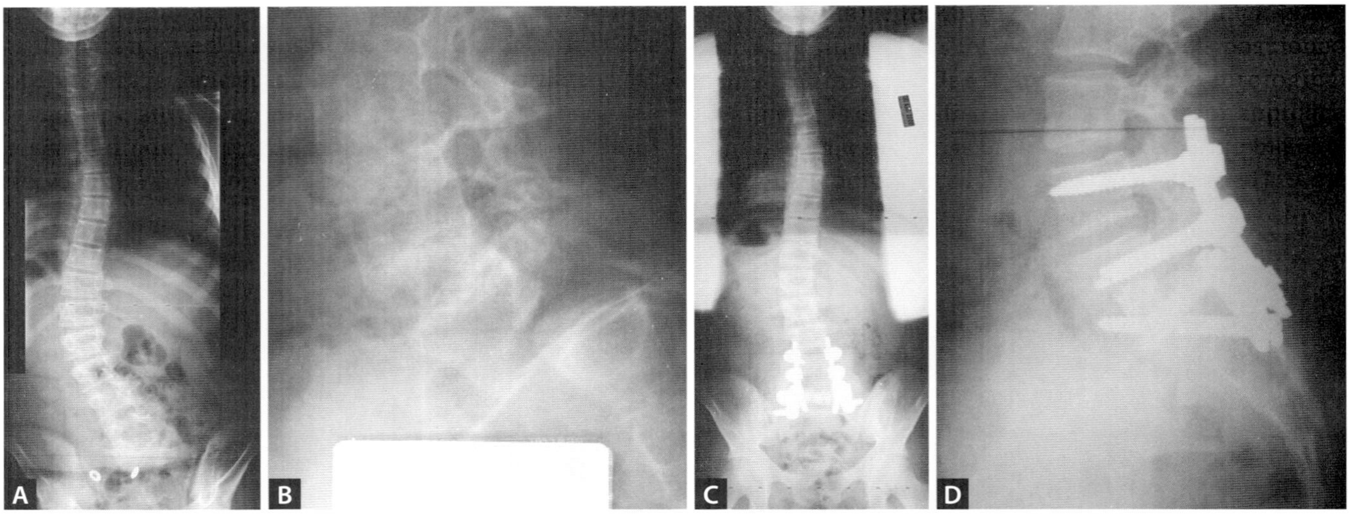

Figs. 11A to D: AP (A) and lateral (B) of a high-grade spondylolisthesis treated with reduction, posterolateral and L5–S1 interbody fusion (C and D).

(L5–S1 mobility), dysplastic lumbosacral anatomy, small lumbar transverse processes, and overall anterior sagittal imbalance. Patients with preoperative L5 radiculopathy or sacral root symptoms who require wide decompression and those individuals with anatomic changes to the vertebral body and sacral dome are at high risk of non-union. These patients with high-grade slips with risk factors for pseudoarthrosis benefit from attempted reduction.[14,65,85-87] Based on findings from the Spine Deformity Study Group, reduction of the L5 vertebral body significantly improves lumbosacral alignment, and they ultimate suggest that reduction might be preferred in certain retroverted pelvic alignments.[74,88,89] Thus, the attempt at the reduction of the slip is indicated to improve the biomechanics of the spin-pelvic alignment and also to reduce the incidence of pseudoarthrosis. The other advantage of reduction is the indirect decompression of the neural elements, thus potentially alleviating the neurological symptoms.[65,87] Attempt at reduction and stabilization of a high-grade slip is also indicated in subjects with a compensatory scoliosis and significant postural abnormalities (Figs. 11A to D).[65,90]

The potential risk associated with the reduction and instrumented fusion procedures is significant. The operation is technically demanding and is associated with longer operative time and higher surgical blood loss. The most common reported complication is injury of the L5 nerve root, which correlates with the degree of reduction achieved.[84,86,91-93] Based on the study by Petraco et al., this risk of L5 nerve root injury is not linear; rather, 75% of the aggregate strain placed upon the L5 root occurs during the final half of the reduction maneuver.[94]

Although several methods of reduction and fusion of high-grade slips have been described in the literature, the ideal choice is still unclear. Current described techniques include preoperative halofemoral traction, AP fusion, a pantaloon hyperextension spica cast, intraoperative closed reduction with posterior fusion, anterior reduction with anterior interbody fusion, and posterior decompression with posterolateral fusion. The ultimate aim of these techniques is to obtain improvement of lumbosacral kyphosis, diminish sagittal translation, and complete solid fusion.[85,91,92,95] Due to the risk of L5 nerve injury as highlighted previously in reduction maneuvers, the acceptable method of treatment includes wide decompression of bilateral L4 roots, partial reduction with posterior lateral fusion, and/or interbody fusion. This method appears to be clinically safe and effective as compared to in-situ fusion while improving lumbosacral alignment parameters simultaneously.[65,87,92,94]

The operative technique for reduction of high-grade spondylolisthesis is as follows. The patient is positioned prone in the standard position and neurological monitoring is established. A midline posterior approach from L4 to the sacrum is performed. A complete bilateral L5 laminectomy (Gill's laminectomy is obtained) to the

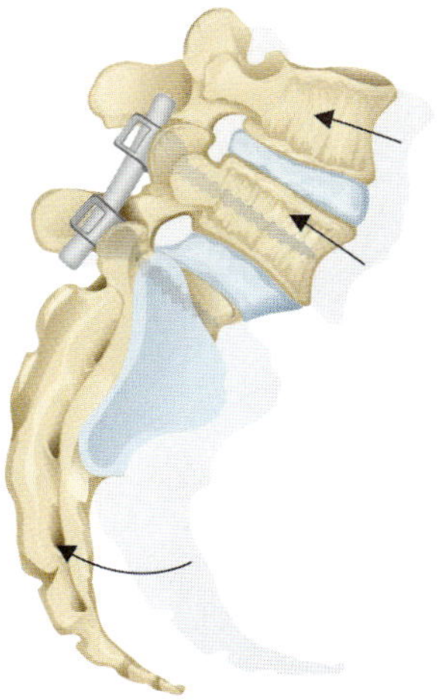

Fig. 12: The corrective forces involved in the reduction of high-grade spondylolisthesis.

pedicles. The L5 and S1 nerve roots are decompressed bilaterally. Pedicle screws are placed bilaterally from L4 to S1 in the standard fashion and reduction is achieved by cantilever flexion of the sacral pelvic unit with a combination of patient positioning that involves extension of the hip and knee and gentle downward force is placed on the sacrum. An interbody device and iliac screws may also be placed depending on the presenting pathology (Fig. 12).[96,97] Reduction-type pedicle screws are also useful to facilitate realignment, taking care to avoid forceful posterior translation of the lumbar segments and screw pull-out.

This realignment is done gradually to take advantage of soft-tissue relaxation and to allow the neurologic structures to accommodate slowly to the new spinal position. Because nerve root strain is highest at the end of the reduction, improvement of high-grade spondylolisthesis to a low-grade slip, confirmed by imaging, is a safe surgical goal. Visual inspection of roots after reduction, neurophysiologic responses, and a wake-up test facilitate assessment of neurologic function immediately after reduction. Decreasing the degree of reduction and/or more extensive root decompression is indicated when neurological dysfunction is seen after correction. Cancellous bone graft is harvested and placed in the posterolateral gutters.[65,86,87,96,97]

SPONDYLOPTOSIS

Spondyloptosis is a term used to describe when the L5 vertebral body has translated completely over the sacral promontory (Figs. 13A and B). Subjects are often symptomatic and can present with severe low back pain, neurological complaints, and postural and gait disturbances. Limited data is available about this condition due to its rarity. Current treatment methods include observation, fusion in situ, decompression and fusion (including posterolateral and circumferential with interbody fusion), or the Gaines procedure.[65,77,80,81,83,85-87,91-93,96,98] Surgical intervention is indicated in patients with persistent symptoms or with development of a neurological deficit. Reduction of the L5 body over the sacrum can result in a significant stretch on the L5 nerve roots and the cauda equina. The Gaines procedure has been described with the intention of correcting the sagittal malalignment without stretching the cauda equina. It involves reduction and AP fusion as a two-stage operation. In the initial stage, a vertebrectomy of the L5 is performed from an anterior spinal approach following by the second stage in 5–7 days with excision of the L5 laminal and pedicles with a fusion from L4 to the sacrum (Figs. 14A and B). Although spinal realignment and fusion are adequately achieved and neurologic improvements are seen, up to one-third of patients may experience iatrogenic nerve injury.[98]

COMPLICATIONS

Neurologic Injury

Neurologic injury represents a potential devastating complication during surgical treatment of high-grade slips. Although it is often associated with reductions, it has also been documented in in-situ fusion.[84,86,91,92,98-100] L5 nerve roots are most commonly affected, although involvement of the cauda equina is known. Majority of the injuries are temporary and improve with time, but permanent deficits including bowel/bladder and sexual dysfunction can occur.[65,86,92,93,98-100]

Schoenecker et al. reported cases of cauda equina syndrome after in-situ fusion for a high-grade slip, with a permanent deficit in 6% of those patients. The authors hypothesized that relaxation of muscle and soft-tissue constraints permits increased mobility of the specific spine segment and subsequent nerve root stretch. To diminish the risk of intraoperative nerve root injury, patient positioning on rolls and decortication with a surgical burr is recommended. For patients diagnosed immediately after surgery with signs and symptoms of cauda equina syndrome, revision surgery for wide and decompression of sacral roots improves outcomes.[65,99]

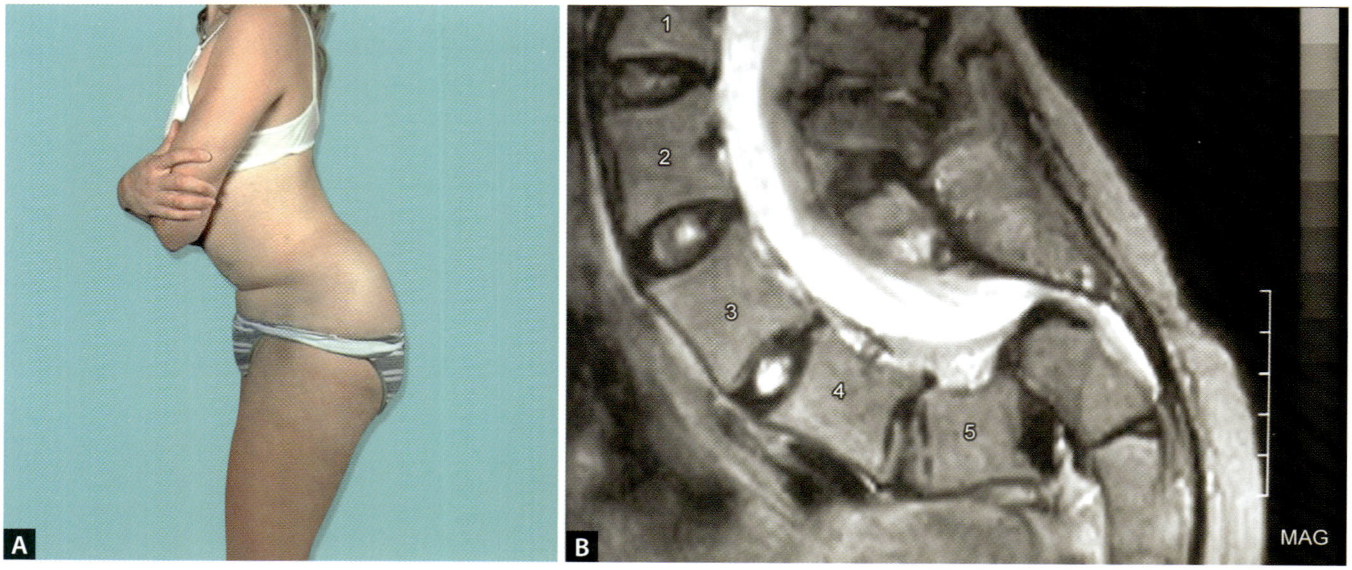

Figs. 13A and B: Clinical (A) and MRI (B) presentation of spondyloptosis.

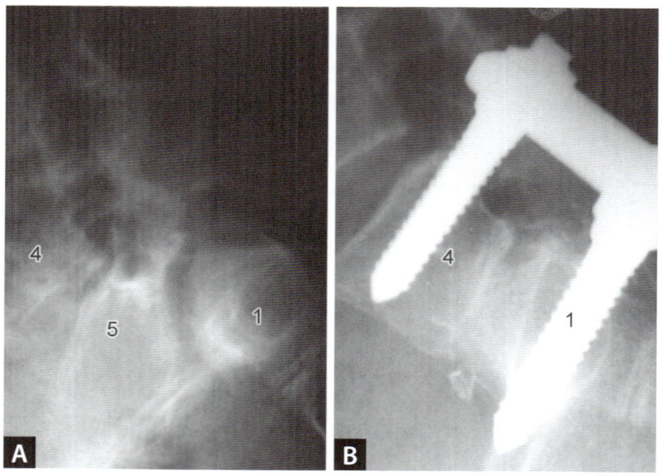

Figs. 14A and B: Preoperative (A) and postoperative (B) lateral X-rays of spondyloptosis treated with L5 vertebrectomy and subsequently posterolateral fusion.

Patients undergoing reduction of the spondylolisthesis are at risk for developing neurological complications. Attempt at partial reduction as opposed to complete reduction in combination with wide compression of bilateral L5 nerve roots can potentially avoid this complication.[65,84,86,87,91,92,94] Use of intraoperative neurological monitoring and wake-up testing can optimize the neurological safety. Partial deficits, when discovered postoperatively, can be observed for improvement with time. On the other hand, patients with complete deficits or bowel/bladder dysfunction should immediately be brought back to the operative room for revision decompression.[65,99]

Vascular Injury

This is a rare but potentially life-threatening complication associated with surgical treatment of the spondylolisthesis, especially by the anterior approach. The complex anterior anatomy associated with high-grade slips does put these patients risk for vascular injury.[101]

Pseudoarthrosis

The incidence of pseudoarthrosis has been described as high as 45% in some studies, making it the most common complication of surgical treatment, particularly with high-grade variants.[14,65,75,86] In in-situ fusion populations, this could be attributed to anatomic factors such as excess junctional mobility, dysplastic anatomy, small lumbar transverse processes, and imbalance.[14,65,85-87] Newton et al. in the analysis of outcomes following in-situ fusion found high slip angles and poor fusion masses related to suboptimal clinical outcomes.[102] Development of radiological pseudoarthrosis may not preclude a good symptomatic relief as progression of slip is unusual and clinically insignificant. Asymptomatic patients with radiological pseudoarthrosis can be managed conservatively with satisfactory outcomes.[14,65,75,86,102]

Presence of persistent back pain, leg pain, hamstring spasm with gait disturbances, and other neurological complaints is an indication for revision surgery.

Progressive slip with back pain in the presence of pseudoarthrosis is an indication for repeat fusion, either in situ or with partial reduction when associated with a high slip angle. Addition of posterior spinal instrumentation is helpful. Patients presenting with hamstring tightness and neurological complaints in addition to back pain need spinal canal decompression by sacroplasty.[65,102]

PROGNOSIS

As highlighted earlier, the natural course of untreated spondylolysis and low-grade isthmic spondylolisthesis is fairly benign with a low incidence progression.[1,14,17,20] Certain radiographic parameters have been discussed that may suggest progression. On the other hand, dysplastic spondylolisthesis has a much higher tendency to progress and develop neurological compromise requiring surgical intervention.[5,17-19] High-grade slips with minimal or no symptoms tend to have positive long-term outcomes with nonoperative measures.[24] Progression of spondylolisthesis has been reported in skeletally immature patients with bilateral pars defect, presentation prior to an adolescent growth spurt, severe slips, and a notable female preponderance.[14,17,20]

Symptomatic patients with spondylolysis and low-grade spondylolisthesis respond well to conservative measures and can expect to lead an active life.[5,53,54,56,57] The small group of patients who fail conservative treatment respond well to either posterolateral segmental fusion or pars repair.[58,59,65-67-69] Symptomatic patients with high-grade slips warrant timely surgical intervention. In-situ fusion as well as partial reduction and fusion have been described to provide satisfactory long-term resu lts.[14,26,59,65,75-81,84,86,87,91,92,94] In-situ fusion may predispose to a higher risk of pseudoarthrosis and potential for further progression of the slip.[14,65,85-87,102] On the contrary, reduction and fusion may increase the incidence of L5 nerve root injury, although accepting partial reduction can significantly mitigate this risk.[14,65,84,86,87,91,92,94]

CONCLUSION

Spondylolysis and spondylolisthesis represent a broad spectrum of pathology that varies from congenital to acquired etiology. Various classification systems have been developed to help understand their etiology, prognosis and potential treatment options. Given the diverse pathophysiology of these conditions, treatment can vary from observation to surgical intervention, depending on a patient's symptoms, radiographic and clinical findings and response to treatment.

REFERENCES

1. Fredrickson BE, Baker D, McHolick WJ, et al. The natural history of spondylolysis and spondylolisthesis. J Bone Joint Surg Am. 1984;66:699-707.
2. Turner RH, Bianco AJ. Spondylolysis and spondylolisthesis in children and teenagers. J Bone Joint Surg Am. 1971;53:1298-306.
3. Rowe GG, Roche MB. The etiology of separate neural arch. J Bone Joint Surg Am. 1953;35:102-10.
4. Stewart TD. The age incidence of neural-arch defects in Alaskan natives, considered from the standpoint of etiology. J Bone Joint Surg Am. 1953;35:937-50.
5. Cavalier R, Herman MJ, Cheung EV, et al. Spondylolysis and spondylolisthesis in children and adolescents: I. Diagnosis, natural history, and nonsurgical management. J Am Acad Orthop Surg. 2006;14:417-24.
6. Wiltse LL. The etiology of spondylolisthesis. J Bone Joint Surg Am. 1962;44:539-60.
7. Albanese M, Pizzutillo PD. Family study of spondylolysis and spondylolisthesis. J Pediatr Orthop. 1982;2:496-9.
8. Rosenberg NJ, Bargar WL, Friedman B. The incidence of spondylolysis and spondylolisthesis in nonambulatory patients. Spine (Phila Pa 1976). 1981;6:35-8.
9. Congeni J, McCulloch J, Swanson K. Lumbar spondylolysis: a study of natural progression in athletes. Am J Sports Med. 1997;25:248-53.
10. Micheli LJ, Wood R. Back pain in young athletes. Arch Pediatr Adolesc Med. 1995;149:15-8.
11. Saraste H. Long-term clinical and radiological follow-up of spondylolysis and spondylolisthesis. J Pediatr Orthop. 1987;7:631-3.
12. Meyerding HW. Spondylolisthesis. Surg Gynecol Obstet. 1932;54:371-7.
13. Wiltse LL Newman PH, Macnab I. Classification of spondylolysis and spondylolisthesis. Clin Orthop Relat Res. 1976;117:23-9.
14. Boxall D, Bradford DS, Winter RB, et al. Management of severe spondylolisthesis in children and adolescents. J Bone Joint Surg Am. 1979;61:479-95.
15. Wiltse LL, Widell EH, Jackson DW. Fatigue fracture: the basic lesion in isthmic spondylolisthesis. J Bone Joint Surg Am. 1975;57:17-22.
16. Marchetti PG, Bartolozzi P. Classification of spondylolisthesis as a guideline for treatment. In: Bridwell KH, DeWald RL (Eds). The Textbook of Spinal Surgery, 2nd edition. Philadelphia: Lippincott-Raven; 1997. pp. 1211-54.
17. McPhee IB, O'Brien JP, McCall IW, et al. Progression of lumbosacral spondylolisthesis. Australas Radiol. 1981;25:91-5.
18. Newman PH. A clinical syndrome associated with severe lumbosacral subluxation. J Bone Joint Surg Br. 1965;47:472-81.

19. Hensinger RN, Lang JR, MacEwen GD. Surgical management of spondylolisthesis in children and adolescents. Spine (Phila Pa 1976). 1976;1:207-16.
20. Sys J, Michielsen J, Bracke P, et al. Nonoperative treatment of active spondylolysis in elite athletes with normal X-ray findings: literature review and results of conservative treatment. Eur Spine J. 2001;10:498-504.
21. Debnath UK, Freeman BJ, Grevitt MP, et al. Clinical outcome of symptomatic unilateral stress injuries of the lumbar pars interarticularis. Spine (Phila Pa 1976). 2007;32:995-1000.
22. Farfan HF, Osteria V, Lamy C. The mechanical etiology of spondylolysis and spondylolisthesis. Clin Orthop Relat Res. 1976;117:40-55.
23. Beutler WJ, Fredrickson BE, Murtland A, et al. The natural history of spondylolysis and spondylolisthesis: 45-year follow-up evaluation. Spine (Phila Pa 1976). 2003;28:1027-35.
24. Harris IE, Weinstein SL. Long-term follow-up of patients with grade-III and IV spondylolisthesis. Treatment with and without posterior fusion. J Bone Joint Surg Am. 1987;69:960-9.
25. Leone A, Cianfoni A, Cerase A, et al. Lumbar spondylolysis: a review. Skeletal Radiol. 2011;40:683-700.
26. Ravichandran G. A radiologic sign in spondylolisthesis. Am J Roentgenol. 1980;134:113-7.
27. Maldague BE. Unilateral arch hypertrophy with spinous process tilt: a sign of arch deficiency. Diagn Radiol. 1976; 121:567-74.
28. Leone A, Guglielmi G, Cassar-Pullicino VN, et al. Lumbar intervertebral instability: a review. Radiology. 2007;245:62-77.
29. Boden SD, Wiesel SW. Lumbosacral segmental motion in normal individuals. Have we been measuring instability properly? Spine (Phila Pa 1976). 1990;15:571-6.
30. Hanley EN. The indications for lumbar spinal fusion with and without instrumentation. Spine (Phila Pa 1976). 1995;20:143-53S.
31. Hession PR, Butt WP. Imaging of spondylolysis and spondylolisthesis. Eur Radiol. 1996;6:284-90.
32. Campbell RS, Grainger AJ, Hide IG, et al. Juvenile spondylolysis: a comparative analysis of CT, SPECT and MRI. Skeletal Radiol. 2005;34:63-73.
33. Dunn AJ, Campbell RS, Mayor PE, et al. Radiological findings and healing patterns of incomplete stress fractures of the pars interarticularis. Skeletal Radiol. 2008;37:443-50.
34. Johnson DW, Farnum GN, Latchaw RE, et al. MR imaging of the pars interarticularis. Am J Roentgenol. 1989;152:327-32.
35. Hollenberg GM, Beattie PF, Meyers SP, et al. Stress reactions of the lumbar pars interarticularis: the development of a new MRI classification system. Spine (Phila Pa 1976). 2002;27:181-6.
36. Jinkins JR, Matthes JC, Sener RN, et al. Spondylolysis, spondylolisthesis, and associated nerve root entrapment in the lumbosacral spine: MR evaluation. Am J Roentgenol. 1992;159:799-803.
37. Saifuddin A, Burnett SJ. The value of lumbar spine MRI in the assessment of the pars interarticularis. Clin Radiol. 1997;52:666-71.
38. Bellah RD, Summerville DA, Treves ST, et al. Low back pain in adolescent athletes: detection of stress injury to the pars interarticularis with SPECT. Radiology. 1991;180:509-12.
39. Raby N, Mathews S. Symptomatic spondylolysis: correlation of CT and SPECT with clinical outcome. Clin Radiol. 1993;48:97-9.
40. Papanicolaou N, Wilkinson RH, Emans JB, et al. Bone scintigraphy and radiography in young athletes with low back pain. Am J Roentgenol. 1985;145:1039-44.
41. Elliot S, Hutson MA, Wastie ML. Bone scintigraphy in the assessment of spondylolysis in patients attending a sports injury clinic. Clin Radiol. 1988;39:269-72.
42. Mettler FA, Huda W, Yoshizumi TT, et al. Effective doses in radiology and diagnostic nuclear medicine: a catalog. Radiology. 2008;248:254-63.
43. Payne WK, Ogilvie JW. Back pain in children and adolescents. Pediatr Clin North Am. 1996;43:899-917.
44. Sakai T, Sairyo K, Mima S, et al. Significance of magnetic resonance imaging signal change in the pedicle in the management of pediatric lumbar spondylolysis. Spine (Phila Pa 1976). 2010;35:E641-5.
45. Fujii K, Katoh S, Sairyo K, et al. Union of defects in the pars interarticularis of the lumbar spine in children and adolescents. The radiological outcome after conservative treatment. J Bone Joint Surg Br. 2004;86:225-31.
46. Sairyo K, Sakai T, Yasui N. Conservative treatment of lumbar spondylolysis in childhood and adolescence: the radiological signs which predict healing. J Bone Joint Surg Br. 2009;91:206-9.
47. Sairyo K, Sakai T, Yasui N, et al. Conservative treatment for pediatric lumbar spondylolysis to achieve bone healing using a hard brace: what type and how long?: Clinical article. J Neurosurg Spine. 2012;16:610-4.
48. Anderson K, Sarwark JF, Conway JJ, et al. Quantitative assessment with SPECT imaging of stress injuries of the pars interarticularis and response to bracing. J Pediatr Orthop. 2000;20:28-33.
49. Ranawat VS, Dowell JK, Heywood-Waddington MB. Stress fractures of the lumbar pars interarticularis in athletes: a review based on long-term results of 18 professional cricketers. Injury. 2003;34:915-9.
50. Sairyo K, Sakai T, Mase Y, et al. Painful lumbar spondylolysis among pediatric sports players: a pilot MRI study. Arch Orthop Trauma Surg. 2011;131:1485-9.
51. Steiner ME, Micheli LJ. Treatment of symptomatic spondylolysis and spondylolisthesis with the modified Boston brace. Spine (Phila Pa 1976). 1985;10:937-43.
52. d'Hemecourt PA, Zurakowski D, Kriemler S, et al. Spondylolysis: Returning the athlete to sports participation with brace treatment. Orthopedics. 2002;25:653-7.
53. Pizzutillo PD, Hummer CD. Nonoperative treatment for painful adolescent spondylolysis or spondylolisthesis. J Pediatr Orthop. 1989;9:538-40.
54. Klein G, Mehlman CT, McCarty M. Nonoperative treatment of spondylolysis and grade I spondylolisthesis in children and young adults: a meta-analysis of observational studies. J Pediatr Orthop. 2009;29:146-56.
55. O'Sullivan PB, Phyty GD, Twomey LT, et al. Evaluation of specific stabilizing exercise in the treatment of chronic low back pain with radiographic diagnosis of spondylolysis or spondylolisthesis. Spine (Phila Pa 1976). 1997;22:2959-67.

56. Herman MJ, Pizzutillo PD, Cavalier R. Spondylolysis and spondylolisthesis in the child and adolescent athlete. Orthop Clin North Am. 2003;34:461-7.
57. Bell DF, Ehrlich MG, Zaleske DJ. Brace treatment for symptomatic spondylolisthesis. Clin Orthop Relat Res. 1988;236:192-8.
58. Helenius I, Lamberg T, Osterman K, et al. Scoliosis research society outcome instrument in evaluation of long-term surgical results in spondylolysis and low-grade isthmic spondylolisthesis in young patients. Spine (Phila Pa 1976). 2005;30:336-41.
59. Frennered AK, Danielson BI, Nachemson AL, et al. Midterm follow-up of young patients fused in situ for spondylolisthesis. Spine (Phila Pa 1976). 1991;16:409-16.
60. Ekman P, Möller H, Tullberg T, et al. Posterior lumbar interbody fusion versus posterolateral fusion in adult isthmic spondylolisthesis. Spine (Phila Pa 1976). 2007;32:2178-83.
61. Sudo H, Oda I, Abumi K, et al. Biomechanical study on the effect of five different lumbar reconstruction techniques on adjacent-level intradiscal pressure and lamina strain. J Neurosurg Spine (Phila Pa 1976). 2006;5:150-5.
62. Barrick WT, Schofferman JA, Reynolds JB, et al. Anterior lumbar fusion improves discogenic pain at levels of prior posterolateral fusion. Spine (Phila Pa 1976). 2000;25:853-7.
63. Lee CK, Vessa P, Lee JK. Chronic disabling low back pain syndrome caused by internal disc derangements. The results of disc excision and posterior lumbar interbody fusion. Spine (Phila Pa 1976). 1995;20:356-61.
64. Mulholland RC, Sengupta DK. Rationale, principles and experimental evaluation of the concept of soft stabilization. Eur Spine J. 2002;11:198-205.
65. Cheung EV, Herman MJ, Cavalier R, et al. Spondylolysis and spondylolisthesis in children and adolescents: II. Surgical management. J Am Acad Orthop Surg. 2006;14:488-98.
66. Bradford DS, Iza J. Repair of the defect in spondylolysis or minimal degrees of spondylolisthesis by segmental wire fixation and bone grafting. Spine (Phila Pa 1976). 1985;10:673-9.
67. Kakiuchi M. Repair of the defect in spondylolysis. Durable fixation with pedicle screws and laminar hooks. J Bone Joint Surg Am. 1997;79:818-25.
68. Buck JE. Direct repair of the defect in spondylolisthesis. Preliminary report. J Bone Joint Surg Br. 1970;52:432-7.
69. Johnson GV, Thompson AG. The Scott wiring technique for direct repair of lumbar spondylolysis. J Bone Joint Surg Br. 1992;74:426-30.
70. Schlenzka D, Remes V, Helenius I. Direct repair for treatment of symptomatic spondylolysis and low-grade isthmic spondylolisthesis in young patients: no benefit in comparison to segmental fusion after a mean follow-up of 14.8 years. Eur Spine J. 2006;15:1437-47.
71. Labelle H, Roussouly P, Berthonnaud E, et al. Spondylolisthesis, pelvic incidence and sagittal spinopelvic balance: a correlation study. Spine (Phila Pa 1976). 2004;29:2049-54.
72. Hresko MT, Labelle H, Roussouly P, et al. Classification of high-grade spondylolistheses based on pelvic version and spine balance: possible rationale for reduction. Spine (Phila Pa 1976). 2007;32:2208-13.
73. Mac-Thiong JM, Labelle H. A proposal for a surgical classification of pediatric lumbosacral spondylolisthesis based on current literature. Eur Spine J. 2006;15:1425-35.
74. Labelle H, Mac-Thiong JM, Roussouly P. Spinopelvic sagittal balance of spondylolisthesis: a review and classification. Eur Spine J. 2011;20:641-6.
75. Lenke LG, Bridwell KH, Bullis D, et al. Results of in situ fusion for isthmic spondylolisthesis. J Spinal Disord. 1992;5:433-42.
76. Pizzutillo PD, Mirenda W, MacEwen GD. Posterolateral fusion for spondylolisthesis in adolescence. J Pediatr Orthop. 1986;6:311-6.
77. Velikas EP, Blackburne JS. Surgical treatment of spondylolisthesis in children and adolescents. J Bone Joint Surg Br. 1981;63:67-70.
78. Johnson JR, Kirwan EO. The long-term results of fusion in situ for severe spondylolisthesis. J Bone Joint Surg Br. 1983;65:43-6.
79. Grzegorzewski A, Kumar SJ. In situ posterolateral spine arthrodesis for grades III, IV, and V spondylolisthesis in children and adolescents. J Pediatr Orthop. 2000;20:506-11.
80. Wiltse LL. The paraspinal sacrospinalis-splitting approach to the lumbar spine. Clin Orthop Relat Res. 1973;91:48-57.
81. Carragee EJ. Single-level posterolateral arthrodesis, with or without posterior decompression, for the treatment of isthmic spondylolisthesis in adults. A prospective, randomized study. J Bone Joint Surg Am. 1997;79:1175-80.
82. Burkus JK, Lonstein LE, Winter RB, et al. Long-term evaluation of adolescents treated operatively for spondylolisthesis. A comparison of in situ arthrodesis only with in situ arthrodesis and reduction followed by immobilization in a cast. J Bone Joint Surg Am. 1992;74:693-704.
83. Smith MD, Bohlman HH. Spondylolisthesis treated by a single-stage operation combining decompression with in situ posterolateral and anterior fusion. An analysis of eleven patients who had long-term follow-up. J Bone Joint Surg Am. 1990;72:415-21.
84. Poussa M, Schlenzka D, Seitsalo S, et al. Surgical treatment of severe isthmic spondylolisthesis in adolescents. Reduction or fusion in situ. Spine (Phila Pa 1976). 1993;18:894-901.
85. Muschik M, Zippel H, Perka C. Surgical management of severe spondylolisthesis in children and adolescents. Anterior fusion in situ versus anterior spondylodesis with posterior transpedicular instrumentation and reduction. Spine (Phila Pa 1976). 1997;22:2036-42.
86. Molinari RW, Bridwell KH, Lenke LG, et al. Complications in the surgical treatment of pediatric high-grade, isthmic dysplastic spondylolisthesis. A comparison of three surgical approaches. Spine (Phila Pa 1976). 1999;24:1701-11.
87. Lenke LG, Bridwell KH. Evaluation and surgical treatment of high-grade isthmic dysplastic spondylolisthesis. Instr Course Lect. 2003;52:525-32.
88. Mac-Thiong JM, Wang Z, de Guise JA, et al. Postural model of sagittal spinopelvic alignment and its relevance for lumbosacral developmental spondylolisthesis. Spine (Phila Pa 1976). 2008;33:2316-25.
89. Labelle H, Roussouly P, Chopin D, et al. Spinopelvic alignment after surgical correction for developmental spondylolisthesis. Eur Spine J. 2008;17:1170-6.

90. Lindholm TS, Ragni R, Ylikoski M, et al. Lumbar isthmic spondylolisthesis in children and adolescents. Radiologic evaluation and results of operative treatment. Spine (Phila Pa 1976). 1990;15:1350-5.
91. Matthiass HH, Heine J. The surgical reduction of spondylolisthesis. Clin Orthop Relat Res. 1986;203:34-44.
92. Bradford DS, Boachie-Adjei O. Treatment of severe spondylolisthesis by anterior and posterior reduction and stabilization. A long-term follow-up study. J Bone Joint Surg Am. 1990;72:1060-6.
93. Dick WT, Schnebel B. Severe spondylolisthesis. Reduction and internal fixation. Clin Orthop Relat Res. 1988;232:70-9.
94. Petraco DM, Spivak JM, Cappadona JG, et al. An anatomic evaluation of L5 nerve stretch in spondylolisthesis reduction. Spine (Phila Pa 1976). 1996;21:1133-8.
95. Dubousset J. Treatment of spondylolysis and spondylolisthesis in children and adolescents. Clin Orthop Relat Res. 1997;337:77-85.
96. Hanson DS, Bridwell KH, Rhee JM, et al. Dowel fibular strut grafts for high-grade dysplastic isthmic spondylolisthesis. Spine (Phila Pa 1976). 2002;27:1982-8.
97. McCord DH, Cunningham BW, Shono Y, et al. Biomechanical analysis of lumbosacral fixation. Spine (Phila Pa 1976). 1992;17:S235-43.
98. Lehmer SM, Steffee AD, Gaines RW. Treatment of L5-S1 spondyloptosis by staged L5 resection with reduction and fusion of L4 onto S1 (Gaines procedure). Spine (Phila Pa 1976). 1994;19:1916-25.
99. Schoenecker PL, Cole HO, Herring JA, et al. Cauda equina syndrome after in situ arthrodesis for severe spondylolisthesis at the lumbosacral junction. J Bone Joint Surg Am. 1990;72:369-77.
100. Honet JC, Ellenberg MR. Cauda equina syndrome after in situ arthrodesis for severe spondylolisthesis at the lumbosacral junction. J Bone Joint Surg Am. 1991;73:629.
101. Fantini GA, Pappou IP, Girardi FP, et al. Major vascular injury during anterior lumbar spinal surgery: incidence, risk factors, and management. Spine (Phila Pa 1976). 2007;32:2751-8.
102. Newton PO, Johnston CE. Analysis and treatment of poor outcomes following in situ arthrodesis in adolescent spondylolisthesis. J Pediatr Orthop. 1997;17:754-61.

CHAPTER 18

Spinal Conditions Associated with Congenital Disorders

Vikram Mehta, Daniel Lubelski, David T Anderson, Edward C Benzel

INTRODUCTION

Spinal disorders associated with skeletal dysplasias and metabolic syndromes represent a rare and diverse group of disorders. The incidence of skeletal dysplasias has been estimated to be as high as 47 affected per 100,000 births.[1] Spinal disorders related to metabolic disorders have an incidence rate of 5.5–8.1 affected per 100,000 births.[2-7] While rare, it is important for the spine surgeon to be aware of the presentation and natural history of these diseases to facilitate earlier diagnosis and treatment. The skeletal dysplasias are typically more easily identified at birth with apparent physical findings, such as disproportionate head to body ratios. In contrast, some of the other metabolic diseases related to spinal disorders are not as apparent, requiring serum or urine analysis. Early recognition and treatment of these syndromes are important particularly when the spinal stenosis or deformity can lead to spinal cord compression. This chapter will highlight some of the notable skeletal dysplasias, mucopolysaccharidoses, and metabolic syndromes that are associated with spinal disorders.

ACHONDROPLASIA

Epidemiology/Genetics

Achondroplasia is a genetic bone growth disease associated with short adult stature that accounts for 90% of all cases of skeletal dysplasias.[8] It has an incidence of approximately 3.6 to 6.0 out of 100,000 births in the United States.[9] There is no known association of achondroplasia with gender, race or geographical distribution.[10]

Achondroplasia displays an autosomal dominant inheritance pattern with full penetrance.[11] Up to 90% of cases are caused by de novo mutations in the fibroblast growth factor receptor 3 (*FGFR3*) gene on the 4p16.3 chromosomal locus in the germline of either normal parent.[9] Only paternal age has been linked to an increased incidence of achondroplasia.[12-14]

Pathological Mechanism

The FGFR3 protein is a receptor expressed on chondrocytes that promotes proliferation, differentiation, and matrix production of articular and growth plate chondrocytes.[15] Accordingly, the resulting mutated protein causes achondroplasia by negatively regulating bone growth, development, and remodeling.[16,17]

Patients with achondroplasia typically have heterozygous *FGFR3* mutations as homozygous mutations cause death within the first year of life.[8,18] Typically, homozygous mutations lead to respiratory insufficiency secondary to rib-cage deformities and a compressed cervicomedullary region.[8,19]

Little is known about the associated risk factors for early morbidity and mortality in this patient population.

Presentation and Diagnosis

Achondroplasia can be detected prenatally. Fetuses with achondroplasia can have short limbs, (rhizomelic), a narrow thorax, and an enlarged head.[8,20] By the 25th week of gestation, femur size is typically in the 3rd percentile and by the 30th week, head size can be described as relative macrocephaly.[21,22] In addition to physical findings, cell-free DNA, chorionic villus sampling, and amniocentesis are considered the gold standard for prenatal screening and can confirm achondroplasia.[8] Other noninvasive methods of diagnosis, such as transvaginal ultrasound, has also been shown to identify achondroplastic fetuses.[21,23]

Achondroplasia is more commonly diagnosed in infants immediately after birth. The neonate can have an enlarged head to body ratio, frontal bossing and nasal bridge depression, short limbs and metacarpals, small thorax, increased joint laxity, thoracolumbar kyphosis, increased lumbar lordosis, bowed legs, and difficulty hearing.[8,14,20]

At birth, computed tomography (CT) or magnetic resonance (MR) imaging can reveal a narrowed foramen magnum, shortened spinal pedicles with spinal canal stenosis, shortened metacarpals with bullet-shaped phalanges, mid-face hypoplasia and frontal bossing, thick tubular bones, irregular epiphyseal plates, and delayed epiphyseal ossification.[14,24,25]

Complications and Treatment

Little medical treatment is available for patients with achondroplasia. Achondroplastics should be closely monitored as this group has a risk of death for the first 14 years of life that is 11.7% greater than the general public, with 7.5% of deaths occurring in the first year due to cervical cord compression.[26,27] Cervical cord compression occurs in approximately 30% of achondroplastics.[28] Somatosensory evoked potential (SSEP) monitoring is useful in diagnosing cervical myelopathy in these patients.[29,30] Medical management typically consists of monitoring the patient for hearing loss, hydrocephalus, and brainstem compression secondary to narrowed foramen magnum, pathological increase or decrease in spinal curvatures, sleep apnea, as well as neurological examinations to identify spinal stenosis.[8,14,31] As with other skeletal disorders, it is crucial to maintain an optimal weight to height ratio.[8,14] Growth hormone is still a potential but unproven treatment for this condition.[14] Data have shown that the increased bone length results in decreased stability, decreased bone strength, and higher rate of complications.[14]

Many of the surgical treatments for achondroplasia are performed for the secondary complications associated with disease progression. The most common complication in patients with achondroplasia is the presence of otitis media, which occurs in 75% of patients due to poor drainage of the ear canal, secondary to mid-face hypoplasia.[8,14] Airway obstruction is also common due to the reduced vital capacity of the lungs, mid-face hypoplasia, and foramen magnum stenosis.[8,25,32] The associated respiratory problems and increased frequency of sleep apnea in infants with achondroplasia can lead to sudden death at an early age.[27] Accordingly, sleep apnea monitors are recommended in the first several months of life if there is an indication of sleep apnea, as well as imaging of the spinal cord at the level of the foramen magnum.[25,33-35]

The foramen magnum is narrowed in 5–10% of patients due to congenital abnormalities, and symptoms can be further exacerbated as the foramen fails to widen with growth.[14,36] CT and MR imaging are both used to identify foramen magnum stenosis and spinal cord impingement, however MR imaging provides better brainstem and cervical spinal cord resolution.[25,32,37-39] A narrowed foramen magnum is a serious complication that can compress the brainstem causing respiratory distress as well as myelopathy and syrinx formation.[14,25,40] This should be closely monitored for 5–7 years of age as sudden death due to brain stem compression secondary to a narrowed foramen magnum can occur.[27,36,37] Foramen magnum stenosis can also lead to an increase in intracranial pressure, requiring a ventriculoperitoneal shunt.[14,20,31,37] On average, cervicomedullary and foramen magnum decompressions are performed on patients at approximately 5 years of age and have been successful regarding the improvement and resolution of correlative symptoms.[37,41]

Among patients with achondroplasia, symptomatic stenosis most commonly develops in the thoracolumbar spine (65%) followed by lumbar spine (20%), cervical spine (8%), cervicothoracic spine (4%), and thoracic spine (2%).[42] Of these patients, 24% require surgical decompression.[43] Symptoms are similar to that of the general population with spinal stenosis including weakness, cramping, numbness or pain in legs.[42] In these patients, however, thoracolumbar spinal stenosis typically becomes symptomatic at an average age of 31 years.[44] Ventral decompression with fusion and dorsal decompression with dorsolateral fusion are recommended in diffuse spinal stenosis covering three or more levels and with a kyphotic angle greater than 40°.[44] Others have recommended decompression with instrumented fusion in skeletally immature achondroplastics undergoing thoracolumbar laminectomies of five levels or more.[45] Thoracolumbar kyphosis can occur in 9% of patients following laminectomy and can warrant further spinal arthrodesis with instrumentation.[45]

Cervical spine stenosis typically presents during the third or fourth decade of life, and up to one-third of achondroplastics require surgical decompression.[46,47] Medical treatment cannot sufficiently reduce the severity of stenosis. Laminoplasty is considered the first surgical intervention warranted with subsequent laminectomy and fusion if needed.[34,47] Diffuse cervical spinal cord stenosis has also been noted and treated with dorsal decompressive laminoplasties or laminectomies of impinging vertebrae.[47,48]

Pediatric thoracolumbar kyphosis is present in 90% of achondroplastic patients.[32] However, it is infrequently associated with significant pathology and typically resolves by age 3 without brace therapy or any other treatment.[37,42,49] In all pediatric cases that require surgical decompression, prophylactic dorsal spinal fusion is also recommended.[50] Furthermore, patients older than 6 years that still have thoracolumbar kyphosis, it will typically be fixed in position, present with a curvature of at least 30° with vertebral wedging, and require surgical intervention.[42,45,49] When the thoracolumbar kyphosis measures greater than 50°, both dorsal and ventral fixation and fusion are recommended.[42,45,49,51] Due to the high rate of revision laminectomy, Shirley and Ain recommended that the first decompression should extend three levels superior to the stenosis and inferior to at least the second sacral vertebrae.[32]

In thoracolumbar kyphosis greater than 50º, dorsal fusion alone can result in pseudoarthrosis in 55% of procedures.[52] Historically, decompression with instrumentation has been found to cause neurological damage through SSEP loss. However, a study by Ain and Brown followed 12 patients that underwent laminectomy with instrumentation and found no iatrogenic neurological loss.[50] Dorsal and ventral spinal fusion with instrumentation has shown a 23–31% reduction in thoracolumbar kyphosis with all patients achieving successful arthrodesis.[53] Pedicle screw instrumentation and fusion has also been shown successful, resulting in an average of 50% reduction in thoracolumbar kyphosis.[50]

It should be noted that decompression without spinal fusion has been shown to increase the risk of thoracolumbar kyphosis later in life due to weakening of the dorsal ligamentous tension band.[42,45,51] To prevent progressive thoracolumbar kyphosis, concurrent fusion should be conducted along with decompressive surgery in skeletally immature achondroplastics.[42] Up to 36% of revision surgeries are due to vertebral stress concentration or junctional kyphosis, therefore fusion site should extend to the terminal kyphotic vertebrae in order to have a better distribution of forces.[42] SSEP can be used to monitor spinal cord integrity before, during, and after surgery.[50]

As a compensatory mechanism to the thoracolumbar kyphosis, a lumbar lordosis associated lumbar stenosis is observed in up to 80% of achondroplastic children. Ultimately, about 10% of achondroplastics will require lumbar decompression.[41,42] There is also a 20% increased risk of lumbar spinal stenosis secondary to degenerative changes and decreased intervertebral foramen spacing.[14] Lumbar lordosis can be improved by bracing.[54] If bracing does not help and subsequent lumbar stenosis occurs, surgical laminectomy with instrumentation has been shown to improve lumbar stenosis significantly more than decompression without instrumentation.[41,50,55] Those without instrumentation showed a 3.5-fold increase in secondary surgery than those with instrumentation.[41] Additionally, those with instrumentation showed up to a 57.5% overall reduction in postoperative symptoms as compared to those without instrumentation.[41]

Long-term Outcomes

A 42 year follow-up study by Wynn et al. showed a 2.3-fold increase in cardiovascular disease-related death and an 8.2-fold increase in neurological disease-related death in achondroplastics when compared to the general population.[56] There is up to a 10-fold increase in heart disease-related mortality in the 25–35 age group.[56] It is unclear if this is related to the involved mutated genes or due to the higher obesity rates in this population. In general, patients with achondroplasia live up to 10 years less than the general population.[56]

Lack of proper surveillance of spinal cord compression will lead to long-term disabilities in many patients.[27] Since achondroplastics are at a higher risk for spinal cord impingement, early identification of neuropathies should trigger the physician to perform imaging studies.[26,57] Furthermore, because there is a lack of elongation with increased radius of the cervicothoracic spinal pedicles, there can be a stenosis of the foramen magnum, spinal canal, and intervertebral foramen leading to compression of the spinal cord and secondary effector degeneration and even paralysis.[8,14,31] The rate of brainstem and cervical spinal cord compression is 5–10% in these patients.[14]

Lutter and Langer[58] categorized achondroplastic neurological involvement into four distinct groups (type I, II, III, and IV). The least severe and most common is type I, which presents with slow, progressive back pain with delayed motor, sensory, or reflex implications.[58] These patients can also show urinary incontinence and the symptoms are highly associated with kyphosis.[58] As a corollary, urologic dysfunction, which can occur in 77% of patients, can be an early indicator of neurologic implications and should prompt imaging studies.[59]

Patients with type II present with intermittent claudication, weakness, numbness, and tingling.[58] These patients tend to prefer squatting, sitting, leaning forward, and lying supine, in order to flex the spine and reduce the pain.[59] If claudication or stenosis is suspected, thoracic and lumbar spinal imaging should be done to determine if decompression is warranted.

Type III patients present with nerve compression, which is usually secondary to disk herniation.[58] Patients can have a positive straight leg test and difficulty ambulating.[58] Thoracic and lumbar spinal imaging should be ordered to determine degree of stenosis.

Type IV is uncommon and patients present with acute and severe back and/or leg pain which is secondary to physical activity or trauma. Usually this is seen in patients with paraparesis or paraplegia. The physical activity or trauma compounds the underlying type I or type II neurological dysfunction, resulting in type IV presentation.[58]

The aforementioned presentation of symptoms associated with spinal stenosis usually occurs between the third to fourth decade of life as a combination of predisposing spinal pedicle characteristics and degenerative changes.[42] Common symptoms of spinal cord impingement include tingling and numbness with eventual muscular atrophy.[42] CT or MR imaging should be ordered as soon as any signs or symptoms of neuropathy are present.

Patients who have had previous spinal correction surgeries, spinal kyphosis, and lordosis should be closely monitored as the integrity of the spinal support ligaments can be stretched and weakened.[42,60]

DYSTROPHIC DYSPLASIA

Epidemiology/Genes

Dystrophic dysplasia (DTD) is a rare disease with an estimated prevalence of 1 in 100,000, though there is about a 3-fold greater prevalence in Finland where it is found among 1 in 30,000 individuals.[61]

Dystrophic dysplasia is caused by alterations of the solute carrier family 26, membrane 2 (*SLC26A2*) gene located on the 5q31-q34 chromosomal locus. Mutations in *SLC26A2* cause a change in sulfate concentrations and thus limit the intracellular availability of sulfate for proteoglycan production.[62] The SLC26A2 protein is widely expressed in cartilage and several epithelial layers such as pancreas, colon, and bronchial tissue.[62] The inheritance is homozygous recessive.[61] There are over 30 identified mutations in the *SLC26A2* gene that result in DTD, all of which result in varying phenotypes.[63]

Pathological Mechanism

The severity varies greatly according to loci of the mutations, which affect the residual transfer activity remaining in the SLC26A2 protein.[63-65] Mutations with less residual sulfate transfer activity correspond with a greater decrease in proteoglycan production and more severe disease states.[63] The Finnish founder mutation typically results in dwarfism.[61]

The decreased proteoglycan production in chondrocytes leads to decreased sulfonification of proteoglycans, which affects cartilage architecture and mechanical properties.[66] This results in bone and joint instabilities, which can result in growth retardation and skeletal dysplasia.[65,66]

Presentation and Diagnosis

Amniocentesis, cell-free DNA, and chorionic villus sampling can be used to test for DTD during pregnancy. Post-birth molecular genetic testing can verify diagnosis of DTD.[61]

In the neonatal period, the infant typically presents with shortened limbs, auricular cystic swelling, cleft palate of variable severity, hitchhiker thumb secondary to shortened first metacarpal and increased joint subluxation, contractures of large joints, spinal deformities or a depressed nasal bridge.[64,65,67-69]

Dystrophic dysplasia can be diagnosed by prenatal ultrasound, however visualization is difficult leading to poor prenatal diagnosis rates of only 40–60%.[23,70] Micromelia can be identified at approximately 20 weeks of gestation.[65] Postpartum X-rays can reveal varying levels of pathological spinal kyphosis or lordosis, with midcervical kyphosis found in 33% of infants with DTD.[65,71,72] In severe cases, spinal cord compression can be seen.[65,72]

Complications and Treatment

The medical treatment of patients with DTD primarily focuses on preventative management.[73] Patients should be closely followed for the first 5 years of life to identify early prognostic factors including changes in joint positioning and mobility, cervical kyphosis with spinal cord impingement, cervical spina bifida, scoliosis, and hip and knee pain.[72-74] Also, careful monitoring of height to weight ratios should be performed in order to limit the amount of stress placed on the weakened joints and bones.[73] Cervical kyphosis is fairly common at a young age in these patients, but progression should be tracked as the kyphosis is frequently corrected spontaneously.[72,75] McKay et al. recommended acquiring imaging at birth, at the 6-month and 1-year intervals, and then proceeding annually; Jalanko et al. recommended imaging every 6 months up to 5 years of life, then proceeding with annual imaging.[72,74] In contrast to other skeletal dysplasias, the foramen magnum is typically not narrowed at birth, however spinal stenosis can progress with age. With exception of rare case-reports, atlantoaxial instability is not seen in patients with DTD.[76] Facial appearance is also distinct in DTD with patients not showing the characteristic depressed nasal bridge.[73]

Cervical kyphosis is common in children with DTD occurring in approximately 37% of patients.[77] In contrast to patients with minimal kyphosis, those with cervical kyphosis with a Cobb angle exceeding 60° are unlikely to have spontaneous correction. If not surgically corrected in the latter cohort, spinal cord damage may ensue.[72,75,78] Ventral-caudal fusion to correct cervical kyphosis has the highest rate of success.[71,74,75] Asymptomatic cervicothoracic spina bifida occulta also occurs at a relatively high rate of 59–79% of patients.[77,79]

Scoliosis is also quite common in patients with DTD, occurring in 49–88% of the DTD population.[77,80] In their own reviewed cohorts, Remes et al. reported an increased rate of scoliosis in females as compared to males, occurring in 49% and 22%, respectively.[77,80] Scoliosis is typically asymptomatic and does not require surgical intervention.[77]

Due to phenotypic variability, as well as limited long-term studies, the postoperative outcomes in patients with DTD are relatively unknown.[74]

Long-term Outcomes

There has been no correlation between genotype and phenotypic disease presentation and outcome.[74] Brace treatment has been shown to have no positive effect on spinal outcomes in patients with DTD.[74,77] Up to 50% of patients will have some spinal deformity of varying severity.[74] If there is any form of spinal impingement, surgical intervention should immediately be considered.[73] However, in contrast with other skeletal dysplasias, there are typically no neurological or spinal cord compression symptoms. Spontaneous spinal correction typically occurs before the age of 5.[77] Early progressive scoliosis should be surgically corrected immediately, whereas surgical intervention for idiopathic scoliosis, which progresses more slowly, can wait until the spinal Cobb angle surpasses 50°.[74] Since these patients are commonly exposed to numerous surgical procedures, there is an associated increase in iatrogenic and neurological complications.[74]

SPONDYLOEPIPHYSEAL DYSPLASIA TARDA AND CONGENITA

Epidemiology/Genes

Spondyloepiphyseal dysplasia (SED) is a disorder affecting the vertebral bones and epiphyseal plates of long bones.[81,82] There are two presentations of this disorder, SED congenita and SED tarda.

Presenting at birth, SED congenita is caused by an autosomal dominant mutation on the 12q13.11 locus which leads to dysfunction of procollagen.[82,83] The prevalence of SED congenita is approximately 3.4 affected per one million individuals and it has an incidence rate of 1 per 100,000 live births.[84,85] SED congenita displays an equal gender distribution.[81,82,84,86,87]

SED tarda is an X-linked inherited disorder.[81,82] The mutation occurs at the Xp22.2 chromosomal locus.[81] SED tarda presents later in life, with symptoms occurring between 5 years and 14 years of age.[81] The prevalence of SED tarda is estimated to be 1.7 affected per one million individuals.[84] SED tarda mostly occurs in males; less than 1% of cases are females with mild disease presentations.[81,82,84,86,87]

Pathological Mechanism

SED congenita and SED tarda are both caused by mutations that lead to dysfunction of proteins that are crucial to

CHAPTER 18

the development and transportation of type 2 collagen, an important structural protein found in cartilage and bone.[83,87-89]

SED congenita is caused by mutations in the procollagen, type II alpha 1chain protein (*COL2A1*) gene, which is important in collagen formation. There are a wide range of phenotypes and severities associated with mutations in the *COL2A1* gene.[82,88-90] The resulting procollagen protein product shows an abnormally high ratio of hydroxylysine to lysine compared to normal collagen.[82,91]

SED tarda is caused by a mutation in sedlin, a component in the tracking protein particle complex (TRAPPC).[81,92] Sedlin is needed for proper exocytosis of procollagen from the rough endoplasmic reticulum to outside the cell.[81,92] Lack of sedlin limits the amount of functional collagen.[81]

Presentation and Diagnosis

SED congenita can be detected prenatally by cell-free DNA testing, chorionic villus sampling, and amniocentesis analysis.[93-95] There is also a novel molecular polymerase chain reaction sequence-specific primer analysis that can be used for rapid detection of SED congenita through identification of known *COL2A1* gene mutations.[96] Infants born with SED congenita usually present with short limbs, cleft palate, club foot, varying degrees of myopia, direct and indirect hernias, hearing loss, detached retina, or a flat mid-face.[82,84,97,98] SED congenita can first be recognized at 20 weeks gestation via ultrasound identifying shortening of all long bones, bowing of femora and humeri, club feet, and a small thoracic cage due to shortened ribs.[99,100] Prenatal femur length consistently measures below the fifth percentile.[93]

SED congenita has very distinct radiological signs that can be present at birth. While CT and MR imaging are both acceptable, MR imaging can better identify spinal cord impingement and spinal canal stenosis in full flexion or extension posture and can identify platyspondyly, coxa vara, fractured epiphyses, absence of pubic bone ossification, lumbar lordosis, atlantoaxial instability secondary to odontoid hypoplasia, and thoracolumbar kyphoscoliosis.[97,99,101,102] While rare in SED congenita, thoracolumbar kyphosis can be severe with reported Cobb angles up to 143° in between T9 and L2.[102] Abnormal cervical flexion and extension in the craniovertebral joint are particularly common due to the complexity of the area.[103] Cervical stenosis has also been noted due to atlantoaxial instability, which is present in 35–60% of patients.[100] Additionally, patients with SED congenita have non-fused atlanto-occiptal joint.[100]

SED tarda can be detected prenatally by genetic testing through cell-free DNA testing, chorionic villus sampling, and amniocentesis analysis. Males with SED tarda are born with normal size proportions with the first signs and symptoms of disease occurring around 5 years of age via cessation of growth patterns.[81,84] Additionally, males often show symptoms of back pain with decreased spinal mobility.[104] Females carrying the SED tarda allele show no early signs or symptoms with the disease, however they are at an increased risk of arthropathy.[81,84,104]

SED tarda is distinct from SED congenita in that patients will present without radiological or clinical abnormalities from birth until approximately 5 years of age.[81,84] Radiological signs of disease include platyspondyly, central vertebral humplike deformities that are most prominent in the lumbar vertebrae, dysplastic changes in femoral head and neck, and narrow configuration of the pelvis.[81,84,104,105] Radiological findings in SED congenita are typically more severe than those in SED tarda.

Complications and Treatment

There are limited data concerning the medical management and treatment of patients with SED congenita. Growth hormone has not been shown to be efficacious in attaining gain in height.[106] Additionally, there are reports of growth hormone treatment in patients with SED congenita leading to worsening of spinal scoliosis, kyphosis, and lordosis.[106,107]

Care must be taken in performing anesthesia in these patients as they could already have impaired neural respiratory control.[107,108] The most common causes of spinal surgery intervention are cervicothoracolumbar kyphoscoliosis and atlantoaxial instability secondary to odontoid hypoplasia, os odontoideum or lax cervical ligaments.[102,109,110] Atlantoaxial instability can cause cervical myelopathy and brainstem compression, which can lead to paralysis and respiratory distress.[110] The most important aspect of surgical intervention in atlantoaxial instability is to enlarge the sagittal canal diameter to at least 10–12 millimeters, as sagittal canal diameters less than this have been shown to cause myelopathy.[110,111]

In patients with cervical myelopathy, presurgical halo cast can be used to generate cervical traction and reduction.[110,112] Atlantoaxial instability with subsequent spinal canal impingement should be resolved with cervical spinal fusion. Dorsal occiput to C3 fusions with instrumentation can resolve instability; foramen magnum decompression and high cervical laminectomies can resolve spinal impingement.[100,103] Midline cervical defects may cause extended instrumentation attachment.103 In severe cases, a C1 laminectomy and C2 laminoplasty can be performed to secure a large enough sagittal canal diameter and sagittal atlas diameter.[110] Surgeons must be cautious when inserting screws into the delicate and small vertebrae. Patients must be placed in a halo cast postoperatively to ensure spinal cord integrity.[72] Halo cast placement should be maintained until solid arthrodesis has been formed and there is no danger of cervical spinal cord damage. Up to 88% of patients will experience improved neurological function after cervical decompression and fusion.[113] However, subsequent fusion surgeries may be necessary in patients with pseudoarthrosis or if neurological symptoms are not resolved.[100]

Milder thoracolumbar kyphoscoliosis can be successfully treated with thoracolumbosacral orthosis. Rarely, severe thoracolumbar kyphoscoliosis can also present in patients with spondyloepiphyseal dysplasia congenital. Soulantis et al. have successfully performed two stage ventral release and dorsal instrumented fusion on these patients.[107] Pediatric kyphoscoliosis can be complicated by progression due to growth, which could result in the need for a repeat fusion.[107] Morita et al. have reported the usefulness of dorsal instrumentation and ventral bone graft to treat thoracolumbar scoliosis.[102]

Due to the progressive nature of spinal disorders in this population, Tolo has recommended that scoliosis in excess of 50° should receive surgical intervention.[51]

Patients with SED tarda usually do not require spinal surgical intervention as their disease state is less severe.

Long-term Outcomes

Studies have shown that the incidence of atlantoaxial instability increases with age in patients with SED congenita; consequently, the risk of spinal cord impingement increases as well.[110,111] Spinal scoliosis and lumbar kyphosis is common in this population and there is evidence supporting the use of bracing to prevent progression.[85]

Patients with SED tarda have been shown to be at an increased risk for scoliosis and kyphosis, and early degenerative joint disease.[90,114,115]

KNIEST SYNDROME

Epidemiology/Genes

Kniest syndrome is caused by mutations in the *COL2A1* gene, resulting in a truncated protein product due to mutations in the exon splicing region.[116-118] The deletion has been seen to occur between exon 12 and 24 in the 12q13.1 locus.[13] This mutation is inherited in an autosomal dominant pattern. There are no known associations of Kniest syndrome with gender, race, or geographical distribution. It is estimated that Kniest syndrome occurs in less than one individual per one million births.[119]

Pathological Mechanism

The dysfunctional COL2A protein product is secreted and incorporated with normal collagen fibers.[117,120] The resulting collagen heterodimers are severely impaired in their structural integrity.

The severity of the disease is not associated with any specific genetic mutation. However, the amount of type II collagen truncation is hypothesized to be associated with worsened disease phenotype.[121,122]

Presentation and Diagnosis

Patients often present at birth with short trunk and limbs, spinal kyphoscoliosis with compensatory lordosis, early onset arthropathy, mid-face hypoplasia, cleft palate, myopia, impaired hearing, and/or small pelvis.[116,119,121,123] Due to these characteristic skeletal changes, patients with Kniest syndrome often have a distinct stiffness presenting with little knee flexion, shuffling, and waddling gait.[124-126] Additionally, patients may be unable to form a fist with their hands due to enlarged metacarpal joint.[116,119]

Confirmatory testing can be made prenatally via amniocentesis, cell-free DNA, or chorionic villus sampling. Molecular genetic testing can confirm disease after birth.[118,122,127] Biopsy sampling of epiphyseal growth plates will show soft, crumbly cartilage, that has been described as similar in appearance to foamy Swiss cheese.[116,117,128]

Patients with Kniest syndrome will have radiological findings similar to those found in Stickler disease and SED congenita.[126] X-rays will show shortened and slender bones with delayed, widened, and abnormal epiphyseal ends.[129,130] Joints can show shortening, most commonly in metacarpal joint contractures.[126] Spinal X-rays can show platyspondyly and kyphoscoliosis.[126,130] Up to 63% of these patients will show abnormal coronal vertebral clefts occurring most frequently in the lumbar spine (60%), followed by the thoracic spine (36%).[130] Vertebral clefts are useful in identifying patients with Kniest syndrome at birth, these clefts tend to disappear at 1 year of age.[124,130]

Complications and Treatment

There is very minimal medical treatment needed with this patient population. Physicians must be aware of myopia with retinal detachment and respiratory distress secondary to tracheomalacia and shortened ribs.[121,127,131-135]

Patients with Kniest syndrome are at a higher risk for cervical spine instability, including atlantoaxial and occipitoatlantal instabilities.[72,136] Cervical extension and flexion that results in greater than 5 mm of subluxation between C1 and C2 is indicative of excessive atlantoaxial instability. Such may indicate that surgical intervention is warranted. Arthrodesis between the occiput and the second cervical vertebrae or the occiput and subaxial levels have been shown to be an effective treatment for cervical instabilities.[72,113] Halo cast should be used postoperatively to facilitate cervical spinal fusion.[136] There are limited data concerning the outcomes following cervical decompression and fusion.

In addition to the cervical spine, the lumbar spine can become hyperlordotic as a compensatory mechanism to abnormal hip flexion or mild thoracolumbar kyphoscoliosis.[124,137]

Long-term Outcomes

Early onset and severe arthropathy has been associated with Kniest syndrome.[126,136]

PSEUDOACHONDROPLASIA

Epidemiology/Genes

Pseudoachondroplasia (PSACH) is an autosomal dominant disorder, which has a prevalence of 4 per one million individuals and an annual incidence of 1 per 30,000 births.[128,138] The mutation can also occur via de novo mutation in the germline of healthy parents, which is perhaps due to germline mosaicism.[139] PSACH is caused by a mutation in the Cartilage Oligomeric Matrix Protein (*COMP*) gene at the 19p13.1 chromosomal locus.[140]

Pathological Mechanism

Cartilage Oligomeric Matrix Protein is mainly expressed by chondrocytes and is secreted into the extracellular matrix. Mutations within COMP cause disruption in the protein's calcium binding affinity. This leads to a decrease in proteoglycan and COMP secretion and increase in sequestration of proteins in the rough endoplasmic reticulum.[138,141-144] As the rough endoplasmic reticulum expands with proteins, it causes death to the chondrocyte.[128,141,145,146] Loss of epiphyseal chondrocytes leads to reduced bone growth and physical stature.[128,140,142]

Presentation and Diagnosis

Pseudoachondroplasia is typically asymptomatic until 1–4 years of age.[147,148] First signs of disease can be abnormally short stature with disproportionally short limbs, joint laxity, pain, and stiffness, bowed legs, and a waddling gait.[142,146,147,149] Adult females with PSACH have an average height of 116 cm and males have an average height of 120 cm.[147] It is similar to achondroplasia in terms of the body proportions, but there are many differences including normal facial structure in PSACH, as well as platyspondyly with normal interpedicular distances, mild lumbar lordosis, and atlantoaxial instability.[128] Common features found in achondroplastics include frontal bossing, mid-face hypoplasia, and normal vertebrae with decreased interpedicular distance.[128] Additionally, severe lumbar lordosis and atlantoaxial instability are rarely seen.[128]

Spinal X-rays can show thoracolumbar kyphosis and scoliosis, lumbar lordosis secondary to hip flexion contracture, ventral spinal projections that disappear by 6–12 years of age.[138,147-149] Cervical spinal radiographs can reveal odontoid hypoplasia with or without atlantoaxial instability.[138,146-148] Long bones tend to be short and broad with metaphyseal flaring. Epiphyseal ossification is significantly delayed.[138,147-149]

Confirmatory testing can be made prenatally via amniocentesis, cell-free DNA, or chorionic villus sampling. Molecular genetic testing can confirm disease after birth.[147,149,150] Bone biopsy can show hypertrophic chondrocyte cells with enlarged rough endoplasmic reticulum and sporadic apoptosis.[145]

Complications and Treatment

Patients with PSACH should be monitored for early onset arthropathy and atlantoaxial instability secondary to odontoid hypoplasia and os odontoideum.[72,150,151] Shetty et al. report that the prevalence of os odontoideum in PSACH is 60% and typically these populations do not present with myelopathy nor require surgical intervention.[151] Ain et al. reported a 75% success rate after first fusion attempt and 100% after two fusion attempts.[113] These patients were in postsurgical halo casts for an average of 3.3 months and all reported improved or normalized neurological function.[113]

The hip joint should be paid special attention as one-third to one-half of all patients with PSACH will need hip replacement by their mid-30s.[146]

Long-term Outcomes

Atlantoaxial instability has been shown to increase with age, requiring careful monitoring.[151] Kyphosis, lordosis, and scoliosis can occur, but is rarely severe enough to warrant surgical intervention.[128,150]

METATROPIC DYSPLASIA

Epidemiology/Genes

Metatropic dysplasia is a rare autosomal dominant disorder, which has a prevalence of 1.7 affected per one million individuals.[152,153] The diseased state occurs via a mutation in transient receptor potential cation channel, subfamily V, member 4 (*TRPV4*) gene, which is located at chromosomal locus 12q24.11.[154] Gene mutations usually occur via de novo germline mutations.[155-157] Prevalence of metatropic dysplasia displays a 3:2 ratio of males to females.[158]

Pathological Mechanism

Mutations in the *TRPV4* gene produce constitutively active calcium channels.[159] While the exact mechanism of disease has not been elucidated, recent studies have shown that calcium is involved with osteoclast differentiation and bone mineralization.[155,160] There is a wide range of metatropic dysplastic phenotypes ranging from lethal to nonlethal mutations and phenotypic severity may be dependent upon degree of misregulated calcium influx.[155,157,161]

Presentation and Diagnosis

Patients with metatropic dysplasia can be born with short limbs and normal trunk size, kyphoscoliosis, narrowed shoulders and thorax, prominent knees, and joint limitations.[158,161,162] In some cases, macrocephaly and a sacrococcygeal tail may be present at birth.[158,161] By the age of 2 years, growth is usually depressed.[161] Later in life, thoracolumbar kyphoscoliosis and cervical instability can become progressively worse and may require surgical intervention.[161] Adult height can range from 107 cm to 146 cm.[158,161]

Confirmatory testing can be made prenatally via amniocentesis, cell-free DNA, or chorionic villus sampling. After birth, molecular genetic testing can confirm disease.[157,163,164]

Prenatal ultrasound can show shortened and "dumbbell" shaped long bones, narrowed thorax, joint contractures, or platyspondyly.[153,161] After birth, spinal imaging can show platyspondyly, wafer-like vertebral bodies, kyphoscoliosis, narrowed interpedicular distance, odontoid hypoplasia with or without atlantoaxial instability, and/or delayed ossification of vertebral bodies.[155,161,162,164,165] Long bones can have metaphyseal flaring resulting in "dumbbell" like appearance.[158,164]

Complications and Treatment

Physicians should monitor patients with metatropic dysplasia for respiratory distress symptoms, which are not due to brainstem compression.[161] This can be due to narrowed thorax, laryngotracheomalacia, restrictive lung disease secondary to chest wall lesion, or chronic pulmonary infection.[161,166]

Spinal kyphoscoliosis occurs in 55–88% of patients with metatropic dysplasia.[161,164] It typically appears early in childhood and is difficult to manage.[161] Vertebral arthrodesis has been performed with varying degrees of success due to postsurgical spinal growth and progression of kyphoscoliosis.[158,161,166]

Shohat et al. reported that atlantoaxial subluxation is present in 73% and odontoid hypoplasia in 92–100% of patients with metatropic dysplasia.[161,165,167] Both conditions can lead to myelopathy. In these cases, cervical arthrodesis is commonly performed, but due to the diseased state, atlantoaxial instability can recur.[158,161]

Long-term Outcomes

Arthropathy has been seen on X-ray imaging, however patients are usually asymptomatic.[161,168] Respiratory capacity and scoliosis should be closely monitored as they are closely linked to the mortality and quality of life in this patient population, respectively.[158,161,164]

CHAPTER 18

CONRADI-HÜNERMANN SYNDROME (CHONDRODYSPLASIA PUNCTATA)

Epidemiology/Genes

Chondrodysplasia punctata disorder is characterized by an abnormal, punctate pattern of cartilage calcium deposits. This disorder, which is also known as Conradi-Hünermann syndrome, or chondrodysplasia punctata 1 X-linked (CPX1), is caused by a mutated gene on the X chromosome at the Xp11.23 locus.[169] This gene codes for the arylsulfatase E (ARSE) protein and mutations are inherited in a sex-linked recessive manner.[170]

Pathological Mechanism

The ARSE protein codes for a steroid sulfatase, with mutations causing a reduction or loss of function in enzymatic activity.[171] ARSE functions to remove sulfate groups and in its absence, there is premature and increased mineralization of the cartilage.[169-172]

Presentation and Diagnosis

There are a wide spectrum of phenotypes associated with mutations in the ARSE protein ranging from varying degrees of physical malformations to neonatal death.[170] Patients with CPX1 can be born with nasal hypoplasia, depressed nasal bridge, shortened nasal septum, deep groove between the nasal alae and tip, short stature, brachytelephalangic (short distal phalanges), mid-face depression or flat facial features, and hearing loss.[169,170,173,174]

Confirmatory testing can be made prenatally via amniocentesis, cell-free DNA, or chorionic villus sampling. After birth, molecular genetic testing can confirm CDPX1 or ARSE protein activity measurements can also confirm disease.[170,171,173]

Prenatal ultrasound can show shortened long bones, hypoplastic nose development, vertebral platyspondyly, or punctate epiphyseal plates.[169,175] Coronal and sagittal vertebral clefts can be found in up to 33% of infants with CPX1.[130] With increasing age, vertebral clefts can be filled and disappear.[130]

Radiographically, the most common sign of CPX1 is the punctate pattern of calcification, most prominent in the tarsals, epiphyseal plates, and vertebrae.[169,174] Other frequently seen pathological features include joint contractures, hypoplastic cervical vertebrae with subsequent kyphosis, platyspondyly, atlantoaxial instability, and a narrowed cervical canal.[169-171,176]

Complications and Treatment

Respiratory problems occur frequently in this population and should be monitored.[177,178] Spinal curvature should be closely monitored to enable early identification of scoliosis, which is commonly seen in early childhood.[179,180] For all chondrodysplasia punctata syndromes, scoliosis can be characterized as either severe with rapid progression or mild with slower progression.[179] Rapid and severe scoliosis is very difficult to manage, requiring an average of 2.5 surgeries as a consequence of a high rate of pseudoarthrosis and curve progression.[179] Ventral strut graft and dorsal fusion have been shown to be effective for this indication.[179] The rarer slowly progressing scoliosis responds well to bracing and if needed, standard dorsal fusion.[179]

Atlantoaxial instability cervical stenosis can also occur in patients with CPX1, although it is less prevalent than kyphoscoliosis.[177,181-183] In a small series, Herman et al. demonstrated that dorsal spinal decompression and fusion is effective in treating atlantoaxial instability and cervical spinal cord impingement.[184]

CAMPOMELIC DYSPLASIA

Epidemiology/Genes

Campomelic dysplasia is a rare disorder affecting seven per one million births with features affecting both the skeletal and reproductive systems.[1,185] Campomelic dysplasia is caused by a mutation in the sex-determining region Y-related high mobility group box gene (*SOX9*) located on the chromosomal locus 17q24.3.[186] Inheritance is autosomal dominant and there is an equal incidence in both males and females.[185,187,188]

Pathological Mechanism

SOX9 is a transcription factor expressed in both the chondrocytes of the skeletal system and within the cells of the gonad.[186,189,190] Mutations in *SOX9* cause a decrease in collagen formation and thus weaken and stunt bone development and growth.[189-195] Additionally, SOX9 is also a transcription factor for the Y-chromosome protein, Sex determining region of the Y-chromosome (SRY), and therefore mutations in SOX9 also decrease SRY protein levels and thus cause a female phenotype in genotypic males.[189,190,196,197] There has been no identified association between the type of SOX9 mutation and severity of camptomelic dysplasia.[198]

Presentation and Diagnosis

At birth, infants with camptomelic dysplasia can present with macrocephaly, depressed nasal bridge, low set ears, club foot, bowed femur and tibia, respiratory distress, narrowed thorax, hypertelorism, Pierre-Robin sequence (micrognathia, glossoptosis, upper airway obstruction, cleft palate), ambiguous genitalia, short limbs, and cone-shaped fingers with or without hypoplastic thumbs.[185-187,198-200]

Confirmatory testing can be made prenatally via amniocentesis, cell-free DNA, or chorionic villus sampling. After birth, molecular genetic testing can confirm campomelic dysplasia.[186,198]

Prenatal ultrasound can show increased nuchal fold, prominent cisterna magna, micrognathia, deviation of the cardiac axis, digit hypoplasia, bowing of femur and tibia, narrowed thorax, hypoplastic scapulae, Pierre Robin sequence, prominent forehead, club feet, and short limbs.[186,198,201]

Spinal X-rays can show hypoplastic cervical vertebrae with kyphosis and instability, and nonmineralized thoracic pedicles.[185,190] Kyphoscoliosis begins in early childhood and becomes more severe later in life.[185,202,203] X-rays can also show pronounced bowing of the femur and tibia as well as only 11 pairs of ribs.[187,199]

Complications and Treatment

In contrast to other skeletal dysplasias, the cause of death in patients with camptomelic dysplasia is usually due to respiratory distress secondary to tracheobronchomalacia or cervical spine instability.[185,204-206] Bracing to stabilize spinal curves has not been proven beneficial.[207] However, Lekovic et al. recommended neonatal bracing until vertebral ossification occurs, typically around 18 months of age.[208] Furthermore, strict bracing compliance has been shown to decrease pathological spinal curvatures.[208]

Early and aggressive surgical intervention with ventral and dorsal fusion has been shown to limit neurological and pulmonary defects due to cervical instability and kyphoscoliosis.[205,207-209] Postoperative halo casts can be used until sufficient spinal fusion has been reached to maintain fusion integrity.[207,209]

Related Complications

Kyphoscoliosis occurs in 100% of patients with camptomelic dysplasia.[207] Despite early and aggressive treatment, pseudoarthrosis occurs in 50% of patients and neurological complications occur in 33% of patients with camptomelic dysplasia.[205,207] Due to the high neonatal lethality of this disease, there are limited data regarding the long-term outcomes.

MUCOPOLYSACCHARIDOSES [HURLER'S SYNDROME (MPS I), SCHEIE SYNDROME (MPS I), HUNTER'S SYNDROME (MPS II), SANFILIPPO SYNDROME (MPS III), MORQUIO SYNDROME (MPS IV), MAROTEAUX-LAMY SYNDROME (MPS IV)]

Overview

Mucopolysaccharidoses (MPS) are genetic mutations in lysosomal enzymes that degrade glycosaminoglycans (GAGs).[210] Incidence ranges from 1.75 to 4.05 affected per 100,000 births.[4-7] With the exception of Hunter's syndrome, which mainly affects males, all of the above MPS disorders show equal distribution across gender.[210]

In normal metabolism, there is the production of GAGs.[211] In patients with lysosomal enzyme deficiencies, GAGs build up intracellularly as the cell is unable to breakdown GAGs into their components.[211-213] A buildup of GAG vesicles in epiphyseal plate chondrocytes leads to immune cell recruitment, inflammation, apoptosis, decreased chondrocyte proliferation, altered growth plate architecture, and osteoclast activation.[211-213] There exists no evidence to support a relationship between genotype mutation and phenotypic severity.[212,214,215]

Prenatally and after birth, genetic testing and lysosomal activity from measurements via amniocentesis sample, chorionic villi tissue can be used to diagnose MPS.[7,214,216] Also, fibroblasts can also be measured to confirm and quantify severity.[7,214,216] Positive urinary GAGs are yet another indication of lysosomal enzymatic disorder and possible MPS diagnosis.[7,214,217]

Epidemiology/Genes

Hurler's Syndrome (MPS I)

Hurler's syndrome is caused by a mutation on chromosomal locus 4p16.3, which codes for iduronidase and is inherited in an autosomal recessive pattern.[210]

Scheie Syndrome (MPS I)

Scheie syndrome is caused by a mutation on chromosomal locus 4p16.4, which codes for iduronidase and is inherited in an autosomal recessive pattern.[210,218]

Hunter's Syndrome (MPS II)

Hunter's syndrome is caused by a mutation on chromosomal locus Xp27.3-28, which codes for iduronate sulfate sulfatase.[210] Hunter's syndrome is inherited in a X-linked inheritance pattern.[210,218] It has an incidence of 0.3–0.71 affected per 100,000 live births.[212]

Sanfilippo Syndrome (MPS III)

Sanfilippo syndrome is caused by mutations in chromosomal loci 17q25.3 that codes for heparan-S-sulfamidase, 17q21.1 that codes for N-acetyl-alpha-glucosaminidase, 8p11-q13 that codes for acetyl-CoA-glucosaminide-N-acetyltransferase, or 12q14 that codes for N-acetyl-glucosamine-6-sulfate sulfatase.[210,218] Sanfilippo syndrome is inherited in an autosomal recessive pattern.[210,218] It has an incidence of 0.78–2.82 affected per 100,000 live births.[212]

Morquio Syndrome (MPS IV)

Morquio syndrome is caused by mutations in chromosomal loci 16q24.3 that codes for N-acetylgalactosamine-6-sulfate sulfatase, or 3p21.33 that codes for beta-galactosidase.[210,218] Morquio syndrome is inherited in an autosomal recessive pattern.[210,218] It has incidence rate of 0.22–1.30 affected per 100,000 live births.[212]

Maroteaux-Lamy Syndrome (MPS VI)

Maroteaux-Lamy syndrome is caused by a mutation on chromosomal locus 5q13q14, which codes for arylsulfatase B.[219] Maroteaux-Lamy syndrome is inherited in an autosomal recessive pattern. It has an incidence rate of 0.36–1.30 affected per 100,000 live births.[212]

Presentation and Diagnosis

Patients with MPS have cessation of growth at 3 to 4 years of age, generally not growing taller than 120 cm.[214] Prenatal ultrasound findings in fetuses with MPS can show cardiac abnormalities.[220] Radiological imaging can find thickened and shortened metacarpal bones with proximal coning, hypoplastic bone development, underdeveloped epiphyseal plates, severe hip dysplasia, and a J-shaped sella in the cranium. Spinal imaging can show ovoid hypoplastic vertebral bodies with platyspondyly and upward hook-like curvatures, ventral wedging, kyphosis, scoliosis, and lumbar lordosis.[212,221-223]

Hurler's Syndrome and Scheie Syndrome (MPS I)

Patients can present with dysostosis multiplex, which is characterized as profound loss of joint range of motion, restricted mobility, growth slowing or arrest in early childhood and short stature.[212] These conditions can result with the hand being claw-shaped and thoracolumbar kyphosis and resulting lumbar lordosis.[212] Unique to MPS I, most patients have progressive corneal clouding, hernias, and gibbus deformities.[216,222] Mild scoliosis can also be seen.[222] Severe cases of MPS I can present with craniocervical and atlantoaxial instability secondary to odontoid hypoplasia.[221] Lastly, children can have cognitive impairment with obvious behavioral and social problems as well.[212,216,217]

Hunter's Syndrome (MPS II)

Patients can present usually at age 2 with dysostosis multiplex similar to MPS I.[212,216,217,222,224] Atlantoaxial instability and cervical spinal cord impingement can be seen secondary to hypertrophy of the dorsal odontoid soft tissue.[221,222,225] Unique to Hunter's syndrome, organomegaly can be present and in severe cases,[212,216,217,224] behavioral and cognitive changes can be seen as well.[212,216,217,224]

Sanfilippo's Syndrome (MPS III)

Sanfilippo syndrome presents with mild bodily changes (with no thoracolumbar kyphosis and mild scoliosis) and most patients have profound mental deterioration and hyperactivity.[212,216,217,222,224] Additionally, the behavioral and cognitive changes occur before any bone and joint manifestations.[212,216,217,224] In early childhood, children can present with developmental delays, behavioral difficulties, sleep disturbances and dementia, as well as mental retardation with underdeveloped social and communication skills.[212,216,217,224] Severe cases can ultimately result with patients entering a vegetative state with a maximum life expectancy of 30–40 years.[212,216,217,224]

Morquio Syndrome (MPS IV)

Patients with Morquio syndrome can present with short trunk dwarfism, fine corneal deposits, and spondyloepiphyseal dysplasia.[216] Craniocervical junction and atlantoaxial instability secondary to odontoid hypoplasia can cause cervical myelopathy.[216,221,224] In Morquio syndrome, cognitive abilities are not impaired and there can be joint hypermobility secondary to ligamentous laxity.[212,217]

Maroteaux-Lamy Syndrome (MPS VI)

Similarly to Morquio syndrome, in Maroteaux-Lamy syndrome, there is no cognitive impairment.[217] There can also be mild to severe corneal clouding, however this typically does not develop as an early sign of disease.[217] Patients can present with dysostosis multiplex similar to MPS I.[212,216,217] Craniocervical junction and atlantoaxial instability secondary to odontoid hypoplasia can cause cervical myelopathy.[216,221,224] Additionally, patients with Maroteaux-Lamy syndrome can present with cardiac valvular disorders, sleep apnea, and decreased pulmonary function.[212,222,224] Patients with severe Maroteaux-Lamy syndrome can present as early as 2 to 3 years of age with decreased ambulation by 10 years of age.[216] On average, patients can survive to 20–30 years of age.[212,216]

Prenatal ultrasound findings in fetuses with MPS can show cardiac abnormalities.[220] Radiological imaging can identify thickened and shortened metacarpal bones with proximal coning, hypoplastic bone development, underdeveloped epiphyseal plates, severe hip dysplasia, and a J-shaped sella in the cranium. Spinal imaging can show ovoid hypoplastic vertebral bodies with platyspondyly and upward hook-like curvatures, ventral wedging, kyphosis, scoliosis, and lumbar lordosis.[212,221-223]

Complications and Treatment

Enzymatic replacement therapy is available for MPS type I and IV. It is crucial to administer therapy early to minimize cellular damage and to avoid irreversible musculoskeletal changes.[214,226-229] Radiological monitoring of the skeletal system is important to ensure integrity.[222] There is no evidence of the efficacy of bracing for spinal cord stabilization in patients with MPS.[222]

Craniocervical and atlantoaxial instability secondary to odontoid hypoplasia with spinal cord impingement is common by age 6, often requiring surgical decompression and fusion, especially in patients with MPS type I and IV.[212,214,218,222,230] Patients with MPS II have been shown to have ventral cervical spine compression secondary to thickening of the dorsal odontoid soft tissue, resulting from GAG deposition.[225] In patients with MPS type IV, prophylactic cervical vertebrae fusion with decompression is recommended as GAG accumulation can occur dorsal to the odontoid process and result in stenosis and subsequent myelopathy.[222,231,232]

Early diagnosis of thoracolumbar kyphotic curves larger than 40° has been shown to be significantly more likely to progress by age 6.[233] Scoliosis is common in MPS, but rarely requires surgical stabilization.[222] In severe kyphosis, ventral and dorsal fusion is commonly performed with postoperative bracing for 3–6 months.[222,234] While scoliosis is rare among patients with MPS, traditional scoliosis surgical criteria should be followed including ventral fusion in prepubescent children to prevent crankshaft phenomenon.[222]

MUCOLIPIDOSES

Epidemiology/Genes

Mucolipidosis is caused by mutations in the N-actyl-glucosamine-1-phosphotransferase subunits alpha and beta (GNPTAB).[3] GNPTAB is coded at chromosomal locus 12q23.3 and these mutations follow an autosomal recessive inheritance pattern.[216,235] The incidence of this disease is 4.05 affected per 100,000 live births.[2,3] Mucolipidosis is equally distributed among males and females.[236]

Pathological Mechanism

There are three types of mucolipidoses—type II, type III, and type III gamma variant.[235] In all subtypes, there is a decrease in activity of the GNPTAB enzyme, which helps traffic enzymes to lysosomal compartments.[237] Intracellularly, there is an accumulation of inclusion bodies as substrates are not degraded by lysosomal enzymes.[238] These cellular changes cause an altered state of chondrocyte differentiation, altered expression of growth factors, and an increase in chondrocyte cathepsin K protease activity, all of which lead to impaired cartilage formation.[239,240]

Presentation and Diagnosis

Mucolipidosis type II is caused by a total absence in GNPTAB enzymatic activity and therefore patients present with symptoms as early as 6 to 12 months of age.[241,242] Mucolipidosis type III is a more mild deficiency in GNPTAB enzymatic activity and patients present with symptoms around age 2 to 3.[241] Mucolipidosis type III gamma is also a mild deficiency in GNPTAB activity and patients present with symptoms around the age of 7.[243] Patients can present with contracted joints with joint stiffness, hypotonia, flat face, depressed nasal bridge, increased skin thickness with wax like texture, or hypertrophied gums.[3,241]

Prenatal amniocentesis, chorionic villus sampling, or cell-free DNA analysis can confirm mucolipidoses. After birth, fibroblast enzymatic activity analysis can confirm mucolipidoses.[243-245]

Prenatal ultrasound can show oligohydramnios, growth retardation, echogenic cardiac foci, or short femurs.[241,246] After birth, radiological findings include generalized osteopenia, inguinal hernia, hepatosplenomegaly, and congenital hip dislocation.[242,247] Spinal imaging can show thoracolumbar kyphosis, lumbar hyperlordosis, ventral-caudal beaking of the vertebra, vertebral subluxation, ovoid-shaped vertebral bodies, and hyperplastic vertebrae.[247-251] Additionally, there have been rare reports of atlantoaxial instability with cervical spinal cord myelopathy secondary to odontoid hypoplasia.[252]

Complications and Treatment

In patients with progressive thoracolumbar kyphosis, dorsal spinal instrumentation with ventral and dorsal fusion is recommended. Mucolipidosis type III rarely compromises spinal cord integrity.[251]

Cardiovascular issues including aortic and mitral valvular thickening and incompetence have been noted in this patient population.[253,254] Cardiac function should be closely monitored.[253,254]

SUMMARY

The advancements in genetic and molecular testing techniques have greatly elucidated the field of genetic disorders. Effective diagnosis plays a key part in the management of patients with skeletal dysplasias and metabolic disorders. While many of these diseases are incurable, early detection and diagnosis allow for the optimization of the treatment regimen and surgical intervention. Understanding the signs and symptoms of each of these diseases can help the surgeon identify, manage, and treat the associated spinal disorders and other complications. This understanding, along with advances in treatment modalities, will further improve patient outcomes and help preserve patient quality of life. To assist with understanding these complex diseases, Table 1 shows the referenced articles with their associated level-of-evidence.

Table 1: Level-of-evidence.

Author, journal, year	*Design*	*LoE*
Goriely, AJHG, 2012	SR	III
Wright, ADC, 2012	SR	III
Laederich, ERMM, 2012	SR	III
Misra, NF, 2003	SR	III
Mckay, Spine, 2012	SR	II
Veeravagu, WN, 2012	SR	III
Bethem, JBJS, 1981+G83A86:J93	SR	III
Vogel, CNS, 2012	SR	III
Simmons, IJPO, 2005	SR	III
Poorthuis, HG, 1999	R	II
Krabbi, GTMB, 2012	R	II
Malm, AP, 2008	R	II
Baehner, JIMD, 2005	R	II
Hecht, AJHG, 1987	R	II
King, JNP, 2009	R	III
Hecht, AJHG, 1989	R	II
Ain, Spine, 2006	R	III
Ain, Spine, 2004	R	III
Wynn, AJMG, 2007	R	II
Schramm, UOG, 2009	R	II
Matsuyama, Spine, 1999	R	III
Jalanko, Spine, 2009	R	III

Contd...

Contd...

Author, journal, year	*Design*	*LoE*
Soultanis, Scoliosis, 2007	R	II
Miyoshi, Spine, 2004	R	III
Nakamura, AOTS, 1998	R	II
Ain, Spine, 2006	R	III
Orioli, JMG, 1986	PC	II
Wilkin, AJHG, 1998	PC	II
Pauli, AJHG, 1995	PC	I
Li, DB, 2008	PC	II
Boor, EJP, 1999	PC	II
Ruiz-Garcia, CNS, 1997	PC	I
Thomas, AJDC, 1988	PC	I
Pauli, JPO, 1997	PC	I
Barbosa, Clin Gen, 2011	PC	II
Murray, AJHG, 1989	PC	II
Xia, CCA, 2008	PC	II
Stevens, JPO, 2007	PC	II
Wynne-Davies, JBJS, 1982	PC	I
Gigliani, GMB, 2012	EO	IV
Lemyre, CARJ, 1990	EO	V
Shirley, JAAOS, 2009	EO	V
Hunter, JM, 1998	EO	V
Tolo, BLF, 1988	EO	V

Contd...

Contd...

Author, journal, year	*Design*	*LoE*
Siebens, APMR, 1987	EO	V
Haga, JOS, 2004	EO	V
Trotter, Ped, 2005	EO	V
Supert-Furga, AJMG, 2007	EO	V
Amirfeyz, Curr Ortho, 2005	EO	V
Berkowitz, Anest, 1990	EO	V
Lachman, AJR, 1975	EO	V
Spranger, AJMG, 1997	EO	V
Nishimura, AJMG, 2012	EO	V
Campbell, Spine, 2009	EO	V
White, Rheum, 2011	EO	V
Wood, JIMD, 2013	EO	V
David, JNS, 1980	CS	IV
Vleggert-Lankamp, JNS, 2012	CS	IV
Ain, JPO, 2004	CS	IV
Lutter, JBJS, 1977	CS	IV
Whyte, Med, 1999	CS	IV
Wilkin, AJHG, 1998	CS	IV
Nagendran, AJMG, 2012	CS	IV
Bogaert, AJHG, 1994	CS	IV
Spranger, Ped Rad, 1994	CS	IV
Westvik, Ped Rad, 1998	CS	IV
Ferguson, AJMG, 1997	CS	IV
Wynee-Davis, JMG, 1986	CS	IV
Geneviève, AJMG, 2008	CS	IV
Kannu, AJMG, 2007	CS	IV
Hall, Ped. Rad, 2004	CS	IV
Shohat, JP, 1989	CS	IV
Andreucci, OJRD, 2011	CS	IV
Krakow, UOG, 2003	CS	IV
Cormier-Daire, Ped Rad, 2001	CS	IV
Casarin, AJMG, 2009	CS	IV
Mason, Spine, 1995	CS	IV
Herman, Ped Rad, 2002	CS	IV
Mansour, JMG, 1995	CS	IV
Velgaleti, AJHG, 2005	CS	IV
Nelson, AORL, 2011	CS	IV
Thomas, Spine, 1997	CS	IV
Schroeder, JIMD Rep, 2013	CS	IV
Schmidt, Ped Rad, 1987	CS	IV
Parsons, Clin Rad, 1996	CS	IV
Cox-Brinkman, JIMD, 2007	CS	IV

Contd...

Contd...

Author, journal, year	*Design*	*LoE*
Hughes, Neurorad., 1997	CS	IV
Siddique, JBJS, 2010	CS	IV
Ransford, JBJS, 1996	CS	IV
Cathey, JMG, 2010	CS	IV
David-Vizcarra, PJCH, 2010	CS	IV
Pazzaglia, Ped Rad,1989	CS	IV
Hetherington, JRSM, 1999	CS	IV
Chitty, UOG, 2011	CS	IV
Khalil, PD, 2011	CS	IV
Ednick, JP, 2009	CS	IV
Bagley, JNP, 2006	CS	IV
Baca, JPO, 2010	CS	IV
Sciubba, JNP, 2007	CS	IV
Horton, JP, 1978	CS	IV
Remes, Spine, 2001	CS	IV
Meizner, AJOG, 1995	CR	V
Jha, JNP, 2008	CR	V
Bauer, NSF, 2005	CR	V
Agabegik, Ortho, 2008	CR	V
Liao, AO, 2006	CR	V
Frigon, Curr Surg, 2000	CR	V
Maeda, AJMG, 2006	CR	V
Dwyer, AJMG, 2010	CR	V
Turner, FPP, 2010	CR	V
Morita, Spine, 2005	CR	V
LeDoux, NS, 1991	CR	V
Unger, AJMG, 2001	CR	V
Al-Awadi, JMG, 1984	CR	V
Fiedler, AO, 2003	CR	V
Winterpacht, MG, 1993	CR	V
Burton, JP, 1865	CR	V
Subramanian, Ind Ped, 2007	CR	V
Cole, COR, 1997	CR	V
Hicks, UP, 2001	CR	V
Yokoyama, AJO, 2003	CR	V
Merrill, JPO, 1989	CR	V
Jackson, HM, 2012	CR	V
Unger, AJMG, 2011	CR	V
Genevieve, AJMG, 2005	CR	V
Leet, JPO, 2006	CR	IV

Contd...

Contd...

Author, journal, year	*Design*	*LoE*
Mundinger, Ped Rad, 2009	CR	V
Yang, JNP, 2006	CR	V
Goodman, MRI, 1990	CR	V
Corbani, MS, 2011	CR	V
Goyal, IJHG, 2011	CR	V
Tongsong, UOG, 2000	CR	V
Ray, COR, 1984	CR	V
Dahdaleh, JCN, 2010	CR	V
Lekovic, CNS, 2006	CR	V
Coscia, JPO, 1989	CR	V
Morishita, Rheum, 2011	CR	V
Gabrielli, Ped, 2010	CR	V
Thomas, JIMD, 2006	CR	V
Tamaki, NS, 1987	CR	V

Contd...

Contd...

Author, journal, year	*Design*	*LoE*
Heo, KJP, 2012	CR	V
Lees, UOG, 2001	CR	V
Melo, OSOMOPORE, 2007	CR	V
Gordon, PMJ, 1973	CR	V
Carl, Spine, 1991	CR	V
Daimon, Card Young, 2005	CR	V
Cripe, Card Young, 2009	CR	V
Radcliff, Spine, 2012	CC	III
Karlstedt, CGDB, 1997	CC	III
Kanazawa, JBM, 2003	CC	III
Mckeand, AJMG, 1996	CC	III
Shetty, JPO, 2007	CC	IV
McGill, Clin Gen, 2010	CC	III

REFERENCES

1. Orioli IM, Castilla EE, Barbosa-Neto JG. The birth prevalence rates for the skeletal dysplasias. J Med Genet. 1986;23:328-32.
2. Poorthuis BJ, Wevers RA, Kleijer WJ, et al. The frequency of lysosomal storage diseases in The Netherlands. Hum Genet. 1999;105:151-6.
3. Leroy JG, Sillence D, Wood T, et al. A novel intermediate mucolipidosis II/IIIαβ caused by GNPTAB mutation in the cytosolic N-terminal domain. Eur J Hum Genet. 2014;22(5):594-601.
4. Krabbi K, Joost K, Zordania R, et al. The live-birth prevalence of mucopolysaccharidoses in Estonia. Genet Test Mol Biomarkers. 2012;16(8):846-9.
5. Malm G, Lund AM, Månsson JE, et al. Mucopolysaccharidoses in the Scandinavian countries: incidence and prevalence. Acta Paediatr. 2008;97(11):1577-81.
6. Baehner F, Schmiedeskamp C, Krummenauer F, et al. Cumulative incidence rates of the mucopolysaccharidoses in Germany. J Inherit Metab Dis. 2005;28(6):1011-7.
7. Giugliani R. Mucopolysacccharidoses: From understanding to treatment, a century of discoveries. Genet Mol Biol. 2012;35(4):924-31.
8. Pauli RM. Achondroplasia: a comprehensive clinical review. Orphanet J Rare Dis 2019;14(1):1.
9. Waller DK, Correa A, Vo TM, et al. The population-based prevalence of achondroplasia and thanatophoric dysplasia in selected regions of the US. Am J Med Genet A. 2008; 146A(18):2385-9.
10. Parikh S, Batra P. Achondroplasia. (2012). [online] Available from https://emedicine.medscape.com/article/1258401-overview [Last Accessed July 2019].
11. Naski MC, Wang Q, Xu J, et al. Graded activation of fibroblast growth factor receptor 3 by mutations causing achondroplasia and thanatophoric dysplasia. Nat Genet. 1996;13(2):233-7.
12. Goriely A, Wilkie AO. Paternal age effect mutations and selfish spermatogonial selection: causes and consequences for human disease. Am J Hum Genet. 2012;90(2):175-200.
13. Wilkin DJ, Szabo JK, Cameron R, et al. Mutations in fibroblast growth-factor receptor 3 in sporadic cases of achondroplasia occur exclusively on the paternally derived chromosome. Am J Hum Genet. 1998;63(3):711-6.
14. Wright MJ, Irving MD. Clinical management of achondroplasia. Arch Dis Child. 2012;97(2):129-34.
15. Davidson D, Blanc A, Filion D, et al. Fibroblast growth factor (FGF) 18 signals through FGF receptor 3 to promote chondrogenesis. J Biol Chem. 2005;280(21):20509-15.
16. Laederich MB, Horton WA. FGFR3 targeting strategies for achondroplasia. Expert Rev Mol Med. 2012;14:e11.
17. Webster MK, Donoghue DJ. Constitutive activation of fibroblast growth factor receptor 3 by the transmembrane domain point mutation found in achondroplasia. EMBO J. 1996;15(3):520-7.
18. Vajo Z, Francomano CA, Wilkin DJ. The molecular and genetic basis of fibroblast growth factor receptor 3 disorders: the achondroplasia family of skeletal dysplasias, Muenke craniosynostosis, and Crouzon syndrome with acanthosis nigricans. Endocr Rev. 2000;21(1):23-39.

19. McKusick VA, Kelly TE, Dorst JP. Observations suggesting allelism of the achondroplasia and hypochondroplasia genes. J Med Genet. 1973;10:11-6.
20. Pauli RM, Horton VK, Glinski LP, et al. Prospective assessment of risks for cervicomedullary-junction compression in infants with achondroplasia. Am J Hum Genet. 1995;56:732-44.
21. Meizner I, Barnhard Y. Achondrogenesis type I diagnosed by transvaginal ultrasonography at 13 weeks' gestation. Am J Obstet Gynecol. 1995;173(5):1620-2.
22. Chitty LS, Griffin DR, Meaney C, et al. New aids for the non-invasive prenatal diagnosis of achondroplasia: dysmorphic features, charts of fetal size and molecular confirmation using cell-free fetal DNA in maternal plasma. Ultrasound Obstet Gynecol. 2011;37(3):283-9.
23. Khalil A, Pajkrt E, Chitty LS. Early prenatal diagnosis of skeletal anomalies. Prenat Diagn. 2011;31(1):115-24.
24. Lemyre E, Azouz E, Teebi A, et al. Bone dysplasia series. Achondroplasia, hypochondroplasia and tanatophoric dysplasia: review and update. Can Assoc Radiol J. 1999; 50(3):185-97.
25. Jha RM, Klimo P, Smith ER. Foramen magnum stenosis from overgrowth of the opisthion in a child with achondroplasia. J Neurosurg Pediatr. 2008;2(2):136-8.
26. Pauli RM, Horton VK, Glinski LP, et al. Prospective assessment of risks for cervicomedullary-junction compression in infants with achondroplasia. Am J Hum Genet. 1995;56(3):732-44.
27. Hecht JT, Francomano C, Horton W, et al. Mortality in achondroplasia. Am J Hum Genet. 1987;41(3):454-64.
28. Morgan DF, Young RF. Spinal neurological complications of achondroplasia. J Neurosurg. 1980;52(4):463-72.
29. Li L, Müller-Forell W, Oberman B, et al. Subcortical somatosensory evoked potentials after median nerve and posterior tibial nerve stimulation in high cervical cord compression of achondroplasia. Brain Dev. 2008;30(8):499-503.
30. Boor R, Fricke G, Brühl K, et al. Abnormal subcortical somatosensory evoked potentials indicate high cervical myelopathy in achondroplasia. Eur J Pediatr. 1999;158(8):662-7.
31. Vleggeert-Lankamp C, Peul W. Surgical decompression of thoracic spinal stenosis in achondroplasia: indication and outcome. J Neurosurg Spine. 2012;17(2):164-72.
32. Shirley ED, Ain MC. Achondroplasia: manifestations and treatment. J Am Acad Orthop Surg. 2009;17(4):231-41.
33. Ednick M, Tinkle BT, Phromchairak J, et al. Sleep-related respiratory abnormalities and arousal pattern in achondroplasia during early infancy. J Pediatr. 2009;155(4):510-5.
34. King JA, Vachhrajani S, Drake JM, et al. Neurosurgical implications of achondroplasia. J Neurosurg Pediatr. 2009; 4(4):297-306.
35. Ruiz-Garcia M, Tovar-Baudin A, Del Castillo-Ruiz V, et al. Early detection of neurological manifestations in achondroplasia. Childs Nerv Syst. 1997;13(4):208-13.
36. Hecht JT, Horton WA, Reid CS, et al. Growth of the foramen magnum in achondroplasia. Am J Med Genet. 1989;32(4): 528-35.
37. Bagley CA, Pindrik JA, Bookland MJ, et al. Cervicomedullary decompression for foramen magnum stenosis in achondroplasia. J Neurosurg. 2006;104(3 Suppl):166-72.
38. Wang H, Rosenbaum AE, Reid CS, et al. Pediatric patients with achondroplasia: CT evaluation of the craniocervical junction. Radiology. 1987;164(2):515-9.
39. Thomas IT, Frias JL, Williams JL, et al. Magnetic resonance imaging in the assessment of medullary compression in achondroplasia. Am J Dis Child. 1988;142(9):989-92.
40. Bauer AM, Mueller DM, Oró JJ. Arachnoid cyst resulting in tonsillar herniation and syringomyelia in a patient with achondroplasia. Case report. Neurosurg Focus. 2005;19(5):E14.
41. Baca KE, Abdullah MA, Ting BL, et al. Surgical decompression for lumbar stenosis in pediatric achondroplasia. J Pediatr Orthop. 2010;30(5):449-54.
42. Sciubba DM, Noggle JC, Marupudi NI, et al. Spinal stenosis surgery in pediatric patients with achondroplasia. J Neurosurg. 2007;106(5 Suppl):372-8.
43. Agabegi SS, Antekeier DP, Crawford AH, et al. Postlaminectomy kyphosis in an achondroplastic adolescent treated for spinal stenosis. Orthopedics. 2008;31(2):168.
44. Liao JC, Chen WJ, Lai PL, et al. Surgical treatment of achondroplasia with thoracolumbar kyphosis and spinal stenosis—a case report. Acta Orthop. 2006;77(3):541-4.
45. Ain MC, Shirley ED, Pirouzmanesh A, et al. Postlaminectomy kyphosis in the skeletally immature achondroplast. Spine (Phila Pa 1976). 2006;31(2):197-201.
46. Hunter AG, Bankier A, Rogers JG, et al. Medical complications of achondroplasia: a multicentre patient review. J Med Genet. 1998;35(9):705-12.
47. Yoshii J, Traynelis VC. Achondroplasia and cervical laminoplasty. J Neurosurg Spine. 2009;11(4):417-20.
48. Frigon VA, Castro FP, Whitecloud TS, et al. Isolated subaxial cervical spine stenosis in achondroplasia. Curr Surg. 2000;57(4):354-6.
49. Pauli RM, Breed A, Horton VK, et al. Prevention of fixed, angular kyphosis in achondroplasia. J Pediatr Orthop. 1997; 17(6):726-33.
50. Ain MC, Browne JA. Spinal arthrodesis with instrumentation for thoracolumbar kyphosis in pediatric achondroplasia. Spine (Phila Pa 1976). 2004;29(18):2075-80.
51. Tolo VT. Surgical treatment of kyphosis in achondroplasia. Basic Life Sci. 1988;48:257-9.
52. Misra SN, Morgan HW. Thoracolumbar spinal deformity in achondroplasia. Neurosurg Focus. 2003;14(1):e4.
53. Ain MC, Shirley ED. Spinal fusion for kyphosis in achondroplasia. J Pediatr Orthop. 2004;24(5):541-5.
54. Siebens AA, Hungerford DS, Kirby NA. Achondroplasia: effectiveness of an orthosis in reducing deformity of the spine. Arch Phys Med Rehabil. 1987;68(6):384-8.
55. Haga N. Management of disabilities associated with achondroplasia. J Orthop Sci. 2004;9(1):103-7.
56. Wynn J, King TM, Gambello MJ, et al. Mortality in achondroplasia study: a 42-year follow-up. Am J Med Genet A. 2007;143A(21):2502-11.
57. Trotter TL, Hall JG; American Academy of Pediatrics Committee on Genetics. Health supervision for children with achondroplasia. Pediatrics. 2005;116(3):771-83.
58. Lutter LD, Langer LO. Neurological symptoms in achondroplastic dwarfs—surgical treatment. J Bone Joint Surg Am. 1977;59(1):87-92.

59. Schkrohowsky JG, Hoernschemeyer DG, Carson BS, et al. Early presentation of spinal stenosis in achondroplasia. J Pediatr Orthop. 2007;27(2):119-22.
60. Radcliff K, Su BW, Kepler CK, et al. Correlation of posterior ligamentous complex injury and neurological injury to loss of vertebral body height, kyphosis, and canal compromise. Spine (Phila Pa 1976). 2012;37(13):1142-50.
61. Hästbacka J, Kerrebrock A, Mokkala K, et al. Identification of the Finnish founder mutation for diastrophic dysplasia (DTD). Eur J Hum Genet. 1999;7(6):664-70.
62. Ohana E, Shcheynikov N, Park M, et al. Solute carrier family 26 member a2 (Slc26a2) protein functions as an electroneutral $SO_4^{2-}/OH^-/Cl^-$ exchanger regulated by extracellular Cl^-. J Biol Chem. 2012;287(7):5122-32.
63. Maeda K, Miyamoto Y, Sawai H, et al. A compound heterozygote harboring novel and recurrent DTDST mutations with intermediate phenotype between atelosteogenesis type II and diastrophic dysplasia. Am J Med Genet A. 2006;140(11):1143-7.
64. Horton WA, Rimoin DL, Lachman RS, et al. The phenotypic variability of diastrophic dysplasia. J Pediatr. 1978;93(4):609-13.
65. Dwyer E, Hyland J, Modaff P, et al. Genotype-phenotype correlation in DTDST dysplasias: Atelosteogenesis type II and diastrophic dysplasia variant in one family. Am J Med Genet A. 2010;152A(12):3043-50.
66. Gualeni B, Facchini M, De Leonardis F, et al. Defective proteoglycan sulfation of the growth plate zones causes reduced chondrocyte proliferation via an altered Indian hedgehog signalling. Matrix Biol. 2010;29(6):453-60.
67. Barbosa M, Sousa AB, Medeira A, et al. Clinical and molecular characterization of Diastrophic Dysplasia in the Portuguese population. Clin Genet. 2011;80(6):550-7.
68. Karlstedt E, Kovero O, Kaitila I, et al. Transverse facial morphology in patients with diastrophic dysplasia. J Craniofac Genet Dev Biol. 1997;17(4):178-83.
69. Superti-Furga A, Unger S. Nosology and classification of genetic skeletal disorders: 2006 revision. Am J Med Genet A. 2007;143A(1):1-18.
70. Schramm T, Gloning KP, Minderer S, et al. Prenatal sonographic diagnosis of skeletal dysplasias. Ultrasound Obstet Gynecol. 2009;34(2):160-70.
71. Matsuyama Y, Robert B, Lonstein JE. The spine in diastrophic dysplasia. The surgical arthrodesis of thoracic and lumbar deformities in 21 patients. Spine (Phila Pa 1976). 1999;24(22):2325-31.
72. McKay SD, Al-Omari A, Tomlinson LA, et al. Review of cervical spine anomalies in genetic syndromes. Spine (Phila Pa 1976). 2012;37(5):E269-77.
73. Bonafé L, Mittaz-Crettol L, Ballhausen D, et al. Achondrogenesis type 1B in GeneReviews® Adam MP, et al. (Eds) University of Washington, Seattle, 1993 1. Bonafé L, et al. A novel mutation in the sulfate transporter gene SLC26A2 (DTDST) specific to the Finnish population causes de la Chapelle dysplasia. J Med Genet. 2008;45:827-31.
74. Jalanko T, Remes V, Peltonen J, et al. Treatment of spinal deformities in patients with diastrophic dysplasia: a long-term, population based, retrospective outcome study. Spine (Phila Pa 1976). 2009;34(20):2151-7.
75. Remes V, Marttinen E, Poussa M, et al. Cervical kyphosis in diastrophic dysplasia. Spine (Phila Pa 1976). 1999;24(19):1990-5.
76. Richards BS. Atlanto-axial instability in diastrophic dysplasia. A case report. J Bone Joint Surg Am. 1991;73(4):614-6.
77. Poussa M, Merikanto J, Ryöppy S, et al. The spine in diastrophic dysplasia. Spine (Phila Pa 1976). 1991;16(8):881-7.
78. Forese LL, Berdon WE, Harcke HT, et al. Severe mid-cervical kyphosis with cord compression in Larsen's syndrome and idastrophic dysplasia: Unrelated syndromes with similar radiologic findings and neurosurgical implications. Pediatr Radiol. 1995;25(2):136-9.
79. Remes VM, Marttinen EJ, Poussa MS, et al. Cervical spine in patients with diastrophic dysplasia—radiographic findings in 122 patients. Pediatr Radiol. 2002;32(9):621-8.
80. Remes V, Poussa M, Peltonen J. Scoliosis in patients with diastrophic dysplasia: a new classification. Spine (Phila Pa 1976). 2001;26(15):1689-97.
81. McKusick V, Hamosh A. Spondyloepiphyseal dysplasia tarda, X-linked; SEDT. OMIM. (1976). Available from https://omim.org/entry/313400 [Last Accessed July 2019].
82. McKusick V, Sobreira N. Spondyloepiphyseal Dysplasia Congenita; SEDC. OMIM. (1986). Available from https://www.omim.org/entry/183900 [Last Accessed July 2019].
83. Cao LH, Wang L, Ji CY, et al. Novel and recurrent COL2A1 mutations in Chinese patients with spondyloepiphyseal dysplasia. Genet Mol Res. 2012;11(4):4130-7.
84. Amirfeyz R, Clark C, Gargan M. Spondyloepiphyseal dysplasia. Current Orthopaedics. 2005;19:309-13.
85. Parikh S. (2011). Spondyloepiphyseal dysplasia. Available from https://emedicine.medscape.com/article/1260836-overview [Last Accessed July 2019].
86. Gedeon AK, Tiller GE, Le Merrer M, et al. The molecular basis of X-linked spondyloepiphyseal dysplasia tarda. Am J Hum Genet. 2001;68(6):1386-97.
87. Christie PT, Curley A, Nesbit MA, et al. Mutational analysis in X-linked spondyloepiphyseal dysplasia tarda. J Clin Endocrinol Metab. 2001;86(7):3233-6.
88. Gedeon AK, Tiller GE, Le Merrer M, et al. The molecular basis of X-linked spondyloepiphyseal dysplasia tarda. Am J Hum Genet. 2001;68(6):1386-97.
89. Gedeon AK, Colley A, Jamieson R, et al. Identification of the gene (SEDL) causing X-linked spondyloepiphyseal dysplasia tarda. Nat Genet. 1999;22(4):400-4.
90. Tiller GE, Polumbo PA, Weis MA, et al. Dominant mutations in the type II collagen gene, COL2A1, produce spondyloepimetaphyseal dysplasia, Strudwick type. Nat Genet. 1995;11(1):87-9.
91. LW Murray, J Bautista, PL James, et al. Type II collagen defects in the chondrodysplasias. I. Spondyloepiphyseal dysplasias. Am J Hum Genet. 1989;45(1):5-15.
92. Venditti R, Scanu T, Santoro M, et al. Sedlin controls the ER export of procollagen by regulating the Sar1 cycle. Science. 2012;337(6102):1668-72.
93. Xia XY, Cui YX, Huang YF, et al. Molecular prenatal diagnosis in 2 pregnancies at risk for spondyloepiphyseal dysplasia congenita. Clin Chim Acta. 2008;387(1-2):153-7.

94. James PA, Shaw J, du Sart D, et al. Molecular diagnosis in a pregnancy at risk for both spondyloepiphyseal dysplasia congenita and achondroplasia. Prenat Diagn. 2003;23(10):861-3.
95. Wang HL, Gao C, Luo Q, et al. Gene diagnosis of X-linked spondyloepiphyseal dysplasia tarda by linkage analysis and DNA sequencing. Zhonghua Er Ke Za Zhi. 2003;41(4):256-9.
96. Cui YX, Xia XY, Bu Y, et al. Rapid molecular prenatal diagnosis of spondyloepiphyseal dysplasia congenita by PCR-SSP assay. Genet Test. 2008;12(4):533-6.
97. Bach C, Maroteaux P, Schaeffer P, et al. Congenital spondyloepiphysial dysplasia with multiple abnormalities. Arch Fr Pediatr. 1967;24(1):23-33.
98. Genetics Home Reference (2013). Spondyloepiphyseal dysplasia congenita. Available from https://ghr.nlm.nih.gov/condition/spondyloepiphyseal-dysplasia-congenita [Last Accessed July 2019].
99. Turner LM, Steffensen TS, Leroy J, et al. Spondyloepiphyseal dysplasia congenita. Fetal Pediatr Pathol. 2010;29(1):57-62.
100. Veeravagu A, Lad SP, Camara-Quintana JQ, et al. Neurosurgical interventions for spondyloepiphyseal dysplasia congenita: clinical presentation and assessment of the literature. World Neurosurg. 2013;80(3-4):437.e1-8.
101. Wynne-Davies R, Hall C. Two clinical variants of spondyloepiphysial dysplasia congenita. J Bone Joint Surg Br. 1982;64(4):435-41.
102. Morita M, Miyamoto K, Nishimoto H, et al. Thoracolumbar kyphosing scoliosis associated with spondyloepiphyseal dysplasia congenita: a case report. Spine J. 2005;5(2):217-20.
103. LeDoux MS, Naftalis RC, Aronin PA. Stabilization of the cervical spine in spondyloepiphyseal dysplasia congenita. Neurosurgery. 1991;28(4):580-3.
104. Whyte MP, Gottesman GS, Eddy MC, et al. X-linked recessive spondyloepiphyseal dysplasia tarda. Clinical and radiographic evolution in a 6-generation kindred and review of the literature. Medicine (Baltimore). 1999;78:9-25.
105. Langer LO. Spondyloepiphyseal dysplasia tarda, hereditary chondrodysplasia with characteristic vertebral configurations in the adult. Radiology. 1964;82:833-9 .
106. Kanazawa H, Tanaka H, Inoue M, et al. Efficacy of growth hormone therapy for patients with skeletal dysplasia. J Bone Miner Metab. 2003;21(5):307-10.
107. Soultanis KC, Payatakes AH, Chouliaras VT, et al. Rare causes of scoliosis and spine deformity: experience and particular features. Scoliosis. 2007;2:15.
108. Berkowitz ID, Raja SN, Bender KS, et al. Dwarfs: pathophysiology and anesthetic implications. Anesthesiology. 1990;73(4):739-59.
109. Unger S, Korkko J, Krakow D, et al. Double heterozygosity for pseudoachondroplasia and spondyloepiphyseal dysplasia congenita. Am J Med Genet. 2001;104(2):140-6.
110. Miyoshi K, Nakamura K, Haga N, et al. Surgical treatment for atlantoaxial subluxation with myelopathy in spondyloepiphyseal dysplasia congenita. Spine (Phila Pa 1976). 2004;29(21):E488-91.
111. Nakamura K, Miyoshi K, Haga N, et al. Risk factors of myelopathy at the atlantoaxial level in spondyloepiphyseal dysplasia congenita. Arch Orthop Trauma Surg. 1998;117(8):468-70.
112. Seller K, Haas S, Raab P, et al. Preoperative halo-traction in severe paralytic scoliosis. Z Orthop Ihre Grenzgeb. 2005;143(5):539-43.
113. Ain MC, Chaichana KL, Schkrohowsky JG. Retrospective study of cervical arthrodesis in patients with various types of skeletal dysplasia. Spine (Phila Pa 1976). 2006;31(6):E169-74.
114. Al-Awadi SA, Fårag TI, Naguib K, et al. Spondyloepiphyseal dysplasia tarda with progressive arthropathy. J Med Genet. 1984;21(3):193-6.
115. Fiedler J, Bergmann C, Brenner R. X-linked spondyloepiphyseal dysplasia tarda Molecular cause of a heritable disorder associated with early degenerative joint disease. Acta Orthop Scand. 2003;74(6):737-41.
116. Weis MA, Wilkin DJ, Kim HJ, et al. Structurally abnormal type II collagen in a severe form of Kniest dysplasia caused by an exon 24 skipping mutation. J Biol Chem. 1998;273(8):4761-8.
117. Fernandes RJ, Wilkin DJ, Weis MA, et al. Incorporation of structurally defective type II collagen into cartilage matrix in kniest chondrodysplasia. Arch Biochem Biophys. 1998;355(2):282-90.
118. Nishimura G, Haga N, Kitoh H, et al. The phenotypic spectrum of COL2A1 mutations. Hum Mutat. 2005;26(1):36-43.
119. Kelnar CJH. Growth hormone therapy for syndromic disorders. Clin Endocrinol (Oxf). 2003;59:12-21.
120. Winterpacht A, Hilbert M, Schwarze U, et al. Kniest and Stickler dysplasia phenotypes caused by collagen type II gene (COL2A1) defect. Nat Genet. 1993;3(4):323-6.
121. Wilkin DJ, Artz AS, South S, et al. Small deletions in the type II collagen triple helix produce kniest dysplasia. Am J Med Genet. 1999;85(2) 105-12.
122. Nagendran S, Richards AJ, McNinch A, et al. Somatic mosaicism and the phenotypic expression of COL2A1 mutations. Am J Med Genet A. 2012;158A(5):1204-7.
123. Bogaert R, Wilkin D, Wilcox WR, et al. Expression, in cartilage, of a 7-amino-acid deletion in type II collagen from two unrelated individuals with Kniest dysplasia. Am J Hum Genet. 1994;55(6):1128-36.
124. Lachman RS, Rimoin DL, Hollister DW, et al. The Kniest syndrome. Am J Roentgenol Radium Ther Nucl Med. 1975;123(4):805-14.
125. Burton BK, Sumner T, Langer LO, et al. A new skeletal dysplasia: Clinical, radiologic, and pathologic findings. J Pediatr. 1986;109(4):642-8.
126. Spranger J, Menger H, Mundlos S, et al. Kniest dysplasia is caused by dominant collagen II (COL2A1) mutations: Parental somatic mosaicism manifesting as Stickler phenotype and mild spondyloepiphyseal dysplasia. Pediatr Radiol. 1994;24(6):431-5.
127. Subramanian S, Gamanagatti S, Sinha A, et al. Kniest syndrome. Indian Pediatr. 2007;44(12):931-3.
128. Herring J (Ed). Tachdjian's Pediatric Orthopaedics, 4th edition. Philadelphia: Saunders Elsevier; 2007. pp. 1677-1794.
129. Spranger J, Winterpacht A, Zabel B. Kniest dysplasia: Dr. W. Kniest, his patient, the molecular defect. Am J Med Genet. 1997;69(1):79-84.
130. Westvik J, Lachman RS. Coronal and sagittal clefts in skeletal dysplasias. Pediatr Radiol. 1998;28(10):764-70.
131. Cole WG. Abnormal skeletal growth in Kniest dysplasia caused by type II collagen mutations. Clin Orthop Relat Res. 1997;(341):162-9.

132. Wilkin DJ, Bogaert R, Lachman RS, et al. A single amino acid substitution (G103D) in the type II collagen triple helix produces Kniest dysplasia. Hum Mol Genet. 1994;3(11):1999-2003.
133. Edwards AO. Clinical features of the congenital vitreoretinopathies. Eye (Lond). 2008;22(10):1233-42 .
134. Hicks J, De Jong A, Barrish J, et al. Tracheomalacia in a neonate with kniest dysplasia: histopathologic and ultrastructural features. Ultrastruct Pathol. 2001;25(1):79-83.
135. Yokoyama T, Nakatani S, Murakami A. A case of Kniest dysplasia with retinal detachment and the mutation analysis. Am J Ophthalmol. 2003;136(6):1186-8.
136. Merrill KD, Schmidt TL. Occipitoatlantal instability in a child with Kniest syndrome. J Pediatr Orthop. 1989;9(3):338-40.
137. Bethem D, Winter RB, Lutter L, et al. Spinal disorders of dwarfism. Review of the literature and report of eighty cases. J Bone Joint Surg Am. 1981;63(9):1412-25.
138. Posey KL, Hayes E, Haynes R, et al. Role of TSP-5/COMP in pseudoachondroplasia. Int J Biochem Cell Biol. 2004; 36(6):1005-12.
139. Ferguson HL, Deere M, Evans R, et al. Mosaicism in pseudoachondroplasia. Am J Med Genet. 1997;70(3):287-91.
140. Briggs MD, Hoffman SM, King LM, et al. Pseudoachondroplasia and multiple epiphyseal dysplasia due to mutations in the cartilage oligomeric matrix protein gene. Nat Genet. 1995;10(3):330-6.
141. Hecht JT, Francomano CA, Briggs MD, et al. Linkage of typical pseudoachondroplasia to chromosome 19. Genomics. 1993;18(3):661-6.
142. Hecht JT, Montufar-Solis D, Decker G, et al. Retention of cartilage oligomeric matrix protein (COMP) and cell death in redifferentiated pseudoachondroplasia chondrocytes. Matrix Biol. 1998;17(8-9):625-33.
143. Vranka J, Mokashi A, Keene DR, et al. Selective intracellular retention of extracellular matrix proteins and chaperones associated with pseudoachondroplasia. Matrix Biol. 2001;20(7):439-50.
144. Hecht JT, Deere M, Putnam E, et al. Characterization of cartilage oligomeric matrix protein (COMP) in human normal and pseudochondroplasia musculoskeletal tissues. Matrix Biol. 1998;17(4):269-78.
145. Hecht JT, Makitie O, Hayes E, et al. Chondrocyte cell death and intracellular distribution of COMP and type IX collagen in the pseudoachondroplasia growth plate. J Orthop Res. 2004;22(4):759-67.
146. Unger S, Hecht JT. Pseudoachondroplasia and multiple epiphyseal dysplasia: New etiologic developments. Am J Med Genet. 2001;106(4):244-50.
147. McKeand J, Rotta J, Hecht JT. Natural history study of pseudoachondroplasia. Am J Med Genet. 1996;63(2):406-10.
148. Wynne-Davies R, Hall CM, Young ID. Pseudoachondroplasia: clinical diagnosis at different ages and comparison of autosomal dominant and recessive types. A review of 32 patients (26 kindreds). J Med Genet. 1986;23(5):425-34.
149. Jackson GC, Mittaz-Crettol L, Taylor JA, et al. Pseudoachondroplasia and multiple epiphyseal dysplasia: a 7-year comprehensive analysis of the known disease genes identify novel and recurrent mutations and provides an accurate assessment of their relative contribution. Hum Mutat. 2012;33(1):144-57.
150. Briggs MD, Wright MJ. Pseudoachondroplasia in GeneReviews.® Adam, MP et al. (Eds). University of Washington, Seattle, 1993.
151. Shetty GM, Song HR, Unnikrishnan R, et al. Upper cervical spine instability in pseudoachondroplasia. J Pediatr Orthop. 2007;27(7):782-7.
152. Wynne-Davies R, Gormley J. The prevalence of skeletal dysplasias. An estimate of their minimum frequency and the number of patients requiring orthopaedic care. J Bone Joint Surg Br. 1985;67(1):133-7.
153. Unger S, Lausch E, Stanzial F, et al. Fetal akinesia in metatropic dysplasia: The combined phenotype of chondrodysplasia and neuropathy? Am J Med Genet A. 2011;155A(11):2860-4.
154. Liedtke W, Choe Y, Martí-Renom MA, et al. Vanilloid receptor-related osmotically activated channel (VR-OAC), a candidate vertebrate osmoreceptor. Cell. 2000;103(3):525-35.
155. Camacho N, Krakow D, Johnykutty S, et al. Dominant TRPV4 mutations in nonlethal and lethal metatropic dysplasia. Am J Med Genet A. 2010;152A(5):1169-77.
156. Jenkins P, Smith MB, McKinnell JS. Metatropic dwarfism. Br J Radiol. 1970;43:561-5.
157. Krakow D, Vriens J, Camacho N, et al. Mutations in the gene encoding the calcium-permeable ion channel TRPV4 produce spondylometaphyseal dysplasia, Kozlowski type and Metatropic dysplasia. Am J Hum Genet. 2009;84(3):307-15.).
158. Geneviève D, Le Merrer M, Feingold J, et al. Revisiting metatropic dysplasia: Presentation of a series of 19 novel patients and review of the literature. Am J Med Genet A. 2008;146A(8):992-6.
159. Loukin S, Su Z, Kung C. Increased basal activity is a key determinant in the severity of human skeletal dysplasia caused by TRPV4 mutations. PLoS One. 2011;6(5):e19533.
160. Masuyama R, Vriens J, Voets T, et al. TRPV4-mediated calcium influx regulates terminal differentiation of osteoclasts. Cell Metab. 2008;8(3):257-65.
161. Kannu P, Aftimos S, Mayne V, et al. Metatropic dysplasia: Clinical and radiographic findings in 11 patients demonstrating long-term natural history. Am J Med Genet A. 2007;143A(21):2512-22.
162. Hall CM, Elçioglu NH. Metatropic dysplasia lethal variants. Pediatr Radiol. 2004;34(1):66-74.
163. Cho TJ, Matsumoto K, Fano V, et al. TRPV4-pathy manifesting both skeletal dysplasia and peripheral neuropathy: A report of three patients. Am J Med Genet A. 2012;158A(4):795-802.
164. Geneviève D, Le Merrer M, Munnich A, et al. Long-term follow-up in a patient with metatropic dysplasia. Am J Med Genet A. 2005;135(3):342-3.
165. Shohat M, Lachman R, Rimoin DL. Odontoid hypoplasia with vertebral cervical subluxation and ventriculomegaly in metatropic dysplasia. J Pediatr. 1989;114(2):239-43.
166. Andreucci E, Aftimos S, Alcausin M, et al. TRPV4 related skeletal dysplasias: a phenotypic spectrum highlighted byclinical, radiographic, and molecular studies in 21 new families. Orphanet J Rare Dis. 2011;6:37.
167. Leet AI, Sampath JS, Scott CI Jr, et al. Cervical spinal stenosis in metatropic dysplasia. J Pediatr Orthop. 2006;26(3):347-52.
168. Nishimura G, Lausch E, Savarirayan R, et al. TRPV4-associated skeletal dysplasias. Am J Med Genet C Semin Med Genet. 2012;160C(3):190-204.

169. Nino M, Matos-Miranda C, Maeda M, et al. Clinical and molecular analysis of arylsulfatase E in patients with brachytelephalangic chondrodysplasia punctata. Am J Med Genet A. 2008;146A(8):997-1008.
170. Brunetti-Pierri N, Andreucci MV, Tuzzi R, et al. X-linked recessive chondrodysplasia punctata: Spectrum of arylsulfatase E gene mutations and expanded clinical variability. Am J Med Genet A. 2003;117A(2):164-8.
171. Parenti G, Buttitta P, Meroni G, et al. X-linked recessive chondrodysplasia punctata due to a new point mutation of the ARSE gene. Am J Med Genet. 1997;73(2):139-43.
172. Daniele A, Parenti G, d'Addio M, et al. Biochemical characterization of arylsulfatase E and functional analysis of mutations found in patients with X-linked chondrodysplasia punctata. Am J Hum Genet. 1998;62(3):562-72.
173. Franco B, Meroni G, Parenti G, et al. A cluster of sulfatase genes on Xp22.3: Mutations in chondrodysplasia punctata (CDPX) and implications for warfarin embryopathy. Cell. 1995;81(1):15-25.
174. Meyer S, Löffler G, Gencik M, et al. Brachytelephalangic chondrodysplasia punctata with a new hemizygous missense mutation in a neonate. Am J Med Genet A. 2013;161A(3):626-9.
175. Krakow D, Williams J 3rd, Poehl M, et al. Use of three-dimensional ultrasound imaging in the diagnosis of prenatal-onset skeletal dysplasias. Ultrasound Obstet Gynecol. 2003;21(5):467-72.
176. Cormier-Daire V, Savarirayan R, Unger S, et al. 'Duplicate calcaneus':a rare developmental defect observed in several skeletal dysplasias. Pediatr Radiol. 2001;31(1):38-42.
177. Krakow D. Skeletal dysplasias. Clin Perinatol. 2015;42:301-19.
178. Casarin A, Rusalen F, Doimo M, et al. X-linked brachytelephalangic chondrodysplasia punctata: A simple trait that is not so simple. Am J Med Genet A. 2009;149A(11):2464-8.
179. Mason DE, Sanders JO, MacKenzie WG, et al. Spinal deformity in chondrodysplasia punctata. Spine (Phila Pa 1976). 2002;27(18):1995-2002.
180. Vogel TW, Menezes AH. Natural history and management of cervical spine disease in chondrodysplasia punctata and coumarin embryopathy. Childs Nerv Syst. 2012;28(4):609-19.
181. Mundinger G, Weiss C, Fishman E. Severe tracheobronchial stenosis and cervical vertebral subluxation in X-linked recessive chondrodysplasia punctata. Pediatr Radiol. 2009;39(6):625-8.
182. Yang BP, Mindea SA, DiPatri AJ Jr. Cervical spinal cord compression in chondrodysplasia punctata. J Neurosurg. 2006;104(3 Suppl):212.
183. Goodman P, Dominguez R. Cervicothoracic myelopathy in conradi-hunermann disease: MRI diagnosis. Magn Reson Imaging. 1990;8(5):647-50.
184. Herman T, Lee B, McAlister W. Brachytelephalangic chondrodysplasia punctata with marked cervical stenosis and cord compression: report of two cases. Pediatr Radiol. 2002;32(6):452-6.
185. Mansour S, Hall CM, Pembrey ME, et al. A clinical and genetic study of campomelic dysplasia. J Med Genet. 1995;32(6):415-20.
186. Velagaleti GV, Bien-Willner GA, Northup JK, et al. Position effects due to chromosome breakpoints that map ~900 kb upstream and ~1.3 mb downstream of SOX9 in two patients with campomelic dysplasia. Am J Hum Genet. 2005;76(4):652-62.
187. Corbani S, Chouery E, Eid B, et al. Mild campomelic dysplasia: Report on a Case and Review. Mol Syndromol. 2011;1(4):163-8.
188. Goyal JP, Gupta A, Shah VB. Campomelic dysplasia. Indian J Hum Genet. 2011;17(3):247-8.
189. Wagner T, Wirth J, Meyer J, et al. Autosomal sex reversal and campomelic dysplasia are caused by mutations in and around the SRY-related gene SOX9. Cell. 1994;79(6):1111-20.
190. Foster JW, Dominguez-Steglich MA, Guioli S, et al. Campomelic dysplasia and autosomal sex reversal caused by mutations in an SRY-related gene. Nature. 1994;372(6506):525-30.
191. Lefebvre V, Li P, De Crombrugghe B. A new long form of Sox5 (L-Sox5), Sox6 and Sox9 are coexpressed in chondrogenesis and cooperatively activate the type II collagen gene. EMBO J. 1998;17(19):5718-33.
192. Lefebvre V, Huang W, Harley VR, et al. SOX9 is a potent activator of the chondrocyte-specific enhancer of the pro alpha1(II) collagen gene. Mol Cell Biol. 1997;17(4):2336-46.
193. Zhang P, Jimenez SA, Stokes DG. Regulation of human COL9A1 gene expression. Activation of the proximal promoter region by SOX9.. J Biol Chem. 2003;278(1):117-23.
194. Bridgewater LC, Walker MD, Miller GC, et al. Adjacent DNA sequences modulate Sox9 transcriptional activation at paired Sox sites in three chondrocyte-specific enhancer elements. Nucleic Acids Res. 2003;31(5):1541-53.
195. Akiyama H, Lefebvre V. Unraveling the transcriptional regulatory machinery in chondrogenesis. J Bone Miner Metab. 2011;29(4) 390-5.
196. Koopman P. Sry and Sox9: mammalian testis-determining genes. Cell Mol Life Sci. 1999;55(6-7):839-56.
197. Knower KC, Kelly S, Harley VR. Turning on the male—SRY, SOX9 and sex determination in mammals. Cytogenet Genome Res. 2003;101(3-4):185-98.
198. Meyer J, Südbeck P, Held M, et al. Mutational analysis of the SOX9 gene in campomelic dysplasia and autosomal sex reversal: lack of genotype/phenotype correlations. Hum Mol Genet. 1997;6:91-8.
199. Harley VR, Clarkson MJ, Argentaro A. The molecular action and regulation of the testis-determining factors, SRY (sex-determining region on the Y chromosome) and SOX9 [SRY-related high-mobility group (HMG) box 9]. Endocr Rev. 2003;24(4):466-87.
200. Becker MH, Finegold M, Genieser NB, et al. Campomelic dwarfism. Birth Defects Orig Artic Ser. 1975;11:113-8.
201. Tongsong T, Wanapirak C, Pongsatha S. Prenatal diagnosis of campomelic dysplasia. Ultrasound Obstet Gynecol. 2000;15(5):428-30.
202. Campbell RM Jr. Spine deformities in rare congenital syndromes: clinical issues. Spine (Phila Pa 1976). 2009;34(17):1815-27.
203. Ray S, Bowen JR. Orthopaedic problems associated with survival in campomelic dysplasia. Clin Orthop Relat Res. 1984;(185):77-82.
204. Unger S, Scherer G, Superti-Furga A. Campomelic Dysplasia in GeneReviews® Adam MP, et al. (Eds). University of Washington, Seattle, 1993.
205. Dahdaleh NS, Albert GW, Hasan DM. Campomelic dysplasia: a rare cause of congenital spinal deformity. J Clin Neurosci. 2010;17(5):664-6.
206. Nelson ME, Griffin GR, Innis JW, et al. Campomelic dysplasia: airway management in two patients and an update on clinical-molecular correlations in the head and neck. Ann Otol Rhinol Laryngol. 2011;120(10):682-5.

207. Thomas S, Winter R, Lonstein J. The treatment of progressive kyphoscoliosis in camptomelic dysplasia. Spine (Phila Pa 1976). 1997;22(12):1330-7.
208. Lekovic G, Rektate H, Dickman C, et al. Congenital cervical instability in a patient with camptomelic dysplasia. Childs Nervous System. 2006;22:1212-4.
209. Coscia MF, Bassett GS, Bowen JR, et al. Spinal abnormalities in camptomelic dysplasia. J Pediatr Orthop. 1989;9(1):6-14.
210. Kliegman R, Stanton B, Geme J, Schor N, Berhman R (Eds). Nelson Textbook of Pediatrics. Philadelphia: Elsevier; 2011.
211. Clarke LA. Pathogenesis of skeletal and connective tissue involvement in the mucopolysaccharidoses: glycosaminoglycan storage is merely the instigator. Rheumatology (Oxford). 2011 Dec;50 Suppl 5:v13-8.
212. Muenzer J. Overview of the mucopolysaccharidoses. Rheumatology (Oxford). 2011;50 Suppl 5:v4-12.
213. Simonaro CM, D'Angelo M, He X, et al. Mechanism of glycosaminoglycan-mediated bone and joint disease: implications for the mucopolysaccharidoses and other connective tissue diseases. Am J Pathol. 2008;172(1):112-22.
214. Valayannopoulos V, Nicely H, Harmatz P, et al. Mucopolysaccharidosis VI. Orphanet J Rare Dis. 2010;5:5.
215. Litjens T, Hopwood JJ. Mucopolysaccharidosis type VI: Structural and clinical implications of mutations in N-acetylgalactosamine-4-sulfatase. Hum Mutat. 2001; 18(4):282-95.
216. Coutinho MF, Lacerda L, Alves S. Glycosaminoglycan storage disorders: a review. Biochem Res Int. 2012;2012:471325.
217. Lehman TJ, Miller N, Norquist B, et al. Diagnosis of the mucopolysaccharidoses. Rheumatology (Oxford). 2011;50 Suppl 5:v41-8.
218. Tebani A, Abily-Donval L, Schmitz-Afonso I, et al. Unveiling metabolic remodeling in mucopolysaccharidosis type III through integrative metabolomics and pathway analysis. J Transl Med. 2018;16(1):248.
219. Garrido E, Chabás A, Coll MJ, et al. Identification of the molecular defects in Spanish and Argentinian mucopolysaccharidosis VI (Maroteaux-Lamy syndrome) patients, including 9 novel mutations. Mol Genet Metab. 2007;92(1-2):122-30.
220. Schroeder L, Orchard P, Whitley CB, et al. Cardiac ultrasound findings in infants with severe (Hurler phenotype) untreated mucopolysaccharidosis (MPS) type I. JIMD Rep. 2013;10:87-94.
221. Morishita K, Petty RE. Musculoskeletal manifestations of mucopolysaccharidoses. Rheumatology (Oxford). 2011;50 Suppl 5:v19-25.
222. White KK. Orthopaedic aspects of mucopolysaccharidoses. Rheumatology (Oxford). 2011;50 Suppl 5:v26-33.
223. Schmidt H, Ullrich K, von Lengerke HJ, et al. Radiological findings in patients with mucopolysaccharidosis I H/S (Hurler-Scheie syndrome). Pediatr Radiol. 1987;17(5):409-14.
224. Simmons MA, Bruce IA, Penney S, et al. Otorhinolaryngological manifestations of the mucopolysaccharidoses. Int J Pediatr Otorhinolaryngol. 2005;69:589-95.
225. Parsons VJ, Hughes DG, Wraith JE. Magnetic resonance imaging of the brain, neck and cervical spine in mild Hunter's syndrome (mucopolysaccharidoses type II). Clin Radiol. 1996;51(10):719-23.
226. McGill JJ, Inwood AC, Coman DJ, et al. Enzyme replacement therapy for mucopolysaccharidosis VI from 8 weeks of age—a sibling control study. Clin Genet. 2010;77(5):492-8.
227. Gabrielli O, Clarke LA, Bruni S, et al. Enzyme-Replacement Therapy in a 5-Month-Old Boy With Attenuated Presymptomatic MPS I: 5-Year Follow-up. Pediatrics. 2010;125(1): e183-e187.
228. Thomas JA, Jacobs S, Kierstein J, et al. Outcome after three years of laronidase enzyme replacement therapy in a patient with Hurler syndrome. J Inherit Metab Dis. 2006;29:762.
229. Cox-Brinkman J, Smeulders MJ, Hollak CE, et al. Restricted upper extremity range of motion in mucopolysaccharidosis type I: no response to one year of enzyme replacement therapy. J Inherit Metab Dis. 2007;30(1):47-50.
230. Hughes DG, Chadderton RD, Cowie RA, et al. MRI of the brain and craniocervical junction in Morquio's disease. Neuroradiology. 1997;39(5):381-5.
231. Stevens PM. Guided growth for angular correction: a preliminary series using a tension band plate. J Pediatr Orthop. 2007;27(3):253-9.
232. Tamaki N, Kojima N, Tanimoto M, et al. Myelopathy due to diffuse thickening of the cervical dura mater in Maroteaux-Lamy syndrome: report of a case. Neurosurgery. 1987;21(3):416-9.
233. Siddique I, Sacho R, Oxborrow NJ, et al. Thoracolumbar kyphosis in mucopolysaccharidosis I (Hurler syndrome). J Bone Joint Surg Br. 2010;92-B:427.
234. Ransford AO, Crockard HA, Stevens JM, et al. Occipito-atlanto-axial fusion in Morquio-Brailsford syndrome. A ten-year experience. J Bone Joint Surg Br. 1996;78(2):307-13.
235. Cathey SS, Kudo M, Tiede S, et al. Molecular order in mucolipidosis II and III nomenclature. Am J Med Genet A. 2008;146A(4):512-3.
236. Roth KS. I-Cell Disease (Mucolipidosis Type II). Medscape. (2012). [online]. Available from https://emedicine.medscape.com/article/945460-overview?pa=fn7Y8bxmBzwQSHEXr8HG5Vypt1JYWYmPfd6lEvpBG%2Bsz3ZtGLeGmhbDQ8a4HIP4ySRmT%2FzVn%2Bt0t8gX%2FkhdSAA%3D%3D%3E [Last Accessed July 2019].
237. Encarnação M, Lacerda L, Costa R, et al. Molecular analysis of the GNPTAB and GNPTG genes in 13 patients with mucolipidosis type II or type III - identification of eight novel mutations. Clin Genet. 2009;76:76-84.
238. Coutinho MF, Prata MJ, Alves S. Mannose-6-phosphate pathway: A review on its role in lysosomal function and dysfunction. Mol Genet Metab. 2012;105(4):542-50.
239. Flanagan-Steet H, Sias C, Steet R. Altered chondrocyte differentiation and extracellular matrix homeostasis in a zebrafish model for mucolipidosis II. Am J Pathol. 2009;175(5):2063-75.

240. Petrey AC, Flanagan-Steet H, Johnson S, et al. Excessive activity of cathepsin K is associated with cartilage defects in a zebrafish model of mucolipidosis II. Dis Model Mech. 2012;5(2):177-90.
241. Cathey SS, Leroy JG, Wood T, et al. Phenotype and genotype in mucolipidoses II and III alpha/beta: a study of 61 probands. J Med Genet. 2010;47(1):38-48 (2010).
242. Heo JS, Choi KY, Sohn SH, et al. A case of mucolipidosis II presenting with prenatal skeletal dysplasia and severe secondary hyperparathyroidism at birth. Korean J Pediatr. 2012;55(11):438-44.
243. Pohl S, Encarnacão M, Castrichini M, et al. Loss of N-acetylglucosamine-1-phosphotransferase gamma subunit due to intronic mutation in GNPTG causes mucolipidosis type III gamma: Implications for molecular and cellular diagnostics. Am J Med Genet A. 2010;152A(1):124-32.
244. Wood TC, Harvey K, Beck M, et al. Diagnosing mucopolysaccharidosis IVA. J Inherit Metab Dis. 2013;36(2): 293-307.
245. Raas-Rothschild A, Spiegel R. Mucolipidosis III Gamma. In: Adam MP, Ardinger HH, Pagon RA, Wallace SE, Bean LJH, Stephens K, Amemiya A (Eds). GeneReviews® [Internet]. Seattle (WA): University of Washington, Seattle; 1993-2019.
246. Lees C, Homfray T, Nicolaides KH. Prenatal ultrasound diagnosis of Leroy I cell disease. Ultrasound Obstet Gynecol. 2001;18(3):275-6.
247. David-Vizcarra G, Briody J, Ault J, et al. The natural history and osteodystrophy of mucolipidosis types II and III. J Paediatr Child Health. 2010;46(6):316-22.
248. Pazzaglia UE, Beluffi G, Campbell JB, et al. Mucolipidosis II: correlation between radiological features and histopathology of the bones. Pediatr Radiol. 1989;19:406-13.
249. Melo MD, Obeid G. Radiolucent lesions of the maxillofacial complex in a patient with mucolipidosis type II (MLSII): case report. Oral Surg Oral Med Oral Pathol Oral Radiol Endod. v2007;104(4):e30-3.
250. Gordon N. I-cell disease—mucolipidosis II. Postgrad Med J. 1973;49:359-61.
251. Hetherington C, Harris NJ, Smith TW. Orthopaedic management in four cases of mucolipidosis type III. J R Soc Med. 1999;92:244-6.
252. Carl A, Waldman J, Malone A. Atlantoaxial instability and myelopathy in mucolipidosis. Spine. 1991;16:215-7.
253. Daimon M, Yamagishi M. Surgical treatment of marked mitral valvar deformity combined with I-cell disease 'Mucolipidosis II.' Cardiol Young. 2005;15:517-9.
254. Cripe LH, Ware SM, Hinton RB. Replacement of the aortic valve in a patient with mucolipidosis III. Cardiol Young. 2009;19:641-3.

CHAPTER 19 Biologics used in Spine Surgery for Fusion

Wellington K Hsu

INTRODUCTION

Spinal arthrodesis is among the most prevalent treatments for various cervical, thoracic, and lumbar disorders. Furthermore, between 1998 and 2008, there was a 137% increase in the number of spinal arthrodesis performed in the United States.[1] In line with the increased spinal fusion rates, the potential bone graft and biologic options available to surgeons has also grown. Yet, even with advances in internal fixation, pseudarthrosis has been reported in 10–15% of spine arthrodesis surgery.[2-5]

Analysis of procedures over the past 20 years demonstrates substantial changes in technique. In spinal fusions, instrumentation increased from 23% to 41%, use of autograft decreased from 82% to 52%, and allograft use increased from 7% to 18%.[6] While the use of autograft bone remains the gold standard, significant morbidity has been associated with iliac crest bone graft (ICBG) harvest. Of all patients undergoing ICBG, literature indicates 30% reported surgical morbidities associated with donor-site pain, neurovascular injury, avulsion fracture, infection, hematoma, abdominal herniation, gait disturbance, sacroiliac joint instability, ureteral injury, and cosmetic defect.[7-16]

The combination of surgical morbidity and pseudarthrosis rates can reduce the success rates of fusion in patients with spinal disorders. Further, reported reoperation rates after primary fusion range from 6% to 40%.[17-21] Histologic study of pseudarthrosis reveals a complex biologic environment composed of dense fibrous soft tissue adjacent to sclerotic bone segments with evidence of microfractures.[22] Fibrous tissue, intervertebral disk, and muscle cells commonly encountered during revision surgery have been found to inhibit host bone regeneration.[23]

In order to address the challenges hindering successful spine fusion, key biologic principles related to bone healing must be understood. Bone regeneration involves four critical processes. First, recruitment and differentiation of osteoprogenitor cells to mature osteoblasts through an osteoinductive signal is required. Second, cells response to an osteoinductive signal must exist at the site of injury, or be provided at the site exogenously by the surgeon. Third, an osteoconductive scaffold must provide a three-dimensional construct facilitating bone formation. Finally, vascular supply allows migration of agents involved in the inflammatory phase of healing including progenitor cells and osteoclasts to the site of injury. Critical assessment of biologic potential for bone regeneration and limitations to fusion formation must be evaluated in order to select an appropriate bone graft strategy.

While autograft bone is currently the only material with inherent capacity for osteoinductivity, osteoconductivity, and neovascularization for bone regeneration, significant pseudarthrosis rates still exist despite the use of instrumentation. Thus, various biologic capacities of bone graft substitutes and adjuncts demand continued research in the application of spine surgery. Effective osteobiologic substitute should be osteogenic, biocompatible, user-friendly, cost-effective, and provide structural support.[24] This chapter reviews the pertinent preclinical and clinical data regarding the use of bone graft substitutes in the induction of spinal arthrodesis (Table 1).

AUTOGRAFT

Autogenous bone graft has historically remained the gold standard material for bone grafting for orthopedic procedures as it uniquely provides all necessary components for bone repair: osteoinductive signals

Table 1: Level-of-evidence.

Author, journal, year	*Design*	*LoE*	*Topic*	*F/U (m)*	*Measures*	*Main results*
Autograft						
Sengupta, Spine, 2006[25]	R	III	Clinical and radiologic outcome of instrumented posterolateral lumbar fusion using local bone versus autogenous ICBG	24	Radiographic evaluation OD	Analyzed according to the number of fusion levels, the local bone group fusion rate (approximately 80%) in single-level fusion but a much smaller fusion rate in multilevel fusion (20% vs. 66%, P = 0.029) compared with the ICBG group
Dimar, Spine J, 2009[26]	R	III	Primary one-level instrumented posterolateral fusion with ICBG	24	Radiographic evaluation with CT scans SF-36 OD	Fusion rates based on radiographs with CTs at 6, 12, and 24 months were 65.3%, 82.5%, and 89.3%, respectively. Fusion rates based on bridging bone on CT scans were 56.1%, 71.5%, 83.9%, respectively
Ohtori, Eur Spine J, 2011[42]	RCT	I	One-level instrumented posterolateral fusion with a local bone graft versus an ICBG	24	Radiographic evaluation VAS OD	Rate and average duration of bone union were 90% and 8.5 months in the local bone graft group, and 85% and 7.7 months in the ICBG group, but without significant difference (P > 0.05)
Allograft						
An, J Spinal Disord, 1995[58]	PC	II	Comparison of autografts, frozen allografts, freeze-dried allografts, and a mixture of allograft and autograft in the same patient with instrumented posterolateral lumbar spine fusion	9	Radiographic evaluation	Autograft sites had 80% solid fusion mix of autograft and freeze-dried 50% solid fusion rate, remaining allograft sites resulted in partial fusion
Jorgenson, Spine, 1994[59]	PC	II	Posterolateral lumbar fusion with control ICBG on one side versus demineralized cancellous chips, demineralized cortical powder, demineralized cortical powder mixed with autograft, or mineralized cancellous chips	12	Radiographic evaluation	Significantly lower fusion grading values when allograft alone or in combination with autograft versus autograft alone
Bishop, J Neurosurg, 1996[62]	PC	II	Anterior cervical discectomy with interbody fusion to compare the efficacy of tricortical iliac crest allograft versus autograft fusion substrates	12	Radiographic evaluation	Tricortical iliac crest autograft substrate for interbody fusion following single- and multiple-level anterior cervical discectomy is superior to allograft tricortical iliac crest material

Contd...

Contd...

Author, journal, year	*Design*	*LoE*	*Topic*	*F/U (m)*	*Measures*	*Main results*
Demineralized bone matrix (DBM)						
Vaccaro, Orthopedics, 2007[89]	PC	II	Instrumented posterolateral lumbosacral spinal fusion with DBM putty enriched with aspirated bone marrow, DBM putty with iliac crest autograft, or autograft alone	24	Radiographic evaluation	63% fusion of DBM bone marrow, 70% fusion of DBM autograft, and 67% fusion of autograft alone group (P = 0.875)
Schizas, Arch Orthop Trauma Surg, 2008[91]	PC	II	One or two-level instrumented posterolateral lumbar fusion with either DBM putty with autograft ICBG/local bone versus ICBG or local bone alone	12	Radiographic evaluation ODI VAS	69.7% fusion with DBM putty plus ICBG/local bone group versus 76.9% fusion in ICBG or local bone alone group (P = 0.57). No statistical difference in preoperative and 12 month follow-up VAS and ODI between the two groups
Kang, Spine, 2012[26]	RC	I	One-level instrumented posterior lumbar fusion with DBM matrix with local bone or autologous ICBG	24	Radiographic evaluation ODI SF-36	Fusion rates were 86% DBM matrix versus 92% ICBG (P = 1.0). No statistical difference between ODI and physical function scores
An, Spine, 1995[94]	PC	II	Anterior cervical interbody fusion with autograft ICBG versus freeze-dried allograft with DBM	12	Radiographic evaluation	Pseudarthrosis developed in 46.2% of patients (33.3% of levels) in the allograft- DBM group compared with 26.3% (22% of levels) in the autograft group (P = 0.11 for patients, P = 0.23 for levels)
Ceramic						
Dai, Spine, 2008[114]	RC	I	One-level instrumented posterolateral lumbar fusion with β-TCP combined with local bone or autogenous iliac crest bone graft plus local bone	36	Radiographic evaluation SF-36	Instrumented posterolateral fusion with β-TCP combined with local autograft achieved same radiographic fusion rates (100%) and similar improvement of clinical outcomes compared with autograft alone
Korovessis, Eur Spine J, 2005[189]	RC	I	Instrumented posterolateral lumbar and lumbosacral fusion using either coralline hydroxyapatite with local bone, ICBG, or both	48	Radiographic evaluation ODI SF-36	Bone fusion began in third month postoperatively in all instrumented spines and all levels posteriorly. However, authors found hydroxyapatite not effective in intertransverse posterolateral fusion. SF-36 and ODI score showed no significant difference

Contd...

Contd...

Author, journal, year	*Design*	*LoE*	*Topic*	*F/U (m)*	*Measures*	*Main results*
Stem cells						
Neen, Spine, 2006[140]	PC	II	Instrumented posterolateral lumbar spine fusions with Type 1 collagen/ hydroxyapatite matrix and BMA versus ICBG	24	Radiographic evaluation Low Back Outcome Score (LBOS) Patient Satisfaction Score Prolo Economic Score	Type 1 collagen/hydroxyapatite matrix and BMA resulted in 84% fusion versus 94% fusion of autograft group. Clinical outcomes for both groups were similar
Ammerman, Clin Neurol Neurosurg, 2013[142]	R	IV	Minimally invasive instrumented transforaminal lumbar interbody fusion with Osteocel Plus (OC+) is an allograft cellular bone matrix containing MSCs and osteoprogenitor cells combined with DBM and cancellous bone	12	Radiographic evaluation	91.3% patients went on to achieve radiographic evidence of solid bony arthrodesis
BMP-2 growth factors						
Baskin, Spine, 2003[172]	RC	I	Anterior cervical discectomy and interbody fusion with fibular allograft and rhBMP-2 collagen versus fibular allograft with cancellous iliac crest autograft	24	Radiographic evaluation	100% fusion in both groups with solid fusions at 6, 12, and 24 months
Boden, Spine, 2000[154]	RC	I	Lumbar interbody fusion with cylindrical threaded fusion cage filled with rhBMP-2/collagen or autologous ICBG	24	Radiographic evaluation SF-36	100% fusion in patients treated with rhBMP-2-filled cages at 6,12, and 24 months versus with autogenous bone graft 67% fused
Dawson, Spine, 2009[162]	RC	I	One-level posterolateral lumbar arthrodesis with instrumentation with rhBMP-2 on an absorbable collagen sponge combined with a ceramic-granule bulking agent versus autogenous ICBG	24	Radiographic evaluation ODI SF-36	Overall success rate was 81% fusion in the investigational rhBMP-2 group and 55% fusion in the ICBG control group (p = 0.345)

(ICBG: iliac crest bone graft; ODI: Oswestry disability index; VAS: visual analog scale)

CHAPTER 19

through associated growth factors, osteoconductive matrix scaffold, and osteogenic cells. Autografts used in spine surgery can be either from cortical or cancellous bone. Cortical bone grafts are primarily used to provide structural support for the spinal column in the application of a wide range of spinal defects (0.5–25 cm). However, cortical grafts show less efficacy and increased time during osteointegration, and increased resorption before host incorporation compared to cancellous bone graft. A recent systematic review of the literature has demonstrated an average posterolateral lumbar fusion rate of 79% with the use of ICBG.[25-28] While significant variations exist in harvest technique, bone volume used, and patient demographics between each study, there is a recognizable failure rate in the formation of bony fusion despite proper surgical treatment.

The most common donor sites include both anterior and posterior iliac crest. Several techniques have been successfully used in bone harvest including curettage allowing inner and outer table harvest,[15] iliac crest-splitting,[15] trapdoor,[29] trephine,[30] and segmental bicortical or tricortical grafts.[31] These procedures commonly access the inner or outer table of the ilium to harvest either corticocancellous or cancellous graft. Anterior ICBG harvest can allow an average of 54.53 cm^3.[32] From a posterior approach, cancellous bone graft may be obtained with trapdoor technique to access the inner tables of the posterior ilium. Posterior ICBG harvest can allow for an average of 55.1 cm^3 of bone.[32]

Complications associated with ICBG have been categorized into major and minor complications. Major complications (reported 1–10% rate) include deep hematoma, incisional hernia, neurovascular injury, sacroiliac joint violation, ureteral injury, Trendelenburg gait, donor-site avulsion fracture, and deep infection.[15,33,34] Minor complications (7–39% rate) include donor-site pain, superficial nerve injury, and superficial hematoma formation.[34]

The most frequently reported complication associated with ICBG harvest is chronic donor site pain, described as high as 60% at 2-year follow-up.[27] A number of techniques have been proposed to reduce the incidence of this postoperative pain. For example, local anesthetic application of continuous postoperative 0.5% Marcaine via infusion catheter at ICBG harvest site for continuous infusion of the reservoir solution at a rate of 2 mL/h for 48 hours demonstrates a significant decrease in harvest site pain VAS score (1.4 vs. 4.8) at minimum 4 year postoperatively P < 0.05).[35] Changes in operative harvest techniques also aim to reduce ICBG-related pain and morbidity. Chau et al. reviewed both randomized controlled trials and nonrandomized controlled trials of iliac crest reconstruction techniques using autologous, allogeneic, and synthetic materials following iatrogenic defect procedure.[36] The authors concluded that while current evidence is suboptimal, iliac crest reconstruction may reduce postoperative pain, minimize functional disability and improve cosmesis. However, further studies are needed to prove the efficacy of "backfilling" techniques as well as others aimed to reduce harvest-related complications such as using a single surgical incision for harvest and fusion procedure.

The accuracy in reporting complication rates associated with ICBG harvest procedure, especially painful iliac crest donor site, recently has been questioned.[37] Contrary to historic belief, recent evidence supports the increased use of local bone autograft (lamina, facet, spinous process, etc.) as a replacement or adjunct to ICBG in lumbar fusions.[25,38-42] A prospective randomized controlled trial showed no significant difference in clinical pain scores, rate and average duration of bone union in a single-level posterolateral lumbar spine fusion between local autograft and ICBG.[42] Subgroup analysis demonstrated decreased operative time, shorter length of hospital stay, and decreased blood loss in the local bone autograft group.[42] Conversely, one limitation of local graft compared to ICBG is the decreased quantity of graft. Carragee et al. found the required mean volume of local bone autograft to be 25 cm^3 (range 12–36 cm^3) during single-level posterolateral lumbar fusion.[43] In comparison, Ahlmann et al. found ICBG autograft harvest can obtain up to approximately 55 cm^3 using either anterior or posterior iliac crest donor sites.[32] Although no clear minimum threshold of autograft exists for the achievement of a successful fusion, a volume of 10 cm^3 or less is suggested to be of limited value in forming a solid fusion mass in single level fusion.[44] In clinical situations when local bone autograft volumes are inadequate, bone graft extenders have been used as an adjunct. These products are utilized with ICBG or local bone autograft, as opposed to replacing autograft. The most commonly used extenders currently include demineralized bone matrix (DBM), allograft, and ceramics.[45]

In summary, autologous bone graft remains the gold standard and primary control group in the setting of spinal arthrodesis. However, ICBG harvest is not without associated morbidity especially with the added challenge of an elderly patient population. This presents a set of clinical problems such as osteoporosis, poor bone stock, and anesthetic risks that can occur with increased operative time. As these limitations already present difficulties in spine fusion rates and long-term functional impairment, clinically significant perioperative and postoperative morbidity of ICBG grafting should be minimized.[46,47]

ALLOGRAFT

Allograft bone, which is obtained through cadaveric sources, has historically been one of the most common bone graft strategies. Both cancellous allograft bone chips and cortical allografts have been widely used in spine fusion surgery. Cortical allograft offers structural stability that is ideal for interbody arthrodesis. Cancellous allograft offers the advantage of a larger surface area for faster integration at a cost of lower initial mechanical strength. Cancellous allografts are most often used in posterior spine fusion, while cortical allograft femoral ring and fibular strut grafts are exclusively used in anterior column procedures.

Several tissue-processing methods are used, aiming to remove antigenic components able to induce host immune response, maintain sterility, and preserve biologic and biomechanical properties. Low-dose (< 20 kGy) irradiation, physical debridement, ultrasonic/pulsatile water washes, ethanol treatment, and antibiotic soaking are used in the treatment of tissues. Preservation of allografts is performed via freezing or lyophilization (freeze-drying). The freeze-drying process decreases antigenicity of allograft, thereby reducing the host's cell-mediated immune response, and ultimately allowing for graft incorporation.[48,49] Conversely, it also decreases osteogenic activity and host vascular invasion attributing to a higher reported incidence of nonunion and delayed union compared with autografts.[50] Freeze-drying preparation involves dehydration and vacuum storage of allografts at room temperature. Subsequent rehydration of allografts may result in 50% loss of mechanical strength.[51] Frozen allografts can be stored at -20°C up to 1 year without change in structural composition.

Allograft bone, which primarily serves as an osteoconductive scaffold, loses its osteoinductive potential with the eradication of donor cells during tissue processing. Allograft bone incorporation into the development of a fusion mass follows the same series of biologic events as hemorrhage, inflammation, vascular invasion, and formation of new bone with remodeling of the original graft. However, allograft remodeling demonstrates delayed vascular penetration, accelerated bone resorption, and delayed or incomplete graft incorporation in comparison to autograft.[52-56] Cancellous allograft chips are incorporated at a faster rate and more completely than cortical allograft due to the ability to revascularize more easily. The increased density of larger cortical allografts contributes to a comparable slower rate of revascularization.[57]

Clinical evidence reporting the efficacy of allograft as a bone graft substitute remains sparse. An et al. performed a prospective investigation comparing autograft to allograft for posterolateral lumbar spine fusion. Autograft bone demonstrated significantly greater bone density of fusion mass than mixture of autograft and allograft, frozen allograft, and freeze-dried allograft ($p < 0.05$).[58] Another prospective analysis comparing autograft and demineralized cancellous allograft chips in posterolateral lumbar fusions demonstrated a high pseudarthrosis rate (92%) leading to the conclusion that ethylene oxide-treated allograft should not be used posterior lumbar fusion.[59] Equivalent fusion rates have been reported with allograft and autograft in posterior spine fusions for thoracolumbar scoliosis in the pediatric population.[53,60]

In anterior cervical procedures, Brown et al. reported equivalent fusion rates with allograft use (94%) compared to iliac crest autograft (97%) through plain roentgenographic evaluation.[61] Other similar studies have reported high fusion rates with allograft bone in single-level fusions (78–90%).[62-64] This has led to a widespread adoption of allograft as a cost-effective bone graft substitute in this anatomic area.

Concerns of disease transmission from the use of allograft are managed by the combined efforts of US Food and Drug Administration (FDA) and the American Association of Tissue Banks (AATB). Blood tests mandated by the FDA for human tissues for transplantation include titers for HIV-1 and HIV-2 antibody, hepatitis B surface antigen, hepatitis B core antibody, hepatitis C antibody, syphilis, human T-lymphotropic virus I antibody, and HIV p24 antigen. As a result until 2007, HIV transmission has only been reported twice, one case of Hepatitis B, and seven cases of Hepatitis C from the musculoskeletal tissue allograft use.[65,66]

To improve the success of allograft incorporation into the formation of bone fusion in the future, delivery of mitigating factors may be one solution. Using an established murine explant bone allograft model, Smith et al. demonstrated that for successful bony incorporation, osteocalcin protein levels peaked at day 4, BMP-2 and transforming growth factor (TGF)-α1 on day 2, VEGF peaking on day 8, and IGF-1 decreasing on day 2 from cultured osteoprogenitor cells.[67] This in-vitro analysis may help determine future applications of exogenous factors to improve fusion rates in allografts.

In summary, cortical allografts have demonstrated comparable fusion rates and outcomes to autograft bone in anterior interbody fusion, in addition to structural support to the anterior column. Cancellous allograft is currently recommended as a bone graft extender only in posterolateral arthrodesis and instrumented thoracolumbar deformity of the spine.

DEMINERALIZED BONE MATRIX

Demineralized bone matrix is created through the acid extraction of the mineralized phase of ground corticocancellous bone. Original preparation of DBM was characterized by Urist et al,[68,69] and subsequently modified by Reddi and Huggins.[70] Allogeneic bone is crushed to a particle size of 74–420 μm followed by demineralization in 0.5 N HCL mEq/g for 3 hours.[83] While these initial steps remain constant, this matrix is then combined with different carrier materials before creating the final composite formulation depending on the product. Commercial preparations use several carriers including glycerol, hyaluronic acid, gelatin, and calcium sulfate powder. DBMs are available in various forms including powder, chips, granules, putty and gel-filled syringes.

Following acid extraction of processed allograft bone, a demineralized matrix remains composed of type 1 collagen and noncollagenous proteins, including numerous signaling molecules. Removal of the mineral phase allows biologically active proteins more accessibility to responsive cells. Furthermore, the bone matrix serves as a scaffold for growth factors. The bone morphogenetic proteins (BMPs) represent a fraction of the proteins present in DBMs, with a composition less than 0.1% of all bone proteins by weight.[71] However, growth factors provide critical signals in the process of osteoinduction, initiating a cascade of cellular events leading to bone formation.

The different processing techniques of DBMs can have a significant effect on their osteoinductivity and osteoconductivity. The osteoconductive efficacy of DBMs is seen through the ability to rapidly induce revascularization, serving as excellent scaffolds.[72] However, osteoinductive capacity depends on a number of factors including the original donor and postharvest commercial sterilization, handling, and processing techniques. The use of ethylene oxide and gamma irradiation during sterilization significantly reduce osteoinductivity of DBMs.[73,74] The wide variety of carriers used in commercial preparations of DBMs also affect biologic properties of DBMs.[75,76] For example, glycerol, which is used to convert the allograft to a putty form, has been shown to induce a dose-dependent lethal toxicity in athymic rats.[74] Despite this, there has never been a reported case of renal toxicity from a glycerol carrier in humans.

Several in vitro and in vivo studies demonstrate osteoinductive variability of DBM with donor age, gender, site of implantation, preparation method used, levels of growth factors, matrix integrity, particle size, geometry, and storage conditions.[77-79] In vitro analysis of 20 different DBM lots from eight different tissue bank sources with alkaline phosphatase assay and in vivo bioassay showed significant variability between samples.[78] In vitro quantification of DBM growth factors, BMP-2, BMP-4, and BMP-7, between nine various commercial DBM products, as well as different lots of each product, detected growth factors concentrations in the order of nanograms per gram of DBMs. Further, because of intra-product variability, donor bone characteristics may play a role in the osteoinductive potency of DBM products.[80] Future application of in vitro ELISA to quantify BMP characteristics may help characterize osteoinductivity potential of individual DBM products.

Despite the wide use of DBMs clinically, relatively few in vivo preclinical studies investigating its efficacy exist. Variability in osteogenic activity of different commercially available DBM preparations has been shown among intramuscular animal model, a rat femoral defect, and a rat spine fusion model.[75,81] In a rat femoral defect model, only 8 of 48 specimens healed at 12 weeks when treated with two different DBMs with either a hyaluronic acid or glycerol carrier. The authors suggested that inherent variability of osteoinductive potential of DBMs led to unpredictable fusion rates.[82] Similar results have been reported in a rat spine fusion model.[75,76] In these studies, histologic analysis of the spines 8 weeks after DBM implantation revealed variations in the rates of fusion, amounts of new bone formation, and presence of residual DBM. The efficacy of DBMs with and without combination of autograft in rabbit and nonhuman primate posterolateral spine fusion models has been reported in several studies.[83-86] The body of evidence from these studies suggests that when used alone, DBMs are unable to induce posterolateral spine fusion in rabbits.[87,88] This range of biologic activity of DBMs is likely influenced by the associated donor, carrier, and the assorted demineralization and sterilization methods used.[75]

Clinical studies utilizing DBM are sparse when taking into account the time span in which these products have been used for spine fusion. Three clinical studies in 192 patients report its use in the posterolateral lumbar spine. A collective fusion rate of 89% (range 62–95%) was calculated in these studies.[89-91] In these clinical scenarios, DBM was used as a bone graft extender when an inadequate amount of autograft for spinal fusion is present. Price et al. investigated DBMs use in 88 patients undergoing segmental instrumented spinal fusion in scoliosis deformity surgery.[92] Three groups of bone graft including autologous ICBG, freeze-dried corticocancellous allograft, and composite graft of autologous bone marrow and DBM were compared. A minimum of 2 year follow-up (mean, 3 years 7 months) with radiographic assessment for pseudarthrosis and loss of correction of 10° or more, both criteria for failure of fusion. A failure rate of 12.5% in the ICBG group, 28% in corticocancellous allograft group, and 11.1% in composite graft of autologous bone marrow and DBM group was observed. The authors concluded fusion rates were comparable for ICBG and composite graft of autologous bone marrow and DBM groups.[92] Kang et al. recently performed a prospective randomized trial comparing outcomes of DBM and local autograft composite versus ICBG in single-level instrumented posterior lumbar fusion.[26] The authors demonstrated an 86% fusion rate in DBM-allograft group compared with 92% in ICBG group at 2-year follow-up, that was not statistically significantly different. These results support the use of DBMs as a bone graft extender in order to achieve similar fusion rates as autograft used in posterolateral spinal fusion.

While DBMs have been reported in the posterolateral space, only a couple of studies have used it with interbody fusion. Thalgott et al. report results of case series study using DBM with coralline hydroxyapatite (HA) in anterior lumbar interbody fusion (ALIF) with autologous posterolateral fusion and rigid fixation.[93] With minimum radiographic long-term follow-up of 36 months, the authors report solid fusion rate of 96%, with mean VAS pain decrease of 60%. A total of 70% of all patients either returned to work or to full home activities at a mean of 8 months after surgery. Based on these results, the authors concluded efficacy of DBMs when used with rigidly instrumented circumferential fusion.[93] Notably, a prospective study comparing allograft and DBM composite versus ICBG in anterior cervical fusion found a higher rate of graft collapse and pseudarthrosis with allograft-DBM composite versus ICBG.[94] This study suggests that use of DBM in this setting will lead to suboptimal patient outcomes.

While the FDA recognizes human tissue products, such as allograft and DBM "minimally manipulated" tissue, the regulatory pathway before clinical use requires less data than comparable products such as a synthetic carrier. However, the addition of carrier components such as sodium hyaluronate, glycerol, or calcium phosphate which are not sterilizing, preserving, or storage agents, requires a more extensive 510(k) predicate process for approval for DBMs.

In summary, clinical studies of DBMs have demonstrated efficacy in lumbar spinal fusion when used as a bone graft extender in combination with autograft or bone marrow. While over 50 DBM products are commercially available for use, few high-level clinical studies report long-term clinical outcomes of DBM. Furthermore, no clinical studies have reported outcomes with the use of DBMs alone in spinal fusion. The variability of osteoinductivity and osteoconductivity between commercially available DBM formulations depends on a number of factors including tissue processing, carrier type, final composite formulation, and donor characteristics. Consistent, standardized techniques to evaluate biologic potential of each DBM product are necessary to guide selection of proper DBM in clinical scenarios.

SYNTHETIC CARRIERS

Ceramic scaffolds are synthetic bone graft substitutes consisting of various materials including HA, β-tricalcium phosphate (β-TCP), calcium sulfate, and natural coral ceramics with calcium carbonate. Hydrothermal chemical exchange technique using high temperatures, called sintering, is used to produce ceramic carriers. This process allows extraction of individual crystals in order to fuse together at crystal-grain boundaries. While all synthetic carriers are primarily osteoconductive matrices, properties of individual materials differ among each type.

Calcium sulfate promotes osteoconductivity through ingrowth of blood vessels and associated fibrogenic and osteogenic cells. Resorption of calcium sulfate typically occurs over 5–7 weeks.[95] Calcium sulfate has a compressive strength that is greater than and tensile strength less than that of cancellous bone. β-TCP is a calcium phosphate compound available in porous, solid, or granule form. The compressive and tensile strength of β-TCP is similar to cancellous bone.[96] β-TCP undergoes slower resorption than sulfate through dissolution and fragmentation over 6–18 month, however the amount of bone formation is less than resorption.[97] HA is also a calcium phosphate material available in porous, solid, blocks, or granules. HA is characterized by strong compressive strength properties but is weak under tension and shear. Synthetic HA resorption occurs at a significantly slower rate of 1–2% of volume per year. Commercially available calcium phosphate materials vary in pore size ranging from 200–500 µm.[95] Pore size and interconnectivity are important factors affecting osteoconductivity through ingrowth of vascularity and integration of osteogenic components. However, significant variation of degree of interconnectivity porosity (12–18%) and pore size (range < 1–1500 µm) do not inhibit formation.[98]

Ceramic carriers have several advantageous qualities as a bone graft substitutes; ceramics are readily available in large quantities, production is inexpensive, and there is no risk of disease transmission. Additionally, ceramics are nontoxic, nonimmunogenic, and easily sterilized. Ceramics also confer greater compressive resistance when compared with DBM materials.[99] The biocompatibility of ceramics allows for biologically active cells such as bone marrow aspirate. The osteoinductive properties of composite β-TCP combined with bone marrow aspirate (BMA) has demonstrated superior biologic potential versus DBM in an athymic rat subcutaneous model.[100] The composite β-TCP combined with BMA group demonstrated more bone filling in implants as well as more rapid bone formation.

The bone formation efficacy of ceramic carriers combined with bioactive cells has been demonstrated through in vitro investigation. Bioactive ceramics uniquely allow recruitment of biomacromolecules and osteogenic cells for bone formation to the surface of the material. Bone formation on the HA surface has been found when seeded with cultured mesenchymal stem cells (MSCs) that further differentiate into osteoblasts.[101] Further, composite biomimetic calcium phosphate has shown significant in vitro osteoinductivity, facilitating differentiation of osteogenic cells and apposition of bone tissue matrix.[102,103] Hsu et al. recently investigated osteoinductivity of several carrier scaffolds including absorbable collagen sponge, ceramic-based carriers of different compositions, mineralized allograft chips, and a phosphoserine-rich nanofiber scaffold using human preosteoblasts.[104] BMP-2 binding/release assay results demonstrated a burst pattern with absorbable collagen sponge, with ceramic and allograft scaffolds inefficiently releasing BMP-2. Interestingly, the experimental nanofiber scaffold showed favorable extended release BMP-2 profile. Optimal osteoinductivity of biologic graft substitutes may require composites and hybrid scaffolds, rather than one type of scaffold alone.

Several animal studies have demonstrated effective osteoconductive potential of ceramic carriers such as calcium sulfate, bioactive glass, highly porous HA.[105-109] In an interbody rabbit model, the use of DBM combined with HA showed earlier development of fusion versus DBM alone, ceramics alone, or autograft alone.[110] Ceramic composite carriers in a New Zealand rabbit noninstrumented posterolateral lumbar fusion investigated efficacy of 100% autograft, 50% autograft, 50% biphasic calcium phosphate 15% HA and 85% β-TCP and 50% autograft, and 50% autograft with 80% highly purified β-TCP and 20% highly purified Type-1 collagen, and 50% autograft with ceramic, and 50% ceramic alone.[111] Fusion rates observed by manual palpation of the 100% and 50% autograft controls were 75% and 12.5%, respectively ($P < 0.01$). In the 50% autograft/80% β-TCP and 20% collagen group and 50% autograft/85% HA and 85% β-TCP group fusion rates were reported at 3/8 and 1/8 of the rabbits to have fused successfully, respectively ($P < 0.01$). This study concluded that neither of the ceramic composite scaffolds enhanced the fusion response compared to an equivalent amount of autograft alone, suggesting that these substances may need to be combined with other osteogenic materials to optimize bone production. Ceramic composites' efficacy in lumbar interbody may be comparable with autograft, while porous calcium phosphate ceramics alone were not suitable as a bone graft substitute for lumbar interbody spinal fusion. The use of combination ceramic carriers such as bone graft material comprising 12% bovine-derived collagen and 88% ceramic in the form of HA and β-TCP has suggested to show equivalent performance as iliac crest autograft in a rabbit model.[112]

Of all the bone graft extenders available, the clinical evidence investigating ceramic carriers in spine fusion is strongest. Case series in patients undergoing one-level or two-level instrumented posterolateral fusion demonstrated use of β-TCP as an bone graft expander resulting in fusion rates of 85% at 6 month follow-up versus 96% using local bone autograft.[113] In a similar randomized controlled trial, ICBG was compared to β-TCP and local autograft bone in posterolateral fusion in a total number of 62 patients. The authors reported a 100% fusion rate using plain radiographs in both groups at 3-year follow-up.[114] A prospective randomized study in patients undergoing posterior spinal fusion for idiopathic scoliosis with either biphasic calcium phosphate ceramic containing HA (60%) and TCP (40%) or ICBG/rib autografts concluded that porous ceramic is an effective and safe bone graft substitute in this setting.[115] In a retrospective study in anterior interbody fusion in both cervical and lumbar regions, coralline HA combined with rigid instrumentation demonstrated efficacious results. However, ceramics are not currently recommended in stand-alone anterior interbody fusion.[93,116,117]

The evidence-based literature supporting the use of ceramic carriers in achieving spinal fusion is stronger than that of allograft or DBM. In vitro studies also demonstrate that ceramics support vascular ingrowth, promote cellular adhesion, and enhance new bone formation. However, because of the lack of osteoinductivity with these products, they are recommended for use as a combination therapy with a stimulus such as BMA. This strategy can lead to a fusion rate of 85% (range 5–100%) in posterolateral lumbar spine fusion.[113]

MESENCHYMAL STEM CELLS

Surgeons have utilized MSCs for fusion in spine surgery for decades. While low in numbers, stromal progenitor cells found in bone marrow from autograft carry osteoinductive potential by stimulating bone formation.[118] Autologous MSCs also confer an even lower risk of communicable disease transmission when compared to allogeneic MSC sources. Other potential sources of MSCs include adipose, muscle, and placental-derived tissues.

Allogeneic transplantation offers the delivery of MSCs without associated morbidity and challenges from harvest procedures. Sources of MSCSs include adipose, umbilical cord blood, peripheral blood, and muscle however the clinically preferred source remains bone marrow aspirate. Of the total nucleated cells in bone marrow, MSCs represent less than 0.01%.[119] Several grafts have been investigated with the use of MSCs including ceramic, DBM, collagen and autograft bone grafts. However, allogeneic sources are associated with concern for disease transmission potential as well as rejection. Allogeneic MSCs have low immunogenicity because these lack the major histocompatibility complex (MHC) I complex and also avoid detection from the complement system. Furthermore, multiple anti-inflammatory and immunosuppressive cytokines are secreted by these cells, potentially further suppressing immune reactions.[120] Consequently, the risk of rejection of allogeneic cells remains minimal.

While MSCs can offer significant osteoinductive capacity through the action of secreted cytokines and growth factors, these do not provide local structural support. As a result, MSCs are often used in combination with biological or synthetic scaffolds such as DBM and ceramics that can promote increased cell adhesion, proliferation, and differentiation.[104,121-127] Currently, MSCs are used only in combination with structural graft support, studies demonstrate successful repair of bone defects in tibial nonunions, bone cysts, and comminuted fracture with associated bone loss.[128-130]

McLain et al. investigated the concentration and prevalence of connective-tissue cells among vertebral body and iliac crest aspirates for posterolateral instrumented lumbar spine fusion.[131] 21 adults (11 men, 10 women mean age of 59 ± 14 years) were included in the study with aspirates obtained from two depths within the vertebral body and were quantified relative to matched, bilateral aspirates from the iliac crest that were obtained from the same patient at the same time. Results of superficial and deep vertebral aspirates revealed a median unadjusted connective-tissue progenitor cell concentration of 237 connective-tissue progenitor cells/cc bone marrow (range 92–517 connective-tissue progenitor cells/cc bone marrow) in superficial aspirates, 260 connective-tissue progenitor cells/cc bone marrow (range 114–567 connective-tissue progenitor cells/cc bone marrow) in deep vertebral aspirates, and 181 connective-tissue progenitor cells/cc bone marrow (range 70–401 connective-tissue progenitor cells/cc bone marrow) in iliac crest aspirates. No significant differences relative to vertebral body level, the side aspirated, the depth of aspiration, or gender between vertebral body aspirates, while an age-related decline in cellularity was suggested for the iliac crest aspirates. The authors suggest suitability of vertebral body aspiration for bone marrow graft augmentation in spinal fusion.

When BMA is used from the iliac crest, MSCs are isolated from the mononuclear layer after density gradient centrifugation. Techniques to concentrate this cell population are highly variable depending on commercial formulation. Concentrating techniques have reported high number of osteogenic progenitor cells ranging between 5,000–10,000 cells of total $1–2 \times 10^6$ cells/mL aspirated bone marrow. Further, cell retention processing techniques may allow for a four-fold expansion of initial number of MSCs harvested. The importance of cell number has been established, as a positive correlation between concentration of cells in aspirate used and amount of mineralized callus formation has been demonstrated in bone grafting for fracture nonunion treatment.[132]

Another principle of centrifugation technique has led to the recommendation of smaller harvest volumes of 2 cc to obtain higher concentration of osteoblast progenitor cells, as larger volumes harvested are associated with contamination with peripheral blood leading to dilution of bone marrow aspirate.[133] In a rabbit posterolateral fusion model, Minamide et al. reported that implantation of one million bone marrow cells resulted in a lower fusion rate and less mature bone formation than 100 million cells.[134] Despite this, the quantity of osteoblast progenitor stem cells needed to promote solid bone fusion in humans is still unknown.

In vitro studies demonstrate variability in the quality of BMA depending on anatomic site. Romih et al. studied the osteogenic potential of MSCs in aspirated cell samples from iliac crest, vertebral body, and lumbar interbody space, and concluded that a significantly lower amount of osteoprogenitor cells from aspirate were collected from the interbody space.[135] The dependence on the performance of BMA to age of patient is yet unclear. Stenderup et al. investigated the in vitro characteristics of MSCs harvested from iliac crests collected from 38 patients. No significant difference was found in number of alkaline phosphatase-positive cell colonies or matrix mineralization between young (ages 22–44 years) and older individuals (age 66–74 years).[136] Conversely, Nishida et al. demonstrated that the highest alkaline phosphatase activity in bone marrow concentrate was in subjects less than 10 years of age, with an inverse relationship with increasing age. The authors suggested that decreased bone formation in the aging population may be caused by a quantitative reduction in number of cells rather than the quality of the existing osteoblasts.[137] In vivo evidence supports the use of autologous stem cells in spinal fusion sites with the most abundant source being iliac crest harvest.[28]

Huang et al. investigated bone formation of a hybrid MSC and HA/type I collagen matrix in a New Zealand rabbit posterolateral fusion model compared to autograft.[138] MSCs harvested from iliac crest and embedded onto the HA/type I collagen matrix graft constructs demonstrated higher alkaline phosphatase activity in osteogenic than in standard media ($p < 0.05$), and no statistical difference between manual palpation scores between MSC composite grafts or autograft. Furthermore, the use of fluorescence-labeled MSCs revealed that new bone formation occurred in the area of the transplanted stem cells.

Evidence suggests that associated carrier with MSCs can lead to improved performance. Kimelman-Bleich et al. reported increased oxygen content when MSCs were cultured on synthetic oxygen carrier-enriched hydrogel scaffolds.[139] The perfluorotributylamine (PFTBA)-treated led to 2.5-fold greater bone formation in subcutaneous ectopic sites, a 1.4-fold increase in bone volume in a posterolateral spinal fusion model when compared to nontreated scaffolds. The authors concluded that a positive effect could be achieved from increased oxygenation with an appropriate osteoconductive scaffold. Other studies have investigated effects on osteoblastic differentiation of stem cells on fusion outcomes.

The best available clinical evidence for the use of autologous MSCs in spinal fusion has studied concentrated BMA. In a prospective case controlled study, Neen et al. compared Healos (Type I collagen /HA matrix) soaked in BMA to iliac crest autograft in either lumbar posterolateral or interbody spinal fusion.[140] Fifty consecutive patients

SECTION 2

(15 posterolateral fusion, 13 posterior lumbar interbody fusion (PLIF), 22 patients with 360° front and back fusion) were matched with historical controls treated with iliac crest autograft. There were equivalent radiographic fusion rates for Healos/BMA versus autograft groups with no significant differences in subjective and objective clinical outcomes. However, the authors recommend against Healos/BMA use with interbody cages, attributing lower fusion rates with an insufficient quantity of osteoinductive and osteoconductive material available.

Gan et al. reported results from a prospective trial in patients with posterior spinal fusion with transpedicular spinal instrumentation and enriched autologous MSCs/β-TCP graft implantation in 41 patients in treatment of degenerative disk disease or thoracolumbar fracture injury.[141] The protocol harvested an average of 45 mL enriched MSC suspension from bilateral iliac crests in each patient and combined them with 15–25 g porous β-TCP granules. There was a positive correlation between the total number of nucleated bone marrow cells and number of MSCs in a given aspirate. Cellular enrichment techniques allowed expansion of MSC colony-forming units by 4.3-fold confirmed by analysis of MSC expression alkaline phosphatase. In this study, subjects less than 40 years of age had more MSCs compared with those older than 40 years. At mean follow-up time of 36.5 months, plain radiographic fusion rate was determined to be 95.1%. The authors concluded the use of enrichment of autologous MSCs combined with porous β-TCP was as effective as autologous bone grafting in instrumented posterior spinal fusion surgery based on the fusion rates of this study, however, this analysis did not have a control autograft group.

The clinical evidence supporting the use of allogeneic stem cells in spine fusion is currently limited. Ammerman et al. performed a retrospective chart review of 23 patients (20 single level, 3 double level) treated with minimally invasive transforaminal lumbar interbody and Osteocel Plus (OC+) (Nuvasive, San Diego, CA), an allograft cellular bone matrix containing MSCs and osteoprogenitor cells combined with DBM and cancellous bone. PEEK interbody devices were used in all cases and packed with 1 cc of OC+ per level. Autograft harvested from the facet joint was placed anterior to the interbody device in all cases. 21 patients (91.3%) and 24 spinal levels (92.3%) went on to achieve radiographic evidence of solid bony arthrodesis by 12 months postoperative by plain radiographs. The authors conclude this fusion rate compares favorably to the reported fusion rates for autograft, allograft and beta-Tricalcium phosphate.[142,143]

Kerr et al. also performed a retrospective study with the use of OC+ in lumbar interbody fusion surgery of 52 patients.[144] The mean age was 50 (range, 27–77) years; 60% were females; 43% were habitual smokers and 21% had previously failed surgery at the index levels, circumferential fusion was performed in 67% of cases, ALIF 17% and transforaminal lumbar interbody fusion (TLIF) 16%. Mean follow-up was 14 months (range 8–27) with 92.3% solid fusion apparent at 5 months follow-up by plain radiographic evaluation ($P < 0.05$). Statistical analysis demonstrated that increasing age (older than 50 years) ($p = 0.017$) and habitual smoking ($p = 0.015$) delayed the fusion time and increased the risk of pseudarthrosis. The authors concluded the use of Osteocel allograft is safe and effective in adult patients undergoing lumbar interbody spinal fusion procedure.

With the development of several stem cell harvesting and enrichment techniques, several ethical and regulatory considerations have been raised. The FDA and European Medicines Agency classify the application of cells processed or expanded ex vivo as advanced therapy medicinal products (ATMPs). The approval for clinical use of these products requires specific quality control and safety criteria of all cell processing based on strict good manufacturing practice (GMP), appropriate conduct of preclinical animal models, and meaningful controlled phase I/II clinical trials.[145] Within the FDA, stem cells treatments can be covered both by the Center for Biologics Evaluation and Research and the Office of Cellular, Tissue and Gene Therapies. When there is no manipulation of human cells in a product, then regulation falls under the Human Cell and Tissue Products pathway. Regulation of tissues falls under section 361 of the Public Health Safety Act, with the aim of preventing the introduction, transmission, and spread of communicable diseases.

Current evidence demonstrates encouraging applicability of MSCs in combination with appropriate carrier scaffolds. Harvesting and processing techniques of osteoprogenitor cells found in BMA have improved in vivo bone formation capacity of these grafts. Studies demonstrate the decreased quantity of MSCs found in older patients, in part contributing to difficultly in achieving high fusion rates. In vitro data continues to demonstrate improved cell viability and function of MSCs implanted on carrier scaffolds, and results from preclinical animal studies show capacity for in vivo bone formation. Future studies investigating enhanced MSC osteoblastic differentiation and ideal delivery carrier characteristics are required to fully realize MSC potential in clinical trials.

BONE MORPHOGENETIC PROTEIN

First described by Dr Marshall Urist[146] in 1965, BMPs and other osteoinductive growth factors have gained a substantial role in bone healing and spinal fusion enhancement. More than 20 different types of BMPs have been identified with BMP-2, -4, -6, -7, -9 having the greatest osteogenic characteristics.[147] Members of TGF-ß superfamily, BMPs promote bone regeneration through initiation of signal transduction through the binding of a membrane-based heterodimeric complex of two transmembrane serine-threonine kinase receptors, BMP receptor (BMPR) type I and II. The activated receptor kinase then phosphorylates transcription factors, Smad 1, 5, and 8 translocates to the nucleus (with Smad 4) and leads to the increased expression of target genes involved in osteogenesis.[148] As a result of extensive preclinical and clinical work, a product containing both recombinant BMP-2 (rhBMP-2) and an absorbable Type I collagen sponge (ACS) (INFUSE™) (Medtronic Sofamor Danek, Memphis, TN) has been FDA-approved for use in anterior spine fusion. Recombinant BMP-7 (or osteogenic protein-1, rhOP-1) has been approved through the humanitarian device exemption for use in treatment of posterior spinal fusion.

In vitro data suggests that BMPs facilitate osteogenic differentiation of MSCs through multiple pathways.[149] BMP-7-treated stem cells show enhanced secretion of osteogenic lineage-specific markers including phosphoprotein 1, osteocalcin, and osterix.[149,150] Furthermore, BMP-7 significantly increased alkaline phosphatase activity with a dose-dependent acceleration of calcium mineralization of osteogenic differentiated MSCs.[149] Similarly, MSCs treated with BMP-2 in vitro demonstrate increased osteocalcin release, while addition of neutralization antibodies of BMP-2 decreased ALP levels.[151]

The efficacy of recombinant BMP has been well established in several preclinical spine fusion models. In single-level ALIFs with rhBMP-2 in a sheep model,[152] Sandhu et al. demonstrated a bony bridge anterior to the titanium cage in all rhBMP-2-treated animals (n = 6) at 6 months postoperatively, whereas it was present in only two animals treated with autogenous bone graft group (n = 5) (P < 0.05). Biomechanically, segments treated with rhBMP-2 were 20% stiffer in flexion than autograft-treated segments at 6 months compared with unoperated spinal column controls. Similarly, Boden et al. reported successful fusion in a laparoscopic anterior lumbar interbody arthrodesis rhesus monkey with rhBMP-2 inside a titanium threaded interbody fusion cage in five animals with computed tomography imaging.[153] The authors also described a dose-response phenomenon; increased bone formation was associated with the higher concentration of rhBMP-2. Based on these results, a recommended concentration of 1.5 mg/mL dose was utilized for interbody fusion implants in subsequent human clinical trials.[154]

Preclinical animal models utilizing posterolateral spinal fusion have also demonstrated enhancement of fusion with rhBMP-2. Schimandle et al. performed posterolateral intertransverse process spinal fusion at L5–L6 in 56 rabbits using different doses of rhBMP-2 with collagen carrier or autogenous bone graft.[155] All rabbits treated with rhBMP-2 achieved solid spinal fusion by manual palpation and radiographic evaluation, whereas 42% of the autograft control achieved fusion (P = 0.01). Fischgrund et al. evaluated the use of rhBMP-2 implanted with various carriers in canine lumbar spines including autogenous bone graft, Type I collagen "sandwich", collagen morsels, polylactic/glycolic acid sponge (PLGA) sandwich, and open-pore polylactic acid morsels.[156] RhBMP-2 significantly increased bone graft volume as noted on CT imaging at 8 weeks. While no significant difference in carrier media for rhBMP-2 could be determined, polylactic/glycolic acid (PLGA) treatment groups were associated with a greater incidence of voids within the fusion mass.

In a study of posterolateral intertransverse process arthrodesis at L4–5 in 29 rhesus monkeys using various doses and carriers of rhBMP-2, Martin et al. demonstrated that tissue compression of the collagen sponge carrier with inadequate binding times could prevent bone induction at standard BMP doses.[157] The authors suggested that premature compression of the collage sponge could cause extravasation of protein and dilution of the osteogenic effect. Suh et al. evaluated biphasic ceramic phosphate granules (60% HA/40% tricalcium phosphate) as an alternative carrier to collagen for rhBMP-2 in a posterolateral spine arthrodesis at L5–L6 in rhesus monkeys.[158] The authors found the biologically compatible biphasic ceramic phosphate carrier matrices of rhBMP-2

SECTION 2

to induce fusion, resulting in stiffer fusion masses than autograft without tissue compression of collagen sponge carriers.

The first clinical prospective, randomized study with BMP was performed in single-level lumbar degenerative disk disease. Boden et al. performed ALIF using a titanium cylindrical cage packed with rhBMP-2 on a collagen sponge (n = 11) or autogenous ICBG (n = 3).[154] All 11 patients treated with rhBMP-2 showed fusion in comparison to two of three patients receiving autologous bone graft fused. Furthermore, the rhBMP-2 treatment group demonstrated improved Oswestry Disability Index (ODI) scores at 3 months than the control, while this difference disappeared at 6 months. This pilot study then led to a multicenter, prospective, randomized study of a total 279 patients treated with rhBMP-2 (n = 143) and control autologous ICBG group (n = 136) undergoing ALIF, which demonstrated an overall fusion rate of 94.5% in the rhBMP-2 treatment group compared to 88.7% in the control ICBG group with CT imaging.[159] Clinical outcome measures (ODI, back pain, and leg pain) were statistically similar at 6, 12, and 24-month follow-up intervals, while 32% of ICBG group patients reported graft site discomfort at 24 months.

As rhBMP-2 is only FDA-approved for ALIF with tapered titanium cages, it is estimated that 85% of current BMP-2 use is off-label, including posterolateral fusions.[160] Boden et al. conducted a prospective, randomized clinical trial of rhBMP-2 used in posterolateral spine fusion with three treatment groups: control group treated with ICBG (n = 5); rhBMP-2 (with tricalcium phosphate/HA granules) and instrumentation (n = 11); and rhBMP-2 (with tricalcium phosphate/HA granules) without instrumentation (= 9).[161] The fusion rate reported in patients treated with rhBMP-2 with or without instrumentation was 100%, while the control group had a fusion rate of only 40%. Dawson et al. performed a prospective randomized study investigating the use of rhBMP-2 combined with a ceramic-granule bulking agent as a replacement for autogenous ICBG in single-level posterolateral lumbar arthrodesis with instrumentation.[162] Fusion rates were reported as 95% in the experimental group compared to 70% in the control group at 24-month follow-up with plain radiographs. Furthermore, the improvement in the mean ODI score, as compared with the preoperative score, was 28.2 points in the investigational group and 23.0 points in the control group at 24 months. These studies support the use of rhBMP-2 as a replacement for autograft in single-level posterolateral lumbar arthrodesis with instrumentation.

In posterior (PLIF) or TLIF, Mummaneni et al.[163] reported higher and faster fusion rates with the use of rhBMP-2 compared to patients treated with only autograft. However, more recent literature has raised concern with the potential complications with use in this anatomic area.[164] Untoward effects of rhBMP-2 have been linked to heterotopic bone formation,[165] transient endplate resorption,[166] and graft subsidence.[167] In a potentially debilitating complication, patients treated with rhBMP-2 in TLIF/PLIF also experience a higher rate of postoperative radiculitis.[168] Mitigating techniques have been suggested to limit the incidence of postoperative pain including using fibrin glue to prevent postoperative radiculitis,[169] and some investigators have postulated that with the use of smaller doses, complications can be minimized.[165,170,171]

In the anterior cervical spine, clinical studies involving rhBMP-2 in the interbody space have reported 100% fusion rates at 6-, 12-, and 24-month follow-up.[172-175] However, a number of series have demonstrated a greater number of devastating complications including post-operative prevertebral swelling, hematoma formation, and dysphagia.[175-178] Furthermore, the reintubation rates for acute airway obstruction are significantly greater in patients with rhBMP-2 than autograft.[179] These and other similar studies have led to an FDA-administered black box warning against the use of rhBMP-2 in the anterior cervical spine. While no study has directly linked the dose-response relationship with the incidence of complications, it is commonly thought among surgeons and scientists alike that use of higher doses increases the likelihood of an adverse event. In any case, the authors here currently recommend against the use of rhBMP-2 in the anterior cervical spine.

Therapeutic applications of rhBMP-2 in the posterior cervical spine may avoid critical anterior structures however complications regarding the safety and efficacy in this use have also been reported. Hamilton et al. report a series of 53 patients undergoing posterior cervical or cervicothoracic-instrumented fusion with rhBMP-2.[180] Surgical indications included basilar invagination (n = 6), fracture (n = 6), atlantoaxial instability (n = 16), kyphosis/kyphoscoliosis (n = 22), osteomyelitis (n = 1), spondylolisthesis (n = 1), cyst (n = 1), and rheumatoid disease (n = 15). The average rhBMP-2 dose was 1.8 mg per level, with a total of 282 levels treated (average, 5.3

levels; SD, 2.8 levels). The authors report 100% fusion at mini-mum 2-year follow-up, suggesting the safety and effectiveness of rhBMP-2 as an adjunct for posterior cervical fusion is safe and effective at an average dose of 1.8 mg per level. While BMP use in the posterior cervical spine may be less devastating than use in the anterior cervical spine, wound complications requiring operative management have been reported in up to 12% of patients undergoing posterior cervical fusions with use of rhBMP-2.[181]

In June of 2011, an issue in The Spine Journal was published that highlighted case series and clinical studies involving rhBMP-2 in the literature. While many of the complications summarized in this issue are known to spine surgeons including osteolysis, ectopic bone formation, and seroma formation, Carragee et al. reported a higher incidence of retrograde ejaculation and a greater risk of new malignancy. Carragee et al. report the rate of retrograde ejaculation in ALIF with rhBMP-2 of approximately 5–7% and possibly two to four times higher than the rate observed without rhBMP-2.[179,182] However, Tepper et al. performed a prospective study evaluating incidence of retrograde ejaculation in 41 males undergoing ALIF with posterior pedicle screw instrumentation and fusion at L4–L5 and/or L5–L1, with preoperative semen and postejaculatory urine analysis, repeat testing 6 months after surgery, and a postoperative standardized questionnaire.[183] The semen analysis consisted of ejaculate volume, total sperm count, concentration, and motility, whereas the urine test reported postejaculatory voided urine for spermatozoa. Of the 21 patients treated with rhBMP-2, two (9.5%) were diagnosed with retrograde ejaculation (RE), based on laboratory analysis, one of which resolved. Of the 20 patients treated without rhBMP-2, two (10.0%) had RE by laboratory analysis, one of which resolved. Based on this data, the authors conclude that use of a questionnaire tends to overestimate the incidence of RE as compared with the quantitative semen and urine analysis.

Data regarding rhBMP-2 effects on induction or mutagenic carcinogenicity in vitro and in vivo remain controversial. It is known that BMP receptors are found on cell membranes of certain cancer lines.[184-186] In a systematic review evaluating rhBMP-2 and its association with primary and metastatic cancer, Thawani et al. found no definitive association between BMPs and the promotion of tumorigenesis or metastasis.[187] The authors also comment on diversity of mechanisms; BMPs act in known existence effecting tumorigenesis or the metastatic process—dysregulation of pathways may suppress or support tumor growth. Furthermore, the majority of studies reviewed provide speculation based on the collective knowledge of downstream effects of intracellular events.[187] Recently Carragee et al. investigated randomized controlled trials of new cancer incidence in patients with degenerative lumbar spine conditions who underwent a single-level instrumented posterolateral arthrodesis with either high-dose 40 mg rhBMP-2 in a compression-resistant matrix (CRM) (rhBMP-2/CRM; n = 239) or autogenous bone graft (control group; n = 224).[188] The incidence rate of new cancer events per 100 person-years was 3.37 [95% confidence interval (CI), 1.89 to 5.56] in the rhBMP-2/CRM group at 2 years compared with 0.50 (95% CI, 0.06 to 1.80) in the control group. From this data, the authors concluded that high dose of 40 mg of rhBMP-2/CRM in lumbar spinal arthrodesis was associated with an increased risk of new cancer.

CONCLUSION

In the development of spine surgery biologics autologous ICBG remains the standard against which substitute and adjunct fusion success are compared. Autograft bone inherently possess the key elements of successful bone formation; osteoinductive signaling and recruitment of osteoprogenitor cells, osteoconductive scaffolding providing three-dimensional bone formation, and capacity of neovascularization. While the morbidity and complications associated with autograft harvest are not insignificant, recent literature suggests the long-term effects are less than previously believed. Advanced bone graft substitutes in the use of spine fusion procedures have proven efficacious in preclinical, animal, and clinical trials including bone allograft, DBM, synthetic carriers, stem cells, and osteoinductive growth factors, chiefly BMP-2. Studies investigating these alternatives, as well as future innovational technology including gene therapy, continue to elucidate the evidence for clinical application of each substitute in spine fusion surgery. Increasing literature examining the biology and specificity of bone graft substitutes and adjuncts remains fundamental in understanding the advantages and limitations regarding decisions regarding their use.

REFERENCES

1. Rajaee SS, Bae HW, Kanim LE, et al. Spinal fusion in the United States: analysis of trends from 1998 to 2008. Spine (Phila Pa 1976). 2012;37(1):67-76.
2. Zdeblick TA. A prospective, randomized study of lumbar fusion. Preliminary results. Spine (Phila Pa 1976). 1993;18(8):983-91.
3. West JL 3rd, Bradford DS, Ogilvie JW. Results of spinal arthrodesis with pedicle screw-plate fixation. J Bone Joint Surg Am.1991;73(8):1179-84.
4. McGuire RA, Amundson GM. The use of primary internal fixation in spondylolisthesis. Spine (Phila Pa 1976). 1993; 18(12):1662-72.
5. Bridwell KH, Sedgewick TA, O'Brien MF, et al. The role of fusion and instrumentation in the treatment of degenerative spondylolisthesis with spinal stenosis. J Spinal Disord. 1993;6(6):461-72.
6. Bono CM, Lee CK. Critical analysis of trends in fusion for degenerative disc disease over the past 20 years: influence of technique on fusion rate and clinical outcome. Spine (Phila Pa 1976). 2004;29(4):455-63; discussion Z5.
7. Banwart JC, Asher MA, Hassanein RS. Iliac crest bone graft harvest donor site morbidity. A statistical evaluation. Spine (Phila Pa 1976). 1995;20(9):1055-60.
8. Goulet JA, Senunas LE, DeSilva GL, et al. Autogenous iliac crest bone graft. Complications and functional assessment. Clin Orthop Relat Res. 1997;339:76-81.
9. Reid RL. Hernia through an iliac bone-graft donor site. A case report. J Bone Joint Surg Am. 1968;50(4):757-60.
10. Coventry MB, Tapper EM. Pelvic instability: a consequence of removing iliac bone for grafting. J Bone Joint Surg Am. 1972;54(1):83-101.
11. Challis JH, Lyttle JA, Stuart AE. Strangulated lumbar hernia and volvulus following removal of iliac crest bone graft. Acta Orthop Scand. 1975;46(2):230-3.
12. Cowley SP, Anderson LD. Hernias through donor sites for iliac-bone grafts. J Bone Joint Surg Am. 1983;65(7):1023-5.
13. Kuhn DA, Moreland MS. Complications following iliac crest bone grafting. Clin Orthop Relat Res. 1986;209:224-6.
14. Kurz LT, Garfin SR, Booth RE Jr. Harvesting autogenous iliac bone grafts. A review of complications and techniques. Spine (Phila Pa 1976). 1989;14(12):1324-31.
15. Ebraheim NA, Elgafy H, Xu R. Bone-graft harvesting from iliac and fibular donor sites: techniques and complications. J Am Acad Orthop Surg. 2001;9(3):210-8.
16. Escalas F, DeWald RL. Combined traumatic arteriovenous fistula and ureteral injury: a complication of iliac bone-grafting. J Bone Joint Surg Am. 1977;59(2):270-1.
17. Brantigan JW. Pseudarthrosis rate after allograft posterior lumbar interbody fusion with pedicle screw and plate fixation. Spine (Phila Pa 1976).1994;19(11):1271-80.
18. Franklin GM, Haug J, Heyer NJ, et al. Outcome of lumbar fusion in Washington state workers' compensation. Spine (Phila Pa 1976). 1994;19(17):1897-904.
19. Hutter CG. Posterior intervertebral body fusion: a 25 year study. Clin Orthop Relat Res.1983;179:86-96.
20. Lehmann TR, LaRocca HS. Repeat lumbar surgery: a review of patients with failure from previous lumbar surgery treated by canal exploration and lumbar spinal fusion. Spine (Phila Pa 1976). 1981;6(6):615-9.
21. Martin BI, Mirza SK, Comstock BA, et al. Are lumbar spine reoperation rates falling with greater use of fusion surgery and new surgical technology? Spine (Phila Pa 1976). 2007; 32(19):2119-26.
22. Heggeness MH, Esses SI, Mody DR. A histologic study of lumbar pseudarthrosis. Spine (Phila Pa 1976). 1993;18(8):1016-20.
23. Bae H, Kanim LEA, Zhao L, et al. Cellular environments alter performance of rhBMP-2 and induce pseudarthrosis. Spine J. 2004;4:52S.
24. Berven S, Tay BK, Kleinstueck FS, et al. Clinical applications of bone graft substitutes in spine surgery: consideration of mineralized and demineralized preparations and growth factor supplementation. Eur Spine J. 2001;10(Suppl 2):S169-77.
25. Sengupta DK, Truumees E, Patel CK, et al. Outcome of local bone versus autogenous iliac crest bone graft in the instrumented posterolateral fusion of the lumbar spine. Spine (Phila Pa 1976). 2006;31(9):985-91.
26. Kang J, An H, Hilibrand A, et al. Grafton and local bone has comparable outcomes to iliac crest bone in instrumented single-level lumbar fusions. Spine (Phila Pa 1976). 2012;37(12):1083-91.
27. Dimar JR II, Glassman SD, Burkus JK, et al. Two-year fusion and clinical outcomes in 224 patients treated with a single-level instrumented posterolateral fusion with iliac crest bone graft. Spine J. 2009;9(11):880-5.
28. Hsu WK, Nickoli MS, Wang JC, et al. Improving the clinical evidence of bone graft substitute technology in lumbar spine surgery. Global Spine J. 2012;2(4):239-48.
29. Brawley SC, Simpson RB. Results of an alternative autogenous iliac crest bonegraft harvest method. Orthopedics. 2006;29(4):342-6.
30. Ilankovan V, Stronczek M, Telfer M, et al. A prospective study of trephined bone grafts of the tibial shaft and iliac crest. Br J Oral Maxillofac Surg. 1998;36(6):434-9.
31. Behairy YM, Al-Sebai W. A modified technique for harvesting full-thickness iliac crest bone graft. Spine (Phila Pa 1976). 2001;26(6):695-7.
32. Ahlmann E, Patzakis M, Roidis N, et al. Comparison of anterior and posterior iliac crest bone grafts in terms of harvest-site morbidity and functional outcomes. J Bone Joint Surg Am. 2002;84(5):716-20.
33. Arrington ED, Smith WJ, Chambers HG, et al. Complications of iliac crest bone graft harvesting. Clin Orthop Relat Res. 1996;329:300-9.
34. Myeroff C, Archdeacon M. Autogenous bone graft: donor sites and techniques. J Bone Joint Surg Am. 2011;93(23):2227-36.
35. Singh K, Phillips FM, Kuo E, et al. A prospective, randomized, double-blind study of the efficacy of postoperative continuous local anesthetic infusion at the iliac crest bone graft site after posterior spinal arthrodesis: a minimum of 4-year follow-up. Spine (Phila Pa 1976). 2007;32(25):2790-6.
36. Chau AM, Xu LL, van der Rijt R, et al. Reconstruction versus no reconstruction of iliac crest defects following harvest for spinal fusion: a systematic review: A review. J Neurosurg Spine. 2012;16(6):565-72.

37. Hu SS. Iliac crest bone graft: are the complications overrated? Spine J. 2011;11(6):538-9.
38. Inage K, Ohtori S, Koshi T, et al. One, two-, and three-level instrumented posterolateral fusion of the lumbar spine with a local bone graft: a prospective study with a 2-year follow-up. Spine (Phila Pa 1976). 2011;36(17):1392-6
39. Ito Z, Matsuyama Y, Sakai Y, et al. Bone union rate with autologous iliac bone versus local bone graft in posterior lumbar interbody fusion. Spine (Phila Pa 1976). 2010;35(21):E1101-5.
40. Kim D-H, Jeong S-S, Lee S-S. Posterior lumbar interbody fusion using a unilateral single cage and a local morselized bone graft in the degenerative lumbar spine. Clin Orthop Surg. 2009;1(4):214-21.
41. Lee S, Chen J, Wu C, et al. In situ local autograft for instrumented lower lumbar or lumbosacral posterolateral fusion. J Clin Neurosci. 2009;16(1):37-43.
42. Ohtori S, Suzuki M, Koshi T, et al. Single-level instrumented posterolateral fusion of the lumbar spine with a local bone graft versus an iliac crest bone graft: a prospective, randomized study with a 2-year follow-up. Eur Spine J. 2011;20(4):635-9.
43. Carragee EJ, Comer GC, Smith MW. Local bone graft harvesting and volumes in posterolateral lumbar fusion: a technical report. Spine J. 2011;11(6):540-4.
44. Cammisa FP Jr, Lowery G, Garfin SR, et al. Two-year fusion rate equivalency between Grafton DBM gel and autograft in posterolateral spine fusion: a prospective controlled trial employing a side-by-side comparison in the same patient. Spine (Phila Pa 1976). 2004;29(6):660-6.
45. Abdullah KG, Steinmetz MP, Benzel EC, et al. The state of lumbar fusion extenders. Spine (Phila Pa 1976). 2011;36(20): E1328-34.
46. Silber JS, Anderson DG, Daffner SD, et al. Donor site morbidity after anterior iliac crest bone harvest for single-level anterior cervical discectomy and fusion. Spine (Phila Pa 1976). 2003;28(2):134-9.
47. Fernyhough JC, Schimandle JJ, Weigel MC, et al. Chronic donor site pain complicating bone graft harvesting from the posterior iliac crest for spinal fusion. Spine (Phila Pa 1976). 1992;17(12):1474-1480.
48. Bos GD, Goldberg VM, Zika JM, et al. Immune responses of rats to frozen bone allografts. J Bone Joint Surg Am. 1983;65(2):239-46.
49. Burwell RG. Studies in the transplantation of bone. V. The capacity of fresh and treated homografts of bone to evoke transplantation immunity. J Bone Joint Surg Br. 1963;45-B:386-401.
50. Goldberg VM, Stevenson S. Natural history of autografts and allografts. Clin Orthop Relat Res. 1987;225:7-16.
51. Hamer AJ, Strachan JR, Black MM, et al. Biomechanical properties of cortical allograft bone using a new method of bone strength measurement: a comparison of fresh, fresh-frozen, and irradiated bone. J Bone Joint Surg Br. 1996;78(3):363-8.
52. Tsuang YH, Yang RS, Chen PQ, et al. Experimental allograft in spinal fusion in dogs. Taiwan Yi Xue Hui Za Zhi. 1989;88(10):989-94.
53. Aurori BF, Weierman RJ, Lowell HA, et al. Pseudarthrosis after spinal fusion for scoliosis. A comparison of autogeneic and allogeneic bone grafts. Clin Orthop Relat Res. 1985;199:153-8.
54. Brooks DB, Heiple KG, Herndon CH, et al. Immunological factors in homogenous bone transplantation. IV. The effect of various methods of preparation and irradiation on antigenicity. J Bone Joint Surg Am. 1963;45:1617-26.
55. Friedlaender GE, Strong DM, Sell KW. Studies on the antigenicity of bone. II. Donor-specific anti-HLA antibodies in human recipients of freeze-dried allografts. J Bone Joint Surg Am. 1984;66(1):107-12.
56. Herron LD, Newman MH. The failure of ethylene oxide gas sterilized freeze-dried bone graft for thoracic and lumbar spinal fusion. Spine (Phila Pa 1976). 1989;14 (5):496-500.
57. Dimitriou R, Jones E, McGonagle D, et al. Bone regeneration: current concepts and future directions. BMC Med. 2011;9:66.
58. An HS, Lynch K, Toth J. Prospective comparison of autograft vs. allograft for adult posterolateral lumbar spine fusion: differences among freeze-dried, frozen, and mixed grafts. J Spinal Disord. 1995;8(2):131-5.
59. Jorgenson SS, Lowe TG, France J, et al. A prospective analysis of autograft versus allograft in posterolateral lumbar fusion in the same patient. A minimum of 1-year follow-up in 144 patients. Spine (Phila Pa 1976). 1994;19(18):2048-53.
60. Dodd CA, Fergusson CM, Freedman L, et al. Allograft versus autograft bone in scoliosis surgery. J Bone Joint Surg Br. 1988;70(3):431-4.
61. Brown MD, Malinin TI, Davis PB. A roentgenographic evaluation of frozen allografts versus autografts in anterior cervical spine fusions. Clin Orthop Relat Res. 1976;119:231-6.
62. Bishop RC, Moore KA, Hadley MN. Anterior cervical interbody fusion using autogeneic and allogeneic bone graft substrate: a prospective comparative analysis. J Neurosurg. 1996;85(2):206-10.
63. Martin GJ Jr, Haid RW Jr, MacMillan M, et al. Anterior cervical discectomy with freeze-dried fibula allograft. Overview of 317 cases and literature review. Spine (Phila Pa 1976). 1999;24(9):852-8; discussion 858-9.
64. Zdeblick TA, Ducker TB. The use of freeze-dried allograft bone for anterior cervical fusions. Spine (Phila Pa 1976).1991;16(7):726-9.
65. Tomford WW, Mankin HJ. Bone banking: update on methods and materials. Orthop Clin North Am. 1999;30(4):565-70.
66. Joyce MJ, Greenwald AS, Boden S, et al. Musculoskeletal allograft tissue safety. American Academy of Orthopaedic Surgeons Annual Meeting 2007.
67. Smith KE, Huang Z, Ma T, et al. Molecular profile of osteoprogenitor cells seeded on allograft bone. J Tissue Eng Regen Med. 2011;5(9):704-11.
68. Urist MR, Silverman BF, Buring K, et al. The bone induction principle. Clin Orthop Relat Res. 1967;53:243-83.
69. Urist MR, Dawson E. Intertransverse process fusion with the aid of chemosterilized autolyzed antigen-extracted allogeneic (AAA) bone. Clin Orthop Relat Res. 1981;154:97-113.
70. Reddi AH, Huggins C. Biochemical sequences in the transformation of normal fibroblasts in adolescent rats. Proc Natl Acad Sci USA. 1972;69(6):1601-5.
71. Sandhu HS, Grewal HS, Parvataneni H. Bone grafting for spinal fusion. Orthop Clin North Am. 1999;30(4):685-98.
72. Finkemeier CG. Bone-grafting and bone-graft substitutes. J Bone Joint Surg Am. 2002;84(3):454-64.

73. Munting E, Wilmart JF, Wijne A, et al. Effect of sterilization on osteoinduction. Comparison of five methods in demineralized rat bone. Acta Orthop Scand. 1988;59(1):34-8.
74. Wang JC, Kanim LE, Nagakawa IS, et al. Dose-dependent toxicity of a commercially available demineralized bone matrix material. Spine (Phila Pa 1976).2001;26(13):1429-35; discussion 1435-6.
75. Peterson B, Whang PG, Iglesias R, et al. Osteoinductivity of commercially available demineralized bone matrix preparations in a spine fusion model. J Bone Joint Surg Am. 2004;86(10):2243-50.
76. Lee YP, Jo M, Luna M, et al. The efficacy of different commercially available demineralized bone matrix substances in an athymic rat model. J Spinal Disord Tech. 2005;18(5):439-44.
77. Becerra J, Andrades JA, Ertl DC, et al. Demineralized bone matrix mediates differentiation of bone marrow stromal cells in vitro: effect of age of cell donor. J Bone Miner Res. 1996;11(11):1703-14.
78. Han B, Tang B, Nimni ME. Quantitative and sensitive in vitro assay for osteoinductive activity of demineralized bone matrix. J Orthop Res. 2003;21(4):648-54.
79. Han B, Yang Z, Nimni M. Effects of moisture and temperature on the osteoinductivity of demineralized bone matrix. J Orthop Res. 2005;23(4):855-61.
80. Bae HW, Zhao L, Kanim LE, et al. Intervariability and intravariability of bone morphogenetic proteins in commercially available demineralized bone matrix products. Spine (Phila Pa 1976). 2006;31(12):1299-306; discussion 1307-8.
81. Schwartz Z, Mellonig JT, Carnes DL Jr, et al. Ability of commercial demineralized freeze-dried bone allograft to induce new bone formation. J Periodontol. 1996;67(9):918-26.
82. Oakes DA, Lee CC, Lieberman JR. An evaluation of human demineralized bone matrices in a rat femoral defect model. Clin Orthop Relat Res. 2003;413:281-90.
83. Choi Y, Oldenburg FP, Sage L, et al. A bridging demineralized bone implant facilitates posterolateral lumbar fusion in New Zealand white rabbits. Spine (Phila Pa 1976). 2007;32(1):36-41.
84. Louis-Ugbo J, Murakami H, Kim HS, et al. Evidence of osteoinduction by Grafton demineralized bone matrix in nonhuman primate spinal fusion. Spine (Phila Pa 1976). 2004;29(4):360-6; discussion Z1.
85. Martin GJ Jr, Boden SD, Titus L, et al. New formulations of demineralized bone matrix as a more effective graft alternative in experimental posterolateral lumbar spine arthrodesis. Spine (Phila Pa 1976). 1999;24(7):637-45.
86. Yee AJ, Bae HW, Friess D, et al. Augmentation of rabbit posterolateral spondylodesis using a novel demineralized bone matrix-hyaluronan putty. Spine (Phila Pa 1976). 2003;28(21):2435-40.
87. Boden SD, Schimandle JH, Hutton WC. 1995 Volvo Award in basic sciences. The use of an osteoinductive growth factor for lumbar spinal fusion. II. Study of dose, carrier, and species. Spine (Phila Pa 1976). 1995;20(24):2633-44.
88. Boden SD, Schimandle JH, Hutton WC. Lumbar intertransverse-process spinal arthrodesis with use of a bovine bone-derived osteoinductive protein. A preliminary report. J Bone Joint Surg Am. 1995;77(9):1404-17.
89. Vaccaro AR, Stubbs HA, Block JE. Demineralized bone matrix composite grafting for posterolateral spinal fusion. Orthopedics. 2007;30(7):567-70.
90. Epstein NE, Epstein JA. SF-36 outcomes and fusion rates after multilevel laminectomies and 1 and 2-level instrumented posterolateral fusions using lamina autograft and demineralized bone matrix. J Spinal Disord Tech. 2007;20(2):139-45.
91. Schizas C, Triantafyllopoulos D, Kosmopoulos V, et al. Posterolateral lumbar spine fusion using a novel demineralized bone matrix: a controlled case pilot study. Arch Orthop Trauma Surg. 2008;128(6):621-5.
92. Price CT, Connolly JF, Carantzas AC, et al. Comparison of bone grafts for posterior spinal fusion in adolescent idiopathic scoliosis Spine (Phila Pa 1976). 2003;28(8):793-8.
93. Thalgott JS, Giuffre JM, Klezl Z, et al. Anterior lumbar interbody fusion with titanium mesh cages, coralline hydroxyapatite, and demineralized bone matrix as part of a circumferential fusion. Spine J. 2002;2(1):63-9.
94. An HS, Simpson JM, Glover JM, et al. Comparison between allograft plus demineralized bone matrix versus auto-graft in anterior cervical fusion. A prospective multicenter study. Spine (Phila Pa 1976). 1995;20(20):2211-6.
95. Bell WH. Resorption rates of bone and bone substitutes. Oral Surg. 1964;17:650-7.
96. Jarcho M. Calcium phosphate ceramics as hard tissue prosthetics. Clin Orthop Relat Res. 1981;157:259-78.
97. Hollinger JO, Brekke J. Role of bone substitutes. Clin Orthop Relat Res. 1996;324:55-65.
98. Liu DM. Influence of porous microarchitecture on the in vitro dissolution and biological behavior of porous CaP ceramics. Mater Sci Forum. 1997;250:183-208.
99. Miyazaki M, Tsumura H, Wang JC, et al. An update on bone substitutes for spinal fusion. Eur Spine J. 2009;18(6):783-99.
100. Gunzburg R, Szpalski M. A highly porous beta tricalcium phosphate/bone marrow graft promotes osteoinductivity in a rat subcutaneous model [poster]. Presented at 3rd Annual Meeting of the Spine Society of Europe; September 4-8, 2001; Gotenburg, Sweden.
101. Ohgushi H, Caplan AI. Stem cell technology and bioceramics: from cell to gene engineering. J Biomed Mater Res. 1999;48(6):913-27.
102. Loty C, Sautier JM, Boulekbache H, et al. In vitro bone formation on a bone-like apatite layer prepared by a biomimetic process on a bioactive glass-ceramic. J Biomed Mater Res. 2000;49(4):423-34.
103. Loty C, Sautier JM, Loty S, et al. The biomimetics of bone: engineered glass-ceramics a paradigm in vitro biomineralization studies. Connect Tissue Res. 2003;43(2-3):524-8.
104. Hsu EL, Ghodasra JH, Ashtekar A, et al. A comparative evaluation of factors influencing osteoinductivity among scaffolds designed for bone regeneration. Tissue Engineering Part A. 2013;19(15-16):1764-72.
105. Hadjipavlou AG, Simmons JW, Tzermiadianos MN, et al. Plaster of Paris as bone substitute in spinal surgery. Eur Spine J. 2001;10(Suppl 2):S189-96.

106. Hile DD, Kandziora F, Lewandrowski KU, et al. A poly (propylene glycol-co-fumaric acid) based bone graft extender for lumbar spinal fusion: in vivo assessment in a rabbit model. Eur Spine J. 2006;15(6):936-43.
107. Kaito T, Mukai Y, Nishikawa M, et al. Dual hydroxyapatite composite with porous and solid parts: experimental study using canine lumbar interbody fusion model. J Biomed Mater Res B Appl Biomater. 2006;78:378-84.
108. Lindfors NC, Tallroth K, Aho AJ. Bioactive glass as bone-graft substitute for posterior spinal fusion in rabbit. J Biomed Mater Res. 2002;63(2):237-44.
109. Motomiya M, Ito M, Takahata M, et al. Effect of hydroxyapatite porous characteristics on healing outcomes in rabbit posterolateral spinal fusion model. Eur Spine J. 2007;16(12):2215-24.
110. Ragni P, Lindholm TS. Interaction of allogeneic demineralized bone matrix and porous hydroxyapatite bioceramics in lumbar interbody fusion in rabbits. Clin Orthop Relat Res. 1991;272:292-9.
111. Miller CP, Jegede K, Essig D, et al. The efficacies of 2 ceramic bone graft extenders for promoting spinal fusion in a rabbit bone paucity model. Spine (Phila Pa 1976). 2012;37(8):642-7.
112. Walsh WR, Vizesi F, Cornwall GB, et al. Posterolateral spinal fusion in a rabbit model using a collagen-mineral composite bone graft substitute. Eur Spine J. 2009;18(11):1610-20.
113. Epstein NE. A preliminary study of the efficacy of Beta Tricalcium Phosphate as a bone expander for instrumented posterolateral lumbar fusions. J Spinal Disord Tech. 2006;19(6):424-9.
114. Dai LY, Jiang LS. Single-level instrumented posterolateral fusion of lumbar spine with beta-tricalcium phosphate versus autograft: a prospective, randomized study with 3-year follow-up. Spine (Phila Pa 1976). 2008;33(12):1299-304.
115. Ransford AO, Morley T, Edgar MA, et al. Synthetic porous ceramic compared with autograft in scoliosis surgery. A prospective, randomized study of 341 patients. J Bone Joint Surg Br. 1998;80(1):13-8.
116. Thalgott JS, Fritts K, Giuffre JM, et al. Anterior interbody fusion of the cervical spine with coralline hydroxyapatite. Spine. 1999;24(13):1295-9.
117. Thalgott JS, Klezl Z, Timlin M, et al. Anterior lumbar interbody fusion with processed sea coral (coralline hydroxyapatite) as part of a circumferential fusion. Spine (Phila Pa 1976). 2002;27(24:E518-25; discussion E526-7.
118. Whang PG LJ. Clinical issues in the development of cellular systems for use as bone graft substitutes. In: Laurencin C (Ed). Bone Graft Substitutes: A Multidisciplinary Approach. West Conshohocken: American Society for Testing and Materials International; 2003. pp. 142-64.
119. Gottfried ON, Dailey A. Mesenchymal stem cell and gene therapies for spinal fusion. Neurosurgery. 2008;63(3):380-92.
120. Aggarwal S, Pittenger MF. Human mesenchymal stem cells modulate allogeneic immune cell responses. Blood. 2005;105(4):1815-22.
121. Ohgushi H, Dohi Y, Tamai S, et al. Osteogenic differentiation of marrow stromal stem cells in porous hydroxyapatite ceramics. J Biomed Mater Res. 1993;27(11):1401-7.
122. Matsushima A, Kotobuki N, Tadokoro M, et al. In vivo osteogenic capability of human mesenchymal cells cultured on hydroxyapatite and on beta-tricalcium phosphate. Artif Organs. 2009;33(6):474-8.
123. Park SH, Tofighi A, Wang X, et al. Calcium phosphate combination biomaterials as human mesenchymal stem cell delivery vehicles for bone repair. J Biomed Mater Res B Appl Biomater. 2011;97(2):235-44.
124. Mauney JR, Jaquiery C, Volloch V, et al. In vitro and in vivo evaluation of differentially demineralized cancellous bone scaffolds combined with human bone marrow stromal cells for tissue engineering. Biomaterials. 2005;26(16):3173-85.
125. Liu G, Sun J, Li Y, et al. Evaluation of partially demineralized osteoporotic cancellous bone matrix combined with human bone marrow stromal cells for tissue engineering: an in vitro and in vivo study. Calcif Tissue Int. 2008;83(3):176-85.
126. Arca T, Proffitt J, Genever P. Generating 3D tissue constructs with mesenchymal stem cells and a cancellous bone graft for orthopaedic applications. Biomed Mater. 2011;6(2):025006.
127. Tsiridis E, Ali Z, Bhalla A, et al. In vitro and in vivo optimization of impaction allografting by demineralization and addition of rh-OP-1. J Orthop Res. 2007;25(11):1425-37.
128. Tiedeman JJ, Garvin KL, Kile TA, et al. The role of a composite, demineralized bone matrix and bone marrow in the treatment of osseous defects. Orthopedics. 1995;18(12):1153-8.
129. Ohgushi H, Goldberg VM, Caplan AI. Repair of bone defects with marrow cells and porous ceramic. Experiments in rats. Acta Orthop Scand. 1989;60(3):334-9.
130. Connolly JF, Guse R, Tiedeman J, et al. Autologous marrow injection as a substitute for operative grafting of tibial nonunions. Clin Orthop Relat Res. 1991;266:259-70.
131. McLain RF, Fleming JE, Boehm CA, et al. Aspiration of osteoprogenitor cells for augmenting spinal fusion: comparison of progenitor cell concentrations from the vertebral body and iliac crest. J Bone Joint Surg Am. 2005;87(12):2655-61.
132. Hernigou P, Poignard A, Beaujean F, et al. Percutaneous autologous bone marrow grafting for nonunions. Influence of the number and concentration of progenitor cells. J Bone Joint Surg Am. 2005;87(7):1430-7.
133. Muschler GF, Boehm C, Easley K. Aspiration to obtain osteoblast progenitor cells from human bone marrow: the influence of aspiration volume. J Bone Joint Surg Am. 1997;79(11):1699-709.
134. Minamide A, Yoshida M, Kawakami M, et al. The use of cultured bone marrow cells in type I collagen gel and porous hydroxyapatite for posterolateral lumbar spine fusion. Spine (Phila Pa 1976). 2005;30(10):1134-8.
135. Romih M, Delécrin J, Heymann D, et al. The vertebral interbody grafting site's low concentration in osteogenic progenitors can greatly benefit from addition of iliac crest bone marrow. Eur Spine J. 2005;14(7):645-8.
136. Stenderup K, Justesen J, Eriksen EF, et al. Number and proliferative capacity of osteogenic stem cells are maintained during aging and in patients with osteoporosis. J Bone Miner Res. 2001;16(6):1120-9.
137. Nishida S, Endo N, Yamagiwa H, et al. Number of osteoprogenitor cells in human bone marrow markedly decreases after skeletal maturation. J Bone Miner Metab. 1999;17(3):171-7.

138. Huang JW, Lin SS, Chen LH, et al. The use of fluorescence-labeled mesenchymal stem cells in poly (lactide-co-glycolide)/hydroxyapatite/collagen hybrid graft as a bone substitute for posterolateral spinal fusion. J Trauma. 2011;70(6):1495-502.
139. Kimelman-Bleich N, Pelled G, Sheyn D, et al. The use of a synthetic oxygen carrier-enriched hydrogel to enhance mesenchymal stem cell-based bone formation in vivo. Biomaterials. 2009;30(27):4639-48.
140. Neen D, Noyes D, Shaw M, et al. Healos and bone marrow aspirate used for lumbar spine fusion: a case controlled study comparing healos with autograft. Spine (Phila Pa 1976). 2006;31(18):E636-40.
141. Gan Y, Dai K, Zhang P, et al. The clinical use of enriched bone marrow stem cells combined with porous beta-tricalcium phosphate in posterior spinal fusion. Biomaterials. 2008;29(29):3973-82.
142. Ammerman JM, Libricz J, Ammerman MD. The role of Osteocel Plus as a fusion substrate in minimally invasive instrumented transforaminal lumbar interbody fusion. Clin Neurol Neurosurg. 2013;115(7):991-4.
143. Lee JH, Chang BS, Jeung UO, et al. The first clinical trial of beta-calcium pyrophosphate as a novel bone graft extender in instrumented posterolateral lumbar fusion. Clin Orthop Surg. 2011;3(3):238-44.
144. Kerr EJ 3rd, Jawahar A, Wooten T, et al. The use of osteo-conductive stem-cells allograft in lumbar interbody fusion procedures: an alternative to recombinant human bone morphogenetic protein. J Surg Orthop Adv. 2011;20(3):193-7.
145. Steinert AF, Rackwitz L, Gilbert F, et al. Concise review: the clinical application of mesenchymal stem cells for musculoskeletal regeneration: current status and perspectives. Stem Cells Transl Med. 2012;1(3):237-47.
146. Urist MR. Bone: formation by autoinduction. Science. 1965;150(3698):893-9.
147. Wozney JM, Rosen V. Bone morphogenetic protein and bone morphogenetic protein gene family in bone formation and repair. Clin Orthop Relat Res. 1998;346:26-37.
148. Hoffmann A, Gross G. BMP signaling pathways in cartilage and bone formation. Crit Rev Eukaryot Gene Expr. 2001;11(1-3):23-45.
149. Shen B, Wei A, Whittaker S, et al. The role of BMP-7 in chondrogenic and osteogenic differentiation of human bone marrow multipotent mesenchymal stromal cells in vitro. J Cell Biochem. 2010;109(2):406-16.
150. Lane JM. Bone morphogenic protein science and studies. J Orthop Trauma. 2005;19(10 suppl):S17-22.
151. Huang Z, Ren PG, Ma T, et al. Modulating osteogenesis of mesenchymal stem cells by modifying growth factor availability. Cytokine. 2010;51(3):305-10.
152. Sandhu HS, Toth JM, Diwan AD, et al. Histologic evaluation of the efficacy of rhBMP-2 compared with autograft bone in sheep spinal anterior interbody fusion. Spine (Phila Pa 1976). 2002;27(6):567-75.
153. Boden SD, Martin GJ Jr, Horton WC, et al. Laparoscopic anterior spinal arthrodesis with rhBMP-2 in a titanium interbody threaded cage. J Spinal Disord. 1998;11(2):95-101.
154. Boden SD, Zdeblick TA, Sandhu HS, et al. The use of rhBMP-2 in interbody fusion cages. Definitive evidence of osteoinduction in humans: a preliminary report. Spine (Phila Pa 1976). 2000;25(3):376-81.
155. Schimandle JH, Boden SD, Hutton WC. Experimental spinal fusion with recombinant human bone morphogenetic protein-2. Spine (Phila Pa 1976). 1995;20(12):1326-37.
156. Fischgrund JS, James SB, Chabot MC, et al. Augmentation of autograft using rhBMP-2 and different carrier media in the canine spinal fusion model. J Spinal Disord. 1997;10(6):467-72.
157. Martin GJ, Boden SD, Marone MA, et al. Posterolateral intertransverse process spinal arthrodesis with rhBMP-2 in a non-human primate: important lessons learned regarding dose, carrier and safety. J Spinal Disord. 1999;12(3):179-86.
158. Suh DY, Boden SD, Louis-Ugbo J, et al. Delivery of recombinant human bone morphogenetic protein-2 using a compression resistant matrix in posterolateral lumbar spine fusion in the rabbit and the non-human primate. Spine (Phila Pa 1976). 2002;27(4):353-60.
159. Burkus JK, Gornet MF, Dickman CA, et al. Anterior lumbar interbody fusion using rhBMP-2 with tapered interbody cages. J Spinal Disord Tech. 2002;15(5):337-49.
160. Ong KL, Villarraga ML, Lau E, et al. Off-label use of bone morphogenetic proteins in the United States using administrative data. Spine (Phila Pa 1976). 2010;35(19):1794-800.
161. Boden SD, Kang J, Sandhu H, et al. Use of recombinant human bone morphogenetic protein-2 to achieve posterolateral lumbar spine fusion in humans: a prospective, randomized clinical pilot trial: 2002 Volvo Award in clinical studies. Spine (Phila Pa 1976). 2002;27(23):2662-73.
162. Dawson E Bae HW, Burkus JK, et al. Recombinant human bone morphogenetic protein-2 on an absorbable collagen sponge with an osteoconductive bulking agent in posterolateral arthrodesis with instrumentation. A prospective randomized trial. J Bone Joint Surg Am. 2009;91(7):1604-13.
163. Mummaneni PV, Pan J, Haid RW, et al. Contribution of recombinant human bone morphogenetic protein-2 to the rapid creation of interbody fusion when used in transforaminal lumbar interbody fusion: a preliminary report. Invited submission from the Joint Section Meeting on Disorders of the Spine and Peripheral Nerves, March 2004. J Neurosurg Spine. 2004;1(1):19-23.
164. Mroz TE, Wang JC, Hashimoto R, et al. Complications related to osteobiologics use in spine surgery: a systematic review. Spine (Phila Pa 1976). 2010;35(9 Suppl):S86-104.
165. Joseph V, Rampersaud YR. Heterotopic bone formation with the use of rhBMP2 in posterior minimal access interbody fusion: a CT analysis. Spine (Phila Pa 1976). 2007;32(25):2885-90.
166. Meisel HJ, Schnoring M, Hohaus C, et al. Posterior lumbar interbody fusion using rhBMP-2. Eur Spine J. 2008;17(12):1735-44.
167. McClellan JW, Mulconrey DS, Forbes RJ, et al. Vertebral bone resorption after transforaminal lumbar interbody fusion with bone morphogenetic protein (rhBMP-2). J Spinal Disord Tech. 2006;19(7):483-6.
168. Mindea SA, Shih P, Song JK. Recombinant human bone morphogenetic protein-2-induced radiculitis in elective

CHAPTER 19

minimally invasive transforaminal lumbar interbody fusions: a series review. Spine (Phila Pa 1976). 2009;34(14):1480-4; discussion 1485.
169. Lubelski D, Abdullah KG, Steinmetz MP, et al. Adverse events with the use of rhBMP-2 in thoracolumbar and lumbar spine fusions: a nine year institutional analysis. J Spinal Disord Tech. 2015;28(5):E277-83.
170. Vaidya R. Transforaminal interbody fusion and the "off label" use of recombinant human bone morphogenetic protein-2. Spine J. 2009;9(8):667-9.
171. Rihn JA, Patel R, Makda J, et al. Complications associated with single-level transforaminal lumbar interbody fusion. Spine J. 2009;9(8):623-9.
172. Baskin DS, Ryan P, Sonntag V, et al. A prospective, randomized, controlled cervical fusion study using recombinant human bone morphogenetic protein-2 with the CORNERSTONE-SR allograft ring and the ATLANTIS anterior cervical plate. Spine (Phila Pa 1976). 2003;28(12):1219-24; discussion 1225.
173. Boakye M, Mummaneni PV, Garrett M, et al. Anterior cervical discectomy and fusion involving a polyetheretherketone spacer and bone morphogenetic protein. J Neurosurg Spine. 2005;2(5):521-5.
174. Lanman TH, Hopkins TJ. Early findings in a pilot study of anterior cervical interbody fusion in which recombinant human bone morphogenetic protein-2 was used with poly (L-lactide-co-D,L-lactide) bioabsorbable implants. Neurosurg Focus. 2004;16(3):E6.
175. Shields LB, Raque GH, Glassman SD, et al. Adverse effects associated with high-dose recombinant human bone morphogenetic protein-2 use in anterior cervical spine fusion. Spine (Phila Pa 1976). 2006;31(5):542-7.
176. Smucker JD, Rhee JM, Singh K, et al. Increased swelling complications associated with off-label usage of rhBMP-2 in the anterior cervical spine. Spine (Phila Pa 1976). 2006;31(24):2813-9.
177. Vaidya R, Carp J, Sethi A, et al. Complications of anterior cervical discectomy and fusion using recombinant human bone morphogenetic protein-2. Eur Spine J. 2007;16(8):1257-65.
178. Perri B, Cooper M, Lauryssen C, et al. Adverse swelling associated with use of rh-BMP-2 in anterior cervical discectomy and fusion: a case study. Spine J. 2007;7(2):235-9.
179. Carragee EJ, Hurwitz EL, Weiner BK. A critical review of recombinant human bone morphogenetic protein-2 trials in spinal surgery: emerging safety concerns and lessons learned. Spine J. 2011;11(6):471-91.
180. Hamilton DK, Smith JS, Reames DL, et al. Safety, efficacy, and dosing of recombinant human bone morphogenetic protein-2 for posterior cervical and cervicothoracic instrumented fusion with a minimum 2-year follow-up. Neurosurgery. 2011;69(1):103-11; discussion 111.
181. Hiremath GK, Steinmetz MP, Krishnaney AA. Is it safe to use recombinant human bone morphogenetic protein in posterior cervical fusion? Spine (Phila Pa 1976). 2009;34(9):885-9.
182. Carragee EJ, Mitsunaga KA, Hurwitz EL, et al. Retrograde ejaculation after anterior lumbar interbody fusion using rhBMP-2: a cohort controlled study. Spine J. 2011;11(6):511-6.
183. Tepper G, Rabbani R, Yousefzadeh M, et al. Quantitative assessment of retrograde ejaculation using semen analysis, comparison with a standardized qualitative questionnaire, and investigating the impact of rhBMP-2. Spine (Phila Pa 1976). 2013;38(10):841-5.
184. Kleeff J, Maruyama H, Ishiwata T, et al. Bone morphogenetic protein 2 exerts diverse effects on cell growth in vitro and is expressed in human pancreatic cancer in vivo. Gastroenterology. 1999;116(5):1202-16.
185. Laitinen M, Jortikka L, Halttunen T, et al. Measurement of total and local bone morphogenetic protein concentration in bone tumours. Int Orthop. 1997;21(3):188-93.
186. Yoshikawa H, Rettig WJ, Lane JM, et al. Immunohistochemical detection of bone morphogenetic proteins in bone and soft-tissue sarcomas. Cancer. 1994;74(3):842-7.
187. Thawani JP, Wang AC, Than KD, et al. Bone morphogenetic proteins and cancer: review of the literature. Neurosurgery. 2010;66(2):233-46.
188. Carragee EJ, Chu G, Rohatgi R, et al. Cancer risk after use of recombinant bone morphogenetic protein-2 for spinal arthrodesis. J Bone Joint Surg Am. 2013;95(17):1537-45.
189. Korovessis P, Koureas G, Zacharatos S, et al. Correlative radiological, self-assessment and clinical analysis of evolution in instrumented dorsal and lateral fusion for degenerative lumbar spine disease. Autograft versus coralline hydroxyapatite. Eur Spine J. 2005;14(7):630-8.

CHAPTER 20 Imaging of the Spine: Types, Strengths and Limitations

Todd M Emch, Michael T Modic

INTRODUCTION

There are many avenues through which patient can enter the care of a spine surgeon from a routine office visit with or without previous imaging to emergent consultation for acute neurologic decline. At any point along this spectrum, decisions regarding appropriate imaging utilization will arise. The role of imaging is to aid diagnostic and therapeutic thinking, not as an end on to itself. To fully appreciate the impact of imaging on this thinking, the prevalence and natural history of altered morphology characterized by imaging is a critical underlying data point. Our intent in what follows is to review options and situational value within a clinical context.

Many options exist for spine imaging each with its own strengths and limitations. This chapter discusses radiography, computed tomography (CT) alone and in conjunction with myelography, and magnetic resonance (MR) imaging. These modalities differ in terms of what they can evaluate and when they should be ideally obtained. Following the discussion of the modalities, their use in specific conditions will be discussed in regards to trauma, degenerative disk disease, the postoperative spine, and in reference to the commonly used anatomic compartments of the spine (extradural including marrow imaging, intradural extramedullary, and intramedullary).

While this chapter clearly cannot discuss every pathologic condition potentially affecting the spine, emphasis is placed on the development of a solid basis for appropriately obtaining imaging studies (or when imaging is not necessary) and also an approach for systematically interpreting the resultant images and arriving at a differential diagnosis that will optimally guide treatment and by extension patient outcome.

RADIOGRAPHY

X-rays were discovered by Wilhelm Röentgen in the late 1800's leading to radiography of the spine with initially only frontal views of the spine available.[1] 30 years later the lateral view was introduced[2] with most indications initially for fracture or foreign body localization. Despite being the first modality in medical imaging, radiography of the spine remains useful in certain cases and is widely used although it has been superseded by CT and MR imaging in many instances. Radiography is readily available, quick to obtain, and relatively inexpensive when compared with advanced cross-sectional imaging. However, while frequently used, its impact rarely supersedes clinical judgment. For instance, conventional radiographs are often ordered on patients when they initially present with symptoms referable to the spine, regardless of the severity of the symptoms or pretest probability for an abnormality. The actual impact on therapeutic thinking has never been well measured. Significant abnormalities detected by conventional radiographs, e.g. fractures, malalignment, and osseous destruction require more advanced imaging prior to diagnosis and management and "normal" radiographs remain insensitive to more common abnormalities such as disk herniation, stenosis, or early metastatic disease. An argument can be made that their value is limited (perhaps to acute significant trauma– however evidence suggests that CT may be the preferred modality) and their deployment should be more judicious.

Technical Issues and Image Evaluation

Radiographs are obtained by placing the patient between the X-ray source and either film or an electronic detector system when digital radiography is being used. The resultant radiograph is the result of the X-ray beam being attenuated to different degrees by the osseous and soft tissue structures of the patient. The duration of the X-ray pulse is less than 1 second however if there is concurrent motion of the patient or difficulty in positioning the patient, the diagnostic quality of the examination will be diminished.[3]

A routine examination of the cervical spine includes anterior-posterior (AP, referring to direction in which the X-ray beam is directed), lateral, and open-mouth odontoid views. To further evaluate the dens, an AP or posterior-anterior view (PA) can be obtained with the patient in extension. The relationship of C7 and T1 should be visualized on the lateral view and if not a swimmer's view should be obtained. Neural foramen in the cervical spine are obliquely oriented by approximately 45°in relation to midline; for evaluation of right neural foramen the patient is imaged with the head turned towards the left or to the right for left neural foramen visualization or alternatively the X-ray tube can be angled in an immobilized patient. In addition to routine views, flexion-extension views can be obtained to evaluate for abnormal motion.

When evaluating any imaging examination, it is paramount to have a systematic routine of viewing images in order to properly identify both expected and unexpected abnormalities. In general, spine images should have the following items evaluated: vertebral body height and alignment, posterior elements, the craniocervical junction, disk spaces, and adjacent soft tissues. The lateral view is used to evaluate vertebral body height and alignment and can clearly visualize the dens on the cervical spine examination. Applicable also to CT and MR imaging, the anterior and posterior margins of the vertebral bodies (the anterior and posterior vertebral lines) should be well aligned as should the spinolaminar junction line which is formed by the junction of the lamina and spinous processes (Fig. 1). The facet joints should be well aligned with no abnormal joint widening. Evaluation of distance between spinous processes should be of uniform distance; widening between two spinous processes of a distance greater than 1.5 times an adjacent level is abnormal. Distance between the dens and anterior arch of C1 should be less than or equal to 3 mm in adults or 5 mm in the pediatric population; if widened, there should be concern for transverse ligament injury (Figs. 2A and B). On the frontal or AP view once again the facets and spinous processes should be normally aligned and the distance between the lateral masses of C1 should be uniformly spaced in relation to the dens. Oblique views demonstrate neural foramen and possible encroachment by uncinate joint hypertrophy.[4,5] Prevertebral soft tissue should be less than 7 mm at level of C2 and less than 22 mm at level of C6.[5]

Similar views are obtained for the thoracic and lumbar spine with the thoracic spine demonstrating a normal kyphosis secondary to minimal normal anterior vertebral body wedging and the lumbar spine should have a slight lordosis. Spondylolisthesis is commonly graded based on the degree of anterior displacement relative to the

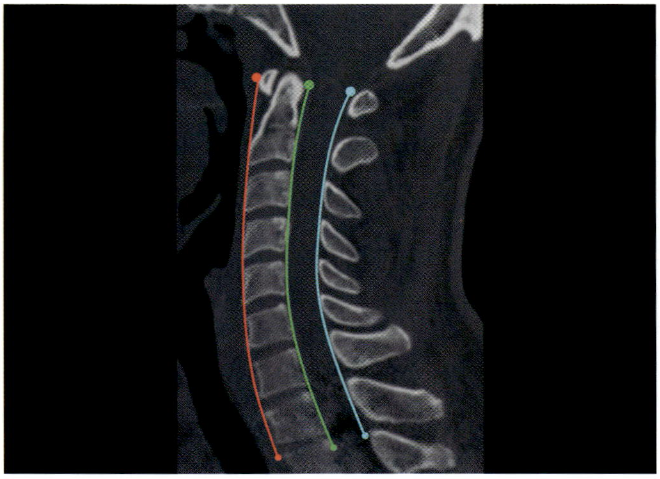

Fig. 1: Sagittal CT image demonstrating the anterior vertebral line (red), posterior vertebral line (green), and spinolaminar junction line (blue).

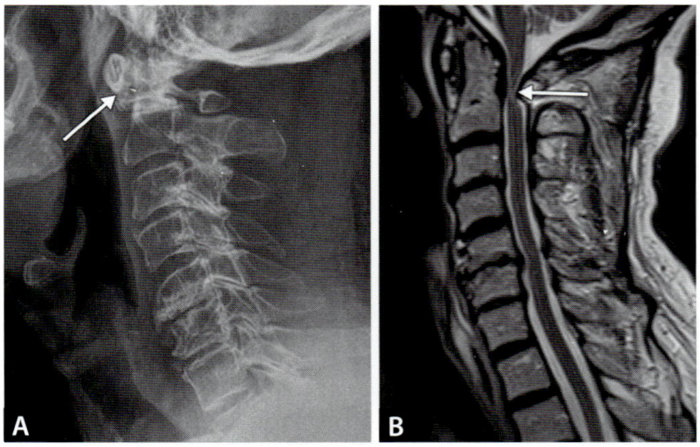

Figs. 2A and B: Lateral radiograph of the cervical spine. (A) Shows increased distance between the dens and anterior arch of C1, white arrow, while sagittal T2 weighted image of the cervical spine; (B) Shows severe narrowing of the spinal canal with cord flattening and edema, white arrow.

adjacent vertebral bodies with grade I displaced up to 25%, grade II 25–50%, grade III 50–75%, and grade IV 75–100%.[6] In addition to findings described in the cervical spine evaluation, pedicles are oriented anterior to posterior and should be evaluated both on the frontal and lateral views. Oblique views of the lumbar spine allow better visualization of the pars interarticularis. Soft tissues of the thorax, abdomen, and pelvis are also partially visualized depending on the region of spine imaged.[5,7]

COMPUTED TOMOGRAPHY

CT imaging of the spine was first described in the mid 1970's and similar to MR imaging has advanced considerably since that time.[8] Currently multidetector CT units are in widespread use which enables faster imaging and thinner sections. With resultant "isotropic voxels", images can be reconstructed into sagittal and coronal reconstructions as well as manipulated in volume rendered technique on postprocessing workstations (Figs. 3A to D).[3] Algorithms are applied to the images which can accentuate osseous structures or soft tissues (Figs. 4A and B). Windowing images can also change the focus from soft tissues to osseous structures. CT imaging allows exquisite bony detail and can also evaluate adjacent soft tissues.

Technical Issues and Image Evaluation

CT imaging is widely available and relatively quick to perform however there are limitations. CT imaging can be suboptimal with the presence of metallic objects, when there is difficulty in positioning the patient, or if there is motion during the image acquisition. CT uses ionizing radiation which should be considered in the pediatric or pregnant patients; many CT manufacturers employ dose reduction protocols however the decision to image should always be on a risk versus benefit basis. Patient size and/or weight can preclude patients from being imaged secondary to gantry diameter and table weight limits. Most CT scanners are able to accommodate patient weights of up to 450 lbs. and have gantry apertures of 70 cm[9] but will differ amongst CT manufacturers.

Exact protocols for spine imaging using CT will vary depending on institution. Following acquisition of the scout image, axial images of the cervical spine are obtained from basiocciput to level of at least T1, of the thoracic spine from C7 through L1, and of the lumbar spine from T12 through S1. It is important for there to be standardization of the reference level for counting vertebral body levels to avoid confusion in cases where there is an intervention. At the authors' institution, the counting reference for the

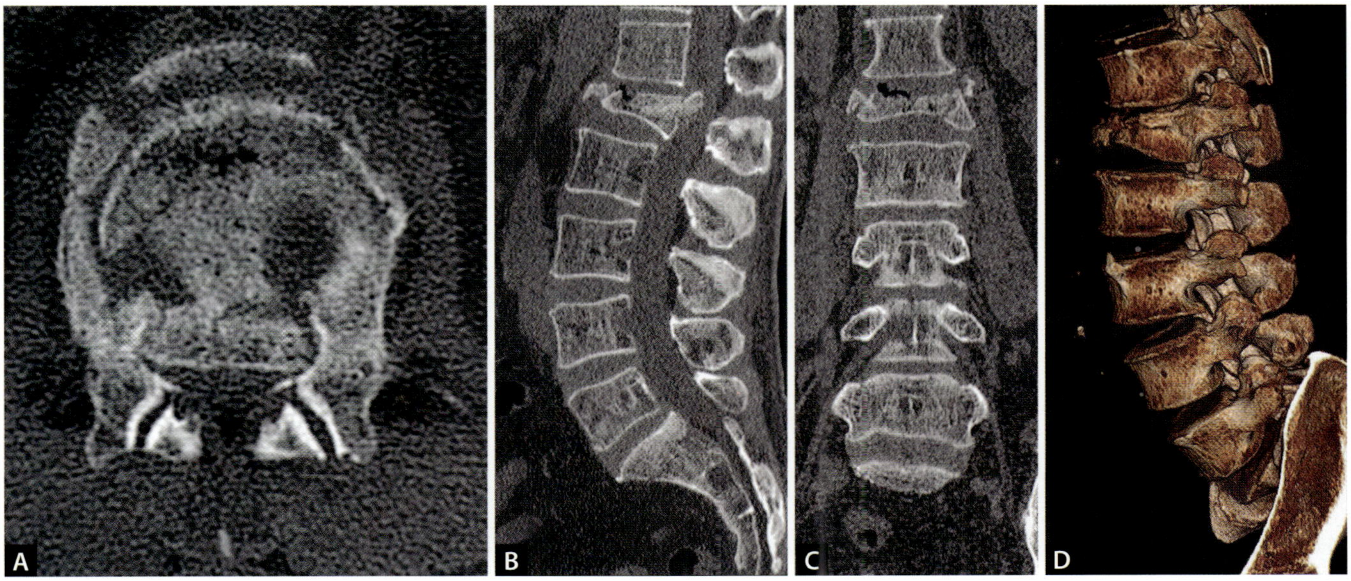

Figs. 3A to D: (A) Axial; (B) Sagittal; (C) Coronal and; (D) Volume rendered technique, of the lumbar spine demonstrates severe compression fracture deformity with retropulsed fragments from L1 vertebral body, demonstrating the multiplanar ability of CT imaging.

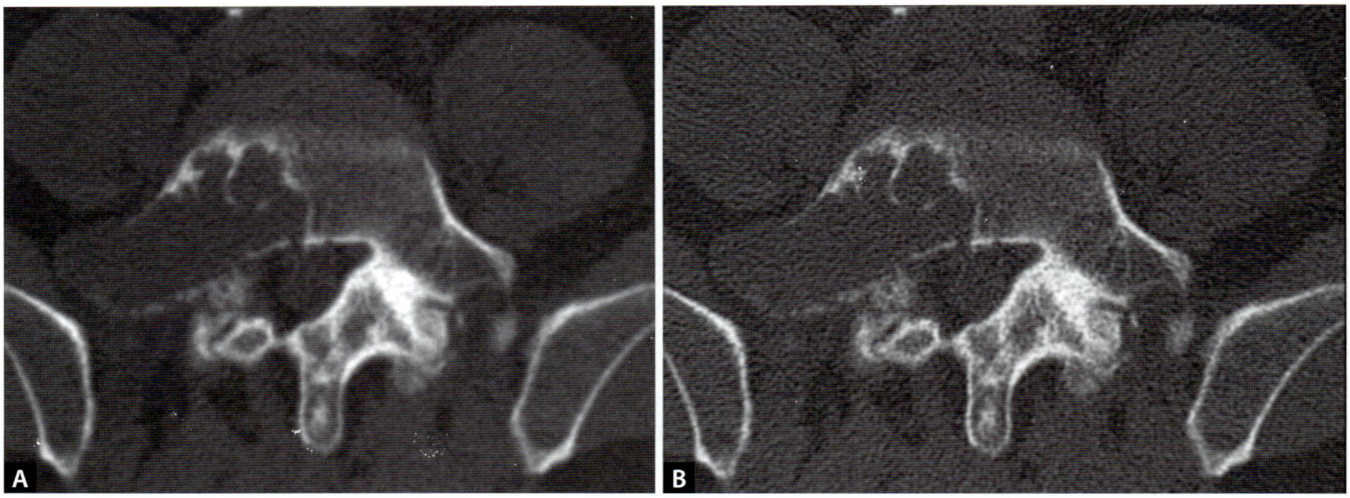

Figs. 4A and B: (A) Processed with a B40 algorithm, accentuates soft tissues; (B) processed with a B70 algorithm, accentuates the osseous structures. Note that both images have the same window width (1800) and level (450). Comparing examinations may be difficult if they are processed with different algorithms.

cervical spine is the craniocervical junction and for the thoracic and lumbar spine the counting reference is the lumbosacral junction which is included on the scout view. Axial images can be reconstructed into various thicknesses, typically 0.6 mm for sagittal and coronal reconstructions and 2–3 mm images for viewing in the axial plane. Bone, soft tissue, or intermediate algorithms can also be applied to the images which can accentuate either bone or soft tissue detail.

In addition to routine spine imaging, tailored protocols may be employed to accentuate a change in spinal alignment or imaging the spine following the administration of exogenous contrast. Dynamic imaging of the cervical spine is typically used for the evaluation of atlantoaxial rotatory subluxation. The upper cervical spine is imaged with the patient in a neutral position, and then with the head turned to either side (Figs. 5A to C).[10] Performing CT imaging of the spine during or after the vascular administration of iodinated contrast may be useful when there is concern for infection or during CT angiography. As with other imaging studies which employ iodinated contrast, if possible, patients should be NPO and renal function and hydration status should be assessed prior to contrast administration. Without risk factors, at the authors' institution a patient with an estimated glomerular filtration rate (eGFR) > 60 requires no intervention prior to contrast administration while those with an eGFR of 30–59 should receive hydration orally. An eGFR of less than 30 should receive intravenous hydration or if additional risk factors are present. Additionally, patients who are allergic to iodinated contrast agents must be premedicated prior to contrast administration. An example of a premedication regimen for patients who are allergic to iodinated contrast includes Prednisone 50 mg orally taken 13, 7, and 1 hour prior to the procedure combined with 50 mg orally of Benadryl. The exact recommendations for patients with impaired renal function and allergy will vary by institution.[11,12]

CT angiography (CTA) can be obtained to evaluate the vasculature of the neck including common carotid arteries, internal carotid arteries, and vertebral arteries for a wide variety of indications including surgical planning when there is vascular encasement by neoplasm or when there is concern for vessel dissection or injury in the setting of trauma (Figs. 6A and B). CTA imaging requires large bore intravenous access, ideally an 18 g IV in the antecubital fossa and precise contrast bolus timing for a diagnostic examination.

The standardized logical assessment of alignment and integrity remains common to all modalities but is complimented in CT by the capability of leveraging attenuation differences between soft tissues and bone (e.g. herniated disks) as well as the skull base and craniocervical junction. The multiplanar ability of both CT and MR imaging allows reformatting into sagittal and coronal planes and allows measuring of skull base angles for evaluation of the craniocervical junction (Figs. 7A and B).[13]

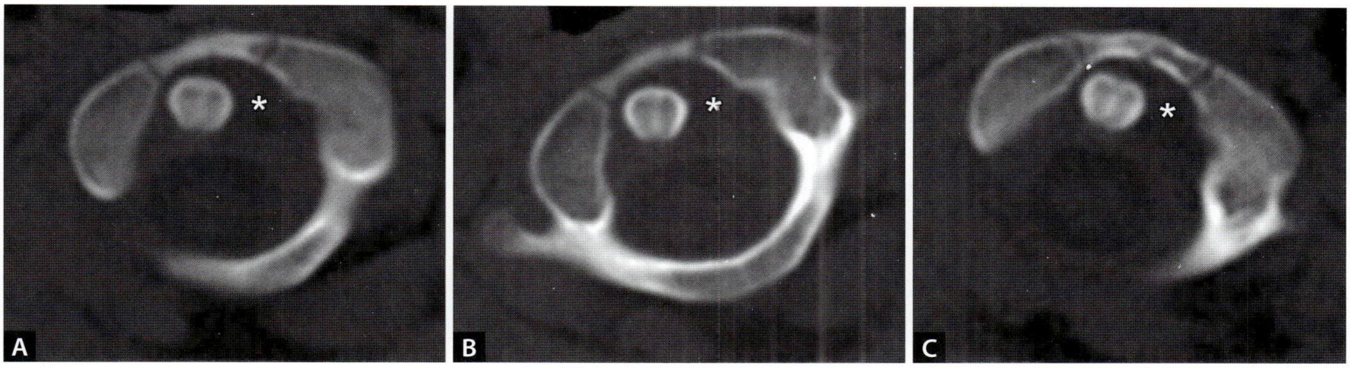

Figs. 5A to C: CT images at level of C1–C2 with the patient (A) Neutrally positioned; (B) Positioned with head turned to the right; and (C) positioned with head turned to the left. All three positions demonstrate persistent rotation of C1 to the right, asterisk, that does not change with positioning.

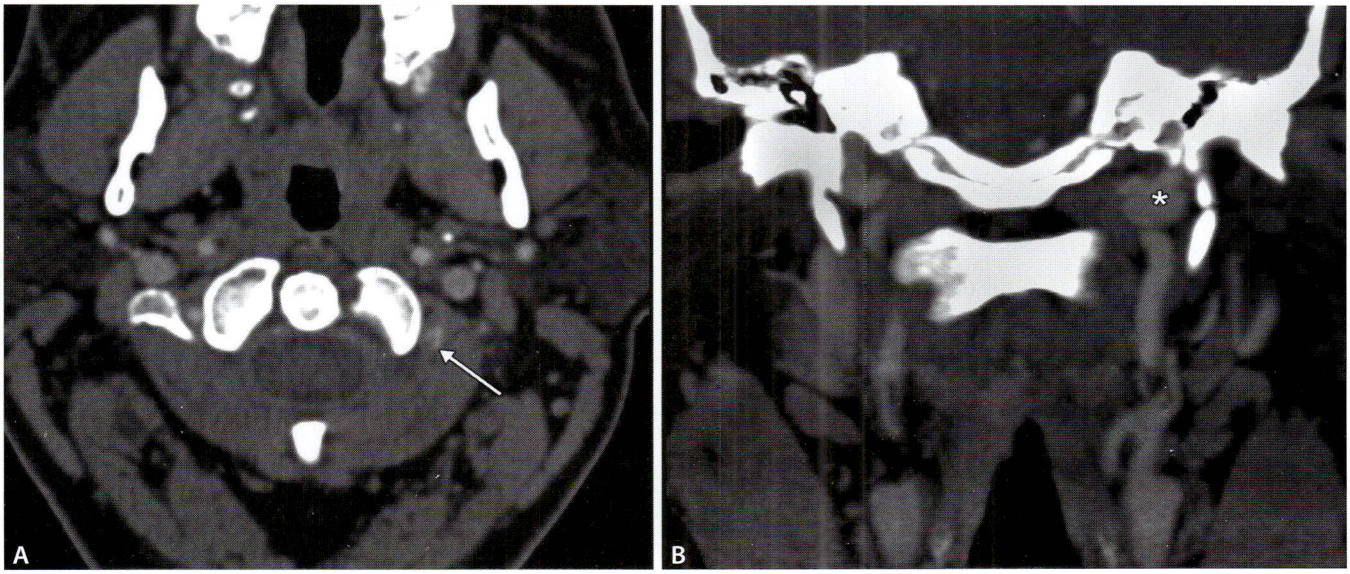

Figs. 6A and B: (A) Axial source CTA image demonstrates focal dissection flap in the distal cervical vertebral artery, white arrow. Coronal reconstruction, (B) shows a large pseudoaneurysm of the distal left cervical internal carotid artery, asterisk, in the same patient who sustained a fall.

MYELOGRAPHY

CT imaging and radiographs alone do not permit direct visualization of the spinal cord, and it is only with the introduction of exogenous intrathecal contrast that the contour of the cord and nerve roots can be visualized. Air was used to localized spinal tumors by Jacobaeus in 1921[14] with many additional contrast agents introduced over time all with differing levels of toxicity ranging from headaches, seizures, arachnoiditis to development of secondary neoplasm.[15-21]

Currently iohexol and iopamidol are available water-soluble nonionic contrast agents associated with significantly less toxicity.[22,23] Adverse reactions with current contrast agents include headache, nausea, vomiting, or pain.[24] Seizure as an adverse reaction are felt to be quite rare with reports largely anecdotal.[25]

Technical Issues and Ordering Considerations

Currently, traditional film myelography has for the most part been replaced by MR and CT. The most common indications for intrathecal contrast in conjunction with CT imaging (CT myelography) include contraindications to MR imaging or when there is beam-hardening artifact on CT from metallic hardware or metallic foreign body.

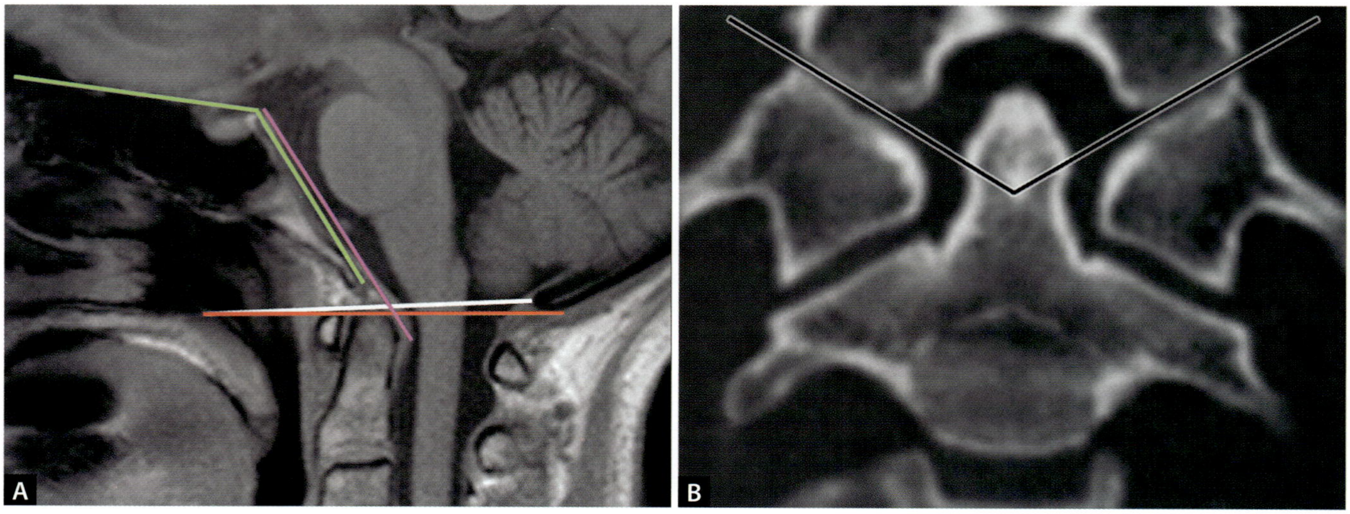

Figs. 7A and B: (A) Sagittal T1-weighted image demonstrating the Welcher basal angle (green line) normally <140°, if widened it represents platybasia. The Wackenheim line (purple line) should lie just posterior to the tip of the dens. The anterior arch of C1 should be below the Chamberlain line (white line) and the McGregor line (red line). The tip of the dens may project up to 5 mm above these lines; (B) Coronal CT shows the atlanto-occipital joint angle which on average should be 125°.

There are many factors to take into account before a myelogram can be performed. Informed consent must be obtained prior to performance of myelography with patients being NPO and having a driver upon discharge if done on an outpatient basis. The procedure is performed under fluoroscopy with the patient prone with access to the subarachnoid space typically achieved at L2–3 or L3–4 or alternatively from a lateral approach at C1–C2. Under local anesthesia, a spinal needle is advanced under intermittent fluoroscopic guidance into the subarachnoid space and then contrast is injected to a maximal dose of 3 g of iodine. If, following access to the subarachnoid space by a lumbar space there is lack of cranial extension of contrast secondary to mass effect (a myelographic block), contrast should be instilled superiorly from a C1–C2 approach to define the superior extent of the pathology. Radiographic images and then CT images are obtained of the requested level of the neural axis. Patients generally tolerate the procedure with local anesthesia however in some situations anxiolysis or general anesthesia may be required. Similar to CT imaging, patient weight and size may prevent the performance of myelography with table weight limits ranging from 350–440 lbs. depending on manufacturers.[9]

Relative to radiographs and cross-sectional imaging, myelography is an invasive procedure with certain considerations that should be taken into account before ordering this examination to maximize patient safety and avoid delays in obtaining the examination or the unfortunate situation where patients arrive for the examination only to be told that it cannot be performed for safety reasons. These factors include allergy to iodinated contrast agents, current anticoagulant therapy, or certain medications which may lower the seizure threshold. Preprocedure laboratory values including platelet levels, prothrombin time PT/international normalized ratio (INR), and partial thromboplastin time (PTT) are not mandatory but are useful in patients who are of advanced age or who are on or have been on anticoagulants. Screening for use of certain medications such as metformin (risk of lactic acidosis with iodinated contrast administration), phenothiazine derivatives, monoamine oxidase (MAO) inhibitors, tricyclic antidepressants, and other psychoactive drugs is recommended but depending on individual practitioner is not mandatory.[26]

The use of aspirin, nonsteroidal inflammatory drugs, or unfractionated subcutaneous heparin at a dose of less than 10,000 units/day is not a contraindication to lumbar puncture or by extension to myelography. Unfractionated heparin administered intravenously should be discontinued 2–4 hours before the procedure. Low molecular weight heparin should be discontinued

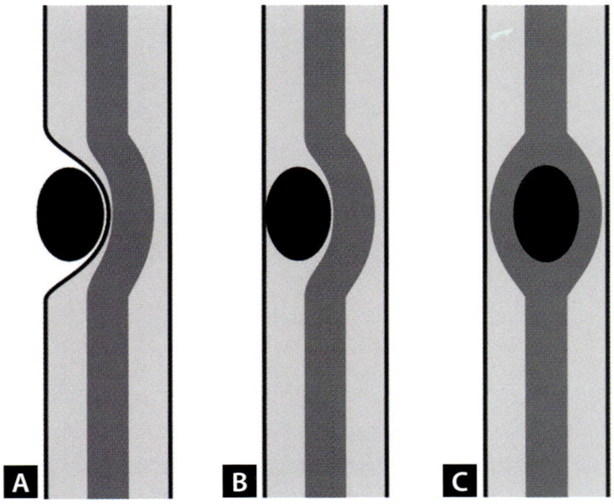

Figs. 8A to C: Diagram demonstrating extradural, (A) intradural-extramedullary, (B) intradural, (C) intramedullary pathology. Dura—vblack lines, spinal cord—dark gray, CSF—light gray, and lesion—solid black oval.

12 hours (low dose) or 24 hours (high dose) before the procedure. Patients on Coumadin need to have the medication stopped and have documentation of a normal INR. Plavix and Ticlid should be held for 5–7 days and 14 days, respectively.[27]

Image Evaluation

Once contrast has been introduced into the thecal sac, neural structures or intrathecal masses are identified as negative relief within the opacified cerebrospinal fluid (CSF). The delineation of the three major spaces–intramedullary, extramedullary intradural, and extradural becomes possible (Figs. 8A to C). Intramedullary masses are identified by enlargement of the spinal cord or nerve root that is surrounded by opacified CSF. Extramedullary intradural masses displace neural structures and have a characteristic border with the dura where there is often an undercut edge or acute angle. Extradural masses produce incursions on the margin of the opacified thecal sac which is usually smooth without acute angles. When a lesion in any of these spaces becomes large enough there can be a resultant block to flow of CSF and contrast, a myelographic block. While one can usually identify the space of origin of the pathology, it can sometimes be impossible. As mentioned previously, the role of myelography in this context is mostly historic and has been replaced entirely by CT and MR imaging except in those rare situations where there is a contraindication to MR or implanted hardware and concomitant beam hardening artifacts on CT.

MAGNETIC RESONANCE IMAGING

In the early 1980's, MR imaging became available for clinical use and has advanced considerably since that time with improved image quality and decreased time for image acquisition.[28,29] MR imaging allows direct evaluation of the bone marrow, spinal cord, nerve roots, the intervertebral disk, evaluation of postoperative scar and does not expose the patient to ionizing radiation.[29-34]

Ordering Considerations

There are many factors to consider before an MR examination can be performed in both a safely and timely manner. Before a patient can be placed into the MR unit a safety screening form is typically filled out by the patient or if the patient is unable then by the patient's family or requesting clinical service. MR safety is paramount, with all patients screened prior the examination for medical implants or metallic foreign bodies. There are multiple resources available for general safety considerations and specific device safety profiles including the free website www.MRIsafety.com and a subscription based website www.magresource.com. A small percentage of patients may require the need for anxiolysis or even general anesthesia to complete the examination depending on level of anxiety or mental status given the configuration of most MR scanners and the relative length of the examination. Table weight limits and gantry size vary but range from 350–550 lbs with gantry size of 55–60 cm.[9]

Prior to administration of gadolinium based contrast agents, eGFR is obtained because of the risk of nephrogenic systemic fibrosis (NSF), a condition characterized by skin thickening and fibrosis, contractions, pain, and multiorgan involvement that has been associated with gadolinium administration in patients with acute and chronic disease.[35] Following evaluation of risks versus benefits for administration of gadolinium in patients with impaired renal function, interventions range from hydration to hemodialysis although the utility of which is not clear.[36]

Imaging Protocols

The MR examination of the spine consists of multiple different pulse sequences, any of which will be variable depending on institution and MR scanner vendors. Below is a description of a typical MR spine examination at the authors' institution.

The examination begins with the scout, typically a HASTE sequence (half-fourier acquisition single-shot

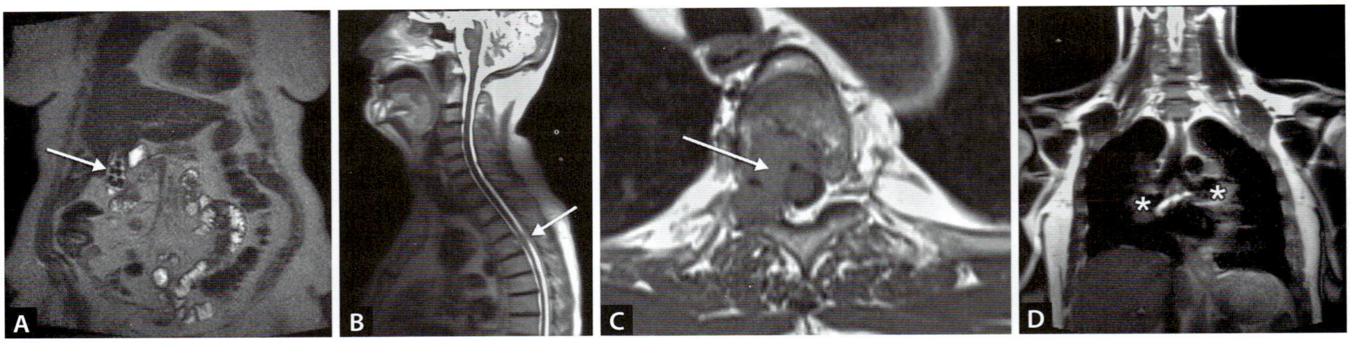

Figs. 9A to D: (A) Coronal HASTE scout demonstrates incidental gallstones, white arrow; (B) Scout image obtained during a lumbar spine MR examination demonstrates slight spinal cord contour irregularity at level of T4, a site of unsuspected osseous metastatic disease, confirmed on later thoracic spine imaging; (C) Axial T1-weighted image; (D) Scout film in a patient with cord signal abnormality and enhancement demonstrates bilateral hilar adenopathy (asterisks), supporting a diagnosis of sarcoidosis.

turbo spine-echo) obtained in the sagittal and coronal plane. For cervical examinations, the counting reference is the craniocervical junction and for both the thoracic and lumbar spines the counting reference is the lumbosacral junction. For the cervical and thoracic spine sagittal T1, turbo-spine echo T2, and short tau inversion recovery (STIR) images are obtained as well as axial T1 and gradient recalled echo (GRE) images. Lumbar spine imaging is similar however axial turbo spine-echo (TSE) T2 images are obtained rather than the axial GRE images. Gadolinium-based contrast can be administered when indicated with both sagittal and axial post contrast T1 images obtained.

Cerebrospinal fluid flow imaging can be obtained for evaluation of flow at level of foramen magnum in patients with Chiari malformation or for further characterizing syrinx formation or tethered cord.[37-40]

Diffusion weighted imaging (DWI) of the vertebral bodies and spinal cord can be performed for a variety of indications but these techniques are not routinely performed. The literature for evaluation of pathologic marrow infiltration in vertebral bodies has produced conflicting evidence for its utility.[41-43] As compared to the brain which is larger and immobile in relation to the spinal cord, DWI of the cord is difficult secondary to the small size of the cord, motion, and potential artifact from adjacent structures.[44,45] MR angiography can also be performed to evaluated the vascular supply of the cord and to evaluate vascular malformations.[46]

Image Evaluation

Evaluation of the MR examination of the spine includes the scout images and dedicated spine images with attention paid to the area of interest as well as to the soft tissues also included in the field of view. Scout images depending on the region of the spine imaged will visualize the neck, thorax, abdomen, and pelvis in an incomplete fashion as will the dedicated spine pulse sequences. While potentially identifying incidental abnormalities, pathologic processes can be visualized which may or may not be related to the primary reason for the examination being obtained (Figs. 9A to D). Aside from the scout images, paravertebral soft tissues are visible on the remainder of the examination to different degrees.

As with conventional radiographs or CT imaging of the spine vertebral body height, alignment, posterior elements, disk spaces, and paravertebral soft tissues should be assessed (Figs. 10A to E). In contrast to CT imaging or radiography, MR imaging allows direct visualization of the marrow; in the adult where marrow is predominantly fatty replaced, the marrow should be hyperintense on T1-weighted images similar to subcutaneous fat.[47] Marrow signal intensity can be heterogeneous but in adults if the marrow is of lower signal intensity compared to the intervertebral disk, it is likely pathologic.[48] Marrow should also be homogenous on T2 and STIR images. The far lateral images allow evaluation of the pedicles and facet joints where bone marrow edema, facet arthropathy, or facet joint effusions can be visualized (Figs. 11A and B). Using both axial and sagittal images the intervertebral disk and spinal cord can be evaluated. Neural foramen in the cervical spine are obliquely oriented and are best visualized on axial images while in the thoracic and lumbar spine the neural foramen are transversely oriented and are best visualized on far sagittal T1 weighted images (Fig. 12).

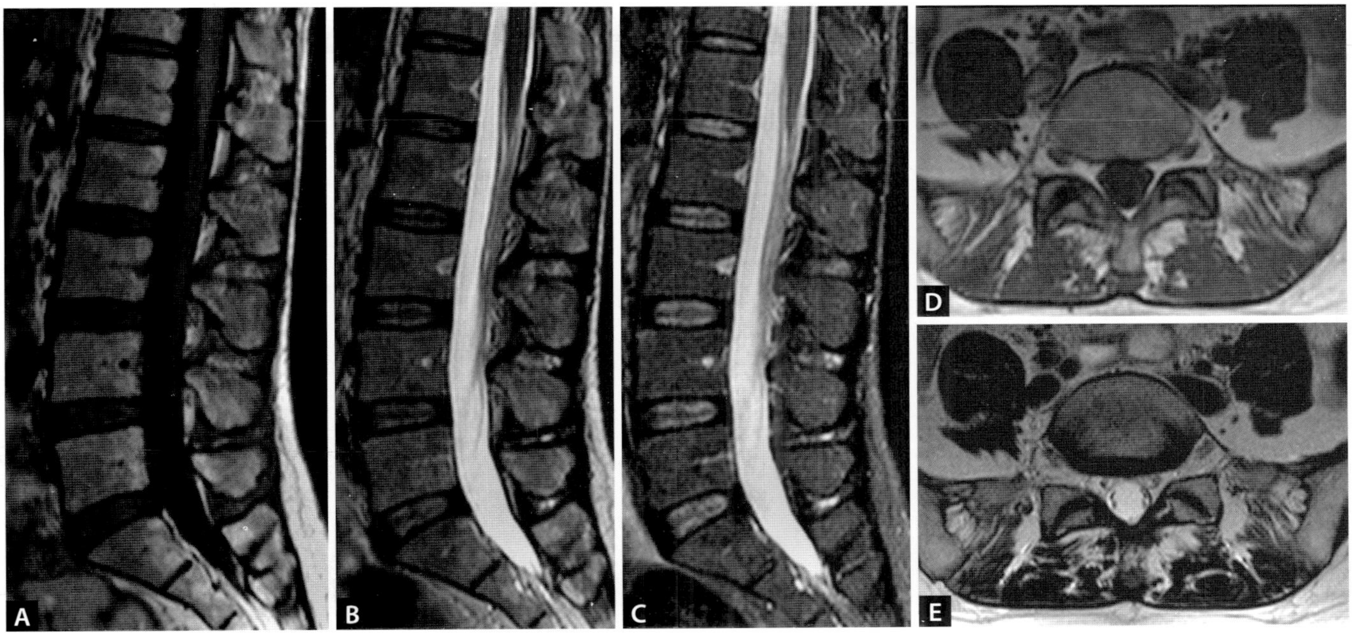

Figs. 10A to E: Routine pulse sequences for a lumbar spine MR examination: (A) Sagittal T1; (B) Sagittal T2; (C) Sagittal STIR; (D) Axial T1; and (E) Axial T2. Evaluation should include vertebral body height, alignment, marrow signal intensity, posterior elements, disk spaces, conus medullaris, canal and neural foramina, and paravertebral soft tissues.

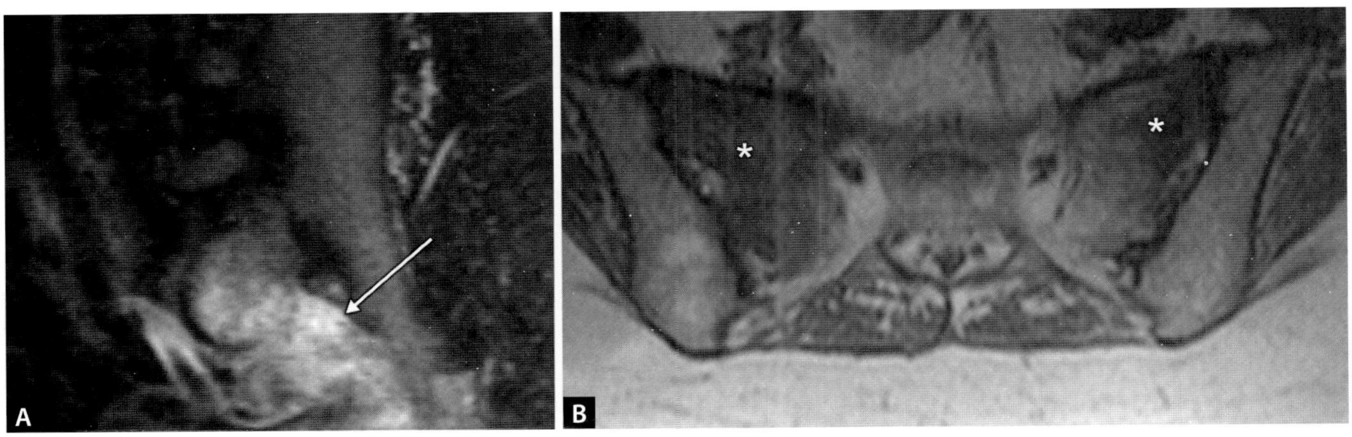

Figs. 11A and B: Far sagittal STIR image demonstrates hyperintensity along the lateral aspect of the sacrum, white arrow (A), with corresponding low T1 signal intensity on an axial T1-weighted image, asterisks (B), representing bilateral sacral insufficiency fractures.

Evaluation of the spinal canal can be made with either axial or sagittal images. The spinal cord should be of uniform signal intensity with no expansion or syrinx formation and the conus medullaris should be normal in position at or above level of L2. CSF should follow the signal intensity of fluid, hyperintense on T2 and FLAIR and hypointense on T1 weighted images (Figs. 13A and B). The main ligaments of the spine are best evaluated with T2-weighted images and should be of uniform low signal intensity.[5]

MR imaging is prone to multiple artifacts which can limit the sensitivity of the examination or in some cases be confused with pathology. Ferromagnetic artifacts from implanted metallic surgical hardware is manifested as a signal void/low signal with peripheral hyperintensity and

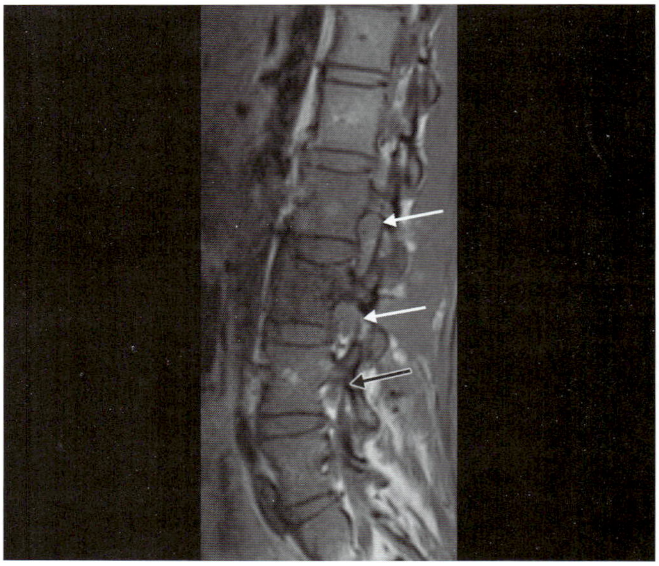

Fig. 12: Sagittal T1-weighted image of the lumbar spine demonstrates a normal appearing neural foramina, black arrow, and effaced neural foramen by epidural disease, white arrows, in a patient with Ewing sarcoma, illustrating the importance of evaluating far lateral images on sagittal T1-weighted images.

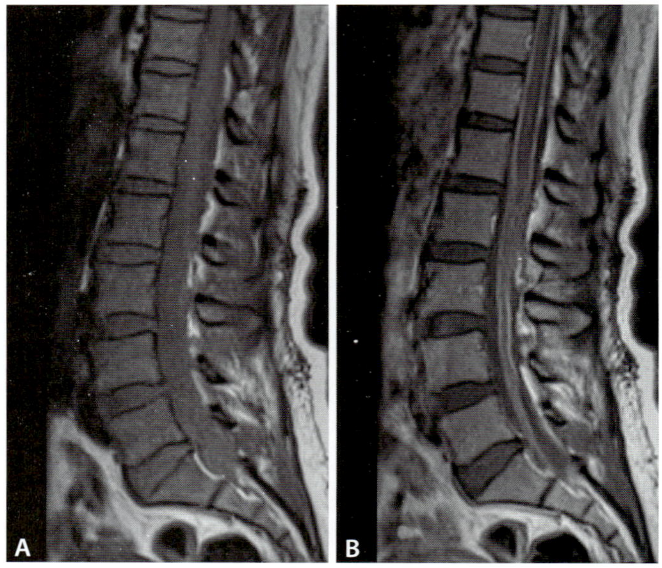

Figs. 13A and B: Sagittal noncontrast T1-weighted image of the lumbar spine, (A) demonstrates relative hyperintensity of the CSF with resultant poor delineation of the conus medullaris. (B) T1-weighted image following contrast administration, demonstrates extensive leptomeningeal enhancement in this patient with Streptococcus meningitis.

is exacerbated with high field strength magnets and use of stainless steel implants (Figs. 14A and B). Inhomogeneity in the magnetic field can result in a zebra stripe artifact, typically peripheral in location in an image with a large field of view. Due to the increased time involved in acquiring individual pulse sequences, patient movement or physiologic motion such as CSF pulsation, breathing, or vascular pulsation can degrade image quality (Figs. 15A to C). Aliasing or wrap around artifact that occurs with the field of view is smaller than the body part being imaged and can result in structures outside the field of view being superimposed on the opposite side of the image (Fig. 16). Gibbs phenomenon can result in the appearance of a syrinx in the spinal cord.[49]

INDICATIONS AND EVIDENCE FOR SPINE IMAGING

Trauma

Given the potential catastrophic complications from traumatic injury to the vertebral column and spinal cord, it is important to identify patients at high risk for injury and perform appropriate imaging based on the strengths and weaknesses of conventional radiographs, CT imaging, and

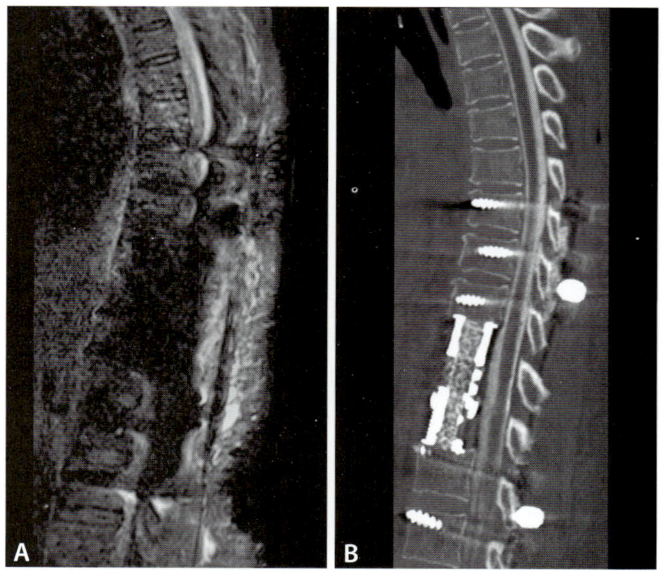

Figs. 14A and B: (A) Sagittal STIR image is essentially uninterpretable secondary to extensive artifact from metallic hardware in a patient with paraplegia following surgery with presumed cord infarct or compression from postoperative fluid collection. (B) Sagittal myelogram CT demonstrates the absence of a compressive fluid collection.

MR imaging. Additional considerations include optimal use of healthcare resources and radiation exposure

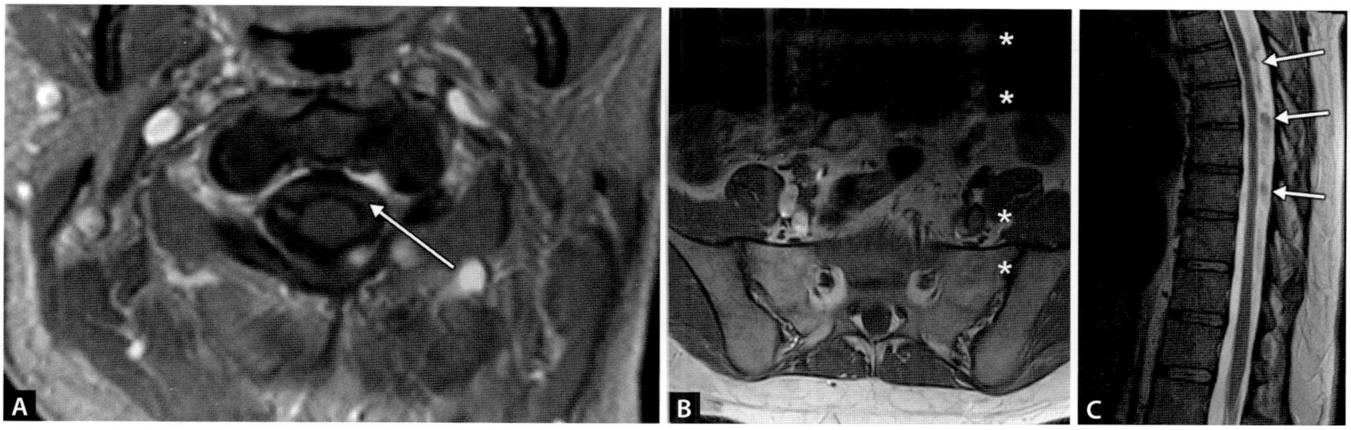

Figs. 15A to C: (A) Demonstrates an apparent intradural extramedullary mass lesion, white arrow, an artifact frequently observed on the first image of a series of images. (B) demonstrates vascular pulsation artifact which is superimposed over the left aspect of the sacrum, simulating pathology, asterisks. CSF pulsation artifact, (C) white arrows, simulates prominent vascularity in the spinal canal which could be confused for an underlying vascular malformation.

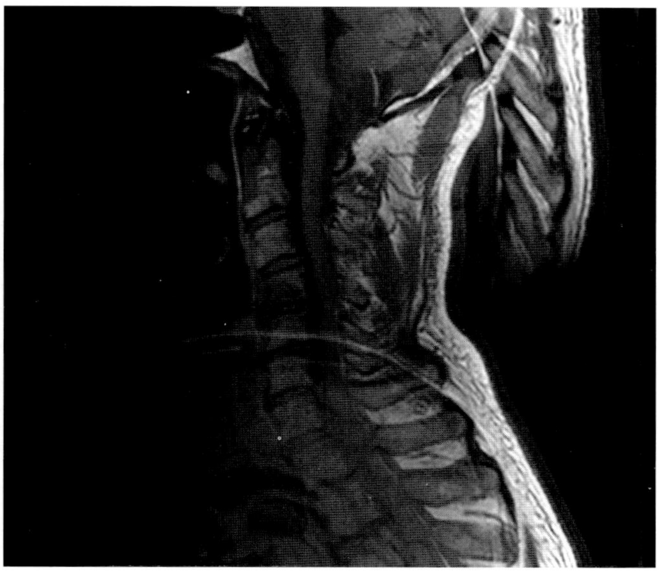

Fig. 16: Wrap-around artifact from a small field-of-view can result in structures outside the field-of-view being superimposed along the opposite end of the image. Note portions of the brain along the inferior aspect of the image and a portion of the thoracic spine along the superior aspect of the image.

specifically targeted towards the decision to not perform advanced imaging in patients who are at low risk of injury and to identify patients who would benefit from CT or MR imaging.

Imaging Findings

Injury to the spine can involve vertebral bodies, posterior elements, or ligaments and soft tissues with the nature of the injury often dependent on the mechanism of injury. Stability of the spine following injury, where the injury results in abnormal mobility during normal biomechanical stresses or motion can be assessed by using the widely accepted 3-column model of the spine described by Denis. The anterior column consists of the anterior half of the vertebral body including the anterior longitudinal ligament and anterior annulus fibrosis. The middle column includes the posterior half of the vertebral body, posterior longitudinal ligament, and posterior annulus. The posterior column includes the posterior elements, facet joints, and posterior ligaments including ligamentum flavum, and the interspinous and supraspinous ligaments. If the injury involves more than one of these columns, the injury is considered unstable.[50] Other radiologic findings suggesting instability include asymmetric increased distance between spinous processes or increased distance between pedicle in the transverse plane, separation of facet joints, disruption of posterior vertebral body line, compression fracture of greater than 50%, or the presence of a kyphosis of greater than 20°.[51]

Cervical spine injury is largely dependent on the mechanism of injury. Hyperflexion injuries can result in malalignment, facet joint dislocations, wedge compression fractures, dens fractures, or fracture of a spinous process (clay-shoveler's fracture). Hyperextension injuries can result in malalignment, avulsion fractures, or hangman's fracture. Axial loading can result in the Jefferson fracture involving C1 vertebral body. Fractures of the thoracic and lumbar spine can include simple compression fractures, considered stable, or burst fractures which are considered unstable.[52]

Ligamentous injury can be inferred from the type of injury or when there is direct visualization of ligamentous disruption or T2 and STIR hyperintensity within the ligaments.[53] Spinal cord injury can be manifested by cord edema and hemorrhage, with hemorrhage having poorer prognosis.[54,55]

Imaging Recommendations

Cervical spine: Conventional radiographic evaluation of the cervical spine should at minimum include frontal/AP, lateral, and open-mouth odontoid views and a swimmer's view as necessary to include the cervical thoracic junction when needed however subsequent CT imaging is frequently performed if the radiographs are suboptimal or if there are questionable abnormalities.

Research into determining the best screening examination for cervical spine trauma takes into account the advantages of varying modalities and the nature of the traumatic event. For evaluation of the spinal cord for contusion or extradural compression from a traumatic disk herniation or epidural hematoma, MR imaging is the preferred modality. Radiographic and CT imaging of the spine are preferred for evaluation of fracture in the appropriate situation. If the initial radiographic examination is technically inadequate, repeat views are frequently performed, leading to the longer examination times for radiographs (average time 22 minutes) as opposed to the average examination time of 12 minutes for CT imaging.[56] An additional study demonstrated similar time savings.[57] Sensitivity of radiographs for cervical spine fractures has been reported as 39.3%[58] to 52% in a large meta-analysis as opposed to the sensitivity for CT imaging which is above 98%.[59] An additional study imaged the cervical spine with both radiographs and CT imaging with CT identifying 100% of fractures as opposed to a sensitivity of 36% for radiographs.[60]

The higher sensitivity of CT imaging for identifying fractures has been established in multiple studies,[58-60] however it is at the expense of increased cost and increased radiation dose that raises the need for proper stratification of which patients should receive CT imaging or alternatively no imaging. The National Emergency X-radiography Use Study (NEXUS) established five clinical criteria consisting of "the absence of tenderness at the posterior midline of the cervical spine, the absence of focal neurologic deficit, a normal level of alertness, no evidence of intoxication, and absence of clinically apparent pain that might distract the patient from the pain of a cervical-spine injury". Meeting these criteria demonstrated sensitivity for excluding cervical spine injury of 99% in all study patients suggesting that when these strict criteria are met that imaging of cervical spine does not need to be obtained. Sensitivity of radiographs in this study was reported as 89% however CT imaging was not performed in all patients.[61] An additional highly sensitive decision based scheme was developed by the Canadian Cervical Spine Group where patients were classified as having either absence of high-risk factors or having low-risk factors for injury.[62] Bailitz et al. performed both radiography and CT imaging in patients at various risk levels as opposed to only those patients at high risk for cervical spine injury and found that CT imaging identified all fractures while radiographs identified only 36%. Out of the 78 patients with imaging findings of injury, 50 were felt to be significant with the distribution of risk stratification being 15 at high-risk, 19 at moderate-risk, and 16 at low-risk which supports the case for screening for cervical spine injury with CT imaging regardless of risk level of injury.[60]

Injury to the soft tissues and ligaments of the spine with potential resultant spinal instability is best evaluated with MR imaging with conflicting evidence for the utility of CT imaging. Flexion extension radiography or dynamic fluoroscopy in the acute setting has been shown to be inferior compared to MR imaging.[63-68] MR imaging can readily detect ligamentous injury, manifested as T2 or STIR signal hyperintensity within the ligaments or by demonstrating ligamentous disruption itself. With the high sensitivity of MR imaging for identifying signal intensity abnormalities in the ligaments it is often uncertain whether these abnormalities are significant.[69,70] It is in these cases that flexion extension radiographs may be of use. MR has been shown to identify additional abnormalities without patient management change. Examination of CT imaging has generated conflicting results as whether the cervical spine can clear based on CT alone.[70,71] A meta-analysis performed by Panczykowski et al. found that the negative predictive value of a negative CT was 100%. Conversely, MR has been shown to demonstrate abnormalities missed by CT that have changed patient management.[72]

Thoracic and lumbar spine: Imaging the thoracic and lumber spine has been recommended by Hsu et al. if any of the following criteria are met: (1) back pain/midline tenderness, (2) local signs of thoracolumbar injury, (3) abnormal neurological signs, (4) cervical spine fractures, (5) GCS < 15, (6) major distracting injury, (7) ETOH/drug intoxication.[73] CT imaging is the preferred modality for trauma patients[74-77] and spine imaging can be obtained as an additional acquisition or alternatively reformatted from the pre-existing CT dataset from the chest, abdomen, and pelvis if performed for evaluation of nonspine traumatic sequelae with sagittal and coronal reconstructions generated without additional radiation exposure.[74,78-82] If there is one fracture identified, imaging the remainder of spine is warranted given the high incidence of additional geographically separate injury.[73,83]

Degenerative Disk Disease

MR imaging is the modality of choice for evaluating the morphologic findings in degenerative disk disease with pain, a common indication for ordering imaging examinations of the spine. The exact etiology of pain in degenerative disk disease is not completely understood but is likely a combination of degenerative disk disease itself including instability, facet and ligamentous hypertrophy, direct neural compression, and biochemical mediators of pain.[84] In addition to the exact mechanism of back pain being poorly understood, further compounding the utility of spine imaging for back pain or degenerative disk disease is the presence of the morphologic alterations in asymptomatic individuals.[85-88] Similar problems exist for neck pain which can be categorized as chronic in nature or secondary to injury/whiplash.[89,90]

Degenerative disk disease and findings in normal aging are similar although degenerative disk disease is thought be a more rapidly progressing process with a predilection for the nucleus pulposus and endplates. Current theories for the development of degenerative disk disease include abnormal mechanical stress, nutritional variables, and genetics. Mechanical stressors result in damage to the endplates and vertebral disk.[91] Alterations in the metabolically active disk result in decreased tensile strength of the disk and loss of differentiation between the annulus fibrosis and nucleus pulposus.[92] Genetic factors have also been described in both humans and in animal models.[93-95]

Imaging Findings

The imaging findings of degenerative disk disease using MR imaging are well-described and include alterations in normal morphology of the intervertebral disk, facet joints, ligaments, vertebral body alignment, marrow signal intensity, and diameter of the spinal canal. Recommendations in 2001 from the Combined Task Forces of the North American Spine Society, American Society of Spine Radiology, and American Society of Neuroradiology presented standardized terminology for the description of disk herniations with emphasis that the terms are purely descriptive and not meant to reflect that the morphologic alteration is causative to the patient's symptoms or that treatment is needed or recommended.[96]

Intervertebral disk and stenosis: The intervertebral disk is composed of the annulus fibrosis peripherally and the nucleus pulposus centrally and forms an amphiarthrodial joint with the adjacent vertebral body endplates. As degenerative disk disease ensues, the disk can develop low T2 signal intensity from alterations in water state and glycosaminoglycan concentration.[29,97] Additional findings include annular tears or fissures of the outer fibers of the annulus fibrosis manifested as focal T2 hyperintensity (Figs. 17A and B),[98,99] disk calcification of variable MR signal intensity,[100] or vacuum disk phenomenon where gas, usually nitrogen, can accumulate within the disk producing low signal intensity on all pulse sequences.[101]

Herniation refers, generally, to extension if disk material is beyond the margin of the disk space which includes the vertebral endplate and the peripheral ring apophyses. A generalized disk herniation is when the disk extends focally more than 50% beyond the margin of the disk space while the term bulging disk is reserved for more diffuse extension of the intervertebral disk of more than 50%, typically no more than a few millimeters beyond the disk space margin.

A localized herniation refers to disk material focally extending less than 50% of the diameter of the disk space margin with a broad-based herniation occupying 25–50%

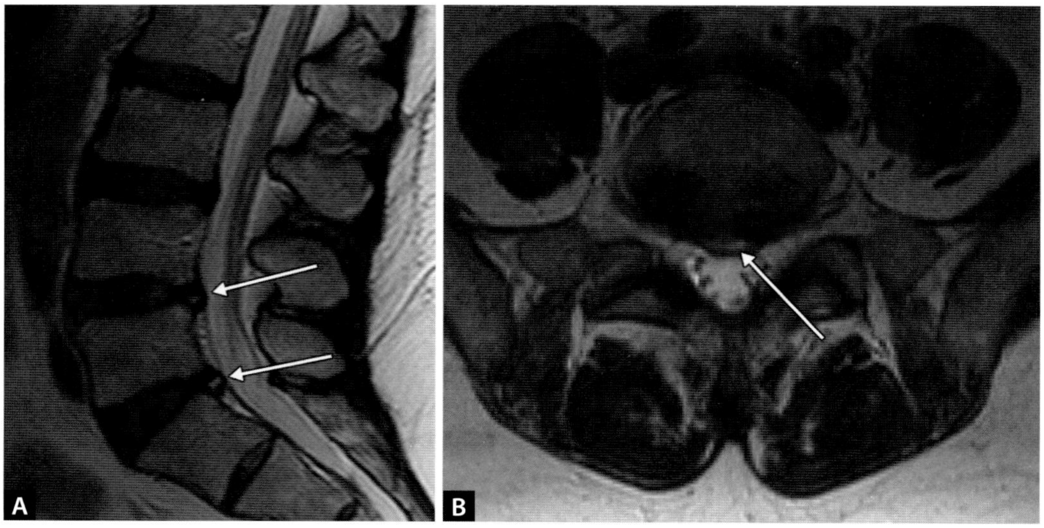

Figs. 17 A and B: Annular tears, focal T2 hyperintensity at level of the disk space at L4–L5 and L5–S1 with superimposed disk protrusions, white arrows (A) and L5–S1, white arrow (B).

the diameter of the disk space and a focal herniation occupying less than 25% of the diameter of the disk space. A protrusion is where the distal herniated disk material is narrowing than the base of the herniated disk material and an extrusion is when the base of the herniated disk material is narrowing than the distal herniated disk material (Figs. 18A to D).

Canal stenosis can result from degenerative disk disease or can be developmental in nature. Symptoms include pain, neurological symptoms, and can change with flexion or extension.[102-104] Degree of spinal canal or neural foraminal compromise can be graded as mild, moderate, or severe. Mild is less than one-third diameter narrowing, moderate is one-third to two-third narrowed, and severe is more than two-third narrowed (Figs. 19A and B).[96]

Facet joints and ligaments: Degenerative changes of the zygoapophyseal type facet joints can occur concurrently or independently of degenerative disk disease (Figs. 20A and B). Facet arthropathy/hypertrophy can contribute to central canal stenosis in conjunction with ligamentous hypertrophy, narrowing of the lateral recesses or neural foramen. Facet joint effusions can occur as well as synovial cysts (Figs. 21A and B) which can narrow the spinal canal or neural foramen.[105,106]

Alignment: Alterations in the normal alignment of the spine can occur with derangement of normal spine biomechanics and can be degenerative, traumatic, or secondary to pars interarticularis defect (Figs. 22A and B).[84]

Marrow changes: Alterations in vertebral body endplate changes in degenerative disk disease have been classified into three types with T1 and T2 characteristics corresponding to edema for type I, fat for type II, and sclerosis for type III. Type I endplate changes demonstrate T1 and T2 signal intensity prolongation (T1 hypointense and T2 hyperintense) and are thought to represent more acute changes (Figs. 23A and B). Enhancement can occur, following gadolinium administration. Type II changes are hyper to isointense on T2 images and hyperintense on T1 weighted images secondary to the presence of yellow marrow (Figs. 24A and B). Type III endplate changes have woven bone histologically and are low in signal intensity on both T2 and T1 images.[107,108]

Dynamic Imaging

Dynamic imaging of the spine refers to imaging the spine in differing positions including flexion, extension, or with axial loading. While standing lateral radiographs can be readily obtained, most CT and MR examinations are performed with the patient supine. There are open MR units in which the patient can be imaged while sitting; however, there is relative low image quality as compared to conventional closed magnets. There are also commercially

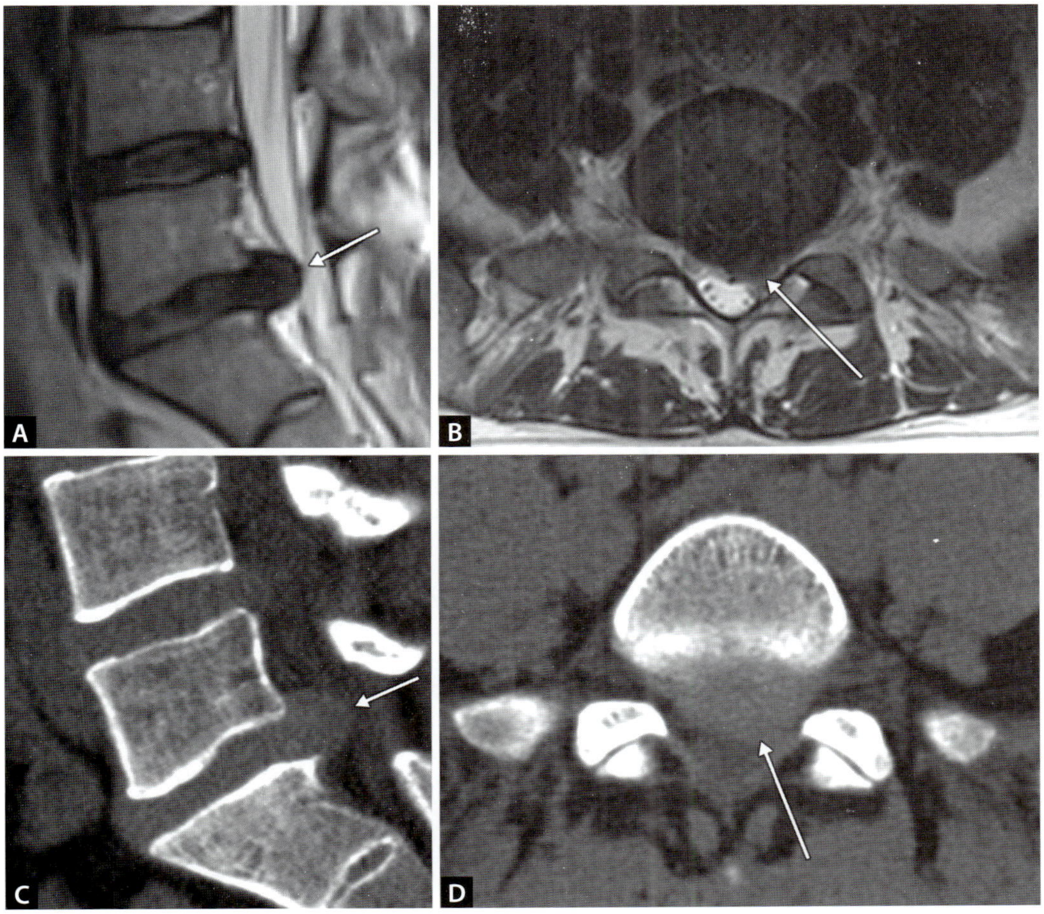

Figs. 18 A to D: Large disk protrusion, white arrows in T2-weighted images (A and B) and CT images (C and D) at L5–S1.

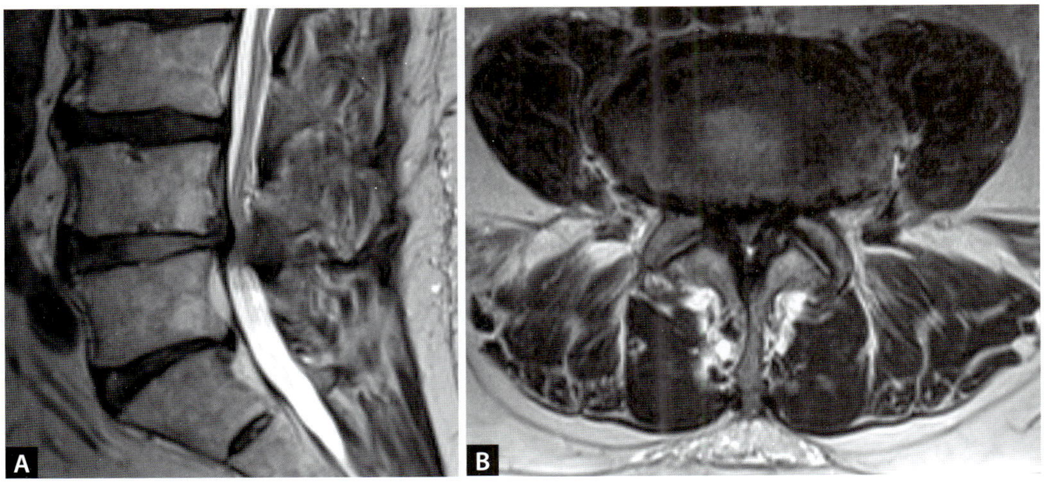

Figs. 19A and B: Severe canal stenosis at L4–L5 on: (A) Sagittal and; (B) Axial T2-weighted images secondary to diffusely bulging disk, facet arthropathy, and ligamentous hypertrophy.

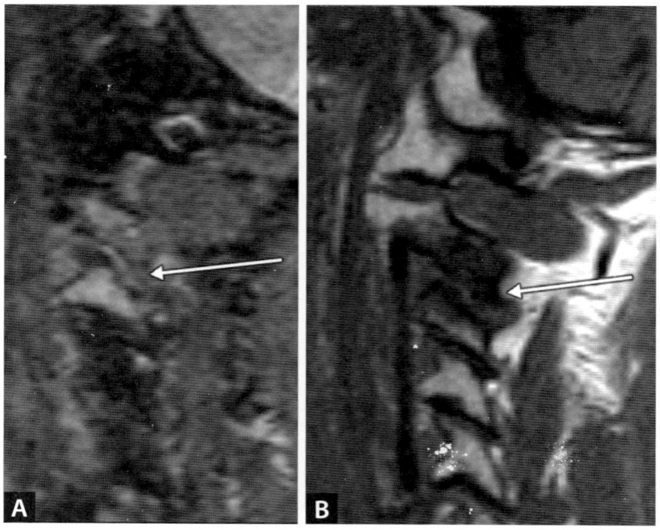

Figs. 20A and B: Facet arthropathy with edema, sagittal STIR (A, white arrow) and sagittal T1-weighted image (B, white arrow) at C2–C3.

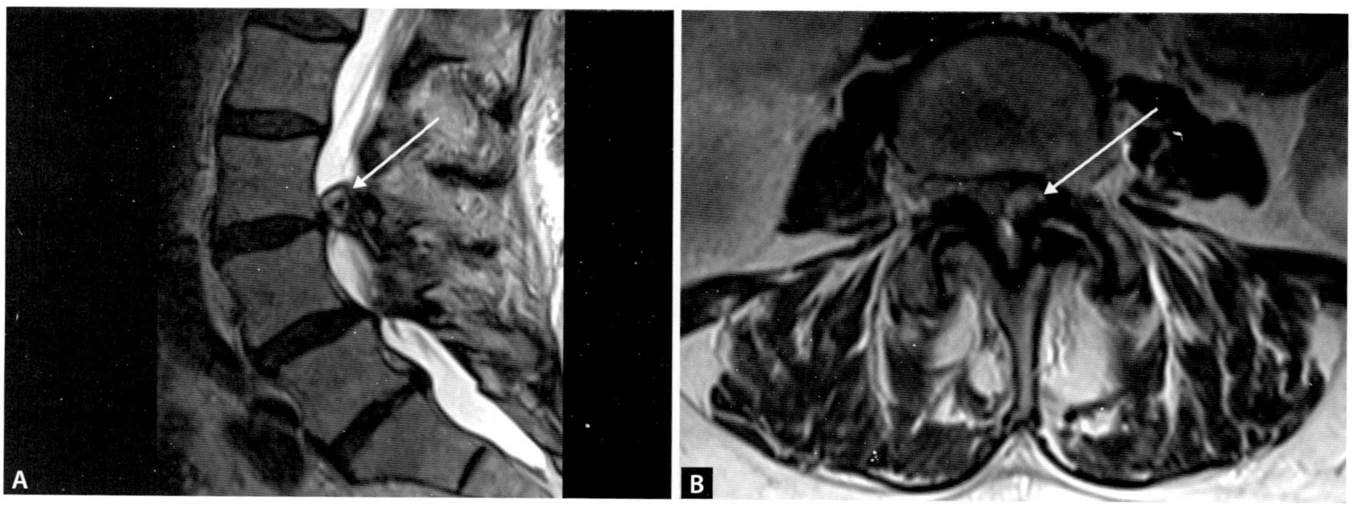

Figs. 21A and B: Large synovial cyst arising from the left L3–L4 facet joint contributes to severe canal stenosis, white arrows in A and B (sagittal and axial T2-weighted images).

available MR compatible axial loading devices (using a load applying harness) and neck flexion devices.

The desire to image the patient in an either flexed or extended state or alternatively with axial loading is secondary to the fact that most symptoms occur in these positions. With patients imaged in extension, there has been documented decreased size of the lumbar spinal canal and neural foramen[109,110] with the decreased measurements more likely in symptomatic individuals rather than healthy controls.[111] Decreasing size of the cervical spine canal is also present with extension.[112-115] Laxity and resultant buckling of ligamentum flavum is felt to be the causative factor in both the cervical and lumbar spine (Figs. 25 and 26). Axial loading demonstrates decreased lumbar spinal canal diameter with a sensitivity of 96.4% and produces similar findings in upright myelography.[116]

Standing lateral radiographs of the lumbar spine can reveal abnormalities not evident on conventional supine images. With standing views, there can be visualization of exaggerated normal lumbar lordosis with an implied narrowed canal[117] or an increase in instability/malalignment.[118] Flexion extension views of the spine can

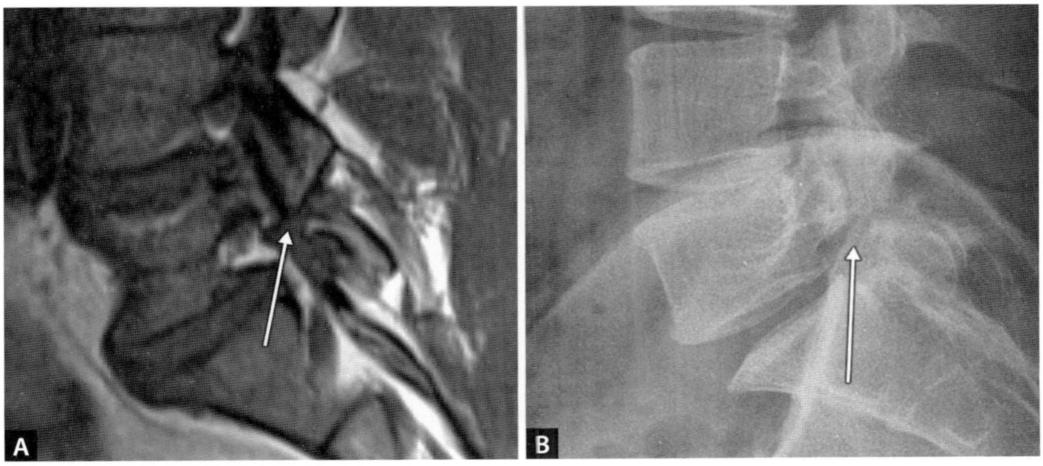

Figs. 22A and B: Pars interarticularis defect of L5, white arrow (A) sagittal T1-weighted image, and white arrow on lateral radiograph (B).

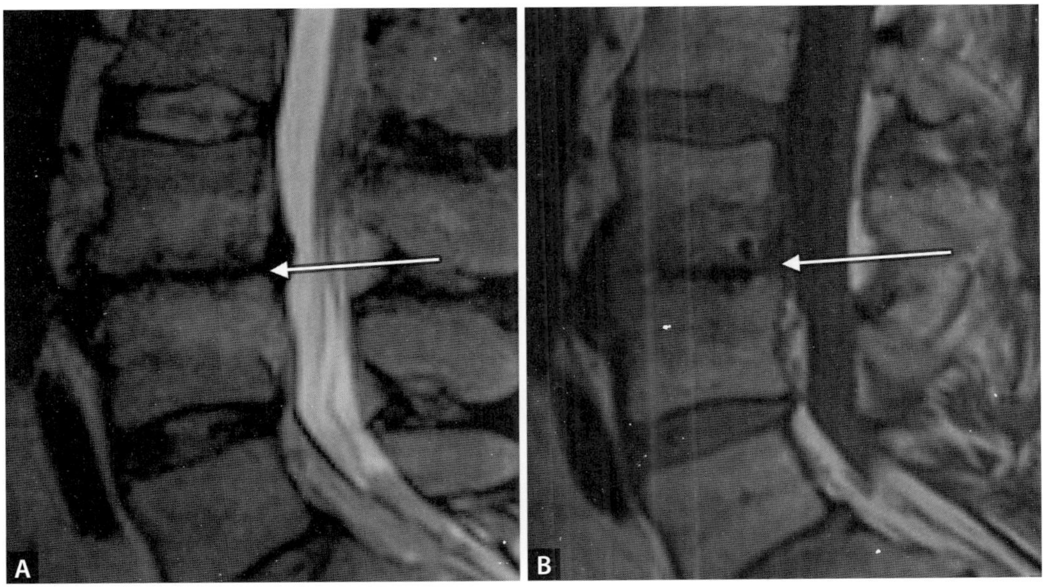

Figs. 23A and B: Type I endplate change, white arrows, at L3–L4, manifested as T2 hyperintensity (A), and T1 hypointensity (B).

also be obtained for evaluation of instability, however there is overall low-yield with patient selection, an important factor before performing this examination.[119] Similar to the potential low yield for flexion extension views of the spine, there is low yield for routine oblique views of both the cervical and lumbar spine.[120,121] Rotational positioned CT imaging can be used to evaluate for atlantoaxial rotatory subluxation where the patient is imaged in the neutral, maximal rotated left, and maximal rotated right positions.[122,123]

There have been many reports demonstrating better delineation of canal stenosis and disk protrusions in the cervical spine.[124-126] Similar findings showing increased disk herniations are also present in the lumbar spine when the patient is imaged in an upright position[125,127] and when imaged in an extended position.[128,129]

While dynamic imaging of the spine has been shown to increase the conspicuity of morphologic alterations in the spine, whether these techniques can positively alter patient outcomes is not clearly defined.

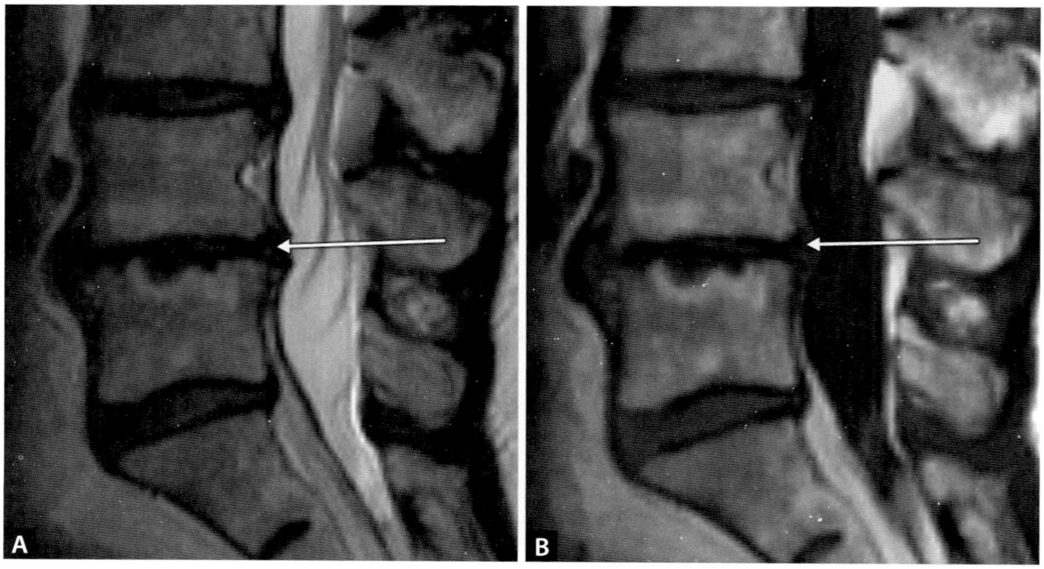

Figs. 24A and B: Type II endplate change: T2 hyperintensity (arrow in A) and T1 hyperintensity (arrow in B) at L4–L5. Schmorl's node present along the superior endplate of L5.

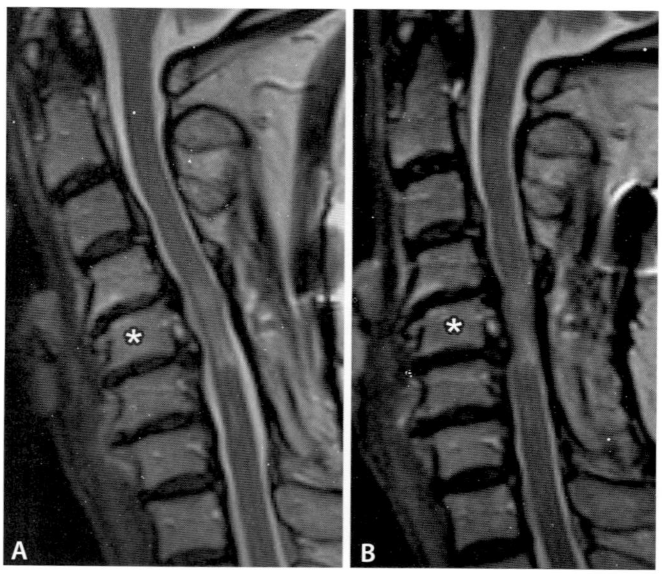

Figs. 25A and B: Dynamic imaging of the cervical spine. (A) T2-weighted image, with patient in neutral position and (B) with patient imaged in extension demonstrating decreased diameter of the canal in this patient with previous laminectomies and cord myelomalacia centered at level of C5, asterisk.
Courtesy: Edward Benzel, MD, Cleveland Clinic, Cleveland, Ohio, USA.

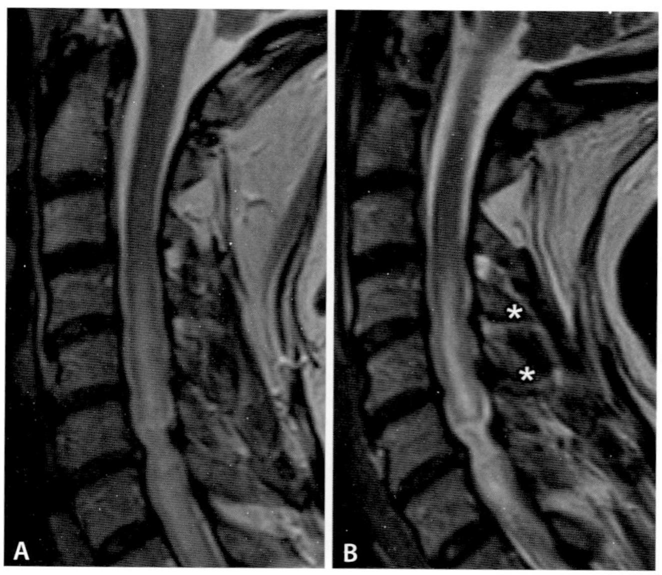

Figs. 26A and B: Patient with pre-existing transverse myelitis is scanned in the neutral position (A) and in extension (B) using sagittal T2-weighted images. Canal stenosis is present at C6–C7 in the neutral position with additional stenosis apparent with extension at C4–C5 and C5–C6, asterisks in B.
Courtesy: Edward Benzel, MD, Cleveland Clinic, Cleveland, Ohio, USA.

Influence of Imaging Findings on Clinical Decision-making

Advanced cross-sectional imaging no doubt demonstrates morphologic alterations; however, does the knowledge to the physician or patient of these abnormalities optimally influence decision-making and, by extension patient, well-being? Abnormalities in imaging studies are common in asymptomatic individuals and the potential resulting treatment, either medical or surgical, which may result from these imaging findings, should be superior to the natural history of the disease process.

Depending on the age of the patient, there can be a 50–57% chance that the CT or MR examination will be abnormal. 50% of asymptomatic patients over the age of 40 had abnormal CT scans consisting of disk herniations, facet arthropathy, or canal stenosis with roughly 20% of patients under the age of 40 showing similar abnormalities.[88] Myelography performed on asymptomatic individuals was abnormal in 24% of patients.[86] MR imaging in asymptomatic individuals demonstrates a similar high prevalence of abnormalities: In patients between 20–39 years of age 22% had abnormalities and in patients 60–80 years of age 57% had abnormalities.[85] In 98 asymptomatic individuals, only 36% of patients had normal examinations. In the abnormal examinations, there tended to be bulging disks and protrusions as opposed to disk extrusions.[87]

Disk herniations, which have a high prevalence, tend to change over time and can resolve completely or decrease in size.[130] Disk extrusions associated with pain have been demonstrated to decrease in size over time (Figs. 27A and B), with one-third of patients improving by 6 weeks and two-third of patients improving by 6 months.[131,132] Additionally, when patients are followed over time, new extrusions could appear and interval changes from baseline to the follow-examinations were not correlated with clinical course.[131]

In terms of whether MR imaging for low back can be predictive, it has been found that genetics, work status, and psychosocial factors tend to be more important.[133-135] The presence of a herniation combined with back pain and Caucasian race were found to be positive predictors of outcome by Modic et al.[131] Other studies have also found that small disk herniations, annulus rupture, and nerve compression are associated with favorable outcome with conservative treatment[136-138] and that foraminal disk protrusions fare better with surgery.[138] In a 7-year follow-up of 50 of the 67 original patients (31% of which had a morphologic abnormality) without back pain studied by Boden et al., MR imaging was shown to not be predictive of who would develop back pain.

For chronic neck pain, multiple studies have shown that psychosocial factors play a great role as opposed to imaging findings.[139,140] When imaging of the cervical spine for whiplash, there is no consensus for what constitutes an abnormal examination.[141,142] However, if underlying degenerative changes are present these can contribute to symptoms.[143]

Although many studies have shown that MR imaging is not predictive and does not offer prognostic information in many cases, morphologic alterations have been shown to correlate with patient symptoms. Beattie et al. have shown that leg pain is associated with disk extrusions and nerve compression while Jarvik et al. have found that canal stenosis can be seen with low back pain.[144,145] Type I endplate changes have been associated with pain[146] and are associated with good clinical outcome if present at baseline following fusion procedure[147] and poor outcome if they persist following fusion.[148]

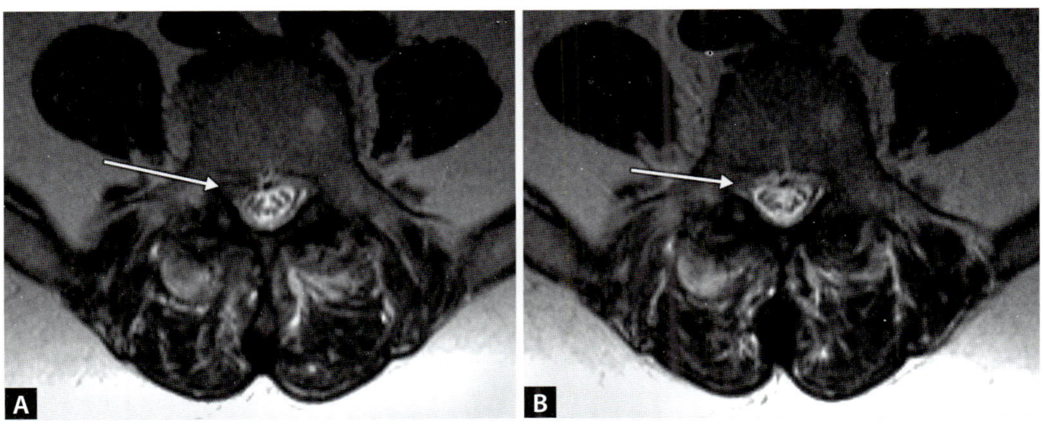

Figs. 27A and B: Axial T2-weighted image (A) shows extruded disk material at level of mid body of L5, white arrow. Two months later (B), there is essentially complete resolution of the extruded disk material, white arrow.

CHAPTER 20

Imaging Decisions

Imaging for low back pain has economic (both direct and indirect) and patient outcome ramifications, hence imaging for low back pain should be obtained in appropriate cases. While the cause of low back pain is frequently unknown, there is concern for excluding other causes such as infection or neoplasm. These cases typically present with trauma, weight loss, advanced age, fever, systemic illness, long duration of symptoms, and history of prior surgery.[149-151]

Nonspecific back pain does not require imaging[131,150,152,153] however if symptoms persist for longer than 6 weeks imaging is recommended.[152] Recommendations from the American College of Physicians recommend radiography combined with erythrocyte sedimentation rate in patients who have major risk factors for cancer and MR imaging in patients with risk factors for infection, cauda equina syndrome, or with severe neurologic symptoms.[150]

Many studies have shown that early imaging does not positively direct patient therapy and can in some instances be harmful. Studies have shown that imaging by radiography, CT, or MR imaging in patients with low back pain and no risk factors had no advantage over conservative care[154] and that clinical treatment was not changed.[155,156] Gillan et al., in contrast, reported that MR imaging provided "diagnostic confidence" in patients who were imaged.[157] Radiography and CT imaging uses ionizing radiation which in itself has risks the most serious of which is carcinogenesis.[158-160] The knowledge of the test results from spine imaging itself has been shown to be associated with poor patient outcome.[161-163] Positive outcome after surgery has been correlated with proper patient selection[164,165] which should be taken into account given that rates of surgery have been shown to increase with increased use of CT and MR imaging.[166-168]

Advanced cross-sectional imaging can be best used in the appropriate clinical setting; in cases of uncomplicated back pain it has not been shown to positively direct conservative treatment but has played a role in patients with "red flags" and in patients who are surgical candidates.

Postoperative Spine

Spine surgery can be performed for both therapeutic and diagnostic aims including decompression from degenerative disk disease, neoplasm, or infection, and also for obtaining tissue diagnosis for directing treatment. There are many available surgical approaches and hardware choices. Imaging of the spine following surgery is frequently performed for many reasons including evaluation of instrumentation/fusion, persistent symptoms, treatment monitoring, and evaluation for potential complications. Imaging choices consist of radiography with or without flexion extension views, CT imaging, and MR imaging.

Instrumentation and Fusion

Imaging of the spine following instrumented fusion is obtained for evaluating the status of osseous fusion and positioning of the instrumentation (Figs. 28A and B), evaluation for complication and for treatment monitoring. Following the spine over time with imaging is valuable to evaluate for subtle changes which may occur over time and not be as apparent on short-term follow-up studies including change in alignment, component positioning, and status of the bony fusion.[169-171] Routine radiographs including AP and lateral views at a minimum are sufficient with conflicting reports as to the utility for obtaining flexion and extension views on a routine basis.[172-174]

One aim of imaging patients following spine surgery is to confirm the presence of spinal fusion, defined as bridging trabecular bone between the adjacent spinal segments (Figs. 29 and 30), include treatment of potentially painful instability. Following surgery, fusion usually

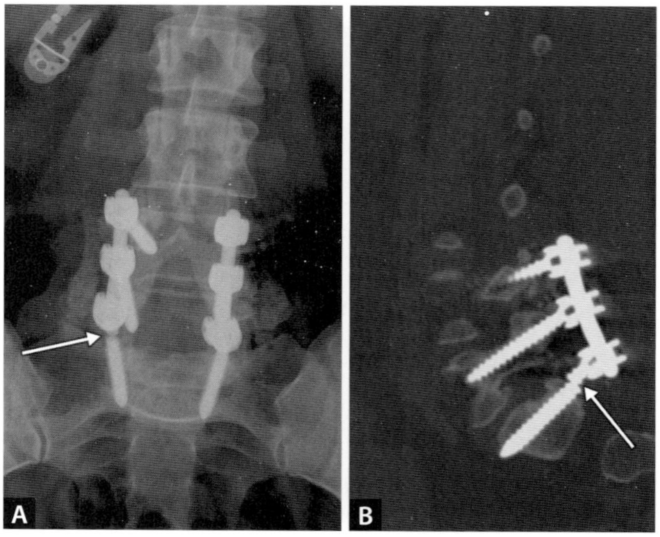

Figs. 28A and B: (A) Frontal radiograph and (B) sagittal CT image, demonstrate fracture of right S1 pedicle screw (white arrows).

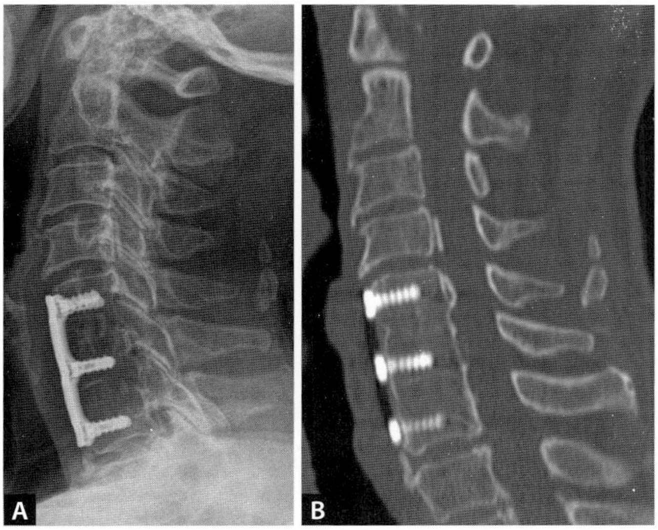

Figs. 29A and B: (A) Lateral radiograph and (B) sagittal CT image, of the cervical spine demonstrates osseous fusion of C5, C6, and C7 vertebral bodies with anterior instrumentation.

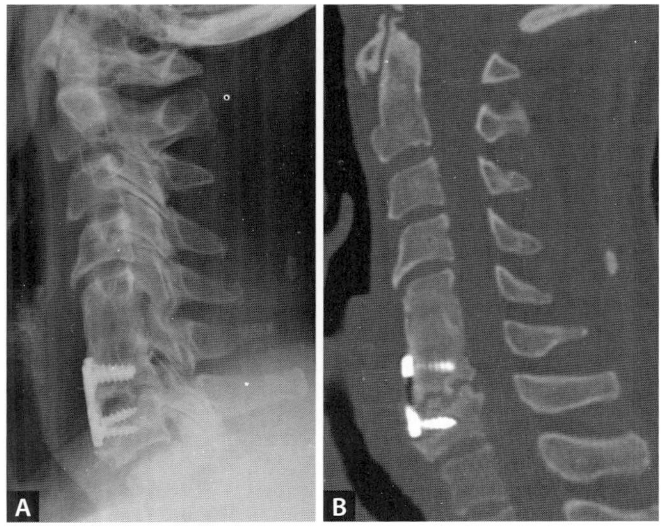

Figs. 30A and B: (A) Lateral radiograph and (B) sagittal CT image of the cervical spine demonstrates fusion of C5 and C6 vertebral bodies, anterior instrumentation of C6 and C7 with no clear bony bridging at this level.

occurs within 6–9 months and can be imaged with either radiographs or with CT imaging.[175] The choice of modality should be based on the clinical presentation of the patient with potential goals being to confirm fusion or to identify symptomatic pseudoarthrosis/nonunion that may require reoperation. Imaging of spinal fusion is overall unreliable with radiographs overestimating fusion.[176] The standard for determining fusion is direct evaluation during surgery.[177,178]

Radiographs for evaluating fusion are easy to obtain, inexpensive, and expose the patient to less radiation when compared with CT imaging. Overall, there is poor accuracy of radiographs for correctly identifying fusion. Tuli et al. found poor agreement between radiologists in evaluating for bony fusion in the cervical spine.[179] In the lumbar spine, radiographs have been reported to be 68% accurate when compared with direct observation during reoperation[180] similar to that seen by Blumenthal et al.[181] Brodsky et al. found discordant findings between imaging results and findings during reoperation with the frequency of disagreement of radiography, dynamic radiography, and CT imaging reported as 36%, 38%, and 43%, respectively.[182] Flexion-extension radiographs can be obtained to evaluate for motion in the fusion which would imply nonunion/pseudoarthrosis, however a degree of motion within the operative site may be normal. Multiples studies have been performed with differing criteria for normal motion with no consensus.[183-185] Radiostereometric analysis attempts to accurately measure motion in three dimensions as opposed to the two dimension available on radiographs. The technique requires implanted markers and its technical demands result in it not being widely used in clinical settings.[186,187]

CT imaging for evaluation of fusion has shown a proclivity for not overestimating bony fusion as compared to radiographs[188,189] however accuracy is improved for dynamic radiographs when quantitative motion analysis (QMA) is employed.[184,185] When CT imaging and dynamic radiography with QMA were used there was up to 100% positive predictive valve (PPV) of fusion.[184] Compared with direct visualization on reoperation in the lumbar spine for posterolateral instrumented fusion, there was 96% chance of fusion when facet joints and posterolateral gutters were fused on CT imaging with percentages decreasing to 89% when only posterolateral gutters and to 74% when only facet joints were fused.[190] While CT imaging is useful for evaluating bony fusion, there is increased radiation exposure to the patient and should be used in select cases.[191] MR imaging and it role in fusion evaluating is a work in progress although there are some reports of its utility.[177,192,193]

Imaging findings can be variable depending on the type of bone graft material used. Either allograft or autograft bone graft material can be used, each with its own advantages and disadvantages[194] and ability to promote fusion. In an attempt to promote bone growth, agents have been developed as either adjuncts to bone grafts or as osteoinducers. Knowledge of the procedure performed and the imaging appearance when these agents have been used is essential to avoid misinterpreting imaging studies. Ceramics are radiopaque and may interfere with visualization of bony fusion in early time frames.[195] Bone morphogenetic protein (BMP) affects all the phases of bone healing and can have an imaging appearance similar to infection or other complications despite good clinical outcome.[196,197] In patients receiving BMP who were followed with CT imaging, 100% of those having cervical level surgery had prevertebral soft tissue swelling which typically resolved by 6 weeks. Endplate resorption, a finding concerning for infection similar to prevertebral soft tissue swelling, occurred in all patients with cervical surgeries and 82% of lumbar levels, occurring by 1.5 months and resolving by 6 months.[198] 50% of patients demonstrated subsidence, which occurred from 3 months to 6 months. Cage migration and heterotopic bone formation are other features associated with the use of BMP.[198] Signal intensity abnormalities/bone marrow edema can also occur on MR imaging.[199]

Potential complications can arise in relation to hardware placement or infection either occurring at time of surgery or postoperatively. Pedicle screws should be evaluated for proper positioning and integrity. Ideal positioning consists of placement in the mid aspect of the pedicle and parallel to the superior endplate.[200] Suboptimal positioning can result in neural compression or vascular injury. Lucency surrounding the pedicle screw is a sign of loosening which can result in instability (Fig. 31).[201] Subsidence of interbody fusion devices of more than 3 mm into the adjacent vertebral body can result in radicular symptoms.[202-204] Following instrumented fusion and the resultant alteration to normal spinal biomechanics, immediate adjacent degenerative changes can occur at an accelerated rate. Infection can involve the osseous structures, disk space, surrounding soft tissues, and can result in epidural abscess formation (Figs. 32A to F).[205] Arachnoiditis is visualized using CT myelography or MR imaging and is manifested from clumping of the nerve roots of the cauda equine, peripheral displacement

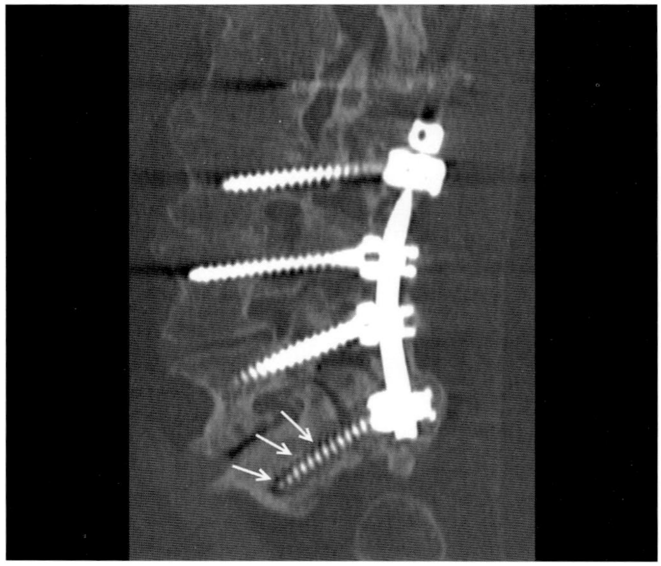

Fig. 31: Sagittal CT image with lucencies (white arrows) surrounding S1 pedicle screw representing hardware loosening. Apparent lucency adjacent to L2–L4 pedicle screws is beam-hardening artifact.

with an apparent empty thecal sac (Fig. 33), to a mass-like conglomerate of clumped nerve roots. Potential etiologies include spine surgery, infection, intradural blood products, and some myelographic agents.[206] It can be difficult to delineate the exact etiology of a postoperative fluid collection given variability of appearance based on age of the collection, protein content with the possibilities including pseudomeningocele (Figs. 34A and B) (varying signal intensity on MR imaging), epidural hematoma (T1 hyperintense in the subacute time-frame on MR imaging), or seroma formation (typically following fluid signal intensity on all pulse sequences).[175]

Vertebral Augmentation

Vertebral augmentation is where under fluoroscopic guidance polymethylmethacrylate is used to treat painful compression fractures.[207,208] The procedure can be performed by only injection (vertebroplasty) or with balloon assistance (kyphoplasty).[209] Methyl methacrylate radiographically is opaque, increased in attenuation on CT imaging, and low on all pulse sequences on MR images (Figs. 35A to D). Relief of pain and height restoration are measures of treatment success.[207-209] Symptomatic complication rate has been reported as 1–6%,[209,210] and include rib fractures, radicular pain, infection, bleeding, and complications relating to cement extravasation such

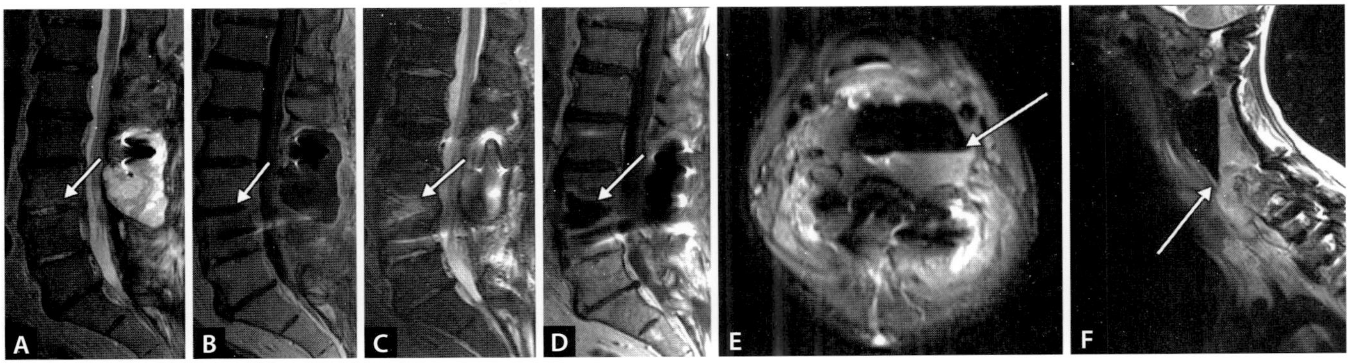

Figs. 32A to F: Sagittal STIR (A) and contrast enhanced sagittal T1 (B) images through lumbar spine show immediate postoperative changes; note appearance of L3–L4 disk space, white arrows, demonstrating minimal STIR hyperintensity. One month later, STIR (C) and contrast enhanced T1 (D) show development of discitis and osteomyelitis, white arrows. (E and F) Different patient operated for spinal neoplasm show a large anterior abscess with air-fluid level (white arrows), secondary to esophageal perforation from a cerclage wire.

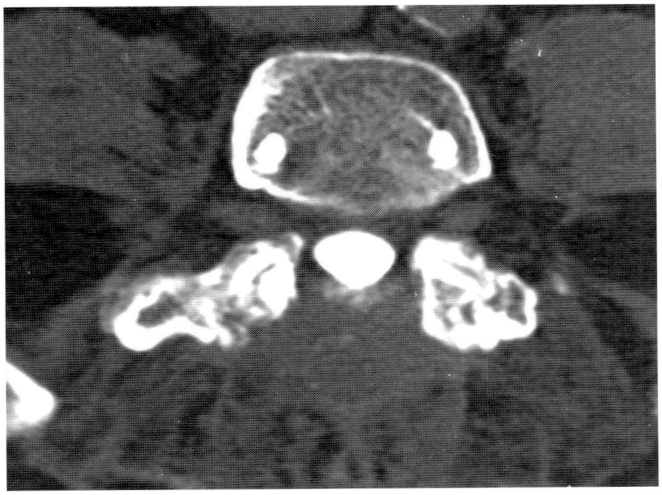

Fig. 33: Axial CT myelogram image lower lumbar spine with previous laminectomy and an apparent "empty thecal sac" representing arachnoiditis.

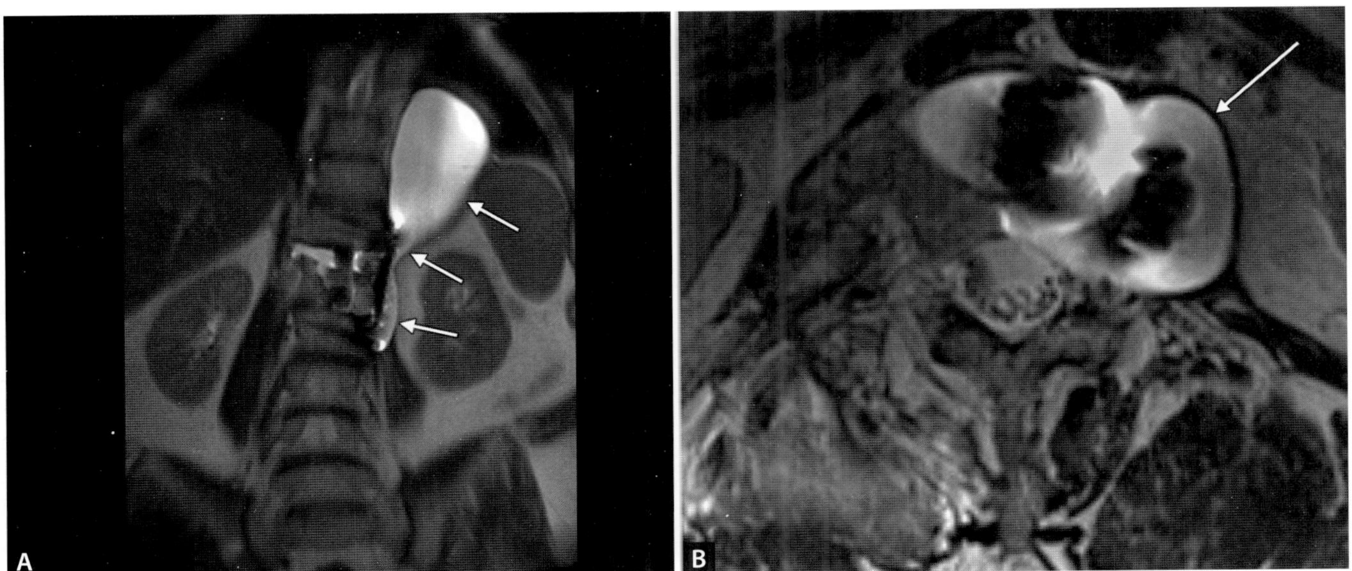

Figs. 34A and B: (A) Localizer; and (B) Axial T2-weighted image in a patient with previous back surgery shows a large pseudomeningocele centered at T12–L1 with superior paravertebral extension, white arrows

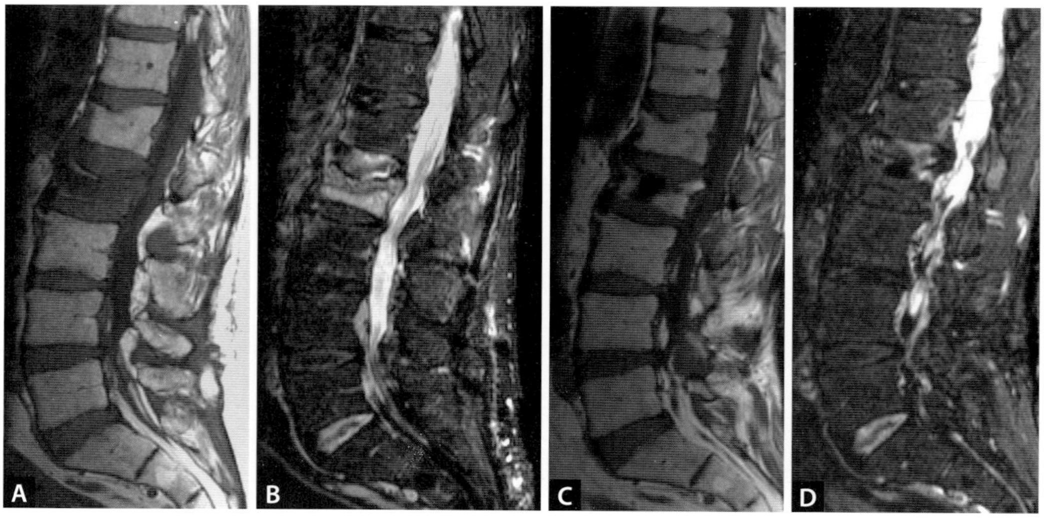

Figs. 35A to D: (A) Sagittal T1-weighted and (B) STIR images demonstrate acute compression deformity of L2 vertebral body. Minimal normal marrow is present on T1-weighted images and there is no posterior bowing of the vertebral body or paravertebral mass to suggest that this is a pathologic fracture. Subsequent imaging performed 18 months later demonstrates the presence of methylmethacrylate, low in signal intensity on both (C) T1; and (D) STIR images. Note return of normal marrow signal intensity on T1-weighted images.

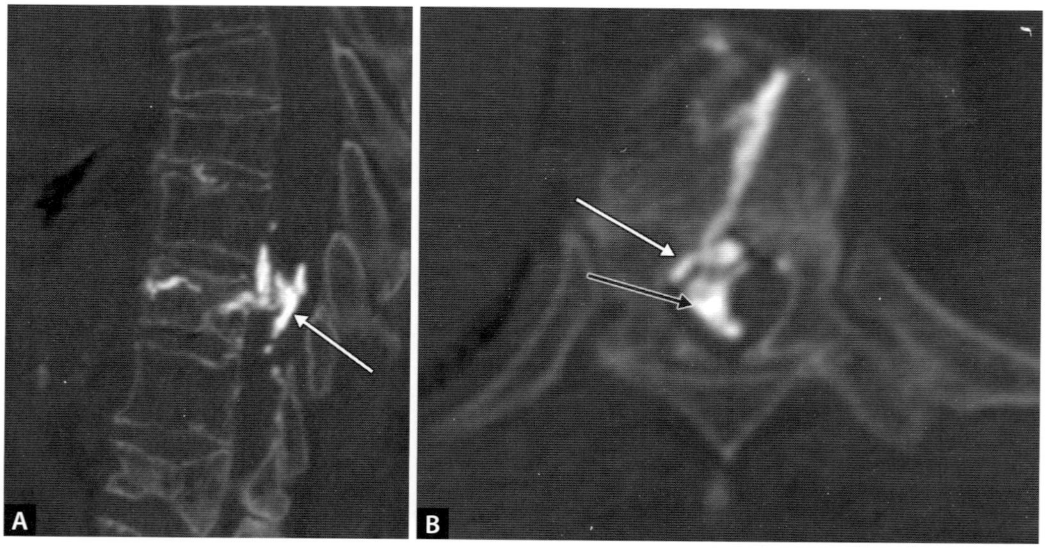

Figs. 36A and B: (A) Sagittal; and (B) Axial CT images through the mid thoracic spine show methylmethacrylate extravasation both into the canal, white arrows (A and B), as well as into the thecal sac, black arrow (B).

as pulmonary embolism and neural element mass effect with neurological deficit (Figs. 36A and B).

Degenerative Disk Disease

Imaging is frequently performed in patients who have undergone surgery for degenerative disk disease. Success rates for the surgical treatment of lumbar disk herniation has been reported to be as high as 90%[211] with success rates falling to 60–82% with repeat surgery.[212-214] Failed back surgery syndrome, resulting in pain and decreased function, can result from residual or recurrent disk herniation, arachnoiditis, stenosis, or incorrect level surgery.[215]

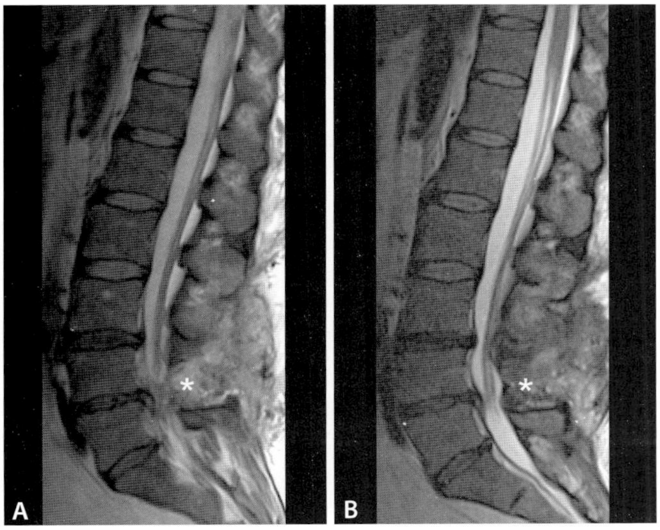

Figs. 37A and B: Sagittal T2-weighted images through the lumbar spine with immediate postoperative change (asterisk in A), which improves in appearance when reimaged 1 month later (asterisk in B) attesting to the difficulty in interpreting MR examinations in the immediate postoperative period.

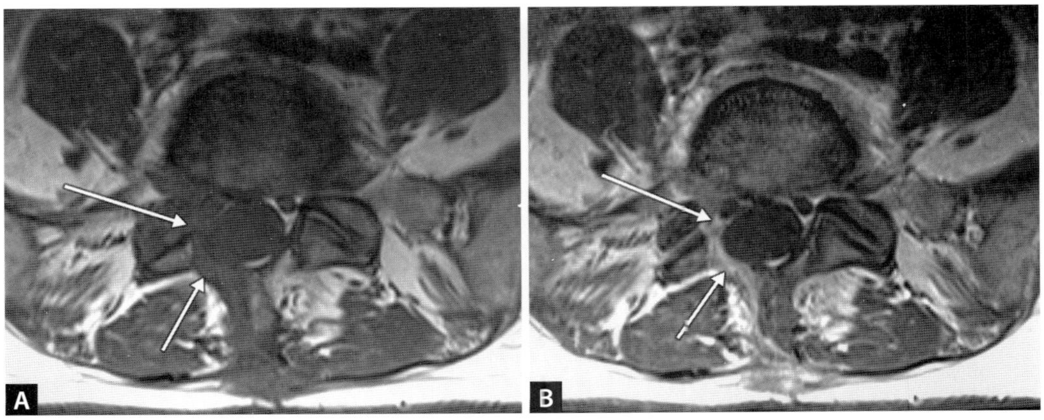

Figs. 38A and B: (A) Axial T1-weighted image with previous hemilaminectomy and low T1 signal intensity material in the right lateral aspect of the canal, arrows, which enhances arrows in (B) representing epidural scar tissue.

Imaging patients immediately or recently postoperative can be problematic as there is disruption of normal tissue planes, postoperative fluid, and enhancement which can be postoperative in nature (Figs. 37A and B). Additionally, enhancement of the intervertebral disk and vertebral endplates has been described.[216] In a study imaging patients following lumbar discectomy with good clinical outcome at 6 weeks and 6 months, initial enhancement was present in paraspinal musculature, facet joints, nerve roots, and disk space with the degree of enhancement decreasing over time. All patients had enhancing epidural scar at baseline with a decrease to 15% of patients by 6 months.[217] In a study by Ross et al., patients were imaged following discectomy at 6 month and 12 months following the procedure and classified scar into the anterior epidural space (96% of patients) and/or the posterior epidural space (86% of patients). At follow-up epidural scar tissue classified as anterior or posterior was unchanged in 85% and 75% of patients respectively with the remaining patients demonstrating a decrease (Figs. 38A and B).[218]

Reports are conflicting as whether enhancing epidural scar can result in pain either by encasement and compression or is physiologic/healing in nature. Psychosocial factors were correlated more with patients symptoms rather than the presence of epidural scar by

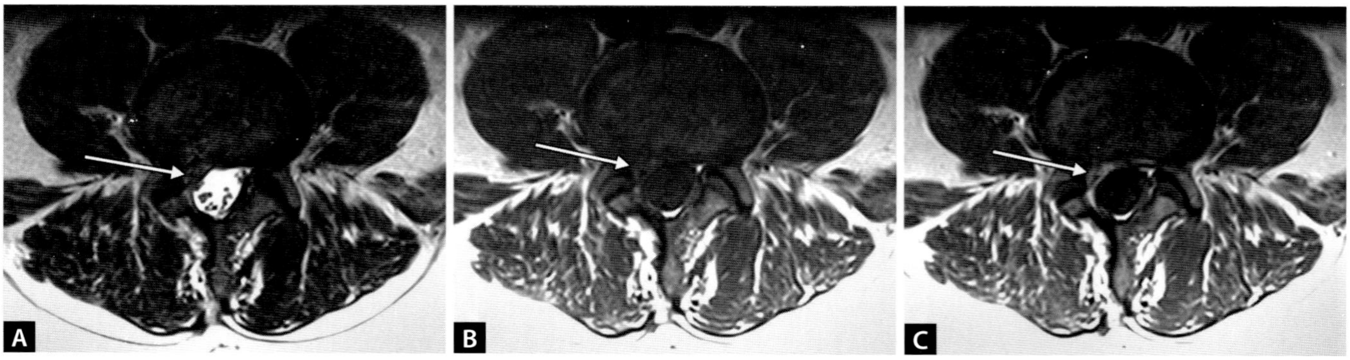

Figs. 39A to C: (A) Axial T2; and (B) Axial T1-weighted images shows low signal intensity extradural material, white arrows, representing either recurrent disk material or scar. (C) T1-weighted image with contrast, demonstrates enhancement, white arrow, representing scar tissue rather than disk material.

Coskun et al.[219] In a study of postoperative patients of which 20 were asymptomatic and 20 were experiencing recurrent pain, no correlation was found between symptoms and degree of epidural scar when imaged by CT.[220] Conversely, epidural scar was found in patients with recurrent radicular pain,[221] its presence was associated with poor outcome following reoperation,[222] and the absence of epidural scar tissue in patients requiring reoperation (along with young age, female gender, and employment status) was associated with good clinical outcome.[223] Nerve root enhancement has been found to correlate with radiculopathy in patients following surgery with a sensitivity of 91.7% and a specificity of 73.2%.[224]

Both CT[225,226] and MR imaging play a role in differentiating residual or recurrent disk herniation from epidural scar tissue however MR is the preferred modality (Figs. 39A to C). When compared with surgical findings in 22 patients undergoing reoperation, CT with intravenous contrast was able to differentiate recurrent herniated disk versus epidural scar in 74% of patients while noncontrast CT imaging was correct 43% of the time.[225]

Compartments

Pathology in spine imaging can be classified based on the anatomical compartments consisting of extradural, intradural extramedullary, and intramedullary. Each compartment possesses a large differential of potential pathologic entities but can be effectively narrowed when combined with the clinical presentation of the patient and laboratory data. The extradural compartment is external to the dura and the pathologic process often extends from the adjacent vertebral body or disk space. The intradural extramedullary compartment contains the contents of the thecal sac excluding the spinal cord. The intramedullary compartment of the spine consists of the spinal cord itself and pia. Following the introduction of MR imaging into clinical use its utility in spine imaging became apparent rapidly.[227-229] Takemoto et al. demonstrated the ability of MR imaging to correctly identify the compartment of origin in 29 patients with spinal neoplasm.[230] Potentially involving more than one compartment, vascular lesions of the spine can be divided into: (1) neoplasms such as hemangioblastoma and cavernoma, (2) aneurysm, and (3) vascular malformation including arteriovenous fistulas and malformations of various spinal compartments.[231]

Extradural and Marrow Imaging

Spine imaging is performed for multiple different indications from evaluating low back pain, screening for metastatic disease, to evaluating neurological symptoms in patients with known malignancies. Regardless of the indication or pre-existing medical conditions that a patient may possess, abnormalities of the marrow or adjacent compartments will inevitably be encountered. While some marrow lesions will be clearly pathologic, other scenarios can be more difficult to interpret including heterogeneous marrow, scattered foci of low T1 signal intensity in a patient without a cancer history, the differentiation of benign versus pathologic compression fracture, or degenerative endplate changes versus early infection.

Although relatively straightforward to compartmentalize in terms of the relationship to the dura and spinal cord, there are rare occasions where it can be difficult to determine the epicenter of the pathologic

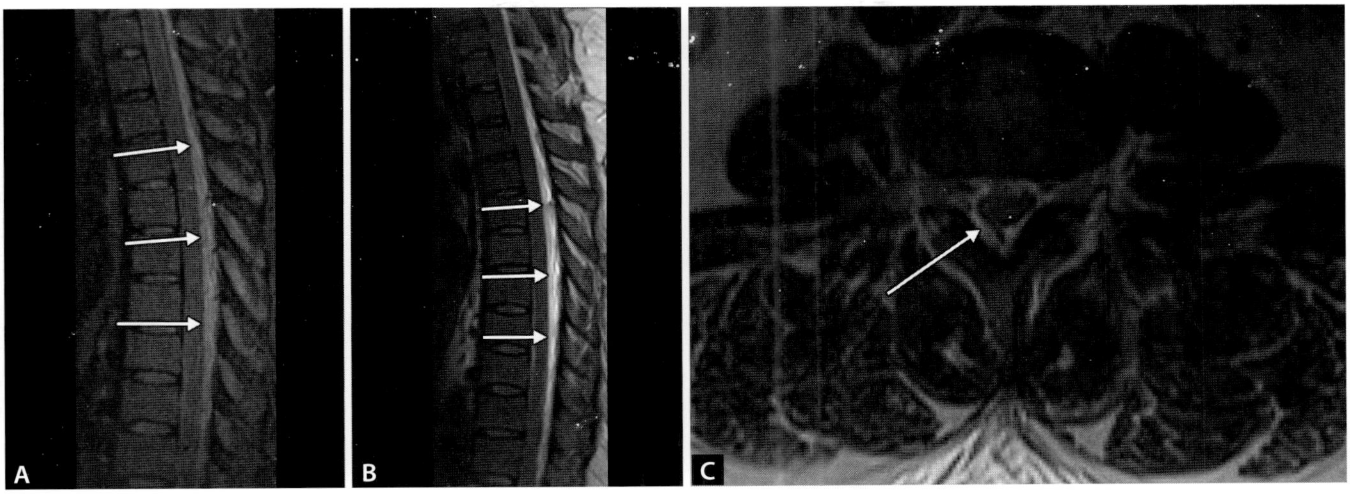

Figs. 40A to C: (A) Sagittal STIR; (B) T2; and (C) Axial T2-weighted images, shows prominence of the epidural plexus (white arrows) in a patient with CSF hypotension.

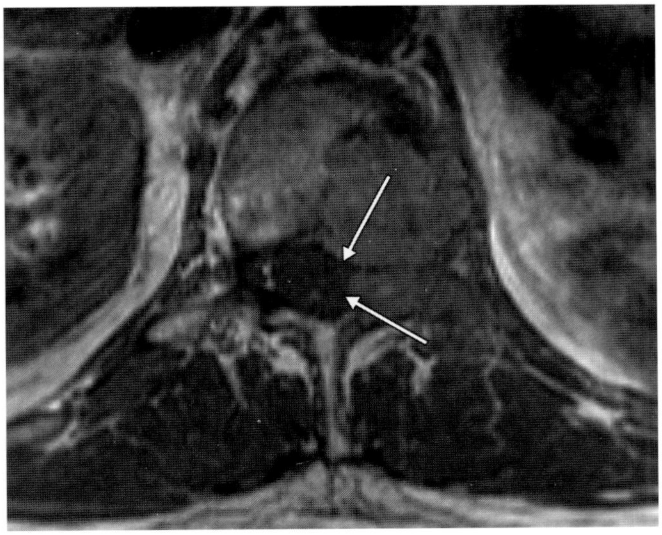

Fig. 41: Axial T1-weighted noncontrast image with anterior epidural extension of osseous metastatic disease, white arrows with mild mass effect on the thecal sac and anterior midline tenting.

process. Also potentially confounding is when a normal structure is accentuated, for example prominence of the epidural venous plexus (Figs. 40A to C).[232] Epidural extension anterior is frequently tented at the midline due to the midline septum which attaches the posterior longitudinal ligament with the adjacent vertebral body (Fig. 41). A lesion located posteriorly in the epidural space can form a curvilinear interface with the adjacent epidural fat and displace the thecal sac in a smooth fashion (Figs. 42A to D). Additionally, a low T2 signal intensity band separating the extradural process from the thecal sac has been described.[230] CT imaging is useful for further defining osseous anatomy and CT myelography can be obtained when MR imaging is contraindicated, suboptimal from metallic artifact, or as an adjunct to MR imaging (*see* Figs. 14A and B).

The epidural space contains fat, connective tissue, and veins and surrounds the dura which extends from the foramen magnum to the coccyx.[5] The anterior epidural space is bordered anteriorly by the posterior longitudinal ligament that is firmly attached to the posterior vertebral bodies by a midline septum that results in a characteristic

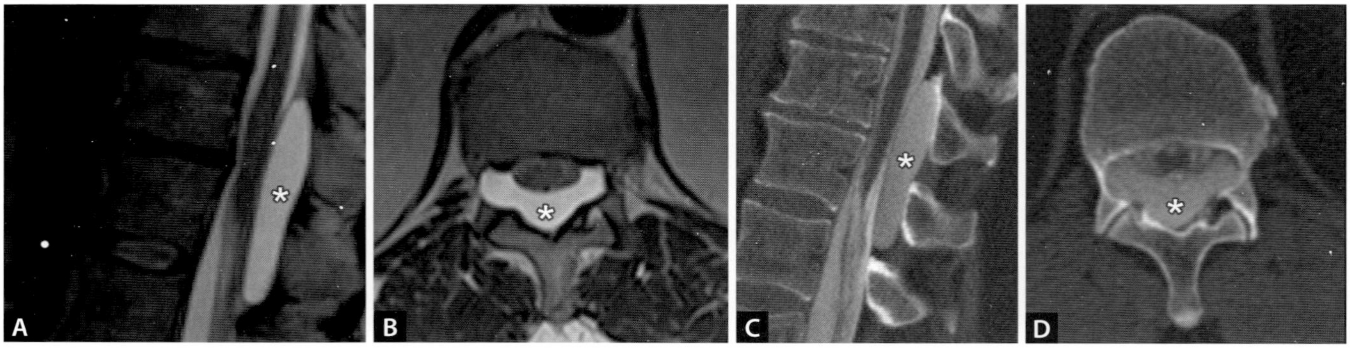

Figs. 42A to D: Posterior epidural/extradural arachnoid cyst, asterisk, on sagittal and axial T2-weighted images (A and B), and sagittal and axial CT myelogram images (C and D) demonstrate capping of the epidural fat which is typical for a posteriorly located epidural process. Filling of the cyst on CT myelogram images can be from a small communication of the cyst with the subarachnoid space or can occur with delayed imaging.

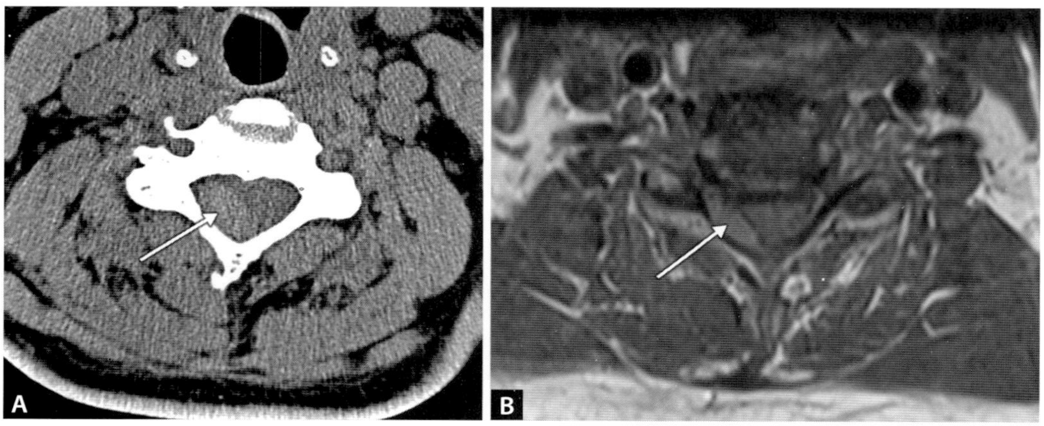

Figs. 43A and B: (A) Axial CT scan of the cervical spine shows faint increased attenuation, white arrow, representing an epidural hematoma, better seen on axial T1-weighted image (white arrow, B).

tented appearance of the epidural process however with infection, epidural hematoma, or advanced metastatic disease this configuration can be altered with resultant extension across the midline.[233,234] Extradural pathology can consist of metastatic disease, infection, hematoma (Figs. 43A and B), degenerative disk disease (including osteophytes and disk protrusions) (Figs. 44A to D), and primary bone neoplasms.[235]

Marrow age-related changes: Before interpreting MR imaging of the spine, it is important to discuss age-related changes that occur given that red marrow has low T1 signal intensity similar to pathologic marrow infiltration. At birth, the spine contains predominantly red marrow which has low signal intensity on T1 weighted images. Over time, there is development of a majority of fatty marrow which is hyperintense on T1 weighted imaging, with this transition typically occurring by the age of 25.[47] Overall, the appearance of marrow signal intensity can vary among different individuals but as a rule marrow on T1 weighted images that is of lower signal intensity than muscle or the disk space is likely pathologic.[236-238]

Normal marrow should be hyperintense on T1-weighted images as compared to disk or muscle, intermediate to hyperintense signal intensity on T2-weighted images compared to muscle, and low in signal intensity on STIR or fat-saturated images although the exact signal intensity is dependent on the ratio of yellow and red marrow elements in the vertebral body.[238] Abnormal marrow generally results in a loss if T1 hyperintensity with the degree ranging from a global loss of T1 signal

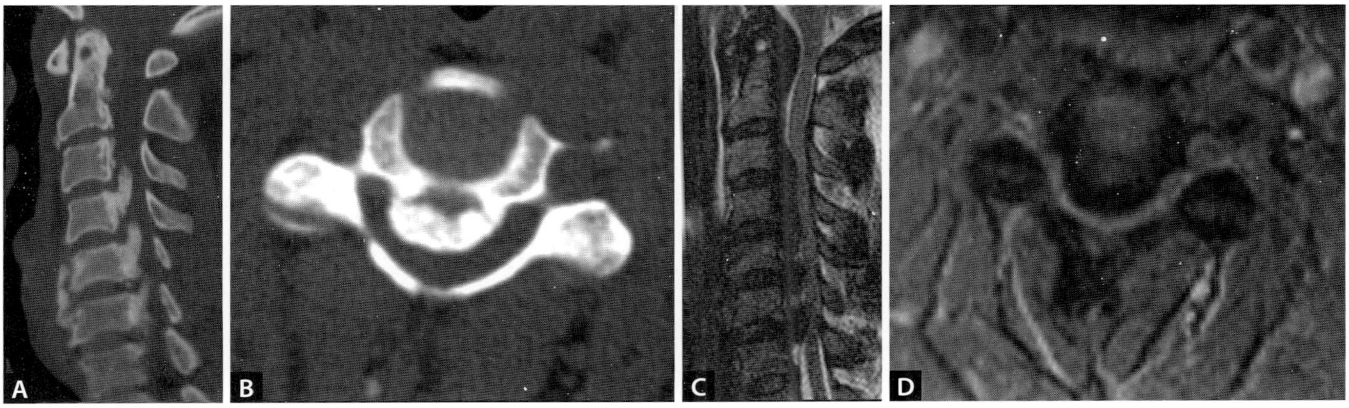

Figs. 44A to D: Sagittal and axial CT (A and B) and T2-weighted MR images (C and D) images demonstrates ossification of the posterior longitudinal ligament with canal compromise and spinal cord flattening.

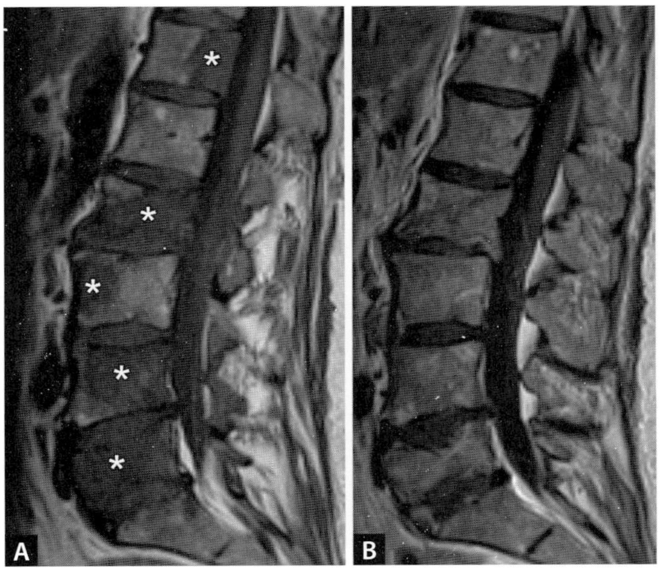

Figs. 45A and B: The necessity of having precontrast images is demonstrated: multiple osseous metastatic foci, asterisks in (A) noncontrast T1-weighted image, are poorly visualized following contrast administration (B).

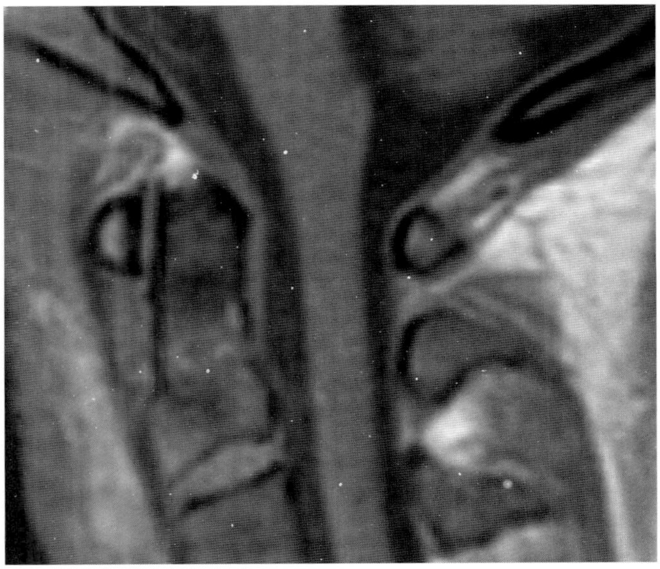

Fig. 46: Sagittal T1-weighted image scanned on a 3T magnet demonstrating low T1 signal of the marrow which can be confused for pathologic marrow infiltration.

intensity to a discreet focus. Accuracy in regards to marrow being abnormal with low T1 signal intensity in relation to disk is 98% and to muscle is 94%. Pathologic marrow infiltration simplistically can be thought of involving increased water content, manifested by both T2 and STIR hyperintensity.[239] Administration of contrast is useful for characterizing intradural and epidural disease however enhancement of a vertebral body lesion can mask its presence if not performed with fat-saturation or if pre-contrast T1-weighted images are also not obtained for comparison (Figs. 45A and B).[240,241] In addition to the age-dependent appearance of bone marrow on MR imaging, technical factors can also result in varying appearances which can be difficult to differentiate from pathology. Higher field strength magnets (3 tesla) can result in lower signal intensity of bone marrow on T1-weighted images which can be mistaken for pathologic marrow infiltration (Fig. 46).[242]

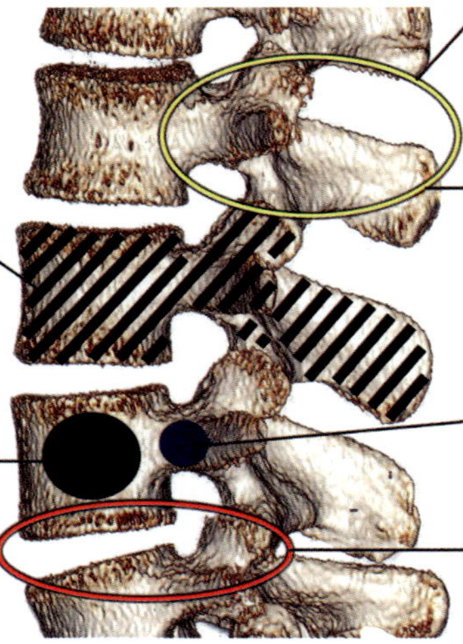

Fig. 47: Location and distribution-based differential of potential pathological entities that can involve vertebral bodies.

Distribution of marrow abnormalities: When faced with an abnormality of the marrow, its distribution, quantity (single or multiple), and geographic location is helpful for forming a differential diagnosis and also for determining the next step be it doing nothing, follow-up imaging to document stability or with a different modality, or obtaining tissue for definitive diagnosis to guide treatment (Fig. 47).[243-245]

Focal T1 hyperintensities are typically benign findings representing fatty marrow or hemangioma (Figs. 48A to D) although melanoma metastases (Fig. 49),[246] blood products,[247] and Paget Disease[248] can be hyperintense on T1-weighted images. Diffuse involvement of the vertebral body by T1 hyperintensity can be from previous radiation therapy (Figs. 50A to C), demineralization, or chronic malnutrition.

Low signal intensity on T1-weighted images when centered at opposing endplates is either degenerative in nature, infectious, or rarely secondary to amyloid infiltration. When focal within the vertebral body possibilities include atypical hemangiomas (Figs. 51A to D), trauma/fracture, neoplasm, or fibrous dysplasia (Figs. 52A to D) and when within the posterior elements consider trauma or primary bone neoplasm. Diffuse low T1 signal intensity within a vertebral body can represent anemia with red marrow replacement (Fig. 53), neoplasm, sarcoid (Figs. 54A and B), and other infiltrative disorders resulting in marrow replacement.[243] Paget disease can have a variable appearance on MR imaging (Figs. 55A to C).[244]

Metastatic disease: There are many options for screening for spinal metastatic disease with patterns of disease consisting of lytic (commonly lung, breast, kidney, thyroid, and renal), blastic (commonly breast and prostate origins), or a combination of both types. Based on these patterns and the mechanisms of detection of the differing modalities, there is no single ideal modality for all clinical scenarios. Radiographs require a 30–75% change in normal appearing osseous structures for visualization of metastatic disease[249,250] potentially resulting in delayed visualization of 4–12 months compared with other modalities.[251] Overlapping structures can simulate pathology (Figs. 56A to C). Bone scans using technetium-99m methylene diphosphonate can visualize a 5–10% change in normal bone[252] however the findings on bone scans are nonspecific and are blood flow and osteoblast dependent. Bone scans are useful for breast, lung, and prostate cancer. Aggressive or lytic metastases (notably from multiple myeloma, kidney, and thyroid cancers) can present as a focal area of lack of radiotracer uptake or "cold" lesion with blastic metastases presenting as focal increased radiotracer uptake or as a superscan in diffuse metastatic disease (Figs. 57A to C).[253] Given the nonspecific nature of bone scans where abnormal uptake can be neoplastic, inflammatory, or traumatic in nature, correlation with additional imaging is frequently necessary.[254,255] CT imaging demonstrates increased body detail and can visualize smaller degrees of osseous destruction as compared with radiography, with sensitivity ranging from 71–100%.[249] MR imaging can directly evaluate bone marrow and can better

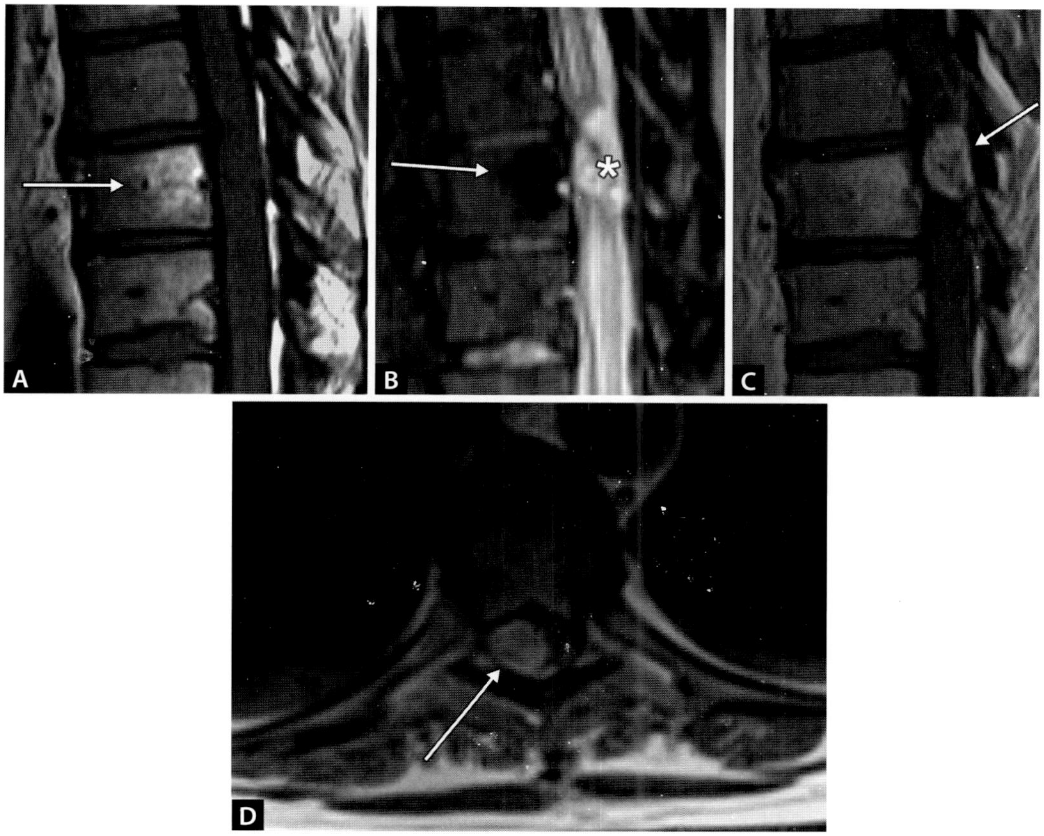

Figs. 48A to D: (A). Noncontrast T1-weighted image shows a T1 hyperintense marrow lesion representing a hemangioma, arrow. Due to fat content, the hemangioma loses signal and becomes hypointense on STIR image (B), arrow. Mixed signal intensity intradural extramedullary mass, asterisk, becomes more apparent. With contrast (C and D), there is enhancement of the intradural extramedullary mass, arrows, which upon resection was a meningioma.

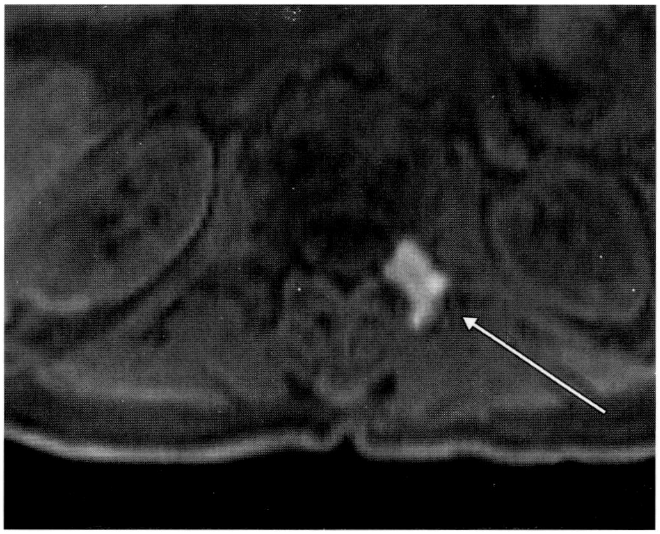

Fig. 49: Fat-saturated noncontrast T1-weighted image in a patient with melanoma and metastatic disease. Increased T1 signal intensity in the left pedicle and facet of L2, white arrow, is concerning for melanoma metastases.

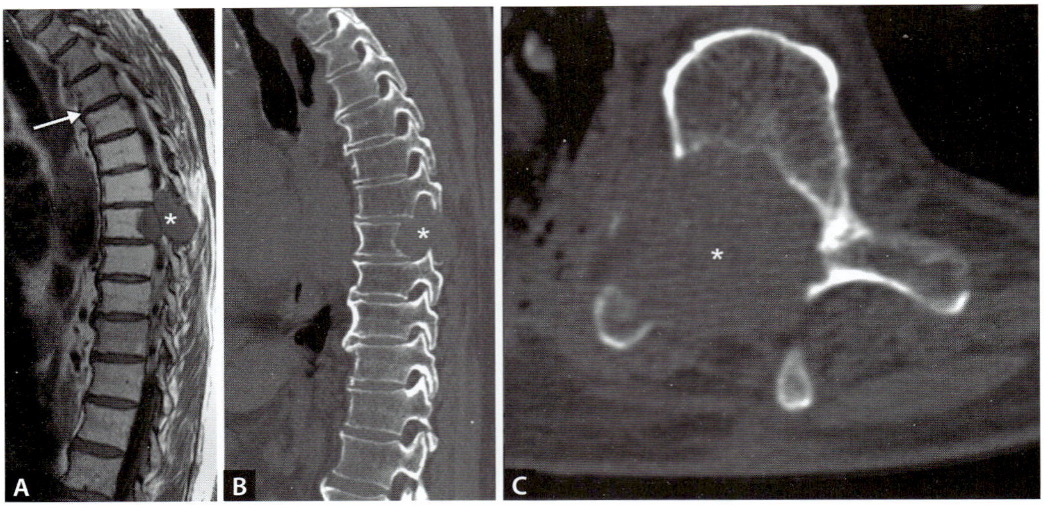

Figs. 50A to C: (A) Sagittal T1-weighted image demonstrates a large metastatic focus in the thoracic spine with posterior element involvement, asterisk. There is a background of T1 hyperintensity of the marrow, superior margin delineated with the white arrow, from previous radiation therapy. (B) Sagittal; and (C) Axial CT images show a large lytic lesion (asterisk), with the soft tissue component better visualized on the MR image.

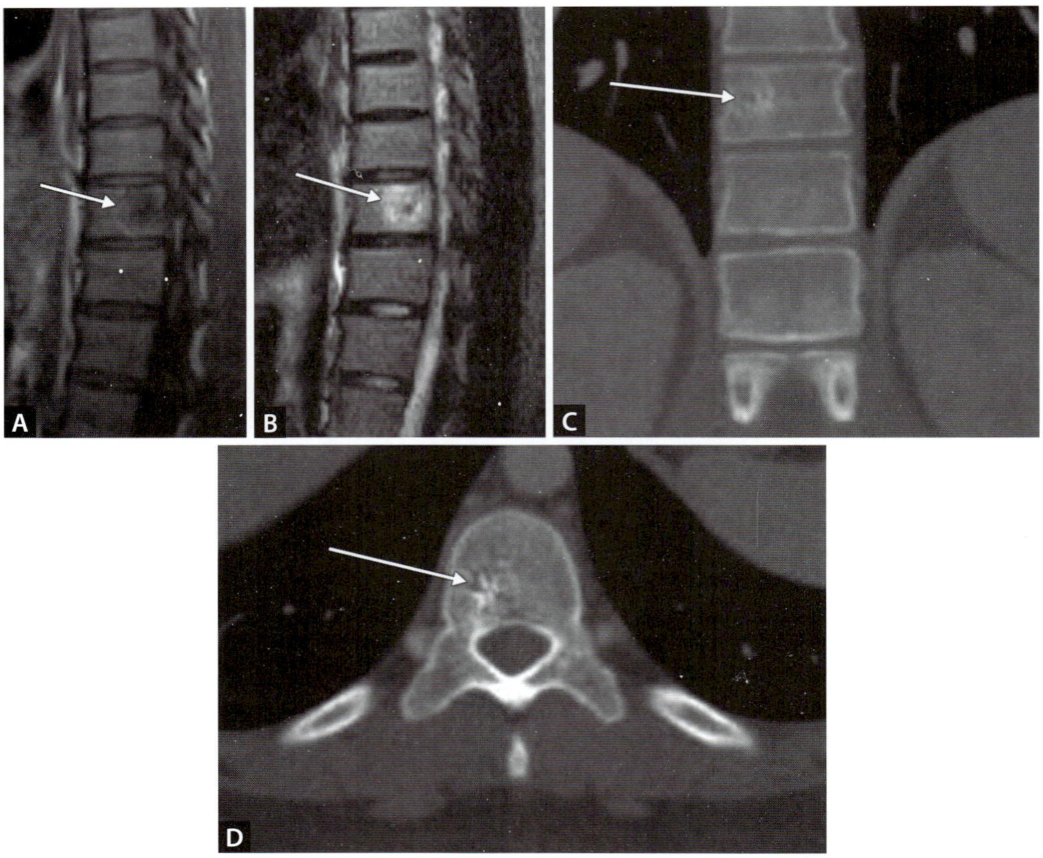

Figs. 51A to D: Sagittal T1-weighted image (A) with a low signal intensity lesion, arrow, that is hyperintense on STIR image (B), arrow, overall concerning for pathologic marrow infiltration. Arrows on CT images (C and D) demonstrate coarsened trabeculae, a characteristic finding for a hemangioma or an atypical hemangioma in this case given its low T1 signal intensity.

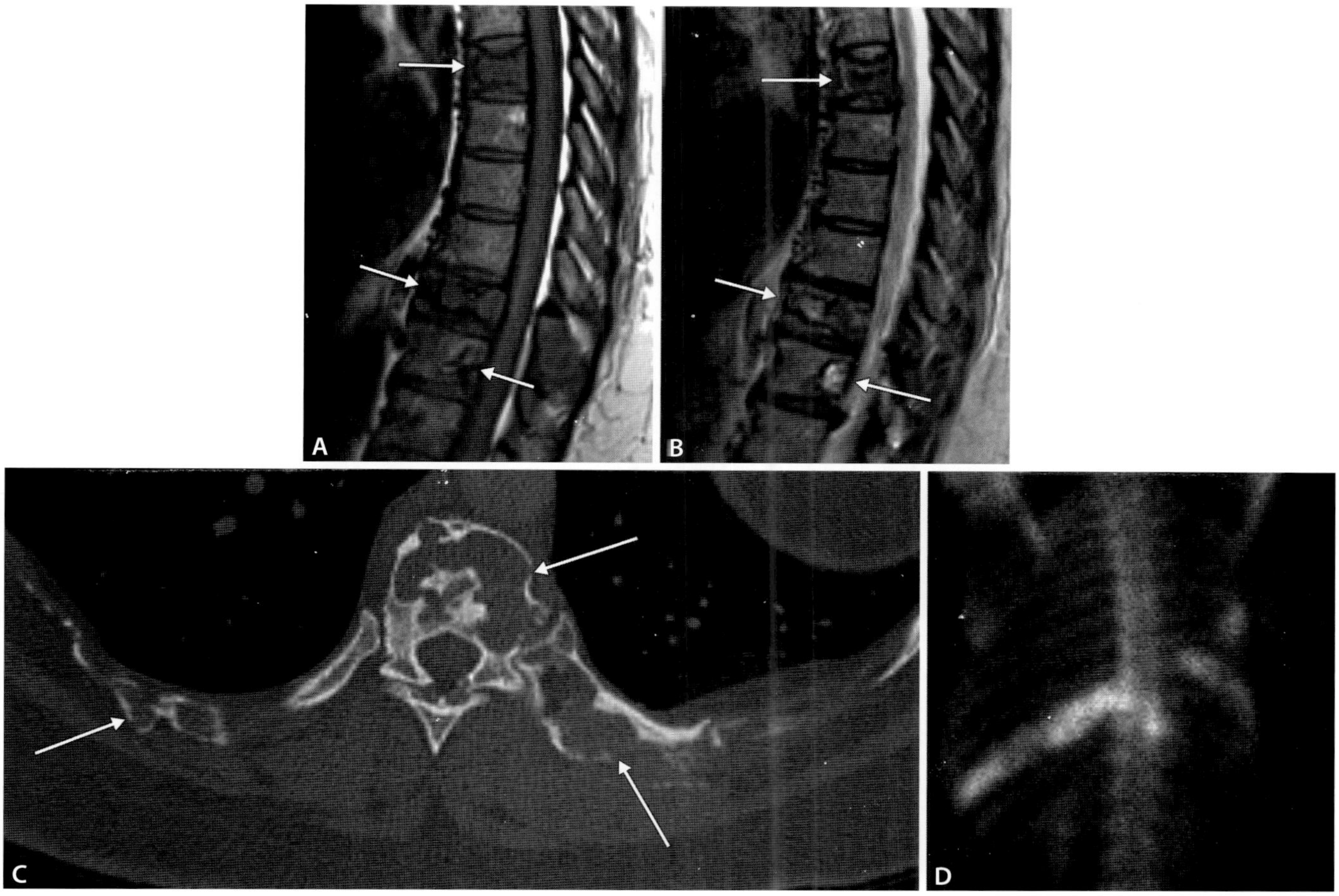

Figs. 52A to D: (A) Sagittal T1 and (B) sagittal T2 images demonstrate multiple foci of abnormal marrow, T1 hypointensity and both T2 hyper and hypointensity, arrows. (C) Axial CT image, demonstrates corresponding bony expansion with a predominantly lytic pattern. (D) Bone scan shows increased radiotracer uptake in this patient with fibrous dysplasia.

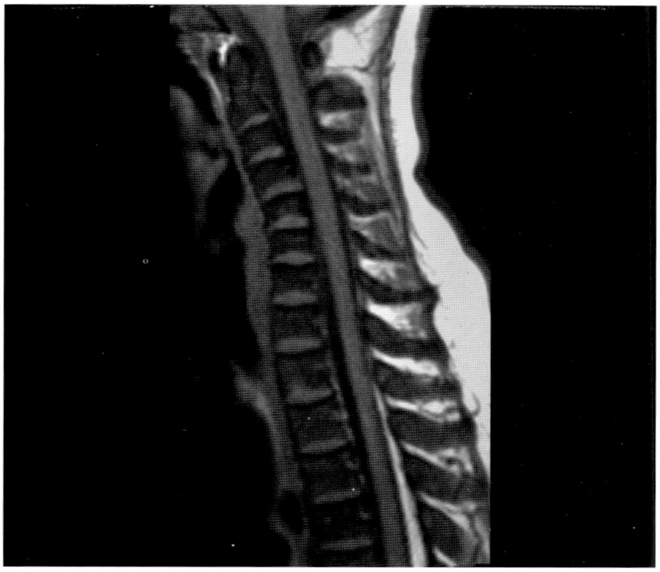

Fig. 53: Sagittal T1-weighted image shows marked decreased signal intensity of the marrow in this patient with sickle cell disease which could otherwise be interpreted as diffuse metastatic disease.

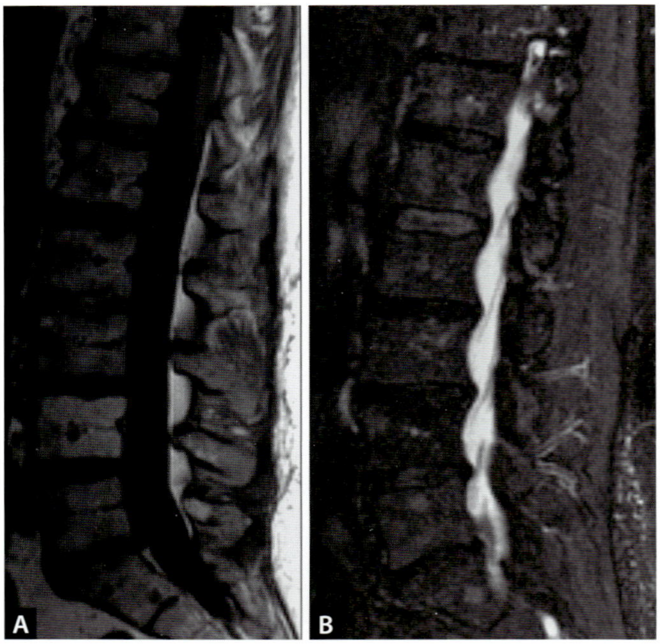

Figs. 54A and B: (A) Sagittal T1 and (B) sagittal STIR show multiple foci of abnormal marrow throughout multiple vertebral bodies. Subsequent biopsy revealed sarcoid.

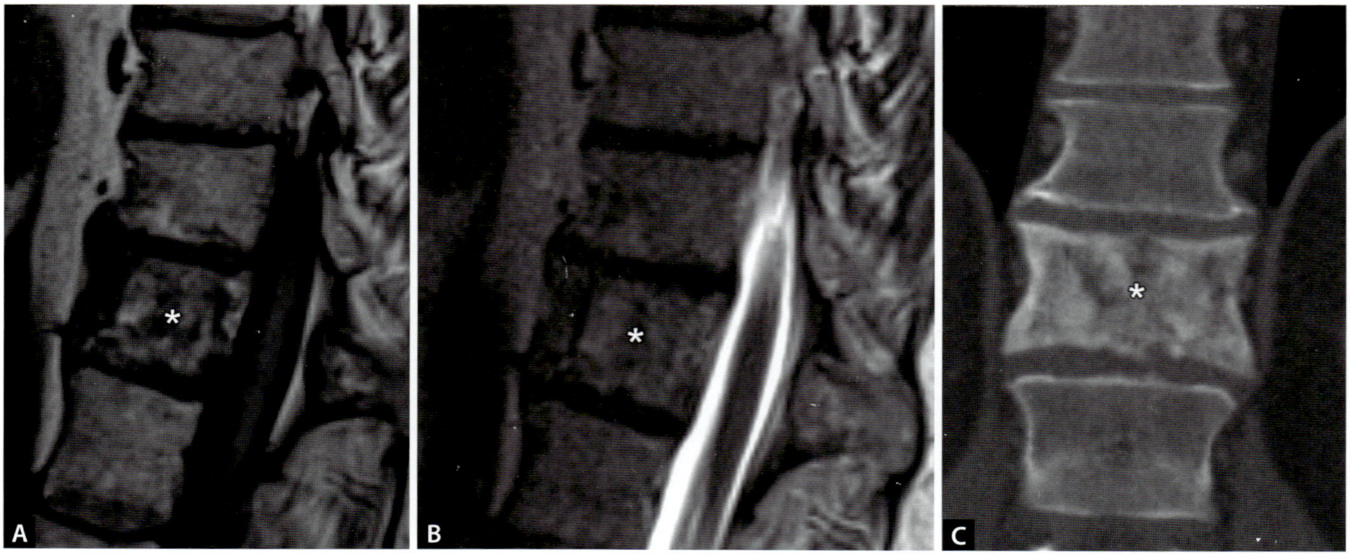

Figs. 55A to C: Sagittal T1-weighted image (A) demonstrates mixed signal intensity, asterisk, in T12 vertebral body. There is only minimal STIR hyperintensity, (B) asterisk. Coronal CT image, (C) demonstrates sclerosis and increased size of the vertebral body, asterisk, supporting a diagnosis of Paget disease.

delineate soft-tissue extension of neoplasm and epidural extension of disease as well as potential mass effect on the spinal cord (Figs. 58 and 59).

Positron emission tomography (PET) imaging can be performed alone or in conjunction with CT (PET/CT). Various tracers can be used for disease localization, the most commonly used being 18F Fluorodeoxyglucose (18F-FDG) which is a glucose analog and taken up in metabolically active processes including neoplasm, infection, inflammation, and degenerative changes.[256,257] There is increased sensitivity for lytic type metastases as opposed to blastic metastases. Red marrow is 18F-FDG avid which may preclude identification of coexisting osseous metastatic disease.[258]

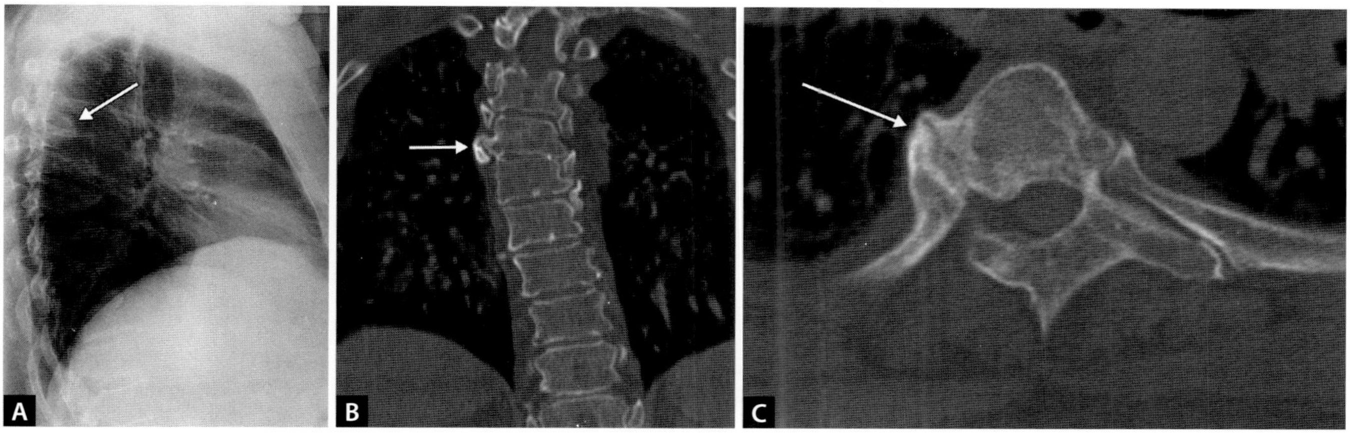

Figs. 56A to C: (A) Lateral chest radiograph, demonstrates an apparent sclerotic lesion upper thoracic spine, white arrow. (B) Coronal; and (C) axial CT images demonstrate that the abnormality was due to overlapping structures (a limitation of radiographs) from degenerative change centered at the costovertebral joint, white arrows.

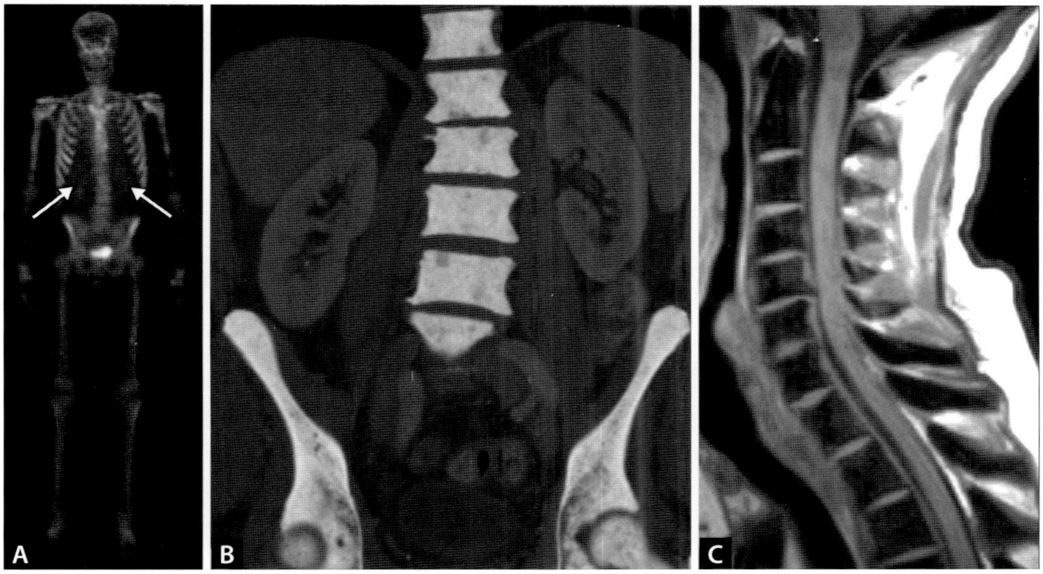

Figs. 57A to C: Bone scan performed in a patient with prostate cancer (A) demonstrating lack of radiotracer uptake in the kidneys, arrows, representing diffuse metastatic disease—a "superscan". In the same patient: Coronal CT scan image (B) demonstrates diffuse sclerosis in all imaged osseous structures. Sagittal T1-weighted image (C) demonstrates diffuse low T1 signal intensity in the marrow, lower than that of the disk space and musculature, representing diffuse metastatic disease.

Multiple studies have compared the sensitivity and specificity of different modalities and different primary neoplasms. Liu et al. compared PET alone with CT imaging in cervical cancer and found sensitivity and specificity of PET at 93.3% and 99.5% respectively as opposed to CT alone with sensitivity and specificity of 33.3% and 99.1% respectively.[259] For breast cancer, PET alone was 87% sensitive and 92% specific as opposed to CT alone which was 67% sensitive and 95% specific.[260] Costelloe et al.[261] performed a review of PET compared with bone scans[260,262-270] and found median sensitivity and specificity for PET of 83.9% and 95.8% respectively and sensitivity and specificity for bone scan of 78% and 91.5%, respectively.[261] Sensitivity and specificity are improved when PET/CT

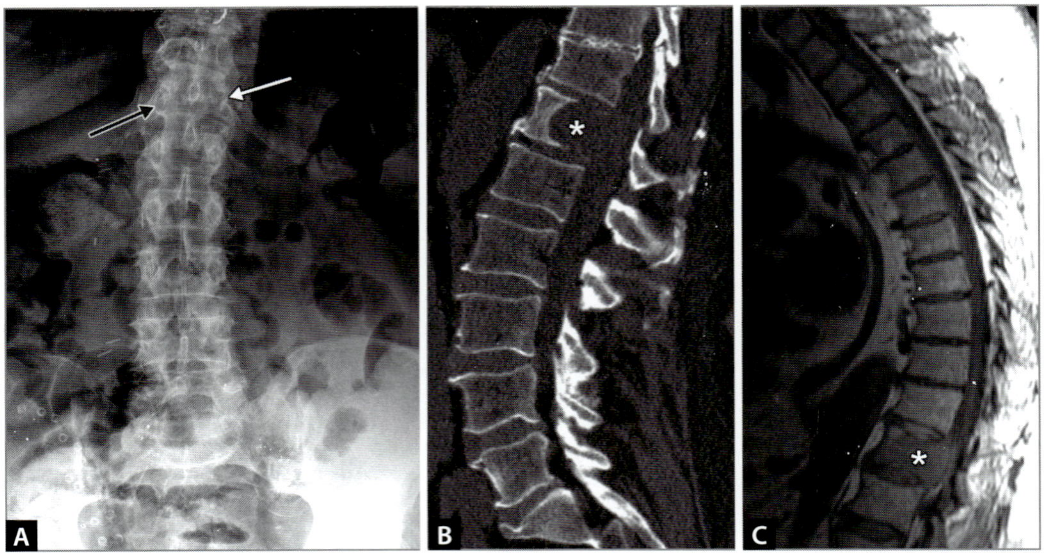

Figs. 58A to C: (A) Frontal radiograph of the lumbar spine in a patient with renal cell carcinoma. Normal pedicle viewed en face, black arrow, and nonvisualized pedicle, white arrow, secondary to metastatic disease. (B) Sagittal CT; and (C) Sagittal T1-weighted image in same patient demonstrate additional vertebral body involvement not readily apparent on the radiograph, asterisks.

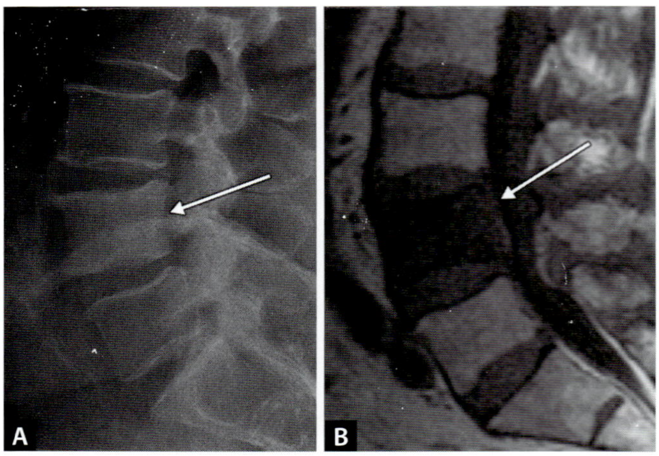

Figs. 59A and B: Lateral radiograph (A) with increased density of L4 vertebral body, arrow, and corresponding low T1 signal intensity, arrow (B), representing blastic metastases.

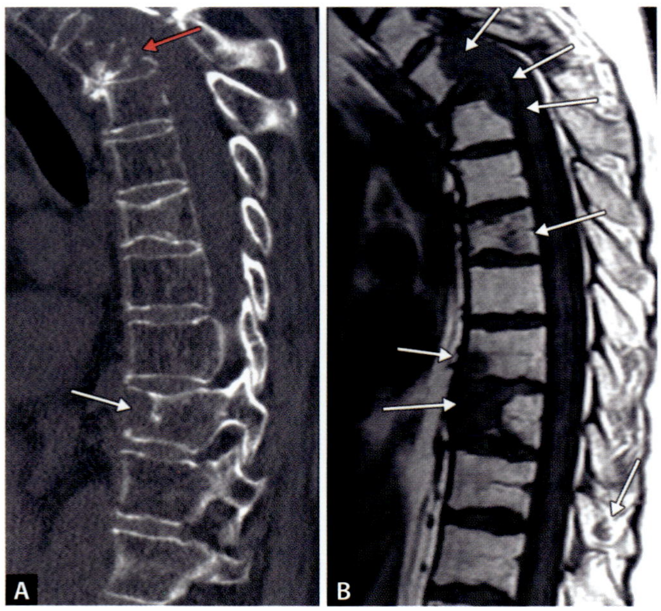

Figs. 60A and B: Pathologic compression fracture of T2 vertebral body, red arrow in image (A) and additional metastases T8, white arrow, on this sagittal CT image. Additional metastasis better visualized with MR imaging, white arrows in image (B).

is used.[271,272] Whole body MR imaging for purposes of evaluation for metastatic disease when compared with PET/CT has comparable specificities and sensitivities.[272-274]

A common scenario is whether a fracture is pathologic or osteoporotic in nature. There is no imaging modality which can answer this question with 100% certainty although there are MR imaging characteristics which can be helpful. Imaging findings favoring a pathologic compression fracture include convex posterior border of the affected vertebral body, posterior element/pedicle involvement, epidural mass, and multiple level involvement (Figs. 60A and B). Findings favoring a benign

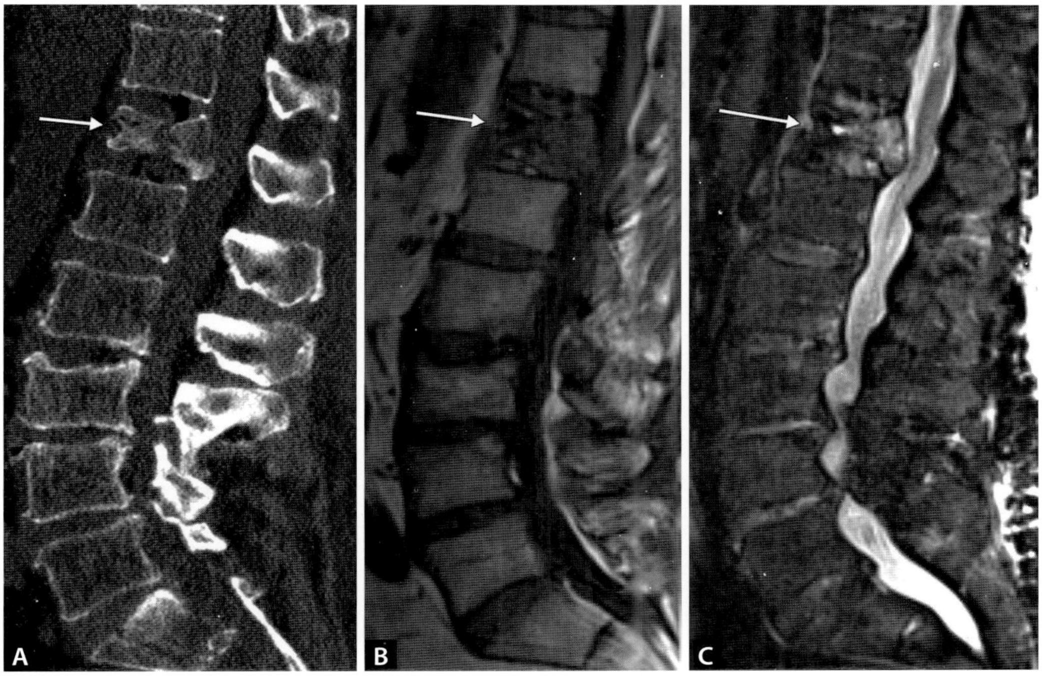

Figs. 61A to C: (A) Sagittal CT image, white arrow, demonstrates an acute compression fracture of T12. Additional remote appearing compression fracture of L3. (B) Sagittal T1; and (C) STIR demonstrates low T1 and increased STIR signal intensity within T12 vertebral body, arrows, with no paravertebral mass or additional focus of marrow signal abnormality. Subsequent biopsy revealed no malignancy.

osteoporotic compression fracture include retropulsed fracture fragments, the presence of normal marrow as opposed to complete marrow replacement in pathologic fracture (Figs. 35 and 61)[275] and the fluid cleft sign (Figs. 62A and B) which is more likely be in osteoporotic compression fractures.[276] Conflicting results have been presented for discriminated benign versus osteoporotic compression fractures with diffusion-weighted images[41,277] and with MR perfusion imaging.[42]

Additionally, once the diagnosis of osseous metastatic disease is made treatment can include radiation therapy which results in alterations in marrow signal intensity and other potential complications. Knowledge of these changes is important for interpreting subsequent treatment monitoring imaging. T1-weighted images gradually progress to fatty replacement/T1 hyperintensity occurring from 3–6 weeks following treatment with the marrow pattern potentially being homogenous or band-like in configuration. Minimal increased T2 signal intensity of the marrow can occur within 3 weeks following therapy which is felt to represent edema. Heterogeneity on T2-weighted images progresses after this time point. STIR

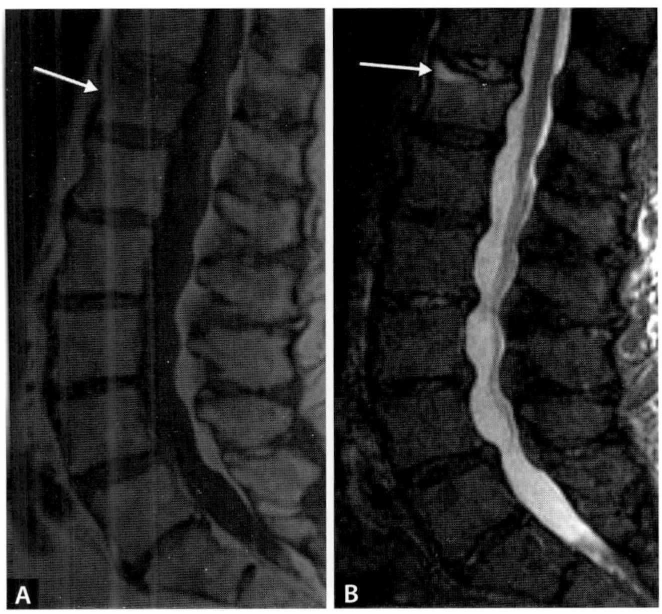

Figs. 62A and B: (A) Sagittal T1-weighted image; and (B) sagittal STIR image, with acute benign superior endplate compression fracture of T12 with fluid cleft sign, arrow in B, supporting diagnosis of a benign fracture.

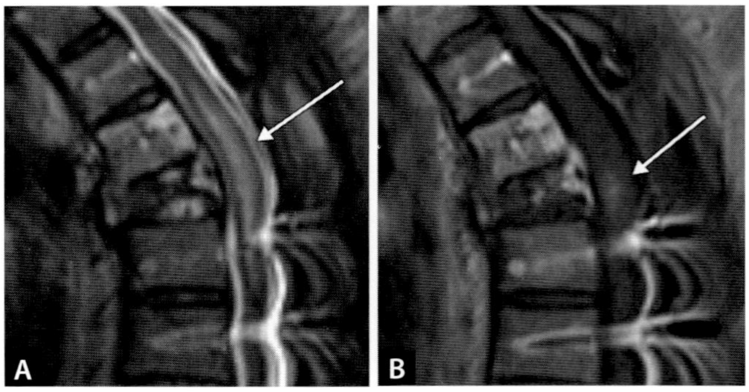

Figs. 63A and B: (A) Sagittal T2-weighted; and (B) Sagittal T1-weighted post-contrast, images of the upper thoracic spine in a patient with breast cancer and history of surgery and radiation therapy for spine metastases. Note cord edema and slight expansion, arrow in A, and faint enhancement, arrow in B, representing radiation myelitis.

hyperintensity felt to represent edema occurs from 7 to 24 days after therapy peaking at 9 days. From 3–6 weeks, there is a gradual decrease in STIR hyperintensity.[278] Radiation osteonecrosis can occur at varying time points following therapy, with report ranging from 10 months to 20 years. There is osseous destruction, vertebral body collapse, and there can be superimposed infection.[279,280] Radiation myelopathy can also occur from months to years following treatment and is largely a diagnosis of exclusion given it nonspecific imaging findings. Findings range from cord edema lasting up to 8 months and ring enhancement which can persist for up to 2 years (Figs. 63A and B) and eventually can progress to volume loss.[281-283]

Infection: In addition to the clinical presentation of low back pain and muscle spasm, leukocytosis, increased erythrocyte sedimentation rate, and increased C-reactive protein levels can suggest the presence of osteomyelitis and discitis.[284] Radiographs are relatively insensitive with findings not present until up to 2 months after symptom onset as opposed to CT imaging which better delineates bony detail. Findings in discitis and osteomyelitis include narrowing of the disk space, poor endplate definition/destruction, and paravertebral soft tissue mass/phlegmon.[285]

MR imaging is the preferred modality and has been demonstrated to be more sensitive than radionuclide imaging.[229,286] The most reliable findings for discitis and osteomyelitis include vertebral body endplate and disk T1 hypointensity and T2 hyperintensity in the disk space, and endplate and disk space enhancement.[287] For treatment monitoring, findings on MR imaging associated with patient improvement include decreasing soft tissue abnormalities[288] and normalization of T1 hyperintensity in the affected marrow[289] however overall imaging findings lag behind the clinical condition of the patient.[290] Degenerative endplate changes, specifically type I changes which have T1 and T2 endplate signal intensity prolongation and potential enhancement can mimic discitis however there should be lack of T2 hyperintensity in the disk space (Figs. 64A to D).[284]

MR imaging is also the preferable modality for evaluation of epidural abscess, manifested as an epidural collection of low T1 signal intensity and T2 hyperintensity with enhancement (Figs. 65A and B). Sensitivity of MR imaging ranges from 91% to 100%.[291,292]

Additional examinations which can be performed for imaging of infection include bone scan, gallium 67 citrate, and indium 111-labeled white blood scans.[284]

Primary bone neoplasm: Primary bone neoplasms are rare as compared to metastatic disease which accounts for greater than 90% of spinal neoplasm.[293] Approach to isolated lesions of the spine should include attention to the location, type of matrix, margins, and extension.[244] Table 1 presents as summary of primary bone neoplasms.

Bone forming tumors demonstrate increased attenuation on CT imaging in an amorphous configuration with areas of ossification low in signal intensity on MR imaging. These tumors include bone islands or enostosis, osteoid osteoma (Figs. 66A to C), osteoblastoma, and osteosarcoma.

Cartilage forming tumors have "punctate comma-like or annular calcifications" when imaging at CT with corresponding low signal on MR imaging. These lesions include osteochondroma, chondroblastoma, and chondrosarcoma.

Other primary neoplasms of spine include eosinophilic granuloma, plasmacytoma, lymphoma, Ewing sarcoma, hemangioma, chordoma (Figs. 67A and B), aneurysmal bone cyst (Figs. 68A and B), and giant cell tumor.[244]

Primary involvement of the spine by lymphoma is rare with metastatic spread from Hodgkin or non-Hodgkin disease being more common.[244] Imaging findings can be nonspecific but lymphoma should be considered when a large paravertebral mass is encountered with marrow infiltration and lack of cortical destruction (Figs. 69A to D).[294]

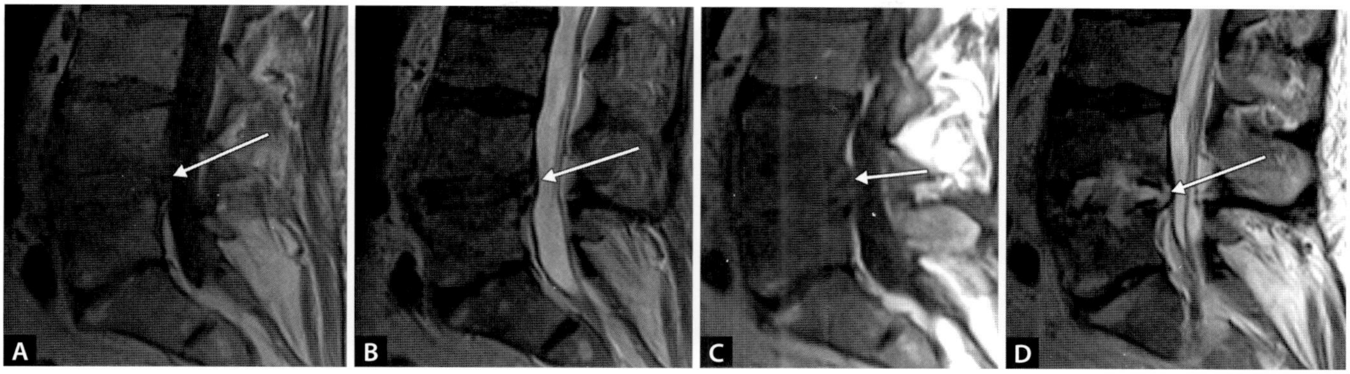

Figs. 64A to D: (A) Sagittal T1 and (B) sagittal T2 images in a patient with low back pain, shows minimal endplate changes centered at L4–L5, arrows. Follow-up imaging obtained 1 month later demonstrates progression of endplate changes and indistinct endplates on T1-weighted imaging, arrow in (C) and development of T2 hyperintensity in the disk space, arrow in (D) representing discitis and osteomyelitis.

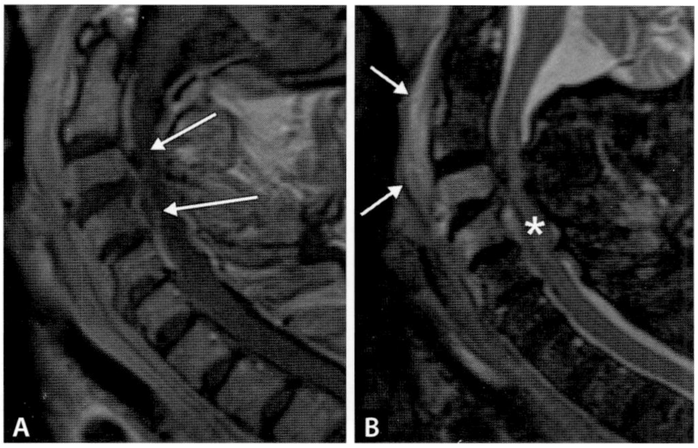

Figs. 65A and B: (A) Sagittal T1-weighted image following contrast administration of the cervical spine with extensive prevertebral soft tissue thickening and epidural abscess, white arrows. (B) Sagittal STIR, demonstrates prevertebral soft tissue thickening (arrows), cord edema (asterisk), and bone marrow edema in C3 and C4 vertebral bodies.

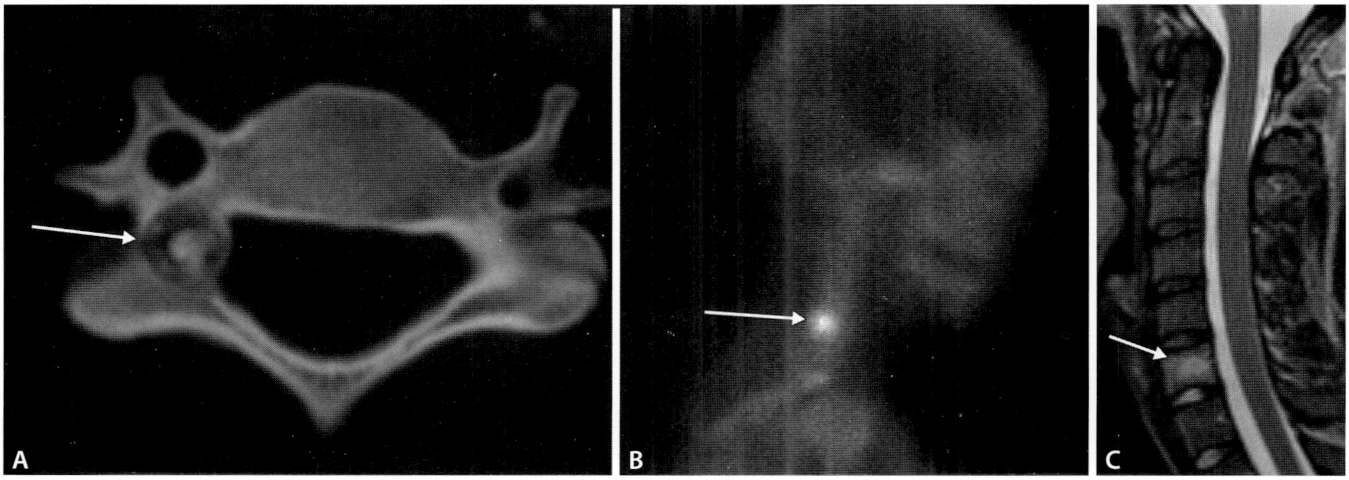

Figs. 66A to C: Well-defined sclerotic nidus of an osteoid osteoma on CT imaging, arrow (A). Bone scan demonstrates intense radiotracer uptake, arrow (B), and sagittal STIR image demonstrates reactive edema extending into C6 vertebral body, arrow (C).

Table 1: Characteristics of primary bone tumors.

Tumor	*Behavior*	*Age range*	*Gender predilection*	*Associated syndromes or diseases*	*Location*	*Histological findings*	*Computed tomography findings*	*Magnetic resonance imaging findings*
Aneurysmal bone cyst	Benign	First to third decades	Female (slight)		Posterior elements	"Blood-filled sponges" of cavernous cysts with walls of woven bone	"Soap bubble," lytic, and multi-lobulated	Variable on T1 and T2; gadolinium enhances
Chondroma/ enchon-dromas	Benign	Second to third decades	Male (2:1)	Ollier syndrome, Maffucci syndrome	Cervical thoracic lumbar	Hypocellular, chondrocytes within lacunae	Calcified, lytic	T1 low to intermediate signal; T2 hyperintense
Eosinophilic granuloma	Benign	Second decade	Male (2–5:1)	Langerhans cell histiocytosis	Thoracic lumbar, vertebral bodies and anterior elements	"Tennis racquet"–shaped Birbeck granules in cytoplasm, stains for CD1a	Lytic destruction of vertebral bodies may cause collapse ("vertebra plana")	T1 isointense, T2 hyperintense with soft-tissue swelling
Fibrous dysplasia	Benign	First to second decades	Equal	McCune-Albright syndrome	No preference	Sheets of broken or retracted fibroblasts with woven bone, foamy macro-phages, cystic changes, hemorrhage	Lytic and expansive with "ground glass" and sclerotic margins	T1 and T2 with variable intensity
Hemangioma	Benign	Fourth to sixth decades	Female (slight)		No preference, vertebral bodies	Multiple small vessels with sclerotic trabeculated bone	"Honeycomb" pattern on plain radiograph, "polka dots" of bone on computed tomography	T1 isointense, T2 hyperintense, gadolinium enhances
Osteoid osteoma	Benign	First to second decades	Male (2–3:1)		Lumbar, posterior elements	"Cloudlike," well-circum-scribed hypodense tumor and surrounding normal trabecula (osteoblas-tomas similar appearing but > 2 cm)	Low attenuation nidus with sclerotic boarder	T1 nidus with intermediate signal intensity, T2 hypointense, gadolinium nidal enhance-ment

Contd...

Contd...

Tumor	*Behavior*	*Age range*	*Gender predilection*	*Associated syndromes or diseases*	*Location*	*Histological findings*	*Computed tomography findings*	*Magnetic resonance imaging findings*
Chordoma	Locally aggressive (malignant)	Fourth to sixth decades	Male (2:1)		Sacrum, cervical	"Physaliphorous," bubble-containing cytoplasm and large, round cells, brachyury, epithelial membrane antigen, S-100 staining	Expansive, lytic, sclerotic	T1 hypointense, T2 hyperintense, gadolinium variable
Giant-cell tumor	Locally aggressive (malignant)	Second to fourth decades	Female (slight)		Sacrum	Multinucleated giant cells in spindle-cell stroma	Lytic, cystic	T1 and T2 hypointense with areas of hemorrhage, gadolinium enhances
Chondrosarcoma	Malignant	Fourth decade	Male (2:1)		Thoracic	Large or binucleated pleomorphic cells with small nucleoli	Expansive and lytic, scalloping of cortext with cortical expansion	Markedly T2 hyperintense, gadolinium "rings and arcs" pattern
Ewing sarcoma	Malignant	First to third decades	Male (slight)		Sacral	Small round cells with uniform nuclei, CD99 is sensitive but not specific	Lytic	T1 isointense, T2 isointense to hyperintense, gadolinium enhances
Multiple myeloma/ solitary plasmacytoma	Malignant	Fifth decade	Male (2:1)		Thoracic	Sheets of plasma cells, cytologic atypia	Lytic, osteoporotic	T1 hypointense, T2 hyperintense, gadolinium enhances
Osteosarcoma	Malignant	Third to sixth decades	Male (slight)		Sacrum	Spindle cells with nuclear pleomorphism; osteoid or bone production within the tumor	Lytic and destructive with matrix mineralization	T1 hypointense, T2 hyperintense

Source: Reprinted with permission; Ropper AE, Cahill KS, McCarthy EF, et al. Primary vertebral tumors: a review of epidemiologic, histological and imaging findings, Part II: locally aggressive and malignant tumors. Neurosurgery. 2012:1(70):211-9.

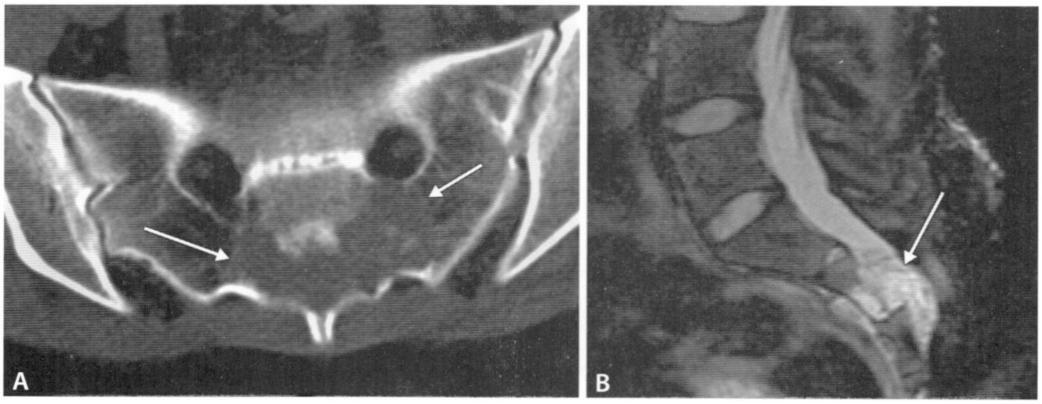

Figs. 67A and B: Axial CT (A) demonstrates a lytic mass in the sacrum, arrows, with soft tissue mass better appreciated on sagittal STIR image, arrows (B), in this patient with a chordoma.

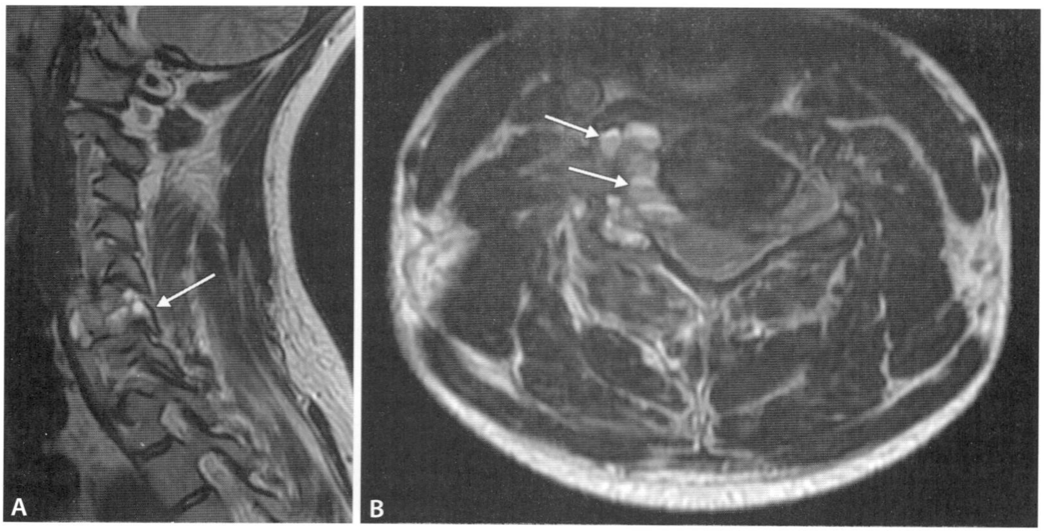

Figs. 68A and B: Aneurysmal bone cyst with its characteristic fluid-fluid levels centered in the posterior elements of C6, arrows (A and B), both T2-weighted images.

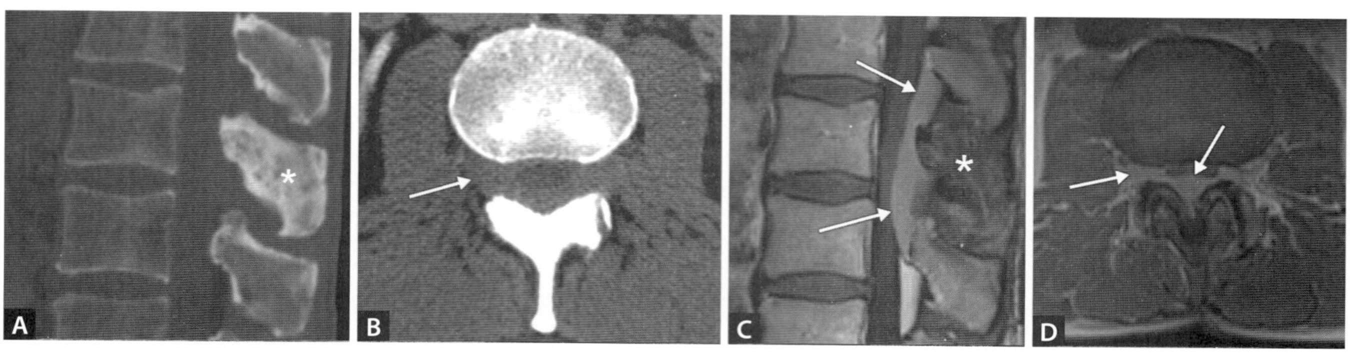

Figs. 69A to D: A sagittal CT (A) in a patient with lymphoma demonstrates a sclerotic spinous process, asterisk. Extensive epidural extension of disease is apparent on axial CT (B, arrow) as well as on contrast-enhanced T1-weighted images (C and D) arrows. Pathologic low T1 signal intensity is present involving the spinous process, asterisk (C), corresponding to sclerosis on CT imaging.

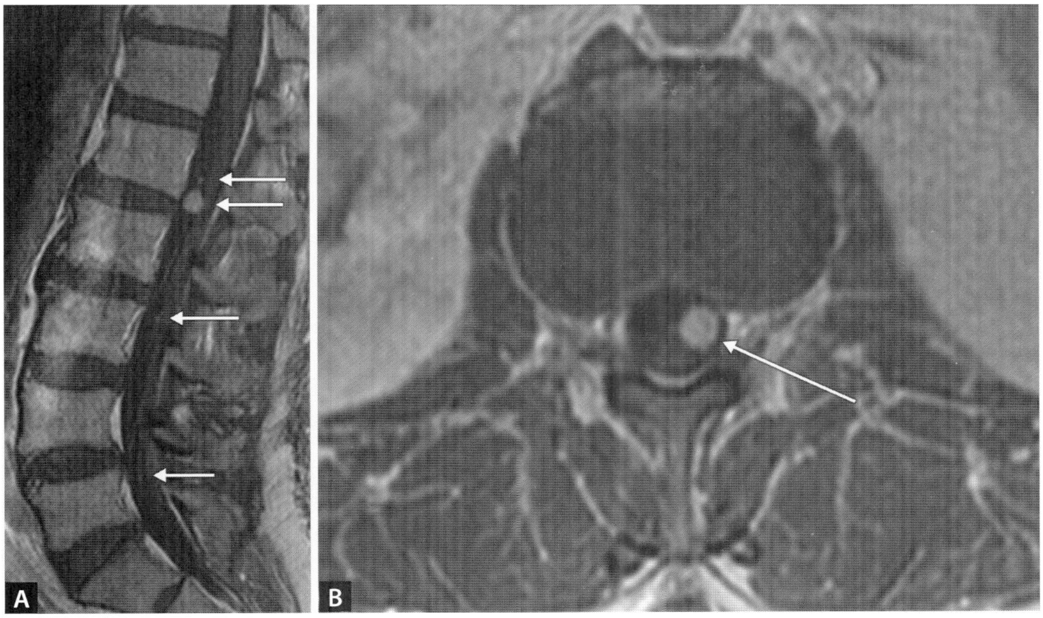

Figs. 70A and B: Multiple schwannomas, arrows in A and B, are well-visualized on these contrast-enhanced T1-weighted images.

Intradural Extramedullary Lesions

Intradural extramedullary lesions can displace and deform the cord.[230] Myelography can demonstrate a myelographic block and distortion or nodularity of the nerve roots[295] however MR imaging has increased sensitivity for more subtle abnormalities and enhancement.

Intradural extramedullary pathology can include meningioma, nerve sheath tumor, lipoma, dermoid, myxopapillary ependymoma (of the conus medullaris or filum terminale), drop metastases, granulomatous disease, infection, and arachnoid cyst.[235,296,297]

Nerve sheath tumors which include schwannomas (Figs. 70A and B) and neurofibromas (Figs. 71A and B) are the most common intradural extramedullary lesions followed by meningiomas (*see* Figs. 48A to D). Other neoplasms are relatively rare as are malignant peripheral nerve sheath tumors.[298] Sarcoidosis can be trans-spacial with involvement of nerve roots or alternatively can present as an intramedullary lesion (Figs. 72A to C).[299] Prominent vascularity with cord edema can be seen with dural arteriovenous fistulas (Figs. 73 and 74).[231] Redundant nerve roots can be present with severe canal stenosis which can be confused for prominent vascularity (Fig. 75).[300] Enhancing nerve roots is nonspecific and can be seen with infection, leptomeningeal metastatic disease, or inflammation (Figs. 76A to D). Enhancement from metastatic disease tends to be more irregular with

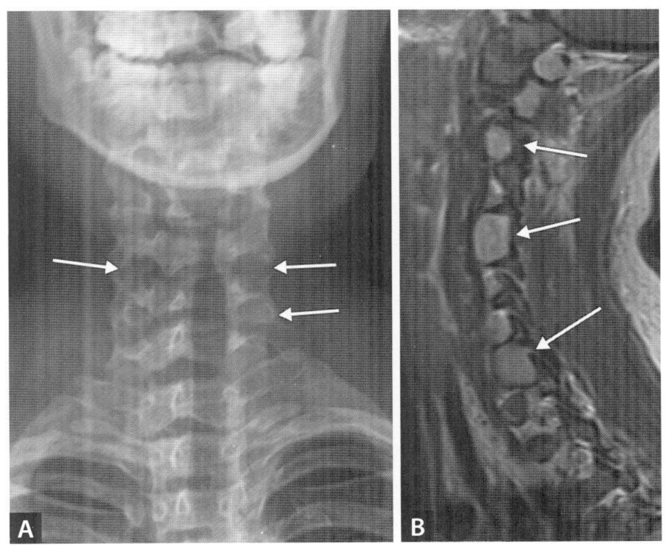

Figs. 71A and B: (A) Frontal radiograph of the cervical spine shows smooth remodeling of multiple neural foramina, arrows. (B) Sagittal contrast-enhanced T1-weighted image shows multiple neurofibromas, arrows, in this patient with neurofibromatosis type 1.

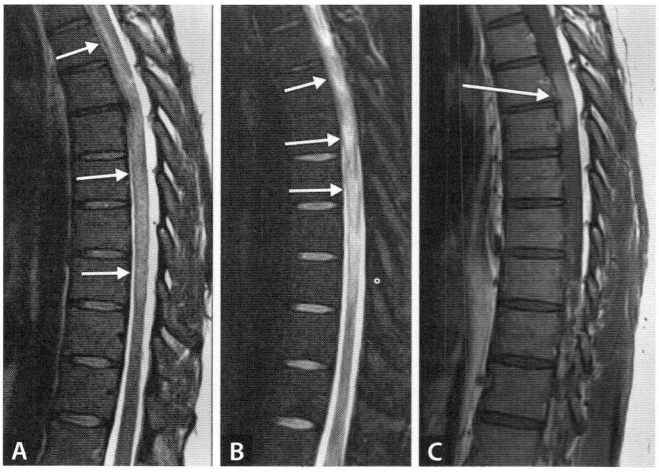

Figs. 72A to C: (A) Sagittal T2, (B) STIR, and (C) T1-weighted with contrast images demonstrate long segment cord edema with enhancement, arrows. There is a superimposed disk protrusion however cord edema is out of proportion to what one would expect. When these imaging findings are combined with the scout of the same patient, Figure 9D, sarcoid is likely and was confirmed with a lymph node biopsy.

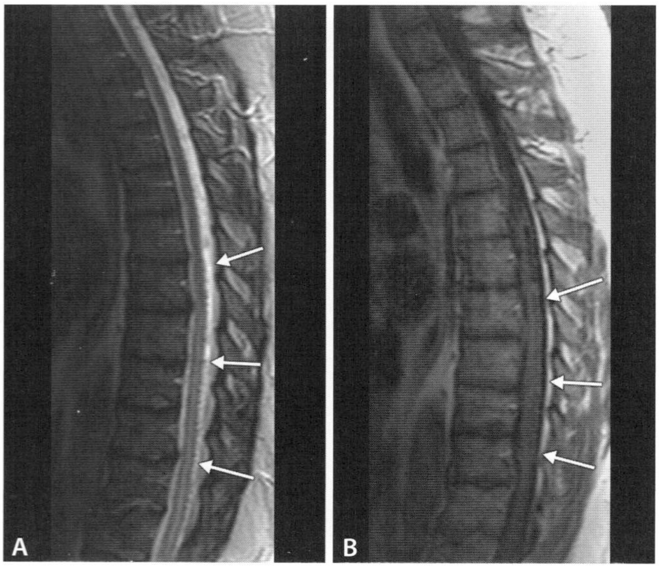

Figs. 73A and B: T2 hyperintensity within the cord and flow voids on the surface of the cord, arrows in A, combined with prominent vascular enhancement, arrows in B (T1-weighted with contrast), represents a dural AV-fistula.

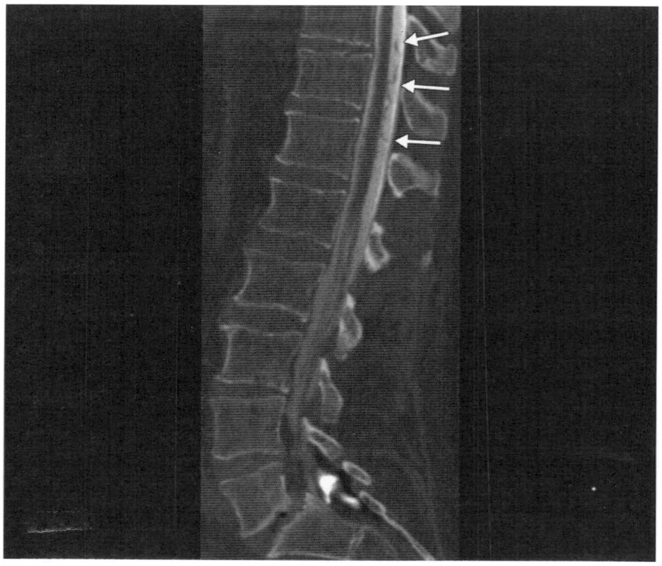

Fig. 74: The presence of a pacemaker precluded MR imaging in this patient with progressive weakness. A CT myelogram was performed which demonstrated prominent tortuous vessels, arrows, with spinal angiography the next appropriate examination.

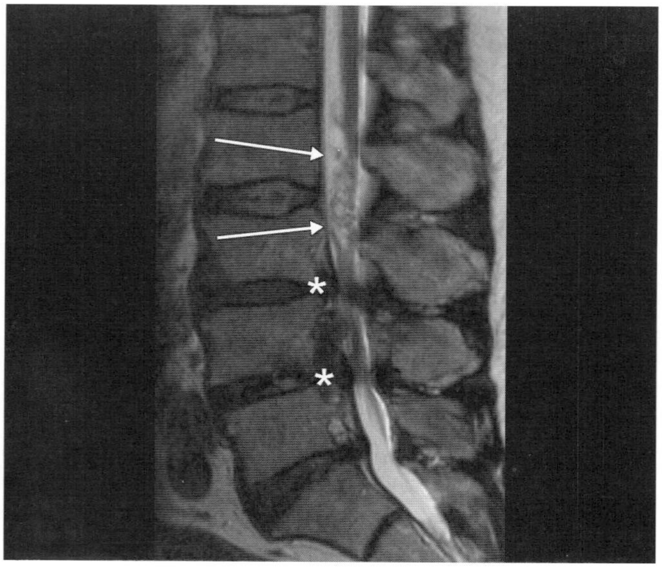

Fig. 75: Degenerative disk disease, worst at levels marked with asterisks, on this sagittal T2-weighted image, results in redundant tortuous nerve roots, arrows, simulating prominent vascularity which can be confused for an underlying vascular malformation.

nerve root clumping.[296] Diffuse enlargement of nerve roots can be seen with the hypertrophic neuropathies (Figs. 77A and B) or with chronic inflammatory demyelinating polyneuropathy.[301,302] Intradural arachnoid cyst resulting in cord compression (Figs. 78 A to E) can have an appearance similar to cord herniation.[297,303]

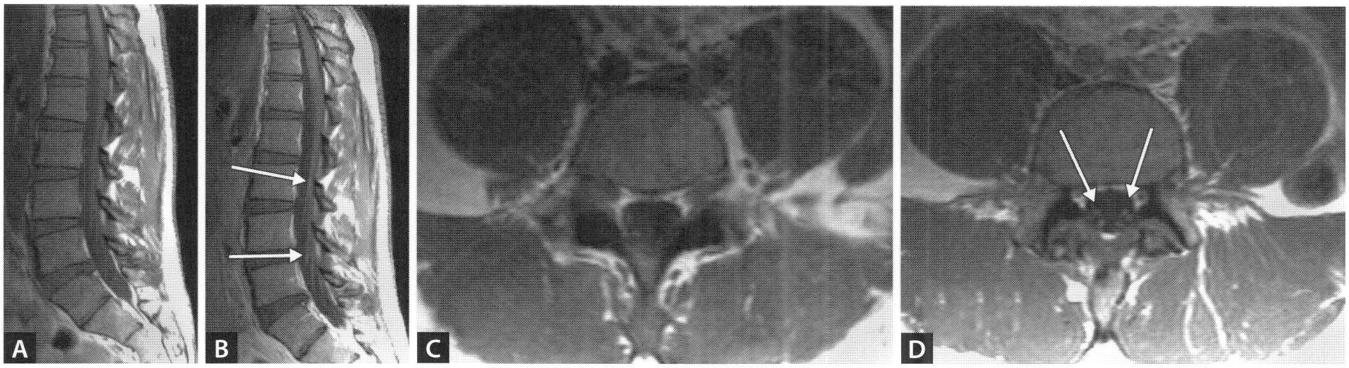

Figs. 76A to D: Sagittal and axial T1-weighted images before (A and C) and after contrast administration (B and D) demonstrates enhancement predominantly of the ventral nerve roots (arrows in B and D) in this patient with ascending paralysis. Guillain-Barré syndrome.

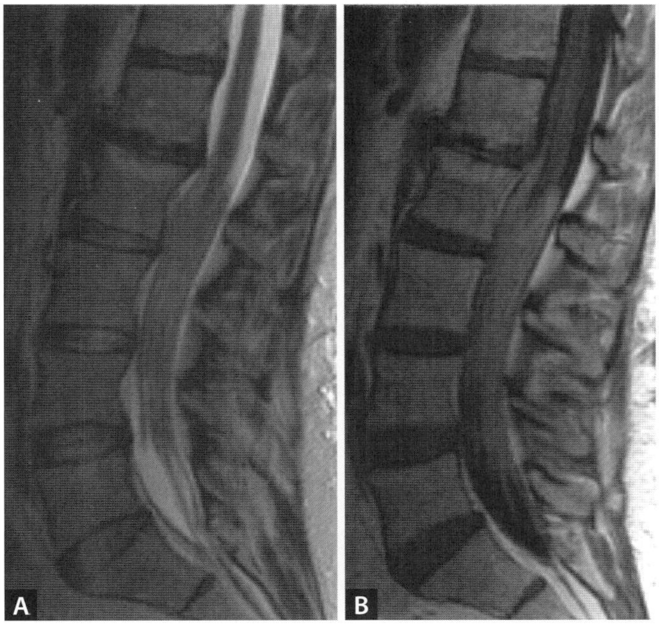

Figs. 77A and B: (A) Sagittal T2-weighted and (B) T1-weighted post contrast images, demonstrate diffuse enlargement and enhancement of the nerve roots of the cauda equina representing a hypertrophic neuropathy such as Charcot-Marie-Tooth or Dejerine-Sottas disease.

Intramedullary Lesions

Intramedullary lesions include neoplasm, syrinx, vascular malformations, infarct, spinal cord contusion, as well as inflammatory and demyelinating conditions.[304-306] Myelography can image cord enlargement and contour abnormalities.[307] The role for conventional radiographs in the diagnosis of spinal tumors is even more limited with findings only visible during later stages of disease. Findings include widening of the canal or increased distance between the pedicles as imaged on a frontal view, increased concavity/remodeling or destruction posterior aspect of a vertebral body, widening of neural foramen, scoliosis, and abnormal soft tissue mass or calcification.[307] MR imaging is the preferred modality as it is the only modality which can directly image the spinal cord.

Potential neoplasms of the spinal cord include ependymoma (Figs. 79A and B), astrocytoma (Figs. 80A and B), hemangioblastoma, subependymoma, ganglioglioma, lymphoma, and metastatic disease (Figs. 81A and B).[308] Primary cord neoplasm typically consists of cord expansion, syrinx formation, and enhancement and is best imaged with MR.[308] Cysts either within the enhancing mass (tumoral cysts) or cysts along the cranial and caudal margins of the mass (polar cysts) can be present[309,310] which have treatment ramifications. A confounding feature of some neoplasms includes the possibility of an exophytic component or when the lesion is of sufficient size that the space of origin is difficult to ascertain (Figs. 82A to D).[311]

Nonexpansile cord abnormalities that involve T2 or STIR hyperintensity, with or without enhancement can present a diagnostic quandary as these findings are ultimately nonspecific. The distribution of findings within cord in terms of transverse and cranial caudal extent, contiguity of the abnormality, degree of enhancement if present, findings elsewhere in the neural axis and remaining body, change over time if, and clinical history can be helpful in determining treatment or need for

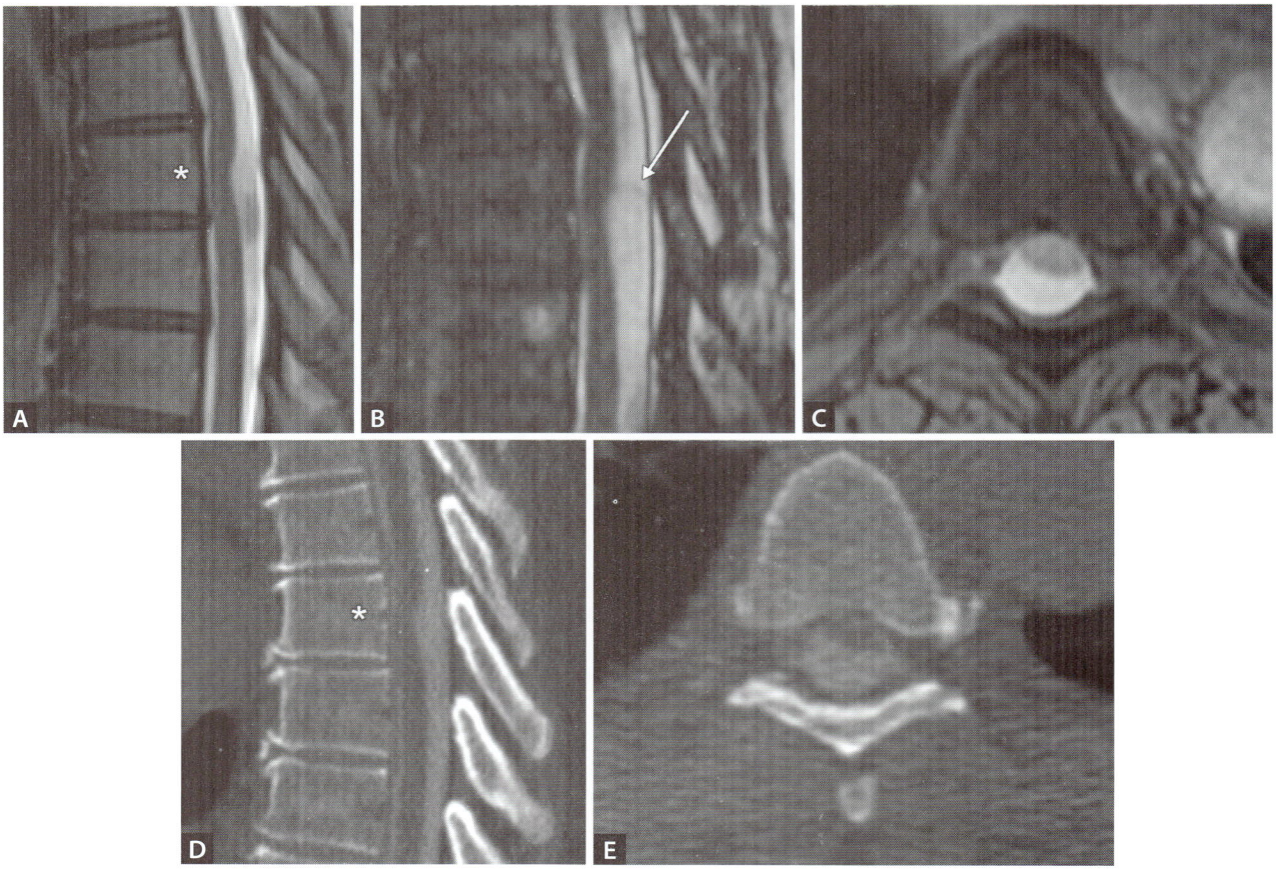

Figs. 78A to E: Sagittal T2 (A) image with focal deformity of the cord, level of asterisk. Sagittal constructive interference in steady state (CISS) reconstruction, (B) shows a thin septation from a likely intradural arachnoid cyst, arrow. (C) Axial T2-weighted image, demonstrates the cord flattening and slight displacement toward the left. CT myelography (D and E) demonstrates the cord flattening but no discreet cyst, however this can be confounding as intradural arachnoid cysts can fill with contrast depending on the size of the communication with the remainder of the subarachnoid space. Cord herniation can have an identical appearance.

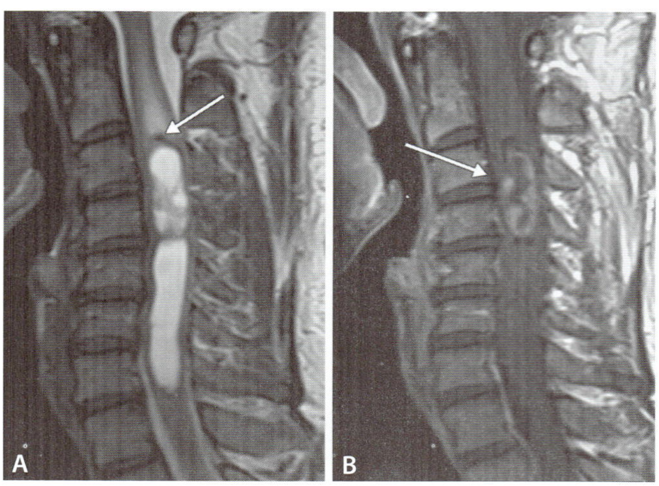

Figs. 79A and B: Typical primary cord neoplasm, in this case an ependymoma, with cord expansion and syrinx formation as well as low T2 signal intensity blood degradation byproducts, arrow (A) (sagittal T2-weighted image). (B) T1 following contrast, demonstrates enhancement, arrow.

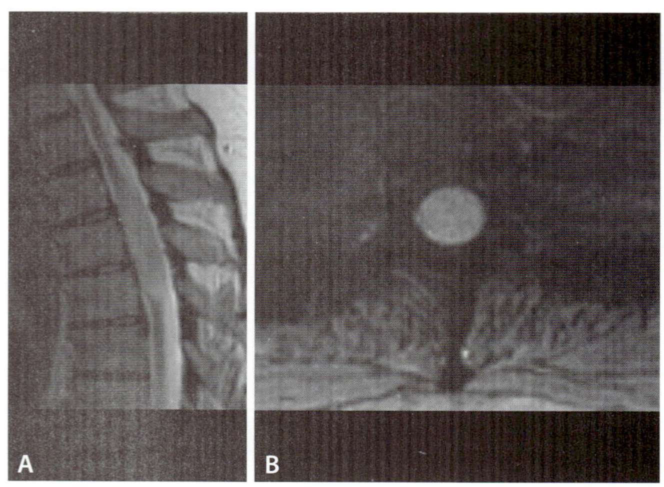

Figs. 80A and B: Cord expansion and T2 hyperintensity in this patient with an astrocytoma.

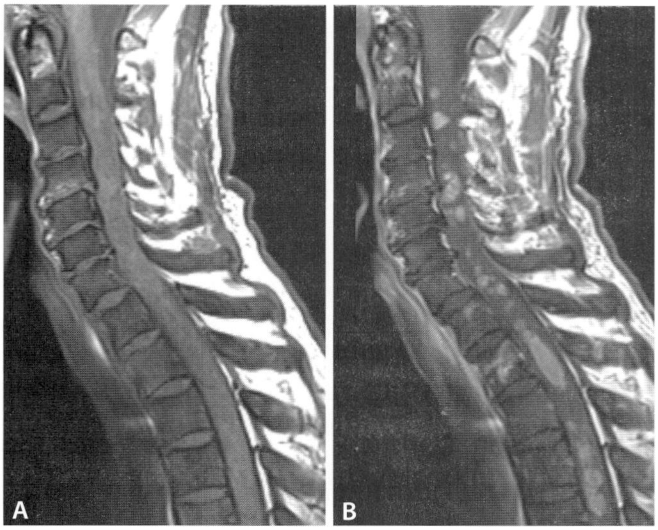

Figs. 81A and B: T1-weighted image without (A) and with contrast (B) in a patient with small cell lung cancer demonstrates diffuse osseous metastasis and extensive intramedullary enhancement representing metastatic disease.

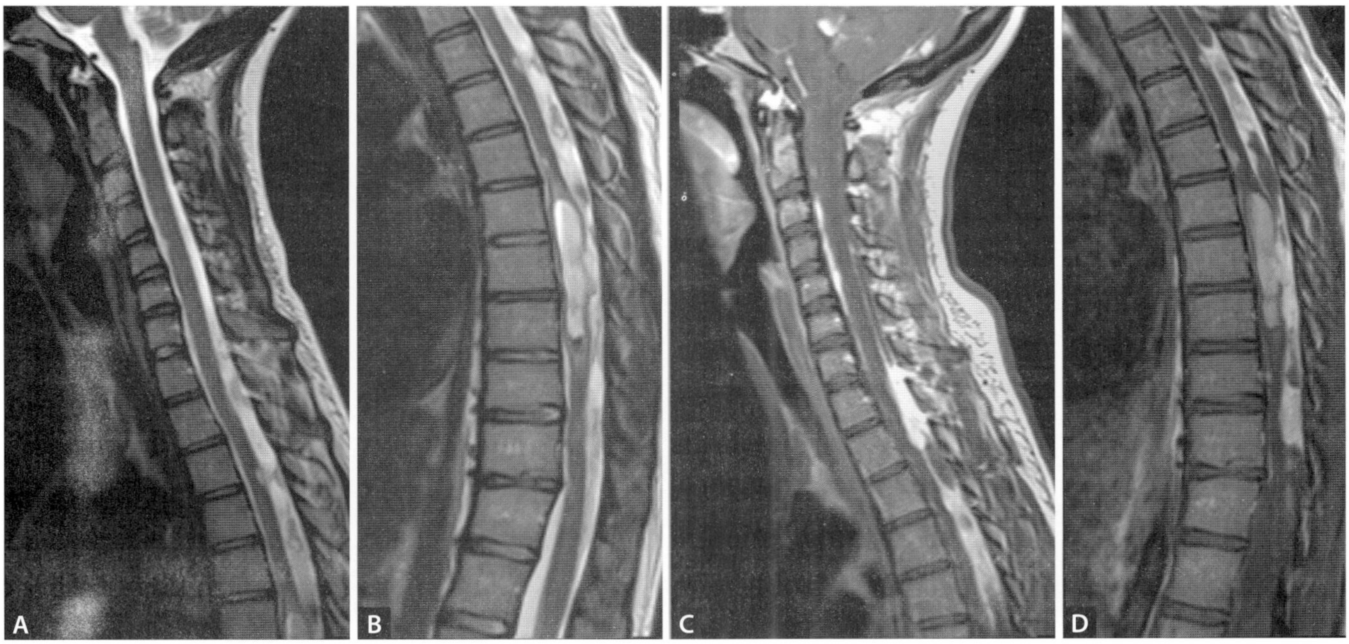

Figs. 82A to D: Sagittal T2-weighted images (A and B) and T1-weighted with contrast images (C and D) demonstrate extensive cord signal abnormality, expansion, and mixed intramedullary and extramedullary enhancement with intracranial involvement. The imaging appearance suggests a primary cord neoplasm, in this case gliofibroma.

surgery either for diagnostic or therapeutic aims. Demyelination tends to involve the dorsal and lateral aspects of the cord with variable enhancement and patchy cranial caudal extent (Figs. 83A to C). Transverse myelitis is centrally located and has cranial caudal extent spanning multiple vertebral bodies and cord infarction is centrally and anteriorly centered (Figs. 84A and B). Subacute combined degeneration from vitamin B_{12} deficiency (Fig. 85) and vacuolar myelopathy of HIV is manifested typically by posteriorly distributed cord signal abnormality.[304]

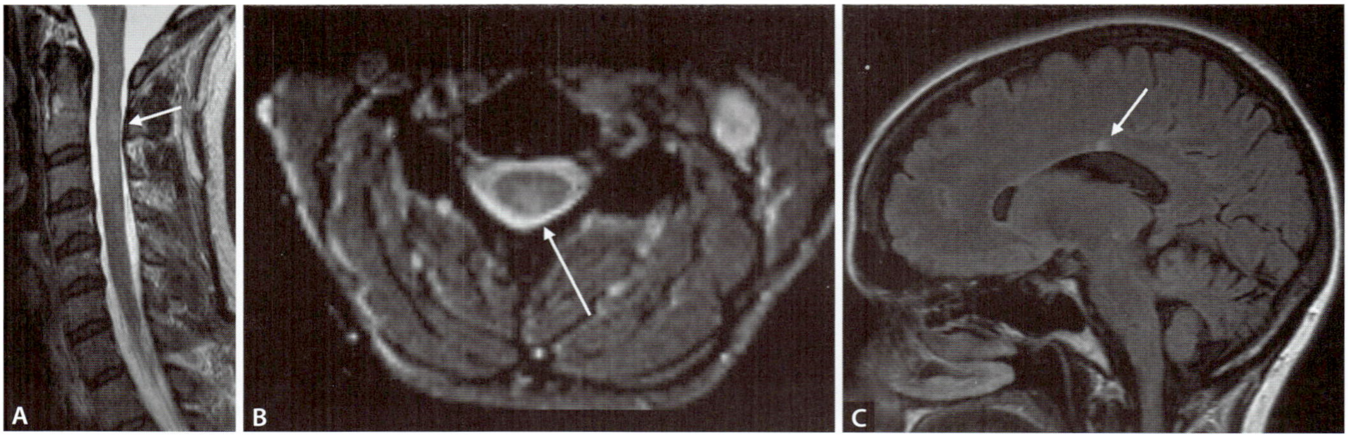

Figs. 83A to C: Sagittal (A) and axial (B) T2-weighted images demonstrate short segment T2 hyperintensity centered dorsally suggestive of demyelination, confirmed by additional finding consisting of FLAIR hyperintensity of the corpus callosum, arrow (C).

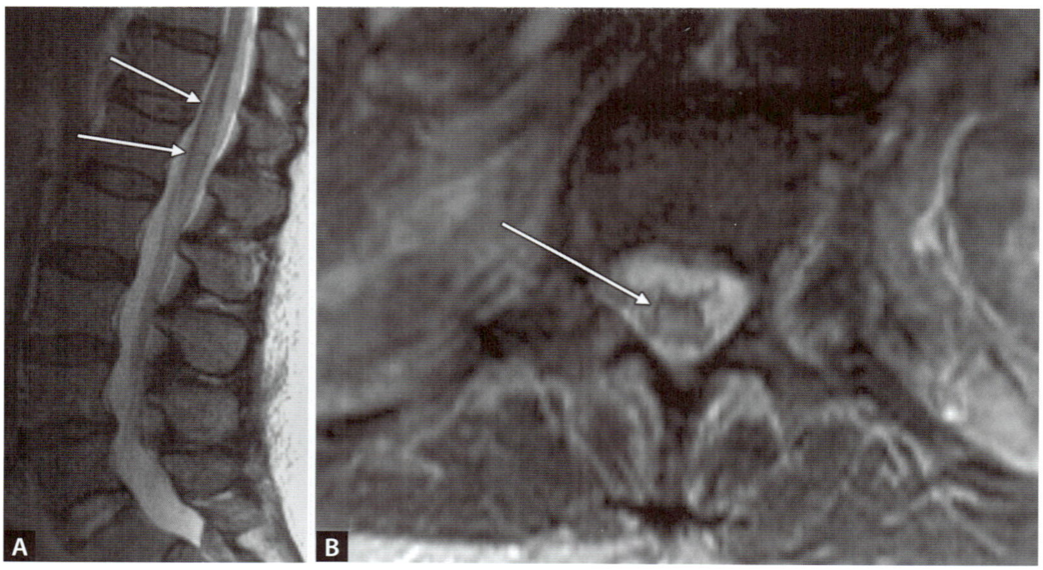

Figs. 84A and B: (A) Sagittal and (B) axial T2-weighted images in a patient who was quadriplegic following abdominal aortic aneurysm repair. T2 hyperintensity centrally in the cord, arrows in A and B, representing spinal cord infarct.

SUMMARY

The decision to perform a diagnostic test is based on four factors. First, what is the probability that the patient has the condition before the test result is known, the pretest probability? Second, the accuracy of the test, third, the therapeutic impact of the test, and fourth, the invasiveness/cost. For instance, if the test is not going to impact the therapeutic decision-making, it has little if any value—even if it is an expectation of the patient or part of the habit of the ordering physician. Unfortunately, this is often a problem in spinal imaging and consequently has become a target in health care reform. A normal examination may provide some but not absolute reassurance relative to suspect pathology—a reassurance which is difficult to measure in terms of value. In spinal imaging, it is the abnormal examination which can produce the greatest diagnostic dilemma. In order to understand the significance of the morphologic alterations noted on imaging, four factors must always be considered. First, the reliability and reproducibility of the imaging findings,

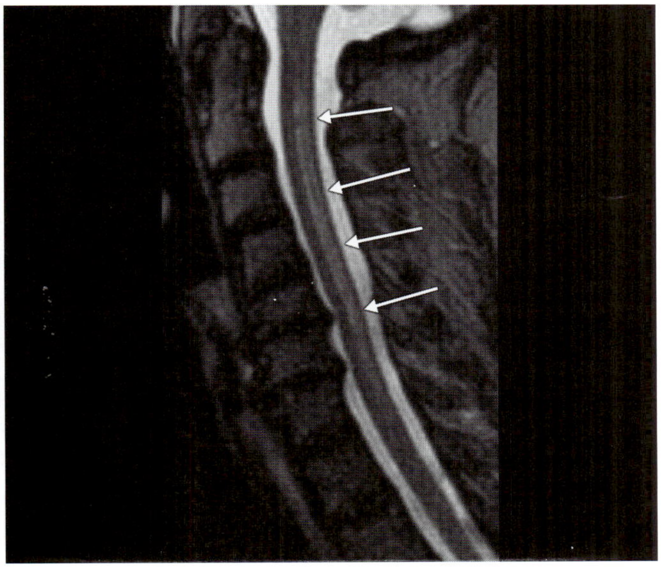

Fig. 85: Sagittal T2-weighted image demonstrates long segment hyperintensity confined to the dorsal aspect of the spinal cord, arrows, representing subacute combined degeneration.

second, the prevalence of the findings in asymptomatic and symptomatic populations over time, third, the natural history of these findings and their behavior over time and lastly, the prognostic value of these findings. Given the high prevalence of asymptomatic morphologic abnormalities it begs the question of relevance and can potentially mistakenly support unwarranted interventions. These are not theoretical consideration: Rates of spinal surgery are increasing and vary significantly over geographic areas with 10–15 fold regional variations for discectomy and fusion across the United States. In parallel, there is moderate to strong correlation between rates of CT/MR use and the volume of spine surgery.[166,168] Clearly, unwarranted imaging can result in unwarranted intervention.

In most cases of back pain, the precise anatomic source of the pain is not identified and in fact the natural history of backpain and even back and leg pain is favorable. Evidence to date would suggest that imaging is not indicated in the routine conservative management of patients with back and leg pain till they have failed conservative management or if there are signs and symptoms of so called "red flag" conditions—malignancy, infection, fracture, and significant neurological symptoms.[131,312,313] Imaging is however an important diagnostic and presurgical tool but must be used and interpreted judiciously, with full knowledge of its strength and weaknesses.

REFERENCES

1. Dewing S. Modern radiology in historical perspective. Springfield: Thomas; 1962.
2. Davis A. Fractures of the spine. J Bone Joint Surg. 1929; 11:133-56.
3. Bushberg JT. The essential physics of medical imaging. 3rd edition 2012, Philadelphia: Wolters Kluwer Health/Lippincott Williams & Wilkins. xii, 1030 p.
4. Lee S, Joyce S, Seeger J. Asymmetry of the odontoid-lateral mass interspaces: a radiographic finding of questionable clinical significance. Ann Emerg Med. 1986;15(10):1173-6.
5. Ross JS. Specialty Imaging: Postoperative Spine, 1st edition. Salt Lake City: Amirsys; 2012.
6. Meyerding H. Spondylolisthesis. Surg Gynecol Obstet. 1932 54:371-7.
7. Bontrager KL, Lampignano JP, Bontrager KL. Bontrager's handbook of radiographic positioning and techniques, 7th edition. St. Louis: Mosby/Elsevier; 2010. p. 323.
8. DiChiro G, Axelbaum SP, Schellinger D, et al. Computerized axial tomography in syringomyelia. N Engl J Med. 1975:292(1):13-6.
9. Uppot RN, Sahani DV, Hahn PF, et al. Impact of obesity on medical imaging and image-guided intervention. Am J Roentgenol. 2007;188(2):433-40.
10. Lustrin ES, Karakas SP, Ortiz AO, et al. Pediatric cervical spine: normal anatomy, variants, and trauma. Radiographics. 2003;23(3):539-60.
11. Nicholas BA, Vricella GJ, Smith M, et al. Contrast-induced nephropathy and nephrogenic systemic fibrosis: minimizing the risk. Can J Urol. 2012;19(1): 6074-80.
12. Thomsen HS. Contrast media safety-an update. Eur J Radiol. 2011;80(1):77-82.
13. Smoker WR. Craniovertebral junction: normal anatomy, craniometry, and congenital anomalies. Radiographics. 1994;14(2):255-77.
14. Jacobæus H. On insufflation of air into the spinal canal for diagnostic purposes in cases of the spinal cord. Acta Med Scand. 1921;21:555-60.
15. Arnell S, Lidstrom F. Myelography with Skiodan (abrodil). Acta Radiol. 1931;12:287-9.
16. Maltby GL. Progressive thorium dioxide myelopathy. N Engl J Med. 1964;270:490-6.
17. Meyer MW. Thorotrast induced adhesive arachnoiditis associated with meningioma and schwannoma. Hum Pathol. 1978;9(3):366-70.
18. Peterson HO. The hazards of myelography. Radiology. 1975;115(1):237-9.
19. Ramsey GH, French JD, Strain WH. Iodinated organic compounds as contrast media for radiographic diagnoses. IV. Pantopaque myelography. Radiology. 1944;43:236-40.
20. Sackett JF, Strother CM, Quaglieri CE, et al. Metrizamide—CSF contrast medium. Analysis of clinical application in 215 patients. Radiology. 1977;123(3):779-82.
21. Sicard J. and F. J, Methode generale d'exploration radiologique par l'huite iodee (Lipidiole). Ann Med Interne, 1922. 46: p. 463-468.

22. Eldevik OP, Nakstad P, Kendall BE, et al. Iohexol in lumbar myelography: preliminary results from an open, noncomparative multicenter clinical study. Am J Neuroradiol. 1983;4(3):299-301.
23. Witwer G, Cacayorin ED, Bernstein AD, et al. Iopamidol and metrizamide for myelography: prospective double-blind clinical trial. Am J Roentgenol. 1984;143(4):869-73.
24. Wang H, Binet EF, Gabrielsen TO, et al. Lumbar myelography with iohexol in outpatients: prospective multicenter evaluation of safety. Radiology. 1989;173(1):239-42.
25. Fedutes BA, Ansani NT. Seizure potential of concomitant medications and radiographic contrast media agents. Ann Pharmacother. 2003;37(10):1506-10.
26. Sandow BA, Donnal JF. Myelography complications and current practice patterns. Am J Roentgenol. 2005;185(3):768-71.
27. Layton KF, Kallmes DF, Horlocker TT. Recommendations for anticoagulated patients undergoing image-guided spinal procedures. Am J Neuroradiol. 2006;27(3):468-70.
28. Hoeffner EG, Mukherji SK, Srinivasan A, et al. Neuroradiology back to the future: spine imaging. Am J Neuroradiol. 2012; 33(6):999-1006.
29. Modic MT, Pavlicek W, Weinstein MA, et al. Magnetic resonance imaging of intervertebral disk disease. Clinical and pulse sequence considerations. Radiology. 1984;152(1): 103-11.
30. Edelman RR, Shoukimas GM, Stark DD, et al. High-resolution surface-coil imaging of lumbar disk disease. Am J Roentgenol. 1985;144(6):1123-9.
31. Hueftle MG, Modic MT, Ross JS, et al. Lumbar spine: postoperative MR imaging with Gd-DTPA. Radiology. 1988;167(3): 817-24.
32. Maravilla KR, Lesh P, Weinreb JC, et al. Magnetic resonance imaging of the lumbar spine with CT correlation. AJNR Am J Neuroradiol. 1985;6(2):237-45.
33. Norman D, Mills CM, Brant-Zawadzki M, et al. Magnetic resonance imaging of the spinal cord and canal: potentials and limitations. Am J Roentgenol. 1983;141(6):1147-52.
34. Nowicki BH, Haughton VM, Schmidt TA, et al. Occult lumbar lateral spinal stenosis in neural foramina subjected to physiologic loading. Am J Neuroradiol. 1996;17(9):1605-14.
35. Sadowski EA, Bennett LK, Chan MR, et al. Nephrogenic systemic fibrosis: risk factors and incidence estimation. Radiology. 2007;243(1):148-57.
36. Kuo PH, Kanal E, Abu-Alfa AK, et al. Gadolinium-based MR contrast agents and nephrogenic systemic fibrosis. Radiology. 2007;242(3):647-9.
37. Levy LM. MR imaging of cerebrospinal fluid flow and spinal cord motion in neurologic disorders of the spine. Magn Reson Imaging Clin N Am. 1999;7(3):573-87.
38. Mauer UM, Freude G, Danz B, et al. Cardiac-gated phase-contrast magnetic resonance imaging of cerebrospinal fluid flow in the diagnosis of idiopathic syringomyelia. Neurosurgery. 2008;63(6):1139-44; discussion 1144.
39. Quigley MF, Iskandar B, Quigley ME, et al. Cerebrospinal fluid flow in foramen magnum: temporal and spatial patterns at MR imaging in volunteers and in patients with Chiari I malformation. Radiology. 2004;232(1):229-36.
40. Rubin JB, Enzmann DR, Wright A. CSF-gated MR imaging of the spine: theory and clinical implementation. Radiology. 1987;163(3):784-92.
41. Castillo M, Arbelaez A, Smith JK, et al. Diffusion-weighted MR imaging offers no advantage over routine noncontrast MR imaging in the detection of vertebral metastases. Am J Neuroradiol. 2000;21(5):948-53.
42. Chen WT, Shih TT, Chen RC, et al. Blood perfusion of vertebral lesions evaluated with gadolinium-enhanced dynamic MRI: in comparison with compression fracture and metastasis. J Magn Reson Imaging. 2002;15(3):308-14.
43. Baur A, Dietrich O, Reiser M. Diffusion-weighted imaging of bone marrow: current status. Eur Radiol. 2003;13(7):1699-708.
44. Ellingson BM, Ulmer JL, Kurpad SN, et al. Diffusion tensor MR imaging of the neurologically intact human spinal cord. Am J Neuroradiol. 2008;29(7):1279-84.
45. Wilm BJ, Gamper U, Henning A, et al. Diffusion-weighted imaging of the entire spinal cord. NMR Biomed. 2009; 22(2):174-81.
46. Bowen BC, Pattany PM. Contrast-enhanced MR angiography of spinal vessels. Magn Reson Imaging Clin N Am. 2000;8(3):597-614.
47. Vogler JB 3rd, Murphy WA. Bone marrow imaging. Radiology. 1988;168(3):679-93.
48. Vande Berg BC, Malghem J, Lecouvet FE, et al. Classification and detection of bone marrow lesions with magnetic resonance imaging. Skeletal Radiol. 1998;27(10):529-45.
49. Tehranzadeh J, Andrews C, Wong E. Lumbar spine imaging. Normal variants, imaging pitfalls, and artifacts. Radiol Clin North Am. 2000;38(6):1207-53, v-vi.
50. Denis F. The three column spine and its significance in the classification of acute thoracolumbar spinal injuries. Spine (Phila Pa 1976). 1983;8(8):817-31.
51. Bohlman HH. Treatment of fractures and dislocations of the thoracic and lumbar spine. J Bone Joint Surg Am. 1985;67(1):165-9.
52. Sundgren PC, Philipp M, Maly PV. Spinal trauma. Neuroimaging Clin N Am. 2007;17(1):73-85.
53. Song J, Mizuno J, Inoue T, et al. Clinical evaluation of traumatic central cord syndrome: emphasis on clinical significance of prevertebral hyperintensity, cord compression, and intramedullary high-signal intensity on magnetic resonance imaging. Surg Neurol. 2006;65(2):117-23.
54. Flanders AE, Schaefer DM, Doan HT, et al. Acute cervical spine trauma: correlation of MR imaging findings with degree of neurologic deficit. Radiology. 1990;177(1):25-33.
55. Marciello MA, Flanders AE, Herbison GJ, et al. Magnetic resonance imaging related to neurologic outcome in cervical spinal cord injury. Arch Phys Med Rehabil. 1993;74(9):940-6.
56. Daffner RH. Cervical radiography for trauma patients: a time-effective technique? Am J Roentgenol. 2000;175(5):1309-11.
57. Daffner RH. Helical CT of the cervical spine for trauma patients: a time study. Am J Roentgenol. 2001;177(3):677-9.
58. Brohi K, Healy M, Fotheringham T, et al. Helical computed tomographic scanning for the evaluation of the cervical spine in the unconscious, intubated trauma patient. J Trauma. 2005;58(5):897-901.

59. Holmes JF, Akkinepalli R. Computed tomography versus plain radiography to screen for cervical spine injury: a meta-analysis. J Trauma. 2005;58(5):902-5.
60. Bailitz J, Starr F, Beecroft M, et al. CT should replace three-view radiographs as the initial screening test in patients at high, moderate, and low risk for blunt cervical spine injury: a prospective comparison. J Trauma. 2009;66(6):1605-9.
61. Hoffman JR, Mower WR, Wolfson AB, et al. Validity of a set of clinical criteria to rule out injury to the cervical spine in patients with blunt trauma. National Emergency X-radiography Utilization Study Group. N Engl J Med. 2000;343(2):94-9.
62. Stiell IG, Wells GA, Vandemheen KL, et al. The Canadian C-spine rule for radiography in alert and stable trauma patients. JAMA. 2001;286(15):1841-8.
63. Bolinger B, Shartz M, Marion D. Bedside fluoroscopic flexion and extension cervical spine radiographs for clearance of the cervical spine in comatose trauma patients. J Trauma. 2004;56(1):132-6.
64. Davis JW, Kaups KL, Cunningham MA, et al. Routine evaluation of the cervical spine in head-injured patients with dynamic fluoroscopy: a reappraisal. J Trauma. 2001;50(6):1044-7.
65. Duane TM, Cross J, Scarcella N, et al. Flexion-extension cervical spine plain films compared with MRI in the diagnosis of ligamentous injury. Am Surg. 2010;76(6):595-8.
66. Duane TM, Scarcella N, Cross J, et al. Do flexion extension plain films facilitate treatment after trauma? Am Surg. 2010;76(12):1351-4.
67. Freedman I, van Gelderen D, Cooper DJ, et al. Cervical spine assessment in the unconscious trauma patient: a major trauma service's experience with passive flexion-extension radiography. J Trauma. 2005;58(6):1183-8.
68. Padayachee L, Cooper DJ, Irons S, et al. Cervical spine clearance in unconscious traumatic brain injury patients: dynamic flexion-extension fluoroscopy versus computed tomography with three-dimensional reconstruction. J Trauma. 2006;60(2):341-5.
69. Muchow RD, Resnick DK, Abdel MP, et al. Magnetic resonance imaging (MRI) in the clearance of the cervical spine in blunt trauma: a meta-analysis. J Trauma. 2008;64(1):179-89.
70. Tomycz ND, Chew BG, Chang YF, et al. MRI is unnecessary to clear the cervical spine in obtunded/comatose trauma patients: the four-year experience of a level I trauma center. J Trauma. 2008;64(5):1258-63.
71. Como JJ, Thompson MA, Anderson JS, et al. Is magnetic resonance imaging essential in clearing the cervical spine in obtunded patients with blunt trauma? J Trauma. 2007;63(3):544-9.
72. Schoenfeld AJ, Bono CM, McGuire KJ, et al. Computed tomography alone versus computed tomography and magnetic resonance imaging in the identification of occult injuries to the cervical spine: a meta-analysis. J Trauma. 2010;68(1):109-13; discussion 113-4.
73. Hsu JM, Joseph T, Ellis AM. Thoracolumbar fracture in blunt trauma patients: guidelines for diagnosis and imaging. Injury. 2003;34(6):426-33.
74. Brandt MM, Wahl WL, Yeom K, et al. Computed tomographic scanning reduces cost and time of complete spine evaluation. J Trauma. 2004;56(5):1022-6; discussion 1026-8.
75. Daffner RH, Sciulli RL, Rodriguez A, et al. Imaging for evaluation of suspected cervical spine trauma: a 2-year analysis. Injury. 2006;37(7):652-8.
76. Mancini DJ, Burchard KW, Pekala JS. Optimal thoracic and lumbar spine imaging for trauma: are thoracic and lumbar spine reformats always indicated? J Trauma. 2010;69(1):119-21.
77. Smith MW, et al. The reliability of nonreconstructed computerized tomographic scans of the abdomen and pelvis in detecting thoracolumbar spine injuries in blunt trauma patients with altered mental status. J Bone Joint Surg Am. 2009;91(10): 2342-9.
78. Gestring ML, Gracias VH, Feliciano MA, et al. Evaluation of the lower spine after blunt trauma using abdominal computed tomographic scanning supplemented with lateral scanograms. J Trauma. 2002;53(1):9-14.
79. Hauser CJ, Visvikis G, Hinrichs C, et al. Prospective validation of computed tomographic screening of the thoracolumbar spine in trauma. J Trauma. 2003;55(2):228-34; discussion 234-5.
80. Inaba K, Munera F, McKenney M, et al. Visceral torso computed tomography for clearance of the thoracolumbar spine in trauma: a review of the literature. J Trauma. 2006;60(4):915-20.
81. Sheridan R, Peralta R, Rhea J, et al. Reformatted visceral protocol helical computed tomographic scanning allows conventional radiographs of the thoracic and lumbar spine to be eliminated in the evaluation of blunt trauma patients. J Trauma. 2003;55(4):665-9.
82. Wintermark M, Mouhsine E, Theumann N, et al. Thoracolumbar spine fractures in patients who have sustained severe trauma: depiction with multi-detector row CT. Radiology. 2003;227(3):681-9.
83. Dai LY, Yao WF, Cui YM, et al. Thoracolumbar fractures in patients with multiple injuries: diagnosis and treatment-a review of 147 cases. J Trauma. 2004;56(2):348-55.
84. Modic MT, Ross JS. Lumbar degenerative disk disease. Radiology. 2007;245(1):43-61.
85. Boden SD, Davis DO, Dina TS, et al. Abnormal magnetic-resonance scans of the lumbar spine in asymptomatic subjects. A prospective investigation. J Bone Joint Surg Am. 1990;72(3):403-8.
86. Hitselberger WE, Witten RM. Abnormal myelograms in asymptomatic patients. J Neurosurg. 1968;28(3):204-6.
87. Jensen MC, Brant-Zawadzki MN, Obuchowski N, et al. Magnetic resonance imaging of the lumbar spine in people without back pain. N Engl J Med. 1994;331(2):69-73.
88. Wiesel SW, Tsourmas N, Feffer HL, et al. A study of computer-assisted tomography. I. The incidence of positive CAT scans in an asymptomatic group of patients. Spine (Phila Pa 1976). 1984;9(6):549-51.
89. Deans GT, Magalliard JN, Kerr M, et al. Neck sprain—a major cause of disability following car accidents. Injury. 1987;18(1):10-2.
90. Gore DR, Sepic SB, Gardner GM, et al. Neck pain: a long-term follow-up of 205 patients. Spine (Phila Pa 1976). 1987;12(1):1-5.
91. Adams MA, Freeman BJ, Morrison HP, et al. Mechanical initiation of intervertebral disc degeneration. Spine (Phila Pa 1976). 2000;25(13):1625-36.

92. Hurri H, Karppinen J. Discogenic pain. Pain. 2004;112(3):225-8.
93. Battie MC, Videman T, Gibbons LE, et al. 1995 Volvo Award in clinical sciences. Determinants of lumbar disc degeneration. A study relating lifetime exposures and magnetic resonance imaging findings in identical twins. Spine (Phila Pa 1976). 1995;20(24):2601-12.
94. Hestbaek L, Iachine IA, Leboeuf-Yde C, et al., Heredity of low back pain in a young population: a classical twin study. Twin Res. 2004;7(1):16-26.
95. Kresina TF, Malemud CJ, Moskowitz RW. Analysis of osteoarthritic cartilage using monoclonal antibodies reactive with rabbit proteoglycan. Arthritis Rheum. 1986;29(7):863-71.
96. Fardon DF, Milette PC. Nomenclature and classification of lumbar disc pathology. Recommendations of the Combined task Forces of the North American Spine Society, American Society of Spine Radiology, and American Society of Neuroradiology. Spine (Phila Pa 1976). 2001;26(5):E93-113.
97. Majors A, MacDevitt CA, Silgalis I, et al. A correlative analysis of T2, ADC and MT ratio with water, hydroxyproline and GAG content in excised intervertebral disk. Orthop Res Soc. 1994:116-20.
98. Sether LA, Yu S, Haughton VM, et al. Intervertebral disk: normal age-related changes in MR signal intensity. Radiology. 1990;177(2):385-8.
99. Yu SW, Sether LA, Ho PS, et al. Tears of the annulus fibrosus: correlation between MR and pathologic findings in cadavers. Am J Neuroradiol. 1988;9(2):367-70.
100. Bangert BA, Modic MT, Ross JS, et al. Hyperintense disks on T1-weighted MR images: correlation with calcification. Radiology. 1995;195(2):437-43.
101. Knutsson F. The vacuum phenomenon in the intervertebral discs. Acta Radiol. 1942;23:173-9.
102. Amundsen T, Weber H, Lilleås F, et al. Lumbar spinal stenosis. Clinical and radiologic features. Spine (Phila Pa 1976). 1995;20(10):1178-86.
103. Arnoldi CC, Brodsky AE, Cauchoix J, et al. Lumbar spinal stenosis and nerve root entrapment syndromes. Definition and classification. Clin Orthop Relat Res. 1976;115:4-5.
104. Inufusa A, An HS, Lim TH, et al. Anatomic changes of the spinal canal and intervertebral foramen associated with flexion-extension movement. Spine (Phila Pa 1976). 1996;21(21):2412-20.
105. Doyle AJ, Merrilees M. Synovial cysts of the lumbar facet joints in a symptomatic population: prevalence on magnetic resonance imaging. Spine (Phila Pa 1976). 2004;29(8):874-8.
106. Schellinger D, Wener L, Ragsdale BD, et al. Facet joint disorders and their role in the production of back pain and sciatica. Radiographics, 1987;7(5):923-44.
107. de Roos A, Kressel H, Spritzer C, et al. MR imaging of marrow changes adjacent to end plates in degenerative lumbar disk disease. Am J Roentgenol. 1987;149(3):531-4.
108. Modic MT, Steinberg PM, Ross JS, et al. Degenerative disk disease: assessment of changes in vertebral body marrow with MR imaging. Radiology. 1988;166(1 Pt 1):193-9.
109. Fujiwara A, An HS, Lim TH, et al. Morphologic changes in the lumbar intervertebral foramen due to flexion-extension, lateral bending, and axial rotation: an in vitro anatomic and biomechanical study. Spine (Phila Pa 1976). 2001;26(8):876-82.
110. Schmid MR, Stucki G, Duewell S, et al. Changes in cross-sectional measurements of the spinal canal and intervertebral foramina as a function of body position: in vivo studies on an open-configuration MR system. Am J Roentgenol. 1999;172(4):1095-102.
111. Danielson B, Willen J. Axially loaded magnetic resonance image of the lumbar spine in asymptomatic individuals. Spine (Phila Pa 1976). 2001;26(23):2601-6.
112. Kitagawa T, Fujiwara A, Kobayashi N, et al. Morphologic changes in the cervical neural foramen due to flexion and extension: in vivo imaging study. Spine (Phila Pa 1976). 2004;29(24):2821-5.
113. Chen IH, Vasavada A, Panjabi MM. Kinematics of the cervical spine canal: changes with sagittal plane loads. J Spinal Disord. 1994;7(2):93-101.
114. Muhle C, Weinert D, Falliner A, et al. Dynamic changes of the spinal canal in patients with cervical spondylosis at flexion and extension using magnetic resonance imaging. Invest Radiol. 1998;33(8):444-9.
115. Zhang L, Zeitoun D, Rangel A, et al. Preoperative evaluation of the cervical spondylotic myelopathy with flexion-extension magnetic resonance imaging: about a prospective study of fifty patients. Spine (Phila Pa 1976). 2011;36(17):E1134-9.
116. Kanno H, Endo T, Ozawa H, et al. Axial loading during magnetic resonance imaging in patients with lumbar spinal canal stenosis: does it reproduce the positional change of the dural sac detected by upright myelography? Spine (Phila Pa 1976). 2012;37(16):E985-92.
117. Wood KB, Kos P, Schendel M, et al. Effect of patient position on the sagittal-plane profile of the thoracolumbar spine. J Spinal Disord. 1996;9(2):165-9.
118. Bendo JA, Ong B. Importance of correlating static and dynamic imaging studies in diagnosing degenerative lumbar spondylolisthesis. Am J Orthop (Belle Mead NJ). 2001;30(3):247-50.
119. Hammouri QM, Haims AH, Simpson AK, et al. The utility of dynamic flexion-extension radiographs in the initial evaluation of the degenerative lumbar spine. Spine (Phila Pa 1976). 2007;32(21):2361-4.
120. Cheh G, Lenke LG, Lehman RA Jr, et al. The reliability of preoperative supine radiographs to predict the amount of curve flexibility in adolescent idiopathic scoliosis. Spine (Phila Pa 1976). 2007;32(24):2668-72.
121. Hall FM. Back pain and the radiologist. Radiology. 1980;137(3):861-3.
122. Been HD, Kerkhoffs GM, Maas M. Suspected atlantoaxial rotatory fixation-subluxation: the value of multidetector computed tomography scanning under general anesthesia. Spine (Phila Pa 1976). 2007;32(5):E163-7.
123. McGuire KJ, Silber J, Flynn JM, et al. Torticollis in children: can dynamic computed tomography help determine severity and treatment. J Pediatr Orthop. 2002;22(6):766-70.
124. Gilbert JW, Wheeler GR, Lingreen RA, et al. Imaging in the position that causes pain. Surg Neurol. 2008;69(5):463-5; discussion 465.
125. Jinkins JR, Dworkin JS, Damadian RV. Upright, weight-bearing, dynamic-kinetic MRI of the spine: initial results. Eur Radiol. 2005;15(9):1815-25.

126. Schlamann M, Reischke L, Klassen D, et al. Dynamic magnetic resonance imaging of the cervical spine using the Neuro Swing System. Spine (Phila Pa 1976). 2007;32(21):2398-401.
127. Zou J, Yang H, Miyazaki M, et al. Dynamic bulging of intervertebral discs in the degenerative lumbar spine. Spine (Phila Pa 1976). 2009;34(23):2545-50.
128. Weishaupt D, Schmid MR, Zanetti M, et al. Positional MR imaging of the lumbar spine: does it demonstrate nerve root compromise not visible at conventional MR imaging? Radiology. 2000;215(1):247-53.
129. Zamani AA, Moriarty T, Hsu L, et al. Functional MRI of the lumbar spine in erect position in a superconducting open-configuration MR system: preliminary results. J Magn Reson Imaging. 1998;8(6):1329-33.
130. Saal JA, Saal JS, Herzog RJ. The natural history of lumbar intervertebral disc extrusions treated nonoperatively. Spine (Phila Pa 1976). 1990;15(7):683-6.
131. Modic MT, Obuchowski NA, Ross JS, et al. Acute low back pain and radiculopathy: MR imaging findings and their prognostic role and effect on outcome. Radiology. 2005;237(2):597-604.
132. Modic MT, Ross JS, Obuchowski NA, et al. Contrast-enhanced MR imaging in acute lumbar radiculopathy: a pilot study of the natural history. Radiology. 1995;195(2):429-35.
133. Carragee E, Alamin T, Cheng I, et al. Are first-time episodes of serious LBP associated with new MRI findings? Spine J. 2006;6(6):624-35.
134. Carragee EJ, Alamin TF, Miller JL, et al. Discographic, MRI and psychosocial determinants of low back pain disability and remission: a prospective study in subjects with benign persistent back pain. Spine J. 2005;5(1):24-35.
135. Elfering A, Semmer N, Birkhofer D, et al. Risk factors for lumbar disc degeneration: a 5-year prospective MRI study in asymptomatic individuals. Spine (Phila Pa 1976). 2002;27(2):125-34.
136. Carragee EJ, Kim DH. A prospective analysis of magnetic resonance imaging findings in patients with sciatica and lumbar disc herniation. Correlation of outcomes with disc fragment and canal morphology. Spine (Phila Pa 1976) 1997;22(14):1650-60.
137. Komori H, Okawa A, Haro H, et al. Factors predicting the prognosis of lumbar radiculopathy due to disc herniation. J Orthop Sci. 2002;7(1):56-61.
138. Vroomen PC, Wilmink JT, de KM. Prognostic value of MRI findings in sciatica. Neuroradiology. 2002;44(1):59-63.
139. Mäkelä M, Heliövaara M, Sievers K, et al. Prevalence, determinants, and consequences of chronic neck pain in Finland. Am J Epidemiol. 1991;134(11):1356-67.
140. van der Donk J, Schouten JS, Passchier J, et al. The associations of neck pain with radiological abnormalities of the cervical spine and personality traits in a general population. J Rheumatol. 1991;18(12):1884-9.
141. Arana E, Martí-Bonmatí L, Montijano R, et al. Relationship between Northwick Park neck pain questionnaire and cervical spine MR imaging findings. Eur Spine J. 2006;15(8):1183-8.
142. Leak AM, Cooper J, Dyer S, et al. The Northwick Park Neck Pain Questionnaire, devised to measure neck pain and disability. Br J Rheumatol. 1994;33(5):469-74.
143. Ichihara D, Okada E, Chiba K, et al. Longitudinal magnetic resonance imaging study on whiplash injury patients: minimum 10-year follow-up. J Orthop Sci. 2009;14(5):602-10.
144. Beattie PF, Meyers SP, Stratford P, et al. Associations between patient report of symptoms and anatomic impairment visible on lumbar magnetic resonance imaging. Spine (Phila Pa 1976). 2000 25(7):819-28.
145. Jarvik JG, Hollingworth W, Heagerty PJ, et al. Three-year incidence of low back pain in an initially asymptomatic cohort: clinical and imaging risk factors. Spine (Phila Pa 1976). 2005 30(13):1541-8; discussion 1549.
146. Kjaer P, Korsholm L, Bendix T, et al. Modic changes and their associations with clinical findings. Eur Spine J. 2006;15(9):1312-9.
147. Esposito P, Pinheiro-Franco JL, Froelich S, et al. Predictive value of MRI vertebral end-plate signal changes (Modic) on outcome of surgically treated degenerative disc disease. Results of a cohort study including 60 patients. Neurochirurgie. 2006;52(4):315-22.
148. Vital JM, Gille O, Pointillart V, et al. Course of Modic 1 six months after lumbar posterior osteosynthesis. Spine (Phila Pa 1976). 2003;28(7):715-20; discussion 721.
149. Bach SM, Holten KB. Guideline update: what's the best approach to acute low back pain? J Fam Pract. 2009;58(12):E1.
150. Chou R, Qaseem A, Owens DK, et al., Diagnostic imaging for low back pain: advice for high-value health care from the American College of Physicians. Ann Intern Med. 2011;154(3):181-9.
151. Chou R, Qaseem A, Snow V, et al. Diagnosis and treatment of low back pain: a joint clinical practice guideline from the American College of Physicians and the American Pain Society. Ann Intern Med. 2007;147(7):478-91.
152. Jarvik JG, Deyo RA. Diagnostic evaluation of low back pain with emphasis on imaging. Ann Intern Med. 2002;137(7):586-97.
153. Jarvik JG, Hollingworth W, Martin B, et al. Rapid magnetic resonance imaging vs radiographs for patients with low back pain: a randomized controlled trial. JAMA. 2003;289(21):2810-8.
154. Chou R, Fu R, Carrino JA, et al. Imaging strategies for low-back pain: systematic review and meta-analysis. Lancet. 2009;373(9662):463-72.
155. Halpin SF, Yeoman L, Dundas DD. Radiographic examination of the lumbar spine in a community hospital: an audit of current practice. BMJ. 1991;303(6806):813-5.
156. Rockey PH, Tompkins RK, Wood RW, et al. The usefulness of X-ray examinations in the evaluation of patients with back pain. J Fam Pract. 1978;7(3):455-65.
157. Gillan MG, Gilbert FJ, Andrew J, et al. Influence of imaging on clinical decision making in the treatment of lower back pain. Radiology. 2001;220(2):393-9.
158. Berrington de Gonzalez A, Mahesh M, Kim KP, et al. Projected cancer risks from computed tomographic scans performed in the United States in 2007. Arch Intern Med. 2009;169(22):2071-7.
159. Fazel R, Krumholz HM, Wang Y, et al. Exposure to low-dose ionizing radiation from medical imaging procedures. N Engl J Med. 2009;361(9):849-57.
160. Smith-Bindman R, Miglioretti DL, Larson EB. Rising use of diagnostic medical imaging in a large integrated health system. Health Aff (Millwood). 2008;27(6):1491-502.

161. Ash LM, Modic MT, Obuchowski NA, et al. Effects of diagnostic information, per se, on patient outcomes in acute radiculopathy and low back pain. Am J Neuroradiol. 2008;29(6):1098-103.
162. Fisher ES, Welch HG. Avoiding the unintended consequences of growth in medical care: how might more be worse? JAMA. 1999;281(5):446-53.
163. Kendrick D, Fielding K, Bentley E, et al. Radiography of the lumbar spine in primary care patients with low back pain: randomised controlled trial. BMJ. 2001;322(7283):400-5.
164. Errico TJ, Fardon DF, Lowell TD. Open discectomy as treatment for herniated nucleus pulposus of the lumbar spine. Spine (Phila Pa 1976). 1995;20(16):1829-33.
165. Keller RB, Atlas SJ, Soule DN, et al. Relationship between rates and outcomes of operative treatment for lumbar disc herniation and spinal stenosis. J Bone Joint Surg Am. 1999;81(6):752-62.
166. Lurie JD, Birkmeyer NJ, Weinstein JN. Rates of advanced spinal imaging and spine surgery. Spine (Phila Pa 1976). 2003;28(6):616-20.
167. Rhodes LA, McPhillips-Tangum CA, Markham C, et al. The power of the visible: the meaning of diagnostic tests in chronic back pain. Soc Sci Med. 1999;48(9):1189-203.
168. Verrilli D, Welch HG. The impact of diagnostic testing on therapeutic interventions. JAMA. 1996;275(15):1189-91.
169. Berquist TH. Imaging of the postoperative spine. Radiol Clin North Am. 2006;44(3):407-18.
170. Lonstein JE, Denis F, Perra JH, et al. Complications associated with pedicle screws. J Bone Joint Surg Am. 1999;81(11):1519-28.
171. Venu V, Vertinsky AT, Malfair D, et al. Plain radiograph assessment of spinal hardware. Semin Musculoskelet Radiol. 2011;15(2):151-62.
172. Bono CM, Khandha A, Vadapalli S, et al. Residual sagittal motion after lumbar fusion: a finite element analysis with implications on radiographic flexion-extension criteria. Spine (Phila Pa 1976). 2007;32(4):417-22.
173. Cleveland M, Bosworth DM, Thompson FR. Pseudarthrosis in the lumbosacral spine. J Bone Joint Surg Am. 1948;30A(2):302-12.
174. Kumar A, Kozak JA, Doherty BJ, et al. Interspace distraction and graft subsidence after anterior lumbar fusion with femoral strut allograft. Spine (Phila Pa 1976). 1993;18(16):2393-400.
175. Thakkar RS, Malloy JP 4th, Thakkar SC, et al. Imaging the postoperative spine. Radiol Clin North Am. 2012;50(4):731-47.
176. Selby MD, Clark SR, Hall DJ, et al. Radiologic assessment of spinal fusion. J Am Acad Orthop Surg. 2012;20(11):694-703.
177. Buchowski JM, Liu G, Bunmaprasert T, et al. Anterior cervical fusion assessment: surgical exploration versus radiographic evaluation. Spine (Phila Pa 1976). 2008;33(11):1185-91.
178. Cook SD, Patron LP, Christakis PM, et al. Comparison of methods for determining the presence and extent of anterior lumbar interbody fusion. Spine (Phila Pa 1976). 2004;29(10):1118-23.
179. Tuli SK, Chen P, Eichler ME, et al. Reliability of radiologic assessment of fusion: cervical fibular allograft model. Spine (Phila Pa 1976). 2004;29(8):856-60.
180. Kant AP, Daum WJ, Dean SM, et al. Evaluation of lumbar spine fusion. Plain radiographs versus direct surgical exploration and observation. Spine (Phila Pa 1976). 1995;20(21):2313-7.
181. Blumenthal SL, Gill K. Can lumbar spine radiographs accurately determine fusion in postoperative patients? Correlation of routine radiographs with a second surgical look at lumbar fusions. Spine (Phila Pa 1976). 1993;18(9):1186-9.
182. Brodsky AE, Kovalsky ES, Khalil MA. Correlation of radiologic assessment of lumbar spine fusions with surgical exploration. Spine (Phila Pa 1976). 1991;16(6 Suppl):S261-5.
183. Cannada LK, Scherping SC, Yoo JU, et al. Pseudoarthrosis of the cervical spine: a comparison of radiographic diagnostic measures. Spine (Phila Pa 1976). 2003;28(1):46-51.
184. Ghiselli G, Wharton N, Hipp JA, et al. Prospective analysis of imaging prediction of pseudarthrosis after anterior cervical discectomy and fusion: computed tomography versus flexion-extension motion analysis with intraoperative correlation. Spine (Phila Pa 1976). 2011;36(6):463-8.
185. Taylor M, Hipp JA, Gertzbein SD, et al. Observer agreement in assessing flexion-extension X-rays of the cervical spine, with and without the use of quantitative measurements of intervertebral motion. Spine J. 2007;7(6):654-8.
186. Johnsson R, Strömqvist B, Axelsson P, et al. Influence of spinal immobilization on consolidation of posterolateral lumbosacral fusion. A roentgen stereophotogrammetric and radiographic analysis. Spine (Phila Pa 1976). 1992;17(1):16-21.
187. Selvik G. Roentgen stereophotogrammetry. A method for the study of the kinematics of the skeletal system. Acta Orthop Scand Suppl. 1989;232:1-51.
188. Epstein NE, Silvergleide RS. Documenting fusion following anterior cervical surgery: a comparison of roentgenogram versus two-dimensional computed tomographic findings. J Spinal Disord Tech. 2003;16(3):243-7.
189. Ploumis A, Mehbod A, Garvey T, et al. Prospective assessment of cervical fusion status: plain radiographs versus CT-scan. Acta Orthop Belg. 2006;72(3):342-6.
190. Carreon LY, Djurasovic M, Glassman SD, et al. Diagnostic accuracy and reliability of fine-cut CT scans with reconstructions to determine the status of an instrumented posterolateral fusion with surgical exploration as reference standard. Spine (Phila Pa 1976). 2007;32(8):892-5.
191. Biswas D, Bible JE, Bohan M, et al. Radiation exposure from musculoskeletal computerized tomographic scans. J Bone Joint Surg Am. 2009;91(8):1882-9.
192. Kroner AH, Eyb R, Lange A, et al. Magnetic resonance imaging evaluation of posterior lumbar interbody fusion. Spine (Phila Pa 1976). 2006;31(12):1365-71.
193. Tohtz SW, Rogalla P, Taupitz M, et al. Inter- and intraobserver variability in the postoperative evaluation of transpedicular stabilization: computed tomography versus magnetic resonance imaging. Spine J. 2010;10(4):285-90.
194. Agarwal R, Williams K, Umscheid CA, et al. Osteoinductive bone graft substitutes for lumbar fusion: a systematic review. J Neurosurg Spine. 2009;11(6):729-40.
195. Lerner T, Bullmann V, Schulte TL, et al. A level-1 pilot study to evaluate of ultraporous beta-tricalcium phosphate as a graft extender in the posterior correction of adolescent idiopathic scoliosis. Eur Spine J. 2009;18(2):170-9.
196. Helgeson MD, Lehman RA Jr, Patzkowski JC, et al. Adjacent vertebral body osteolysis with bone morphogenetic protein

use in transforaminal lumbar interbody fusion. Spine J. 2011;11(6):507-10.

197. Vaidya R, Sethi A, Bartol S, et al. Complications in the use of rhBMP-2 in PEEK cages for interbody spinal fusions. J Spinal Disord Tech. 2008;21(8):557-62.
198. Sethi A, Craig J, Bartol S, et al. Radiographic and CT evaluation of recombinant human bone morphogenetic protein-2-assisted spinal interbody fusion. Am J Roentgenol. 2011;197(1):W128-33.
199. Glassman SD, Howard JM, Sweet A, et al. Complications and concerns with osteobiologics for spine fusion in clinical practice. Spine (Phila Pa 1976). 2010;35(17):1621-8.
200. Rutherford EE, Tarplett LJ, Davies EM, et al. Lumbar spine fusion and stabilization: hardware, techniques, and imaging appearances. Radiographics. 2007;27(6):1737-49.
201. Tehranzadeh J, Ton JD, Rosen CD. Advances in spinal fusion. Semin Ultrasound CT MR. 2005;26(2):103-13.
202. Barsa P, Suchomel P. Factors affecting sagittal malalignment due to cage subsidence in standalone cage assisted anterior cervical fusion. Eur Spine J. 2007;16(9):1395-400.
203. Bartels RH, Donk RD, Feuth T. Subsidence of stand-alone cervical carbon fiber cages. Neurosurgery. 2006;58(3):502-8; discussion 502-8.
204. Gercek E, Arlet V, Delisle J, et al. Subsidence of stand-alone cervical cages in anterior interbody fusion: warning. Eur Spine J. 2003;12(5):513-6.
205. Van Goethem JW, Parizel PM, van den Hauwe L, et al. The value of MRI in the diagnosis of postoperative spondylodiscitis. Neuroradiology. 2000;42(8):580-5.
206. Ross JS, Masaryk TJ, Modic MT, et al. MR imaging of lumbar arachnoiditis. Am J Roentgenol. 1987;149(5):1025-32.
207. Evans AJ, Jensen ME, Kip KE, et al. Vertebral compression fractures: pain reduction and improvement in functional mobility after percutaneous polymethylmethacrylate vertebroplasty retrospective report of 245 cases. Radiology. 2003;226(2):366-72.
208. Jensen ME, Evans AJ, Mathis JM, et al. Percutaneous polymethylmethacrylate vertebroplasty in the treatment of osteoporotic vertebral body compression fractures: technical aspects. Am J Neuroradiol. 1997;18(10):1897-904.
209. Lieberman IH, Dudeney S, Reinhardt MK, et al. Initial outcome and efficacy of "kyphoplasty" in the treatment of painful osteoporotic vertebral compression fractures. Spine (Phila Pa 1976). 2001;26(14):1631-8.
210. Kobayashi K, Shimoyama K, Nakamura K, et al. Percutaneous vertebroplasty immediately relieves pain of osteoporotic vertebral compression fractures and prevents prolonged immobilization of patients. Eur Radiol. 2005;15(2):360-7.
211. Davis RA. A long-term outcome analysis of 984 surgically treated herniated lumbar discs. J Neurosurg. 1994;80(3):415-21.
212. Herron L. Recurrent lumbar disc herniation: results of repeat laminectomy and discectomy. J Spinal Disord. 1994;7(2):161-6.
213. Bernard TN Jr. Repeat lumbar spine surgery. Factors influencing outcome. Spine (Phila Pa 1976). 1993;18(15):2196-200.
214. Fandino J, Botana C, Viladrich A, et al. Reoperation after lumbar disc surgery: results in 130 cases. Acta Neurochir (Wien). 1993;122(1-2):102-4.
215. Van Goethem JW, Parizel PM, van den Hauwe L, et al. Imaging findings in patients with failed back surgery syndrome. J Belge Radiol. 1997;80(2):81-4.
216. Ross JS, Zepp R, Modic MT. The postoperative lumbar spine: enhanced MR evaluation of the intervertebral disk. Am J Neuroradiol. 1996;17(2):323-31.
217. Van Goethem JW, Van de Kelft E, Biltjes IG, et al. MRI after successful lumbar discectomy. Neuroradiology. 1996;38(Suppl 1):S90-6.
218. Ross JS, Obuchowski N, Zepp R. The postoperative lumbar spine: evaluation of epidural scar over a 1-year period. Am J Neuroradiol. 1998;19(1):183-6.
219. Coskun E, Süzer T, Topuz O, et al. Relationships between epidural fibrosis, pain, disability, and psychological factors after lumbar disc surgery. Eur Spine J. 2000;9(3):218-23.
220. Cervellini P, Curri D, Volpin L, et al. Computed tomography of epidural fibrosis after discectomy: a comparison between symptomatic and asymptomatic patients. Neurosurgery. 1988;23(6):710-3.
221. Ross JS, Robertson JT, Frederickson RC, et al. Association between peridural scar and recurrent radicular pain after lumbar discectomy: magnetic resonance evaluation. ADCON-L European Study Group. Neurosurgery. 1996;38(4):855-61; discussion 861-3.
222. Hurme M, Katevuo K, Nykvist F, et al. CT five years after myelographic diagnosis of lumbar disk herniation. Acta Radiol. 1991;32(4):286-9.
223. North RB, Campbell JN, James CS, et al. Failed back surgery syndrome: 5-year follow-up in 102 patients undergoing repeated operation. Neurosurgery. 1991;28(5):685-90; discussion 690-1.
224. Lee YS, Choi ES, Song CJ. Symptomatic nerve root changes on contrast-enhanced MR imaging after surgery for lumbar disk herniation. Am J Neuroradiol. 2009;30(5):1062-7.
225. Braun IF, Hoffman JC Jr, Davis PC, et al. Contrast enhancement in CT differentiation between recurrent disk herniation and postoperative scar: prospective study. Am J Roentgenol. 1985;145(4):785-90.
226. Teplick JG, Haskin ME. Intravenous contrast-enhanced CT of the postoperative lumbar spine: improved identification of recurrent disk herniation, scar, arachnoiditis, and diskitis. Am J Roentgenol. 1984;143(4):845-55.
227. DeLaPaz RL, Brady TJ, Buonanno FS, et al. Nuclear magnetic resonance (NMR) imaging of Arnold-Chiari type I malformation with hydromyelia. J Comput Assist Tomogr. 1983;7(1):126-9.
228. Modic MT, Weinstein MA, Pavlicek W, et al. Magnetic resonance imaging of the cervical spine: technical and clinical observations. Am J Roentgenol. 1983;141(6):1129-36.
229. Modic MT, Weinstein MA, Pavlicek W, et al. Nuclear magnetic resonance imaging of the spine. Radiology. 1983;148(3):757-62.
230. Takemoto K, Matsumura Y, Hashimoto H, et al. MR imaging of intraspinal tumors—capability in histological differentiation and compartmentalization of extramedullary tumors. Neuroradiology. 1988;30(4):303-9.
231. Spetzler RF, Detwiler PW, Riina HA, et al. Modified classification of spinal cord vascular lesions. J Neurosurg. 2002;96(2 Suppl):145-56.

232. Rabin BM, Roychowdhury S, Meyer JR, et al. Spontaneous intracranial hypotension: spinal MR findings. Am J Neuroradiol. 1998;19(6):1034-9.
233. Kim DH, Rosenblum JK, Panghaal VS, et al. Differentiating neoplastic from non-neoplastic processes in the anterior extradural space. Radiology. 2011;260(3):825-30.
234. Schellinger D. Patterns of anterior spinal canal involvement by neoplasms and infections. Am J Neuroradiol. 1996; 17(5):953-9.
235. Wald JT. Imaging of spine neoplasm. Radiol Clin North Am. 2012;50(4):749-76.
236. Shah LM, Hanrahan CJ. MRI of spinal bone marrow: part I, techniques and normal age-related appearances. Am J Roentgenol. 2011;197(6):1298-308.
237. Vande Berg BC, Lecouvet FE, Galant C, et al. Normal variants of the bone marrow at MR imaging of the spine. Semin Musculoskelet Radiol. 2009;13(2):87-96.
238. Carroll KW, Feller JF, Tirman PF. Useful internal standards for distinguishing infiltrative marrow pathology from hematopoietic marrow at MRI. J Magn Reson Imaging. 1997;7(2):394-8.
239. Mirowitz SA, Apicella P, Reinus WR, et al. MR imaging of bone marrow lesions: relative conspicuousness on T1-weighted, fat-suppressed T2-weighted, and STIR images. Am J Roentgenol. 1994;162(1):215-21.
240. Georgy BA, Hesselink JR. Evaluation of fat suppression in contrast-enhanced MR of neoplastic and inflammatory spine disease. Am J Neuroradiol. 1994;15(3):409-17.
241. Meyer JS, Siegel MJ, Farooqui SO, et al. Which MRI sequence of the spine best reveals bone-marrow metastases of neuroblastoma? Pediatr Radiol. 2005;35(8):778-85.
242. Gold GE, Suh B, Sawyer-Glover A, et al. Musculoskeletal MRI at 3.0 T: initial clinical experience. Am J Roentgenol. 2004;183(5):1479-86.
243. Hanrahan CJ, Shah LM. MRI of spinal bone marrow: part 2, T1-weighted imaging-based differential diagnosis. Am J Roentgenol. 2011;197(6):1309-21.
244. Rodallec MH, Feydy A, Larousserie F, et al. Diagnostic imaging of solitary tumors of the spine: what to do and say. Radiographics. 2008;28(4):1019-41.
245. Ropper AE, Cahill KS, Hanna JW, et al. Primary vertebral tumors: a review of epidemiologic, histological, and imaging findings, Part I: benign tumors. Neurosurgery. 2011;69(6):1171-80.
246. McMenamin DS, Stuckey SL, Potgieter GJ. T1 hyperintense vertebral column melanoma metastases. Am J Neuroradiol. 2007;28(9):1817-8.
247. Baker LL, Goodman SB, Perkash I, et al. Benign versus pathologic compression fractures of vertebral bodies: assessment with conventional spin-echo, chemical-shift, and STIR MR imaging. Radiology. 1990;174(2):495-502.
248. Hayes CW, Jensen ME, Conway WF. Non-neoplastic lesions of vertebral bodies: findings in magnetic resonance imaging. Radiographics. 1989;9(5):883-903.
249. Hamaoka T, Madewell JE, Podoloff DA, et al. Bone imaging in metastatic breast cancer. J Clin Oncol. 2004;22(14):2942-53.
250. Rybak LD, Rosenthal DI. Radiological imaging for the diagnosis of bone metastases. Q J Nucl Med. 2001;45(1):53-64.
251. Cook GJ, Fogelman I. Skeletal metastases from breast cancer: imaging with nuclear medicine. Semin Nucl Med. 1999;29(1):69-79.
252. Blake GM, Park-Holohan SJ, Cook GJ, et al. Quantitative studies of bone with the use of 18F-fluoride and 99mTc-methylene diphosphonate. Semin Nucl Med. 2001;31(1):28-49.
253. Even-Sapir, E. Imaging of malignant bone involvement by morphologic, scintigraphic, and hybrid modalities. J Nucl Med. 2005;46(8):1356-67.
254. Braunstein EM, Kuhns LR. Computed tomographic demonstration of spinal metastases. Spine (Phila Pa 1976). 1983;8(8):912-5.
255. Smoker WR, Godersky JC, Knutzon RK, et al. The role of MR imaging in evaluating metastatic spinal disease. Am J Roentgenol. 1987;149(6):1241-8.
256. Metser U, Lerman H, Blank A, et al. Malignant involvement of the spine: assessment by 18F-FDG PET/CT. J Nucl Med. 2004;45(2):279-84.
257. Metser U, Miller E, Lerman H, et al. Benign nonphysiologic lesions with increased 18F-FDG uptake on PET/CT: characterization and incidence. Am J Roentgenol. 2007; 189(5):1203-10.
258. Clamp A, Danson S, Nguyen H, et al. Assessment of therapeutic response in patients with metastatic bone disease. Lancet Oncol. 2004;5(10):607-16.
259. Liu FY, Yen TC, Chen MY, et al. Detection of hematogenous bone metastasis in cervical cancer: 18F-fluorodeoxyglucose-positron emission tomography versus computed tomography and magnetic resonance imaging. Cancer. 2009;115(23):5470-80.
260. Mahner S, Schirrmacher S, Brenner W, et al. Comparison between positron emission tomography using 2-[fluorine-18] fluoro-2-deoxy-D-glucose, conventional imaging and computed tomography for staging of breast cancer. Ann Oncol. 2008;19(7):1249-54.
261. Costelloe CM, Chuang HH, Madewell JE. FDG PET for the detection of bone metastases: sensitivity, specificity and comparison with other imaging modalities. Pet Clin. 2010;5(3):281-95.
262. Abe K, Sasaki M, Kuwabara Y, et al. Comparison of 18FDG-PET with 99mTc-HMDP scintigraphy for the detection of bone metastases in patients with breast cancer. Ann Nucl Med. 2005;19(7):573-9.
263. Dose J, Bleckmann C, Bachmann S, et al. Comparison of fluorodeoxyglucose positron emission tomography and "conventional diagnostic procedures" for the detection of distant metastases in breast cancer patients. Nucl Med Commun. 2002;23(9):857-64.
264. Gallowitsch HJ, Kresnik E, Gasser J, et al. F-18 fluorodeoxy-glucose positron-emission tomography in the diagnosis of tumor recurrence and metastases in the follow-up of patients with breast carcinoma: a comparison to conventional imaging. Invest Radiol. 2003;38(5):250-6.
265. Gayed I, Vu T, Johnson M, et al. Comparison of bone and 2-deoxy-2-[18F]fluoro-D-glucose positron emission tomography in the evaluation of bony metastases in lung cancer. Mol Imaging Biol. 2003;5(1):26-31.
266. Ito S, Kato K, Ikeda M, et al. Comparison of 18F-FDG PET and bone scintigraphy in detection of bone metastases of thyroid cancer. J Nucl Med. 2007;48(6):889-95.

267. Kato H, Miyazaki T, Nakajima M, et al. Comparison between whole-body positron emission tomography and bone scintigraphy in evaluating bony metastases of esophageal carcinomas. Anticancer Res. 2005;25(6C):4439-44.
268. Kim MR, Roh JL, Kim JS, et al. 18F-fluorodeoxyglucose-positron emission tomography and bone scintigraphy for detecting bone metastases in patients with malignancies of the upper aerodigestive tract. Oral Oncol. 2008;44(2):148-52.
269. Liu FY, Chang JT, Wang HM, et al. [18F]fluorodeoxyglucose positron emission tomography is more sensitive than skeletal scintigraphy for detecting bone metastasis in endemic nasopharyngeal carcinoma at initial staging. J Clin Oncol. 2006;24(4):599-604.
270. Ohta M, Tokuda Y, Suzuki Y, et al. Whole body PET for the evaluation of bony metastases in patients with breast cancer: comparison with 99Tcm-MDP bone scintigraphy. Nucl Med Commun. 2001;22(8):875-9.
271. Min JW, Um S-W, Yim J-J, et al. The role of whole-body FDG PET/CT, Tc 99m MDP bone scintigraphy, and serum alkaline phosphatase in detecting bone metastasis in patients with newly diagnosed lung cancer. J Korean Med Sci. 2009;24(2):275-80.
272. Takenaka D, Ohno Y, Matsumoto K, et al. Detection of bone metastases in non-small cell lung cancer patients: comparison of whole-body diffusion-weighted imaging (DWI), whole-body MR imaging without and with DWI, whole-body FDG-PET/CT, and bone scintigraphy. J Magn Reson Imaging. 2009;30(2):298-308.
273. Luboldt W, Küfer R, Blumstein N, et al. Prostate carcinoma: diffusion-weighted imaging as potential alternative to conventional MR and 11C-choline PET/CT for detection of bone metastases. Radiology. 2008;249(3):1017-25.
274. Schmidt GP, Schoenberg SO, Schmid R, et al. Screening for bone metastases: whole-body MRI using a 32-channel system versus dual-modality PET-CT. Eur Radiol. 2007;17(4):939-49.
275. Jung HS, Jee WH, McCauley TR, et al. Discrimination of metastatic from acute osteoporotic compression spinal fractures with MR imaging. Radiographics. 2003;23(1):179-87.
276. Baur A, Stäbler A, Arbogast S, et al. Acute osteoporotic and neoplastic vertebral compression fractures: fluid sign at MR imaging. Radiology. 2002;225(3):730-5.
277. Baur A, Stäbler A, Brüning R, et al. Diffusion-weighted MR imaging of bone marrow: differentiation of benign versus pathologic compression fractures. Radiology. 1998;207(2):349-56.
278. Stevens SK, Moore SG, Kaplan ID. Early and late bone-marrow changes after irradiation: MR evaluation. Am J Roentgenol. 1990;154(4):745-50.
279. Donovan DJ, Huynh TV, Purdom EB, et al. Osteoradionecrosis of the cervical spine resulting from radiotherapy for primary head and neck malignancies: operative and nonoperative management. Case report. J Neurosurg Spine. 2005;3(2):159-64.
280. Mut M, Schiff D, Miller B, et al. Osteoradionecrosis mimicking metastatic epidural spinal cord compression. Neurology. 2005;64(2):396-7.
281. Hirota S, Yoshida S, Soejima T, et al. Chronological observation in early radiation myelopathy of the cervical spinal cord: gadolinium-enhanced MRI findings in two cases. Radiat Med. 1993;11(4):154-9.
282. Koehler PJ, Verbiest H, Jager J, et al. Delayed radiation myelopathy: serial MR-imaging and pathology. Clin Neurol Neurosurg. 1996;98(2):197-201.
283. Wang PY, Shen WC, Jan JS. Serial MRI changes in radiation myelopathy. Neuroradiology. 1995;37(5):374-7.
284. DeSanto J, Ross JS. Spine infection/inflammation. Radiol Clin North Am. 2011;49(1):105-27.
285. Golimbu C, Firooznia H, Rafii M. CT of osteomyelitis of the spine. Am J Roentgenol. 1984;142(1):159-63.
286. Modic MT, Feiglin DH, Piraino DW, et al. Vertebral osteomyelitis: assessment using MR. Radiology. 1985;157(1):157-66.
287. Dagirmanjian A, Schils J, McHenry M, et al. MR imaging of vertebral osteomyelitis revisited. Am J Roentgenol. 1996; 167(6):1539-43.
288. Gillams AR, Chaddha B, Carter AP. MR appearances of the temporal evolution and resolution of infectious spondylitis. Am J Roentgenol. 1996;166(4):903-7.
289. Sharif HS. Role of MR imaging in the management of spinal infections. Am J Roentgenol. 1992;158(6):1333-45.
290. Carragee EJ. The clinical use of magnetic resonance imaging in pyogenic vertebral osteomyelitis. Spine (Phila Pa 1976). 1997;22(7):780-5.
291. Hlavin ML, Kaminski HJ, Ross JS, et al. Spinal epidural abscess: a ten-year perspective. Neurosurgery. 1990;27(2):177-84.
292. Rigamonti D, Liem L, Sampath P, et al. Spinal epidural abscess: contemporary trends in etiology, evaluation, and management. Surg Neurol. 1999;52(2):189-96; discussion 197.
293. Hsu W, Kosztowski TA, Zaidi HA, et al. Multidisciplinary management of primary tumors of the vertebral column. Curr Treat Options Oncol. 2009;10(1-2):107-25.
294. Mulligan ME, McRae GA, Murphey MD. Imaging features of primary lymphoma of bone. Am J Roentgenol. 1999; 173(6):1691-7.
295. Sze G, Abramson A, Krol G, et al. Gadolinium-DTPA in the evaluation of intradural extramedullary spinal disease. Am J Roentgenol. 1988;150(4):911-21.
296. Georgy BA, Snow RD, Hesselink JR. MR imaging of spinal nerve roots: techniques, enhancement patterns, and imaging findings. Am J Roentgenol. 1996;166(1):173-9.
297. Khosla A, Wippold FJ 2nd. CT myelography and MR imaging of extramedullary cysts of the spinal canal in adult and pediatric patients. Am J Roentgenol. 2002;178(1):201-7.
298. Beall DP, Googe DJ, Emery RL, et al. Extramedullary intradural spinal tumors: a pictorial review. Curr Probl Diagn Radiol. 2007;36(5):185-98.
299. Hamasaki T, Noda M, Kamei N, et al. Intradural extramedullary mass formation in spinal cord sarcoidosis: case report and literature review. Spine (Phila Pa 1976). 2003;28(20):E420-3.
300. Hacker DA, Latchaw RE, Yock DH Jr, et al. Redundant lumbar nerve root syndrome: myelographic features. Radiology. 1982;143(2):457-61.
301. Maki DD, Yousem DM, Corcoran C, et al. MR imaging of Dejerine-Sottas disease. Am J Neuroradiol. 1999;20(3):378-80.

302. Thawait SK, Chaudhry V, Thawait GK, et al. High-resolution MR neurography of diffuse peripheral nerve lesions. Am J Neuroradiol. 2011;32(8):1365-72.
303. Watters MR, Stears JC, Osborn AG, et al. Transdural spinal cord herniation: imaging and clinical spectra. Am J Neuroradiol. 1998;19(7):1337-44.
304. Thurnher MM, Cartes-Zumelzu F, Mueller-Mang C. Demyelinating and infectious diseases of the spinal cord. Neuroimaging Clin N Am. 2007;17(1):37-55.
305. Bowen BC, Pattany PM. Vascular anatomy and disorders of the lumbar spine and spinal cord. Magn Reson Imaging Clin N Am. 1999;7(3):555-71.
306. Krings T, Lasjaunias PL, Hans FJ, et al. Imaging in spinal vascular disease. Neuroimaging Clin N Am. 2007;17(1): 57-72.
307. Shapiro JH, Och M, Jacobson HG. Differential diagnosis of intradural (extramedullary) and extradural spinal canal tumors. Radiology. 1961;76:718-32.
308. Koeller KK, Rosenblum RS, Morrison AL. Neoplasms of the spinal cord and filum terminale: radiologic-pathologic correlation. Radiographics. 2000;20(6):1721-49.
309. Epstein F, Epstein N. Surgical treatment of spinal cord astrocytomas of childhood. A series of 19 patients. J Neurosurg. 1982;57(5):685-9.
310. Epstein FJ, Farmer JP, Schneider SJ. Intraoperative ultrasonography: an important surgical adjunct for intramedullary tumors. J Neurosurg. 1991;74(5):729-33.
311. Brotchi J, Dewitte O, Levivier M, et al. A survey of 65 tumors within the spinal cord: surgical results and the importance of preoperative magnetic resonance imaging. Neurosurgery. 1991;29(5):651-6; discussion 656-7.
312. Chou R, Deyo RA, Jarvik JG. Appropriate use of lumbar imaging for evaluation of low back pain. Radiol Clin North Am. 2012;50(4):569-85.
313. Gilbert FJ, Grant AM, Gillan MG, et al. Low back pain: influence of early MR imaging or CT on treatment and outcome—multicenter randomized trial. Radiology. 2004;231(2):343-51.

CHAPTER 21

Navigation and Robotics in Spine Surgery

Xiaobang Hu, Christopher Bonsignore, Isador H Lieberman

INTRODUCTION

Optimizing the accuracy of instrumentation has always been of great interest to spine surgeons. Traditionally, spine surgeons relied solely on their knowledge of spine anatomy and plain radiography to identify the proper anatomical level and confirm the position of spinal implants. However, even with experienced surgeons, the implant malposition rate could range from 6% up to 54% with these conventional techniques and such malposition may lead to serious vascular and neurologic complications.[1-5]

Since 1990s, significant progresses have been made in navigation technology with the integration of computer technology, imaging systems and robotics. In 1995, Nolte et al. reported the first successful clinical application of an image guidance system for the placement of pedicle screws in lumbar spine.[6,7] Since then, image guidance has been progressively integrated into spine surgery. Today, a variety of navigation technologies are available in spine surgery and some have even become routine in many centers.

Surgical robotics also emerged during the 1990s and since then much progress has been made to optimize the use of robotic technology in the operating room. Surgical robots aim to enhance and complement the surgeon's free-hand abilities during surgery. The recently developed robotic systems span the spectrum of surgical disciplines and include the ROBDOC, which is used to bore the medullary cavity of bones for hip implants, the Computer Assisted Surgery Planning and Robotics (CASPAR) system for hip replacement, the URS AESOP system for endoscopic camera support, and the Da Vinci (Intuitive Surgical) and Zeus (Computer Motion) systems for remotely manipulated minimally invasive procedures.[8,9] With the significant advances in the image-guidance field, several robotic systems have been developed to address challenges in spine surgeries, especially for the accurate placement of spinal instrumentation.[10-12]

TECHNICAL ASPECTS OF NAVIGATION-ASSISTED SPINE SURGERY

Currently, there are several commonly used methods for spinal navigation such as preoperative CT-based image guidance and intraoperative 3D fluoroscopy-based guidance. Although there are a variety of approaches, the underlying concepts are similar.

There are two essential steps for spinal navigation: image acquisition and processing followed by intra-operative navigation. The image acquisition and processing can be done preoperatively or intraoperatively. It can be a preoperative computed tomography (CT) scan or an intraoperative fluoroscopy. Then reference will be performed with remote tracking technologies such as infrared light-based optoelectronic tracking or electromagnetic tracking with the aim to form a relationship between the patient's intraoperative position and the orientation of navigation tools. A dynamic reference array (DRA) is attached to the bony structure such as spinous process to allow constant location tracking and accurate navigation. Then a matching of the anatomical landmarks with the preoperative or intraoperative imaging will be conducted.

When using preoperative CT-based registration, there could be a difference between the patient's preoperative CT position and the patient's intraoperative position. This problem could be alleviated by using single-level

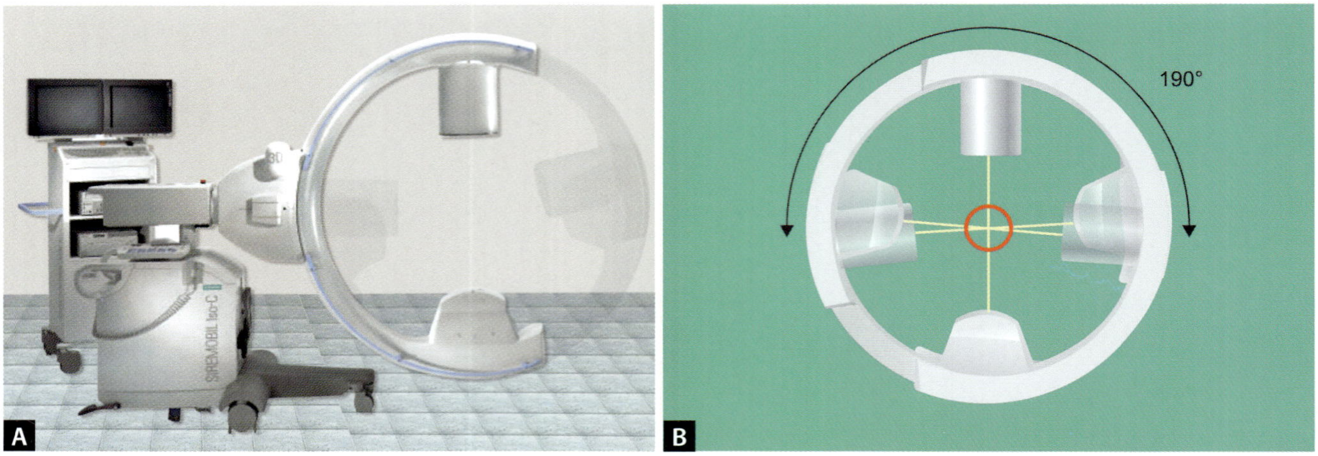

Figs. 1A and B: The Isocentric C navigation system. (A) Siemens SIREMOBIL® Iso-C3D C-arm with 3D imaging capabilities; (B) The Siemens SIREMOBIL® Iso-C3D is automatically rotated through a 190° arc about the patient to obtain 3D images.

registration; however, this is very time-consuming. An isocentric motorized C-arm could also help to solve this problem (Figs. 1A and B). The isocentric motorized C-arm can obtain multiplanar images as the fluoroscope rotates around the patient. These images can then be transferred to a workstation and reformatted into sagittal, coronal, and axial views. The intraoperative images are acquired while the DRA is attached to the bony anatomy. The registration process is automatic as an electro-optical camera is used to track the position of DRAs while the images are obtained. Then the placement of spinal instrumentation can be tracked real time based on the reconstructed images of the patients' intraoperative position.

One of the most recently developed spinal navigation system combines intraoperative CT (O-arm) with infrared tracking (Stealth) system (Medtronic Surgical Technologies, Louisville, CO). This system incorporates a flat-panel detector and can provide standard fluoroscopic images or volumetric CT scans. The X-ray source and detector are contained within a cylindrical bore which can open laterally. This allows the imaging device to be placed around a patient while he or she is lying on an operating table. The source and detector can move in a 360° arc and multiplanar (axial, coronal and sagittal) images can be obtained (Fig. 2A). An integrated LED tracker in the O-arm allows for its tracking with the navigation system (Fig. 2B). The registration process is automated as the images are obtained with the DRAs attached to the bony anatomy such as the spinous process. Navigated instrumentation can then be performed by using instruments such as the long drill guide (LDG). The length of the screws and their trajectory can also be planned directly on the computer station (Fig. 2C). After all levels are instrumented, a final scan can be obtained to verify optimal screw position and incorrect screw placements can thus be corrected immediately.

Using the isocentric motorized C-arm and the O-arm systems, any navigation inaccuracy due to inter-vertebral alignment differences between the preoperative CT scan and the intraoperative images can be eliminated. Also, the need for anatomical registration is obviated as navigation can start immediately after the images been transferred to the workstation. However, these systems are costly and can only be used with narrow radiolucent specially designed operating table.

TECHNICAL ASPECTS OF ROBOTIC-ASSISTED SPINE SURGERY

Currently, there is one robotic system approved and commercially available for spine surgeries (Renaissance, Mazor Robotics Ltd.). This system is based on a bone mounted hexapod miniature robot. It consists of the cylindrical robot composed of two endplates and six pistons which maneuver the endplates over six degrees-of-freedom (Fig. 3A), as well as a workstation that runs an interface software. Details of the system and related surgical techniques have been described previously.[12-15] Briefly, robotic-assisted spine surgery with this system includes the following steps:

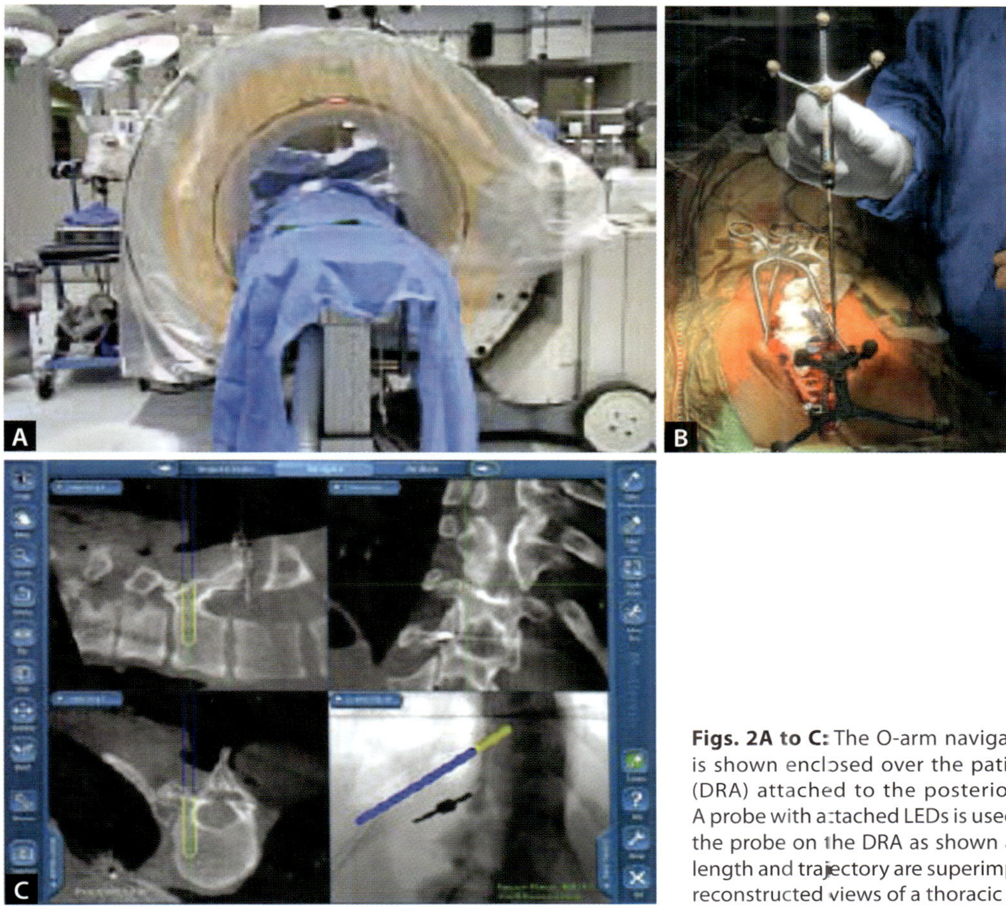

Figs. 2A to C: The O-arm navigation system. (A) The draped O-arm is shown enclosed over the patient; (B) A dynamic reference array (DRA) attached to the posterior elements of the exposed spine. A probe with attached LEDs is used to complete registration by placing the probe on the DRA as shown above; (C) The estimated screw size, length and trajectory are superimposed over axial, sagittal and coronal reconstructed views of a thoracic vertebra.

- *Preoperative planning (Figs. 3B and C)*: A standard CT (1 mm cuts) is performed and uploaded to the planning software. Preoperatively, the surgeon simulates different implants by selecting length, diameter, orientation and the angle of insertion, on a virtual 3D model of the spine. At the start of the operation, the surgeon uploads the preoperative plan into the workstation connected both to the robotic guidance system device and to the operating room C-arm.
- *Mounting the stabilization platform (Fig. 3D)*: The surgeon mounts a stabilization platform from either a bed mounted bracket or a clamp applied to the spinous process in the region of the surgery. A bridge is then secured onto the bracket or clamp and further secured with percutaneous K-wires to a bony prominence (spinous process or posterior superior iliac spine).
- *Automatic image registration*: Once the platform is secured, a reference frame is mounted to it and two fluoroscopic images are taken and transferred directly to the workstation software from the C-arm. Based on the images, the software performs a fully automatic image registration without the need for user intervention. The system then integrates the fluoroscopic images with the preoperative plan. The surgeon then verifies the system's accuracy in a segmental fashion (vertebrae to vertebrae).
- *Implant placement (Fig. 3E)*: Once registration is achieved and accuracy is verified, the robotic guidance device is mounted onto the frame and dispatched to the respective position from which the robot positions its arm in the trajectory planned by the surgeon, pinpointing the starting location of the planned implant insertion. The surgeon then drills and places the desired implant through a series of trocars attached to the robot arms.

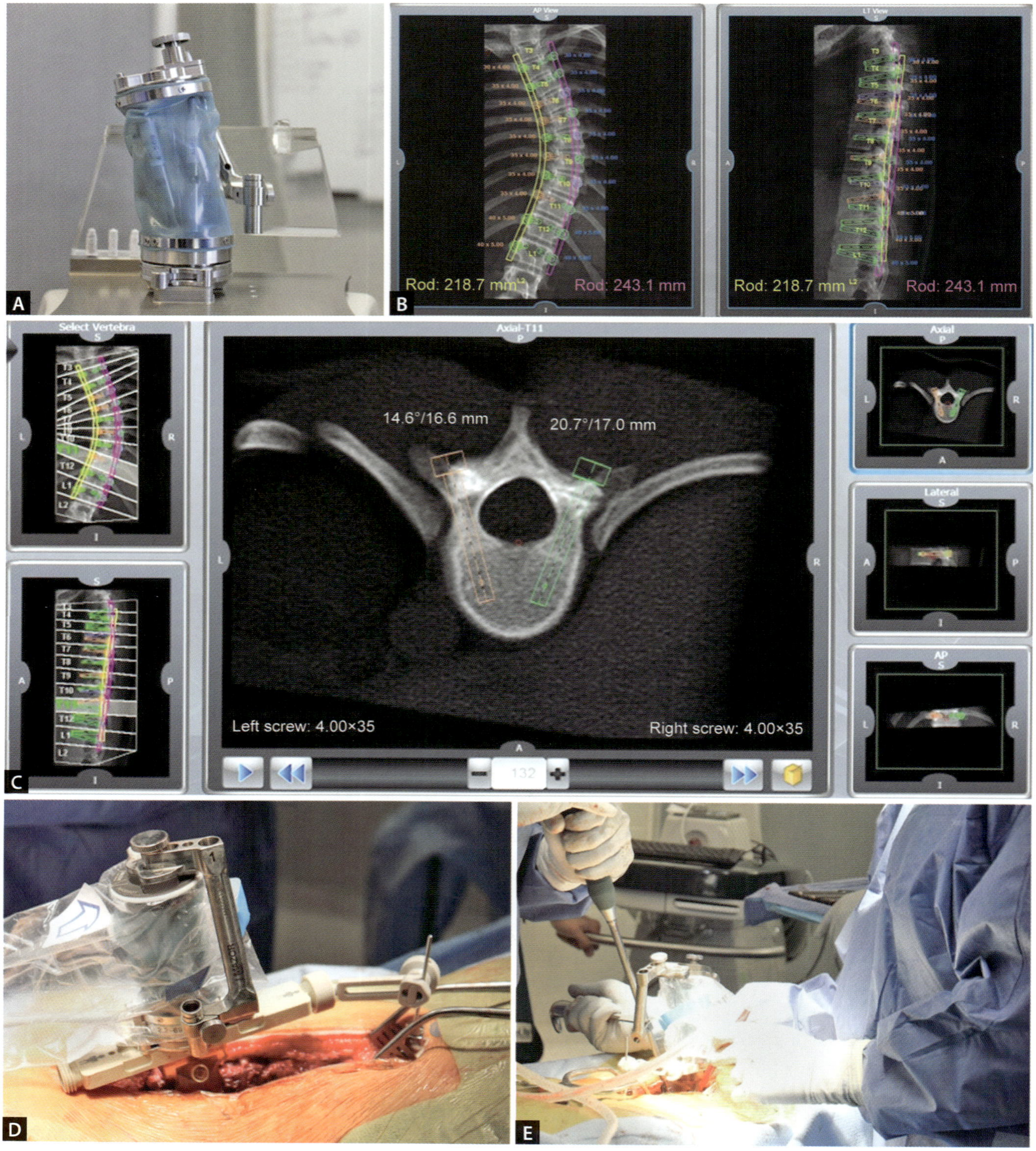

Figs. 3A to E: Robotic assisted pedicle screw placement. (A) The miniature robot; (B) Anteroposterior and lateral demonstration of the preoperative planning; (C) Axial view showing the position of planned screws; (D) Mounting the stabilization platform on patient; (E) Placing pedicle screw with robotic guidance.

GENERAL RESULTS OF NAVIGATION AND ROBOTIC-ASSISTED SPINE SURGERY

Accuracy

Various studies have shown that there is improved accuracy of pedicle screws implantation with navigation-assisted spine surgery. Preoperative CT-based image guidance is the first generation of navigation applied to spine surgery. Laine et al. in a prospective, randomized controlled study compared the pedicle screw insertion accuracy between preoperative CT-based navigation and conventional implantation methods. The authors found that the pedicle perforation rate was significantly lower in the navigation group (4.6% comparing to 13.4% in the conventional group).[16] Tian et al. in 2011 reported a meta-analysis and verified that the majority of studies showed improved implant accuracy with the preoperative CT-based navigation.[2] For 3D fluoroscopy-based navigation, the reported screw misplacement rates range from 2% to 2.5%.[17,18] This is in comparison with a 6–54% malposition rate with conventional techniques.[1-5]

For robotic-assisted pedicle screw placement, the reported misplacement rates range from 1.1% to 4% which is also superior to the conventional techniques.[13,19,20] However, a recent prospective randomized study compared pedicle screw placement in lumbar and sacral spine and the authors found that more screws in the robotic group were in suboptimal position comparing to the free-hand group. This result is surprising as most prior cadaveric and retrospective studies reported improved screw placement accuracy with robotic assistance. However, several technique factors such as the fixation method used in this study could have a negative influence on the performance of the robotic system.[21,22] Further studies will thus be necessary to compare the robotic system to free-hand and other guidance techniques.

Minimal and Less Invasive Surgical Techniques

Standard open spine surgery is associated with significant paraspinal muscle dissection and retraction which can result in significant intraoperative blood loss and postoperative pain. For properly selected patients, minimal and less invasive surgical techniques have the advantages of reducing the degree of soft tissue dissection and damage, decreasing intraoperative bleeding and faster postoperative recovery. However, there is reduced sensory feedback to the surgeon regarding the accuracy of pedicle screw placement as the surgeon has very limited visualization of the position of screws relative to the patient's anatomical structures. It has been shown that the navigation and robotic system can improve the accuracy of pedicle screw placement in these minimal and less invasive spine surgeries. Intraoperative real-time fluoroscopy-based navigation system and the robotic guidance system may provide the surgeon more confidence while performing percutaneous pedicle screw placement without directly viewing the anatomic landmarks.

In a prospective, comparative, multicenter study, Yang et al. found that with CT and fluoroscopy-based navigation for percutaneous placement of lumbar pedicle screws, the screw breach rate in the guidance group is less than half of the control group (3% compared with 7.2%).[23] Several authors also reported that intraoperative 3D navigation can provide a high accuracy of percutaneous lumbar pedicle screw placement.[24-27] Wood et al. compared the accuracy of minimally invasive lumbar pedicle screw placement using two different CT-based image-guidance techniques. They found that use of an intraoperative 3D fluoroscopy system with an image-guidance system results in greater accuracy of pedicle screw placement comparing to preoperative CT-based navigation.[27]

To date, there are two studies reporting the use of robotic-assisted percutaneous pedicle screw placement and both reported improved placement accuracy.[15,28]

Spinal Deformity Surgeries

Pedicle screw implantation can be especially challenging in patients with severe spinal deformity (such as scoliosis) and those patients who need revision surgeries where the anatomical landmarks were altered. Overall, it appears that the use of navigation and robotic assisted placement of pedicle screws in deformity surgery has a relatively low screw malposition rate. With the use of 2D or 3D navigation, the reported pedicle screw perforation rates vary between 2% and 4%.[4,29] Similar results were also reported in adolescent idiopathic scoliosis and congenital spinal deformity patients.[30,31]

For robotic assisted pedicle screw placement, Devito et al. reported a perforation rate of 4.1% in adolescent scoliosis patients.[32] We recently reported that with robotic navigation, the screw malposition rates were between 0.7% and 2.9% for the patients who had spinal deformity and/or previous spine surgery.[33]

CHAPTER 21

Surgical Time

The amount of time taken to insert a pedicle screw using navigation varies among different reports and it can be affected by many factors, such as the navigation technique, the surgeon's experience, the surgeon's familiarity with the navigation system and accuracy of the registration process.[34]

Sasso et al. retrospectively reviewed the operative time for posterior L5–S1 spine fusion between spinal navigation and conventional fluoroscopy techniques. They reported that the spinal navigation group has shorter mean operative time.[35] In a randomized clinical trial, Rajasekaran et al. reported that a significantly shorter time is required to insert a pedicle screw using the 3D isocentric fluoroscopy based navigation in thoracic spine deformities. The authors attributed this to the rapid registration process.[4] A prospective comparative study also showed that spinal navigation expedites the placement of guidewires for percutaneous placement of lumbar pedicle screws.[23] However, two studies including one prospective randomized study showed that the use of intra-operative CT navigation system increases the preparation time for screw placement and the actual time taken to insert pedicle screws.[36,37] More prospective randomized studies will help to better address the time issue associated with spinal navigation.

The amount of time taken to place an instrument using the robot system also varies. In a controlled, cadaveric implantation study, Lieberman et al. found that comparing to the conventional group, the robotic assisted surgery group has shorter procedure time and shorter time per screw.[38] However, in a retrospective review of 112 clinical cases, Kantelhardt et al. found that the average time per screw was not significantly different between the robotic-guided group and the conventional group.[28]

Radiation Exposure

Spine surgeries require thorough knowledge of the anatomy and the orientation of vertebrae, and its relation to the spinal column. As such, traditionally, spine surgeons rely heavily on intraoperative fluoroscopy or image guidance to achieve optimal screw/guidewire position. However, these conventional fluoroscopy-assisted techniques result in significant radiation exposure to the patient, surgeon and operating room staff.[14,20,39-44] Some studies have shown that there is less intraoperative radiation exposure time and total radiation dose with the use of spinal navigation.[45-50] A cadaver study showed that with spinal navigation, there is a significant reduction in ionizing radiation exposure to the torso of the operating surgeon.[41] However, for CT-based navigation system, the overall radiation exposure to the patient could be higher because of the need of high-resolution CT scans.[47,51,52] Nottmeier et al. shown that if the registration of spinal navigation can be performed on multiple vertebral levels, the amount of radiation could be significantly reduced.[53] In addition, Fransen found that the fluoroscopy time and radiation exposure differs between surgeons for the same procedure and simple awareness and training may help to reduce perioperative radiation exposure.[54]

Studies using the robotic system have shown a substantial decrease in the radiation exposure compared with conventional fluoroscope-assisted pedicle screw implantation surgeries.[28,38] The mean fluoroscopic image taken during robotic vertebroplasty was also significantly less than conventional vertebroplasty.[55,56] Meanwhile, because the robotic system requires a thin-sliced, high resolution CT scan, it is not clear whether the overall radiation to the patient is different from conventional fluoroscope-assisted surgeries.

Learning Curve

The learning curve of a novel surgical procedure is considered as the process for a surgeon to gain knowledge and improve skills about the novel procedure. It is an objective assessment of technical ability and a benchmark to compare different surgical techniques. Bai et al. found that the learning curve of spinal navigation dropped sharply after 6 months and it plateaued after 12 months which was shown by the improvement in screw perforation rate and operative time.[57] A recent study showed that the learning curve of navigation-assisted pedicle screw placement is not prolonged and experience with less than 10 patients was adequate to provide familiarity with the system.[58] However, the actual learning curve of spinal navigation may vary among different systems and different spinal procedures. It may also vary among different surgeons.

We recently assessed the learning curve of the robotic-assisted pedicle screw placement and it appears that surgeons will achieve consistent results after 30 cases especially in the setting of spinal deformity and/or revision spine surgery.[59]

Clinical Outcome and Cost-effectiveness

To date, there are no true studies comparing the long-term functional outcome of spinal implantation with or without navigation. Kantelhardt et al. reported that the patients required less opioids, had a shorter hospitalization and lower rate of adverse events in the perioperative period with robotic-assisted pedicle screw placement comparing to the conventional technique. These benefits are even greater for those patients who had robotic-assisted percutaneous procedures.[28]

It is generally agreed that spinal navigation adds to the cost of surgery. Increased utilization of navigation systems as well as development of novel and affordable navigation technique may help to improve its cost-effectiveness.[60,61] Considering the high cost of revision surgery for misplaced pedicle screws, utilization of navigation in difficult surgeries (such as patients with deformity) may be cost-effective in those spine practices who have heavy volume of challenging cases.[62]

CONCLUSION

Navigation and robotics has been revolutionizing surgery in a growing number of medical disciplines, such as neurosurgery, urology, gynecology, cardiology, and others. As importantly, they have the potential to change many aspects of the way we practice spinal surgery. The potential advantages of navigation and robotic-assisted surgery are increased implant placement accuracy and decreased malposition related complications, reduced invasiveness of the procedure, and reduced radiation exposure to the surgeons and operating staff. Successful application of the navigation and robotic system require careful planning, an adequate study of the spinal anatomy, and sound surgical experience. The navigation and robotic-assisted spine surgery systems are continuously evolving and only through careful clinical evaluation their successful applications, limitations, and areas for improvement can be defined (Table 1).

Table 1: Level-of-evidence.

Author, journal, year	*Design*	*LoE*	*Topic*	*F/U (m)*	*Measures*	*Main results*
Laine, European Spine Journal, 2000	RCT	I	Conventional vs. computer-assisted pedicle screw placement	NA	Time taken for screw insertion, pedicle perforation rate and complications	Improved accuracy with image-guided computer navigation, statistical analysis reported
Gebhard, Spine, 2006	PC	III	CT-based vs. Iso-C based navigation vs. non-navigation	NA	Duration of radiation time, radiation doses	Spinal navigation reduces the duration of radiation time and radiation dose, statistical analysis reported
Rajasekaran, Spine, 2007	RCT	I	Non-navigation vs. Iso-C based navigation	NA	Screw placement accuracy, screw insertion time, and the number of times the C-arm had to be brought into the field	Iso-C navigation increases accuracy, reduces surgical time and radiation in thoracic deformity correction surgeries, statistical analysis reported
Sasso, Journal of Spinal Disorders and Techniques, 2007	R	III	Computer-assisted guidance vs. intraoperative serial radiography technique	NA	Operative time	Image-guided spinal surgery did not cause an increase in operative time, statistical analysis reported
Nakashima, Journal of Spinal Disorders and Techniques, 2009	R	III	Iso-C 3D navigation vs. conventional fluoroscopy	NA	Screw placement accuracy	Improved accuracy with Iso-C 3D navigation, statistical analysis reported

Contd...

Contd...

Author, journal, year	*Design*	*LoE*	*Topic*	*F/U (m)*	*Measures*	*Main results*
Fraser, Minimally Invasive Neurosurgery, 2010	R	III	Iso-C/stereotactic 3D neuronavigation (3D NAV) vs. standard AP/lateral fluoroscopy (2D) NAV	NA	Screw placement accuracy	3D NAV for percutaneous or mini-open lumbar screw placement during the early learning curve for MISS was associated with higher screw accuracy, statistical analysis reported
Kraus, Clinical Orthopaedics and Related Research, 2010	Prospective + Retrospective	II	Conventional fluoroscopy-assisted vs. computer (3D)-navigated procedures	NA	Radiation dose to the patient	The patient's effective radiation dose can be reduced by 3D computer-assisted spinal and pelvic surgery, statistical analysis reported
Bai, Chinese Medical Journal, 2010	PC	II	Computer-assisted navigation vs. conventional fluoroscopy	NA	Pedicle screw accuracy and operative time	Computer-assisted navigation decreased the lumbar screw cortical perforation rate and operative time. The learning curve showed a sharp drop after 6 months, statistical analysis reported
Watkins, The Open Orthopaedics Journal, 2010	Prospective + Retrospective	III	Spinal navigation vs. non-navigation	NA	Rate of revision surgery, cost savings of spinal navigation	Image guidance for the placement of pedicle screws may be cost effective in spine practices with heavy volume, that perform surgery in difficult cases, and that require long surgical times for the placement of pedicle screws, statistical analysis reported
Allam, European Spine Journal, 2012	PC	II	Freehand vs. a generic 3D-based navigation	NA	Screw placement accuracy	3D navigation-assisted pedicle screw placement is superior to freehand technique in the thoracic spine, statistical analysis reported
Van de Kelft, Spine, 2012	Prospective, postmarketing clinical registry	IV	O-arm with StealthStation navigation	NA	Screw placement accuracy	High accuracy of pedicle screw placement, statistical analysis not reported
Yang, Spine, 2012	PC	II	Computer-assisted fluoroscopic navigation vs. conventional fluoroscopic placement	NA	Screw placement accuracy, fluoroscopy times and guidewire insertion times	Use of navigation reduces fluoroscopy and insertion times with increased accuracy in percutaneous lumbar pedicle screw insertion, statistical analysis reported
Larson, Spine, 2012	R	IV	O-arm with StealthStation navigation	NA	Screw placement accuracy	High accuracy of pediatric pedicle screw placement using intraoperative CT and a 3D navigation system, statistical analysis reported
Ughwanogho, Spine, 2012	R	III	CT-guided navigation vs. conventional freehand technique	NA	Accuracy and safety of thoracic pedicle screw placement, the frequency of intraoperative screw removal	CT navigation resulted in more optimally placed thoracic pedicle screws, fewer potentially unsafe screws, and fewer screw removals in patients with adolescent idiopathic scoliosis (AIS), statistical analysis reported

Contd...

Contd...

Author, journal, year	*Design*	*LoE*	*Topic*	*F/U (m)*	*Measures*	*Main results*
Larson, Journal of Pediatric Orthopedics, 2012	R	IV	O-arm with StealthStation Navigation	NA	Screw placement accuracy	High accuracy of pedicle screw placement in patients with significant congenital spine deformity and altered anatomy, statistical analysis not reported
Shin, Journal of Korean Neurosurgical Society, 2012	R	III	O-arm vs. C-arm fluoroscopy	NA	Screw placement accuracy, preparation and screwing time	O-arm guidance has higher accuracy, but the preparation and screwing time is longer than C-arm fluoroscopy, statistical analysis reported
Abdullah, Spine, 2012	Prospective case series	IV	O-arm navigation	NA	Radiation exposure to the spine surgeon	Radiation exposure is minimal to the surgical team during routine use of the O-arm imaging system in lumbar and thoracolumbar fusions, statistical analysis not reported
Lee, Journal of Spinal Disorders and Techniques, 2012	R	IV	Intraoperative CT (iCT) navigation	NA	Screw breach rate and screw revision rate, screw insertion time and screw revision time	The iCT navigation system is clinically feasible for thoracolumbar pedicle screw surgery. The learning curve was not steep. Statistical analysis not reported
Pechlivanis, Spine, 2009	Prospective case series	IV	Robotic-guided percutaneous pedicle screw placement	NA	Accuracy of pedicle screws placement	Robotic-guidance has high accuracy of percutaneous pedicle screw placement in lumbar spine, statistical analysis not reported
Devito, Spine, 2010	R	IV	Robotic-guided spinal implants	NA	Accuracy of pedicle screws and guide-wires placement	Robotic-guidance increases placement accuracy and reduces neurologic risks, statistical analysis not reported
Kantelhardt, European Spine Journal, 2011	R	III	Robot-assisted vs. conventional pedicle screw placement	3	Accuracy of pedicle screw placement, intraoperative X-ray exposure, duration of surgery, postoperative administration of opioid analgesics, adverse events, postoperative hospitalization, revision surgery	Robotic-guidance increases placement accuracy, reduces intraoperative X-ray exposure, decreases postoperative administration of opioid analgesics, decreases intraoperative adverse events and shortens postoperative hospitalization. Statistical analysis reported
Hu, European Spine Journal, 2012	R	IV	Robotic-guided pedicle screw placement	NA	Accuracy of pedicle screws placement	High accuracy of pedicle screw placement, statistical analysis not reported
Ringel, Spine, 2012	RCT	I	Robot-assisted vs. freehand pedicle screw placement	NA	Screw position, radiation exposure, duration of surgery/ planning, and hospital stay	Robotic guidance decreased placement accuracy of lumbar and sacral pedicle screws, statistical analysis reported

(F/U: follow-up; LoE: level-of-evidence; MISS: minimally invasive spine surgery; PC: prospective cohort; R: retrospective; RCT: randomized controlled trial; CT: computed tomography; NAV: Navigation)

REFERENCES

1. Jutte PC, Castelein RM. Complications of pedicle screws in lumbar and lumbosacral fusions in 105 consecutive primary operations. Eur Spine J. 2002;11(6):594-8.
2. Tian NF, Huang QS, Zhou P, et al. Pedicle screw insertion accuracy with different assisted methods: a systematic review and meta-analysis of comparative studies. Eur Spine J. 2011;20(6):846-59.
3. Kosmopoulos V, Schizas C. Pedicle screw placement accuracy: a meta-analysis. Spine. 2007;32(3):E111-20.
4. Rajasekaran S, Vidyadhara S, Ramesh P, et al. Randomized clinical study to compare the accuracy of navigated and non-navigated thoracic pedicle screws in deformity correction surgeries. Spine. 2007;32(2):E56-64.
5. Lou E, Zhang C, Le L, et al. Using ultrasound to guide the insertion of pedicle screws during scoliosis surgery. Studies in health technology and informatics. Stud Health Technol Inform. 2010;158:44-8.
6. Nolte LP, Zamorano L, Visarius H, et al. Clinical evaluation of a system for precision enhancement in spine surgery. Clinical biomechanics (Bristol, Avon). 1995;10(6):293-303.
7. Nolte LP, Visarius H, Arm E, et al. Computer-aided fixation of spinal implants. J Image Guid Surg. 1995;1(2):88-93.
8. Lanfranco AR, Castellanos AE, Desai JP, et al. Robotic surgery: a current perspective. Ann Surg. 2004;239(1):14-21.
9. Shoham M, Burman M, Zehavi E, et al. Bone-mounted miniature robot for surgical procedures: concept and clinical applications. IEEE Transactions on Robotics and Automation. 2003;19(5):893-901.
10. Lee J, Kim K, Chung W, et al. Human-guided surgical robot system for spinal fusion surgery: CoRASS. IEEE International Conference on Robotics and Automation. 2008.
11. Ortmaier T, Weiss H, Hagn U, et al. A hands-on-robot for accurate placement of pedicle screws. Proceedings of the 2006 IEEE International Conference on Robotics and Automation. 2006.
12. Lieberman IH, Togawa D, Kayanja MM, et al. Bone-mounted miniature robotic guidance for pedicle screw and translaminar facet screw placement: Part I--Technical development and a test case result. Neurosurgery. 2006;59(3):641-50; discussion 641-50.
13. Devito DP, Kaplan L, Dietl R, et al. Clinical acceptance and accuracy assessment of spinal implants guided with SpineAssist surgical robot: retrospective study. Spine. 2010;35(24):2109-15.
14. Togawa D, Kayanja MM, Reinhardt MK, et al. Bone-mounted miniature robotic guidance for pedicle screw and translaminar facet screw placement: part 2--Evaluation of system accuracy. Neurosurgery. 2007;60(2 Suppl 1):ONS129-39; discussion ONS39.
15. Pechlivanis I, Kiriyanthan G, Engelhardt M, et al. Percutaneous placement of pedicle screws in the lumbar spine using a bone mounted miniature robotic system: first experiences and accuracy of screw placement. Spine. 2009;34(4):392-8.
16. Laine T, Lund T, Ylikoski M, et al. Accuracy of pedicle screw insertion with and without computer assistance: a randomised controlled clinical study in 100 consecutive patients. Eur Spine J. 2000;9(3):235-40.
17. Allam Y, Silbermann J, Riese F, et al. Computer tomography assessment of pedicle screw placement in thoracic spine: comparison between free hand and a generic 3D-based navigation techniques. Eur Spine J. 2013;22(3):648-53.
18. Van de Kelft E, Costa F, Van der Planken D, et al. A prospective multicenter registry on the accuracy of pedicle screw placement in the thoracic, lumbar, and sacral levels with the use of the O-arm imaging system and StealthStation Navigation. Spine (Phila Pa 1976). 2012;37(25):E1580-7.
19. Hu X, Ohnmeiss DD, Lieberman IH. Robotic-assisted pedicle screw placement: lessons learned from the first 102 patients. Eur Spine J. 2013;22(3):661-6.
20. Sukovich W, Brink-Danan S, Hardenbrook M. Miniature robotic guidance for pedicle screw placement in posterior spinal fusion: early clinical experience with the SpineAssist. Int J Med Robot. 2006;2(2):114-22.
21. Ringel F, Stuer C, Reinke A, et al. Accuracy of robot-assisted placement of lumbar and sacral pedicle screws: a prospective randomized comparison to conventional freehand screw implantation. Spine (Phila Pa 1976). 2012;37(8):E496-501.
22. Cahill KS, Wang MY. Evaluating the accuracy of robotic assistance in spine surgery. Neurosurgery. 2012;71(2):N20-1.
23. Yang BP, Wahl MM, Idler CS. Percutaneous lumbar pedicle screw placement aided by computer-assisted fluoroscopy-based navigation: perioperative results of a prospective, comparative, multicenter study. Spine (Phila Pa 1976). 2012;37(24):2055-60.
24. Nakashima H, Sato K, Ando T, et al. Comparison of the percutaneous screw placement precision of isocentric C-arm 3-dimensional fluoroscopy-navigated pedicle screw implantation and conventional fluoroscopy method with minimally invasive surgery. J Spinal Disord Tech. 2009;22(7):468-72.
25. Fraser J, Gebhard H, Irie D, et al. Iso-C/3-dimensional neuronavigation versus conventional fluoroscopy for minimally invasive pedicle screw placement in lumbar fusion. Minim Invasive Neurosurg. 2010;53(4):184-90.
26. Wood MJ, Mannion RJ. Improving accuracy and reducing radiation exposure in minimally invasive lumbar interbody fusion. J Neurosurg Spine. 2010;12(5):533-9.
27. Wood M, Mannion R. A comparison of CT-based navigation techniques for minimally invasive lumbar pedicle screw placement. J Spinal Disord Tech. 2011;24(1):E1-5.
28. Kantelhardt SR, Martinez R, Baerwinkel S, et al. Perioperative course and accuracy of screw positioning in conventional, open robotic-guided and percutaneous robotic-guided, pedicle screw placement. Eur Spine J. 2011;20(6):860-8.
29. Larson AN, Santos ER, Polly DW Jr, et al. Pediatric pedicle screw placement using intraoperative computed tomography and 3-dimensional image-guided navigation. Spine (Phila Pa 1976). 2012;37(3):E188-94.
30. Ughwanogho E, Patel NM, Baldwin KD, et al. Computed tomography-guided navigation of thoracic pedicle screws for adolescent idiopathic scoliosis results in more accurate placement and less screw removal. Spine (Phila Pa 1976). 2012;37(8):E473-8.

31. Larson AN, Polly DW Jr, Guidera KJ, et al. The accuracy of navigation and 3D image-guided placement for the placement of pedicle screws in congenital spine deformity. J Pediatr Orthop. 2012;32(6):e23-9.
32. Devito DP, Gaskill T, Erickson M. Robotic-based guidance for pedicle screw instrumentation of the scoliotic spine. Spine Arthroplasty Society (SAS) 10th Annual Global Symposium on Motion Preservation Technology. 2010.
33. Hu X, Lieberman IH. Use of robotic assisted pedicle screw placement in deformity and revision spine surgery. The 19th International Meeting on Advanced Spine Techniques (IMAST), Istanbul, Turkey. 2012.
34. Purushothamdas S, Meir AR. Computer-assisted Spinal Surgery for Deformity-A Review. European Musculoskeletal Review. 2011;6(1):48-54.
35. Sasso RC, Garrido BJ. Computer-assisted spinal navigation versus serial radiography and operative time for posterior spinal fusion at L5-S1. J Spinal Disord Tech. 2007;20(2):118-22.
36. Shin MH, Ryu KS, Park CK. Accuracy and safety in pedicle screw placement in the thoracic and lumbar spines: comparison study between conventional C-arm fluoroscopy and navigation coupled with O-arm(r) guided methods. J Korean Neurosurg Soc. 2012;52(3):204-9.
37. Ryu K, Park C, Lee K, et al. Accuracy and safety in pedicle screw placement in the thoracic and lumbar spines: prospective randomized comparison study between conventional C-arm fluoroscopy and navigation coupled with O-arm guided methods. The International Society for the Advancement of Spine Surgery (ISASS) 11th Annual Conference Las Vegas, Nevada, April 26-29. 2011.
38. Lieberman IH, Hardenbrook MA, Wang JC, et al. Assessment of pedicle screw placement accuracy, procedure time, and radiation exposure using a miniature robotic guidance system. J Spinal Disord Tech. 2012;25(5):241-8.
39. Rampersaud YR, Foley KT, Shen AC, et al. Radiation exposure to the spine surgeon during fluoroscopically assisted pedicle screw insertion. Spine (Phila Pa 1976). 2000;25(20):2637-45.
40. Singer G. Occupational radiation exposure to the surgeon. J Am Acad Orthop Surg. 2005;13(1):69-76.
41. Smith HE, Welsch MD, Sasso RC, et al. Comparison of radiation exposure in lumbar pedicle screw placement with fluoroscopy vs computer-assisted image guidance with intraoperative three-dimensional imaging. J Spinal Cord Med. 2008;31(5):532-7.
42. Takahashi J, Hirabayashi H, Hashidate H, et al. Accuracy of multilevel registration in image-guided pedicle screw insertion for adolescent idiopathic scoliosis. Spine (Phila Pa 1976). 2010;35(3):347-52.
43. Ul Haque M, Shufflebarger HL, O'Brien M, et al. Radiation exposure during pedicle screw placement in adolescent idiopathic scoliosis: is fluoroscopy safe? Spine (Phila Pa 1976). 2006;31(21):2516-20.
44. Wu H, Gao ZL, Lü ZW, et al. [Radiation exposure to spine surgeon: a comparison of computer-assisted navigation and conventional technique]. Zhongguo gu shang. 2009;22(11):874-6.
45. Gebhard FT, Kraus MD, Schneider E, et al. Does computer-assisted spine surgery reduce intraoperative radiation doses? Spine (Phila Pa 1976). 2006;31(17):2024-7; discussion 2028.
46. Kim CW, Lee YP, Taylor W, et al. Use of navigation-assisted fluoroscopy to decrease radiation exposure during minimally invasive spine surgery. Spine J. 2008;8(4):584-90.
47. Bandela JR, Jacob RP, Arreola M, et al. Use of CT-based intraoperative spinal navigation: management of radiation exposure to operator, staff, and patients. World Neurosurg. 2013;79(2):390-4.
48. Nottmeier EW, Bowman C, Nelson KL. Surgeon radiation exposure in cone beam computed tomography-based, image-guided spinal surgery. Int J Med Robot. 2012;8(2):196-200.
49. Abdullah KG, Bishop FS, Lubelski D, et al. Radiation exposure to the spine surgeon in lumbar and thoracolumbar fusions with the use of an intraoperative computed tomographic 3-dimensional imaging system. Spine (Phila Pa 1976). 2012;37(17):E1074-8.
50. Kraus MD, Krischak G, Keppler P, et al. Can computer-assisted surgery reduce the effective dose for spinal fusion and sacroiliac screw insertion? Clin Orthop Relat Res. 2010;468(9):2419-29.
51. Park MS, Lee KM, Lee B, et al. Comparison of operator radiation exposure between C-arm and O-arm fluoroscopy for orthopaedic surgery. Radiat Prot Dosimetry. 2012;148(4):431-8.
52. Giordano BD, Baumhauer JF, Morgan TL, et al. Cervical spine imaging using mini--C-arm fluoroscopy: patient and surgeon exposure to direct and scatter radiation. J Spinal Disord Tech. 2009;22(6):399-403.
53. Nottmeier EW, Crosby T. Timing of vertebral registration in three-dimensional, fluoroscopy-based, image-guided spinal surgery. J Spinal Disord Tech. 2009;22(5):358-60.
54. Fransen P. Fluoroscopic exposure in modern spinal surgery. Acta Orthop Belg. 2011;77(3):386-9.
55. Boris S, ALIK B, Vitaly A. Robot guided surgery in treatment of osteoporotic fractures. European Federation of National Associations of Orthopaedics and Traumatology (EFORT) 2011 Annual Congress. 2011;abstract 1097.
56. Zaulan Y, Alexandrovsky V, Khazin F, et al. Robotic assisted vertebroplasty: our experience with a novel approach to the treatment of vertebral compression fractures. World Society for Endoscopic Navigated and Minimal Invasive Spine Surgery (WENMISS) Annual Congress; London, UK. 2008.
57. Bai YS, Zhang Y, Chen ZQ, et al. Learning curve of computer-assisted navigation system in spine surgery. Chin Med J (Engl). 2010 Nov;123(21):2989-94.
58. Lee MH, Lin MH, Weng HH, et al. Feasibility of Intra-operative Computed Tomography Navigation System for Pedicle Screw Insertion of the Thoraco-lumbar Spine. J Spinal Disord Tech. 2013;26(5):E183-E187.
59. Hu X, Lieberman IH. The learning curve of robotic assisted pedicle screw placement in spine surgery. The International Society for the Advancement of Spine Surgery (ISASS) 13th Annual Conference, April 3-5, 2013, Vancouver, Canada. 2013;Accepted as poster presentation.
60. Uhl E, Zausinger S, Morhard D, et al. Intraoperative computed tomography with integrated navigation system in a multidisciplinary operating suite. Neurosurgery. 2009;64(5 Suppl 2):231-9; discussion 239-40.
61. Abe Y, Ito M, Abumi K, et al. A novel cost-effective computer-assisted imaging technology for accurate placement of thoracic pedicle screws. J Neurosurg Spine. 2011;15(5):479-85.
62. Watkins RG, Gupta A, Watkins RG. Cost-effectiveness of image-guided spine surgery. Open Orthop J.. 2010;4:228-33.

CHAPTER 22 Evidence in Spinal Surgery

Daniel K Resnick

INTRODUCTION

Evidence-based practice is a practice where the available medical evidence is considered along with a consideration of available resources, physician experience, and patient wants and needs. In the ideal world, all medical decisions would be based upon irrefutable evidence demonstrating that a particular treatment decision was the most likely to result in a favorable outcome for an individual patient with a particular diagnosis. In reality, this situation will never exist. There is no piece of evidence so irrefutable, there is no diagnosis so specific, and there is no patient so generic that such a model could exist even in theory. As physicians, we are required to make decisions based on an incomplete understanding of faulty data on a daily basis. Patients with similar symptoms may respond completely differently to similar treatment strategies based on differences in the underlying etiology of their symptoms or individual idiosyncrasies. Further complicating the situation is that patients may have completely different definitions of "favorable outcome" than their caregiver. Despite these limitations, the pursuit of evidence-based practice is worthwhile as it forces a critical examination of treatment strategies and will eventually result in more effective, more efficient, and more appropriate care at the level of the individual patient.

In order to truly appreciate the worth of medical information for decision making, it is important to understand the strengths and limitations of the evidence considered. The purpose of this chapter is to discuss common sources of evidence used to make medical decisions in the treatment of patients with spinal disorders. By understanding the intrinsic strengths and limitations of evidence sources, the practitioner or policy maker will be better able to incorporate useful knowledge into everyday patient care.

SOURCES OF EVIDENCE

Physicians and policy makers are inundated with "evidence" from many sources. Administrative databases are frequently used to make sweeping indictments of medical care despite the fact that little or no patient outcome information is contained in such databases (with the exception of some complications data). Randomized trials are held up as the "gold standard" for development of medical evidence despite the fact that the methodology employed for such trials significantly limits the applicability of information gained. Case series are frequently criticized as an evidence source as they provide only descriptive information but may be the only possible way to gather information about certain disease states and treatments. Registries are being touted as a possible solution to fill perceived gaps in medical evidence yet critics note that registries are really not much more than a collection of case series! The remainder of this chapter will consist of a discussion of each of these evidence sources with a provided case example. Hopefully, the reader will gain an understanding about which evidence source is appropriate to answer which questions and how much "stock" to place in those answers based on methodology.

RANDOMIZED CLINICAL TRIALS

Randomized trials are truly the gold standard when a comparison is being made between two competing treatment strategies. The reason that this methodology is so powerful is simply the fact that randomization eliminates the influence of known or unknown confounding factors. For example, diabetes, smoking, and depression are important predictors of outcome in many studies looking at interventions for low back pain. If one were to do a comparison of outcomes achieved between two different treatment strategies and did not account for these factors, an apparent beneficial effect could be seen in one group simply because of differences in the prevalence of these predictors between the groups. If we knew all of the potential confounding factors and kept track of them, we might be able to control for them in a cohort study. The Spinal Outcomes Research Trial (SPORT) was designed as a randomized clinical trial (RCT) but suffered due to methodological issues which resulted in a loss of randomization[1-4] (discussed below). The data from the study is presented as a "well-controlled cohort study" because the authors kept track of many known risk factors for poor outcomes in spine care and were able to demonstrate that the treatment groups were comparable with regard to most of those risk factors. The quality of information derived from the study is downgraded, or considered of lower quality, because of the potential role of unknown confounding factors which may not be comparable between the groups. As it turns out, there were important differences detected between the groups with regard to disease severity and socioeconomic variables.

Another benefit of randomization is the elimination of treatment bias. In an examination of the database from the degenerative spondylolisthesis arm of the SPORT study, Abdu et al. were not able to demonstrate any significant differences in patient outcome when patients were stratified by fusion technique.[5] One potential interpretation of this information is that fusion technique is not important when treating degenerative spondylolisthesis. This interpretation would likely be very popular with third party payers who could use this interpretation as a justification for limiting access to more expensive fusion techniques—why pay for caviar if peanut butter has the same nutritional value? This interpretation is almost certainly false however based upon the fact that surgeons and patients agreed upon techniques on an individual basis and the biases of both the patients and surgeons influenced the choice of fusion procedure. For example, elderly patients with stable spondylolisthesis may have been disproportionately selected for noninstrumented posterolateral fusion compared to younger working patients with mobile slips. Anatomical and other functional details relevant to the choice of fusion technique were not collected as part of the initial database, so the role of this type of bias cannot be accurately quantified. If patients had been randomized to different fusion techniques, then such biases would be removed and the data would be of higher quality.

When interpreting an RCT, there are a number of quality indicators that need to be paid attention to. There are numerous factors that influence the quality of information derived from a clinical trial. A thorough discussion of all potential factors is beyond the scope of this chapter but there are a few which are easy to discern and important. One important factor to consider is the trial size. Were there enough patients included to be able to definitively state whether or not there was a difference between the groups compared? There should always be a description of a power calculation in the methodology. This is a mathematical calculation of the likelihood of accidentally missing a treatment effect. It is based on a preselected estimate of the size of a relevant treatment effect and a preselected estimate of the variability of outcome measurement (*see* http://statpages.org/#Power for a list of calculators and more information). If a trial is too small (underpowered) and fails to show a significant effect, then the importance of the negative trial is diminished. A second factor to consider is the fidelity of the randomization process. In simple terms, did the patients stay randomized? In the SPORT studies,[1-4] there was significant patient crossover between the treatment groups which resulted in a complete loss of randomization (patient selecting treatments based on their own bias). Choice of outcomes measures is also an important consideration. The outcome measure should be reliable, valid, and responsive (all of which can be measured mathematically) but should also make sense. For example, in the low back pain literature, measures of psychological distress are sometimes used as outcomes measures for surgical intervention.[6,7] While psychological distress is clearly an important factor in ultimate outcome, is it really logical to expect back surgery to alleviate psychological issues?

Perhaps the most important piece of information to consider is the nature of the treatment and control groups—is the comparison being made reasonable and reflective of actual practice? For example, there have been several RCTs evaluating the role of vertebral augmentation for osteoporotic compression fractures.[8-10] The results of these studies vary depending upon the selection criteria for inclusion into the study (the main difference being the methods used to identify the painful fracture and the time interval between presumed fracture and treatment) and the control group selected (standard nonoperative care versus anesthetic injection into the periosteum of the painful vertebra). Therefore, it is possible to influence the results of the study through patient selection and through choice of control groups. The usefulness of information gained from RCT's is limited to patients who are substantially similar to those selected for the study and who are offered treatment options similar to those utilized in the study. If, e.g. the study population was drawn from a very small group of "ideal" candidates, and your patient is not necessarily "ideal," it is not reasonable to expect similar results from similar interventions.

Despite these limitations (and others), the highest quality medical information is derived from RCT's. Why then are there so few high quality RCT's to guide spine care? There are practical as well as theoretical challenges to performing RCT's. First of all, RCT's are very difficult to run and are expensive. They require extensive preparatory work to determine the optimum study design and size, review by (usually multiple) institutional review boards (IRB), the employment of study coordinators (to administer the consent forms mandated by the IRBs, to assess for eligibility in the study and to collect outcomes data), and patient incentives (i.e. bribes) to encourage participation. In the absence of the possibility of a major return on investment, a private party (such as an instrumentation company) is unlikely to invest in such an enterprise and funding through public enterprises (such as the National Institutes of Health) is very limited. More important than these practical concerns however, are theoretical and ethical barriers.

The most important ethical barrier is equipoise. If a caregiver firmly believes in the superiority of a particular treatment strategy, is it ethical of that caregiver to withhold that strategy from a patient for the sake of a clinical trial? Many believe that it is not. An interesting example comes from the head trauma literature concerning the use of intracranial pressure (ICP) monitoring for the treatment of patients with severe head injuries. The American Association of Neurological Surgeons in conjunction with the Brain Trauma Foundation developed Guidelines for the Management of Severe Head Injury (Brain Trauma Foundation, 1995).[11] Among these guidelines was the recommendation for ICP monitoring for all severely head injured patients. This recommendation was based on observations that high ICP was associated with poor outcomes in a prospective registry (Traumatic Coma Databank).[12] The authors of the guideline reasoned that treating intracranial hypertension should improve outcome based on animal research and a number of clinical case series. They openly acknowledged that definitive evidence for ICP monitoring as a means to improve patient outcome was lacking, however they stated that a definitive trial would be impossible for both practical (greater than $5,000,000 in cost and more than 5 years to complete) as well as ethical reasons as follows: "(1) ICP monitoring has become an integral part of the management of severe head injury in virtually all head injury research centers. Hence, it would be difficult to design a study in which a group of patients would not be monitored; (2) The ethical basis for such a study may be questionable; (3) with several promising drugs becoming available for clinical trials, enthusiasm is limited for embarking on a study of a technique that is considered to be indispensable by most experts in the field; and (4) such a study was proposed ....but was not funded by the National Institutes of Health."

These guidelines remained unchallenged until 2012, when Randy Chestnut et al. performed a RCT in Latin America (where there was equipoise regarding the utility of ICP monitoring) evaluating the outcomes of patients with severe head injuries treated with or without ICP monitoring.[13] Compared to a standardized protocol of ICP management which did not employ an intracranial monitor, patients treated with the aid of an intracranial monitor did not enjoy a survival benefit or improvements in functional outcome. When the results of this study were presented at the 2012 meeting of the Congress of Neurological Surgeons, the only sound in the room was that of chins hitting the floor (DKR unpublished observation). This example shows the power of a RCT to radically alter our concepts of what is "considered to be indispensable by experts in the field."

Another barrier to RCT performance is a lack of patient equipoise. As we saw in the SPORT study, patients often have very strong preconceived notions about what they consider effective intervention and will resist randomization. In the previously referenced trials looking at vertebroplasty for osteoporotic compression fractures,[8-10] patient recruitment was ridiculously slow because the vast majority of patients treated by the investigators refused randomization because they had already decided that they wanted the procedure. This led to a highly select patient population in the study who may have had symptoms or other characteristics different from the majority of patients treated with the procedure. In trials of new technology, patients enroll in the study specifically so that they may have a chance to get the "latest and greatest" innovation. Patients who are randomized to the control group often are disappointed by their assignment and this disappointment may well affect scores for subjective patient reported outcomes measures.

Because of these barriers, RCT is not usually a good mechanism for evaluating established procedures and technologies where there is a strong bias for or against the procedure amongst patients and practitioners. Realistically, because of cost and effort, RCT's are not practical for evaluating the breadth of practice and are best reserved (in the author's opinion) for the evaluation of new or highly controversial procedures. They are absolutely essential when such procedures are associated with increased risk or expense compared to existent practices.

ADMINISTRATIVE DATASETS

The use of administrative datasets to evaluate healthcare utilization has grown in prevalence over the last decade and such studies have caused many to ask profound questions regarding the variability in consumption of healthcare resources based on geographic location. The large size of these datasets and the ease of statistical manipulation of their elements have made them popular fodder for healthcare economists. Unfortunately, many proponents of these methodologies have overstepped their data and offer "answers" without any relevant information to backup their assertions. The standard approach goes something like this: The rate of procedure X being performed in county A is much higher than the rate of the same procedure being performed in neighboring county B. There does not appear to be a major difference in overall wellness between counties A and B. Therefore, the utilization of procedure X in county A is too high. This argument would carry weight if in fact health outcomes were measured and found to be equivalent (and if numerous other methodological problems were addressed related to patient travel, access to care issues, and dozens of other potential confounds). As it turns out, at least in the spine literature, no such equivalence has been demonstrated or even investigated.

Because of this, the standard conclusions regarding overutilization of procedure X can be just as easily reversed. Consider the case for lumbar fusion. Christiansen et al. have determined that lumbar fusion is an effective and cost effective treatment for lower back pain.[14-18] This is not because lumbar fusion is exquisitely effective or cheap, it is because nothing (with the possible exception of long-term intensive cognitive therapy performed at select centers in Europe) else works at all for these very difficult patients who continue to consume resources during decades of ineffective care. If lumbar fusion is in fact more effective than nonoperative alternatives, then the utilization of lumbar fusion in county B may be inappropriately low. Now, every practicing spine surgeon has seen patients who were treated over aggressively with likely inappropriate surgery—this does happen and is a major issue that is being and must continue to be addressed through multiple mechanisms. However, every practicing spine surgeon has also seen patients with clear operative indications who have wasted years of their lives and countless thousands of dollars receiving ineffective and costly injections and who are now dependent upon narcotics and disability insurance to make it through the day. The goal of evidence-based practice is to operate on appropriate patients—not more or fewer patients. Administrative datasets do not contain patient outcomes measures relevant to spinal surgery and do not allow for the determination of "appropriate" rates. Therefore, analysis of these datasets generally does not contribute to the formulation of practice guidelines.

In 2010, Deyo and Martin published a report based upon an examination of the Medicare administrative database dealing with the operative treatment of Medicare patients with spinal stenosis. They reported that the overall rate of surgical intervention was fairly stable over a 5 year time period but that the utilization of fusion surgery, particularly "complex" fusion surgery increased significantly.[19,20] These authors indicated that this information indicated the over utilization of fusion in the elderly, leading to increased costs and complications.

The authors failed to note that during the time course of their study, the Center for Medicare Services changed the coding procedure for lumbar fusion resulting in classification of fusions which were "simple" during the first year or so of the accrual period as "complex" during the latter 2 years of the accrual period. This fact in and of itself probably explains the entire observed increase in reporting of "complex" fusion. Ignoring this obvious error, we are left with the fact that more patients were treated with fusion as an adjunct to decompression in 2007 than in 2002. Unfortunately, the proportion of patients who had spondylolisthesis, scoliosis, or sagittal plane deformity was not reported so the influence of spinal deformity and a widely acknowledged increase in aggressiveness in the treatment of deformity over the last decade could not be assessed. Critically, no information was provided on how the patients responded to the surgery. Given the increasing lifespan of the elderly and increasing demands for functional independence, the increased application of an effective technology would seem to be completely appropriate. If the increased application of the new technology did not result in improved outcomes, then the utilization is likely inappropriately high. We have no way of knowing what the answer is without clinical outcomes measures for the patients treated during the study period. This paper poignantly illustrates the limitations of administrative dataset analysis for making healthcare decisions. We have absolutely no way to tell if reported rates are too high, too low, or appropriate for the patient population treated.

Administrative datasets are useful for asking interesting and important questions such as "why is there such a disparity in utilization between neighboring counties." They are generally unable to provide answers to these questions because they do not contain patient reported outcomes relevant to the disorder being treated.

COHORT STUDIES, CASE SERIES, AND OTHERS

The vast majority of the literature in the field of spine care consists of case series and comparative cohort studies of varying quality. These studies may in fact contain valuable information, and for rare disease processes may be the only possible resource available for evidence gathering. Critics of evidence-based medicine frequently point out that a religious reliance on RCT's can force some pretty ridiculous conclusions. An early and very well done critique of EBM published in the British Medical Journal advocated the participation of evidence-based medicine zealots in a randomized controlled study of the use of parachutes when jumping out of planes.[21-23] The rationale being that since there are reports (e.g. case series) of survival after falling out of planes without parachutes and reports of death associated with parachute use, higher quality evidence is required to justify the costs and inconvenience of parachute use in skydiving. The author's point is very well taken, and a valid critique of the Cochrane review process is the complete reliance on RCTs, a practice that sometimes, in this author's opinion, results in a missing of the forest for the trees.[24,25]

Case series and most cohort studies provide descriptive information which may be valuable. Properly done prospective case series in fact provide the highest quality evidence regarding the prognosis of disease states and the influence of baseline characteristics on long-term outcomes. However, such studies do not generally provide high quality evidence when it comes to treatment decisions. The reason for this is bias. Patients are chosen for inclusion in a case series or inclusion in one arm or another of a cohort study for specific reasons. Often these reasons are very important all by themselves in terms of predicting outcome. For example, Fehlings et al. recently published a large prospective cohort study looking at the potential benefit of early surgical decompression for acute spinal cord injury.[26] They found that patients who were operated upon earlier did in fact have better outcomes than patients whose surgery was delayed. One interpretation of this (the authors interpretation) is that early surgery should be performed in patients with acute spinal cord injury.

This interpretation must be taken with a grain of salt because of confounds introduced by the study design. In this case, patients who were operated on earlier were in fact those who were available for operation earlier. These patients were the ones who arrived at a specialized treatment center promptly, were hemodynamically stable, and were examined within a few hours of injury. These patients did not have long transports, did not have medical comorbidities precluding operation, and did not have the opportunity for spontaneous improvement (frequently seen between the trauma bay and the ICU a few hours later) prior to entry into the study. Therefore, the "early surgery" group were healthier, at the nadir of their neurological function, and at the best possible place for treatment earlier than the "late surgery" patients. Any of these factors could have been important in the ultimate outcome. A randomized study would have eliminated these confounds and would have made the author's conclusions much more convincing. In fairness, the author group has tried heroically to get a randomized trial funded and performed, thus far without success (an illustration of the difficulty of performing RCTs).

Case series provide information on what happens to patients who are treated a certain way by certain practitioners. This information may be valuable, especially for prognosis as mentioned before. Treatment decisions for rare diseases or for the application of new technologies may be illuminated to some extent by these studies when there is little other background information available to guide treatment decisions. Case series do not, however, provide any information regarding the relative worth of one treatment strategy versus another for similar disease processes. Comparing case series in crude "meta-analyses" is not generally useful. Because the caregiver and the patient are free to select the treatment, substantial bias is introduced at the outset and it is not valid to assume that patients in different case series are drawn from the same patient population. For example, if we wanted to compare the management of cervical radiculopathy through surgical decompression versus transforaminal epidural steroid injection we could pull a fairly large number of case series and we would find that pretty much every case series reports good results with the author's intervention. Lumping this data together and stating that the results of the interventions are equivocal is not valid unless we are able to demonstrate that the patients selected for treatment in the various studies were substantially similar. It is pretty much the rule that patients selected for different interventions are at different stages in their disease process (that is generally why they selected one procedure over another). It is also pretty much the rule that there is not enough information provided to allow reasonable comparison of treatment groups.

In summary, the use of case series and cohort studies to make treatment decisions is problematic. Since this type of information is often all that is available, it should not be ignored but should be viewed with appropriate skepticism. Well-controlled cohort studies may be the best possible evidence available for well-accepted treatment modalities and case series' may be all that will ever be available to guide treatment of rare disorders. When higher quality evidence becomes available, the new information must supersede previous dogma.

REGISTRIES

Since the passage of the Affordable Care Act (ACA), there has been a tremendous amount of emphasis on the concept of comparative effectiveness research. The idea is that by collecting large volume of data concerning the characteristics and outcomes of patients treated for a variety of pathologies, meaningful information can be generated which will allow more effective and cost effective treatments tailored to individual patients. The most commonly cited mechanism for this type of research is through the use of registries. Registries are simply data repositories where information derived from clinical practice can be collated. The key difference between a registry and an administrative database is that a registry contains clinical information about patients linked to outcomes measures. This information can, potentially, permit the acquisition of meaningful data regarding who gets treated with which modality and what happens to these patients.

Depending upon the design of the registry, different types of information can be collected. The most common type of registry currently in use is a procedure based registry. The Neuropoint Alliance, a subsidiary of the American Association of Neurological Surgeons, has hosted two procedure based registries, Neuropoint SD and Neurosurgery quality and outcomes database (N2QOD). The Neuropoint SD registry[27] was a grant supported research project that tracked the results of microdiscectomy and single level fusion for spondylolisthesis at approximately 15 sites over a 1-year time frame. Through the employment of highly motivated site investigators, clinical coordinators, and patient incentives, a greater than 90% follow-up rate was achieved. The authors were able to demonstrate substantial improvements in patient reported outcomes measures for both procedures (Figs. 1 to 3) and established the feasibility of registry reporting across a reasonably sized consortium of practices. N2QOD is a similar project differing from Neuropoint SD, in that participating centers were required to fund the project and a mechanism for auditing of the reported outcomes measures was employed. At the present time, only 3 month data is available which appears to be very similar to that obtained by the Neuropoint SD study except on a larger scale, with several thousand patients enrolled as opposed to a few hundred.[28]

An astute reader might at this point question the quality of the data derived from a procedure based registry—how is this evidence any better than a case series? The answer is that for the purposes of establishing the relative worth of the index procedures, the information is a case series and of very little use for guiding treatment decisions. The value

CHAPTER 22

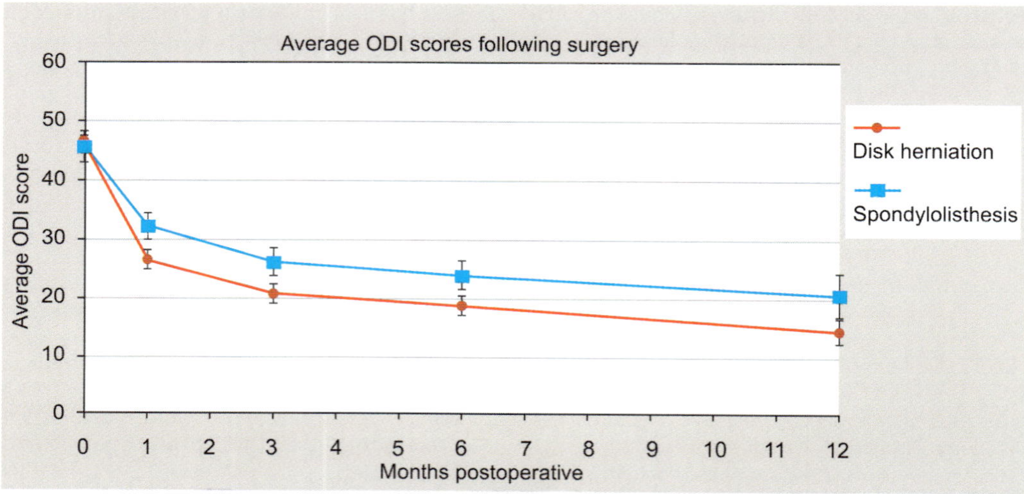

Fig. 1: Significant and sustained decrease in functional disability following surgical intervention for radiculopathy due to lumbar disk herniation or for neurogenic claudication associated with spondylolisthesis. The Oswestry disability index (ODI) is a disease specific measure and provides information regarding the effectiveness if an intervention for a specific disease process. This information was generated quickly through the use of a multicenter registry, illustrating the power of a registry to accumulate large amounts of patient reported outcomes data in a relatively limited time period.

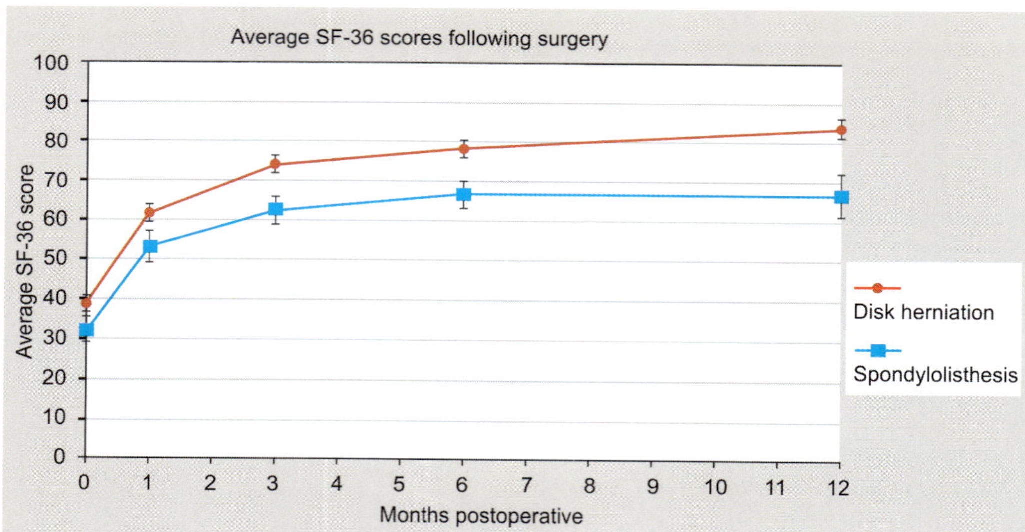

Fig. 2: Significant and sustained improvement in health status as measured by the SF-36 following surgical intervention for radiculopathy due to lumbar disk herniation or for neurogenic claudication associated with spondylolisthesis. The recording of health utility scores with generic instruments such as the SF-36 allows for the calculation of quality adjusted life years. If costs are known, then the value of an intervention and its relative cost-effectiveness compared to other treatments for similar or different disease processes can be determined.

of the registry design in this situation lies in the ability to collect large amounts of data quickly and to use this data to describe the characteristics of patients and surgeons which may predict better or worse outcomes.[14,29] The data can also be used to establish normative values for improvement that can be very useful for patient education, establishment of cost effectiveness (degree of improvement per unit cost), and for comparing participating centers against each other with regard to degree of patient improvement and complication rates.

In order to begin to determine the relative effectiveness of competing treatment strategies in any given patient

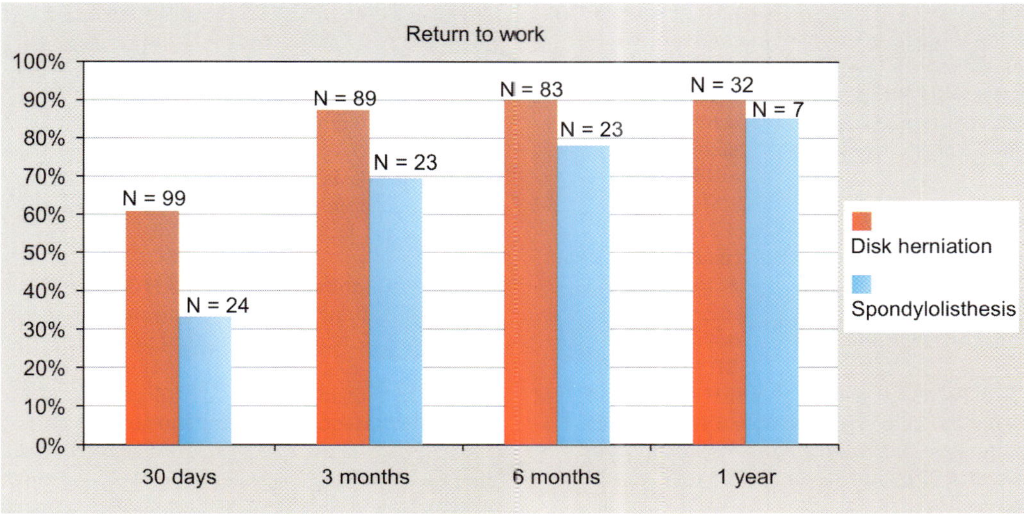

Fig. 3: By keeping track of demographic and socioeconomic variables, a registry can provide valuable information regarding the financial impact of an illness and potential treatments. Again, this information was gathered quickly through the use of a multicenter registry.

population, a "diagnosis" based registry is necessary. Instead of enrolling patients upon the performance of a particular procedure, patients are enrolled once they are demonstrated to have a particular diagnosis. The North American Spine Society is currently developing such a registry focused on common lumbar spine disorders such as disk herniation with radiculopathy, lumbar stenosis with neurogenic claudication, and lumbar spondylolisthesis with neurogenic claudication. Patients are entered into the registry upon the establishment of one of these diagnoses and are followed regardless of what treatment modality they choose. Through careful analysis of demographic variables, concomitant morbidity, and individual disease characteristics, the use of such a registry will allow the comparison of different treatment modalities in relatively similar patient populations. Information derived from this type of registry can be used for comparative effectiveness research. This is because in addition to providing rich descriptive information regarding which patients choose which procedures and when, the registry can provide information regarding the outcomes of these interventions, the pattern of use of these interventions, and the relative effectiveness of the interventions with evidence potentially consistent with well-controlled cohort studies. More importantly, high quality prognostic information can be gained which should enable a more rationale and evidence based selection of patients for interventions.

Another type of registry currently in use are complications registries, such as the Society for Thoracic Surgeons registry or the American College of Surgeons National Surgical Quality Improvement Program (NSQIP) which collect data regarding complications following index procedures. These registries are very valuable for helping to improve patient safety as it has been repeatedly demonstrated that simply the act of measuring an outcome can improve performance. Both of these registries have demonstrated measurable improvements in certain complication rates across the spectrum of care settings in North America. This success is in stark contrast to the failure of the most common government mandated "quality improvement" programs which use financial incentives to drive adherence to process measures. These programs by and large have not been shown to improve quality or reduce costs.[30] Therefore, even the most simple registries can provide information that is useful for quality improvement. Well-designed registries can provide high quality information regarding prognostic factors which may predict positive or negative outcomes after certain interventions. This information should be useful for improving the outcomes of patients subjected to those procedures by improving patient selection. Finally, the use of registries can provide useful, if not irrefutable, evidence regarding the relative value of different procedures in similar patient populations.

CLINICAL PRACTICE GUIDELINES

Clinical practice guidelines consist of a series recommendations regarding use of medical or surgical strategies for the treatment of patients with particular disorders. Guidelines can cover the utility of diagnostic tests, the efficacy of competing treatment strategies, the role of patient and disease characteristics in determining prognosis, and in some cases may touch upon cost effectiveness. These recommendations are based on a systematic review of the literature and a predetermined grading system for strength of evidence.[31] The quality of a guideline is directly related to the transparency of the search strategy and the rigorousness with which the grading strategy is adhered to. Another important factor is the make up and expertise of the author group. It is very important to have members of the author group expert in methodology in order to understand how the literature is to be evaluated and how the grading system is applied. It is also critically important for the author group to include subject matter experts who are better able to recognize the importance of conclusions drawn from the literature. Both the Institute of Medicine and the Council of Medical Specialty Societies have developed "quality criteria" for the production of clinical practice guidelines and many of their recommendations are broadly applicable.[32]

The quality and utility of an individual recommendation is directly related to the strength of evidence supporting the recommendation. Recommendations supported by multiple high quality RCT's are generally offered with a great deal of confidence, whereas recommendations supported by lower quality evidence or conflicting evidence will be offered with substantially less confidence. The first recommendation may be designated as a "Level I, A, or Strong" recommendation depending on the grading system whereas the second recommendation may be labeled as a "Level III/IV/V, C, or inconclusive." The reader is strongly encouraged to pay close attention to the scientific rationale offered in support of lower level recommendations, as these recommendations are most vulnerable to bias. We discussed the risks of intrinsic bias based on study design earlier, however publication bias and the opinions of the writing group can also substantially influence the final recommendation.

Publication bias results from the fact that a study with a positive result is much more likely to be published than a study with a negative result. A "positive" result may be defined here as a result that is consistent with the author's hypothesis. In extreme cases, multiple studies or statistical tests may be performed with mixed results yet only the results consistent with the author's hypothesis are presented (whenever a post hoc analysis is performed, be wary!). Recently, the government has required that ALL randomized trials be registered at a central website in order to allow interested reviewers the opportunity to see how many studies on a particular topic go unpublished.

Author group bias is operant during multiple phases of guideline formation. The first is the initial selection of the question to be answered by the literature review. It is necessary for a question to be specific enough to be answered, yet generalizable enough to be useful. Take, e.g. the question "Are epidural steroid injections effective for the alleviation of low back pain?" Depending upon the time frame and measure of efficacy chosen, the same evidence can lead to apparently opposite conclusions.

The next opportunity for author bias to occur is during grading of the quality of evidence from a particular reference. The most common reason for downgrading a piece of evidence is because of methodological flaws in the study. Perhaps the patient population was too small to rule out a potential treatment effect, perhaps a nonvalidated outcomes measure was used, or perhaps there was substantial crossover between treatment groups. These studies are downgraded and there is usually little controversy as there are fairly well-accepted standards for these parameters. A paper may be methodologically pure, however, and downgraded because it does not precisely fit the question asked. For example, if the patient population enrolled or the treatment groups assigned do not match the clinical scenario that the guideline is meant to influence, then the evidence may be downgraded. An example of this would be the potential downgrading of the previously discussed Buchbinder study.[8] This study compared vertebroplasty to anesthetic injection in a population of patients who were a very small minority of the patients treated at the center and who were treated across a large time interval following injury. If the question addressed by the guideline was "what is the benefit of vertebroplasty versus anesthetic injection in patients willing to be randomized," then the paper would provide definitive evidence that vertebroplasty does not provide benefit compared to anesthetic injection. If however, the question addressed is "what is the benefit of vertebroplasty versus usual medical management of patients with subacute osteoporotic compression fractures," then the paper does not provide as much useful information and the evidence would be downgraded. This type of analysis requires clinical expertise as a methodologist may not appreciate the difference between no treatment and sham treatment or may not appreciate the importance of the interval between injury and intervention. Depending upon who is in the room, these factors may or may not be accounted for and are a source of bias. This factor is what is most likely for observed differences in clinical practice guidelines on similar topics produced by different organizations.[33,34]

SUMMARY

The "evidence" used for clinical decision making in the medical literature in general and the spine literature in particular is made up of interpretations of a wide variety of evidence sources. When translating these interpretations into clinical treatment decisions, it is important to recognize the strengths and limitations of evidence sources. While it is difficult to defend treatment choices which subject patients to risk without strong evidence of efficacy, it is also unreasonable to expect a RCT to be performed to evaluate every variation of care within the currently accepted range of practice. Clinical practice guidelines represent systematic "snapshots" of the current knowledge base and these guidelines may be very valuable when combined with local expertise and patient desires.

REFERENCES

1. Weinstein JN, Lurie JD, Tosteson TD, et al. Surgical vs nonoperative treatment for lumbar disk herniation: the Spine Patient Outcomes Research Trial (SPORT) observational cohort. JAMA. 2006;296(20):2451-9.
2. Weinstein JN, Lurie JD, Tosteson TD, et al. Surgical versus nonoperative treatment for lumbar disc herniation: four-year results for the Spine Patient Outcomes Research Trial (SPORT). Spine (Phila Pa 1976). 2008;33(25):2789-800.
3. Weinstein JN, Lurie JD, Tosteson TD, et al. Surgical compared with nonoperative treatment for lumbar degenerative spondylolisthesis. four-year results in the Spine Patient Outcomes Research Trial (SPORT) randomized and observational cohorts. J Bone Joint Surg Am. 2009;91(6):1295-304.
4. Weinstein JN, Tosteson TD, Lurie JD, et al. Surgical vs nonoperative treatment for lumbar disk herniation: the Spine Patient Outcomes Research Trial (SPORT): a randomized trial. JAMA. 2006;296(20):2441-50.
5. Abdu WA, Lurie JD, Spratt KF, et al. Degenerative spondylolisthesis: does fusion method influence outcome? Four-year results of the spine patient outcomes research trial. Spine (Phila Pa 1976). 2009;34(21):2351-60.
6. Brox JI, Reikerås O, Nygaard Ø, et al. Lumbar instrumented fusion compared with cognitive intervention and exercises in patients with chronic back pain after previous surgery for disc herniation: a prospective randomized controlled study. Pain. 2006;122(1-2):145-55.
7. Brox JI, Sorensen R, Friis A, et al. Randomized clinical trial of lumbar instrumented fusion and cognitive intervention and exercises in patients with chronic low back pain and disc degeneration. Spine (Phila Pa 1976). 2003;28(17):1913-21.
8. Buchbinder R, Osborne RH, Ebeling PR, et al. A randomized trial of vertebroplasty for painful osteoporotic vertebral fractures. N Engl J Med. 2009;361(6):557-68.
9. Kallmes DF, Comstock BA, Heagerty PJ, et al. A randomized trial of vertebroplasty for osteoporotic spinal fractures. N Engl J Med. 2009;361(6):569-79.
10. Wardlaw D, Cummings SR, Van Meirhaeghe J, et al. Efficacy and safety of balloon kyphoplasty compared with non-surgical care for vertebral compression fracture (FREE): a randomised controlled trial. Lancet. 2009;373(9668):1016-24.
11. Bullock R, Chesnut RM, Clifton G, et al. Guidelines for the management of severe head injury. Brain Trauma Foundation. Eur J Emerg Med. 1996;3(2):109-27.
12. Aldrich EF, Eisenberg HM, Saydjari C, et al. Predictors of mortality in severely head-injured patients with civilian gunshot wounds: a report from the NIH Traumatic Coma Data Bank. Surg Neurol. 1992;38(6):418-23.
13. Carney N, Lujan S, Dikmen S, et al. Intracranial pressure monitoring in severe traumatic brain injury in latin america: process and methods for a multi-center randomized controlled trial. J Neurotrauma. 2012;29(11):2022-9.
14. Soegaard R, Bünger CE, Christiansen T, et al. Determinants of cost-effectiveness in lumbar spinal fusion using the net benefit framework: a 2-year follow-up study among 695 patients. Eur Spine J 2007;16(11):1822-31.
15. Adogwa O, Parker SL, Davis BJ, et al. Cost-effectiveness of transforaminal lumbar interbody fusion for Grade I degenerative spondylolisthesis. J Neurosurg Spine. 2011;15(2):138-43.
16. Adogwa O, Parker SL, Shau DN, et al. Cost per quality-adjusted life year gained of revision neural decompression and instrumented fusion for same-level recurrent lumbar stenosis: defining the value of surgical intervention. J Neurosurg Spine. 2012;16(2):135-40.
17. Glassman SD, Polly DW, Dimar JR, et al. The cost effectiveness of single-level instrumented posterolateral lumbar fusion at 5 years after surgery. Spine (Phila Pa 1976). 2012;37(9):769-74.
18. Polly DW Jr, Glassman SD, Schwender JD, et al. SF-36 PCS benefit-cost ratio of lumbar fusion comparison to other surgical interventions: a thought experiment. Spine (Phila Pa 1976). 2007;32(11 Suppl):S20-6.
19. Deyo RA, Mirza SK, Martin BI. Error in trends, major medical complications, and charges associated with surgery for lumbar spinal stenosis in older adults. JAMA. 2011;306(10):1088.
20. Deyo RA, Mirza SK, Martin BI, et al. Trends, major medical complications, and charges associated with surgery for lumbar spinal stenosis in older adults. JAMA. 2010;303(13):1259-65.
21. McGuire W. Parachute approach to evidence based medicine: arguments are easily refuted. BMJ. 2006;333(7572):807.

22. Potts M, Prata N, Walsh J, et al. Parachute approach to evidence based medicine. BMJ. 2006;333(7570):701-3.
23. Reeves BC. Parachute approach to evidence based medicine: as obvious as ABC. BMJ. 2006;333(7572):807; discussion 807-8.
24. van Tulder M, Furlan A, Bombardier C, et al. Updated method guidelines for systematic reviews in the cochrane collaboration back review group. Spine (Phila Pa 1976). 2003;28(12):1290-9.
25. van Tulder MW, Assendelft WJ, Koes BW, et al. Method guidelines for systematic reviews in the Cochrane Collaboration Back Review Group for Spinal Disorders. Spine (Phila Pa 1976). 1997;22(20):2323-30.
26. Fehlings MG, Vaccaro A, Wilson JR, et al. Early versus delayed decompression for traumatic cervical spinal cord injury: results of the Surgical Timing in Acute Spinal Cord Injury Study (STASCIS). PloS one. 2012;7(2):e32037.
27. Ghogawala Z, Shaffrey CI, Asher AL, et al. The efficacy of lumbar discectomy and single level fusion for spondylolisthesis. Results from the NeuroPoint-SD registry. J Neurosurg Spine. 2013;19(5):555-63.
28. McGirt MJ, Speroff T, Dittus RS, et al. The National Neurosurgery Quality and Outcomes Database (N(2)QOD): general overview and pilot-year project description. Neurosurg Focus. 2013;34(1):E6.
29. Schoenfeld AJ, Ochoa LM, Bader JO, et al. Risk factors for immediate postoperative complications and mortality following spine surgery: a study of 3475 patients from the National Surgical Quality Improvement Program. J Bone Joint Surg Am. 2011;93(17):1577-82.
30. Cima RR, Lackore KA, Nehring SA, et al. How best to measure surgical quality? Comparison of the Agency for Healthcare Research and Quality Patient Safety Indicators (AHRQ-PSI) and the American College of Surgeons National Surgical Quality Improvement Program (ACS-NSQIP) postoperative adverse events at a single institution. Surgery. 2011;150(5):943-9.
31. Resnick DK, Choudhri TF, Dailey AT, et al. Guidelines for the performance of fusion procedures for degenerative disease of the lumbar spine. Part 1: introduction and methodology. J Neurosurg Spine. 2005;2(6):637-8.
32. Institute of Medicine (U.S.). Committee on Standards for Developing Trustworthy Clinical Practice Guidelines. Graham R, Mancher M, Miller Wolman D, Greenfield S, Steinberg E (Eds). Clinical practice guidelines we can trust. Washington, DC: National Academies Press; 2011.
33. Chou R, Baisden J, Carragee EJ, et al. Surgery for low back pain: a review of the evidence for an American Pain Society Clinical Practice Guideline. Spine (Phila Pa 1976). 2009;34(10):1094-109.
34. Resnick DK, Choudhri TF, Dailey AT, et al. Guidelines for the performance of fusion procedures for degenerative disease of the lumbar spine. Part 7: intractable low-back pain without stenosis or spondylolisthesis. J Neurosurg Spine. 2005;2(6):670-2.

SECTION 3

Cervical

CHAPTER 23 Cervical Spine: History and Physical Examination

Marzena Buzanowska

INTRODUCTION

The cervical spine history and physical examination should be comprehensive on the first visit and if the patient reports similar symptoms in follow-up, a focused, problem oriented history and examination is appropriate. Evaluation of the cervical spine is incomplete without a history and examination including the craniomandibular complex as well as the glenoscapular region of the shoulder, as there is significant overlap in symptoms between the spine and adjacent joint structures, and one might come to incorrect conclusions without a complete assessment.

While evaluating the cervical spine it is important to consider neck pain within the biopsychosocial model (biological, psychological, and social factors) that may contribute to disorder and influence recovery; this fits within the framework of World Health Organization's International Classification of Functioning, Disability and Health domains, where impairments, activity and participation limitations are considered within the context of a person's overall health and quality of life.[1] This is especially important in some conditions of the neck where impairments may persist after resolution of symptoms.[2]

HISTORY

History taking relies on the knowledge of conditions of the cervical spine and their respective presentations. It focuses on eliciting the location and nature of patient's symptoms, type of onset, mechanism of injury, time course and duration, factors that may modify the symptoms (alleviate or exacerbate) as well as any associated findings, with special attention to "red flags".

As with assessment of any organ system; age, past medical, family and social history are important starting points because the differential diagnosis may be expanded in the setting of other underlying medical conditions. A young child with radicular upper extremity pain is more likely to have a tumor, while a middle-aged person with the same symptoms is most likely to have root compression due to a disk osteophyte complex. Inquiring about social history, such as patient's occupation, hobbies, recreational activities such as sports, may provide crucial information about the likely etiology of the patient's symptoms. It is vital however, to always keep an open mind while taking history, to not miss less likely but ominous conditions (Table 1).

Nature

The most common presenting symptom is pain. The choice of descriptors the patient uses to define their pain may give clues about the pathoanatomical source or its physiological mechanism. Pain that is dull and achy is more likely related to a problem of the bone, joint or muscle. Pain that is numb and tingly in nature is more likely related to nerve compression or irritation.

Location

The precise location of pain in the cervical spine sometimes cannot be discerned but when it can, it is very useful. Pain that is midline suggests a bony, ligamentous or disk etiology. Pain that is unilateral or bilateral may indicate the zygapophyseal joint or myofascial structures as the pain generator. Once the main location of pain is established, the next step is to determine pain referral patterns. Does the pain or paresthesia radiate into the arm/forearm or

Table 1: Cervical spine related diseases.

Common	*Less common*	*Not to be missed*
Myofascial neck pain	Whiplash	Metastatic/primary bone tumor
Degenerative disk disease	Stingers or burners	Compression fracture
Intervertebral disk herniation	Thoracic outlet syndrome	Cervical myelopathy
Zygapophyseal joint arthropathy	Referred pain from the glenoscapular or craniomandibular joints	Spondylolisthesis with instability
Cervical radiculopathy		Vertebrobasilar insufficiency
		Motor neuron disease
		Osteomyelitis/discitis
		Inflammatory arthritis

hand, and if so, is there a dermatomal pattern to it? If there is, it may indicate nerve root compression or irritation as etiology. If the pain radiates down the arm but without a clear dermatomal distribution, an intramedullary or peripheral nerve etiology needs to be considered. In addition to the widely accepted dermatomal pain distribution patterns, there are also well established pain referral patterns related to the cervical zygapophyseal joints. Dwyer et al. in 1990 published a study in which they reported results of pain referral patterns after cervical facet joint capsule distension in normal volunteers.[20] They found that the C2–C3 joint refers pain to the posterior scalp and suboccipital region and can produce a headache. The C3–C4 joint produces pain in the neck and suboccipital area. The C4–C5 joint related pain is in the entire neck and extends to the upper trapezius. C5–C6 joint produces pain in the lower neck, top of the shoulder and upper scapula. The C6–C7 joint refers pain to the upper trapezius and entire periscapular area.

Onset

The onset of symptoms can be sudden, delayed or insidious. The type of onset may be related to the mechanism of injury and includes trauma (sudden or delayed onset) or overuse injuries (abnormal posture, repetitive movements). If there was trauma, whether minor or major, further details need to be elicited, such as whether there were any associated bony fractures, ligamentous tears, loss of consciousness, etc.

Modifying Factors

Aggravating and relieving factors inform about the possible source of the patient's symptoms. If the symptoms improve with neck extension but worsens with flexion, this may indicate that the etiology is intervertebral disk or fatigue of cervical spine extensor muscles. If extension provokes pain, the most likely etiology is the zygapophyseal joint. If cervical rotation and extension combined together provokes distal symptoms, it may be related to compression of the neural structures, while if it provokes axial symptoms, it is likely related to the zygapophyseal joints.

Time Course

With few exceptions, patients will not present with cervical spine conditions immediately after the onset of pain or symptoms. While obtaining historical information, the clinician must find out how the symptom first started, how long it has been going on and what kind of progression there has been. Pain that lasts more than 6 months warrants further evaluation. If the pain has a progressively worsening course without pain free episodes, a more ominous etiology such as neoplasm is suspected. It is important to find out whether the symptoms are episodic or intermittent. Most of the benign cervical spine disorders are intermittent. If there were previous episodes with the same symptoms, it is helpful to know how the previous episodes resolved. Episodic pattern may suggest instability of the affected structure and may point towards the etiology as intervertebral disk versus arthritic changes. If the patient was pain free in between episodes, it is more likely that it can be accomplished again. A diurnal pattern of symptoms can also point to a specific source of pain. Pain that is worse in the morning or at night may have an inflammatory component (osteoarthritic, discogenic, infectious, rheumatologic), while pain that is worse at the end of the day and is best in the morning is more likely due to mechanical overuse, muscle fatigue or postural.

Associated Findings

While the cervical spine is a complex structure, a dysfunction or injury of different anatomical structures may present in a similar manner. Sometimes, the only distinguishing factor is an additional symptom, such as a headache, dizziness, dysphagia, dysarthria, nausea, fever, weight loss, muscle weakness or atrophy; presence of one or more of these symptoms may indicate a more serious pathology and are referred to as "red flags". Vertebrobasilar insufficiency from arterial stenosis or dissection may present initially as achy pain at the base of the skull. It may be associated with 5 "D"s for dizziness, dysphagia, dysarthria, diplopia, drop attacks. Craniovertebral ligament instability due to trauma, inflammatory or genetic conditions may also present with one of the 5 "D"s as well. In addition, there may be nausea, perioral paresthesia, tinnitus or syncope with neck rotation and extension. Muscle weakness in the neck or in the upper extremity, especially when it is not associated with pain, but associated with dysphagia or dysarthria requires consideration of a motor neuron disease or myopathy. Any mention of headache requires further questions. Even a subtle complaint of incoordination should raise a suspicion of injury to the spinal cord. In contrast to "red flag", a term "yellow flag" has been coined to indicate presence of factors that are predictive of poor long-term recovery or disability. These factors include high score on Pain Catastrophizing Scale, presence of depression and psychosocial factors.[3]

PHYSICAL EXAMINATION

Physical examination of the cervical spine follows the typical structure of a musculoskeletal examination and includes observation, palpation, range of motion, neurologic examination and special tests. The goal of physical examination is to confirm or reject the hypothesis and narrow or expand the differential diagnosis that the clinician has formed based on the history of the patient's symptoms. It is imperative that the examination of cervical spine includes the examination of the craniomandibular complex as well as the glenoscapular region and the evaluation will be incomplete without it.

Observation

The examination begins by observing the patient as she/he walks into the room. This includes analysis of the gait pattern, posture, use of assistive devices, quality of movement and ease of functional tasks such as removing coat/sitting in the chair. A closer observation of the affected area is ideally done with the patient in a gown. It should include a detailed posture evaluation—is there a loss of normal cervical lordosis, are shoulder forward flexed and rounded instead of slightly retracted, is there an increase in thoracic kyphosis. Also, note should be taken if the patient is guarding a certain body part, whether there are skin changes or rash, or if there is evidence of muscle wasting or hypertrophy.

Palpation

The palpation portion of the examination includes soft tissue as well as bony palpation. Bony palpation includes palpation of the cervical spinous processes as well as bilateral zygapophyseal joints. Tenderness of the spinous processes may be due to soft tissue injury, such as in a whiplash or a spinous process fracture if there is a history of trauma. Gwendolen Jull et al. reported that in cervical zygapophyseal joint arthritic pain, the precise level can be accurately identified on palpation.[19] Palpation of the zygapophyseal joints is best done with the patient in supine position and head comfortably resting on the examination table, ensuring that the neck musculature is completely relaxed. The examiner will start with finding the spinous process of C2, then the examiner will move each hand laterally about one inch to find the zygapophyseal joints. This is done most accurately by finding each spinous process first.

In cervical myofascial pain, palpation is a key component of evaluation. The examination will reveal trigger points, characterized by palpable nodules in skeletal muscle with associated taut bands of muscle fibers. Palpation of a trigger point will characteristically produce a twitch response with radiation of pain. Trigger points are most commonly noted in the upper trapezius, supraspinatus, infraspinatus, rhomboids, and levator scapulae muscles. Soft tissue examination is best done with the patient in sitting position and the examiner standing behind the patient. The examiner would begin by palpating the trapezius from its origin to insertion. The superior portion of the trapezius is frequently stretched in flexion injuries of the cervical spine, such as motor vehicle accidents. The examiner can then palpate the attachment of trapezius on the spinous processes and up to its origin on the superior nuchal line. Both sides should be palpated for comparison. When palpating the trapezius at the base of the skull, the examiner can move a fingerbreadth laterally on each side to palpate the greater occipital nerves, which may provoke pain and headache if it is inflamed (as in whiplash injuries).

Range of Motion

The orientation of the cervical zygapophyseal joints determines the amount and direction of motion that occurs between each segment of the cervical spine. The atlanto-occipital (AO) and atlanto-axial (AA) joints are not true synovial joints. The AO joint is composed of the articulation of each occiput with the superior articular surface of atlas. This joint allows about 13° of flexion and extension, lateral bending of about 8° and negligible rotation. The AA joint articulates at three locations, creating a medial atlantodental and two lateral AA joints. The AA joint allows about 47° of rotation, which accounts for 50% of the total rotation of the cervical spine.[4] Distal to C2, the superior articular processes of the zygapophyseal joints are oriented in a posterior and superior direction, at a 45° angle from the horizontal plane. Flexion and extension is greatest at the C5–C6 and C6–C7 joints, which amounts to 17° and 16°, respectively. The overall cervical flexion is generally between 50–69°, with extension between 73 and 93°. Lateral bending ranges between 11 and 38°, while rotation ranges between 26 and 74°.[5] Cervical spine range of motion is restricted in cervical myofascial pain, zygapophyseal joint arthropathy and in cervical radiculopathy. In 2003, Wainner et al. published a blinded, prospective study of 82 patients and found that a four test item cluster including a positive upper limb tension test A, involved side restriction in range of motion to less than 60° of rotation, positive distraction and Spurling's test had a positive likelihood ration of 30.3 in predicting cervical radiculopathy.[13]

Neurologic Examination

Neuromuscular evaluation should be performed on every patient, even if the patient does not endorse radicular pain or neurological symptoms. This is because patients tend to under-report symptoms that are not painful and certain conditions such as cervical myelopathy or motor neuron disease in early stages may present with subtle neurological deficits. The neurologic examination includes testing of muscle strength, muscle stretch reflexes, upper motor neuron signs (Hoffmann's sign, Babinski reflex, Lhermitte's sign, clonus), sensory examination, balance and coordination testing and on occasion cranial nerve examination. Both upper and lower extremity strength and reflexes should be examined. Description of a detailed neurological examination is beyond the scope of this chapter.

Special Tests

There are many special tests that can be performed in evaluating the cervical spine. Not all of them must be done for every patient and the selection of examination maneuvers will depend on the suspected etiology of patient's symptoms. These include:

Spurling's Neck Compression Test

Spurling's test is also known as foraminal compression test or neck compression test. It was first described in 1944 by Spurling and Scoville based on their observation of 12 patients who presented with radicular upper extremity symptoms and had surgically proven "ruptured cervical disks".[6] The test was originally described as "tilting the head and neck toward the painful side may be sufficient to reproduce the characteristic pain and radicular features of the lesion. Pressure on the top of the head in this position may greatly intensify the symptoms." The test is currently performed by neck extension and rotation to the symptomatic side, axial compression can be added. The test is considered positive if it reproduces radicular pain on ipsilateral side. Viikari-Juntura performed a prospective validity study of Spurling's compression test, axial manual traction and shoulder abduction test in evaluation for cervical radiculopathy.[7] Forty three patients who were referred for cervical myelography were interviewed and examined. The results were compared against findings of root compression on myelography with neurologic signs. The results were reported for roots from C6 to C8 and found that sensitivity of Spurling's compression test ranged from 40% to 60% while specificity ranged from 92% to 100%.

Shoulder Abduction Test

Shoulder abduction test is also known as Bakody's sign and is used in evaluation of cervical radiculopathy. It is described as "active or passive abduction of the ipsilateral shoulder so that the hand rests on top of the head. Relief or reduction of ipsilateral cervical radicular symptoms is indicative of a positive test".[8] This test was first reported by Spurling and described by Davidson et al.[9] Davidson et al. in 1981 published a prospective study of 22 patients with cervical radicular symptoms who presented for a myelogram. All of these patients were found to have an extradural compressive lesion. Fifteen (68%) of the 22 patients had a positive shoulder abduction test which led to the conclusion that shoulder abduction led to relief of the nerve root compression. In his 1989 study, Viikaru-Juntura assessed the validity of the shoulder abduction test in 22 patients.[7] It was reported that sensitivity ranged from 43% to 50% and specificity ranged from 80% to 100%. Ellenberg and Honet described the shoulder abduction test helpful in distinguishing cervical radiculopathy from shoulder pathology, when present.[10]

Neck Distraction Test

This test is also known as manual traction or cervical traction maneuver. This test is performed in supine position and is described as follows: "The examiner places on hand under the patient's chin and the other hand around the occiput, then slowly lifts the patient's head. The test is positive if the pain is relieved or decreased when the head is lifted or distracted".[8] The test is used in evaluation of cervical radiculopathy caused by discogenic pathology. In the same validity study by Viikaru-Juntura[7] the test's specificity was reported as 100%, while sensitivity was 40–43%.

Upper Limb Tension Test A

The upper limb tension test A or upper limb neural tension test with median nerve bias (also known as Elvey test) was originally described by Elvey in 1983 and was meant to serve a role similar to what the straight leg test does in evaluation of lumbar nerve root tension. There are three types of upper limb tension tests—(1) one with median, (2) radial, and (3) ulnar nerve bias. McLellan and Swash reported in 1976 that movements of the upper limb apply stress on the neural tissues.[11] It was later added by others that additional glenohumeral movements place tension on the cervical roots. The test is currently described as follows:[12] "With the patient positioned supine, the examiner performs the following movements in this order—scapular depression, shoulder abduction, forearm supination, wrist and finger extension, elbow extension followed by cervical contralateral then ipsilateral side bending." The test is positive if the arm symptoms are reproduced with cervical contralateral side bending and relieved with ipsilateral side bending. Wainner et al. in 2003 published a clinical prediction rule for cervical radiculopathy.[13] In a blinded, prospective study of 82 patients they found that a four test item cluster including a positive upper limb tension test A, involved side restriction in range of motion to less than 60°, positive distraction and Spurling's test had a positive likelihood ration of 30.3 in predicting cervical radiculopathy. Furthermore, the upper limb tension test was found to be the most useful test for ruling out cervical radiculopathy.

Vertebrobasilar Insufficiency Test

When history taking reveals presence of associated symptoms such as dizziness, nausea, vision changes, etc. it raises suspicion of involvement of the vertebrobasilar artery system. Vertebrobasilar insufficiency can be a result of arterial occlusion or dissection and may be intermittently symptomatic with transient changes in blood pressure and sometimes due to mechanical forces. The vertebrobasilar artery system can be occluded with neck in the end range of rotation and extension. Because the vertebrobasilar arteries deliver blood flow to the posterior circulation of the brain (midbrain, pons, medulla, cerebellum, thalamus, occipital cortex), the symptoms of insufficiency may include vertigo, double vision, blurry vision, nausea, dysarthria, dysphagia, paralysis or sudden onset of generalized weakness ("drop attack"). Often, patients may present with neck pain only. The test for vertebrobasilar insufficiency is performed with the patient lying supine on the table and the patient's head extending beyond the end of the table. The examiner then takes the patient's head in her/his hands and passively extends and rotates the head to the symptomatic side until end range or until patient reports symptoms. If this maneuver reproduces the patient's symptoms, it is considered positive. The test can also be performed in a sitting position with the patient actively extending and rotating the head to end range.[14] The value of this test however is questionable and it's thought to have poor validity and low sensitivity.[15]

Flexion-Rotation Test

This flexion-rotation test is used to assess for dysfunction at the C1–C2 motion segment. The C1–C2 segment is responsible for 50% of cervical rotation and motion of this segment can be isolated with the neck in flexion.[17] Normal range of motion at C1–C2 in end range flexion has been shown to be 44° to each side, while in subjects suffering from headache with C1–C2 dysfunction it is reduced on average by 19°.[16] The test can be performed actively with the patient in a sitting position or passively with the patient supine. The goal is to have the patient's neck maximally flexed and then rotated to both sides. If this motion reproduces pain on the ipsilateral side or there is restriction of range of motion on the ipsilateral side, the test is considered positive. This test has been shown to have a sensitivity of 90%, specificity of 88% and kappa of 0.85 for intertester reliability.[18]

SUMMARY

Neck pain is a very common complaint. While most of the time it is of benign etiology, due to vital organs passing through the neck, there are ominous processes that may present in a benign fashion. It is thus imperative that a knowledgeable clinician performs a thorough history and physical examination prior to administering a treatment plan.

TAKE HOME POINTS

- History taking is guided by clinician's knowledge of the most likely pathology as well as serious conditions that cannot be missed.
- Physical examination is partially dependent on the clinician's suspected diagnosis but a thorough examination should be performed in every new patient.
- Physical examination of the cervical spine must include examination of the craniocervical junction as well as the glenoscapular joint.

REFERENCES

1. Childs JD, Cleland JA, Elliott JM, et al. Neck pain: Clinical practice guidelines linked to the International Classification of Functioning, Disability, and Health from the Orthopedic Section of the American Physical Therapy Association. J Orthop Sports Phys Ther. 2008;38(9):A1-A34.
2. Sterling M, Jull G, Vicenzino B, et al. Physical and psychological factors predict outcome following whiplash injury. Pain. 2005;114(1-2):141-8.
3. Lentz TA, Beneciuk JM, Bialosky JE, et al. Development of a yellow flag assessment tool for orthopaedic physical therapists: results from the optimal screening for prediction of referral and outcome (OSPRO) cohort. J Orthop Sports Phys Ther. 2016;46(5):327-43.
4. White AA, Panjabi MM. Clinical Biomechanics of the Cervical Spine. Philadelphia: JB Lippincott; 1978.
5. Youdas JW, Garrett TR, Suman VJ, et al. Normal range of motion of the cervical spine: an initial goniometric study. Phys Ther. 1992;72(11):770-80.
6. Spurling RG, Scoville WB. Lateral rupture of the cervical intervertebral discs: a common cause of shoulder and arm pain. Surg Gynecol Obstet. 1944;78:350-8.
7. Viikari-Juntura E, Porras M, Laasone EM. Validity of clinical tests in the diagnosis of root compression in cervical disease. Spine (Phila Pa 1976). 1989;14(3):253-7.
8. Magee DJ. Cervical spine. In: Orthopedic Physical Assessment, 3rd edition. Philadelphia: WB Saunders; 1997.
9. Davidson RI, Dunn EJ, Metzmaker JN. The shoulder abduction relief test in the diagnosis of radicular pain in cervical extradural compressive monoradiculopathies. Spine (Phila Pa 1976). 1981;6(5):441-6.
10. Ellenberg M, Honet JC. Clinical pearls in cervical radiculopathy. Phys Med Rehabil Clin N Am. 1996;7(3):487-508.
11. McLellan DL, Swash M. Longitudinal sliding of the median nerve during movements of the upper limb. J Neurol Neurosurg Psychiatry. 1976;39(6):566-70.
12. Flynn TW, Cleland JA, Whitman JM. Users' Guide To The Musculoskeletal Examination. Evidence in Motion; 2008.
13. Wainner RS, Irrgang JJ, Boninger ML, et al. Reliability and diagnostic accuracy of the clinical examination and patient self-report measures for cervical radiculopathy. Spine (Phila Pa 1976). 2003;28(1):52-62.
14. Grant R. Vertebral Artery Testing–the Australian Association protocol after 6 years. Man Ther. 1996;1(3):149-53.
15. Côté P, Kreitz BG, Cassidy JD, et al. The validity of the extension-rotation test as a clinical screening procedure before neck manipulation: a secondary analysis. J Manipulative Physiol Ther. 1996;19(3):159-64.
16. Ogince M, Hall T, Robinson K, et al. The diagnostic validity of the cervical flexion-rotation test in C1/2 related cervicogenic headache. Man Ther. 2007;12(3):256-62.
17. Panjabi M, Dvorak J, Duranceau J, et al. Three-dimensional movements of the upper cervical spine. Spine (Phila Pa 1976). 1988;13(7):726-30.
18. Hall TM, Robinson KW, Fujinawa O, et al. Intertester reliability and diagnostic validity of the cervical flexion-rotation test. J Manipulative Physiol Ther. 2008;31(4):293-300.
19. Jull G, Bogduk N, Marsland A. The accuracy of manual diagnosis for cervical zygapophyseal joint pain syndromes. Med J Aust. 1988;148(5):233-6.
20. Dwyer A, Aprill C, Bogduk N. Cervical zygapophyseal joint pain patterns. I: A study in normal volunteers. Spine (Phila Pa 1976).1990;15(6):453-7.

CHAPTER 24

Spine Surgery: Current Concepts and Evidence Neck Pain

Zachary L Gordon, James D Kang

INTRODUCTION

Neck pain, as a result of degenerative disease of the cervical disks and facet joints, is a nearly universally experienced problem in the adult population. The changes associated with cervical disk degeneration are largely age-related, and often times are asymptomatic. For the purposes of this chapter, the term *spondylosis* will refer to age-related degenerative changes found within the spine.[1,2] These changes can subsequently manifest themselves into the distinct entities of axial neck pain, upper extremity radicular pain, myelopathy, or a combination of the three.[2]

This chapter will focus on the clinical entity of axial neck pain. Axial neck pain refers to pain along the spinal column and its related paraspinal muscles.[1] The epidemiology, natural history, physical examination and workup, medical treatment, surgical treatment, and prognosis will be discussed (Table 1).

EPIDEMIOLOGY AND NATURAL HISTORY

Axial neck pain affects adults of all ages, and both of the sexes nearly equally, however, there are very few population-based studies examining the prevalence of neck pain on which this claim is made.[1] There are three large, population-based studies that attempt to determine the prevalence of axial neck pain in the general population. These studies were conducted in Saskatchewan, Finland, and Norway.[3-5] In the Saskatchewan study,[5] the Saskatchewan Health and Back Pain Survey was mailed to 2,184 adults between the ages of 20 years and 69 years old. They received a response rate of 55% and the results were analyzed. The authors found that the lifetime prevalence of neck pain was 66%, with 5% of those being highly disabled by their pain. They also found that women were more likely to experience highly disabling neck pain than their male counterparts. According to the Finnish registry,[4] which incorporated survey results from 7,200 respondents at least 30-year-old, 9.5% of men and 13.5% of women were severely affected by a chronic neck pain syndrome. The affected individuals had a history of injury to the neck, back, or shoulders; or a history of mental or physical stress in the workplace. Between those aged 30 years and 64 years in their study, being overweight was also predictive of disabling neck pain. The Norwegian study found that 34% of the adult population surveyed had experienced neck pain within the past year and that 14% of those had symptoms lasting greater than 6 months.[3] Furthermore, a follow-up analysis of the Saskatchewan study found that the prevalence of neck pain was increased in individuals who were highly educated, or who had low-back pain or other medical comorbidities, including cardiovascular and digestive disorders.[6]

Unfortunately, no true natural history studies of neck pain exist.[1] In published studies examining the natural history of neck pain, most individuals had some kind of treatment precluding a true natural history without treatment. In fact, examining what happens to patients with axial neck pain who undergo no treatment at all in a large population would be a nearly impossible feat. However, there are still conclusions that can be drawn from these larger studies. DePalma and Subin[7] found that most patients suffering from axial neck pain resulting from cervical spondylosis will respond favorably to nonoperative treatment. In their study, 49% of patients had some improvement, and 29% of patients had complete

Table 1: Evidentiary table.

Author, journal, year	*Design*	*LoE*	*Topic*	*F/U*	*Measures*	*Main results*
Gore, Spine, 1987	RR	IV	Axial neck pain	15 years	Patient-reported pain, radiographic parameters	Long term F/U of patients with neck pain. 2/3 with the improvement of symptoms, 1/3 residual pain. No correlation of presence/severity of pain with radiographic findings
Grubb, Spine, 2000	RR	IV	Cervical discography	N/a	Patient-reported pain	Cervical discography is safe. Reproducible pain patterns are produced depending on levels injected
Dwyer, Spine, 1990	PC	IV	Cervical facet pain patterns	N/a	Patient-reported pain	Provocative injection of facet joints at different levels creates pain referred to distinct regions
Okada, Spine, 2009	PC	II	Cervical spine magnetic resonance imaging (MRI) correlation with symptoms	10 years	Patient-reported pain, MRI findings	In this longitudinal study, over 80% of patients had MRI evidence of cervical spondylosis progression, but only 34% developed pain
Gennis, Acad Emerg Med, 1996	RCT	II	Soft collar treatment for whiplash injuries	6 weeks	Patient-reported pain	Most patients with whiplash-associated pain have pain for 6 weeks. Soft collars do not affect the duration or degree of persistent pain
Rosenfeld, Spine, 2003	RCT	II	Active versus passive therapy for whiplash injuries	3 years	Patient-reported pain, cervical range of motion	Pain relief and length of sick leave significantly improved for active exercises versus passive treatment. Early active ROM improved final cervical ROM
Graham, Cochrane Database Syst Rev, 2008	SR	II	Cervical traction	N/a	N/a	Evidence regarding traction is highly biased. The available body of evidence does not support or refute the use of traction
Peloso, Cochrane Database Syst Rev, 2007	SR	II	NSAID, analgesic, and muscle relaxant medication for axial neck pain	N/a	N/a	There are limited evidence and unclear benefits of these types of medication in the treatment of axial neck pain
Pettersson, Spine, 1978	RCT	I	IV steroids for treatment of whiplash injuries	6 months	Patient-reported symptoms, duration of sick leave, sick-leave profile	Administration of IV methylprednisolone within 8 hours of whiplash injury significantly reduced pain, duration of sick leave, and improved the sick-leave profile
Andersen, Arthritis Rhem, 2008	RCT	II	Muscle-specific exercise versus general conditioning	10 weeks	VAS pain	Both general and muscle-specific exercise reduce neck pain, but muscle-specific exercise has a greater effect and provides longer-lasting relief
Bronfort, Spine, 2001	RCT	I	Compares neck exercise with spinal manipulation	1 year	Patient-reported pain, SF-36, patient satisfaction	Exercise combined with manipulation was superior to manipulation alone for patient satisfaction only at 1 year. No difference in SF-36.

Contd...

SECTION 3

Contd...

Author, journal, year	*Design*	*LoE*	*Topic*	*F/U*	*Measures*	*Main results*
Stav, Acta Anaesthesiol Scand, 1993	RCT	II	Epidural steroid injections	1 year	VAS pain	Significantly better pain relief at 1 week, and at 1 year, when steroid/local mixture injected in epidural space as opposed to posterior muscles
Manchikanti, Pain Physician, 2010	RCT	I	Epidural injections with or without steroid	1 year	Numeric rating scale, NDI	Significant improvements in pain and function with epidural injection of local anesthetic with or without steroids. No significant difference between the two groups
Cicala, Clin J Pain, 1989	CS, RR	IV	Epidural steroid injections	6 months	Patient-reported pain	70% of patients in this series had >50% relief of their pain for at least 6 weeks following treatment
Manchikanti, Pain Physician, 2004	PC	I	Medial branch blocks	1 year	Numeric rating scale, ODI, work status, persistent pain profile	Showed >50% pain relief at 3, 6, and 12 months. Improved physical function, work status, and psychological function at 12 months
Manchikanti, Pain Physician, 2010	RCT	II	Medial branch blocks with or without steroid	2 years	Numeric rating scale, NDI, employment status, opioid use	Showed >50% pain relief in over 85% of patients in both groups, no difference between the two groups. Significant improvement in function in both groups at 2 years
Barnsley, NEJM, 1994	RCT	II	Intra-articular facet injection local or local + steroid	20 weeks	VAS pain, McGill pain questionnaire, symptom checklist	No benefit to intra-articular steroid injection. Both groups had minimal pain lasting only 3 days. Recommended against intra-articular facet injection
Garvey, Spine, 2002	CS, RR	IV	Surgical treatment of axial neck pain	4.4 years	VAS pain, NASS satisfaction questionnaire, ODI, modified Roland-Morris disability index	Improvement in all outcomes measures with surgery. 82% of patients reported good, very good, or excellent outcomes. 93% reported improved pain, on average >50%

(CS: case series; F/U: follow-up; IV: intravenous; LoE: level-of-evidence; NDI: neck disability index; NSAID: nonsteroidal anti-inflammatory drug; PC: Prospective cohort; RCT: randomized control trial; ROM: range-of-motion; RR: retrospective review; SR: systematic review; VAS: visual analog scale; ODI: Oswestry Disability Index)

relief of their symptoms, while 22% did not improve at all after 3 months of conservative treatment.

Gore et al.[8] found similar results inf their long-term study of 205 individuals with axial neck pain and an average of 15.5 years of follow-up. In their study, all patients had at least 10 years of clinical and radiographic follow-up. They found that 79% of patients had a decrease in their pain and 43% of patients were pain-free. Unfortunately, 32% of the patients they followed had moderate or severe residual pain. Patients who had severe pain at presentation, and patients who suffered from neck pain as a result of an injury, were the most likely to have persistent symptoms and an unsatisfactory outcome. This is the closest study to a true natural history of neck pain that currently exists.

Rothman and Rashbaum[9] followed a group of patients with "predominantly" axial neck pain who were managed

CHAPTER 24

without surgery. About 23% of their patients remained partially or totally disabled from their symptoms after 5 years. They also found no significant differences between this group of patients and another similar group who underwent surgery for their neck pain. They went on to recommend nonoperative treatment of axial neck pain that was "nonneurogenic" in nature.

Taking all of these long-term studies into account, it is reasonable to assume that most patients will experience at least some decrease in their pain with little or no intervention. However, it is clear that a minority of patients, albeit a significantly large percentage, will continue to experience debilitating pain to some degree.

HISTORY, PHYSICAL EXAMINATION, AND WORKUP

History and Physical Examination

Axial neck pain is a very common presenting symptom and is usually nonspecific in nature. Pain or soreness may be felt in the paraspinal neck muscles posteriorly just off the midline, on one or both sides. The pain may radiate upward toward the occiput or out toward the shoulders and periscapular regions.[10] Headaches are often an accompanying symptom.[11] Patients may also report stiffness in motion in one or more directions. Fatigue is another symptom that may accompany axial neck pain. Generally speaking, most acute cases of neck pain are a result of soft tissue sprains or muscular injuries. These instances of neck pain will be accompanied by a history of injury, including twisting mechanisms, falls, or whiplash-type injuries. Soft tissue sprains are typically accompanied by localized tenderness and pain in the posterior musculature. Cases of axial neck pain with an insidious onset of pain that is longer-lasting in nature is more likely due to underlying cervical spondylosis.[12]

Referred pain into the shoulders or periscapular region may have a burning or tingling sensation, and may also be accompanied by autonomic phenomena including piloerection and diaphoresis.[10] This radiating pain typically occurs in a nondermatomal pattern. Burning pain in a dermatomal distribution should raise concern for cervical radiculopathy, which is a different clinical entity from axial neck pain, although the two are not exclusive of one another. Several studies suggest that nondermatomal pain can be attributed to degeneration of the cervical disks and facet joints.[13-17] A particularly important finding of pain distributions relating to degenerative disks was made by Grubb and Kelly in a review of their 12-year experience of cervical diskography.[17] They found that the stimulation of each subaxial cervical disk produced consistent and predictable patterns of pain. The pain patterns included the occipital, neck, and periscapular pain, some of which are overlapping depending on the levels involved (Figs. 1A to E). Dwyer et al.[16] performed a similar study, instead of using provocative injections into the cervical facet joints of asymptomatic volunteers. They also found a consistent and reproducible pattern of pain involving the suboccipital, neck, and periscapular regions (Fig. 2).

Determining a position of maximal discomfort is often helpful in determining the source of the underlying pain.[1,10] When pain is elicited along the sternocleidomastoid muscle that is made worse by rotation of the head to the opposite side, a muscular strain is most often responsible. Pain in the posterior neck muscles that is made worse with flexion of the neck suggests a myofascial cause. Pain in the posterior neck that is exacerbated by extension and rotation of the neck may point toward a diskogenic source of pain. Limited rotation of the neck to one side or pain localizing to the back of the ear or occiput with rotation strongly suggests atlantoaxial pathology.

After visual inspection and palpation of the cervical spine for areas of tenderness, the examination continues with determining the range of motion of the cervical spine. Range of motion of the cervical spine in all directions (flexion, extension, rotation, and lateral bending) should be quantified and compared from side-to-side, as well as normal values. Normal extension is the ability to gaze upward at the ceiling, and normal flexion is the ability to lower one's chin to the chest. Normal rotation is the ability to place one's chin nearly in line with the ipsilateral shoulder. Lateral bending is normal when the head is 45° from the shoulder without having to raise the shoulder upward toward the head.[18]

As is the case with any type of musculoskeletal complaint, performing a complete neurologic examination is an important next step. Motor and sensory examinations should include all of the nerve roots of the subaxial cervical spine from C5 through T1 and should be compared from side-to-side. Deep tendon reflexes of the biceps, triceps, and brachioradialis should also be evaluated. Weakness,

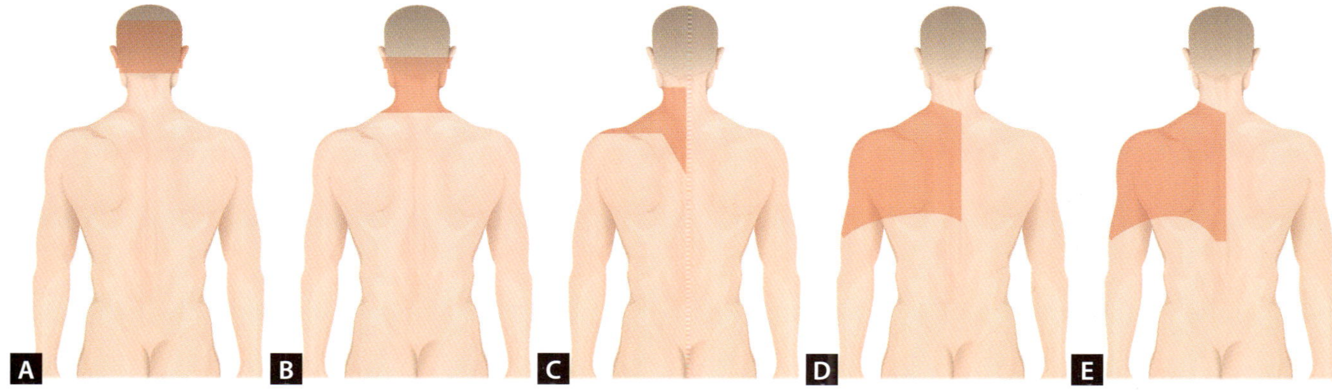

Figs. 1A to E: Axial pain patterns provoked during discography at each cervical level. (A) C2–3; (B) C3–4; (C) C4–5; (D) C5–6; (E) C6–7.
Source: Grubb SA, Kelly CK, Bogduk N. Cervical discography: clinical implications from 12 years of experience. Spine. 2000;25:1382-9.

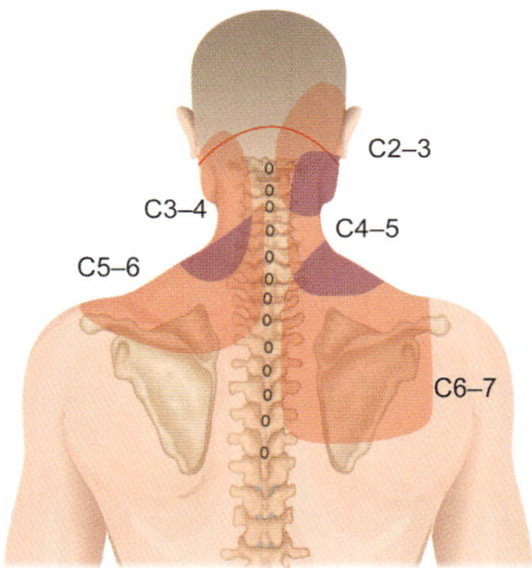

Fig. 2: Composite map of axial pain patterns from facet joints at C2–3 to C6–7.
Source: Dwyer A, Aprill C, Bogduk N. Cervical zygapophyseal joint pain patterns. I: A study in normal volunteers. Spine. 1990;15(6):453-7.

sensory deficits, or loss of deep tendon reflexes in one or more distributions may signify the presence of cervical radiculopathy, and its subsequent treatment differs somewhat from axial neck pain.

Other special tests may also be performed to rule out signs of radiculopathy. Signs of cervical radiculopathy include the Spurling maneuver, Valsalva test, and shoulder abduction sign.[1,18] The shoulder abduction sign is relief of shoulder and arm pain with the positioning of the head rotated toward the contralateral side and the ipsilateral shoulder held abducted over the patient's head. A positive Spurling maneuver is an exacerbation of shoulder and arm pain when the patient's neck is extended, rotated to the ipsilateral side, and an axial load is placed on the neck. A positive Valsalva maneuver is a demonstration of the typical shoulder and arm pain with a sustained Valsalva by the patient. The presence of one or more of these signs should tip the examiner toward a diagnosis of cervical radiculopathy. Although technically, a symptom rather than a test, the presence of the Lhermitte sign, electric shock sensations down the arms or legs with cervical spine flexion, should concern the physician for cervical myelopathy rather than the more common axial neck pain. One must keep in mind, though, that such electrical discharge can occur with extension. Thus, there is a correlation with the region (i.e. anterior, posterior, combined) of compression and pathobiomechanics of the spine.

Patients with overlapping shoulder pain should be carefully examined. A history of pain localizing to the lateral and anterior arm and radiating to the neck may suggest a glenohumeral or coracoacromial arch impingement process. A history of pain with overhead use of the hands and a physical examination with positive impingement tests can help delineate the shoulder girdle as the source of pain rather than the neck. Pain in the neck and shoulder can also be referred from processes involving the heart, lungs, other viscera, and even the temporomandibular joint. Neck stiffness occurring in the morning, the involvement of other joints, rigidity, and skin lesions may suggest an autoimmune or inflammatory-type process.

It is also important to differentiate mechanical neck pain from nonmechanical neck pain. The typical *mechanical* axial neck pain described above is a result of maintaining an upright posture and performing varying degrees of physical activity. *Nonmechanical* neck pain occurs while at rest and while lying flat. Nonmechanical pain coupled with fevers, weight loss, pain mostly at night, and other constitutional symptoms may represent an infectious or neoplastic process. When these symptoms are present, extra attention to the physical examination and imaging studies is warranted to differentiate these more urgent conditions from typical axial neck pain.

Imaging

The most basic, and least costly, imaging studies include an anteroposterior (AP) and lateral X-ray of the cervical spine. AP and lateral radiographs should be evaluated for signs of cervical disk degeneration and facet arthrosis, including narrowing of disk spaces with or without osteophyte formation, the reversal of the normal cervical lordosis, spondylolisthesis, uncovertebral joint hypertrophy, and apophyseal joint osteoarthrosis. The canal diameter can also be approximated on plain films. An open mouth odontoid view should be obtained in individuals when atlantoaxial pathology is suspected. Lateral flexion and extension radiographs may also be obtained to evaluate for dynamic instability, but are typically more helpful in the evaluation of cervical radiculopathy or myelopathy as they may demonstrate hypermobility of the cervical spine when dynamic spinal cord compression is suspected.

Typically plain radiography alone is sufficient when evaluating axial neck pain, especially the first time the patient is presenting to a physician. In cases where the pain has been present for a long duration, or if conservative management is not progressing as expected, advanced imaging may be obtained. The imaging study of choice in this setting is magnetic resonance imaging (MRI). Using MRI, the physician can evaluate the neural elements and soft tissues without radiation in a noninvasive setting.[19] Osseous anatomy can also be assessed, and the dimension of the spinal canal can be more accurately measured. Additionally, infiltrative soft tissue and vertebral abnormalities such as infection, sarcoma, and metastatic disease may also be recognized. Computed tomography (CT) myelography can be used instead for patients who cannot undergo MRI examination, although extraspinal soft tissue lesions may not be as easily assessed.

The cornerstone of evaluating patients with axial neck pain, and ruling out radiculopathy and myelopathy, continues to remain a thorough history and physical examination. In the cases of advanced imaging such as CT myelography and MRI, any findings must be correlated with the clinical evaluation of the patient. Boden et al.[20] reported MRI findings consistent with cervical spondylosis were present in 25% of asymptomatic patients under the age of 40 and in nearly 60% of patients older than 60 years. A 10-year longitudinal study of healthy volunteers performed by Okada et al.[21] showed that degenerative changes on MRI progressed in 81% of individuals, but only 34% developed clinical symptoms. Age was the only factor associated with progression of the radiographic disease.

Laboratory Evaluation

When evaluating patients for neck pain, laboratory studies are generally not needed when the history, physical examination, and imaging is consistent with mechanical axial neck pain. It is only when the neck pain is long-lasting and associated with other findings suggestive of inflammatory arthropathy, infection, or neoplasm that laboratory examinations may become useful.

In the setting of infection, a complete blood count may reveal an elevated white blood cell count. Thrombocytosis may also be another sign that systemic infection is present.[22] Typical systemic markers for infection include the erythrocyte sedimentation rate (ESR) and C-reactive protein (CRP). The leukocyte count may be elevated in only 42% of patients with spinal infection, but the ESR may be elevated in over 90%.[23-26] The ESR is a nonspecific test and may be elevated in other conditions such as pregnancy, malignancy, connective tissue disorders, and is influenced by serum globulin and fibrinogen.[25,26] Additionally, in infections with low-virulence organisms, the ESR may be normal.[27] The CRP test has largely supplanted the ESR as the study of choice for assessing for the presence of infection.[26] The CRP is an acute-phase reactant that increases within the first 4–6 hours and doubles every 8 hours, reaching a peak within 36–50 hours.[28,29] The degree of increase of CRP can be 10,000-fold, while the degree of increase of ESR is only 100-fold.[29] Additionally, the ESR only begins to increase after the onset of infection, and peaks around 7–8 days,[28] making it less useful in the very early stages of infection. Similar to ESR, CRP values are also nonspecific, and both values are typically elevated in the setting of an acute infection or inflammatory process.[30]

Inflammatory arthropathies such as ankylosing spondylitis or rheumatoid arthritis may also be associated with abnormal laboratory values.[31] Mild anemia with an elevated ESR and CRP, along with presence HLA-B27 and absence of rheumatoid factor and antinuclear antibodies is characteristic, although not entirely diagnostic, of ankylosing spondylitis. HLA-B27 is also present in other spondyloarthropathies such as psoriatic arthritis, reactive arthritis, and arthritis associated with inflammatory bowel disease. In the setting of rheumatoid arthritis, nonspecific markers such as ESR and CRP are elevated, rheumatoid factor is typically present, antinuclear antibodies are variably present (in up to 30% of patients), and serum globulin levels may also be increased.

Neoplastic or metastatic disease as the cause of neck pain is typically observed on advanced imaging of the cervical spine,[32] and should be investigated in cases of nonmechanical neck pain or in those with a history of malignancy. Laboratory abnormalities differ depending on the underlying neoplasm. For example, one would expect to see a monoclonal spike on serum protein electrophoresis (SPEP) in the setting of multiple myeloma. In metastatic disease, tumor-specific markers may also be elevated and can be used to follow the course of the disease.

MEDICAL MANAGEMENT

Once a diagnosis of axial neck pain is made, and other conditions such as spondylotic myelopathy and radiculopathy have been ruled out, the next step in management is to initiate a course of conservative treatment. The physician should keep in mind the goals of the treatment prescribed, as well as the patient's own goals.[12] The immediate goal is to control the patient's pain and allow them to continue with their daily activities with as little limitation as possible. Additionally, educating the patient on their condition, and what the trajectory of their symptoms is likely to be, is critical in designing an effective strategy to help them cope with their pain.

For patients suffering from acute pain, pain control is going to be the most important factor initially addressed. While some form of medication is usually prescribed, this should not be viewed as a permanent solution. A painful cervical spine can limit the return to normal activities, and the recuperation process can often be a lengthy one. The longer the period of inactivity, the more deconditioned the patient becomes, further inhibiting their return to normal activities. A comprehensive plan, centered on the goals of treatment and the patient's expectations, is the most effective way to ensure that a cycle of pain and inactivity does not develop. If the cervical degenerative disease is left untreated, and this cycle persists, the patient may be left with a chronic pain syndrome.[12]

There is a multitude of nonoperative treatments at the physician's disposal, and they will each be discussed individually with attention to the best available evidence. These conservative therapies include rest and bracing, passive modalities such as heat or ice, traction, medication, exercise and physical therapy, cervical manipulation, and steroid injections.

Bracing, Immobilization, and Rest

As is the case with lumbar strain and a short period of rest, many physicians have treated acute axial neck pain with a short period of immobilization in a soft cervical collar. It is thought that immobilization for a short period can help to diminish inflammation in the soft tissues surrounding the neck, and may help to alleviate spasm.[12] Disadvantages of immobilization in the neck are similar to those of immobilizing any other part of the body, namely the risk of muscle atrophy and deconditioning. Cervical spine soft collar use may be slightly different, as some motion is still maintained while in the soft collar.[33]

The use of cervical orthoses in the treatment of axial neck pain remains a controversial subject. There is very little reported on their use in the literature.[33,34] Results of a survey published in the British Journal of Rheumatology[35] found anecdotal evidence that 76% of patients found some benefit in wearing a collar, and that 78% found that their pain was somewhat relieved. Common complaints in their population were that the collar was too hot or uncomfortable to wear. This study had no control group and no validated outcome measures, so any conclusions may be invalid and may not justify the cost of the soft collar itself. Furthermore, a prospective, randomized trial

CHAPTER 24

comparing the use of soft collars in whiplash injuries to no collar showed that the duration of neck pain and overall recovery were not influenced by the use of a collar.[36]

Ice, Heat, and Passive Modalities

It is not uncommon for patients to attempt to treat their pain with ice or heat prior to seeking medical attention. Cold therapy may be effective in reducing spasm and pain in the immediate period after the onset of pain. Heat may initially worsen the pain but may be beneficial once motion has started to return.[12] Again, there is a paucity of literature regarding the efficacy of ice or heat on soft tissue injury, and most evidence is anecdotal. A meta-analysis evaluating the use of ice in soft tissue injuries (including areas other than the cervical spine) concluded that ice may be effective in reducing pain.[37] The authors also discuss that the mechanism by which ice helps has not been fully elucidated and that the quality of the studies included in their review were poor to begin with.

Other passive modalities such as massage, ultrasound, and iontophoresis (the use of electrical stimulation to deliver medication, usually steroid, transdermally) have also been shown to have little long-term efficacy in the treatment of axial neck pain.[38] These treatments are still prescribed by physicians because they pose little to no risk to patients. A Cochrane Review of massage for the treatment of neck pain found that only four published studies noted adverse effects.[39] These side effects were pain and hypotension following treatment, with hypotension occurring in 22% of patients. The authors found no long-term benefits of massage but noted some short-term relief of pain and tenderness. The use of passive modalities should be reserved as a compliment to treatments that actively involve the patient, as several other studies suggest that active rather than passive modalities are more effective in relieving symptoms.[40,41]

TRACTION

Cervical traction, particularly home-based traction therapies, have been said to provide temporary relief of pain in patients with axial neck pain or radiculopathy. Again, the majority of this evidence is anecdotal.[12] There has been some short-term benefit reported using at-home traction, however, these studies do not include long-term follow-up.[42-44] The study by Swezey et al.[44] demonstrated 81% of patients with mild to moderately severe spondylotic syndromes improved with a simple home traction system for 5 minutes twice daily. This study was retrospective and lacked a control group, so it is difficult to draw a valid conclusion on the efficacy of home traction. The authors called for more prospective, randomized studies.

A Cochrane review of traction for the treatment of neck pain with or without radiculopathy identified only seven randomized control trials of traction in the literature.[45] The study populations and indications for treatment varied. Only one study reviewed was identified as "low-bias", and the results suggested there was no benefit for the use of traction. The authors concluded that there are no randomized studies that either support or refute the use of traction, and that better studies which limit bias are needed to make that determination.

Medications

A number of medications have been used for the treatment of neck pain. These most commonly include nonsteroidal anti-inflammatory drugs (NSAIDs), narcotic pain medications, antidepressants, anticonvulsants, oral corticosteroids, and muscle relaxers.[46] These medications act by different mechanisms to affect the pain cascade at different points. All of them have been used with varying degrees of success.

Nonsteroidal Anti-inflammatory Drugs

Nonsteroidal anti-inflammatory drugs are widely used to treat musculoskeletal problems, including axial neck pain. They are used for both their anti-inflammatory and analgesic effects.[47] Most studies evaluating the efficacy of NSAIDs are for acute low-back pain, and there are few that address their use specifically for neck pain.[48-51] Generally speaking, these medications are safe and are easily available at a low cost to patients. Patients who take these medications for prolonged periods of time should be monitored for renal, gastrointestinal, and liver problems.[12] There is the availability of selective cyclooxygenase-2 inhibitors that may limit gastrointestinal and platelet inhibiting side effects, however, in controlled studies for osteoarthritis they do not appear to have improved efficacy over nonselective NSAIDs.[52-54] Although selective COX-2 inhibitors are well-tolerated by those with gestrointestinal (GI) upset issues, they have been implicated in cardiovascular complications including acute myocardial infarction and death.[55]

A Cochrane review article examining the evidence for the use of various medical and injection therapies for neck pain found only five studies related to the use of NSAIDs for axial neck pain.[50] These studies were graded as an indeterminate benefit since none were comparing the use of NSAIDs to a control group. Only two of the five published studies had similar groups where one of the treatment differences was the presence or absence of NSAIDs in the treatment plan,[56,57] and in only one of the five was the single difference the use of NSAIDs.[56] In this study, the authors found no difference in pain at 4 weeks when patients underwent a trial of manipulation with or without concomitant use of ibuprofen. The clear takeaway here is that there is severely limited evidence for the use of NSAIDs as they relate specifically to mechanical neck pain, and further studies are warranted. To quote the authors, "systematic evaluation of medicines for neck pain yielded disappointing results".

Narcotic Pain Medication

Narcotic pain medication may be reasonable or even necessary to control severe pain in the acute setting. They should not be prescribed for the long-term management of symptoms due to the potential for abuse, tolerance, and addiction. The ideal setting for narcotic pain medication use would be only for breakthrough pain for patients who are relying on more traditional type medications such as NSAIDs, or for patients who are intolerant of NSAIDs.[12] The side effect profile of narcotics is well established and includes sedation, constipation, and possibilities for abuse. Additionally, there is little attention paid to the depressant qualities of narcotic pain medication,[12] which can be a problem in a population of patients where rates of depression are high.[58] A truly multidisciplinary approach must be undertaken for patients suffering from chronic neck pain, including psychological support and counseling. These types of programs are typically run by anesthesiologists or physiatrists and are increasing in popularity for patients with chronic neck pain and other chronic pain disorders.

Unfortunately, the rate of narcotic pain medication being prescribed by primary care practitioners in the United States is on the rise.[59] As is the case with other treatment modalities discussed so far, there is little or no evidence that narcotic pain medication is of any benefit for the treatment of axial neck pain.[50,60] There have been some benefits reported for the use of narcotics in the treatment of low-back pain,[61] and this has been extrapolated to other spine conditions. Additionally, the studies conducted on the use of opioid medications do not adequately address the long-term harms associated with their use.[60,61]

Antidepressants and Anticonvulsants

Antidepressants and anticonvulsants are more typically used in the treatment of neuropathic pain disorders.[12] The most commonly prescribed medication of this class prescribed for the treatment of cervical spondylotic disease is amitriptyline.[46] The mechanism by which these medications may be beneficial is unknown. They have been used to treat depression and other mood disorders, which can be an accompanying problem for patients with chronic neck pain and may also have an analgesic and sedative effect helping with sleep patterns. No studies on their use specifically for neck pain exist, but there has been at least one study where there was a beneficial effect for low-back pain and lumbar radiculopathy.[62]

Oral Corticosteroids

Oral corticosteroids are a commonly prescribed class of medications used to treat patients with acute neck or arm pain.[46] They may be beneficial in reducing short-term pain. Only one study involving corticosteroids for the treatment of acute neck pain secondary to whiplash demonstrates a short-term benefit if administered within the first 8 hours, but no long-term effects of administration of intravenous steroids were noted.[63] No studies exist that show any relationship between improved neck pain and the use of corticosteroids. There are rare side effects that must also be considered when using this class of drugs including avascular necrosis of the femoral head and perforated ulcers when used in conjunction with other anti-inflammatory medications. Corticosteroids can also cause acute rises in blood glucose levels, and should be used cautiously in diabetic patients and with appropriate patient counseling.[12]

Muscle Relaxants

Muscle relaxants are a class of medication that is often prescribed for axial neck pain. They may cause significant sedation and fatigue, and do have a potential for abuse.[12]

There have been five studies examining the use of cyclobenzaprine or diazepam for the treatment of neck pain.[64-68] Two of these studies showed a small short-term benefit of muscle relaxers,[66,67] while the remaining three showed no difference over placebo.[64,65,68] All five of these studies involved small numbers of patients and often more than one intervention besides the medication. As a result of the limited number of studies investigating muscle relaxants, this class of medications was also deemed to have unclear evidence of benefit by a recent Cochrane Systematic Review.[50]

Physical Therapy and Exercise

After the initial onset of neck pain, a short period of rest is generally prescribed. This is usually followed by a course of physical therapy. Historical studies have shown that physical therapy does not alter the natural history of axial neck pain or radiculopathy.[69,70] A combination of active and passive modalities are typically prescribed, although passive treatments have also been shown to be ineffective in the long term.[71] There are several studies examining the effects of exercise for the treatment of neck pain. These studies focus on stretching, strengthening, or a combination of the two. The quality of these studies, however, varies significantly and there is often more than one intervention being studied.[72]

General aerobic conditioning has been thought to improve the symptoms of axial neck pain and treating physicians typically make this recommendation. There are some randomized trials regarding general aerobic conditioning in the literature. A study conducted by Takala et al.[73] examined the effects of a gymnastics program in the workplace targeting women who suffered from neck pain. Forty-five women were enrolled in a randomized study where the treatment group was randomized to perform 45 minutes of gymnastics once per week for 10 weeks. Both the treatment and control groups were matched for the frequency of symptoms, age, and work tasks. Their results showed no clear effects of the gymnastics on neck pain. Both groups had equal and significant reductions in pain in the springtime, with recurrence of symptoms in the fall. A second intervention in the fall did not produce the same effects as in the springtime suggesting a seasonal variation in symptoms independent of any intervention. Another randomized study comparing muscle-specific exercise to general conditioning with an exercise bicycle found a larger magnitude of pain relief in the muscle-specific exercise group.[74] General conditioning did produce a significant relief in acute pain, but its effects were transient and small in magnitude in comparison. There has been a difficulty with compliance of these types of physical exercise programs, and Anderson et al.[75] have found that as little as 2 minutes daily of resistance exercise can provide significant relief of neck and shoulder pain for chronic sufferers.

Perhaps, the most common exercise regimen for treating axial neck pain involves a combination of exercises targeting cervical and scapulothoracic stretching and strengthening. There is some evidence to support the use of these types of programs.[76-78] Franca et al.[77] compared this type of exercise program alone to an exercise with acupuncture, and acupuncture alone in a randomized trial. The authors found that all groups had a significant decrease in pain that was sustained at 6 months, and that acupuncture may be a beneficial adjunct to an exercise program in the treatment of neck pain. Chiu et al.[76] found a significant decrease in pain and an increase in neck muscle strength when a strengthening program was added to infrared irradiation treatment in a randomized trial of 218 patients with chronic neck pain. These results were maintained at 6-month follow-up. Bronfort et al.[78] found that patient satisfaction was significantly higher when a home exercise program was combined with spinal manipulation therapy in a randomized trial. Additionally, the authors found that all patient-rated outcomes were significantly better in the home exercise and directed physical therapy groups compared to spinal manipulation alone. However, Martel et al.[79] found no additional difference in visual analog scale neck pain when an exercise program was added to spinal manipulation therapy in another prospective, randomized trial. A recent Cochrane review article[72] pooled the data from these four studies with comparable exercise programs,[76-79] and found that there was moderate evidence to suggest long-term benefits of an exercise program combining cervical and scapulothoracic stretching and strengthening.

Another focus of exercise treatment has been on cervical stretching exercises. Again, there are few studies of quality addressing the usefulness of this type of regimen.[72] One such study examined the effects of a cervical stretching program used either before or after chiropractic manipulation of the neck.[80] In this randomized study, the authors found no difference in pain or function after treatment with a manipulation if the patient also performed cervical stretching prior to, or after, the treatment. A different randomized study performed by Kjellman and Oberg[81] showed a trend toward better pain improvement at 3 weeks and at 6 months for patients who performed a stretching program versus a sham ultrasound treatment, although their results were not statistically significant. The stretching group also demonstrated a trend toward fewer healthcare visits at 1-year follow-up.

The treating physician should follow some basic principles when prescribing exercise in the treatment of axial neck pain.[12] The passive motion should be avoided, especially early in the course of treatment, to limit the possibility of injury from the patient's inability to protect their self, past the endpoint of comfortable motion. General conditioning may be started early in the course of treatment, but the goal should be to transition the patient to a home exercise program focusing on cervical and scapulothoracic stretching and strengthening. Patients should also be monitored for any self-limiting side effects of exercise treatment such as headaches, thoracic pain, or worsening of symptoms.[75,78,82-85]

Cervical Manipulation

There is no high-quality evidence to suggest that manipulation of the cervical spine has any clinical effectiveness in the treatment of axial neck pain.[86] Several theories exist as to why this may be beneficial, including manipulation's effects on primary afferent neurons from paraspinal tissues, the motor control system, and pain processing.[87] There are some studies that do suggest there is some benefit to a spinal manipulation in combination with exercise programs.[78,80] Other studies have shown that manipulation alone offers some pain relief, however, none have used an effective sham manipulation group, making it difficult to interpret the role of the placebo effect.[88]

Although they are rare, there are several catastrophic complications that have been associated with manipulation of the cervical spine. These adverse events include radiculopathy, myelopathy, spinal cord injury, and vertebrobasilar artery injuries. They occur with an estimated incidence of 5–10 per 10 million manipulations.[89] The actual incidence of complications related to manipulation is unknown but is likely very low. Careful evaluation for cervical spine instability is warranted prior to referring any patient for manipulation.[12] Cervical manipulation is contraindicated in cases of vertebral fracture or dislocation, infection, malignancy, spondylolisthesis, myelopathy, vertebral hypermobility, Marfan and Ehlers-Danlos syndromes, osteoporosis, spondyloarthropathies, severe diabetes mellitus, anticoagulation therapy, and objective signs of spinal nerve root compromise.[86]

Cervical Steroid Injections

Steroid injections are commonly prescribed in the treatment of lumbar spondylosis and stenosis. There are several mechanisms that are suggested for why steroid injections may work in the lumbar spine: (1) an anti-inflammatory effect, with inhibition of prostaglandin synthesis; (2) interruption of nociceptive input from somatic nerves; (3) a direct membrane-stabilizing effect; (4) blockade of neuropeptide synthesis; (5) sympathetic blockade; (6) the mechanical effect of the injectant breaking up epidural adhesions; and (7) blockade of C-fiber activity in the dorsal root ganglion.[12] Presumably, the sources of pain in the cervical spine are similar to those in the lumbar spine, and cervical steroid injections should be effective. There is some evidence to support the use of cervical epidural injections and cervical facet blocks in the treatment of axial neck pain, however, there are few high-quality studies in the literature.[12,90]

Stav et al. performed a randomized, prospective study of 42 patients who received an injection of steroid and lidocaine into the epidural space or into the posterior neck musculature.[91] These patients were suffering from neck pain with or without radicular symptoms. They were surveyed at 1 week following the last injection and at 1 year regarding their pain relief. The group receiving the epidural injection rather than the intramuscular injection had significantly more pain relief after 1 week (76% vs. 35%) and at 1 year (68% vs. 12%). The epidural injection group also had more range of motion, decreased their daily analgesic use, and had a higher recovery capacity for returning to work. This study was not blinded, and the patients were not separated by the neck or arm pain.

More recently, in 2010, Manchikanti and colleagues published a prospective, randomized, double-blinded, and controlled study of epidural steroid injections for the treatment of diskogenic neck pain.[92] Patients with facet joint pain (diagnosed by relief with medial branch blocks) and patients with radiculopathy were excluded from this study. In total, 70 patients were randomized to receive either local anesthetic combined with a steroid (nonparticulate betamethasone) or local anesthetic alone. Significant pain relief was noted in 80% of patients in

CHAPTER 24

each group, and significant improvement in function was found in 69% of the local anesthetic only group and 80% in the group who received steroids (the difference was not statistically significant). Over the course of the year, each group received an average of four treatments and reported pain relief for more than 40 of the 52 weeks they were followed for. The authors concluded that either local anesthetic with or without steroid is an effective treatment. This study had several weaknesses, including relatively small numbers of patients and the lack of a placebo group.

There are several pertinent retrospective studies that have also examined the effects of epidural injections for neck pain. Shulman reported on a group of 96 patients who were treated with cervical epidural steroid injections for axial neck pain and found overall improvement in 41% of patients, with 38% experiencing relief lasting more than 1 month. Cicala et al. followed a group of 58 patients who received epidural steroid injections for the treatment of neck pain with or without arm pain.[93] Six months following injection of steroid into the epidural space via a translaminar approach at C7–T1, 41% of patients had greater than 50% improvement in their pain lasting for the duration of the 6-month follow-up period. An additional 29% reported relief lasting for more than 6 weeks, but less than 6 months. The results of these two studies mirror the natural history of axial neck pain, and without a control group are difficult to interpret in and of themselves.

Two other retrospective analyses attempt to predict which patients will improve with cervical epidural injections. Ferrante et al. evaluated 100 patients who underwent cervical epidural steroid injections and found that patients older than 50 years and those with radicular symptoms did better in contrast to those who suffered from axial neck pain at a follow-up of 13.5 months.[94] Kwon et al. retrospectively evaluated 91 patients who underwent cervical epidural steroid injections and found similar results.[95] In their study, 72% of all patients experienced significant pain relief. The only predictive factor for an improved outcome was a radiographic diagnosis of a herniated disk, rather than cervical stenosis caused by spondolytic changes. Similar to the Ferrante study, there was a trend for improved outcome in patients who suffered from radicular pain versus neck pain combined with radicular pain, although the difference was not statistically significant.

Other types of cervical steroid injection involve articular facets. The medial branches of the dorsal cervical rami innervate the facet joints, which may be a pain generator in cases of axial neck pain.[1] Two types of injections target the cervical facets—(1) intra-articular injections and (2) medial branch blocks. The effects of medial branch blocks have been well-documented in several high quality, prospective studies conducted by Manchikanti and colleagues.[96-98] Using comparative diagnostic blocks to rule out diskogenic neck pain (i.e. pain that does respond to local anesthetic medial branch blocks), 100 patients who met the criteria for facet pain were enrolled in a prospective clinical outcome study.[97] This initial study found that there was a significant decrease in pain at 3, 6, and 12 months. Functional improvement was significantly better, and there was a significant increase in employment among eligible participants at 12 months as well. In a prospective, randomized, double-blinded study of local anesthetic injections versus local anesthetic plus steroid injections, Manchikanti and colleagues again found significant relief of pain in both groups, with no significant differences between the two, at 1 year after treatment.[96] On average, each patient received 3.5 treatments per year and had relief for a time period of 13–16 weeks. A second prospective, randomized, double-blinded study of similar design by the same author followed patients out to 24 months.[98] Again, significant pain relief and functional improvement were found in both the steroid and local anesthetic groups for up to 2 years, with the average patient receiving six treatments over the course of the study. However, there are limitations to these studies. Most notably, there is no true placebo group in any study, as steroid injections were compared to local anesthetic alone. These studies are active-controlled studies as opposed to placebo-controlled, and injection of steroid or local anesthetic may be equally as effective as the injection of a saline solution.

Cervical facet pain has also been treated by intra-articular injection of steroid, similar to other degenerative conditions. There is little high-quality evidence to support the use of this type of treatment.[99] Barnsley et al. in a prospective, randomized, double-blinded study comparing intra-articular injection of steroid versus local anesthetic for chronic axial neck pain associated with whiplash found no benefit of steroid injection.[100] In fact, in both groups pain had returned to greater than 50% of baseline pain within 3 days. Again, this is an active-controlled study rather than placebo-controlled, however, the pain relief was so short in both groups that it is likely to be clinically insignificant if compared to a placebo control. A more recent examination of the effects of intra-articular injection was carried out by Park and Kim.[101] The authors studied a group of 400 patients suffering from myofascial pain syndrome with "referral pain patterns of cervical facet joint syndrome." All patients were prescribed identical medication and an exercise program, and half were randomized to receive bilateral facet joint injections of local anesthetic combined with steroid at C5–6 and C6–7. The group receiving the steroid injections had better pain improvement and a longer symptom-free period, particularly in the patients younger than 45 years. The results of this study are difficult to apply to all patients suffering from axial neck pain due to the underlying diagnosis of myofascial pain syndrome in their series. Additionally, some patients in the injection group also received trigger point injections and botulinum toxin injections into the paraspinal muscles, further confounding the results.

Recent systematic reviews examining cervical epidural injections[90] and cervical facet blocks[99] have also been reported on in the literature. In regards to applications of these techniques for axial neck pain, the literature reviewed in totality (including the high-quality studies previously discussed) was graded as only fair for both cervical epidural injections as well as cervical facet medial branch blocks. The evidence for intra-articular injections is highly limited, and it is difficult to draw any meaningful conclusion.

Although cervical steroid injections may be beneficial in treating axial neck pain, there are serious complications that have been reported. These complications include spinal cord trauma, spinal cord or epidural hematoma formation, nerve injury, subdural or subarachnoid injection, intravascular entry either venous or arterial, vascular injury or vascular embolism, and injection leading to an abscess.[12,90] Several strategies exist to reduce the incidence of serious complications. These include interlaminar injections at the C6–7 or C7–T1 level due to increased space available for the cord, use of fluoroscopic guidance, interlaminar rather than a transforaminal injection, and avoidance of injection at a level where there is a large herniated disk.[12,90] Fortunately, these are rare events and it is difficult to quantify their true incidence. Other minor complications associated with epidural injections include increase in the neck pain, vasovagal reactions, headache, insomnia, increase in temperature, and dural puncture.[90]

SURGICAL INDICATIONS AND TREATMENT

Once a patient has undergone extensive conservative treatment for axial neck pain with a combination of any of the options discussed previously, the only remaining treatment maybe surgery. There are no high-quality, prospective, randomized studies that seek to answer the question of whether or not surgery is an effective treatment for neck pain. Much of the information available in the literature is based on case series without any control groups. There is a large variability in the outcomes measured by these studies, and often they rely on the patient's self-reported level of satisfaction. While this measure should not be discounted, there are many factors that may contribute to patient satisfaction and they are difficult to measure objectively.[102]

The first step in deciding on whether surgery may be effective for treating axial neck pain is to localize the level or levels that are the primary pain generators. This is typically done by performing diagnostic cervical diskography, although this method remains controversial.[103] Contrast diskography relies on mapping the presence of tears in the disks and also aims to reproduce the pain typically experienced by the patient. A concordant diskogram represents typical pain patterns reproduced in the patient when a degenerative disk is injected with contrast, and when neighboring normal disks do not reproduce the patient's typical pain. These circumstances may be difficult to reproduce. and the procedure itself can produce pain even in asymptomatic individuals making a diagnosis of a culprit level or levels difficult.[17,104] Analgesic diskography was introduced by Roth in 1976 and may be more effective in determining the level responsible for pain.[105] In this type of diskography, a local anesthetic is injected into the disk and a concordant, or positive, test is indicated by transient pain relief and restoration of normal cervical range of motion.

Once the decision to proceed with the surgery is made, the necessary question to answer is whether or not surgery offers a higher rate of improvement in pain and function than would be observed with continued conservative treatment or no treatment at all. To adequately answer this question comparative studies are needed, although none exist specifically for axial neck pain. What little information that can be assessed is a product of case series.

The largest such series of patients with the longest follow-up period was conducted by Garvey and colleagues.[106] This study was a retrospective review of 87 patients who answered an extensive survey relating to pain and function at a mean of 4.4 years after surgery for predominantly axial neck pain. Patients reported on the improvement of pain using visual analog scales, on function using modified Oswestry and modified Roland-Morris disability indexes, and on satisfaction using the North American Spine Society outcome tool. The authors found that 82% of patients rated their outcome as good, very good, or excellent. 93% of patients reported pain improvement, and their visual analog pain scores dropped from an average of 8.4 to 3.8 after surgery. Their functional status according to the Oswestry Disability Index and the modified Roland-Morris index improved about 50%. Additionally, there was no negative correlation observed in the outcomes with pending litigation or tobacco use. The authors concluded that surgery for axial neck pain is a viable option in properly selected patients and that self-reported improvements in pain and function are likely.

Other case series of surgery for axial neck pain report similar results. In his series of patients undergoing analgesic diskography followed by surgery, Roth reported 93% good or excellent results.[105] Palit and colleagues reported prospectively on 38 consecutive patients who underwent operative treatment for axial neck pain and found a significant decrease in pain, a significant increase in function, and 79% of patients who were satisfied at 53 months of follow-up.[107] Ratliff and Voorhies retrospectively reported on 20 patients who underwent surgery for chronic axial neck pain over a 4-year period and found that 85% of patients were satisfied with their pain relief and that 95% of those surveyed would repeat the procedure.[108] Zheng and colleagues reported a 76% patient satisfaction rate when cervical diskectomy and fusion was performed for axial neck pain and concordant diskograms.[109]

The pioneers of cervical diskectomy also noted some benefits of surgery when it came to self-reported neck pain improvement by their patients. Robinson et al.[104] reported on their early experience with anterior cervical diskectomy and fusion as it related to axial neck pain. In this series, 80% of patients reported neck pain preoperatively and 46% had interscapular radiation. They noted 73% of patients had marked pain improvement during a follow-up period ranging from 2 months to 73 months. Riley et al. had similar findings in their review of 93 consecutive patients, with 72% of patients reporting good or excellent results after surgery.[110]

Although the only evidence to support surgical treatment of axial neck pain is derived from case series and patient-reported outcomes, there is no doubt that patient satisfaction with their treatment is ultimately very important. Skolasky et al. examined the relationship between clinical and functional outcomes with patient satisfaction in 428 patients undergoing cervical spine surgery.[102] The Cervical Spine Outcomes Questionnaire was utilized in all cases, and the association between patient satisfaction and 3 months of clinical and functional outcome was tested. The authors concluded that patient satisfaction is an unobservable outcome, but it can be assessed through self-report. They also found that clinical improvement in neck pain after surgery correlates with higher patient satisfaction. So while data from case series has difficulties with bias and a lack of control groups, it is impossible to ignore the self-reported improvement in neck pain following surgery. For this reason, surgical treatment may be a reasonable option to treat axial neck pain in appropriately selected patients. It is clear that further investigation with higher quality studies is lacking, and future efforts to determine surgery's true effect should include a randomized patient population as well as self-reported satisfaction rates.

PROGNOSIS

In general, patients who present with axial neck pain can be reassured that their symptoms are likely self-limited and will resolve with little or no conservative treatment.[1-9] Approximately, one-quarter of patients with axial neck pain will have persistent symptoms that will affect their quality of life to some degree, while the remainder will have a decrease or complete resolution of their symptoms. The group with persistent pain and disability should be considered differently, and a more comprehensive evaluation may be warranted to further delineate reasons for their continued symptoms.

Nonoperative treatment should be the first line of treatment for axial neck pain without radiculopathy or myelopathy; however, it still remains unclear whether nonoperative treatment will significantly alter the natural history. There are no controlled studies comparing conservative treatment to no treatment at all,[1] making a true comparison of the effects of treatment impossible. It also is not clear whether surgery is truly helpful in reducing the symptoms of axial neck pain for the same reasons.

The body of evidence for particular individual treatments for axial neck pain is lacking in high-quality studies. There are even fewer prospective, randomized control trials that are generally considered the gold standard for studies examining treatment effects. Additionally, in the available literature regarding medical and surgical treatment of axial neck pain, the results universally mirror the outcomes of population-based studies with minimal intervention. That is, the majority of patients will experience resolution or improvement of their symptoms regardless of what is recommended, and that one-quarter to one-third of patients will continue to have symptoms of varying degrees.

REFERENCES

1. Jurek S, Rao R. Cervical spondylosis: pathophysiology, natural history, and clinical syndromes of neck pain, radiculopathy, and myelopathy. In: Herkowitz HN, Garfin S, Eismont F, Bell G, Balderston R (Eds). Rothman-Simeone: The Spine, 6th edition. Philadelphia: Saunders Elsevier; 2011.
2. Roh JS, Teng AL, Yoo JU, et al. Degenerative disorders of the lumbar and cervical spine. Orthop Clin North Am. 2005;36(3):255-62.
3. Bovim G, Schrader H, Sand T. Neck pain in the general population. Spine. 1994;19(12):1307-9.
4. Mäkelä M, Heliövaara M, Sievers K, et al. Prevalence, determinants, and consequences of chronic neck pain in Finland. Am J Epidemiol. 1991;134(11):1356-67.
5. Côté P, Cassidy JD, Carroll L. The Saskatchewan Health and Back Pain Survey. The prevalence of neck pain and related disability in Saskatchewan adults. Spine. 1998;23(15):1689-98.
6. Côté P, Cassidy JD, Carroll L. The factors associated with neck pain and its related disability in the Saskatchewan population. Spine. 2000;25(9):1109-17.
7. DePalma AF, Subin DK. Study of the cervical syndrome. Clin Orthop Relat Res. 1965;38:135-42.
8. Gore DR, Sepic SB, Gardner GM, et al. Neck pain: a long-term follow-up of 205 patients. Spine. 1987;12(1):1-5.
9. Rothman RH, Rashbaum RF. Pathogenesis of signs and symptoms of cervical disc degeneration. Instr Course Lect. 1978;27:203-15.
10. Rao R. Neck pain, cervical radiculopathy, and cervical myelopathy: pathophysiology, natural history, and clinical evaluation. J Bone Joint Surg Am. 2002;84(10):1872-81.
11. Travell JG, Simmons DG. Myofascial Pain and Dysfunction: The Trigger Point Manual. Baltimore: Williams and Wilkins; 1983.
12. Dean CL, Rhee JM. Nonoperative management of cervical disc and degenerative disorders. In: Herkowitz HN, Garfin S, Eismont F, Bell G, Baldersion R (Eds). Rothman-Simeone: The Spine, 6th edition. Philadelphia: Saunders Elsevier; 2011.
13. Aprill C, Dwyer A, Bogduk N. Cervical zygapophyseal joint pain patterns. II: a clinical evaluation. Spine. 1990;15(6): 458-61.
14. Bogduk N, Marsland A. The cervical zygapophysial joints as a source of neck pain. Spine. 1988;13(6): 610-7.
15. Bogduk N, Windsor M, Inglis A. The innervation of the cervical intervertebral dscs. Spine. 1988;13(1):2-8.
16. Dwyer A, Aprill C, Bogduk N. Cervical zygapophyseal joint pain patterns. I: a study in normal volunteers. Spine. 1990;15(6):453-7.
17. Grubb SA, Kelly CK. Cervical discography: clinical implications from 12 years of experience. Spine. 2000;25(11):1382-9.
18. Hoppenfeld S. Physical Examination of the Spine and Extremities. New York: Appleton-Century-Crofts; 1976.
19. Crowder TT, Fischgrund JD. Cervical radiculopathy: anterior surgical approach. In: Herkowitz HN, Garfin S, Eismont F, Bell G, Balderston R (Eds). Rothman-Simeone: The Spine, 6th edition. Philadelphia: Saunders Elsevier; 2011.
20. Boden SD, McCowin PR, Davis DO, et al. Abnormal magnetic-resonance scans of the cervical spine in asymptomatic subjects. A prospective investigation. J Bone Joint Surg Am. 1990;72(8):1178-84.
21. Okada E, Matsumoto M, Ichihara D, et al. Aging of the cervical spine in healthy volunteers: a 10-year longitudinal magnetic resonance imaging study. Spine. 2009;34(7):706-12.
22. Rose SR, Petersen NJ, Gardner TJ, et al. Etiology of thrombocytosis in a general medicine population: analysis of 801 cases with emphasis on infectious causes. J Clin Med Res. 2012;4(6):415-23.
23. Garcia A Jr, Grantham SA. Hematogenous pyogenic vertebral osteomyelitis. J Bone Joint Surg Am. 1960;42-A:429-36.
24. Goldman AB, Freiberger RH. Localized infectious and neuropathic diseases. Semin Roentgenol. 1979;14(1):19-32.
25. Sapico FL, Montgomerie JZ. Pyogenic vertebral osteomyelitis: report of nine cases and review of the literature. Rev Infect Dis. 1979;1(5):754-76.
26. Kim CW, Currier BL, Eismont FJ. Infections of the spine. In: Herkowitz HN, Garfin S, Eismont F, Bell G, Balderston R (Eds). Rothman-Simeone: The Spine, 6th edition. Philadelphia: Saunders Elsevier; 2011.
27. Schofferman L, Schofferman J, Zucherman J, et al. Occult infections causing persistent low-back pain. Spine. 1989;14(4):417-9.
28. Jaye DL, Waites KB. Clinical applications of C-reactive protein in pediatrics. Pediatr Infect Dis J. 1997;16(8):735-46.
29. Saez-Llorens X, Lagrutta F. The acute phase host reaction during bacterial infection and its clinical impact in children. Pediatr Infect Dis J. 1993;12(1):83-7.
30. Lin Z-Y, Chuang WL, Dai CY, et al. Clinical application of serum C-reactive protein measurement in the detection of

CHAPTER 24

bacterial infection in patients with liver cirrhosis. Kaohsiung J Med Sci. 2002;18(3):121-6.
31. Borenstein DG. Arthritic disorders. In: Herkowitz HN, Garfin S, Eismont F, Bell G, Balderston R (Eds). Rothman-Simeone: The Spine, 6th edition. Philadelphia: Saunders Elsevier; 2011.
32. Lewandrowski K-U, Anderson ME, Mclain RF. Tumors of the spine. In: Herkowitz HN, Garfin S, Eismont F, Bell G, Balderston R (Eds). Rothman-Simeone: The Spine, 6th edition. Philadelphia: Saunders Elsevier; 2011.
33. Johnson RM, Hart DL, Simmons EF, et al. Cervical orthoses. A study comparing their effectiveness in restricting cervical motion in normal subjects. J Bone Joint Surg Am. 1977;59(3):332-9.
34. Muzin S, Isaac Z, Walker J, et al. When should a cervical collar be used to treat neck pain? Curr Rev Musculoskelet Med. 2008;1(2):114-9.
35. Naylor JR, Mulley GP. Surgical collars: a survey of their prescription and use. Br J Rheumatol. 1991;30(4):282-4.
36. Gennis P, Miller L, Gallagher EJ, et al. The effect of soft cervical collars on persistent neck pain in patients with whiplash injury. Acad Emerg Med. 1996;3(6):568-73.
37. Hubbard TJ, Denegar CR. Does cryotherapy improve outcomes with soft tissue injury? J Athl Train. 2004;39(3): 278-9.
38. Philadelphia Panel. Philadelphia Panel evidence-based clinical practice guidelines on selected rehabilitation interventions for neck pain. Phys Ther. 2001;81(10):1701-17.
39. Patel KC, Gross A, Graham N, et al. Massage for mechanical neck disorders. Cochrane Database Syst Rev. 2012;9:CD004871.
40. Rosenfeld M, Seferiadis A, Carlsson J, et al. Active intervention in patients with whiplash-associated disorders improves long-term prognosis: a randomized controlled clinical trial. Spine. 2003;28(22):2491-8.
41. Verhagen AP, Scholten-Peeters GG, van Wijngaarden S, et al. Conservative treatments for whiplash. Cochrane Database Syst Rev. 2007;2:CD003338.
42. Pain in the neck and arm: a multicentre trial of the effects of physiotherapy, arranged by the British Association of Physical Medicine. Br Med J. 1966;1(5482):253-8.
43. Moeti P, Marchetti G. Clinical outcome from mechanical intermittent cervical traction for the treatment of cervical radiculopathy: a case series. J Orthop Sports Phys Ther. 2001;31(4):207-13.
44. Swezey RL, Swezey AM, Warner K. Efficacy of home cervical traction therapy. Am J Phys Med Rehabil. 1999;78(1):30-2.
45. Graham N, Gross A, Goldsmith CH, et al. Mechanical traction for neck pain with or without radiculopathy. Cochrane Database Syst Rev. 2008;3:CD006408.
46. Dillin W, Uppal GS. Analysis of medications used in the treatment of cervical disk degeneration. Orthop Clin North Am. 1992;23(3):421-33.
47. Aslan TE, Karaduman A. Effects of three different conservative treatments on pain, disability, quality of life, and mood in patients with cervical spondylosis. Rheumatol Int. 2012;32(4):1033-40.
48. Beebe FA, Barkin RL, Barkin S. A clinical and pharmacologic review of skeletal muscle relaxants for musculoskeletal conditions. Am J Ther. 2005;12(2):151-71.
49. Douglass AB, Bope ET. Evaluation and treatment of posterior neck pain in family practice. J Am Board Fam Pract. 2004;(17-Suppl):S13-22.
50. Peloso P, Gross A, Haines T, et al. Medicinal and injection therapies for mechanical neck disorders. Cochrane Database Syst Rev. 2007;3:CD000319.
51. Van Tulder MW, Assendelft WJ, Koes BW, et al. Method guidelines for systematic reviews in the cochrane collaboration back review group for spinal disorders. Spine. 1997;22(20):2323-30.
52. Bensen WG. Antiinflammatory and analgesic efficacy of COX-2 specific inhibition: from investigational trials to clinical experience. J Rheumatol Suppl. 2000;60:17-24.
53. Bensen WG, Zhao SZ, Burke TA, et al. Upper gastrointestinal tolerability of celecoxib. A COX-2 specific inhibitor, compared to naproxen and placebo. J Rheumatol. 2000;27(8):1876-83.
54. Day R, Morrison B, Luza A, et al. A randomized trial of the efficacy and tolerability of the COX-2 inhibitor rofecoxib vs ibuprofen in patients with osteoarthritis. Rofecoxib/Ibuprofen Comparator Study Group. Arch Intern Med. 2000;160(12):1781-7.
55. Graham DJ, Campen D, Hui R, et al. Risk of acute myocardial infarction and sudden cardiac death in patients treated with cyclo-oxygenase 2 selective and non-selective non-steroidal anti-inflammatory drugs: nested case-control study. Lancet. 2005;365(9458):475-81.
56. Dosta C, Pavelka K, Lewit K. Ibuprofen in the treatment of the cervicocranial syndrome in combination with manipulative therapy. Fysiatr Revmatol Vestn. 1978;56(5):258-63.
57. Koes BW, Bouter LM, Knipshild PG, et al. The effectiveness of manual therapy, physiotherapy and continued treatment by the general practitioner for chronic nonspecific back and neck complaints: design of a randomized clinical trial. J Manipulative Physiol Ther. 1991;14(9):498-502.
58. Chen X, Cheng HG, Huang Y, et al. Depression symptoms and chronic pain in the community population in Beijing, China. Psychiatry Res. 2012;200(2–3):313-7.
59. Olsen Y, Daumit GL, Ford DE. Opioid prescriptions by U.S. primary care physicians from 1992 to 2001. J Pain. 2006;7(4):225-35.
60. Goode AP, Freburger J, Carey T. Prevalence, practice patterns, and evidence for chronic neck pain. Arthritis Care Res. 2010;62(11):1594-601.
61. Chou R, Huffman LH. Medications for acute and chronic low back pain: a review of the evidence for an American Pain Society/American College of Physicians clinical practice guideline. Ann Intern Med. 2007;147(7):505-14.

62. Atkinson JH, Slater MA, Williams RA, et al. A placebo-controlled randomized clinical trial of nortriptyline for chronic low back pain. Pain. 1998;76(3):287-96.
63. Pettersson K, Toolanen G. High-dose methylprednisolone prevents extensive sick leave after whiplash injury. A prospective, randomized, double-blind study. Spine. 1998;23(9):984-9.
64. Basmajian J. Cyclobenzaprine hydrochloride effect on skeletal muscle spasm in the lumbar region and neck: two double-blind controlled clinical and laboratory studies. Arch Phys Med Rehabil. 1978;59:58-63.
65. Basmajian J. Reflex cervical muscle spasm: treatment by diazepam, phenobarbital or placebo. Arch Phys Med Rehabil. 1983;64:121-4.
66. Bose K. The efficacy and safety of eperisone in patients with cervical spondylosis: results of a randomized, double-blind, placebo-controlled trial. Methods Find Exp Clin Pharmacol. 1999;21(3):209-13.
67. Nasswetter G, de los Santos AR, Di Girolamo G, et al. Asociacion De Clonixinato De Lisina Con Ciclobenzaprina En Afecciones Dolorosas Del Raquis Con Contractura Muscular. Prensa Medica Argentina. 1998;85:507-14.
68. Thomas M, Eriksson SV, Lundeberg T. A comparative study of diazepam and acupuncture in patients with osteoarthritis pain: a placebo controlled study. Am J Chin Med. 1991;19(2):95-100.
69. Levine MJ, Albert TJ, Smith MD. Cervical radiculopathy: diagnosis and nonoperative management. J Am Acad Orthop Surg. 1996;4(6):305-16.
70. Tan JC, Nordin M. Role of physical therapy in the treatment of cervical disk disease. Orthop Clin North Am. 1992;23(3):435-49.
71. Santiesteban AJ. The role of physical agents in the treatment of spine pain. Clin Orthop Relat Res. 1983;79:24-30.
72. Gross A, Kay TM, Paquin JP, et al. Exercises for mechanical neck disorders. Cochrane Database Syst Rev. 2012;8:CD004250.
73. Takala EP, Viikari-Juntura E, Tynkkynen EM. Does group gymnastics at the workplace help in neck pain? A controlled study. Scand J Rehabil Med. 1994;26(1):17-20.
74. Andersen LL, Kjaer M, Søgaard K, et al. Effect of two contrasting types of physical exercise on chronic neck muscle pain. Arthritis Rheum. 2008;59(1):84-91.
75. Andersen LL, Saervoll CA, Mortensen OS, et al. Effectiveness of small daily amounts of progressive resistance training for frequent neck/shoulder pain: randomised controlled trial. Pain. 2011;152(2):440-6.
76. Chiu TT, Hui-Chan CW, Chein G. A randomized clinical trial of TENS and exercise for patients with chronic neck pain. Clin Rehabil. 2005;19(8):850-60.
77. França DL, Senna-Fernandes V, Cortez CM, et al. Tension neck syndrome treated by acupuncture combined with physiotherapy: a comparative clinical trial (pilot study). Complement Ther Med. 2008;16(5):268-77.
78. Bronfort G, Evans R, Nelson B, et al. A randomized clinical trial of exercise and spinal manipulation for patients with chronic neck pain. Spine. 2001;26(7):788-97.
79. Martel J, Dugas C, Dubois JD, et al. A randomised controlled trial of preventive spinal manipulation with and without a home exercise program for patients with chronic neck pain. BMC Musculoskelet Disord. 2011;12:41.
80. Allan M, Brantingham JW, Menezes A. Stretching as an adjunct to chiropractic manipulation of chronic neck pain: before, after or not at all? A prospective randomized controlled clinical trial. Eur J Chiropractic. 2003;50:41-52.
81. Kjellman G, Oberg B. A randomized clinical trial comparing general exercise, mckenzie treatment and a control group in patients with neck pain. J Rehabil Med. 2002;34(4):183-90.
82. Rendant D, Pach D, Lüdtke R, et al. Qigong versus exercise versus no therapy for patients with chronic neck pain: a randomized controlled trial. Spine. 2011;36(6):419-27.
83. Jull G, Trott P, Potter H, et al. A randomized controlled trial of exercise and manipulative therapy for cervicogenic headache. Spine. 2002;27(17):1835-43.
84. Stewart MJ, Maher CG, Refshauge KM, et al. Randomized controlled trial of exercise for chronic whiplash-associated disorders. Pain. 2007;128(1-2):59-68.
85. von Trott P, Wiedemann AM, Lüdtke R, et al. Qigong and exercise therapy for elderly patients with chronic neck pain (QIBANE): a randomized controlled study. J Pain. 2009;10(5):501-8.
86. Laban MM, Taylor RS. Manipulation: an objective analysis of the literature. Orthop Clin North Am. 1992;23(3):451-9.
87. Pickar JG. Neurophysiological effects of spinal manipulation. Spine J. 2002;2(5):357-71.
88. Vernon HT, Triano JJ, Ross JK, et al. Validation of a novel sham cervical manipulation procedure. Spine J. 2012;12(11):1021-8.
89. Haldeman S, Kohlbeck FJ, Mcgregor M. Unpredictability of cerebrovascular ischemia associated with cervical spine manipulation therapy: a review of sixty-four cases after cervical spine manipulation. Spine. 2002;27(1):49-55.
90. Diwan S, Manchikanti L, Benyamin RM, et al. Effectiveness of cervical epidural injections in the management of chronic neck and upper extremity pain. Pain Phys. 2012;15(4):405-34.
91. Stav A, Ovadia L, Sternberg A, et al. Cervical epidural steroid injection for cervicobrachialgia. Acta Anaesthesiol Scand. 1993;37(5):562-6.
92. Manchikanti L, Cash KA, Pampati V, et al. Cervical epidural injections in chronic discogenic neck pain without disc herniation or radiculitis: preliminary results of a randomized, double-blind, controlled trial. Pain Physician. 2010;13(4):265-78.
93. Cicala RS, Thoni K, Angel JJ. Long-term results of cervical epidural steroid injections. Clin J Pain. 1989;5(2):143-5.
94. Ferrante FM, Wilson SP, Iacobo C, et al. Clinical classification as a predictor of therapeutic outcome after cervical epidural steroid injection. Spine. 1993;18(6):730-6.

95. Kwon JW, Lee JW, Kim SH, et al. Cervical interlaminar epidural steroid injection for neck pain and cervical radiculopathy: effect and prognostic factors. Skeletal Radiol. 2007;36(5):431-6.
96. Manchikanti L, Damron K, Cash K, et al. Therapeutic cervical medial branch blocks in managing chronic neck pain: a preliminary report of a randomized, double-blind, controlled trial: clinical trial NCT0033272. Pain Physician. 2006;9(4):333-46.
97. Manchikanti L, Manchikanti KN, Damron KS, et al. Effectiveness of cervical medial branch blocks in chronic neck pain: a prospective outcome study. Pain Physician. 2004;7(2):195-201.
98. Manchikanti L, Singh V, Falco FJ, et al. Comparative outcomes of a 2-year follow-up of cervical medial branch blocks in management of chronic neck pain: a randomized, double-blind controlled trial. Pain Physician. 2010;13(5):437-50.
99. Falco F, Manchikanti L, Datta S, et al. Systematic review of the therapeutic effectiveness of cervical facet joint interventions: an update. Pain Physician. 2012;15(6):E839.
100. Barnsley L, Lord SM, Wallis BJ, et al. Lack of effect of intraarticular corticosteroids for chronic pain in the cervical zygapophyseal joints. N Engl J Med. 1994;330(15):1047-50.
101. Park S-C, Kim K-H. Effect of adding cervical facet joint injections in a multimodal treatment program for long-standing cervical myofascial pain syndrome with referral pain patterns of cervical facet joint syndrome. J Anesth. 2012;26(5):738-45.
102. Skolasky RL, Albert TJ, Vaccaro AR, et al. Patient satisfaction in the cervical spine research society outcomes study: relationship to improved clinical outcome. Spine J. 2009; 9(3):232-9.
103. Garvey TA. Surgical management of axial pain. In: Herkowitz HN, Garfin S, Eismont F, Bell G, Balderston R (Eds). Rothman-Simeone: The Spine, 6th edition. Philadelphia: Saunders Elsevier; 2011.
104. Riley LH Jr, Robinson RA, Johnson KA, et al. The results of anterior interbody fusion of the cervical spine. J Bone Joint Surg Am. 1962;44:1569-87.
105. Roth DA. Cervical analgesic discography. a new test for the definitive diagnosis of the painful-disk syndrome. JAMA. 1976;235(16):1713-4.
106. Garvey TA, Transfeldt EE, Malcolm JR, et al. Outcome of anterior cervical discectomy and fusion as perceived by patients treated for dominant axial-mechanical cervical spine pain. Spine. 2002;27(17):1887-95.
107. Palit M, Schofferman J, Goldthwaite N, et al. Anterior discectomy and fusion for the management of neck pain. Spine. 1999;24(21):2224-8.
108. Ratliff J, Voorhies RM. Outcome study of surgical treatment for axial neck pain. South Med J. 2001;94(6):595-602.
109. Zheng Y, Liew SM, Simmons ED. Value of magnetic resonance imaging and discography in determining the level of cervical discectomy and fusion. Spine. 2004;29(19):2140-5; discussion 2146.
110. Riley LH, Robinson RA, Johnson KA, et al. The results of anterior interbody fusion of the cervical spine. J Neurosurg. 1969;30:127-33.

CHAPTER 25

Spine Surgery: Current Concepts and Evidence Cervical Radiculopathy

Abhishek Ray, Michael P Steinmetz

EPIDEMIOLOGY

Cervical radiculopathy is a neurologic syndrome characterized by pain and/or sensorimotor deficit caused by compression of a cervical nerve root. The pain typically localizes to the neck, trapezial and/or periscapular region, and/or the ipsilateral arm. There may also be a combination of sensory loss, loss of motor function, and/or reflex changes in the affected nerve-root distribution. The compression of the nerve root can be caused by disk herniation, osteophyte formation instability, and rarely by infection, trauma, or neoplastic processes.[1,2] The symptoms typically develop insidiously but may develop after trauma.[3,4]

Radhakrishnan and colleagues performed a population-based study in Rochester, Minnesota between 1976 and 1990 that included 561 patients. They found the average annual age-adjusted incidence rate to be 83.2 per 100,000 for cervical radiculopathy in this population.[5] A door-to-door survey done in a Sicilian municipality of 7,653 subjects found 27 of these patients to be affected by cervical radiculopathy, giving a prevalence of 3.5 cases per 1,000 population.[6] They found cervical radiculopathy to be most prevalent at age 50–59. This is consistent with the increased incidence of 202.9 per 100,000 in a similar age group of 50–54 in the Rochester study.[5]

NATURAL HISTORY

Cervical radiculopathy appears to be self-limited in the majority of patients. Typical symptom duration is variable in the literature. Anecdotally, symptoms abate or resolve by 3 months (authors' experience) but may persist for up to a year. However, Lees and Turner were the first to delineate the natural history of cervical radiculopathy in 1963, and they concluded that it rarely progressed to myelopathy. While 45% of patients had only a single pain episode without recurrence, 25% had persistent or worsening symptoms.[7] Others have demonstrated a more favorable long-term outcome for those with radiculopathy. Radhakrishnan et al. demonstrated that at a mean follow-up of 5.9 years (median 4.9 years) the majority of patients (90.5%) were normal or only mildly incapacitated by pain.[5] It is significant to note that approximately one-third of these patients experienced a recurrence of their symptoms during the study.

Despite persistent or recurrent symptoms, cervical radiculopathy rarely progresses to myelopathy.[8] In one study, 24 of 26 patients were successfully treated with aggressive nonsurgical means. Twenty-one patients returned to their preinjury employment and no patient demonstrated progressive neurologic loss.

Cervical radiculopathy may be incapacitating in a number of patients, however, as detailed above, the natural history is favorable. The majority do not progress and require surgical intervention. Therefore, surgery is reserved for those patients that do not improve over time or develop a progression in their neurological symptoms (i.e. weakness).

WORK-UP (CLINICAL FINDINGS)

The patient history alone can make one diagnose cervical radiculopathy in over 75% of cases,[2] however, to be able to diagnose this condition correctly, one must understand cervical spinal anatomy. The cervical nerve roots are named by the corresponding vertebral body below a particular nerve. Specifically, the nerve exits above its corresponding pedicle. The C8 nerve root exits between

C7 and T1 vertebral bodies. The neural foramen is comprised of the corresponding pedicles of the vertebral bodies superiorly and inferiorly, by the facet joint posteriorly, and the intervertebral disk anteriorly. The most common cause of cervical radiculopathy is cervical spondylosis, accounting for 70–75% of cases. Herniation of the nucleus pulposus is responsible for 20–25% of cases and other causes such as tumors are rare.[1] Cervical spondylosis results in foraminal narrowing and nerve root impingement by a combination of degenerative changes of the intervertebral disk and by hypertrophy of the uncovertebral joints anteriorly and the facet joints posteriorly. With age, there is a progressive reduction in water content in the intervertebral disk from approximately 88% at infancy to 70% at age 72. As a result, the disk loses height, the annulus fibrosis begins to bulge, anterior osteophytes form, and the facet joints hypertrophy. This collective process results in progressive narrowing of the foraminal dimensions, and in a minority of people, to a clinical radicular syndrome (Fig. 1). The nerve root most commonly affected in cervical radiculopathy is the C7 nerve root, followed by C6.[1] This is most likely related to the fact that the cervical foramina are largest in the upper cervical spine and gradually narrow as you progress more caudal.[2]

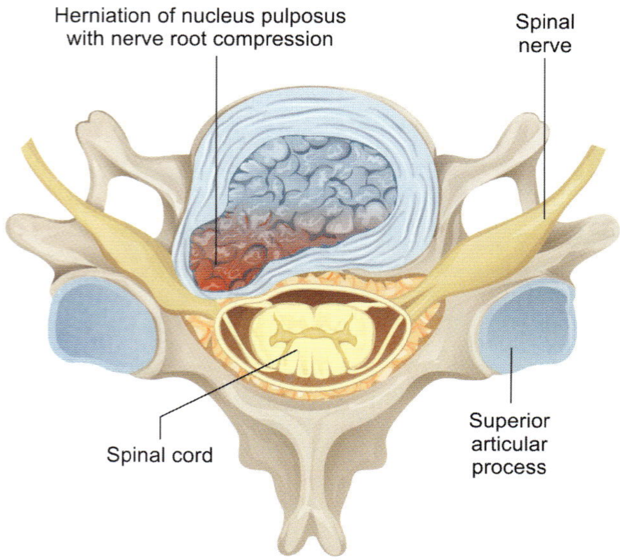

Fig. 1: Cross-sectional diagram showing spinal cord and spinal nerve roots. The left spinal nerve is being compressed by the cervical disk herniation.

History and Presentation

The most common symptom of cervical radiculopathy is arm pain. Specifically, there is a pain in the distribution of a particular nerve root. Patients typically also complain of paresthesias in the same dermatomal location. Although neck pain is not universally present, it is also a common associated presenting symptom. Symptom onset is acute in about half of instances and subacute or insidious in the other half.[4] Patients may report pain and/or spasm in the cervical and trapezius muscles, or the periscapular region, as well as limited or painful neck movements. In the majority of cases, complaints are unilateral. Lastly, patients may report weakness in the affected limb.[5] Classically, this follows the myotome associated with the involved nerve root. For example, with C6 radiculopathy, patients may describe weakness in holding items with the elbow flexed, such as difficulty lifting a gallon of milk off of a shelf.

The location of pain and paresthesias and their associated nerve root are detailed in Table 1. It is fairly easy to describe and correlate these symptoms for cervical roots C5–C8. Henderson et al. reported findings in 736 patients that were treated with posterolateral foraminotomy for cervical radiculopathy and found the correlation between pain/paresthesia, motor deficit, deep tendon reflex (DTR) changes, and the primary operative level to be 73.8%, 84.8%, and 83.5%, respectively.[9] There was an overall 71.5% incidence of correlation between

Table 1: Physical findings associated with cervical radiculopathy.

Disc level	*Root*	*Pain pattern*	*Weakness*	*Sensory loss*	*Reflex loss*
C4–5	C5	Suprascapular, lateral upper arm	Deltoid	Lateral upper arm	
C5–6	C6	Suprascapular, lateral forearm, first two digits	Biceps, brachioradialis, wrist extensors	First two digits	Biceps reflex
C6–7	C7	Interscapular, posterior forearm, third digit	Triceps, wrist flexors, finger extensors	Posterior forearm, third digit	Tricep reflex
C7–T1	C8	Scapula, ulnar side of the forearm, fifth digit	Finger abductors, grip	Fifth digit	

preoperative clinical findings and operative findings. The same cannot be said for cervical roots, C1–4. Symptoms associated with these roots tend to be vague and not easily ascribed to a specific dermatome. Patients often describe pain only without paresthesias. Pain may be located in the occipital region and/or ear (C2) or upper shoulder lateral neck (suprascapular region/trapezius muscle) with C3 and 4 pathologies.[2]

As detailed above, sensory symptoms such as burning and tingling typically follow a dermatomal distribution, however, pain is often referred outside the dermatomal maps and more in a myotomal pattern. Specifically, pain may be located in a body region not described in Table 1 or classic dermatomal maps. Authors have demonstrated that C5 or C6 radiculopathy caused suprascapular pain, C7 or C8 radiculopathy caused interscapular pain, and C8 radiculopathy caused scapular pain.[10] This was further confirmed by Slipman and colleagues.[11] The investigators studied symptoms provoked by fluoroscopically guided stimulation of cervical nerve roots and found a distinctive difference between the distribution of pain provoked by each nerve root and the classic dermatomal maps created by Keegan and Garrett.[11]

Physical Examination

The physical examination should begin with an inspection. The patient should be observed with the shirt off and comparisons made right to left. Possible observations may include winging of the scapula, muscle atrophy (i.e. deltoid, biceps, intrinsic muscles of the hand).[12] This not only may aid in the diagnosis of radiculopathy but also ruling in or out of masqueraders (see below). The examination should proceed in a standard format as to not skip or miss any key aspects of the examination. The order of the examination is less important. Following inspection and observation, the authors proceed with examining all key motor groups of the upper extremities and grading power (0–5); a grade of 0 being complete paralysis, while a 5 is considered normal. Table 1 may be used as a reference to associate motor weakness and its associated nerve roots. Key muscle groups include shoulder abduction (deltoid), elbow flexion and pronation (biceps brachii), elbow extension (triceps), wrist extension (extensor carpi radialis and ulnaris), finger abduction (dorsal interossei), grip [palmar interossei (finder adduction), flexor digitorum muscles, and others]. A more detailed examination may be included as well as indicated specifically for ruling in or out of peripheral nerve injuries. A comprehensive detailing of the upper extremity neurologic examination is beyond the scope of this chapter, but the reader is directed to *Examination of Peripheral Nerve Injuries: An Anatomical Approach* by Stephen M. Russel for more information.[13] The sensory examination may proceed next. The examination should include light touch, pain (pinprick) and proprioception, or 2-point discrimination. The aforementioned sensory modalities should be tested in all major dermatomes of the upper extremity. Sensation (light touch and pinprick) should be noted as present and normal usually comparing right to left, diminished, or absent in each dermatome. Table 1 details specific upper extremity regions in which sensation may be altered or lost and its corresponding nerve root. Reflexes are examined next. These include the biceps, triceps, and brachioradialis. Reflexes are graded 0–4, with 0 being absent, 2—normal, and 4—hyperactive. Absence or diminution of the reflex may correspond to a specific nerve root (Table 1). The examiner should investigate abnormal reflexes including testing for Hoffman's sign or reflex. Its presence may be seen in a normal person, but its acute onset or being seen in an asymmetric fashion may indicate pathology. It raises suspicion of the pathology of the corticospinal tract (spinal cord pathology vs. nerve root). For this examination, the examiner flicks the terminal phalanx of the index finder and observes for a flexion of the terminal phalanx of the thumb, which indicates a positive response. The findings of the motor, sensory, and reflex examinations may aid in identifying the involved nerve root. As with all neurological examinations, a complete test should be performed. Specifically, a motor, sensory, and reflex examination should be performed in the lower extremities. A cranial nerve examination should be performed and gait observed. Hyperreflexia in the upper and lower extremities in someone with an abnormal gait may indicate myelopathy and not radiculopathy. Tongue atrophy and fasciculations in someone with painless motor weakness in the upper extremities may indicate amyotrophic lateral sclerosis (ALS) and not radiculopathy. These two pathologies are used as examples of why a complete neurological examination is required in all patients.

Provocation tests can strengthen the diagnosis. There are five of these tests that are well-documented including the Spurling's test, the Valsalva maneuver, the shoulder abductor sign, neck distraction, and the upper limb tension test. These, however, should be relied upon with caution because the reliability and diagnostic accuracy of any one of these tests alone is poor.[14] In the Spurling's test, the patient is seated and the neck extended and passively tilted laterally toward the symptomatic side and pressure is applied to the patient's head by the examiner. A positive test results if the patient's symptoms in the arm are reproduced. In the Valsalva maneuver, the patient is asked to breathe in and hold his/her breath while trying to exhale for 2–3 seconds. A positive test results if symptoms in the arm are reproduced. The shoulder abduction sign is symptom diminution when the patient places his hand of the symptomatic side on the head. Often, this sign can be apparent by the position of most comfort that a patient assumes in the office. The neck distraction test involves placing gradual distraction of up to approximately 14 kg by grasping under the chin and occiput while the patient is supine and the neck flexed to a comfortable position. A positive test results from radicular symptom diminution. The upper limb tension test was found to be the most useful for ruling out cervical radiculopathy; however, it is also the most complicated. With the patient supine and the shoulder abducted to 30°, the examiner gradually performs the following: scapular depression, shoulder medial rotation, full elbow extension, wrist and finger flexion, contralateral, and then ipsilateral cervical side-bending. A positive test results from symptoms reproduced from any of the maneuvers other than ipsilateral side-bending which reduces symptoms.

Differential Diagnosis (Table 2)

There are several conditions that have overlapping symptoms or signs with cervical radiculopathy and should be ruled out. These peripheral nerve syndromes include suprascapular nerve entrapment, supinator entrapment, carpal tunnel syndrome (CTS), cubital tunnel syndrome (ulnar neuropathy), posterior interosseous nerve entrapment, and less commonly thoracic outlet syndrome (TOS) and acute brachial neuritis (i.e. Parsonage-Turner syndrome). These entities usually can be distinguished from the history and physical examination alone, but electrodiagnostic studies [electromyography/nerve conduction velocity (EMG/NCV)] can be helpful in cases that are unclear. The clinical distinguishing features will be discussed here while the electrodiagnostic differences will be discussed later in the "Laboratory Findings" section.

When distinguishing radiculopathy from entrapment neuropathies, it is important to remember that entrapment of a peripheral nerve causes the motor and sensory dysfunction in the muscles and sensory area in a distribution that is quite specific to the effected nerve usually in a sharply defined and discrete manner. Cervical nerve root compression, on the other hand, affects muscles and sensory areas in a much more shared fashion. The group of muscles and the sensory area affected by the axons from a single cervical nerve root is called a myotome and a dermatome, respectively. In radiculopathy, weakness is found in muscles innervated by one cervical nerve root but by multiple peripheral nerves. In addition, unlike peripheral nerves, myotomes and dermatomes of adjacent cervical nerve roots exhibit overlap. Thus, the weakness and sensory loss in cervical radiculopathy are usually partial or incomplete. With peripheral nerve entrapment, there is no neck pain, nor scapular pain that usually accompanies cervical radiculopathy. Provocation tests such as the Spurling test described above do not alleviate pain associated with peripheral nerve entrapment.

In TOS, the lower trunk of the brachial plexus is compressed within the scalene triangle either by a cervical rib or a fibrous band from an elongated C7 transverse process. The lower trunk is composed of motor fibers from the C8 and T1 nerve roots, and thus intrinsic muscles of the hand innervated by the ulnar and median nerves are affected. Patients can occasionally have a deep aching pain on the medial surface of the forearm that extends to the hand. It is easy to see, therefore, how these symptoms could be mistaken for a C8 radiculopathy. Paresthesias, pain, and sensory changes demonstrate significant overlap with C8 radiculopathy. However, some differences should be noted when evaluating TOS in the differential diagnosis. Patients with TOS typically have no neck pain and provocative tests are negative. Patients with TOS often present with hand weakness and atrophy, especially of the thenar and hypothenar eminences. This not only differentiates this condition from C8 radiculopathy but also ulnar neuropathy. Significant overlap may still exist, therefore findings on EMG/NCV are often needed for definitive diagnosis. Apical chest radiographs and oblique cervical spine X-rays can delineate both a cervical rib or the elongated C7 process which, if present, help to confirm the diagnosis of TOS.[15]

Acute brachial neuritis is a rare disease process that can be mistaken for cervical radiculopathy. This disease

Table 2: Level-of-evidence.

Author, journal, year	*Study design and methods*	*Level of evidence*	*Main results*
Henderson, Neurosurgery, 1983	Retrospective, 736 pts underwent PLF for CR	II	71.5% of the time, the surgical site can be accurately predicted on the basis of clinical findings
Tanaka, Spine, 2006	Prospective, 50 pts w neck or scapular pain underwent single-root dcm	I	Pain in the suprascapular region suggests C5 or C6 CR, pain in the interscapular region suggests C7 or C8 CR, and scapular pain suggests C8 CR
Alrawi, Eur Spine J, 2007	Prospective case series, comparison of ACDF outcomes of 8 pts who had EMG evidence of CR versus 12 that did not preoperatively	III	Pts with CR and MRI showing foraminal stenosis have better clinical outcome with ACDF if preoperative EMG testing showed evidence of radiculopathy
Bartlett, Br J Radiol, 1998	Prospective, 20 pts comparison of MRI T2, MRI w gad, and CTM	II	MRI has a 90% accuracy in detecting foraminal encroachment in pts w CR and gad enhancement does not add any benefit in the investigation
Modic, Radiology, 1986	Prospective, comparison of MRI, myelography, and CTM in 28 pts who underwent surgical confirmation	III	Diagnostic accuracy rates confirmed in surgery were 74% for MRI, 85% for CTM, and 67% for myelography. MRI is a viable alternative for CTM and together with CT if needed, provides a thorough exam for cervical nerve root compression
Cyteval, AJNR, 2004	Prospective case series of 30 pts who underwent CT-guided transforaminal epidural steroid injections	IV	60% of patients can gain good or excellent pain relief (pain diminished by 50% or more) at 2 wk after injection without any rebound at 6 mo
Anderberg, Eur Spine J, 2007	Prospective randomized control trial of 40 pts treated w TEI w either steroid/ local anesthetic or local anesthetic/ saline	II	Addition of steroids to local anesthetic in TEI provides no additional therapeutic benefit in pts w CR at 3 wk post-injection follow-up
Anderberg, Eur Spine J, 2005	Prospective case series assessed the utility of TSNRB in 30 pts w CR and MRI findings at 2 levels ipsilateral to the patient's symptoms	III	TSNRB may be useful in the preoperative evaluation of pts w CR and MRI findings at 2 levels ipsilateral to the patient's symptoms
Persson, Eur Spine J, 1997	Prospective randomized control trial compared CI, PT, and ACDF in 81 pts with 4 mo and 1 yr follow-up	II	Surgical treatment results in better outcomes at 4 mo, but outcomes are similar for surgery and conservative measures at 1 yr
Sampath, Spine, 1999	Prospective, multicenter, compared surgery to medical intervention for CR in 51 and 104 pts, respectively	III	Surgery results in improved outcomes compared to medical treatment on short-term follow-up
Hauerberg, Spine, 2008	Prospective randomized control trial comparing ACD versus ACDF in 86 pts w 2-yr follow-up	II	In pts w CR from single-level degenerative disease, clinical outcomes, fusion rates, and incidence of adjacent level disease are similar with ACD and ACDF
Xie, Neurosurgery, 2007	Prospective randomized control trial comparing ACD, ACDF, and ACDF with instrumentation in 42 pts w 2-yr follow-up	II	In pts w CR from single-level degenerative disease, clinical outcomes are similar for ACD and ACDF with or without plating, however ACD has worse fusion rates and significant segmental kyphosis, although the clinical consequences of this are unknown
Korinth, Spine, 2006	Retrospective study comparing ACDF in 124 pts to PLF in 168 pts w mean follow-up of 72.1 mo	III	Pts w CR from single-level disc herniation improve w both ACDF and PLF, but ACDF results in statistically significant better outcomes and lower reoperation rates. ACDF is associated w higher risk of complications primarily related to dysphagia or hoarseness
Uribe, Eur Spine J, 2009	Retrospective study comparing ACDF in 42 pts to ACCF in 38 pts w multilevel spondylosis w least 1-yr follow-up	III	Both multilevel ACDF and ACCF have equivalent high fusion rates and good clinical outcomes, but ACCF has higher level of early hardware failure and pseudoarthrosis

Contd...

Contd...

Author, journal, year	*Study design and methods*	*Level of evidence*	*Main results*
Jawahar, Spine J, 2010	Prospective randomized trial comparing ACDF and CDA in 93 pts w 1 or 2-level cervical DDD, median 37 mo follow-up	II	CDA and ACDF are equivalent in providing relief from symptoms and there is no difference in risk of ASD. Risk of ASD is higher in pts who have concurrent DDD in lumbar spine
Grobb, Eur Spine J, 2001	Prospective randomized trial comparing ACDF and ACDFP in 50 pts w 1 or 2-level cervical fusion, average 37 mo follow-up	II	There is no significant difference in improvement of pain, range of motion, nor rate of pseudoarthrosis, however, ACDFP is better at maintaining graft height/sagittal alignment
Mobbs, J Clin Neurosci, 2007	Retrospective study comparing ACDFP to ACDF in 242 pts	III	ACDFP leads to lower rates of poor outcomes that require revision surgery for nonunion, kyphosis, graft extrusion or collapse (1.8% compared to 10% in ACDF group) and higher rate of fusion, but no difference in the rate of good or excellent outcomes
Wang, Spine, 2000	Retrospective review comparing ACDF to ACDFP in 2-level fusions; 60 pts, avg 2.7 yr follow-up	III	Pseudoarthrosis rate drops from 25% to 0% with the addition of an anterior cervical plate in two-level ACDF
Wang, Spine, 2001	Retrospective review comparing ACDF to ACDFP in 3-level fusions, 59 pts, avg 3.2 yr follow-up	III	Pseudoarthrosis rated drops from 37% to 18% with the addition of an anterior cervical plate in three-level ACDF

[ACD: anterior cervical discectomy (without interbody fusion); ACDF: anterior cervical discectomy and fusion; ASD: adjacent segment disease; CDA: cervical disc arthroplasty; CI: collar immobilization; CR: cervical radiculopathy; CTM: computed tomography-assisted myelography; Dcm: decompression; DDD: degenerative disc disease; EMG: electromyography; Gad: gadolinium; Mo: months; MRI: magnetic resonance imaging; PLF: posterior cervical laminoforaminotomy; PT: physical therapy; Pts: patients; TEI: transforaminal epidural injection; TSNRB: transforaminal selective nerve root block; W: with; Wk: weeks; Yr: years; ACDFP: anterior cervical discectomy and fusion plate; ACCF: anterior cervical corpectomy and fusion]

process has many names including brachial plexitis, acute brachial plexus neuropathy, neuralgic amyotrophy, and Parsonage-Turner syndrome. The etiology is unclear but symptoms are discrete and very typical to this process. There is a sudden onset of severe pain classically located in the shoulder girdle. The pain persists for hours to weeks and as the pain subsides, the patient experiences sudden and simultaneous near-total weakness in the muscles that are innervated by the upper cervical trunk. These include the deltoid, the supraspinatus, the infraspinatus, the serratus anterior, and the biceps brachii. Visible changes in muscle bulk occur in 2–4 weeks in these muscles; the atrophy may be significant. Sensory symptoms are less common and if present, usually involve the distribution of the axillary nerve. The acute onset and eventual subsidence of pain in the shoulder region, followed by profound weakness and atrophy in the muscles supplied by the upper trunk of the brachial plexus typifies this condition and is rarely seen in cervical radiculopathy. The diagnosis may be made by these signs and symptoms. Although there is no proof of causation, brachial neuritis follows a viral illness in 25% of cases and immunization in 15% of cases. There is bilateral involvement in 33% of cases. Despite such a fulminant course and no specific treatment options, the prognosis is generally favorable in the long run. Strength is gradually recovered but may be incomplete. Recovery has been estimated to be 90% by 3 years and this should be explained to patients.[1]

The suprascapular nerve may be confused with C5 radiculopathy. With both, patients may present with pain localized to the shoulder and weakness of shoulder muscles. Patients with suprascapular nerve entrapment typically have a dull pain in the top but also the posterior aspect of the shoulder, which is rare in C5 palsy. C5 compression may result in a sensory disturbance on the lateral aspect of the shoulder (deltoid), which is not seen in suprascapular entrapment. Involvement of the suprascapular nerve results in weakness in the abduction of the arm at the shoulder (first 30°) and also the external rotation of the shoulder, which differentiates this pathology from a C5 palsy. Lastly, patients with suprascapular entrapment classically present with atrophy of the supraspinatus and infraspinatus muscles, which is not seen with C5 nerve root involvement.

Carpal tunnel syndrome (CTS) may be confused with C6 radiculopathy. In CTS, patients typically present with pain and paresthesias in the hand, classically located in the thumb, index, and middle fingers. The symptoms worsen with activities such as typing on a keyboard or holding a phone to the ear. A very typical complaint is waking up with a worsening of the parenthesis necessitating shaking of the affected hand to relieve the symptoms. Subjective weakness may be present, but objective weakness is most often absent. Sensory changes may be seen in the thumb and first two digits but not in the arm. Pain may radiate from the wrist *proximally* into the arm but this may be absent. Tapping the wrist above the carpal tunnel may elicit paresthesias in the first three digits (Tinel's sign); symptoms may also worsen by hyperflexion of the wrist (Phalen's sign). C6 radiculopathy may also present with paresthesias in the thumb and index finger. Patients often have associated cervical pain. Pain in the arm radiates from the cervical region *down* the arm and often localizes in the forearm. There may be both subjective and objective weakness. Classically, there is a weakness in elbow flexion and especially pronation. Sensory changes may be seen along the C6 dermatome in the arm, while the biceps reflex may be diminished or lost. Lastly, provocative maneuvers detailed above will typically exacerbate the symptoms.

Ulnar neuropathy (cubital tunnel syndrome) can be particularly challenging to distinguish from C8 radiculopathy because both can cause paresthesias in the 4th and 5th digits. A careful history and physical examination can help differentiate. Patients with ulnar nerve compression classically only have symptoms in the hand. Most troubling are paresthesias in the 4th and 5th digits, but hand weakness, especially grip, may be the predominant complaint. Pain may be present in the arm, especially the elbow. There may be hypothenar atrophy as well as atrophy of the first dorsal web space. Sensory changes are demonstrated in the 5th and ulnar half of the 4th digits as well as the dorsal aspect of the medial hand. The patient may note weakness in the 5th digit; the finger may deviate from the hand when attempting to hold the fingers together. A C8 radiculopathy will involve the 4th and 5th digits in their entirety. In addition, aC8 radiculopathy will cause weakness in hand intrinsic innervated by the median nerve.[2,15] This helps to differentiate this from weakness due to ulnar nerve compression. Reflexes are normal and tapping over the ulnar nerve in the cubital tunnel may elicit paresthesias along the nerve especially in the 4th and 5th digits. Lastly, patients with C8 radiculopathy often complain of neck pain while this is rare in cases of ulnar neuropathy.

Amyotrophic lateral sclerosis (ALS) should also be considered in cases of suspected cervical radiculopathy, mainly in males over the age of 60. There is overlap with those cases in which patients present with primarily motor weakness and little or no sensory findings. Both may present with progressive weakness and atrophy, typically in the hands. Both may demonstrate a lack of reflexes. ALS may be differentiated from cervical radiculopathy by close observation and examination. Classically, motor symptoms predominate, often with atrophy in the hands; however, this disease process usually extends beyond single myotomes. There are mixed lower and upper motor signs. Patients may have loss of reflexes in the upper extremities while displaying hyperreflexia in the lower extremities. Additionally, tongue fasciculation should be sought and may be considered a distinguishing hallmark of the disease.

Imaging

Cervical radiculopathy may be diagnosed by history and physical examination. Moreover, most pathologies in the differential diagnosis may be eliminated with this detailed history and examination. The vast majority of patients do not require imaging because the condition is self-limited. Typically imaging is required when: (1) the patient fails to have improvement in symptoms after some predetermined time, often 8 weeks of conservative treatment; (2) evidence of neurological deficit, especially if progressive; or (3) the presence of red flags (examples include fever, pain out of proportion to expectations, pain while at rest, progressive neurological decline, bowel or bladder incontinence).

Cervical Radiographs

Weight-bearing cervical radiographs, including anteroposterior, lateral, and oblique views should be obtained during the initial evaluation of radiculopathy. These studies are most helpful in defining cervical alignment and any evidence of instability. These variables carry considerable weight when deciding interventional strategies and may not be seen on a supine magnetic resonance imaging (MRI). If oblique radiographs are ordered, foraminal stenosis may be visualized. Cervical radiographs are considered complimentary with more advanced imaging such as MRI in the diagnosis of cervical radiculopathy.

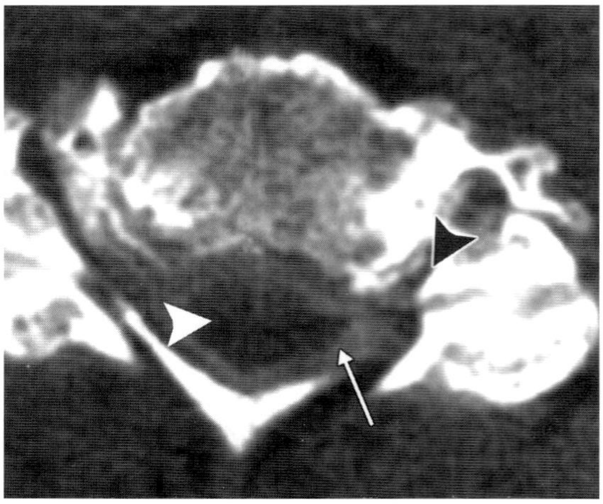

Fig. 2: Axial computed tomography (CT) myelogram of the cervical spine showing bilateral foraminal narrowing with nerve root impingement secondary to spondylosis. The white arrow points to the subarachnoid space. The white arrowhead points to the spinal cord. The black arrowhead points to the left nerve root in the cervical foramen compressed by the degenerated uncovertebral joint anteriorly and the facet joints posteriorly.

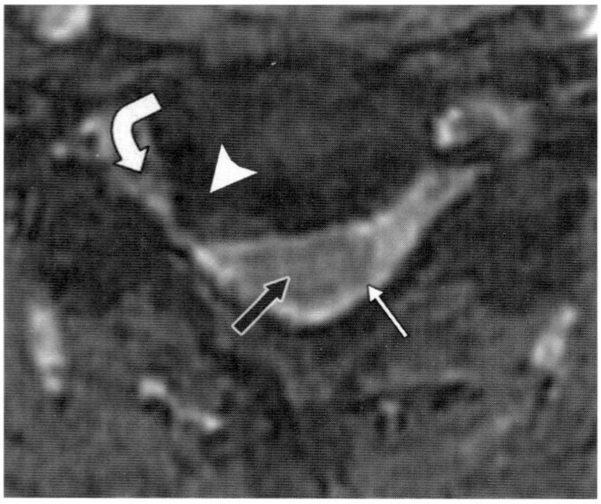

Fig. 3: Axial magnetic resonance imaging (MRI) of the cervical spine showing right foraminal narrowing and nerve root impingement (curved white arrow) secondary to cervical disk herniation (white arrowhead). The straight white arrow points to the subarachnoid space. The black arrow points to the spinal cord.

X-ray and Computed Tomography Myelography

Plain X-ray myelography is performed by obtaining plain X-rays after administering water-soluble contrast into the subarachnoid space. This allows visualization of the nerve roots and spinal cord. Lateral films are useful for evaluating spinal cord compression, while anteroposterior views are better at detecting nerve root compression. The latter is seen as cervical root sleeve dye-filling defects, which may represent nerve root compression by an osteophyte or disk. Plain computed tomography (CT) is the most sensitive test for assessing the bony elements of the spine; however, its utility is also limited in the setting of cervical radiculopathy. This is because the soft tissue abnormalities that are most commonly responsible for this disease process are not well visualized on plain CT. However, CT with coronal and sagittal reconstructions can help demonstrate osteophytes, ossification of the posterior longitudinal ligament (PLL), and facet joint hypertrophy. CT combined with myelography greatly enhances the ability to detect nerve root compression and best delineates the nerve root in relation to surrounding bony structures (Fig. 2). In a retrospective case series of 734 patients who underwent computed tomography myelography (CTM) for cervical disk disease, 280 patients underwent surgery for cervical radiculopathy. CTM corresponded to surgical findings in 260 of these 280 patients and the authors concluded that CTM can identify 90% of cervical extruded disk herniations confirmed by surgery.[16] Karnaze et al. found that CTM was superior to MRI in depicting cases of spondylosis.[17] However, in another retrospective case series reviewing the surgical and CTM findings in 95 patients with foraminal stenosis, the authors found that the diagnosis on the basis of CTM is difficult because stenosis was evident as a bone spur in only 13% of cases, could not be distinguished from prolapsed disk in 39%, had to be differentiated from a congenitally narrow foraminal canal in 27%, and was missed in 20% of the cases.[18] In addition, myelography, whether done with CT or X-rays, is an invasive procedure and subjects the patient to ionizing radiation.

Magnetic Resonance Imaging

Magnetic resonance imaging allows passive imaging of the cervical spine with high definition of the neural anatomy and soft tissues (Fig. 3). It is the most commonly employed higher-order imaging used in the United States for patients with cervical radiculopathy. As stated previously, MRI should only be ordered in the face of red flags or following completion of conservative treatment with the persistence of symptoms. This is highlighted by the fact that there is a high frequency of abnormalities detected on MRI in asymptomatic patients. Disk protrusion was seen in 57% of patients over 64-year-old in a study where patients had

MRIs done of the neck for suspected laryngeal pathology without any symptoms referable to the cervical spine.[19]

The value of MRI is its ability to define soft tissue. Specifically, MRI is able to demonstrate disk bulges, herniations, and ligamentum flavum hypertrophy, all of which may be compressing a nerve root. The evidence supporting MRI for diagnosing the cause of cervical radiculopathy is strong. When radiologic nerve root compression was compared with clinical radiculopathy, CT myelography and MR had similar sensitivity and accuracy in the setting of cervical spondylosis and disk herniation.[17,20-22] Bartlett et al. compared T2 and gadolinium-enhanced MRI with CT myelography in cervical radiculopathy prospectively in 30 patients and found that MRI T2 images had an accuracy approaching 90% for the diagnosis of foraminal encroachment.[23] MRI with gadolinium conferred no additional benefit in this study; however, in the appropriate setting gadolinium enhancement can accurately display soft-tissue compression from infection or tumor. Modic et al. found in a prospective study comparing the predictive value of MRI, myelography, and CTM in patients that subsequently underwent surgery that MRI was as sensitive as CTM for identification of disease level, but not as specific for type of disease.[21] Plain X-ray myelography was the least sensitive and specific of the modalities. A more recent retrospective study of 50 patients who underwent anterior cervical diskectomy showed no significant difference in intraobserver or interobserver agreement between MRI and CTM.[22] They found that MRI was better for identifying disk abnormality and nerve root compression while CTM was better for foraminal stenosis and bony changes. It is important to remember that when compared to the lumbar spine, the cervical foramina are much smaller and lack the epidural fat present in the lumbar foramina. This makes detecting foraminal stenosis and the nature of the stenosis to be either bony or not more difficult on MRI. This is why many surgeons choose to get CT imaging in addition to MRI much more readily when it comes to cervical radiculopathy.

The downsides of MRI are costs and the MRI itself. MRI is costly and is overused in the diagnosis of cervical radiculopathy. The test is, therefore, highly scrutinized currently by payer policies and the US Government. Many people are not able to undergo an MRI. This may be due to claustrophobia or the presence of an implanted pacemaker, deep brain or spinal stimulator, or the presence of ferromagnetic metal in the body such as bullet fragments or old cerebral aneurysm clips. CT myelography is an appropriate alternative in such cases.

Without any strict guidelines of whether to get MRI, X-rays, plain CT, CTM, or a combination of these imaging modalities, in patients without a contraindication to MRI, it is appropriate to get MRI as the initial imaging modality in addition to plain radiographs. As mentioned above, plain upright radiographs can provide useful information about alignment and potential instability which may not be evident on a supine MRI. Since the quality of MRI has continued to improve, it is usually sufficient for surgical planning. Plain CT should then be performed in addition to the MRI for cases where the ossified posterior longitudinal ligament (OPLL) is suspected, the foraminal stenosis is suspected to be caused by a bony lesion, the nature or degree of nerve root compression is unclear on MRI, or when symptoms are incongruent with MRI findings. It may also be appropriate to get a plain CT in addition to an initial MRI when there is multilevel disease and the surgeon needs additional information to make a decision about the main causing level and the extent of the operation. Because of the invasive nature of the test and lack of evidence supporting its diagnostic superiority to MRI, CTM should be reserved for patients who cannot get an MRI because they have an implanted device such as a cardiac pacemaker.

Diagnostic Testing

Laboratory Values

Blood work is of limited value in the diagnosis of degenerative cervical radiculopathy, but elevated inflammatory markers in this setting including C-reactive protein (CRP) and erythrocyte sedimentation rate (ESR) may be red flags for intraspinal infection or cancer. At times, it may be useful to order blood tests evaluating for the diagnosis of a rheumatologic condition such as rheumatoid factor (RF) in the diagnosis of rheumatoid arthritis.

Electromyography and Nerve Conduction Velocity

Electromyography and nerve conduction velocity testing are very valuable for making a diagnosis of cervical radiculopathy. Moreover, it has greater value in the authors' opinion of ruling in or out of masqueraders. There are limitations of this diagnostic testing that must be noted.

EMG/NCV has been shown to have a variable correlation with neuroimaging and surgical localization. Patient with only radicular pain and sensory symptoms usually do not have measurable electrophysiologic correlates with these standard techniques. Specifically, their test may be interpreted as "normal" despite true nerve compression and root irritation. This is because pain and paresthesias are mediated by c-type fibers, which are too small to be evaluated by EMG/NCV. EMG/NCV testing is, therefore, most useful in patients with focal motor weakness and/or asymmetric changes in deep tendon reflexes. The aforementioned should be carefully considered before EMG/NCV is ordered in the clinical setting of cervical radiculopathy. If one is attempting to rule out a peripheral nerve compression, it may be an excellent test to order. However, in the face of an accurate clinical diagnosis of radiculopathy in the absence of motor findings, the test may likely be "normal." The utility of the test is then in questions and moreover, appropriate treatment may not be rendered even in the face of true pathology.

Sensory Nerve Action Potentials

Sensory nerve action potentials (SNAPs) are recorded by stimulating a peripheral nerve and recording along a pure sensory portion of the nerve, like the finger. Amplitude and latency are recorded. SNAPs are typically normal in cervical radiculopathy. The dorsal root ganglion (DRG) is distal to the nerve root compression or irritation and is therefore intact. Because the DRG (location of sensory cell body) is intact, the sensory axon remains intact (unaltered), and the SNAP amplitude and latency are normal. However, one can see how this test could be helpful in ruling in peripheral nerve entrapment. In peripheral nerve pathology, the compression is distal to the DRG and the SNAP amplitude and latency will be effected and helping rule out radiculopathy. A slight caveat should be explained in that the C5 and C6 DRGs, however, have been shown to reside in a relative intraspinal location in cadaveric studies, therefore, more vulnerable to injury and resulting in SNAP amplitude changes. However, this is not very common.

Compound Muscle Action Potential

Compound muscle action potentials (CMAPs) are part of the conduction motor testing performed during the NCV part of the EMG/NCV testing. Similar to SNAPs, the peripheral nerve is stimulated and the CMAP is recorded in the muscle of interest. Unlike SNAPs, motor conduction cannot discern between central and peripheral lesions (i.e. proximal or distal to the DRG) in that the motor cell body resides in the spinal cord. Moreover, a significant number of motor axons (>50%) is required to impart a significant decrement to the CMAP. Most radiculopathies interrupt only a fraction of the total number of motor root fibers and hence the compound muscle action potential (CMAP) would typically be normal. In addition, the myotome from which the CMAP amplitude is generated must match that of the injured root. Muscles in the C6 and C7 myotomes are not discretely isolated from muscles of other myotomes, and thus CMAPs cannot be reliably correlated to these nerve roots.[24] Similar to SNAPs, however, the CMAP is better served to rule in or out masquerading pathologies rather than diagnosing a cervical radiculopathy.

Unlike nerve conduction studies, needle electrode examination (NEE) only assesses the motor component of radiculopathy, however, it is the most specific and sensitive of the electrodiagnostic tests for diagnosing acute axon loss radiculopathy. NEE can give information not only about the nerve root level that is involved, but also about the degree of axon loss, and the chronicity of this process. In acute radiculopathy, fibrillation potentials are the abnormality most likely to be seen; however, these rarely develop before 2 weeks have elapsed since the onset of weakness. For this reason, physicians are recommended to delay ordering NEE testing until at least 3 weeks after the onset of motor symptoms. Although there is no high-level evidence that EMG is effective in clinical diagnosis of cervical radiculopathy like there is in lumbosacral radiculopathy, a systematic evidence-based review found that EMG testing provided confirmatory evidence of cervical radiculopathy in 30–72%, that EMG abnormalities were highly correlated with weakness, and that there was good agreement between imaging studies and needle EMG in 65–85% of cases.[25]

As previously stated, EMG/NCV testing may be normal in cervical radiculopathy. In most cases, the diagnosis is made by history and physical examination and correlated with imaging (i.e. MRI). *EMG/NCV is rarely used to diagnose cervical radiculopathy.* It is, however, invaluable for the evaluation of other conditions in the differential diagnosis such as peripheral nerve entrapment or compression. Some important findings should be noted when using EMG/NCV for the evaluation of cervical radiculopathy.

The classic EMG (NEE) findings in radiculopathy are fibrillations at rest in the muscles supplied by the nerve root (i.e. its myotome). The more muscles identified as abnormal in the myotome, the more reliable the diagnosis is for a single-root lesion. EMG changes should be found in at least two muscles in myotome that do not share the same peripheral nerve innervation.[24] Because the posterior division of the nerve, which supplies these muscles, arises in the lateral part of the neural foramina, paraspinal denervation or fibrillations will be demonstrated as well. This finding distinguishes a radiculopathy from a more distal lesion. Sensory and motor conduction velocities are typically normal. However, decreased amplitude and increased latencies may be seen in severely affected individuals. Entrapment neuropathies, such as carpal tunnel syndrome, typically have normal NEE findings with evidence of denervation seen only in severe cases. If seen, however, the findings are seen only in the muscles of that particular nerve root. NEE of the paraspinal muscles will be normal (hallmark finding). NCV testing classically demonstrates increased sensory latency (conduction delay) at the site of the compression.

TREATMENT

Nonsurgical Treatment

The outcomes of conservative management are deficient and contrasting in the literature. Studies which were written by surgeons often demonstrate a significant failure rate of conservative treatment and make an argument for aggressive surgical intervention. DePalma and Subin found that only 29% of patients treated conservatively had complete resolution of symptoms,[8] while Gore et al. demonstrated in their study, which followed 205 patients with neck and referred pain for 15 years, that one-third of patients treated conservatively had moderate to severe pain that interfered with their lifestyle.[26] Physiotherapy-based studies, however, have reported much better outcomes. These studies have typically found that between 77% and 92% of patients respond favorably to conservative therapy including cervical traction and/or physical therapy.[27-30] The largest of these studies was a multicenter trial of the effect of physiotherapy for neck and arm pain sponsored by the British Association of Physical Medicine.[28] Of the 493 patients that were divided into different conservative treatment arms including traction, collar, positioning, instructions in posture, or placebo tablets, three-fourths were assessed as cured or with only mild symptoms at the end of 4 weeks of treatment. Nonetheless, compared to lumbar radiculopathy which is well recognized to be in most cases self-limiting with symptoms resolving in weeks to months,[31] the natural history of cervical radiculopathy is less clear. The condition appears to be self-limited in the majority of patients, but less predictable as compared to its correlate in the lumbar spine.

Patients are often initially given a trial of nonsteroidal anti-inflammatory drugs (NSAIDs), muscle relaxants, or a tapered dose of oral steroids. Nonpharmacologic treatments include collar immobilization, rest from activities that aggravate the condition, ergonomic neck instructions, use of a cervical pillow, and intermittent cervical traction. Patients undergoing more active treatments including an aggressive physical medicine rehabilitation program with a combination of treatment modalities seem to improve more quickly and have the most effective results.[32,33] There is insufficient evidence for or against the efficacy of manipulation or chiropractic treatments for cervical radiculopathy from degenerative disorders. There may be, however, major complications with these maneuvers including but not limited to vertebral artery dissection or worsening of symptoms and therefore careful consideration should be made regarding this therapy.[12]

Patients are also often referred for transforaminal epidural steroid injections for cervical radiculopathy; however, there is insufficient evidence to show that these injections provide long-term relief of symptoms. The reported results are in fact variable. One prospective case series measured the intensity of radicular pain scored on a visual analog scale in 30 patients who underwent CT-guided transforaminal steroid injections with follow-up at 2 weeks and 6 months. About 60% of patients had good or excellent pain relief (pain diminished by 50% or more) at 2 weeks and no rebound of pain at the 6-month follow-up.[34] Two additional studies further demonstrated the benefit of injections noting that between 25% and 63% of patients opted to cancel surgery because of clinical improvement from their epidural steroid injections.[35,36] However, other studies have not found such a positive benefit. A prospective randomized controlled trial of 40 patients compared transforaminal epidural steroid injection with transforaminal injections of local anesthetic alone in the treatment of cervical radiculopathy. Interestingly, they found that there was no statistically significant difference in pain improvement at 3-week follow-up between the two groups.[37] Transforaminal injections may be helpful, however, as a diagnostic means before surgery. In the setting of cervical radiculopathy where MRI shows positive findings at multiple levels ipsilateral to the patient's symptoms, transforaminal selective nerve root blocks may be helpful in the preoperative evaluation and surgical planning.[38]

SURGICAL INDICATIONS AND TREATMENT

In general, surgery is indicated in patients with spondylotic cervical radiculopathy who have disabling pain that is refractory to nonoperative management, progressive muscular weakness, or when red flags are present (i.e. incontinence). The duration of nonoperative care required prior to surgical intervention is unclear. Typically surgeons advocate 8–12 weeks of sufficient conservative therapy prior to recommending surgical intervention (absent red flags). A prospective randomized controlled trial compared outcomes in 81 patients equally divided into three groups: (1) cervical bracing; (2) physical therapy; and (3) anterior cervical diskectomy and fusion (ACDF).[39] At 4 months, the surgery group reported less pain, less sensory loss, and had better muscle strength compared to the two conservative treatment groups. The authors concluded that patients have better outcomes within a few months after surgery, while those in the other two groups demonstrated much slower improvement. Some in the ACDF arm had evidence of recurrent symptoms after initial improvement, leading the authors to conclude that all three treatment modalities resulted in similar outcomes at 1 year. Sampath et al. reported an additional prospective, multicenter study, which compared surgical to nonoperative management.[40] Of the 155 patients on whom there were follow-up data, 51 underwent surgery and 104 received medical treatment. Both groups improved significantly, but there was a greater improvement in the surgical group including patient satisfaction, neurological improvement, and functional improvement in activities of daily living. It is worth noting that with only short follow-up, 26% still had bothersome symptoms at the latest evaluation.

When patients fail nonoperative management or otherwise meet inclusion criteria for surgery, the options for surgical interventions include anterior cervical diskectomy (ACD) without fusion, anterior cervical diskectomy with fusion, posterior cervical foraminotomy, and cervical disk arthroplasty. Each procedure has its unique indication for use, each modality has demonstrated near equal and positive outcomes.

Hauerberg et al. performed a prospective randomized controlled trial comparing the clinical and radiologic outcomes of ACD versus ACDF in 86 patients with follow-up at 3, 12, and 24 months after surgery.[41] Two years after the operation, 86.1% of patients treated with ACDF reported good outcomes, compared to 76.7% in the ACD group. This was not a statistically significant difference. Additionally, the rates for fusion and adjacent level disease were the same as well for the two groups. Xie and Hurlbert also performed a prospective randomized controlled trial comparing ACD, ACDF, and ACDF with instrumentation (plate and screw fixation) in 42 patients with 2-year follow-up.[42] Although patients in all groups had similar significant improvement in arm and neck pain, fusion rates on radiographs were 67%, 93%, and 100% for the ACD, ACDF, and ACDF with instrumentation groups, respectively. Additionally, ACD alone resulted in segmental kyphosis compared to the ACD and ACDF with instrumentation groups. Segmental kyphosis occurred in 75% of the ACD patients postoperatively compared with 17% preoperatively, while there was no change in sagittal balance in the ACDF or ACDF with instrumentation groups. Thus, without knowing the long-term effects of kyphosis after anterior cervical diskectomy, the addition of an interbody graft for fusion is suggested to improve sagittal alignment and maintain the foraminal opening. There are several choices to the surgeon for the graft material and the cages that contain the graft and these will be discussed later.

Another surgical option for cervical radiculopathy is posterior cervical laminoforaminotomy (PLF). This has the advantage of avoiding the well-recognized risks associated with an anterior approach including recurrent laryngeal nerve injury and dysphagia. In addition, a posterior foraminotomy maintains spinal alignment and spares the motion segment, avoiding the risk of adjacent level disease. Korinth et al. studied 292 patients retrospectively comparing anterior and posterior surgery for cervical monoradiculopathy caused by soft disk disease. One hundred twenty-four patients underwent ACDF with polymethyl methacrylate interbody fusion and 168 patients underwent PLF.[43] The authors found that although patients improved with both ACDF and PLF, ACDF results in statistically better outcomes, with a success rate of 93.6% for the ACDF group and 85.1% in the

PLF group. One reason for this may be because the amount of bony decompression that can be attained by a posterior foraminotomy is limited without jeopardizing the facet joint. If there is a large amount of bony foraminal stenosis, it may not be possible to adequately decompress the nerve root without destabilizing the facet joint and require an additional fusion procedure. Korinth et al. found in their study, that is described above, that patients with cervical radiculopathy from a mixture of soft and hard disks had lower success rates than patient with pure soft disks.[43] The success rates in the cases with a mixture of soft and hard disks were 90.6% and 80% for ACDF and PLF, respectively. This difference, however, was not statistically significant. Nonetheless, PLF can be performed safely as an outpatient procedure with good outcomes in 75–98% of patients with a lower risk of complications than anterior surgery,[44] the latter of which has a significant risk of dysphagia and hoarseness. In addition, PLF may be more cost-effective than ACDF. A retrospective review of 38 patients who either underwent PLF or ACDF found that both the direct cost of the surgery as well as the long-term indirect cost, including the time required to return to active-duty service, were higher for the ACDF group.[45] Posterior cervical laminoforaminotomy should be considered as an acceptable alternative to ACDF especially in patients where the nerve root compression is from soft disk fragments.

Cervical disk arthroplasty (CDA) is a newer technique that has been met with mixed sentiment. The most important feature of this procedure, which is also sometimes referred to as total disk replacement, is the ability to preserve motion while maintaining stability.[46] One of the reasons that the enthusiasm for this procedure has been tempered is because ACDF has been successfully performed for decades with highly predictable and largely favorable results. There are concerns, however, that cervical interbody arthrodesis alters spinal kinematics and leads to accelerated degeneration of adjacent segments. The incidence of adjacent segment disease is reported to be as high as 2.9% per year, potentially affecting more than a quarter of all patients undergoing anterior cervical arthrodesis.[47] This can lead to a significant number of reoperations, which carries a higher risk of complications. Preserving the motion segment with total disk arthroplasty (TDA) has been proposed to reduce the risk of adjacent segment disease. Whether this truly is the case, however, is controversial. Song et al. compared degenerative changes in adjacent segments to nonadjacent segments in 87 patients who underwent ACDF and found that although fusion can accelerate the severity of adjacent level degeneration, there was no significant difference between adjacent and nonadjacent segments in terms of the incidence of symptomatic disease.[48] The authors concluded that adjacent segment disease is more a result of the natural history of cervical spondylosis than the presence of fusion. Additionally, a more recent retrospective study using an 11-year nationwide database to analyze the incidence of adjacent segment disease found the annual incidence of repeat ACDF for adjacent segment disease to be only 0.8%.[49] Nonetheless, cervical disk arthroplasty has been shown to be a viable surgical alternative to ACDF in treatment of patient with cervical radiculopathy caused by degenerative disk disease. Recently, multiple prospective, randomized trials have shown that single-level arthroplasty produces clinical results that are equivalent to and in some instances better than those reported for cervical fusion.[50-54]

Anterior Cervical Diskectomy and Fusion

History and Technique

The current surgical options for cervical disk disease are the result of continuous innovations in surgical approaches, minimally invasive techniques, bone-grafting techniques, nonfusion technologies, and instrumentation. There is no doubt that there will be further advances in surgery of the cervical spine even by the time this book is published, however, continuing innovations require an understanding of the past advances and the history of how we came to the surgical approaches that are available to us today. Posterior approaches to the spine were the first described and anterior surgery developed independently of spinal surgery to address nonspinal diseases in the late nineteenth century, e.g. the drainage of tuberculous abscesses of the posterior wall of the pharynx.[55] Anterior approaches, especially transoral approaches were first met by an overwhelming number of postoperative infections. It was not until the widespread use of antibiotics that there was more widespread use of this approach. In the 1950s, surgeons started shifting from posterior to anterior techniques. Smith and Robinson were the first to describe the anterolateral approach to cervical spine in 1955, that is the high presternocleidomastoid, retropharyngeal, and precarotid approach.[56] Smith and Robinson adjoined the adjacent vertebrae using a horseshoe graft harvested from the iliac crest. They published the success of this procedure later with more patients and longer follow-up in 1958.[57] That same year, Cloward reported a similar technique using a large-bore hand drill and guard to remove disk material and a dowel-shaped autogenous bone graft for fusion.[58] In 1960, Baily and Badgley described a fusion technique involving the onlay of a strut graft in patients with neoplasms and instability of the cervical spine.[59] This is the same concept now used in cervical corpectomy. The Smith-Robinson exposure is the fundamental technique utilized to this day for anterior approaches to the cervical spine and this approach along with the current technique used for diskectomy and fusion is described next. While the original surgery described by Smith and Robinson preserved the endplate and PLL, surgeons have modified this technique to achieve more extensive decompression and to enhance the rate of fusion.

After general endotracheal anesthesia, the patient is put supine and the neck is positioned in a neutral position avoiding hyperextension. Landmarks can be used for localization of the appropriate level. C3 is at the level of the hyoid bone, C4–5 disk space at the thyroid cartilage, and C6 at the cricoid. However, lateral fluoroscopic images should be checked to ensure the incision is made at the appropriate level. After the level to be treated is confirmed by fluoroscopy and marked, the patient is prepped and draped in a sterile fashion. A transverse incision is then made at the marked level from the midline to the posterior border of the sternocleidomastoid muscle (SCM). The plastysma is then exposed and incised. The deep cervical fascia is then exposed between the anterior belly of the SCM laterally and the strap muscles (sternohyoid and sternothyroid muscles) medially. After palpating the carotid pulse and staying medial to it, the surgeon uses blunt dissection to separate the carotid from the medial structures, including the esophagus, trachea, and thyroid, until the cervical spine can be palpated. The vertebra can be visualized as covered by the longus colli, the prevertebral fascial and anterior longitudinal ligament when the carotid and SCM are retracted laterally and the medial structures described above retracted medially. The midline of the cervical spine is defined as the middle of the gap created by the medial borders of the longus colli muscles. This can be confirmed radiographically as well if there is any uncertainty. The longus colli muscles are elevated laterally off the anterior vertebral body with cauterization and self-retaining retractors are placed such that the teeth of the retractors are under the muscle. This avoids excessive retraction of the esophagus and carotid artery. Then Caspar distracting pins are placed at the midlevel of the vertebral bodies above and below the disk space for craniocaudal distraction.

The microscope is then brought into the surgical field and used for the diskectomy. The anterior aspect of the annulus fibrosis is removed circumferentially with a sharp knife. The superficial disk is removed with curettes and pituitary rongeurs. Any osteophytic ridges removed as well with a high-speed drill with a small-diameter burr down to the PLL. The uncovertebral joint, also known as the Luschka joint, is a good landmark for how far lateral to carry the diskectomy. The PLL is identified and removed by first separating it from the dura with a blunt nerve hook. This is done best at the most lateral aspect of the canal where the PLL is thinnest. A combination of Kerrison punches and up-biting curettes are used to resect the PLL. The surgeon checks for any subligamentous disk material and removes these segments as well. Epidural bleeding can be controlled with bipolar cauterization and thrombogenic agents such as Floseal Hemostatic Matrix (Baxter Health Care Corporation, Deerfield, IL). After the diskectomy is performed, the endplates are prepared with the high-speed drill to create bleeding surfaces and enhance fusion across the graft. The use of autograft from the iliac crest or fibula or allograft is surgeon preference and grafting options are discussed later. The graft is placed in the disk space while the endplates are distracted and the distraction is removed slowly to provide compression along with the graft site.

Then if the surgeon chooses to use instrumentation including plate and screw fixation, the Caspar screws are removed and the anterior surface of the vertebral bodies are prepared with the high-speed drill to create a flat surface such that the plate will make flush contact. The plate is fixed to the vertebral bodies above and below the disk space with screws pointed slightly medially and away in the craniocaudal direction from the disk space (Figs. 4A to C). The screws should be placed in dense bone tissue without breaching the endplates. The position of the graft, as well as the screws, can be confirmed radiographically.

The side the surgeon chooses to operate is also surgeon-dependent. In general, right-handed surgeons like to do this procedure from the patient's right, while left-handed surgeons prefer the patient's left side. Both sides have their disadvantages. On the right side, the recurrent

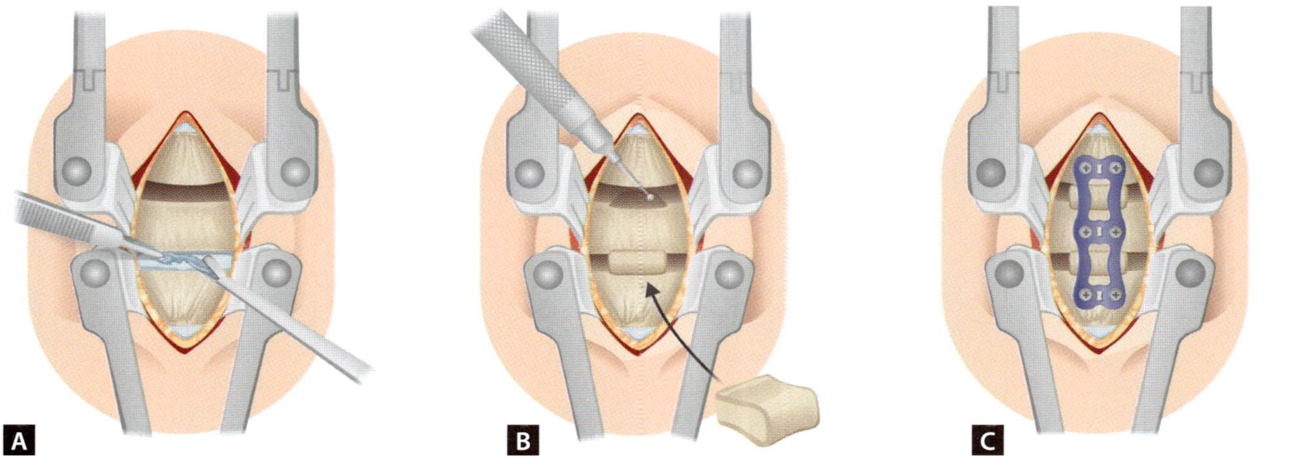

Figs. 4A to C: (A) After the self-retaining retractor is in place and the correct level is identified, a scalpel is used to incise the disk annulus and a combination of curettes and pituitary rongeurs are used to remove the bulk of the disk; (B) Osteophytes and the endplates are removed to expose blood-rich cancellous bone with a high-speed burr. Then a graft is contoured and tapped into the shelf space; (C) The shortest plate possible is fixed to the vertebral body with superior screws angled upward and inward and inferior screws angled inward and posterior.

laryngeal nerve has a more aberrant course and is thus more susceptible to injury. On the left side, the thoracic duct may be in the surgical field, especially in surgery of the lower cervical spine. With patients that have vocal cord paralysis, one must enter on the side of the paralysis.

Evolution and Evidence for Plates

The use of instrumentation after ACDF involving plates and screws is still controversial for one level ACDF but is generally recommended for multilevel ACDF. There are a variety of plates that are available for the cervical spine and some of the advantages these plates provide include increased segmental stiffness, prevention of graft displacement, and restoration of cervical lordosis. One prospective randomized controlled trial compared the clinical and radiographic outcomes of ACDF and ACDF with plating (ACDFP) in 50 patients.[60] Twenty-four patients were randomized to the ACDFP group and 24 patients to the ACDF group. At an average of 34-month follow-up, both groups had good improvement in pain and range of motion without a statistical difference between the groups. There was also no difference in the frequency of pseudoarthrosis/nonunion, however, there was better maintenance of graft height in the ACDFP group. Mobbs et al., however, found that plating reduced the number of poor clinical outcomes and led to a significantly higher rate of fusion. In this retrospective study comparing ACDF to ADCF plus plate, clinical and radiographic outcomes were reported on 212 patients with radiculopathy.[61] There was no significant difference in good to excellent outcomes between the two groups, however, the instrumented group had a statistically significant higher frequency of poor outcomes at 10% compared to 1.8% in the ACDFP group. Patients with poor outcomes required revision surgery for nonunion, kyphosis, graft extrusion, and graft collapse with foraminal stenosis.[61] Additional studies comparing ACDF to ACDFP showed improved fusion rates, improved sagittal alignment, and no significant increase in complications with the use of a cervical plate.[62-65] The use of a plate is especially compelling in the setting of multilevel fusion. Wang et al. reported the results of a retrospective study comparing ACDF and ACDFP in patients surgically treated at two levels.[63] The pseudoarthrosis rates were 0% for the ACDFP group and 25% for the ACDF group ($P = 0.003$). There was also significantly less graft collapse and less amount of kyphotic deformity in the ACDFP group. Thus, although there is insufficient evidence that the addition of a cervical plate results in significant improvement in clinical outcomes, plate stabilization is recommended for multilevel fusions and for a single-level disease where there may be increased instability, insufficient bone quality, or inappropriate graft placement. More recently, dynamic anterior plates that allow angular motion between the screws and plate have been proposed. This was theorized to promote cervical fusion by allowing controlled settling, thereby promoting load sharing across the construct, however, a recent study failed to confirm any clinical or radiographic advantage over traditional static plates.[66]

Evolution, Options, and Evidence of Grafting Options

Once the decision is made to proceed with ACDF, the surgeon must choose which graft to use. Graft incorporation into the adjacent bony vertebral bodies occurs through the process of hematoma formation, inflammation, vascularization, and creeping substitution.[67] The ideal bone graft is osteogenic (creates new bone), osteoinductive [stimulates progenitor cells to differentiate into osteoblasts, and osteoconductive (provides a scaffold for bone deposition)]. The only autograft possesses all of these features. Autograft can be accessed from the anterior iliac crest, fibula, or rib. The anterior iliac crest is the most common site from which autogenous bone graft is harvested. Tricorticocancellous graft from the iliac crest has a fusion rate of over 97%,[68-70] and this is the gold standard against which all other fusion material must be compared. Unfortunately, the harvesting of autogenous bone graft is associated with both short- and long-term morbidity. Schnee et al. reported the complications of harvesting autologous iliac bone graft for anterior cervical fusion in 144 procedures.[70] A second procedure was performed in four patients (2.8%). Superficial wound infection or dehiscence occurred in 5.6% of patients. Protracted wound symptoms of pain and poor cosmesis were reported in 2.8% and 3.5% of patients, respectively. The wound problems were found in a disproportionate number of women and obese patients. There is also increased operative time, hospital stay, and postoperative recovery with autograft harvest.

There are several options of synthetic bone graft material, which allows the surgeon to avoid these donor site morbidities and surgical disadvantages. None of these materials are, however, superior to autograft. Fresh frozen allogenic bone grafts, the most commonly used allograft today, are harvested from a human cadaver and preserved to remove some of its antigenicity. It is stored at –60°F to prevent enzymatic breakdown. Although this freeze-drying process reduces the antigen load, it also decreases the graft strength. Donor bone is screened by evaluating the donor's medical history and serology for human immunodeficiency virus (HIV), hepatitis B, and hepatitis C, making the disease transmission from allograft extremely low. Bishop et al. compared freeze-dried allograft to autograft in 132 patients who underwent ACDF.[68] Of the patients that underwent single-level fusion, X-rays performed at 1 year showed incomplete union in 6% of patients with autograft and 27% of patients with allograft ($P = 0.004$). Of the patients that underwent multilevel fusion, 13% had nonunion using autograft and 47% in cases using allograft. None of the patients in either group, however, had symptoms of pseudoarthrosis nor radiographic evidence of instability. Cigarette consumption had a significant adverse effect on successful fusion for both autograft and allograft groups, an effect that was most pronounced among smokers treated with allograft bone ($P = 0.004$).[68] Samartzis et al., however, reported comparable excellent outcomes in a retrospective study comparing allograft to autograft in multilevel ACDFP 80 patients: 94.3% of allograft patients and 100% of autograft patients achieved successful bone fusion, a difference that was not statistically significant.[69]

Another substitute for autograft used today for interbody fusion is the synthetic interbody spacer. These are either made from metal or polyetheretherketone (PEEK). The interest in the use of these synthetic spacers stemmed from the theoretical risk of allograft disease transmission and the potentially limited supply of allografts. Additionally, these spacers illicit minimal to no inflammatory response. PEEK is a semicrystalline polyaromatic polymer that is nonabsorbable and has a modulus of elasticity similar to bone.[71] The advantages to the PEEK cage over the metallic cage for interbody fusion include radiolucency allowing for bridging bone within the cage to be demonstrated on plain X-rays and MRI compatibility with minimal or no MRI image artifact. Synthetic cages have the potential for maintaining foraminal height and better sagittal alignment over the long term when compared to allograft or autograft, however, these same properties also cause increased stress shielding and thus decreased contact surface, leading to higher rates of pseudoarthrosis. This is especially a problem with the metallic cages, which was shown in a prospective randomized study by Vavruch et al.[72] The authors in this study randomized 52 patients to ACDF with a carbon fiber intervertebral fusion cage and 51 patients to ACDF with autograft. They found that except for reduced donor site pain in the synthetic spacer group, the clinical outcomes were the same for both groups. Use of the spacer resulted in more lordotic alignment and increased disk height, but this also resulted in a higher pseudoarthrosis rate. This, however, seems not be the case for PEEK cages, which have fusion rates reported to be over 95%.[73] PEEK, however, is not osteoinductive and must be used in conjunction with an osteoinductive agent. Cancellous autograft, cancellous allograft, or demineralized bone matrix can be used inside the cage. The PEEK spacer is an acceptable alternative to autograft and allograft for anterior one-level interbody fusion for cervical radiculopathy. The rate of successful fusion for multilevel surgery with this material is yet to be seen.

Recombinant human bone morphogenetic protein-2 (rhBMP-2) is a very osteoinductive material and its use in the lumbar spine has shown considerable promise. This has sparked significant interest in its use in other areas such as the cervical spine. Baskin and colleagues were the first to show that this material can be used safely with a perfect fusion rate in the cervical spine.[74] In this study, 33 patients with degenerative cervical disk disease were randomly assigned to either the investigational group, which received a fibular allograft with an rhBMP-2-laden collagen carrier inside the graft along with an anterior cervical plate, or the control group, which received a fibular allograft with cancellous iliac crest autograft placed inside it. All patients had solid fusion at 6, 12, and 24 months after surgery. There were no device-related adverse events and at 24 months, the investigational group had significantly better improvement in neck and arm pain than the control group. But rhBMP-2 does not guarantee fusion in all situations as was shown in a consecutive case series published by Shen and colleagues.[75] In this study, 127 patients underwent three- to five-level anterior cervical fusion with rhBMP-2, structural allograft, and plate fixation with a minimum of 2-year follow-up. The pseudoarthrosis rate was 10.2% at 6 months and the authors concluded that a long fusion lever arm may biomechanically overwhelm the biologic advantage of rhBMP-2. Additionally, there may be ectopic bone formation[76] and two studies have reported high complication rates with the use of rhBMP-2.[77,78] Shields et al. reported a complication rate of 23.2%, including hematoma requiring surgical evacuation, swallowing, and breathing difficulty requiring readmission, and dramatic swelling without hematoma.[77] Smucker et al. performed a retrospective review of 234 patients who underwent anterior spinal fusion, 69 of whom had rhBMP-2 used for fusion. About 27.5% of those patients in the rhBMP-2 group had a clinically significant swelling event versus only 3.6% of patients in the non-rhBMP-2 group ($P < 0.0001$).[78] This difference remained statistically significant even after controlling for other significant predictors of swelling. In 2008, the US Food and Drug Administration (FDA) gave a formal warning on the use of rhBMP-2 in anterior cervical spine surgery. Thus, the surgeon should be very cautious with the use of rhBMP-2 in the cervical spine and a detailed discussion regarding the risks and benefits of its use should be held with the patient preoperatively.

Outcomes

Single versus multilevel pseudoarthrosis: Most patients with radiculopathy suffer from one level, and sometimes two-level disease. The incidence of multilevel disease-causing polyradiculopathy without myelopathy is rare but can occur. The goal of anterior surgery for multiple levels is decompression of the neurologic elements, restoration of spinal alignment, and achievement of fusion. Of these, fusion is usually the most difficult part. Pseudoarthrosis, or the failure of bony fusion, can occur in up to 44% of patients with multilevel anterior cervical arthrodesis.[79] Pseudoarthrosis can cause significant postoperative pain, sometimes requiring revision surgery. And although not all pseudoarthroses are symptomatic, superior clinical results are achieved with a solid fusion.[80] Historically, anterior cervical corpectomy and fusion (ACCF) has been advocated for patients with two-level disease, however, data suggests that there are worse outcomes with ACCF when compared to ACDF. Uribe et al. reported the results of a retrospective comparative study of 80 consecutive patients who either underwent ACCF or ACDF with clinical and radiographic follow-up at 6 and 12 weeks, 6 months, 1 year, and 2 years (if necessary).[81] Titanium mesh cages filled with autograft and anterior cervical plates were used in both procedures. The fusion rates were high for both procedures, 97.6% in the ACDF group and 92.1% in the ACCF group, a difference that was not statistically significant. Patients in both groups also had an equivalent improvement in their clinical symptoms at a minimum of 1-year follow-up. However, there was a higher rate of hardware failure in the ACCF group, 2.6% versus 0% in the ACDF group. Thus, with a higher rate of early hardware failure in ACCF compared to ACDF, it is generally recommended that multilevel ACDF be performed instead of ACCF for multilevel degenerative disk disease causing symptoms of polyradiculopathy or myelopathy. ACCF is still appropriate in other instances where there is specific pathology requiring removal of the vertebral body.

Unfortunately, as the number of operative levels increases, the fusion rates for ACDF decrease. Bohlman et al. reported clinical and radiographic results in their retrospective study of 122 patients who underwent the Robinson technique of ACDF with autogenous iliac crest bone graft in one-to-four levels.[80] A one-level procedure was performed in 62 patients, a two-level procedure in 48, a three-level procedure in 11, and a four-level procedure in 1. The average follow-up was 6 years. Pseudoarthrosis was found at 24 of 195 segments, and the risk of pseudoarthrosis was significantly greater after a multiple-level arthrodesis. At most recent follow-up, 96.3% of patients who had a motor deficit had a complete recovery, while the rest had a partial recovery, and 92.2% of patients who had sensory loss regained sensation. No patients had increased neurologic deficits after surgery. In another retrospective study where the authors compared multiple interbody grafting to long segment strut grafting following multilevel anterior cervical decompression, they found that only 48 of 69 patients who underwent multiple interbody grafting achieved solid fusion.[82] That gives a pseudoarthrosis rate of 30.4%, and the authors reported that patients with pseudoarthrosis whether in the strut grafting group or in the multiple interbody grafting group had significantly poorer outcomes. Additionally, 81.1% of patients who underwent multiple interbody grafting had "good" or "excellent" clinical outcomes, a success rate that is significantly lower than that reported for single-level anterior arthrodesis. In this study, the surgeon did not use a plate for neither the strut grafting group nor the multiple interbody grafting group. In another study that retrospectively looked at only three-level ACDF without plating in 16 patients found unacceptably high pseudoarthrosis rates.[79] With an average of 37-month follow-up, only 9 of the 16 patients (56%) achieved solid fusion at all three levels. Of the seven patients with pseudoarthrosis, two had severe pain and required revision, two had moderate pain, and three had no pain. Of the nine patients with solid fusion, three had mild pain, and six had no pain, a spastically significant difference in clinical outcome between the fusion and pseudoarthrosis groups. The authors concluded that the fusion rate in three-level ACDF without plating is unacceptably low and recommended that these patients undergo additional or alternative measures to achieve arthrodesis more consistently.

The addition of an anterior cervical plate (ACDFP), however, has increased the fusion rates for multilevel anterior cervical arthrodesis. Samartzis et al. reported excellent radiographic outcomes in a retrospective study comparing allograft to autograft in 80 patients who underwent ACDFP.[69] Radiographic fusion was assessed in all patients with a mean follow-up of 16 months and the authors found that 94.3% of allograft patients and 100% of autograft patients achieved successful bony fusion, a difference that was not statistically significant. Clinical outcome at 20 months was "excellent" or "good" in 88.8% of patients and the rest had a "fair" clinical outcome. Wang and associated published two retrospective reviews on multilevel ACDF and the effect on fusion with addition of an anterior cervical plate.[62,63] For two-level ACDF without a plate, the pseudoarthrosis rate was 25% and dropped to 0% with the addition of a plate.[63] For three-level ACDF without a plate, the pseudoarthrosis rate was 37% and dropped to 18% with the addition of a plate.[62] The results of these studies show that even though there is a higher chance of pseudoarthrosis and lower success rates with multilevel ACDF compared to single-level ACDF, it is still a relatively safe procedure that can relieve pain and lead to resolution of neurologic deficits in a high percentage of patients, especially with the addition of an anterior cervical plate. When symptomatic pseudoarthrosis occurs with anterior cervical fusion, a posterior cervical fusion is more effective than anterior repair with better fusion rates and clinical outcomes.[83]

Foraminotomy

Indications

Posterior cervical laminoforaminotomy was first described by Frykholm and then popularized by Spurling and Scoville in the 1940s.[84,85] This technique is indicated for relief of cervical radiculopathy secondary to nerve root compression from disk herniation or osteophyte encroachment. PLF has little effect if there is spinal cord compression or spinal canal stenosis and is indicated only when there are focal radicular symptoms. PLF avoids the well-recognized risks associated with an anterior approach including recurrent laryngeal nerve injury and dysphagia. This procedure also maintains spinal alignment and spares the motion segment, avoiding the risk of adjacent level disease.

Technique

Posterior cervical laminoforaminotomy was traditionally done in the sitting position to minimize epidural bleeding, however, with the advent of new thrombotic agents, it can be done safely with the patient prone and the head of the bed kept elevated at 30°. The neck is kept in a slightly flexed position after the patient is put prone in cranial three-point fixation with the Mayfield head holder. The medial portion of the cervical facet can be approached by either the midline or a paramedian muscle-splitting approach. In an open PLF, the simpler midline approach is more common, while the paramedical muscle splitting approach is utilized in a minimally invasive approach. Lateral fluoroscopy is used to locate the surgical level. The skin is marked, prepped, and draped in the usual sterile fashion and the dermal layer is infiltrated with lidocaine and epinephrine.

In the open technique,[86,87] a midline skin incision is made 4-5 cm centered over the interspace to be operated on. The incision is deepened through the ligamentum nuchae until a spinous process is exposed and a lateral X-ray is again obtained to confirm the level with a metal clamp on the exposed spinous process. Then, the posterior cervical musculature of the affected side is detached from the lateral spinous processes, lamina and facet joints above and below the pathologic disk space with a Cobb periosteal elevator and unipolar cautery. Once the dorsal surface of the facet joint is exposed, a hemilaminectomy retractor is placed between the spinous process and the muscle, exposing the facet joint and both laminae.

With the aid of a microscope or loop magnification, the foraminotomy is then performed using a high-speed drill with a 4-6 mm cutting burr. First, the superficial cortical bone is drilled off to define the perimeter of bony removal, which is the lateral third of superior and inferior hemilaminae and medial third to half of the descending facet. The decompression is carried out deeper to remove the cancellous bone, exposing the inner cortical bone of the laminae and facet. This thin osseous layer and underlying ligamentum flavum are then removed with an angled curette and Kerrison Rongeur initially over the laminae to expose the thecal sac. Then the exposure is followed laterally over the exiting nerve root, where a plexus of

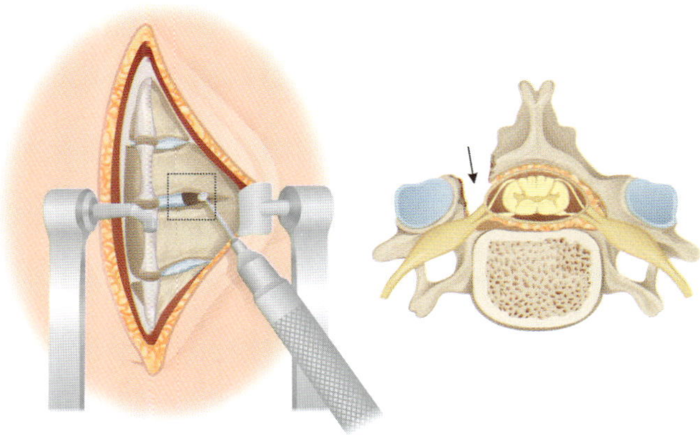

Fig. 5: The left diagram shows the hemilaminectomy retractor in place to expose the lamina facet junction, which is drilled using a 4–6 mm cutting burr to expose the underlying ligament flavum. The diagram on the right shows the angle of exposure and extent of bony removal including the small laminotomy medially and lateral decompression of the nerve root up to where the cervical pedicle can be felt with a small nerve hook.

epidural veins usually covers the nerve root. These can be coagulated using bipolar cautery and controlled further with the use of thrombin-soaked gelfoam. The lateral extent of the surgical decompression is complete when the cervical pedicle can be palpated using a small nerve hook.

After the nerve root has been exposed, the surgeon should discern whether the dorsal sensory and ventral motor roots are combined in a single dural sleeve, or if there is a smaller motor portion inferiorly and anteriorly. The root is gently teased away from the underlying disk or spur using a small Penfield dissector and nerve hook. Free disk fragments may be removed with a small pituitary rongeur and anterior osteophytes above or below the root can be carefully drilled. This latter maneuver should be performed only when there is marked root deformation or compression after the foramen is unroofed. Once the root is freed and dissection deemed complete, hemostasis is obtained with the use of thrombin-soaked gelfoam and/or Floseal Hemostatic Matrix (Baxter Health Care Corporation). The wound is then irrigated and the fascia, subdermal layer, and skin are closed in layers (Fig. 5).

Open and Minimally Invasive Options

Outcomes: The success rate for PLF ranges from 75% to 98%.[44] Herkowitz et al. compared PLF to ACDF in a prospective study.[88] Of 33 patients who had cervical radiculopathy secondary to single level anterolateral disk herniations, 17 patients underwent ACDF while 16 patients underwent PLF. About 94% of patients in the ACDF group and 75% of patients in the PLF group reported good or excellent outcomes, a difference that was not statistically significant. The authors concluded that both surgical procedures were effective in improving pain and weakness. In a retrospective comparative study, Korinth et al. compared ventral microdiskectomy and polymethyl methacrylate interbody stabilization in 124 to PLF in 168 patients.[43] The authors found the success rate to be higher for the anterior diskectomy and interbody stabilization group (93.6%) than the PLF group (85.8%). Although patients who underwent PLF had less hoarseness and dysphagia and operative time was significantly shorter, the reoperation rate was 7.1% compared to 2.4% for the ACDF group.

In order to minimize incision, periosteal muscle dissection, postoperative neck pain, and postoperative recovery, minimally invasive procedures have been developed for posterior foraminotomy. With the minimally invasive technique, a small stab skin incision is made approximately 5 mm off the midline ipsilateral and at the target level. Then a K-wire is slowly advanced through the musculature and docked on the bone at the inferomedial edge of the rostral lateral mass at the target level under fluoroscopic guidance. The incision is lengthened above and below the K-wire entry point to a total of 2 cm and the fascia is incised to the equivalent length. The tubular muscle dilators are then placed serially. After this is complete, a final working tubular retractor is placed over the dilators and fixed over the laminofacet junction with a table-mounted retractor arm. The level is again confirmed using fluoroscopy. Under the surgical microscope, a partial hemilaminectomy, foraminotomy, and partial facetectomy of the target level are performed using the high-speed drill as described above.

Richard Fessler first described this technique of microendoscopic foraminotomy (MEF) and their initial clinical experience with this procedure in 2002.[89] They found that MEF had comparable success rates to the open procedure. MEF resulted in symptomatic improvement in 87% of patients with neck pain and 92% of patients with radiculopathy. The authors found that with the minimally invasive procedure, there was less blood loss, patients recovered more rapidly, had a shorter postoperative stay, and used less narcotics. Multiple other studies have reported similar success rates and benefits to the minimally invasive technique since then.[90-92]

Disk Arthroplasty

Indications

The indications for TDA are similar to that of ACDF. These include cervical radiculopathy refractory to conservative management, objective evidence of motor weakness, progressive neurologic deficit, cervical myelopathy, or myeloradiculopathy with ventral compression. In addition, TDA has the benefit of preserving motion at the treated level and theoretically reducing the risk of adjacent level disease. Hillibrand et al. (1999) reported the results of 374 patients who underwent anterior cervical arthrodesis for the treatment of cervical spondylosis with radiculopathy, myelopathy, or both and found that there was an incidence of symptomatic adjacent segment disease, of 2.9% per year. The authors predicted that symptomatic adjacent-segment disease may affect more than one-fourth of all patients undergoing anterior cervical arthrodesis within 10 years of surgery, leading to a significant number of reoperations. Thus, preserving the motion segment with arthroplasty could potentially lead to fewer reoperations for adjacent segment disease. In cases of advanced degeneration where there is a significant loss of disk height, significant osteophyte formation, or facet arthrodesis, or ankylosis, ACDF may be preferable to TDA. Posterior column instability, retrovertebral stenosis, diffuse skeletal hyperostosis, ossification of the PLL, infection, osteoporosis, and axial neck pain without radiculopathy or myelopathy are also relative contraindications for TDA. These patients would theoretically benefit more from anterior arthrodesis or posterior decompression with or without fusion than arthroplasty.

Technique

The fundamental surgical technique for TDA is largely based on the traditional techniques used for ACDF. Access to the anterior cervical spine is gained via the Smith-Robinson technique as described above in the ACDF section. After the disk space is properly identified by intraoperative fluoroscopy and the longus colli muscle are elevated bilaterally, craniocaudal distracting Caspar-type pins are placed. Compared to an ACDF, a wider decompression of the disk space is performed with generous bilateral foraminotomies including the resection of the uncovertebral joints bilaterally. This is one of the key differences between TDA and ACDF. Unlike ACDF, the motion will continue with TDA, so complete direct foraminal decompression is crucial to relieve radicular symptoms. The PLL is usually removed for adequate positioning of the prosthesis since contractures of this ligament can limit the distraction of the vertebral endplates. Another major difference between TDA and ACDF is when carrying out a TDA, the endplates should be preserved to avoid heterotopic ossification, which may later cause the prosthesis to lose function. A combination of curettes and Kerrison rongeurs are used for decompression, while a burr should be avoided to preserve vertebral endplates as much as possible. After the endplates are prepared and a wide decompression is performed, an implant of proper height and width is obtained using trial spacers. The widest width able to be safely implanted and the shortest height that is stable in the disk space should be used to reduce the risk of subsidence and allow for maximal motion at the operative segment, respectively. The TDA implant should be placed strictly in the center and more posteriorly to allow for normal kinematics (Fig. 6). Anteroposterior and lateral X-rays are obtained afterward to ensure that this step is performed correctly.

Outcomes

Implant options: Since 2007, three TDA devices have been approved by the FDA to treat cervical disk disease. The Prestige cervical disk replacement (Medtronic Sofamor Danek Inc., Memphis, TN) is a two-piece metal device that is attached to adjacent vertebral bodies with bone screws. The superior and inferior metal parts move with respect to one another by a ball and trough mechanism.[93] The Bryan Cervical Disc System (Medtronic Sofamor Danek, Inc., Memphis, TN) is a one-piece, biarticulating implant with two titanium pieces separated by a polyurethane part.[94] The ProDisc-C Total Disc Replacement (Synthes Spine, Inc., West Chester, Pennsylvania) consists of two cobalt-chrome alloy endplates that are anchored to the top and bottom surfaces of the adjacent vertebral bodies and a plastic ultra-high molecular weight polyethylene inlay that fits between the two endplates.[95] The superior endplate can slide over the domed part of the plastic inlay allowing movement at the level where it is implanted.

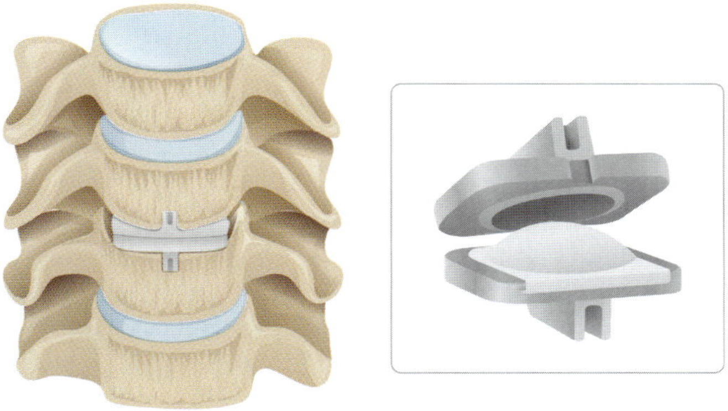

Fig. 6: The total disk arthroplasty implant is placed strictly in the center and posteriorly as possible to preserve normal kinematics. The endplates are preserved to avoid heterotopic ossification. The implant illustrated here is the ProDisc-C Total Disc Replacement. *Source*: Synthes Spine Inc., West Chester, Pennsylvania.

Clinical and radiographic outcomes: Each of the above approved FDA devices for TDA has been compared to traditional ACDF techniques in randomized controlled trials with at least equivalent and in some cases improved statistical outcomes at 2 years.[50,51,53] More recently, 4-year outcomes were reported on the Bryan Cervical Disc System (Medtronic Sofamor Danek, Inc.), which showed an overall success rate of 85.1% at 4 years with a mean range of motion of 8.08° and 8.48° at 24 and 48 months, respectively.[52]

Whether TDA truly reduced the risk of symptomatic adjacent segment disease still remains in question. Jawahar et al. conducted a prospective, randomized controlled trial to compare TDA to ACDF in 93 patients with symptomatic one- or two-level cervical disk disease who failed to respond to conservative therapy.[96] Fifty-nine patients were randomized to the TDA arm and 34 to the ACDF arm. Clinical and radiographic follow-up was performed at 6 weeks and at 3, 6, 12, 24, 36, and 48 months after surgery. About 16% of TDA patients and 18% of ACDF patients developed adjacent segment degeneration, which was not statistically different. Interestingly, the authors found that concurrent lumbar degenerative disk disease significantly increased the risk of adjacent segment degeneration. Thus, ACDF and TDA were found to be equivalent in both relief of symptoms and risk of adjacent segment disease.

A recent systemic review and meta-analysis of nine randomized controlled trials comparing TDA to ACDF (1,778 participants) found that TDA is associated with a statistically significant improvement in functionality as

CHAPTER 25

measured by the neck disability index, neck and arm pain as measured by the visual analog scale, and quality of life as measured by the SF-36 physical component score.[97] There was no statistically significant difference between the two groups with respect to surgery for the adjacent level disease, reoperation, dysphagia, or dysphonia. The authors concluded that the TDA is an option for single-level cervical spondylosis, but without any strong evidence of reduced symptomatic adjacent segment disease compared to ACDF, the use of TDA increases healthcare costs, is a technically more difficult operation, and has a potential for greater harm if performed by a nonexpert surgeon.

Multilevel cervical arthroplasty has also been shown to be a safe and effective alternative to fusion for the management of cervical radiculopathy and myelopathy,[98] however, there is currently no strong evidence to support the routine use of TDA over ACDF for either single or multilevel cervical spondylosis.

COMPLICATIONS

Knowledge of the complications associated with the above surgeries allows for their recognition in the perioperative setting and proper management. A retrospective review of 1,015 patients undergoing the first-time ACDF for cervical radiculopathy and/or myelopathy due to degenerative disk disease using the standard Smith-Robinson approach resulted in overall morbidity of 19.3%.[99] The most common complication was the development of postoperative dysphagia, which was observed in 9.5%. Postoperative hematoma occurred in 5.6%, but required surgical intervention in only 2.4%. Symptomatic recurrent laryngeal nerve injury occurred in 3.1%. Other rare complications that occurred at a rate of 0.5% or less included dural tear, esophageal perforation, worsening of pre-existing myelopathy, Horner's syndrome, instrumentation back out, and superficial wound infection.

Dysphagia is by far the most common postoperative complication and is reported to have high as 50% at 1 month postoperatively, but decreases significantly by 6 months to 12.5%.[100] In another prospective study of 384 patients undergoing anterior cervical spine surgery, at 2 years postoperatively, the prevalence of dysphagia was found to be significantly higher in women (18.3%) than men (9.9%), in revision surgery patients (27.7%) than primary surgery (11.3%) patients, and in patients who underwent more than two-level surgery (19.3%) than patients who had two or less levels (9.7%) operated on.[101] Vertebral artery injury is a rare complication of anterior cervical surgery and maybe caused during decompression or screw tapping.[102] Injury to the vertebral artery can be avoided by preoperative identification of anomalous arteries and meticulous intraoperative attention to the midline. As mentioned above, there is a risk of failure of fusion with ACDF, or pseudoarthrosis, with a higher risk with each additional segment fused. The pseudoarthrosis rate is as high as 44% in multilevel ACDF. The incidence of symptomatic adjacent segment disease is reported to be anywhere from 0.8% to 2.9% per year with ACDF,[47,49] however, this may be a result of the natural history of cervical spondylosis rather than the fusion procedure.

The complications associated with TDA are similar to that of ACDF and the theoretical risk deduction of clinically significant adjacent level disease with TDA has not been proven. The key complication difference with arthroplasty is the formation of heterotopic bone formation. While in ACDF, the goal is bony fusion, the goal in TDA is the preservation of the motion segment. If the end plates are not adequately preserved, heterotopic ossification can occur and cause the prosthesis to lose function. The prevalence of this in cervical arthroplasty is 44.6% at 12 months and 58.2% at 24 months, although this is reported to be unrelated to the clinical improvement.[103]

The main complications of posterior cervical foraminotomy are that patients often complain of radiculopathy that lasts for up to 6 weeks postoperatively. And although the idea of this procedure is to avoid a fusion, if more than 50% of the facet joint has been compromised, it may become unstable and warrant a second surgery for fusion. A reoperation rate as high as 27% has been reported.[104] The intraoperative complication rate, including excessive bleeding, is 2.2%. Air embolus can occur with the sitting position. Although rare, vertebral artery injury can occur if the dissection is carried out too far laterally.[105] Cerebrospinal fluid leakage, postoperative wound infection and dehiscence, and persistence of cervical radiculopathy symptoms may occur in cervical foraminotomy as with anterior cervical decompression.

PROGNOSIS

In summary, cervical radiculopathy has an unclear natural history. Although there are physiotherapy-based studies that show up to 92% of patients benefit favorably to conservative therapy,[27-30] there are also long-term investigations that show up to a third of patients can have persistent pain over a decade from their diagnosis.[106] There are surgical options, however, when medical therapy fails and these procedures all have relatively high success rates especially for the single-level disease. Both anterior and posterior cervical decompression procedures have reported to have good or excellent outcomes in greater than 90% of patients. Additionally, there is good evidence that surgery gives greater relief of neck and/or arm pain, weakness, and sensory loss at 3–4 months when compared to conservative therapy.[107]

REFERENCES

1. Carette S, Fehlings MG. Clinical practice. Cervical radiculopathy. N Engl J Med. 2005;353(4):392-9.
2. Caridi JM, Pumberger M, Hughes AP. Cervical radiculopathy: a review. HSS J. 2011;7(3):265-72.
3. Ahlgren BD, Garfin SR. Cervical radiculopathy. Orthop Clin North Am. 1996;27:253-63.
4. Dillin W, Booth R, Cuckler J, et al. Cervical radiculopathy. Spine. 1986;11:988-91.
5. Radhakrishnan K, Litchy WJ, O'Fallon WM, et al. Epidemiology of cervical radiculopathy. A population-based study from Rochester, Minnesota, 1976 through 1990. Brain. 1994;117(Pt 2):325-35.
6. Salemi G, Savettieri G, Meneghini F, et al. Prevalence of cervical spondylotic radiculopathy: a door-to-door survey in a Sicilian municipality. Acta Neurol Scand. 1996;93(2-3):184-8.
7. Lees F, Turner JW. Natural history and prognosis of cervical spondylosis. Br Med J. 1963;2(5373):1607-10.
8. Saal JS, Saal JA, Yurth EF. Nonoperative management of herniated cervical intervertebral disc with radiculopathy. Spine. 1996;21(16):1877-83.
9. Henderson CM, Hennessy RG, Shuey HM Jr, et al. Posterior-lateral foraminotomy as an exclusive operative technique for cervical radiculopathy: a review of 846 consecutively operated cases. Neurosurgery. 1983;13(5):504-12.
10. Tanaka Y, Kokubun S, Sato T, et al. Cervical roots as origin of pain in the neck or scapular regions. Spine. 2006;31(17): E568-73.
11. Slipman CW, Plastaras CT, Palmitier RA, et al. Symptom provocation of fluoroscopically guided cervical nerve root stimulation. Are dynatomal maps identical to dermatomal maps? Spine. 1998;23(20):2235-42.
12. Bono CM, Ghiselli G, Gilbert TJ, et al. An evidence-based clinical guideline for the diagnosis and treatment of cervical radiculopathy from degenerative disorders. Spine J. 2011;11(1):64-72.
13. Russell SM. Examination of Peripheral Nerve Injuries: An Anatomical Approach. Thieme: New York; 2006.
14. Wainner RS, Fritz JM, Irrgang JJ, et al. Reliability and diagnostic accuracy of the clinical examination and patient self-report measures for cervical radiculopathy. Spine. 2003;28(1):52-62.
15. McGillicuddy JE. Cervical radiculopathy, entrapment neuropathy, and thoracic outlet syndrome: how to differentiate? Invited submission from the Joint Section Meeting on Disorders of the Spine and Peripheral Nerves, March 2004. J Neurosurg Spine. 2004;1(2):179-87.
16. Houser OW, Onofrio BM, Miller GM, et al. Cervical disk prolapse. Mayo Clin Proc. 1995;70(10):939-45.
17. Karnaze MG, Gado MH, Sartor KJ, et al. Comparison of MR and CT myelography in imaging the cervical and thoracic spine. Am J Roentgenol. 1988;150(2):397-403.
18. Houser OW, Onofrio BM, Miller GM, et al. Cervical neural foraminal canal stenosis: computerized tomographic myelography diagnosis. J Neurosurg. 1993;79(1):84-8.
19. Teresi LM, Lufkin RB, Reicher MA, et al. Asymptomatic degenerative disk disease and spondylosis of the cervical spine: MR imaging. Radiology. 1987;164(1):83-8.
20. Larsson EM, Holtås S, Cronqvist S, et al. Comparison of myelography, CT myelography and magnetic resonance imaging in cervical spondylosis and disk herniation. Pre- and postoperative findings. Acta Radiol. 1989;30(3):233-9.
21. Modic MT, Masaryk TJ, Mulopulos GP, et al. Cervical radiculopathy: prospective evaluation with surface coil MR imaging, CT with metrizamide, and metrizamide myelography. Radiology. 1986;161(3):753-9.
22. Song KJ, Choi BW, Kim GH, et al. Clinical usefulness of CT-myelogram comparing with the MRI in degenerative cervical spinal disorders: is CTM still useful for primary diagnostic tool? J Spinal Disord Tech. 2009;22(5):353-7.
23. Bartlett RJ, Hill CR, Gardiner E. A comparison of T2 and gadolinium enhanced MRI with CT myelography in cervical radiculopathy. Br J Radiol. 1998;71(841):11-9.
24. Levin KH. Approach to the patient with suspected radiculopathy. Neurol Clin. 2012;30(2):581-604.
25. American Association of Electrodiagnostic Medicine, So YT. Guidelines in electrodiagnostic medicine. Practice parameter for needle electromyographic evaluation of patients with suspected cervical radiculopathy. Muscle Nerve Suppl. 1999;8:S209-21.
26. Gore DR, Sepic SB, Gardner GM, et al. Neck pain: a long-term follow-up of 205 patients. Spine. 1987;12(1):1-5.
27. Rubin D. Cervical radiculitis: diagnosis and treatment. Arch Phys Med Rehabil. 1960;41:580-6.
28. Pain in the neck and arm: a multicentre trial of the effects of physiotherapy, arranged by the British Association of Physical Medicine. Br Med J. 1966;1(5482):253-8.
29. Martin GM, Corbin KB. An evaluation of conservative treatment for patients with cervical disk syndrome. Arch Phys Med Rehabil. 1954;35(2):87-92.
30. McCormack BM, Weinstein PR. Cervical spondylosis. An update. West J Med. 1996;165(1-2):43-51.

31. Casey E. Natural history of radiculopathy. Phys Med Rehabil Clin N Am. 2011;22(1):1-5.
32. Jette DU, Jette AM. Physical therapy and health outcomes in patients with spinal impairments. Phys Ther. 1996; 76(9):930-41; discussion 942-5. Erratum in: Phys Ther. 1997;77(1):113.
33. Dreyer SJ, Boden SD. Nonoperative treatment of neck and arm pain. Spine. 1998;23(24):2746-54.
34. Cyteval C, Thomas E, Decoux E, et al. Cervical radiculopathy: open study on percutaneous periradicular foraminal steroid infiltration performed under CT control in 30 patients. Am J Neuroradiol. 2004;25(3):441-5.
35. Kolstad F, Leivseth G, Nygaard OP. Transforaminal steroid injections in the treatment of cervical radiculopathy. A prospective outcome study. Acta Neurochir. 2005;147(10):1065-70.
36. Lin EL, Lieu V, Halevi L, et al. Cervical epidural steroid injections for symptomatic disc herniations. J Spinal Disord Tech. 2006;19(3):183-6.
37. Anderberg L, Annertz M, Persson L, et al. Transforaminal steroid injections for the treatment of cervical radiculopathy: a prospective and randomised study. Eur Spine J. 2007;16(3):321-8.
38. Anderberg L, Annertz M, Rydholm U, et al. Selective diagnostic nerve root block for the evaluation of radicular pain in the multilevel degenerated cervical spine. Eur Spine J. 2006;15(6):794-801.
39. Persson LC, Moritz U, Brandt L, et al. Cervical radiculopathy: pain, muscle weakness and sensory loss in patients with cervical radiculopathy treated with surgery, physiotherapy or cervical collar. A prospective, controlled study. Eur Spine J. 1997;6(4):256-66.
40. Sampath P, Bendebba M, Davis JD, et al. Outcome in patients with cervical radiculopathy. Prospective, multicenter study with independent clinical review. Spine. 1999;24(6):591-7.
41. Hauerberg J, Kosteljanetz M, Bøge-Rasmussen T, et al. Anterior cervical discectomy with or without fusion with ray titanium cage: a prospective randomized clinical study. Spine. 2008;33(5):458-64.
42. Xie JC, Hurlbert RJ. Discectomy versus discectomy with fusion versus discectomy with fusion and instrumentation: a prospective randomized study. Neurosurgery. 2007;61(1):107-16.
43. Korinth MC, Krüger A, Oertel MF, et al. Posterior foraminotomy or anterior discectomy with polymethyl methacrylate interbody stabilization for cervical soft disc disease: results in 292 patients with monoradiculopathy. Spine. 2006;31(11):1207-14.
44. Heary RF, Ryken TC, Matz PG, et al. Cervical laminoforaminotomy for the treatment of cervical degenerative radiculopathy. J Neurosurg Spine. 2009;11(2):198-202.
45. Tumialán LM, Ponton RP, Gluf WM. Management of unilateral cervical radiculopathy in the military: the cost effectiveness of posterior cervical foraminotomy compared with anterior cervical discectomy and fusion. Neurosurg Focus. 2010;28(5):E17.
46. Baaj AA, Uribe JS, Vale FL, et al. History of cervical disc arthroplasty. Neurosurg Focus. 2009;27(3):E10.
47. Hilibrand AS, Carlson GD, Palumbo MA, et al. Radiculopathy and myelopathy at segments adjacent to the site of a previous anterior cervical arthrodesis. J Bone Joint Surg Am. 1999;81(4):519-28.
48. Song KJ, Choi BW, Jeon TS, et al. Adjacent segment degenerative disease: is it due to disease progression or a fusion-associated phenomenon? Comparison between segments adjacent to the fused and non-fused segments. Eur Spine J. 2011;20(11):1940-5.
49. Wu JC, Liu L, Huang WC, et al. The incidence of adjacent segment disease requiring surgery after anterior cervical discectomy and fusion: estimation using an eleven-year comprehensive nationwide database in Taiwan. Neurosurgery. 2012;70(3):594-601.
50. Mummaneni PV, Burkus JK, Haid RW, et al. Clinical and radiographic analysis of cervical disc arthroplasty compared with allograft fusion: a randomized controlled clinical trial. J Neurosurg Spine. 2007;6(3):198-209.
51. Heller JG, Sasso RC, Papadopoulos SM, et al. Comparison of BRYAN cervical disc arthroplasty with anterior cervical decompression and fusion: clinical and radiographic results of a randomized, controlled, clinical trial. Spine. 2009;34(2):101-7.
52. Sasso RC, Anderson PA, Riew KD, et al. Results of cervical arthroplasty compared with anterior discectomy and fusion: four-year clinical outcomes in a prospective, randomized controlled trial. J Bone Joint Surg Am. 2011;93(18):1684-92.
53. Garrido BJ, Taha TA, Sasso RC. Clinical outcomes of Bryan cervical disc arthroplasty a prospective, randomized, controlled, single site trial with 48-month follow-up. J Spinal Disord Tech. 2010;23(6):367-71.
54. Murrey D, Janssen M, Delamarter R, et al. Results of the prospective, randomized, controlled multicenter Food and Drug Administration investigational device exemption study of the ProDisc-C total disc replacement versus anterior discectomy and fusion for the treatment of 1-level symptomatic cervical disc disease. Spine J. 2009;9(4):275-86.
55. Denaro V, Di Martino A. Cervical spine surgery: an historical perspective. Clin Orthop Relat Res. 2011;469(3):639-48.
56. Robinson R, Smith G. Anterior lateral disc removal and interbody fusion for cervical disc syndrome. Bull Johns Hopkins Hosp. 1955;69:223-4.
57. Smith GW, Robinson RA. The treatment of certain cervical-spine disorders by anterior removal of the intervertebral disc and interbody fusion. J Bone Joint Surg Am. 1958;40-A(3):607-24.
58. Cloward RB. The anterior approach for removal of ruptured cervical disks. J Neurosurg. 1958;15(6):602-17.
59. Bailey RW, Badgley CE. Stabilization of the cervical spine by anterior fusion. J Bone Joint Surg Am. 1960;42-A:565-94.
60. Grob D, Peyer JV, Dvorak J. The use of plate fixation in anterior surgery of the degenerative cervical spine: a comparative prospective clinical study. Eur Spine J. 2001;10(5):408-13.

61. Mobbs RJ, Rao P, Chandran NK. Anterior cervical discectomy and fusion: analysis of surgical outcome with and without plating. J Clin Neurosci. 2007;14(7):639-42.
62. Wang JC, McDonough PW, Kanim LE, et al. Increased fusion rates with cervical plating for three-level anterior cervical discectomy and fusion. Spine. 2001;26(6):643-6.
63. Wang JC, McDonough PW, Endow KK, et al. Increased fusion rates with cervical plating for two-level anterior cervical discectomy and fusion. Spine. 2000;25(1):41-5.
64. Wang JC, McDonough PW, Endow K, et al. The effect of cervical plating on single-level anterior cervical discectomy and fusion. J Spinal Disord. 1999;12(6):467-71.
65. Kaiser MG, Haid RW Jr, Subach BR, et al. Anterior cervical plating enhances arthrodesis after discectomy and fusion with cortical allograft. Neurosurgery. 2002;50(2):229-36.
66. DuBois CM, Bolt PM, Todd AG, et al. Static versus dynamic plating for multilevel anterior cervical discectomy and fusion. Spine J. 2007;7(2):188-93.
67. Chau AM, Mobbs RJ. Bone graft substitutes in anterior cervical discectomy and fusion. Eur Spine J. 2009;18(4):449-64.
68. Bishop RC, Moore KA, Hadley MN. Anterior cervical interbody fusion using autogeneic and allogeneic bone graft substrate: a prospective comparative analysis. J Neurosurg. 1996;85(2):206-10.
69. Samartzis D, Shen FH, Matthews DK, et al. Comparison of allograft to autograft in multilevel anterior cervical discectomy and fusion with rigid plate fixation. Spine J. 2003;3(6):451-9.
70. Schnee CL, Freese A, Weil RJ, et al. Analysis of harvest morbidity and radiographic outcome using autograft for anterior cervical fusion. Spine. 1997;22(19):2222-7.
71. Hee HT, Kundnani V. Rationale for use of polyetheretherketone polymer interbody cage device in cervical spine surgery. Spine J. 2010;10(1):66-9.
72. Vavruch L, Hedlund R, Javid D, et al. A prospective randomized comparison between the cloward procedure and a carbon fiber cage in the cervical spine: a clinical and radiologic study. Spine. 2002;27(16):1694-701.
73. Song KJ, Choi BW, Kim GH, et al. Usefulness of polyetheretherketone (PEEK) cage with plate augmentation for anterior arthrodesis in traumatic cervical spine injury. Spine J. 2010;10(1):50-7.
74. Baskin DS, Ryan P, Sonntag V. A prospective, randomized, controlled cervical fusion study using recombinant human bone morphogenetic protein-2 with the CORNERSTONE-SR allograft ring and the ATLANTIS anterior cervical plate. Spine. 2003;28(12):1219-24.
75. Shen HX, Buchowski JM, Yeom JS, et al. Pseudarthrosis in multilevel anterior cervical fusion with rhBMP-2 and allograft: analysis of one hundred twenty-seven cases with minimum two-year follow-up. Spine. 2010;35(7):747-53.
76. Boakye M, Mummaneni PV, Garrett M, et al. Anterior cervical discectomy and fusion involving a polyetheretherketone spacer and bone morphogenetic protein. J Neurosurg Spine. 2005;2(5):521-5.
77. Shields LB, Raque GH, Glassman SD, et al. Adverse effects associated with high-dose recombinant human bone morphogenetic protein-2 use in anterior cervical spine fusion. Spine. 2006;31(5):542-7.
78. Smucker JD, Rhee JM, Singh K, et al. Increased swelling complications associated with off-label usage of rhBMP-2 in the anterior cervical spine. Spine. 2006;31(24):2813-9.
79. Emery SE, Fisher JR, Bohlman HH. Three-level anterior cervical discectomy and fusion: radiographic and clinical results. Spine. 1997;22(22):2622-4.
80. Bohlman HH, Emery SE, Goodfellow DB, et al. Robinson anterior cervical discectomy and arthrodesis for cervical radiculopathy. Long-term follow-up of one hundred and twenty-two patients. J Bone Joint Surg Am. 1993;75(9):1298-307.
81. Uribe JS, Sangala JR, Duckworth EA, et al. Comparison between anterior cervical discectomy fusion and cervical corpectomy fusion using titanium cages for reconstruction: analysis of outcome and long-term follow-up. Eur Spine J. 2009;18(5):654-62.
82. Nirala AP, Husain M, Vatsal DK. A retrospective study of multiple interbody grafting and long segment strut grafting following multilevel anterior cervical decompression. Br J Neurosurg. 2004;18(3):227-32.
83. Brodsky AE, Khalil MA, Sassard WR, et al. Repair of symptomatic pseudoarthrosis of anterior cervical fusion. Posterior versus anterior repair. Spine. 1992;17(10):1137-43.
84. Frykholm R. Deformities of dural pouches and strictures of dural sheaths in the cervical region producing nerve-root compression: a contribution to the etiology and operative treatment of brachial neuralgia. J Neurosurg. 1947;4:403-13.
85. Scoville WB, Whitcomb BB. Lateral rupture of cervical intervertebral disks. Postgrad Med. 1966;39:174-80.
86. Farin A, Wang MY. Posterior keyhold cervical foraminotomy. In: Kim DH, Henn JS, Vaccaro AR, Dickman CA (Eds). Surgical Anatomy & Techniques to the Spine. Philadelphia, PA: Saunders Elsevier; 2006. pp. 164-7.
87. Russell SM, Benjamin V. Posterior surgical approach to the cervical neural foramen for intervertebral disc disease. Neurosurgery. 2004;54(3):662-5, discussion 665-6.
88. Herkowitz HN, Kurz LT, Overholt DP. Surgical management of cervical soft disc herniation. A comparison between the anterior and posterior approach. Spine. 1990;15(10):1026-30.
89. Fessler RG, Khoo LT. Minimally invasive cervical micro-endoscopic foraminotomy: an initial clinical experience. Neurosurgery. 2002;51(5 Suppl):S37-45.
90. Kim KT, Kim YB. Comparison between open procedure and tubular retractor assisted procedure for cervical radiculopathy: results of a randomized controlled study. J Korean Med Sci. 2009;24(4):649-53.
91. Ruetten S, Komp M, Merk H, et al. A new full-endoscopic technique for cervical posterior foraminotomy in the treatment of lateral disc herniations using 6.9-mm endoscopes: prospective 2-year results of 87 patients. Minim Invasive Neurosurg. 2007;50(4):219-26.

92. Winder MJ, Thomas KC. Minimally invasive versus open approach for cervical laminoforaminotomy. Can J Neurol Sci. 2011;38(2):262-7.
93. Traynelis VC. The Prestige cervical disc replacement. Spine J. 2004;4(6 Suppl):310S-4S.
94. Papadopoulos S. The Bryan cervical disc system. Neurosurg Clin N Am. 2005;16(4):629-36.
95. Chi JH, Ames CP, Tay B. General considerations for cervical arthroplasty with technique for ProDisc-C. Neurosurg Clin N Am. 2005;16(4):609-19.
96. Jawahar A, Cavanaugh DA, Kerr EJ 3rd, et al. Total disc arthroplasty does not affect the incidence of adjacent segment degeneration in cervical spine: results of 93 patients in three prospective randomized clinical trials. Spine J. 2010;10(12):1043-8.
97. Fallah A, Akl EA, Ebrahim S, et al. Anterior cervical discectomy with arthroplasty versus arthrodesis for single-level cervical spondylosis: a systematic review and meta-analysis. PLoS One. 2012;7(8):e43407.
98. Cardoso MJ, Rosner MK. Multilevel cervical arthroplasty with artificial disc replacement. Neurosurg Focus. 2010;28(5):E19.
99. Fountas KN, Kapsalaki EZ, Nikolakakos LG, et al. Anterior cervical discectomy and fusion associated complications. Spine. 2007;32(21):2310-7.
100. Bazaz R, Lee MJ, Yoo JU. Incidence of dysphagia after anterior cervical spine surgery: a prospective study. Spine. 2002;27(22):2453-8.
101. Lee MJ, Bazaz R, Furey CG, et al. Risk factors for dysphagia after anterior cervical spine surgery: a two-year prospective cohort study. Spine J. 2007;7(2):141-7.
102. Golfinos JG, Dickman CA, Zabramski JM, et al. Repair of vertebral artery injury during anterior cervical decompression. Spine. 1994;19(22):2552-6.
103. Chen J, Wang X, Bai W, et al. Prevalence of heterotopic ossification after cervical total disc arthroplasty: a meta-analysis. Eur Spine J. 2012;21(4):674-80.
104. Wirth FP, Dowd GC, Sanders HF, et al. Cervical discectomy. A prospective analysis of three operative techniques. Surg Neurol. 2000;53(4):340-6, discussion 346-8.
105. Epstein NE. A review of laminoforaminotomy for the management of lateral and foraminal cervical disc herniations or spurs. Surg Neurol. 2002;57(4):226-33, discussion 233-4.
106. DePalma AF, Subin DK. Study of the cervical syndrome. Clin Orthop Relat Res. 1965;38:135-42.
107. Matz PG, Holly LT, Groff MW, et al. Indications for anterior cervical decompression for the treatment of cervical degenerative radiculopathy. J Neurosurg Spine. 2009; 11(2):174-82.

CHAPTER 26 Cervical Spondylotic Myelopathy

Sean Barry, Michael G Fehlings

EPIDEMIOLOGY AND NATURAL HISTORY

Myelopathy occurs as a result of any process leading to functional impairment of the spinal cord. Similarly, radiculopathy results from the pathological disturbance of the neural circuitry within a spinal nerve root. Myeloradiculopathy implies concurrent involvement of both spinal cord and nerve root(s). All three terms are nonspecific and may be the result of a myriad of clinical entities including degenerative, infectious, neoplastic, traumatic, vascular, rheumatologic, or other causes. This chapter will focus on the most common cause of cervical myeloradiculopathy, cervical spondylotic myelopathy (CSM). CSM refers to age-related degenerative osteoarthritic changes of the disks, facet joints, ligaments, and connective tissues of the cervical spine resulting in myelopathy.

The exact prevalence and incidence of cervical myeloradiculopathy are unknown, although based on rates of imaging and surgery for a cervical spine condition, it can certainly be considered a common condition. Cervical spondylosis is the most frequent cause of myeloradiculopathy in patients over the age of 55. CSM is also the most common cause of nontraumatic spinal cord injury (SCI) overall, resulting in high rates of functional disability and decreased quality of life.[1] Due to the unique pathobiology of CSM, it is predominantly a disease of the elderly. Ossification of the posterior longitudinal ligament (OPLL), which also results in spinal cord compression and dysfunction, is another important cause of CSM. OPLL is more common in the Asian population. CSM more often affects men than women, at a ratio of 2.7:1.[2]

In a prospective series of 585 patients with nontraumatic SCI, CSM was responsible for 23.6% of cases. The average age at diagnosis in this series was 64 years. The multilevel disease was most commonly seen, with C5–6 being the single most common level involved.[3] Other common causes of cervical myeloradiculopathy include trauma, primary and metastatic malignancy, infection, and ossification of the ligamentum flavum.

The pathophysiology of CSM involves a combination of both static and dynamic mechanical components. This mechanical trauma, in turn, activates a complex cascade of biomolecular alterations in the spinal cord with resultant ischemia, excitotoxicity, and apoptosis.[4] The resulting hallmark neuropathological features include cystic cavitation, gliosis, Wallerian degeneration of descending and ascending fiber tracts, and anterior horn cell loss.[5] Although there is currently only limited understanding of the biomechanical and molecular mechanisms involved in the development of CSM, it is an active area of research. Defining these mechanisms may allow for the development of therapeutic neuroprotective agents which could be used in conjunction with surgical decompressive management strategies. It has recently been reported that Fas/Fas ligand-mediated apoptosis of neurons and oligodendrocytes and the resultant inflammation contributes to the pathobiology of spinal cord degeneration and affects neuronal function and survival in CSM.[6]

Cervical spondylosis with resultant osteophytic spurring and disk degeneration is a natural consequence of aging. Age is repeatedly seen as the most common risk factor for the development of CSM. As our population continues to age, the incidence of CSM will reflect this phenomenon. In males, the radiographic prevalence of cervical spondylosis has been reported to be 13% in the third decade of life and approaches 100% by the seventh decade. In females, there is a 5% prevalence by 40 years of age, which increases to 96% by age 70.[7] Men present more commonly than women with CSM and their radiographic changes tend to be more severe.[8]

A genetic predisposition to the development of CSM has been suggested by several authors. Studies linking genetics with the development of CSM have historically been twin studies or case reports of families harboring unusually high incidences of the disease.[9,10] While these studies effectively demonstrate the potential role of genetics in the development of CSM, they remain speculative. It has also been well-documented that patients with Down syndrome have both an increased prevalence as well as a risk of the early development of cervical spondylosis. Other less common genetic syndromes such as Kniest syndrome (a collagenopathy associated with complex skeletal manifestations) and fibrodysplasia ossificans progressiva can result in varied cervical stenosis leading to life-threatening myelopathy.[11] Recently, a large population-based study using genealogic data from over 2 million Utah residents has demonstrated excessive familial clustering to both close and distant relatives of patients with symptomatic CSM.[12] Identifying the specific responsible genes for this predisposition and direct biological targeting to both prevent and treat CSM are current areas of research.

The natural history of CSM can be variable but has been classically described as following a prolonged stepwise progression in neurological dysfunction. Some patients' symptoms may stabilize for periods of time but rarely do they improve spontaneously.[13] The quality of the evidence defining the true natural history is low, however, and many questions remain unanswered. This is in part due to the heterogeneity of the patient population and the trend toward more aggressive surgical management of CSM, which negates the ability to longitudinally analyze many patients. The true natural history of CSM can only be studied in the absence of surgical intervention. Additionally, most natural history studies lack validated objective outcome measures, relying instead on qualitative data. An excellent summary of the literature pertaining to the natural history of the condition by Matz et al.[14] offers some guidance for the treatment of patients with mild CSM. There is evidence to suggest that clinical stability may be expected in patients under the age of 75 observed over a 3-year period.[14] However, this course of action cannot be entirely recommended. Mild myelopathy may be the source of significant functional disability for an individual. Likewise, clinical stability cannot always be equated with a good clinical outcome.[15]

As the spine ages, cervical disk degeneration progresses which leads to both anterior and posterior osteophyte formation. Ligamentum flavum and facet hypertrophy then ensue. These processes frequently result in the narrowing of the spinal canal and subsequent compression of the neural elements. This natural aging process is nearly ubiquitous in the general population but may be exacerbated in individuals with congenitally narrow spinal canals. Early spondylosis is generally asymptomatic. One magnetic resonance imaging (MRI) study of the subaxial spine in asymptomatic subjects found an 86% rate of degenerative disk disease in men and 89% in women over the age of 60. The authors also found a linear relationship between age and degenerative changes seen on imaging. Spinal cord compression was seen in nearly 8% of cases.[16] Autopsy findings support the accepted belief that the majority of cervical spondylosis remains asymptomatic. One series of 200 autopsies demonstrated cervical spondylosis in 53.5% with evidence of spinal cord compression in 7.5% of specimens. The mean age of those with spondylosis was significantly greater (70.2) than those without (57.3).[17] CSM is rare in patients below the age of 40.

WORK-UP (CLINICAL FINDINGS)

Symptoms and Signs

The clinical presentation of CSM is highly variable and its course unpredictable. There are no pathognomonic findings. The onset is generally insidious in nature but it is not uncommon for patients to present with sudden neurologic deterioration following a fall or other mild traumatic event resulting in acute SCI. Hyperextension is the most common mechanism for such an injury with a central cord syndrome being a frequent pattern of injury.

Signs and symptoms are dependent on the involved neurological elements. This most commonly results in multilevel compression of both spinal cord and cervical nerve roots, often resulting in an asymmetric pattern of mixed upper and lower motor neuron disease symptoms. In our experience, subtle gait disturbance is the most common initial symptom. Patients will frequently complain of leg stiffness and resulting imbalance. Numbness and paresthesias of the extremities are frequent complaints. Additional symptoms follow unpredictably and include upper and lower extremity weakness and discoordination. A decrease in hand dexterity is a very common early feature with patients describing difficulty with buttoning clothing and other activities requiring fine motor skills. More often than not, axial neck pain is not a dominant complaint. Significant neck pain should raise the suspicion of tumor or infectious etiology. Similarly, pain dominant presentations, and a history of trauma may herald instability, which must be ruled out.

Sphincter impairment is also a relatively common finding. In one series of 269 patients, bladder dysfunction was seen in 18% and bowel dysfunction in 15%.[18]

On physical examination, the earliest motor signs include hand extrinsic and triceps weakness.[19] Hyperactive deep tendon reflexes are expected findings below the level of stenosis. Hoffman's reflex, Babinski's sign, and clonus are commonly present. Classic objective examination findings are absent, however, in approximately 20% of myelopathic patients.[20] As with other causes of myelopathy, L'Hermittes phenomenon may be present. This sign is characterized by an "electric shock-like" sensation radiating from the neck down the center of the spine and is classically elicited with neck flexion.

A useful screening test is that of the jaw jerk. This reflex is mediated by the fifth cranial nerve and may be indicative of ALS or MS. Hyperactivity suggests corticobulbar disease resulting from a lesion above the level of the cervical spinal cord. However, it is not normally present and therefore of limited value if absent.[21]

Nerve conduction studies and electromyelography (EMG) are important adjunctive diagnostic tests in the evaluation of CSM. Because they predominantly evaluate lower motor neuron function distal to the spinal cord, they are inadequate in and of themselves for assessing spinal cord compression. They are usually reserved for cases in which other differential diagnostic causes of radiculopathy must be excluded, such as ulnar or median nerve entrapments or ALS.

Although neurophysiological monitoring is often used in patients with CSM during surgery, preoperative motor evoked potentials (MEPs), somatosensory evoked potentials (SEPs) and other forms of neurophysiological testing are not routinely performed preoperatively. Lyu et al. performed SEPs and MEPs in 39 patients with clinical and radiographically diagnosed CSM and found that upper extremity MEP was the most sensitive test for detecting myelopathy.[22] Medial and tibial SEPs correlated with the severity of myelopathy as measured by the modified Japanese Orthopaedic Association scale (mJOA). Patients with normal median nerve SEPs had better surgical outcomes than those with abnormal ones. A thorough understanding of the clinical features predicting surgical outcomes in patients with CSM will undoubtedly aid in determining the optimal treatment plan. Factors influencing prognosis in this patient population are becoming more apparent, but many questions remain unanswered. A recent systematic review of clinical factors predicting surgical outcomes in patients undergoing cervical decompression for CSM recommended that preoperative SEPs be considered to provide supplementary objective data in patients where clinical factors are unclear.[23]

A review of EMG for assessment in patients with CSM by Mummaneni et al. recommends that preoperative EMG be performed to evaluate patients with atypical or unusual symptoms or in those whose disease is felt to be multifactorial. They conclude that EMG has poor sensitivity in detecting cervical radiculopathy. Furthermore, there is little available evidence supporting the utility of EMG for predicting outcome after surgical decompressive surgery.[24]

Grading and Functional Outcome Measures

Appropriate objective functional outcome parameters to measure both conservatively treated and surgically managed patients are critical to record temporal functional disability in patients with CSM. The two most commonly used systems are the mJOA and the Nurick grading scheme (Tables 1 and 2). These scales assess, to some degree, distinct realms of disability. The Nurick grade is a nonspecific scale which emphasizes impairment as it

Table 1: Nurick grade.

Grade	Description
0	Signs or symptoms of root involvement but without evidence of spinal cord disease
1	Signs of spinal cord disease but no difficulty walking
2	Slight difficulty in walking which did not prevent full-time employment
3	Difficulty in walking which prevented full-time employment or the ability to do all housework but was not so severe as to require someone else's help to walk
4	Able to walk only with someone else's help or with the aid of a frame
5	Chair bound or bedridden

CHAPTER 26

Table 2: Modified Japanese Orthopaedic Association scoring system.

Score	*Definition*
Motor dysfunction	
Upper extremities:	
0	Unable to move hands
1	Unable to eat with a spoon but able to move hands
2	Unable to button shirt but able to eat with a spoon
3	Able to button shirt with great difficulty
4	Able to button shirt with slight difficulty
5	No dysfunction
Lower extremities:	
0	Complete loss of motor and sensory function
1	Sensory preservation without ability to move legs
2	Ability to move legs but unable to walk
3	Able to walk on flat floor with a walking aid (cane or crutch)
4	Able to walk up and/or downstairs w/aid of a handrail
5	Moderate-to-significant lack of stability but able to walk up and/or downstairs without handrail
6	Mild lack of stability but able to walk unaided with smooth reciprocation
7	No dysfunction
Sensory dysfunction	
Upper extremities:	
0	Complete loss of hand sensation
1	Severe sensory loss or pain
2	Mild sensory loss
3	No sensory loss
Sphincter dysfunction	
0	Unable to micturate voluntarily
1	Marked difficulty in micturition
2	Mild-to-moderate difficulty in micturition
3	Normal micturition

relates to an individual's ambulatory ability and ability to work.[25] The mJOA is a validated and reliable system, which considers both sensory and motor impairment in the upper and lower extremities as well as sphincter function (Table 2). Neither is a comprehensive scale that assesses all facets of an individual's impairment.

The Neck Disability Index (NDI) is another commonly used outcome measure to evaluate the patient's perceived disability and the impact of the disease on an individual's daily life. The NDI contains 10 items, 7 of which relate to activities of daily living, 2 of which are related to pain, and 1 item related to concentration. The NDI has shown to be a reliable and valid self-reported questionnaire for patients with neck pain.[26]

Gait analysis has proven to be a practical, valid, and reliable outcome measure in the assessment of patients undergoing surgical decompression for CSM.[27] Singh and Crockard have developed a simple, 30-meter walking test which serves as a quantifiable measure of CSM severity. They performed gait analysis in 41 patients treated surgically for CSM and demonstrated statistically significant variations in pre- and postoperative walking time.[28]

The Berg Balance Scale (BBS) is a widely used test to measure both static and dynamic balancing abilities in the elderly. It is a well-validated and easily reproducible scale containing 14 items and is considered the "gold-standard" for functional assessment of balance. In a study by Furlan et al., the BBS was found to be significantly improved in 81 patients treated surgically for CSM at both 6 months and 1 year postoperatively.[29]

In order to assess upper extremity function after SCI, the Graded Redefined Assessment of Strength, Sensibility, and Prehension (GRASSP) measure was developed. This objective clinical research tool includes three domains which are important in characterizing hand function; strength, sensibility, and prehension. It is an important clinical outcome measure that can be administered routinely along the continuum of a patient's diagnosis, treatment, and recovery. GRASSP has recently been found to demonstrate reliability, construct validity, and concurrent validity for use as a standardized upper-limb impairment measure for individuals with complete or incomplete tetraplegia.[30]

Laboratory Findings

Beyond routine preoperative blood work, laboratory investigations are generally reserved for cases in which alternative diagnoses are suspected or need to be ruled out. In subspecialty spine practice, nearly all patients will present with most relevant imaging already performed. Given the high rate of cervical spondylosis in the general population, this may lead clinicians to presume that all neurologic impairment is a result of radiographically apparent compression. A high index of suspicion for alternative diagnoses should be maintained. The most common entities mimicking CSM, which may not be evident radiographically, include MS, motor neuron disease [particularly amyotrophic lateral sclerosis (ALS)], compressive peripheral neuropathy, carpal tunnel syndrome (CTS), and ulnar neuropathy. The clinical manifestations of CSM are usually bilateral and, therefore, clinicians should maintain a healthy degree of skepticism whenever the diagnosis of bilateral CTS is made.

Amyotrophic lateral sclerosis is a particularly important differential diagnosis to entertain. It is the most common of all the motor neuron disorders. Pathologically, it can be recognized by the gliosis and neuronal loss within the motor cortex and the anterior horns of the spinal cord. Clinically, it most commonly manifests as focal atrophic extremity weakness or dysarthria, which then progresses in both severity and location to involve both upper and lower motor neurons. It is not generally an easy diagnosis to make and neurologists may take months ruling out other possible causes of presenting signs and symptoms. Importantly, sensory signs are conspicuously absent and bulbar signs may be present in ALS. EMG is useful if ALS is a diagnostic consideration. Classic findings include diffuse fibrillation and fasciculation potentials and large complex motor unit potentials, all of which are absent in CSM. Diagnostic electrophysiological criteria for ALS have been established according to what is known as the El Escorial criteria.[31]

Any patient who is immunocompromised or displays evidence of systemic infection requires a septic workup. Demyelinating and noninfectious inflammatory conditions are relatively common causes of myelopathy and should be considered. Cerebrospinal fluid (CSF) sampling should be performed and investigated in cases of suspected MS. Rheumatologic conditions such as ankylosing spondylitis, diffuse idiopathic skeletal hyperostosis (DISH), and OPLL are often noted on radiographic investigations and can be confirmed with serologic markers, such as HLA-B27.

In patients presenting with primarily sensory symptoms and radiographic evidence of cervical spondylosis, dual pathology should be considered. Nutritional and metabolic disorders may often coexist with cervical spondylosis, particularly in the elderly. Detection and correction of these abnormalities should be completed prior to surgical intervention.[32]

Imaging

An MRI is warranted in all patients with established cervical myelopathy. It is the noninvasive, high resolution, and multiplanar modality of choice to assess neural and ligamentous structures. MRI is sensitive in delineating both the size and contour or the spinal cord. It is also able to depict internal signal intensity and intramedullary processes such as edema, demyelination, hemorrhage, tumor, syringomyelia, and infarction. Intradural extramedullary and extradural pathology such as hematoma, tumors, and vascular malformations are also well-visualized and may be ruled out as diagnostic considerations. The foramen magnum should be evaluated for Chiari malformation.

In patients for whom MRI is contraindicated, computed tomography (CT) myelography is the favored alternative. There is Level II evidence recommending preoperative imaging with MRI or CT myelography to confirm the presence of compressive pathology for those patients undergoing elective surgery for CSM.[24]

The ability of specific MRI findings to predict clinical outcomes has been extensively studied. The most commonly investigated finding is that of intramedullary T2-weighted hyperintensity at single or multiple levels on preoperative imaging. T1 hypointensity has also been studied but to a lesser extent. One study of 121 patients with surgically treated CSM demonstrated that patients with no intramedullary signal changes or signal changes only on T2-weighted images had improved outcomes compared with patients with signal changes on both T1- and T2-weighted images. The patients where regression of spinal cord signal change was seen had significantly better outcomes.[33] Other studies have reported the finding that postoperative resolution of preoperative T2 hyperintensity correlates with better functional outcome.[34] A systematic review by Holly et al. summarizing the literature on the subject concludes that multisegmental high signal on T2 MRI is predictive of poor outcome following surgery. The literature is less concordant regarding focal T2 hyperintensity, with some studies demonstrating this finding to predict a more negative outcome and others not. Combined demonstration of T1 hypointensity with T2 hyperintensity seems to be a consistent predictor of a worse outcome.[35] The absence of spinal cord re-expansion following decompression has also been correlated with a worse postoperative outcome.[36] Other findings specific to CSM on MRI include a reduced transverse area of the

CHAPTER 26

spinal cord (TASC) with a resultant "banana-shaped" cord deformity at the level of maximum compression.

In patients with spondylotic syndromes causing symptoms of radiculopathy, Ashkan et al. examined the ability of MRI to predict surgical outcome. Preoperative MRI demonstrated foraminal compression in 45 patients, all of whom improved symptomatically after surgery. MRI had a higher sensitivity in detecting nerve root compression (92%) then did EMG (42%).[37]

When calcified pathology is suspected, CT is the modality of choice. CT should also be performed in any case where trauma is suspected. CT allows optimal imaging of osteophytes and calcified disk or ligaments. It is particularly helpful in the workup of OPLL. CT also allows detailed views of planned osseous trajectories for cervical instrumentation thus decreasing screw-related complications.

Plain X-rays are important for assessing spinal alignment. Dynamic flexion and extension views are important to investigate for unstable motion. X-rays allow for the measurement of the absolute diameter of the spinal canal. The average A-P diameter of the cervical spinal canal on lateral plain films is 17 mm, however, significant variation exists according to sex and race.[38] A more accurate indicator of stenosis is defined by the Pavlov ratio, which avoids inaccuracies inherent to direct measurements from radiographs. These include different target distances and magnification errors. The Pavlov ratio is calculated by dividing the AP diameter of the spinal canal at the mid-vertebral body to the sagittal diameter of the corresponding vertebral body. A ratio of less than 0.8 is indicative of stenosis.[39]

MR tractography and diffusion tensor imaging (DTI), while promising modalities to depict discrete ascending and descending fiber tracts, generally remain experimental and preclinical. The sensitivity of MRI remains both its greatest strength as well as its major limitation. As emphasized above, clinically silent spinal cord compression is a relatively common incidental finding. Any imaging findings should strongly correlate and support clinical signs and symptoms if surgery is to be considered.

MEDICAL MANAGEMENT

The pathophysiological mechanisms that underlie CSM are believed to be threefold. These include both static and dynamic physical compressive injury as well as spinal cord ischemia.[5] This combined pattern of injury often results in spinal cord damage beyond the confines of the directly compressive pathology. A greater understanding of the cellular and molecular events involved in CSM has led to the development of promising preclinical pharmacotherapeutics. No pharmacological agents have yet proven effective enough in either acute or subacute SCI to be fully translated into the clinic and used as neuroprotective agents. An important ongoing clinical trial is the CSM-Protect (efficacy of riluzole in surgical treatment for cervical spondylotic myelopathy) study. Riluzole is an FDA-approved medication for the treatment of ALS. As mentioned above, ALS has several similar clinical features to CSM. Preclinical evidence of traumatic and nontraumatic SCI strongly suggests that this sodium-glutamate antagonist may confer a neuroprotective benefit to patients. CSM-Protect is a randomized, double-blind, placebocontrolled multicenter trial studying the potential neurological benefits of riluzole as an adjunctive treatment to surgical decompression in patients with CSM (http://clinicaltrials.gov/ct2/show/NCT01257828?term=riluzole+CSM&rank=1).

Cervical spondylotic myelopathy remains a condition treated predominantly by surgical decompression. Conservative management is the initial and preferred course of therapy in patients presenting with axial or radicular pain in the absence of objective neurologic findings. Ultimately, the optimal treatment paradigm must be fitted to each individual patient. There is little debate, however, that patients with signs of myelopathy should be offered surgical decompression if no medical contraindication exists. It may be reasonable to initially observe mild, slowly progressive cases of patients with subjective complaints. Pharmacological agents and nonpharmacological modalities of treatment may be employed independently or in conjunction with surgery. Currently, the role of pharmacotherapy is limited to the management of neck pain, neuropathic pain from radiculopathy, and muscle spasm secondary to spondylosis. Medical management also has an important role in the acute, subacute, and chronic rehabilitation postoperative phases.

Clinical studies investigating the efficacy of both pharmacological and nonpharmacological modalities are lacking. Those that exist are generally of low quality. Prospective randomized trials comparing surgical therapy versus conservative management for radicular or axillary neck pain have not been done. Despite this, a myriad of modalities is used empirically in isolation or in combination in nearly every patient treated for CSM. The medications most commonly used are nonsteroidal anti-inflammatory drugs, opioids or other analgesics, muscle relaxants, and neuromodulating medications (tricyclic antidepressants and antiepileptics). Nonpharmacological methods most commonly employed include physical therapy, manual therapy, and cervical traction.

SURGICAL INDICATIONS AND TREATMENT

Despite being the most common cause of acquired disability in those above the age of 50, there remains a lack of high-quality evidence guiding surgical management of cervical degenerative myelopathy. This is due to the absence of large, prospective studies using consistent and validated outcome measures to support any single surgical approach over another. The lack of Level 1 and II evidence is compounded by the diversity of both the patient population and the surgical modalities with which they are treated.[15] This methodological heterogeneity also makes the interstudy evaluation of the literature difficult to interpret. Expert opinion and general consensus support the notion that all methods that effectively decompress the affected segments of spinal cord and nerve roots are equally efficacious in the short-term. Retrospective analysis of anterior versus posterior surgical decompression demonstrates variable yet similar functional outcomes in both cohorts.[40] Options include posterior approaches in the form of laminectomy, laminectomy plus instrumented arthrodesis, or laminoplasty. Anterior approaches include anterior cervical diskectomy and fusion (ACDF) and corpectomy. A third category encompasses circumferential decompression with both anterior and posterior reconstructive techniques employing combinations of the abovementioned approaches.

The surgical strategy elected is dependent upon multiple factors including the cause of compression, the primary site of compression, the number of levels involved, the sagittal alignment of the spine and the patient's age, general medical status, and comorbidities. Last but not least, the surgeon's familiarity and comfort level with each technique must be considered. Degenerative ventral pathology generally results in stretching of the spinal cord during flexion. Conversely, extension results in buckling of the ligamentum flavum and spinal cord distension.[41] Either movement may result in repetitive dynamic microtrauma. Foraminal stenosis will result in pain and discrete sensorimotor findings depending on the nerve root involved. Taking these factors into account, a single optimal surgical approach can usually be chosen. The primary objective of surgery is the decompression of the spinal cord and nerve roots. Secondary objectives include spinal stabilization in order to prevent deformity and/or restore normal alignment.

Intuitively, advanced patient age, as well as both duration of symptoms and degree of their preoperative neurological impairment, would seem to be expected factors in predicting surgical outcome. A large prospective study involving 146 consecutive patients with CSM over a 2-year period found that patients younger than 40 years of age fared significantly better in short-term follow-up, as compared to patients above the age of 40, as graded by the Nurick scoring system. Duration of myelopathic symptoms greater than 2 years was also found to be a significant outcome predictor.[33] The literature is, however, inconsistent with regards to the use of age and duration of symptoms as prognostic indicators of surgical outcomes.[23]

There remains insufficient evidence to make strong recommendations regarding the timing of surgical intervention for CSM. In the setting of an acute SCI secondary to spondylosis without fracture or instability but with persistent spinal cord compression, urgent surgical decompression is reasonable and safe and should be considered in patients with profound neurologic deficits (ASIA C).[42]

Ventral Approaches

In general, ventral approaches are opted for when the primary site of compression is anterior to the spinal cord. Loss of cervical lordosis also favors ventral surgery. When compression exists at more than three levels, however, the risk of surgical complications from approaching anteriorly must be considered.

Anterior approaches for the management of cervical myeloradiculopathy include both fusion and nonfusion procedures. By far, the most commonly employed modern-day ventral approach is ACDF. When more extensive compression exists beyond the region accessible via the disk-space, anterior cervical corpectomy and fusion (ACCF) is the ventral approach of choice. Nonfusion techniques employed less frequently include the oblique corpectomy and cervical disk arthroplasty (CDR). There are significant disadvantages to fusing motion

CHAPTER 26

segments. Adjacent segment degeneration is the primary concern, which in theory may be obviated by CDR. Unexpectedly, however, a decrease in adjacent segment disease has not been consistently found following CDR.[43] Currently, CDR may be indicated in select patients with cervical radiculopathy, however, myelopathy remains a relative contraindication. There remains no Level I data supporting the superiority of CDR over ACDF, although a review of the literature suggests equivalency in patients with symptomatic cervical radiculopathy.[44]

Anterior Cervical Diskectomy and Fusion

Case

A 46-year-old female presents with progressive subacute onset of left arm pain and weakness. Over the past 3 days, she had difficulty with ambulation. MRI reveals spondylosis at C4/5 and C5/6 with spinal cord and nerve root compression. Early signal change can be appreciated within the cord parenchyma at C5–6. The patient underwent ACDF of C4/5 and C5/6. Postoperatively, she awoke with the resolution of radicular pain and return of full power in the left arm (Figs. 1A to C).

Anterior cervical diskectomy and ACDF are proven and extremely successful methods of ventral spinal decompression.[45] There is an abundance of literature on the matter yet there is no Level 1 evidence to support the efficacy of adding either instrumented fusion or plate fixation to anterior cervical diskectomy. In a systematic review of techniques for anterior cervical decompression, Matz et al. recommended ACD and ACDF as equivalent treatment strategies for single-level cervical disk degeneration with respect to clinical outcomes. ACDF with plating is recommended for multilevel disk degeneration over ACD and ACDF without the use of a plate.[44] In modern-day clinical practice, it is relatively uncommon to encounter a surgeon who would perform even a single-level anterior cervical diskectomy without the use of an interbody graft and plate.

Interbody graft options include autologous iliac crest bone graft (ICBG), the cadaveric iliac crest of the fibula, or synthetic implants (PEEK, titanium cages, etc.). Autologous bone or substitutes are often employed if synthetic fusion devices are implanted. Although less commonly employed currently than in the past, ICBG is considered the gold standard in anterior cervical arthrodesis, with fusion rates approaching 100%.[46] A meta-analysis on the subject by Floyd and Ohnmeiss included 310 patients who underwent 1 and 2 level cervical interbody fusions. Of patients who underwent single-level fusion, they report a 6% radiographic pseudoarthrosis rate in the autograft group versus a 14.7 in the allograft group. For 2 level fusions, the pseudoarthrosis rate was much higher at 20% in the autograft group compared with 46% in the allograft group.[47] With respect to osteobiologics, BMP-2 is discouraged for use in anterior cervical spine surgery based on evidence demonstrating extremely high rates of adverse events, most commonly local edema.[48]

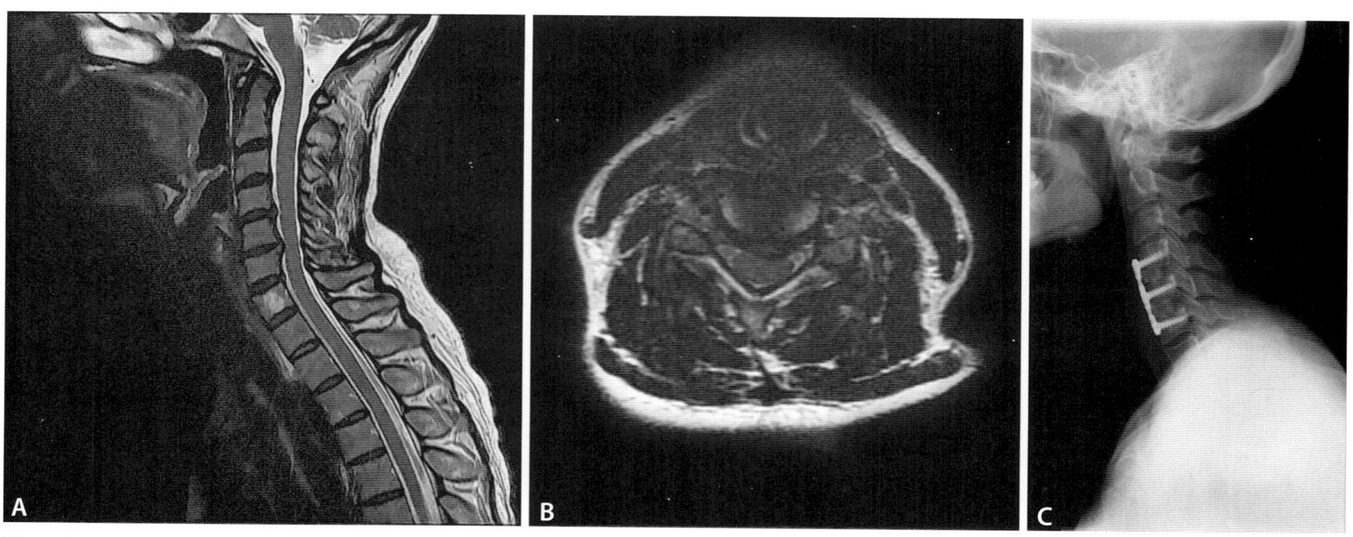

Figs. 1A to C: (A) Sagittal T2 magnetic resonance imaging (MRI); (B) Axial T2 MRI at the level of C5/6; (C) Postoperative lateral X-ray.

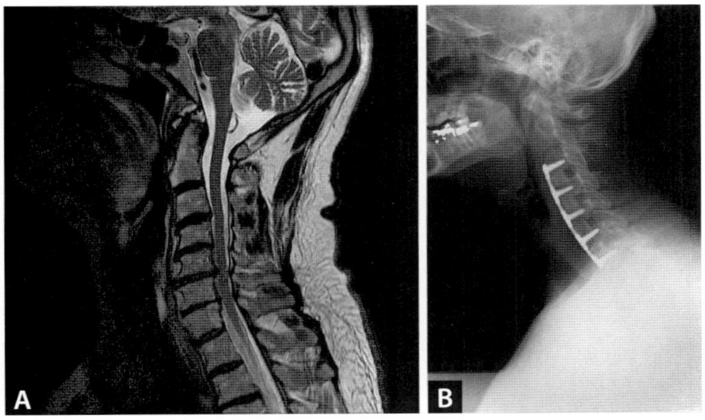

Figs. 2A and B: Four-level anterior cervical discectomy and fusion (ACDF): (A) Preoperative sagittal T2 magnetic resonance imaging (MRI); (B) Postoperative lateral X-ray.

Four level ACDF is occasionally performed for severe, multisegmental disk disease. Extension of the construct greater than three levels, however, results in the increased risks of complications in the form of pseudoarthrosis, fracture, and graft extrusion.[49,50] Although not absolutely contraindicated, alternatives to a 4 level ACDF should be entertained prior to embarking on such a course. Additional posterior supplementation should be strongly considered in such cases (Figs. 2A and B).

Corpectomy

Anterior cervical corpectomy and fusion may be indicated for the treatment of degenerative disease when multiple, contiguous levels of spondylosis or OPLL exist or when ventral pathology exists posterior to the vertebral body which is not accessible via the disks-pace. Existing evidence suggests that multilevel ACDF and ACCF are comparable treatment strategies and offer equivalent outcomes in the anterior surgical treatment of CSM. If fixation is not used anteriorly, ACCF may offer better fusion rates.[51]

There is no current Level I evidence to evaluate the efficacy of anterior surgery for CSM. Several Level II studies composed of small randomized trials have compared anterior surgery to conservative therapy, suggesting both may be effective options for mild to moderate CSM in the short term (3 years).[52,53] Current evidence suggests that multilevel ACDF and ACCF offer equivalent functional outcomes in the management of CSM.

Posterior Approaches

Laminectomy

Multilevel cervical laminectomy is a historically proven and safe technique for spinal decompression. Prior to the widespread use of instrumentation in spinal surgery, multisegmental laminectomy was the most commonly employed surgical strategy. A systematic literature review assessing laminectomy for the treatment of CSM included only retrospective single-arm studies. The majority of these studies were published in the 1970s. Summarized as a whole, they describe positive outcomes ranging from 42% to 92%.[54]

The central concern with laminectomy as a standalone procedure is the increased risk of development of postoperative kyphosis when compared to laminectomy and fusion, laminoplasty, and anterior surgical approaches. Guigui et al. reported a retrospective study in 58 patients with multilevel laminectomy followed for a mean of 3.6 years. 18 patients (31%) developed postoperative kyphosis. Of these 18, 15 were deemed to be unstable and 3 patients required reoperation.[55] The above-mentioned review by Ryken et al. found the occurrence of reported radiographic postoperative kyphosis to range from 14% to 47%. The implications of this deformity regarding patient's clinical symptoms and quality of life have not been clearly demonstrated.[54]

Laminectomy and Fusion

Case

This 74-year-old male presents with early progressive cervical myeloradiculopathy. Anatomically C2 and C3 are fused. Imaging demonstrates severe compression at the C2/3 level with multilevel spondylosis with subaxial compression. Increased signal change can be appreciated within the cord parenchyma. He underwent C2–T1 posterior cervical laminectomy and instrumented reconstruction from C2 to T1, which resulted in moderate improvement in his symptoms (Figs. 3A to D).

Laminectomy and instrumented arthrodesis is another technique often employed in the surgical management of CSM. The addition of instrumentation and bone graft effectively negates the instability which may exist preoperatively or when iatragenically introduced via posterior decompression. The most commonly employed

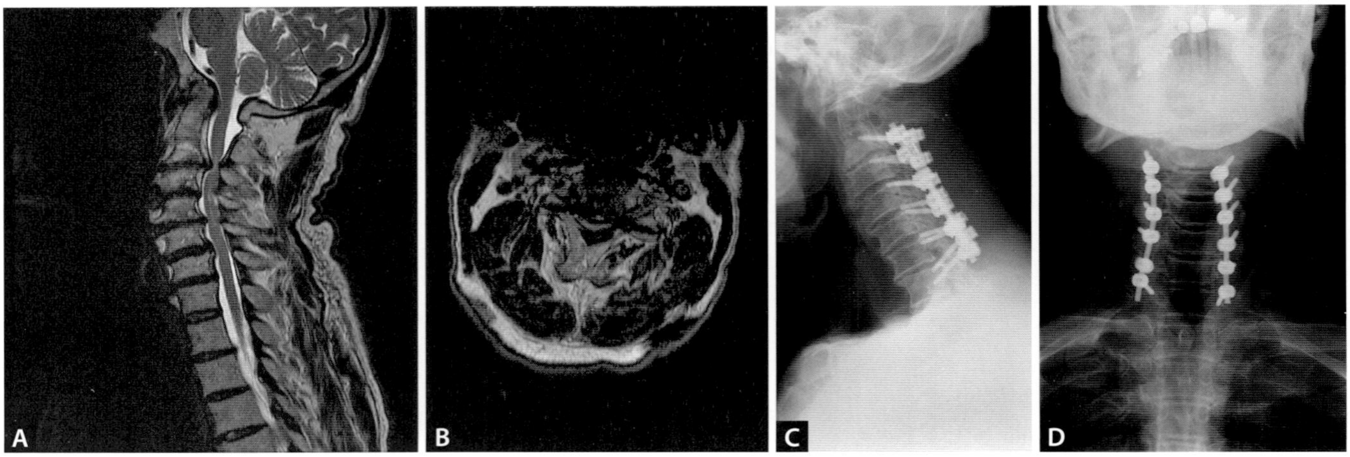

Figs. 3A to D: (A) Preoperative sagittal T2 magnetic resonance imaging (MRI); (B) Axial T2 at the C2/C3 level; (C) Postoperative lateral X-ray; (D) Postoperative anterior-posterior (AP) X-ray.

modern method for subaxial cervical spinal fusion is using lateral mass screws and rods. If the surgical plan necessitates incorporating C7 or the upper thoracic spine in the reconstruction, pedicle screws are often employed. Although many surgeons feel that C7 is anatomically unfavorable for lateral mass instrumentation, the authors routinely place lateral mass screws at the C7 level with very low rates of complications.

This technique allows for adequate expansion of the spinal canal without the risk of postlaminectomy kyphosis. It is felt to be best suited to patients with lordotic or neutral cervical spinal alignment. Although the use of internal posterior fixation can be used to provide some degree of reduction from kyphosis to lordosis, anterior approaches should be first considered in patient's harboring kyphotic cervical curvature.

Hamanashi et al. demonstrated equivalent functional outcomes between patients undergoing either laminectomy or laminectomy and fusion, with both arms of the study improving on average 50% by 3.5 years.[56] A systematic review by Mummanemi et al. concluded that there is insufficient evidence to date to recommend laminectomy and fusion over laminectomy alone or over other decompressive techniques. Both laminectomy and fusion and laminectomy alone produce equivalent clinical outcomes in the short-term but the authors caution that laminectomy alone is associated with higher rates of the development of late kyphotic deformity.[51]

Posterior Laminoforaminotomy

Herniated cervical disks and/or spondylosis resulting in radiculopathy confined to a distribution involving a single nerve root may be treated by either an anterior or a posterior approach. Occasionally, stenosis of multiple neural foramina may occur simultaneously resulting in compression of multiple roots. Concurrent myelopathy may uncommonly exist as well, resulting in myeloradiculopathy.

Posterior keyhole laminoforaminotomy may be indicated for lateral or foraminal pathologic compression. More broad based, ventral or centrally located pathology is probably best approached anteriorly. Advantages of laminoforaminotomy include the preservation of the cervical motion segment and the ensuing adjacent segment degeneration associated with fusion.

There are many clinical studies supporting the effectiveness of laminoforaminotomy in the treatment of radiculopathy, all of which are of a low level of evidence and most lacking validated outcome measures. The largest of these is by Henderson et al., who reviewed 846 surgical cases performed in 736 consecutively treated patients with cervical radiculopathy using the laminoforaminotomy technique. They reported a 96% improvement in arm pain and paresthesia and a 98% resolution of preoperative motor deficits. Subjectively, 91.5% of patients rated their outcomes as good or excellent. All patients were investigated with myelography as this study was done in the pre-MRI era. There was no statistically significant variation between the clinical outcomes for patients with hard or soft disk herniation or cervical spondylosis.[57]

An evidence-based review of the subject by Heary et al. concludes that foraminotomy improves clinical outcome in radiculopathy. This review of the current literature was unable to support the recommendation of either anterior versus posterior approaches regarding short- or long-term outcomes.[58]

Laminoplasty

Cervical laminoplasty was developed as a surgical alternative to laminectomy in the early 1970s in Japan for the treatment of CSM and OPLL.[59] By maintaining the bony neural arch, laminoplasty allows preservation of the attachments for the posterior paraspinal musculature. This theoretically improves stability and results in decreased postoperative kyphosis. Maintenance of the arch also has been advocated to prevent the formation of a "laminectomy membrane" or epidural adhesions, which is felt by some authors to be a compressive cause of late deterioration.[60]

There have been various described laminoplasty techniques including the "open-door", "French-door," and Z-plasty techniques.[61] All involve hinging of the lamina in some form to achieve multisegmental decompression by increasing the diameter of the spinal canal.[62] Numerous modifications for reattaching the posterior spinal musculature or reconstructing the posterior elements have also been described.

A commonly implicated association with laminoplasty is that of decreased range of motion (ROM) and neck pain. However, the clinical significance of these findings is a matter of debate. The most common complication of laminoplasty is C5 palsy, with a reported incidence of 5–8%.[60]

A thorough systematic review of the literature by Matz et al. includes 46 studies dealing with cervical laminoplasty and outcome. 10 studies reviewed used the mJOA outcome scale. Patients improvement was on average 55–60%, however, none of the studies included had a nonoperated control arm for comparison. There is no Level I or II evidence suggesting that laminoplasty is superior to other posterior decompressive techniques.[60]

Case

This 59-year-old man presents with neck pain and bilateral arm numbness and tingling, worse on left than on right. The examination demonstrated positive Hoffman and Babinsky signs. Preoperative MRI demonstrates multilevel spondylosis with compression of the spinal cord at multiple subaxial levels. He was treated with C3–C7 open-door instrumented laminoplasty (Figs. 4A to C).[63]

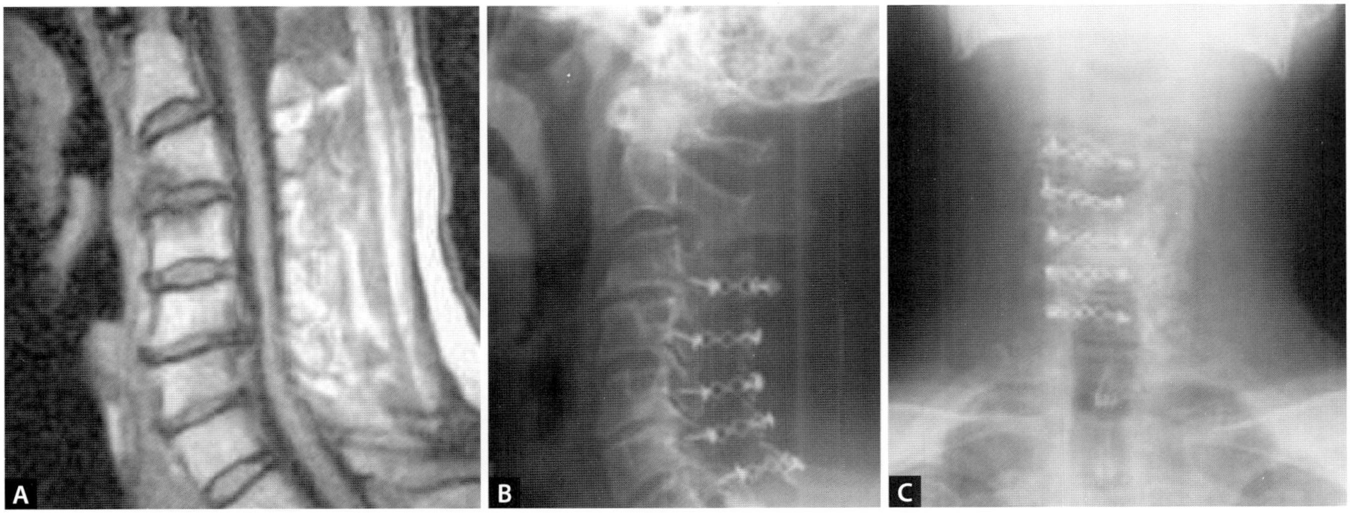

Figs. 4A to C: Preoperative magnetic resonance imaging (MRI) demonstrates multilevel spondylosis with compression of the spinal cord at multiple subaxial levels. (A) Preoperative sagittal T2 MRI; (B) Postoperative lateral X-ray; (C) Postoperative anterior-posterior (AP) X-ray.
Source: Dimar JR 2nd, Bratcher KR, Brock DC, et al. Instrumented open-door laminoplasty as treatment for cervical myelopathy in 104 patients. Am J Orthop. 2009;38(7):E123-8.

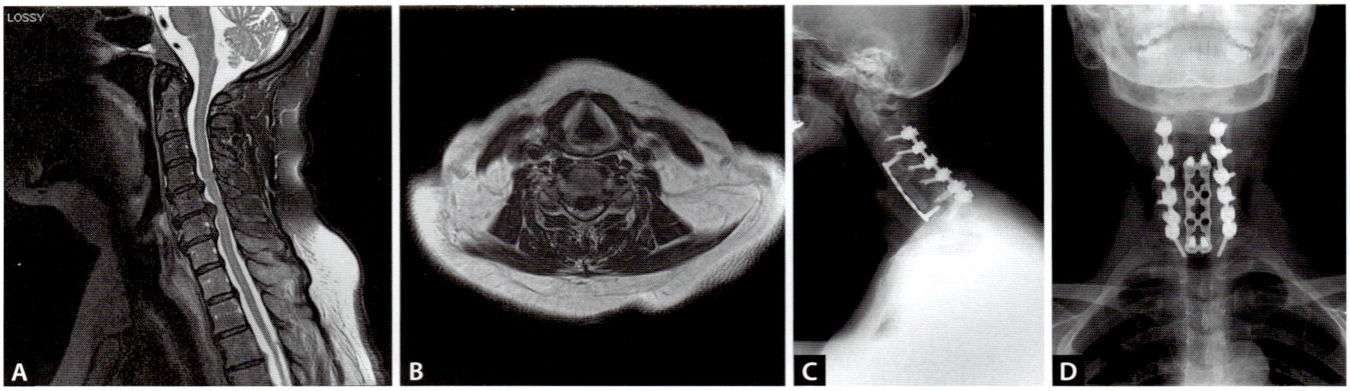

Figs. 5A to D: (A) Preoperative sagittal T2 magnetic resonance imaging (MRI); (B) Preoperative axial T2 MRI at C5/6 level; (C) Postoperative lateral X-ray; (D) Postoperative anterior-posterior (AP) X-ray.

Circumferential Surgery

Circumferential decompression and fusion is a technique normally reserved for patients with severe myelopathy or gross multilevel instability. Circumferential reconstruction has become more commonplace as spine surgeons have become increasingly aware of the issue of nonunion following complex deformity correction and multilevel corpectomy. A review by Witham et al. of 67 cases of CSM treated with anterior surgery concluded that ACDF of three levels or less, or single-level corpectomy, do not require supplementary stability with posterior instrumentation.[64]

Circumferential cervical decompression and fusion are performed in one stage if possible, but the procedure may be staged if required due to patient-specific factors.

Case

A 65-year-old woman presents with progressive cervical myelopathy. MRI demonstrates marked multilevel anterior spondylosis with a large extruded calcified disk at C5/6. There is increased signal change within the spinal cord at this level. The patient was treated with a multilevel anterior cervical decompression and reconstruction incorporating C4/5, C5/6, and C6/7 ACDF and C6 corpectomy with fibular strut graft. This was supplemented with a second stage posterior decompression and reconstruction from C3 to T1 (Figs. 5A to D).

COMPLICATIONS

Although CSM is a condition that is most often treated surgically until recently the associated perioperative and delayed complications were not well defined. Important data has been generated from a prospective, multi-center, externally monitored clinical study of more than 300 patients surgically treated for CSM. The overall perioperative complication rate was 15.6%. The vast majority of complications were minor and treatable, with no long-term impact on patient outcome. The overall rate of perioperative neurological complications was low. The rate of c5 palsy was 1.7% and only 1.3% of patients had a clinical worsening of their myelopathy. The overall delayed complication rate was 4.4%. The study highlights that the factors associated with perioperative complications are predominantly surgical in nature. These include blood loss, duration of surgery, and combining anterior-posterior procedures. No associations could be identified from comorbidity scores, BMI, the severity of myelopathy, or smoking status. Patient age was the only preoperative factor associated with a higher rate of complications. The rates of complications did not significantly differ between anterior and posterior approaches, or between specific techniques of these two approaches.[65]

There are distinct concerns and complications associated with both anterior and posterior approaches. The literature has consistently shown a significantly higher risk of postoperative infection posterior cervical surgery as compared to anterior surgery.[66] The reported rates of dysphagia and dysphonia following anterior surgery vary markedly in the literature. Fehlings et al. report a 3% rate of clinically significant dysphagia from anterior fusion, which increases to 21.3% when combined with a posterior approach.[65]

The development of pseudoarthrosis is a common additional surgical concern whenever instrumented arthrodesis is included in any procedure. The presence of a solid arthrodesis is often secondary only to neurological outcome in determining surgical success. Factors influencing fusion rates are multiple and include the surgical approach, the levels involved, and choice of graft. Patient factors such as smoking history and whether or not it is a revision case may also influence the ability to obtain adequate fusion. Due to these factors, the reported pseudoarthrosis rates in the literature vary greatly. Although often reported in the literature and commonly encountered in clinical practice, there remains a lack of definitive data linking fusion failure to poor clinical outcomes. A systematic review of radiographic imaging to assess pseudoarthoris by Kaiser et al. suggests that a measurement of interspinous distance on dynamic radiographs of >2 mm is an accurate indicator of pseudoarthrosis. They also emphasize that the identification of increased interspinous distance and of bone trabeculations by the treating surgeon may be unreliable indicators of adequate fusion. They recommend blinded interpretations of radiographs.[67]

Symptomatic pseudarthrosis may manifest as mechanical neck pain or neurologic symptoms. It is one of the most common indications for revision surgery. This can usually be addressed by choosing an alternative second surgical approach. Current evidence supports correction by either anterior or posterior approaches, with a higher fusion rate reported, yet no definite difference in outcome seen, in patients undergoing revision posterior procedures.[48]

OUTCOMES

Surgery in patients with CSM most often results in an improvement in neurological function. Many patients will not improve, however, and very uncommonly patients will worsen neurologically. Classic conventional wisdom holds that decompressive surgery results in preservation of preoperative functional status with the goal of surgery being to halt the progression of the disease. Recent clinical trials, however, depict a more optimistic view of postoperative outcomes. One study involving 81 cases resulted in significant postoperative clinical improvement, which was found to plateau at 6 months after surgery. Functional outcomes were assessed using the Nurick grading system and the mJOA and Berg Balance scales.[29]

An evidence-based review of the management of CSM underscores the shortcomings of the literature on this topic. Any recommendations regarding specific treatment options are only as strong as the literature on which they are based. These issues are currently being addressed through ongoing large, multicenter, controlled clinical trials.[15]

For radiculopathy patients presenting with a combination of arm pain, sensory abnormalities, and motor dysfunction, there is strong data supporting the notion that surgery is superior to conservative therapy in the short term. A randomized trial by Persson and Lilja of surgical management versus conservative therapy for the treatment of cervical radiculopathy found that patients in the surgical arm had an improvement in their pain faster than those managed conservatively, but the results were similar after a year.[68] Similarly, a Cochrane review by Fouyas et al. concluded that ACDF or ACD improved pain and neurologic deficits more quickly at 3 months than did nonoperative management, but the results were equal in both groups at 1 year.[69]

CONCLUSION

Cervical spondylotic myelopathy remains a common yet challenging condition. It is one that is ubiquitous in aging adults. As a preventable disease, it unnecessarily disables a large number of patients. In spite of the prevalence of the disease, there remains a lack of firm evidence regarding the timing of surgery as well as prognostic factors associated with its management. Future prospective longitudinal data is needed to further define optimal timing for surgical intervention. We encourage early surgery for myelopathic patients, as the duration of disease clearly has a negative impact on prognosis. MRI is the imaging modality of choice both for diagnostic and prognostic purposes. The surgical technique employed to decompress the spinal cord, be it anterior or posterior, is of less importance, but certain basic principles should be adhered to. These include consideration of the presence of kyphosis and addressing the region of maximal stenosis. With an increased understanding of the pathophysiological mechanisms involved in cervical myelopathy, we expect there will be improved reparative and regenerative strategies that can be developed to relieve spinal cord and nerve root compression. Defining the goals of surgery and evaluating each patient factor's comprehensively may decide upon an optimal management strategy. This will result in the best possible functional outcome for each individual patient.

REFERENCES

1. Wada EM, Suzuki SM, Kanazawa AM, et al. Subtotal corpectomy versus laminoplasty for multilevel cervical spondylotic myelopathy: a long-term follow-up study over 10 years. Spine. 2001;26(13):1443-7, discussion 1448.
2. Kalsi-Ryan S, Karadimas SK, Fehlings MG. Cervical spondylotic myelopathy: the clinical phenomenon and the current pathobiology of an increasingly prevalent and devastating disorder. Neuroscientist. 2013;19(4):409-21.
3. Moore AP. A prospective survey of the causes of non-traumatic spastic paraparesis and tetraparesis in 585 patients. Spinal Cord. 1997;35(6):361-7.
4. Baptiste DC, Fehlings MG. Pathophysiology of cervical myelopathy. Spine J. 2006;6(6 Suppl):190S-7S.
5. Fehlings MG, Skaf GM. A review of the pathophysiology of cervical spondylotic myelopathy with insights for potential novel mechanisms drawn from traumatic spinal cord injury. Spine. 1998;23(24):2730-7.
6. Yu WR, Liu T, Kiehl T-R, et al. Human neuropathological and animal model evidence supporting a role for Fas-mediated apoptosis and inflammation in cervical spondylotic myelopathy. Brain. 2011;134(Pt 5):1277-92.
7. Irvine DH, Foster JB, Newell DJ, et al. Prevalence of cervical spondylosis in a general practice. Lancet. 1965;1(7395):1089-92.
8. Rahim KA, Stambough JL. Radiologic evaluation of the degenerative cervical spine. Orth Clin North Am. 1992; 23(2):395-404.
9. Yoo K, Origitano TC. Familial cervical spondylosis. Case report. J Neurosurg. 1998;89(1):139-41.
10. Sambrook PN, MacGregor AJ, Spector TD. Genetic influences on cervical and lumbar disc degeneration: a magnetic resonance imaging study in twins. Arthritis Rheum. 1999;42(2):366-72.
11. McKay SD, Al-Omari A, Tomlinson LA, et al. Review of cervical spine anomalies in genetic syndromes. Spine. 2012;37(5):E269-77.
12. Patel AA, Spiker WR, Daubs M, et al. Evidence of an inherited predisposition for cervical spondylotic myelopathy. Spine. 2012;37(1):26-9.
13. Lees F, Turner JWA. Natural history and prognosis of cervical spondylosis. BMJ. 1963;2(5373):1607-10.
14. Matz PG, Anderson PA, Holly LT, et al. The natural history of cervical spondylotic myelopathy. J Neurosurg Spine. 2009;11(2):104-11.
15. Fehlings MG, Arvin B. Surgical management of cervical degenerative disease: the evidence related to indications, impact, and outcome. J Neurosurg Spine. 2009;11(2):97-100.
16. Matsumoto M, Fujumura Y, Suzuki N, et al. MRI of cervical intervertebral discs in asymptomatic subjects. J Bone Joint Surg Br. 1998;80(1):19-24.
17. Hughes JT, Brownell B. Necropsy observations on the spinal cord in cervical spondylosis. Riv Patol Nerv Ment. 1965;86(2):196-204.
18. Hukuda S, Mochizuki T, Ogata M, et al. Operations for cervical spondylotic myelopathy. A comparison of the results of anterior and posterior procedures. J Bone Joint Surg Br. 1985;67(4):609-15.
19. Chiles BW 3rd, Leonard MA, Choudhri HF, et al. Cervical spondylotic myelopathy: patterns of neurological deficit and recovery after anterior cervical decompression. Neurosurgery. 1999;44(4):762-9, discussion 769-70.
20. Rhee JM, Heflin JA, Hamasaki T, et al. Prevalence of physical signs in cervical myelopathy: a prospective, controlled study. Spine. 2009;34(9):890-5.
21. Pearce JMS. The jaw jerk: an instance of misattribution. J Neurol Neurosurg Psychiatry. 2011;82(3):351-2.
22. Lyu RK, Tang LM, Chen CJ, et al. The use of evoked potentials for clinical correlation and surgical outcome in cervical spondylotic myelopathy with intramedullary high signal intensity on MRI. J Neurol Neurosurg Psychiatry. 2004;75(2):256-61.
23. Holly LT, Matz PG, Anderson PA, et al. Clinical prognostic indicators of surgical outcome in cervical spondylotic myelopathy. J Neurosurg Spine. 2009;11(2):112-8.
24. Mummaneni PV, Kaiser MG, Matz PG, et al. Preoperative patient selection with magnetic resonance imaging, computed tomography, and electroencephalography: does the test predict outcome after cervical surgery? J Neurosurg Spine. 2009;11(2):119-29.
25. Nurick S. The natural history and the results of surgical treatment of the spinal cord disorder associated with cervical spondylosis. Brain. 1972;95(1):101-8.
26. Vernon H, Mior S. The neck disability index: a study of reliability and validity. J Manipulative Physiol Ther. 1991;14:409-15.
27. Holly LT, Matz PG, Anderson PA, et al. Functional outcomes assessment for cervical degenerative disease. J Neurosurg Spine. 2009;11(2):238-44.
28. Singh A, Crockard HA. Quantitative assessment of cervical spondylotic myelopathy by a simple walking test. Lancet. 1999;354(9176):370-3.
29. Furlan JC, Kalsi-Ryan S, Kailaya-Vasan A, et al. Functional and clinical outcomes following surgical treatment in patients with cervical spondylotic myelopathy: a prospective study of 81 cases. J Neurosurg Spine. 2011;14(3):348-55.
30. Kalsi-Ryan S, Curt A, Verrier MC, et al. Development of the graded redefined assessment of strength, sensibility and prehension (GRASSP): reviewing measurement specific to the upper limb in tetraplegia. J Neurosurg Spine. 2012;17(1 Suppl):65-76.

31. Sorensen EJ. The electrophysiology of the motor neuron diseases. Neurol Clin. 2012;30(2):605-20.
32. Patel MS, Rasul Z, Sell P. Dual pathology as a result of spinal stenosis and vitamin B12 deficiency. Eur Spine J. 2011;20(12):2247-51.
33. Suri A, Chabbra RP, Mehta VS, et al. Effect of intramedullary signal changes on the surgical outcome of patients with cervical spondylotic myelopathy. Spine J. 2003;3(1):33-45.
34. Mastronardi L, Elsawaf A, Roperto R, et al. Prognostic relevance of the postoperative evolution of intramedullary spinal cord changes in signal intensity on magnetic resonance imaging after anterior decompression for cervical spondylotic myelopathy. J Neurosurg Spine. 2007;7(6):615-22.
35. Vedantam A, Rajshekhar V. Does the type of T2-weighted hyperintensity influence surgical outcome in patients with cervical spondylotic myelopathy? Eur Spine J. 2013;22(1):96-106.
36. Arvin B, Kalsi-Ryan S, Karpova A, et al. Postoperative magnetic resonance imaging can predict neurological recovery after surgery for cervical spondylotic myelopathy: a prospective study with blinded assessments. Neurosurgery. 2011;69(2):362-8.
37. Ashkan K, Johnston P, Moore, AJ. A comparison of magnetic resonance imaging and neurophysiological studies in the assessment of cervical radiculopathy. Br J Neurosurg. 2002;16(2):146-8.
38. Tatarek NE. Variation in the human cervical neural canal. Spine J. 2005;5(6):623-31.
39. Pavlov H, Torg JS, Robie B, et al. Cervical spinal stenosis: determination with vertebral body ratio method. Radiology. 1987;164(3):771-5.
40. Ebersold MJ, Pare MC, Quast LM. Surgical treatment for cervical spondylitic myelopathy J Neurosurg. 1995;82(5):745-51.
41. Yuan QB, Dougherty LP, Margulies SSP. In vivo human cervical spinal cord deformation and displacement in flexion. Spine. 1998;23(15):1677-83.
42. Lenehan B, Fisher CG, Vaccaro A, et al. The urgency of surgical decompression in acute central cord injuries with spondylosis and without instability. Spine. 2010;35(21 Suppl):S180-6.
43. Yang B, Li H, Zhang T, et al. The incidence of adjacent segment degeneration after cervical disc arthroplasty (CDA): a meta analysis of randomized controlled trials. PloS One. 2012;7(4):e35032.
44. Matz PG, Ryken TC, Groff MW, et al. Techniques for anterior cervical decompression for radiculopathy. J Neurosurg Spine. 2009;11(2):183-97.
45. Papadopoulos EC, Huang RC, Girardi FP, et al. Three-level anterior cervical discectomy and fusion with plate fixation: radiographic and clinical results. Spine. 2006;31(8):897-902.
46. Gore DRM, Sepic SBM. Anterior discectomy and fusion for painful cervical disc disease: a report of 50 patients with an average follow-up of 21 years. Spine. 1998;23(19):2047-51.
47. Floyd T, Ohnmeiss, D. A meta-analysis of autograft versus allograft in anterior cervical fusion. Eur Spine J. 2000;9(5):398-403.
48. Kaiser MG, Mummaneni PV, Matz PG, et al. Management of anterior cervical pseudarthrosis. J Neurosurg Spine. 2009;11(2):228-37.
49. Vaccaro AR, Falatyn SP, Scuderi GJ, et al. Early failure of long segment anterior cervical plate fixation. J Spinal Disord. 1998;11(5):410-5.
50. Wang JCM, Hart RAM, Emery SEM, et al. Graft migration or displacement after multilevel cervical corpectomy and strut grafting. Spine. 2003;28(10):1016-21, discussion 1021-2.
51. Mummaneni PV, Kaiser MG, Matz PG, et al. Cervical surgical techniques for the treatment of cervical spondylotic myelopathy. J Neurosurg Spine. 2009;11(2):130-41.
52. Kadaňka Z, Bednařík J, Voháňka S, et al. Conservative treatment versus surgery in spondylotic cervical myelopathy: a prospective randomised study. Eur Spine J. 2000;9(6):538-44.
53. Bednarik JD, Kadanka ZD, Vohanka SM, et al. The value of somatosensory- and motor-evoked potentials in predicting and monitoring the effect of therapy in spondylotic cervical myelopathy: prospective randomized study. Spine. 1999;24(15):1593-8.
54. Ryken TC, Heary RF, Matz PG, et al. Cervical laminectomy for the treatment of cervical degenerative myelopathy. J Neurosurg Spine. 2009;11(2):142-9, 55.
55. Guigui PM, Benoist MM, Deburge AM. Spinal deformity and instability after multilevel cervical laminectomy for spondylotic myelopathy. Spine. 1998;23(4):440-7.
56. Hamanishi C, Tanaka S. Bilateral multilevel laminectomy with or without posterolateral fusion for cervical spondylotic myelopathy: relationship to type of onset and time until operation. J Neurosurg. 1996;85(3):447-51.
57. Henderson CM, Hennessy RG, Shuey HM, Jr, et al. Posterior-lateral foraminotomy as an exclusive operative technique for cervical radiculopathy: a review of 846 consecutively operated cases. Neurosurgery. 1983;13(5):504-12.
58. Heary RF, Ryken TC, Matz PG, et al. Joint section on disorders of the spine and peripheral nerves of the American Association of Neurological Surgeons and Congress of Neurological Surgeons. Cervical laminoforaminotomy for the treatment of cervical degenerative radiculopathy. J Neurosurg Spine. 2009;11(2):198-202.
59. Hirabayashi K, Satomi K. Operative procedure and results of expansive open-door laminoplasty. Spine. 1988;13(7):870-6.
60. Matz PG, Anderson PA, Groff MW, et al. Cervical laminoplasty for the treatment of cervical degenerative myelopathy. J Neurosurg Spine. 2009;11(2):157-69.
61. Ratliff JK, Cooper PR. Cervical laminoplasty: a critical review. J Neurosurg Spine. 2003;98(3):230-8.
62. Kohno K, Kumon Y, Oka Y, et al. Evaluation of prognostic factors following expansive laminoplasty for cervical spinal stenotic myelopathy. Surg Neurol. 1997;48(3):237-45.

63. Dimar JR, 2nd, Bratcher KR, Brock DC, et al. Instrumented open-door laminoplasty as treatment for cervical myelopathy in 104 patients. Am J Orthop. 2009;38(7):E123-8.
64. Gok B, Sciubba DM, McLoughlin GS, et al. Surgical treatment of cervical spondylotic myelopathy with anterior compression: a review of 67 cases. J Neurosurg Spine. 2008;9(2):152-7.
65. Fehlings MG, Smith JS, Kopjar B, et al. Perioperative and delayed complications associated with the surgical treatment of cervical spondylotic myelopathy based on 302 patients from the AOSpine North America Cervical Spondylotic Myelopathy Study. J Neurosurg Spine. 2012;16(5):425-32.
66. Smith JS, Shaffrey CI, Sansur CA, et al. Rates of infection after spine surgery based on 108,419 procedures: a report from the Scoliosis Research Society Morbidity and Mortality Committee. Spine. 2011;36(7):556-63.
67. Kaiser MG, Mummaneni PV, Matz PG, et al. Radiographic assessment of cervical subaxial fusion. J Neurosurg Spine. 2009;11(2):221-7.
68. Persson LC, Lilja A. Pain, coping, emotional state and physical function in patients with chronic radicular neck pain. A comparison between patients treated with surgery, physiotherapy or neck collar–a blinded, prospective randomized study. Disabil Rehabil. 2001;23(8):325-35.
69. Fouyas IP, Statham PF, Sandercock PA, et al. Surgery for cervical radiculomyelopathy. Cochrane Database Syst Rev. 2001;3:CD001466.

CHAPTER 27 Revision Cervical Spine Surgery

Justin K Scheer, Jessica A Tang, Christopher P Ames, Robert A Hart

INDICATIONS

Given the complexity surrounding the nature of revision surgery, especially in a region as intricate as the cervical spine, it is of utmost importance to recognize the underlying problem and understand the failures of the initial procedure in order to guide management and avoid repeat revision. Thorough history-taking, physical examination, appropriate imaging, and other relevant studies should be employed when identifying the fundamental issues that necessitated revision; as discussed below.

The indications for revision of cervical spine surgery are numerous and dictate the appropriate workup and management. The primary indications for revision are well described in the literature and include pseudarthrosis, adjacent segment disease (ASD), recurrent stenosis, postoperative deformity, and infection.[1-7]

Pseudarthrosis

Pseudarthrosis is one of the more common indications for revision surgery with an incidence rate following anterior cervical diskectomy and fusion (ACDF) of 0–50% depending on the technique used and the number of levels fused.[4,8-11] Pseudarthrosis, or nonunion of bone either following surgery or fracture is affected by both patient-specific (e.g. osteoporosis, smoking, diabetes, previous history of pseudarthrosis) and surgical factors (e.g. inadequate decompression of endplate, type of internal fixation, surgical approach, grafting material, number of levels fused).[1,12] Among the most described risk factors are multiple-level cervical fusions[8,13,14] with greater rates reported at the caudal-most level of fusion.[15]

As many as one-third of patients with pseudarthrosis are asymptomatic, but those that have symptoms commonly present with radiculopathy and/or neck pain.[8,15] Plain radiography and computed tomography (CT) are methods of choice when evaluating for the presence of pseudarthrosis.[16,17] Features of flexion-extension radiographs suggesting nonunion include continued segmental motion, migration of instrumentation, and screw or rod failure. Although static, CT has advantages for assessing pseudarthrosis in showing greater bony detail, as well as evidence of structures or devices that may be causing neurologic symptoms in patients. However, surgical exploration remains the gold standard and pseudarthrosis is confirmed intraoperatively by examining motion at the affected spinal level and visualization of the lack of bony bridging.[1,16,17]

Adjacent Segment Disease

Adjacent segment disease of the cervical spine continues to be a controversial topic. The clinical definition of ASD is the development of new symptomatic spinal stenosis at motion segment adjacent to the site of a previous arthrodesis (either superior or inferior).[7,18-22] It is often confused with the radiographic definition of adjacent segment *degeneration* in which disk degeneration is observed at adjacent motion segments to the fusion but without associated symptoms of neurologic compromise. However, studies have not demonstrated a strong correlation between the radiographic changes of adjacent segment degeneration and the clinical presentation of ASD.[18,23,24] The prevalence of ASD has been reported to range from 9% to 17% with an annual incidence ranging from 1.5% to 4% and a 10-year incidence of 25% for the patients undergoing ACDF.[18,24]

There is a plethora of evidence for the existence for both ASD and degeneration; however, controversy remains regarding its etiology, especially whether ASD is the natural course of the spine, or if spinal fusion contributes directly to ASD.[18-21,25,26] However, biomechanical studies have suggested a possible mechanism of ASD due to increased loading and motion at segments adjacent to cervical.[27-33]

Adjacent segment disease may be related to cervical alignment, especially cervical kyphosis. The cervical spine maintains a natural lordotic curvature that allows distribution of load through the posterior columns (about 64% of the total load) and the anterior column (about 36% of the total load).[34] When the cervical spine has a kyphotic deformity, the load shifts from the posterior columns to the anterior column leading to a potential increase in the mechanical load of the disk and possible acceleration of the development of ASD. This concept has been studied in the lumbar spine suggesting that postoperative sagittal malalignment of the lumbar spine and pelvis may promote ASD with up to a fourfold increased incidence.[35-38] Thus, maintaining sagittal alignment may reduce the development of ASD. At the time of this chapter, there appears to be only one study investigating postoperative cervical kyphosis and ASD. Katsuura et al.[39] performed a retrospective radiographic analysis of 42 patients who underwent ACDF with a minimum of 5-year follow-up. The authors found that postoperative kyphosis of the cervical spine may contribute to the development of ASD.[39] Of the 42 patients, 21 (50%) had radiographic evidence of ASD. Of the normal group (without ASD), physiologic cervical lordosis was preserved in 18 cases (85.7%).[39] However, normal physiological lordosis was only present in nine cases (42.8%) in the group with adjacent level degeneration, which was significantly different compared to the nonaffected group.[39] Despite the small sample size of this study, the results suggest that cervical malalignment may contribute to ASD and this study sets up the groundwork for further investigation of this complicated topic.

Despite the controversy regarding the etiology, symptomatic ASD remains an indication for revision cervical surgery. Patients with clinical ASD may present with signs and symptoms of myelopathy and/or radiculopathy referable to the level adjacent to the arthrodesis.[7,18,20] Plain radiographs may demonstrate adjacent level degeneration or spondylosis such as disk space narrowing, osteophyte formation, subchondral endplate sclerosis, and instability. The imaging modality of choice is magnetic resonance imaging (MRI) due to its ability to evaluate the disks, ligamentous structures, and neural compression for patients with signs and symptoms of neurological compression.

Postoperative Deformity

Cervical kyphosis is the most prevalent iatrogenic cervical spinal deformity and is most commonly caused by posterior decompressive surgical procedures that disrupt the posterior ligamentous complex, and paraspinal muscles, or include extensive capsulectomy and/or facetectomy. This phenomenon is referred to as postlaminectomy kyphosis.[5,40-46]

Cervical spinal stability has been described by dividing the bony anatomy of the cervical spine into three primary columns; one anterior and two posteriors.[34,47] The anterior column consists of the vertebral bodies and disks while the two posterior columns consist of the articulating facet joints.[34,47] Performing extensive multilevel laminectomies does not immediately destabilize an intact spine. However, loss of the posterior arch-facet complex causes a shift in load-bearing from the posterior column to the anterior column and over time this shift places added stress on the cervical musculature in order to maintain an upright head posture. As cervical kyphosis develops, the load is further shifted anteriorly and the disks and vertebral bodies erode, leading to yet greater imbalance. The incidence of cervical kyphosis following multilevel laminectomy is reported to range from 21% to 37% with the pediatric population being the most susceptible.[40,41,48-50]

Progressive cervical kyphosis has been shown to contribute to myelopathy as the spinal cord becomes draped against the vertebral bodies, creating both compression and longitudinal tension of the spinal cord due to its tethering by the dentate ligaments and cervical nerve roots.[5,40] As the curve progresses over time, the spinal cord becomes flattened[51] leading to compression of its anterior and posterior margins. This compression leads to neuronal loss and demyelination of the cord.[51] Furthermore, the small feeder blood vessels on the cord are also flattened, leading to the reduced blood supply. There is a large reduction in the number of vessels, the network size, as well as interruption and abnormal arrangement of the blood vessels.[51] Greater cord tension also increases intramedullary cord pressure[52-55] and has been shown to lead to apoptosis in animal models.[51] Thus, kyphosis of the cervical spine may play a substantial role in the development of cervical myelopathy.

Patients typically present with neck pain, muscular fatigue, inability to maintain a horizontal gaze, a kyphotic sagittal appearance, and possible neurologic symptoms and signs, including myelopathy or radiculopathy.[5,40,41,43,49,56] Radiographic evaluation aids in the diagnosis and can confirm the severity of the deformity as well as its flexibility. MRI is best for patients with signs and symptoms of neurologic compromise in order to determine the need for future decompression and to assess the amount of myelomalacia, cord atrophy, and syringomyelia, which can complicate as well as increase risk of treatment.[40,43] CT scans can also be very helpful in surgical planning by demonstrating the bony anatomy available for the placement of instrumentation.

Recurrent Stenosis

Unlike ASD, recurrent stenosis pertains to the development of new radiculopathy or myelopathy following decompression with or without arthrodesis, however, as the name suggests, the site of the disease is located at the same level that arthrodesis was performed. Recurrent stenosis has been characterized as having a 5-year risk of developing of 3.2% and 10-year risk rate of 5.0% after posterior cervical foraminotomy compared to a 0.7% annual rate and 6.7% 10-year rate of developing ASD.[57]

Commonly, the recurrent same-segment disease is the result of incomplete ACDF or disk arthroplasty in which decompression of treated level is inadequate,[1,58,59] but in some cases, redevelopment of stenosis precipitates same-segment disease. Since patients with inadequate decompression during index surgery present with symptoms similar to their preoperative complaints of radiculopathy or myelopathy, it is important for surgeons to exclude the possibility of an initial misdiagnosis or other causes of neurological impingement. A comprehensive preoperative workup will help to identify the etiology of the same-segment disease. If imaging fails to disclose persistent stenosis, assessment with electrodiagnostic studies and neurological consultation will help to exclude diagnoses such as carpal tunnel syndrome, multiple sclerosis, amyotrophic lateral sclerosis, or Parsonage-Turner syndrome. As with most revision surgeries, the revision itself is often more technically difficult than the index procedure because of the presence of scar tissue and, in some cases, previously failed instrumentation.

Instrumentation failure including graft dislodgment is another contributor to the same-segment disease of the cervical spine that may require revision surgery.[60,61] The revising surgeon should consider what led to the prior failure. Often this implies that the original construct was mechanically insufficient. For example, corpectomies spanning greater than two levels without posterior stabilization are associated with a threefold increase in incidences of graft or instrumentation failure than single-level corpectomies.[62]

As part of the preoperative assessment, spinal imaging is critical for determining the etiology of same-segment disease as well as the specific location of inadequate decompression. CT myelography and MRI are especially valuable in providing different types of information for better surgical planning. In particular, CT myelography may be useful for distinguishing inadequate decompression in the presence of hardware[22,63] while signal changes on MRI are helpful in identifying the state of the spinal cord, whether atrophy has occurred or whether changes to the cord are reversible or irreversible.[64,65]

Infection

While the development of infection following cervical spine surgery is relatively infrequent, it more commonly occurs following posterior than anterior cervical surgery. It is impossible to completely eliminate bacteria from the operative setting, but a combination of higher bacterial loads, spinal implants, and postoperative hematomas can increase susceptibility to infection. Risk factors for infection can be subdivided into preoperative, intraoperative, and postoperative risk factors.

Preoperative risk factors for infection include a history of prior spine surgery or prior infections and lifestyle contributors such as obesity, smoking, and severe acne. Inappropriately timed administration of prophylactic antibiotics may also precipitate infection. Patients with a past medical history of hypothyroidism, cardiomyopathy, steroid use, immunosuppression, sickle cell disease, and immune thrombocytopenic purpura are also at increased risk of developing infections.

Intraoperatively, procedures that are staged or last longer than 5 hours have an increased risk of infection.

Blood loss is also a factor to be mindful of as blood loss greater than 80 mL/kg remains a risk factor. Details of the procedure itself such as the number of vertebrae fused (if >10), or the use of instrumentation and allografts are considered significant risk factors. Having more than two assistants participating in a procedure also increases the risk of infection.

Blood transfusions, lack of postoperative drains, wound contamination, or focal wound pressure confer the postoperative risk factors for infection.

Both laboratory tests and imaging are important in diagnosing postoperative infections. Specifically, C-reactive protein (CRP) levels are most sensitive in testing for acute infection along with erythrocyte sedimentation rate (ESR), and white blood cell count. The use of MRI can also be particularly helpful in detecting abscesses and diskitis/osteomyelitis. Typical clinical presentations for infection due to surgery include fever, wound drainage, erythema, increased pain, and new neurologic symptoms.

PRINCIPLES OF SURGICAL MANAGEMENT

History and Physical Examination

Patient history and physical examination are key elements for informing surgical decision-making, particularly in cases of cervical revision. History taking should focus on questions relating to the index procedure while a complete examination should include wound assessment, range-of-motion testing, and a full neurological evaluation. The nature and characteristics of symptoms prior to and following index surgery may shed light on whether the initial problem was appropriately treated or if symptoms may be due to recurrence of the disease. The evaluation should also exclude the possibility of the occurrence of an entirely different disease entity in order to avoid unnecessary operations.

Patient complaints indicating myelopathy and/or radiculopathy following earlier improvement in these symptoms after the index procedure may suggest the development of pseudarthrosis, ASD, or progressive deformity such as postlaminectomy kyphosis. With progressive kyphosis, patients may also present with muscular fatigue, neck pain, difficulty with maintaining horizontal gaze or pronounced sagittal kyphosis with head leaning forward.[40] Patients with pseudarthrosis or nonunion of the fusion site, on the other hand, are only symptomatic two-thirds of the time,[8] but when symptomatic, their symptoms often manifest as axial neck pain and radiculopathy symptoms.

Imaging

While history and examination are instrumental in guiding further assessment of potential revision surgery, imaging is critical to diagnosis and surgical decision-making. Among imaging modalities, radiographic plain films, CT, and MRI are most widely used to further assess concrete parameters that may be helpful in identifying pertinent pathoanatomical features.

Plain radiographs are often the first-line agent for evaluating deformity or changes to the spinal anatomy. If progressive deformity is suspected following index procedure, plain radiographs can be used to assess parameters such as coronal and sagittal malalignment, the presence of fixed versus flexible deformity, and static versus dynamic changes of the bony spine anatomy. Spondylosis or disk degeneration, which may be seen in cases of ASD, are well evaluated with radiographic plain films which can detect disk space narrowing, endplate sclerosis, and osteophyte formation.

For thoracolumbar adult spinal deformity, the initial imaging evaluation generally begins with lateral 36-inch X-rays to provide an assessment of global and regional spinopelvic alignment.[66,67] It is critical to also assess the cervical spine using these films as compensatory mechanism may be occurring. Primary cervical deformity may induce a secondary thoracolumbar deformity as a compensatory mechanism to maintain horizontal gaze.[68,69] Similarly, the converse may occur in the cervical spine as a result of thoracolumbar deformity.[68,69] In order to evaluate the effect of cervical alignment in relation to the overall alignment of the spine it is very helpful to obtain 36-inch radiographs.

While plain film radiography has traditionally been the default method for assessing bony anatomy, CT has been shown to be superior in its sensitivity and ability to diagnose spinal fractures.[62] For detailed inspection of bony structures and instrumentation of the spine, CT is the imaging modality of choice. In suspected pseudarthrosis, instrumentation failure or migration can be captured by CT scans. CT scans can also be important for detecting ankylosis, as might be present in cases of progressive deformity, or gauging the adequacy of decompression, which may be insufficient in same-segment disease. Especially for cases requiring deformity correction, surgeons will often use CT for surgical planning purposes.

Magnetic resonance imaging is often complementary to CT scans, providing the most useful evaluation of soft

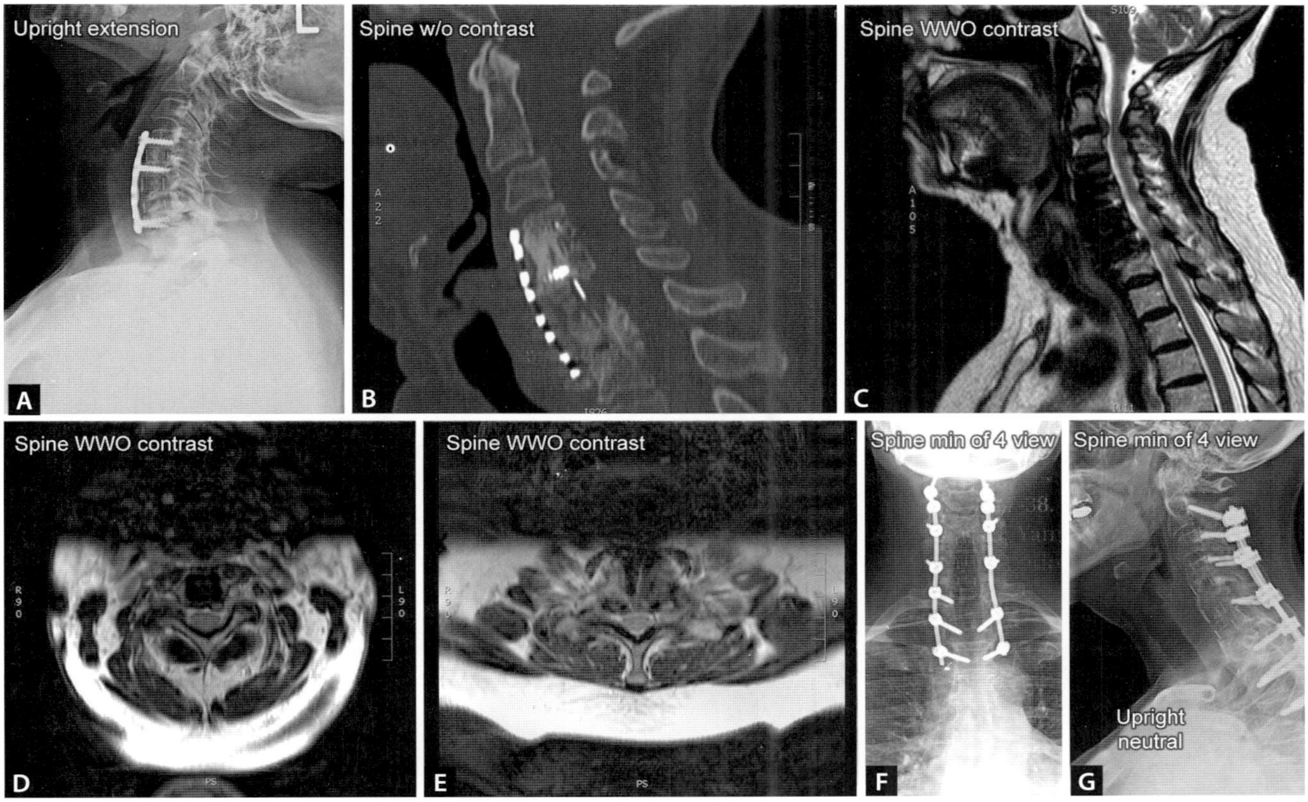

Figs. 1A to G: Pseudarthrosis and adjacent segment stenosis. (A) Lateral radiograph of a 63-year-old female psychologist that had undergone diskectomy at C4–5 and corpectomy of C6 with anterior fusion from C4 to C7 2 years prior. Although she had had early relief of myelopathic symptoms she had developed progressive cervical and radicular arm pain due to recurrent stenosis; (B) Computed tomography (CT) scan shows solid fusion at C4–5 but nonunion within the cage from C5 to C7. In addition, there is profound degeneration of the C7–T1 disk, potentially related to the inferior position of the anterior plate and screws; (C) Magnetic resonance imaging (MRI) shows recurrent stenosis at C2–3 and C7–T1, both of which correlated with anatomic pain distribution; (D) Large left-sided herniation is present at C2–3; (E) Central and lateral stenosis at C7–T1 adjacent to inferior hardware; (F and G) 2 years following revision hardware removal and diskectomy at C7–T1 along with posterior decompression of C2–3 and C7–T1 with fusion from C2 to T3, the patient had returned to her practice and was essentially pain free.
(w/o: without contrast; WWO: with and without contrast)

tissues. Cord compression, atrophy of the spinal cord, and syringomyelia are among the common neurologic conditions potentially implicating revision surgery in which MRI can be beneficial. Disk extrusion and infections are also best imaged with MRI. Same segment disease and progressive deformity can often manifest with neurological symptoms that may necessitate further imaging with MRI.

Preoperative Planning and Considerations

Revision surgery is often more technically complicated than the original procedure. Dissection through scar tissue can be challenging, and considerations should be taken regarding complications that may arise based on the selected approach. General principles to keep in mind during preoperative planning are to avoid the approach of the original operation and to avoid prior areas of cord exposure if possible. Voice evaluation should be obtained before revision anterior surgery as damage to the recurrent laryngeal nerve and dysphagia may be complications during anterior approaches.[70] An ENT surgeon may be enlisted to assist if an esophageal injury is suspected. If posterior wound infection or dehiscence has occurred, then a plastic surgeon may be helpful in definitive wound management.

Pseudarthrosis

Treatment of pseudarthrosis does not always require revision surgery, even if symptomatic. Revision surgery is indicated for patients who demonstrate radiculopathy or myelopathy, have evidence of unstable or failed hardware, or remain severely symptomatic with regard to neck pain despite extended conservative treatment.[71]

Pseudarthrosis can manifest either anteriorly or posteriorly, the former of which is more common. Posterior pseudarthrosis is often more complicated due to the risk of durotomy during surgical dissection if a prior laminectomy has been performed. Approaches for posterior pseudarthrosis, whether dorsal, ventral, or circumferential, depend to a large degree on the biomechanical stability required.[1]

Anterior pseudarthrosis has been successfully repaired with both anterior and posterior approaches. However, a number of studies have shown that despite an increased blood loss and longer recovery time, posterior approaches do demonstrate higher fusion rates than anterior approaches.[72-74] Posterior approaches also have the additional advantage of avoiding the risk of dissection through anterior scar tissue.[72]

Adjacent Segment Disease

Adjacent segment disease has long been a topic of controversy. More research has investigated methods to prevent ASD rather than treatment of ASD. Motion-sparing techniques such as posterior laminoforaminotomy and devices such as cervical disk replacement have been advocated over ACDF to prevent ASD, but evidence remains equivocal regarding which technique yields better outcomes.[63,75-77]

Regardless of the cause of ASD, surgical management of ASD usually requires further fusion.[78] While ACDF is perhaps the more common surgical technique employed, patients undergoing corpectomy for ASD may have improved outcomes compared to those receiving ACDF.[79,80]

Total disk replacement (TDR) has also been employed as a strategy to revise ASD. In fact, health-related outcome measures such as visual analog pain scale (VAS), neck disability index (NDI), and Oswestry disability index (ODI) have been shown to not only be comparable to ACDF for ASD revision but also improve following TDR for ASD revision.[81-83] The combination of TDR and fusion has also been suggested as a possible effective means for revision surgery for ASD based on biomechanical evidence.[84] Patients should be informed that combination approaches remain experimental at this time.

Posterior decompression and fusion approaches are less well-recognized for treatment of ASD but are nonetheless advocated by some surgeons. The specific method of open-door laminoplasty has been suggested for patients with myelopathy and preserved lordosis as the approach also avoids high risk from the initial anterior cervical surgery.[59,61,85]

Anecdotally, the approach for ASD revision surgery also depends to some degree on the number of fusion segments indicated. Specifically, an isolated anterior approach may be preferred for shorter segments while a combined anterior-posterior or posterior approach can be employed for patients with three or more disk levels of involvement, kyphosis, or pronounced instability. Revision may be approached through the same incision site as the index ACDF procedure for single-level ASD. However, combined anterior-posterior approaches have a high complication rate with dysphagia and airway edema requiring intubation being the most common.[86] In an attempt to combat the airway complications of combined anterior-posterior approaches, Hart and colleagues developed a fluid management protocol that reduced the incidence of prolonged intubation and reintubation.[87] The protocol consisted of limiting crystalloid fluid resuscitation intraoperatively with maintenance of blood pressure with vasopressors.[87] When planning for a combined anterior-posterior procedure, one may consider using this protocol to reduce the risk of reintubation.

Postlaminectomy Kyphosis

Postoperative deformity, most frequently manifested as postlaminectomy kyphosis, is the most common etiology of cervical spine deformity.[5,40,88] In biomechanical terms, the cervical spine relies on the lordotic curvature to distribute most of the load posteriorly. Following laminectomy, during which the posterior neural arch is removed, significant loss of stability can result. The shift from posterior to anterior column load bearing over time not only leads to muscular fatigue in order to maintain an upright posture but eventual cervical kyphosis and sagittal malalignment. The goals of surgical management are to simultaneously correct deformity and achieve decompression while preserving neurologic function and long-term stability through arthrodesis.

For rigid deformities, preoperative traction may be helpful in preparing for deformity correction and

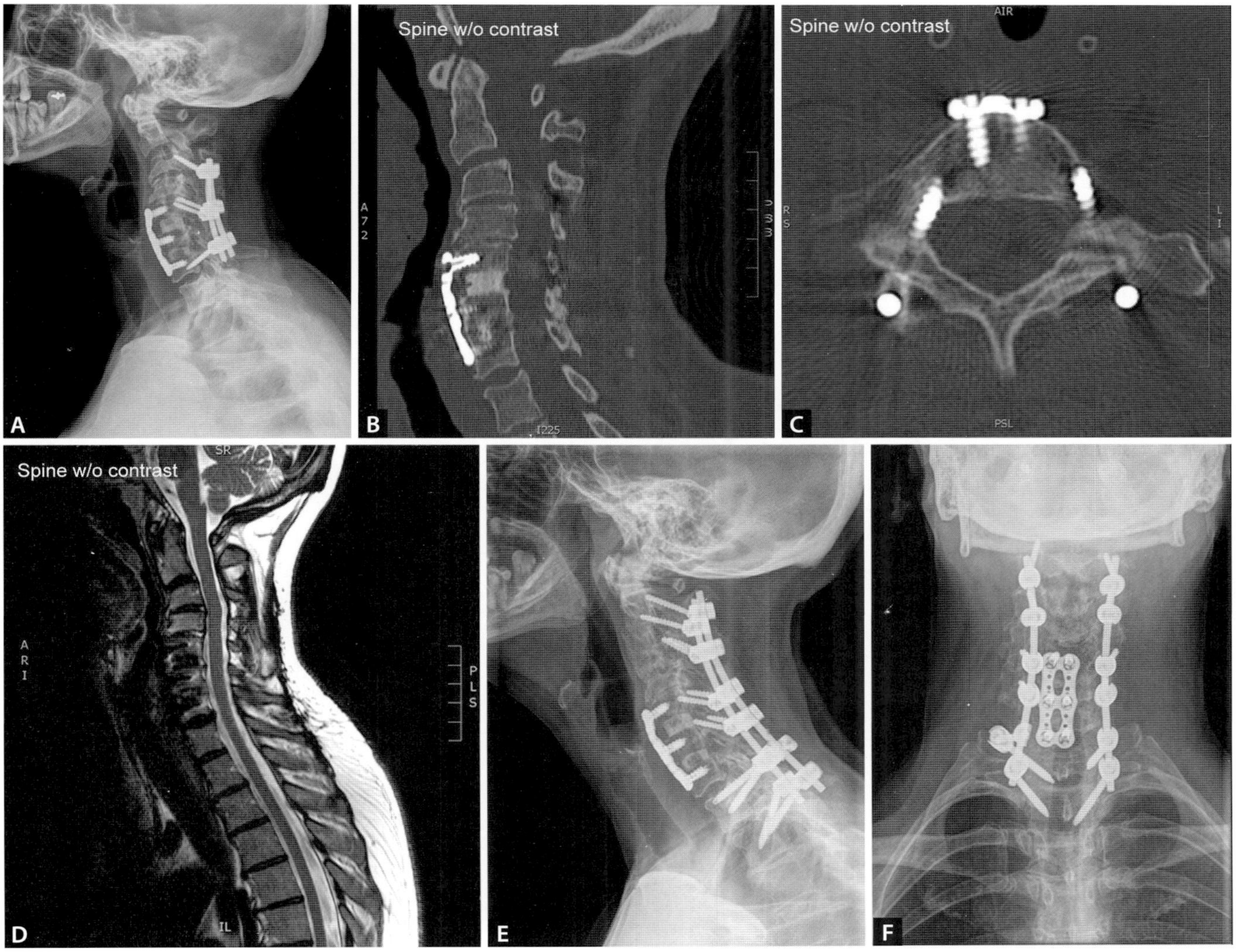

Figs. 2A to F: Postoperative kyphosis and hardware malposition. (A) A 53-year-old woman status post anterior and second posterior spinal fusion from C3 to C7. Symptoms include shoulder and neck pain, as well as persistent right arm C8 radiculopathy; (B) CT shows solid fusion with significant kyphosis from C2 to C4; (C) Inferior and medial C7 pedicle screw may explain persistent radiculopathy; (D) MRI shows flattening of the cord over the kyphosis at C3–4; (E) Lateral and anteroposterior (AP, F) views 2 years after anterior corpectomy of C3 with posterior facet-based osteotomies at C2–3 and C3–4. Right C7–T1 foraminotomy was also performed after screw removal. Solid fusion in much better alignment was obtained from C2 to T2. Though the patient did complain about the impact of cervical stiffness, preoperative symptoms were much improved. (w/o: without contrast)

determining levels to treat.[56] The determination of fixed versus flexible deformity is important when selecting a surgical approach, which can vary from posterior-only, anterior-only, combined anterior-posterior, or even posterior-anterior-posterior. In flexible deformity in which patients are able to correct to passively neutral, anterior- or posterior-only approaches may be suitable. If ventral decompression is not necessary in a patient with a flexible deformity, a posterior arthrodesis with lateral mass and pedicle instrumentation often results in good outcomes.[1]

In instances of fixed deformity in which patients must be extended intraoperatively to obtain a neutral position, it is important to prevent iatrogenic compression of the nerve roots by performing additional laminoforaminotomies. Anterior approaches with interbody spacers whether through ACDF or corpectomies may be necessary to

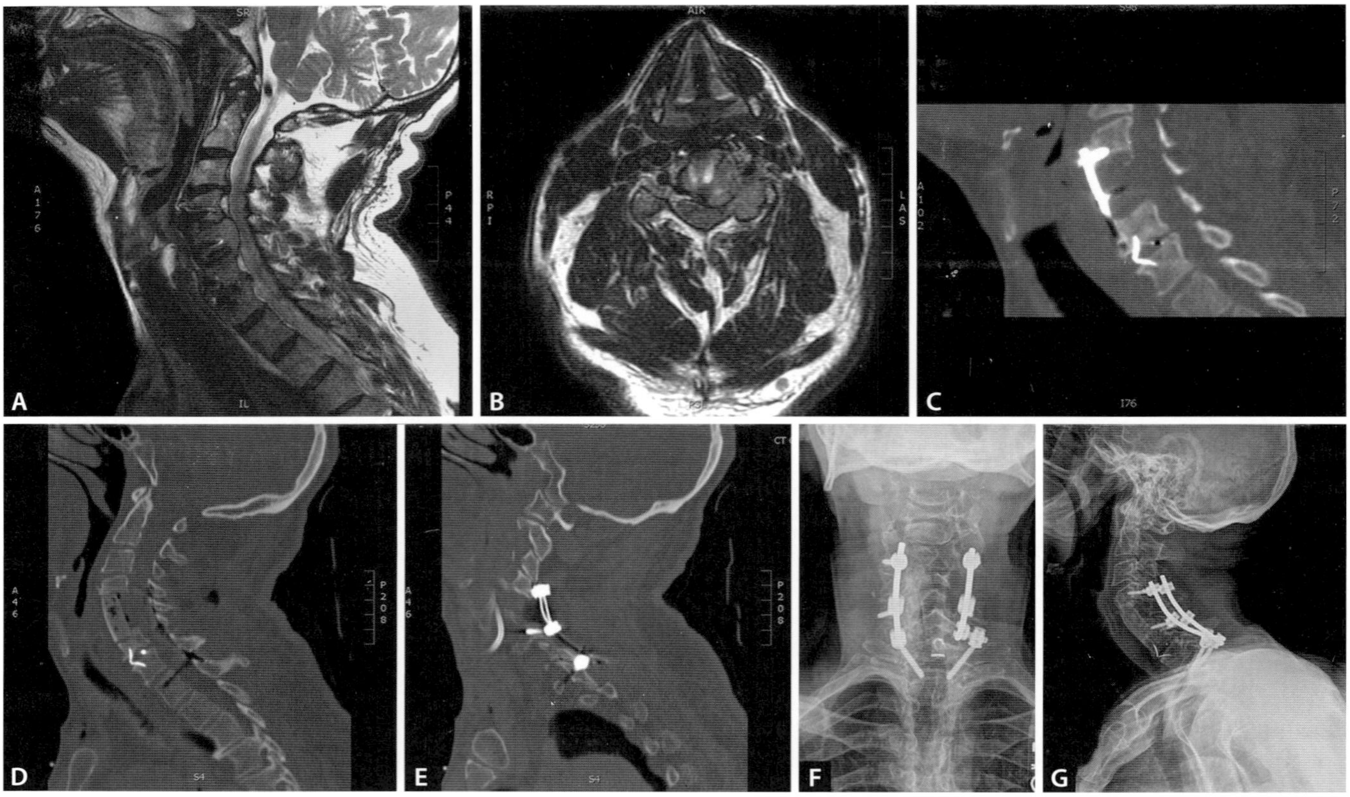

Figs. 3A to G: Misdiagnosis and incomplete tumor resection. (A) A 65-year-old man with metastatic gastrointestinal (GI) tumor. He had undergone anterior cervical discectomy and fusion (ACDF) at C6–7 2 years after an initial 2 level ACDF from C4 to C6. No updated preoperative imaging was obtained based on the assumption of adjacent segment stenosis. Examination was remarkable for profound weakness in left deltoid. Magnetic resonance imaging (MRI) was obtained at 6 weeks postoperatively when symptoms failed to improve; (B) Marked stenosis of the C4–5 foramen and recess due to metastatic involvement of vertebral body and lateral mass; (C) CT shows the extent of bony erosion at the vertebral body of C4; (D) The patient underwent removal of the anterior locking plate and vertebrectomy of C4. The lateral mass on the left was completely resected exposing the vertebral artery and the C5 nerve root; (E) Lateral CT image shows posterior resection of the C4 lateral mass as well; (F and G) One year postoperatively, the patient was pain-free and had recovered functional activity in left deltoid with ability to perform overhead activities with the left hand.

restore the natural lordotic curvature of the cervical spine with a correction as great as 20°.[89] Some have advocated anterior-only approaches regardless of fixed or flexible deformity as it addresses aspects of stiff cervical kyphosis for which a posterior-only approach may be insufficient.[60]

When multiple segments of cervical kyphosis are involved, combined anterior-posterior approaches are recommended with multilevel ACDF preferred over corpectomy. The greater number of fixation points in ACDF allows for a greater ability to achieve lordosis that may ultimately decrease the likelihood of graft dislodgement.[40,56,90] Prevention of graft dislodgement is also a benefit of multilevel ACDF as opposed to corpectomy. Incidences of graft-related complications as high as 82% have also been seen in corpectomy with struts.[60]

Same-Segment Disease

Surgical management for inadequate decompression, a frequent cause of same-segment disease, is largely dependent on the structures causing persistent or recurrent neurologic compression, along with the alignment of the cervical spine. For anterior compression of one or two levels in the presence of cervical kyphosis, ACDF can be employed with good outcomes. For anterior compression greater than two levels, both multilevel ACDF and corpectomies have been advocated, as previously discussed. The advantages of ACDF include greater biomechanical stability and increased lordosis, but ACDF also comes with a higher risk of pseudarthrosis up to 47–56%.[9,14,91] Corpectomies spanning multiple levels have higher fusion rates of 86–99% relative to ACDF, but also a higher rate of graft dislodgement for which simultaneous posterior fixation is also advised.[92,93]

For anterior compression without cervical kyphosis, surgical management may depend on the presence or absence of instability and/or axial neck pain. If instability or severe neck pain is present, laminectomy with fusion is typically a better choice. Without such issues, laminoplasty with or without foraminotomies may be successfully performed. Both these approaches have yielded excellent outcomes more than 90% of the time.[94,95]

Adequate decompression of neurological elements remains critical for successful surgical management regardless of whether minimally invasive and motion-sparing techniques are employed. Posterior osteophytes are an important factor to consider for decompression in those undergoing cervical disk replacement.[57,96] Because cervical disk replacement aims at preserving motion, recurrence or persistence of osteophytes, and cord compression can be seen in the same segment if not adequately addressed at the index surgery.

Since instrumentation failure is often a concern in same-segment disease, CT myelography can be beneficial in diagnosis. Especially for multisegment corpectomy constructs, adding posterior instrumentation can reduce rates of pseudarthrosis and graft dislodgement. Revision surgery is not always necessary for instrumentation failure if there is limited pain without neurologic compression and positioning remains satisfactory. Sometimes, a halo vest and continued observation are sufficient. However, when significant displacement of instrumentation or subsequent development of kyphosis is observed, revision surgery is mandated.[97]

Infection

When an infection is suspected due to clinical, laboratory, and imaging evidence, reoperation may be indicated for irrigation and drainage. More often than not, removal of instrumentation is not indicated unless loosening is detected upon irrigation and drainage. In fact, it is generally recommended to attempt preservation of instrumentation if as possible even with postoperative infection in order to obtain solid fusion and prevent future occurrence of cervical spine instability.

The main goal of surgical management for infection is to achieve healthy, definitive closure of wound which may require multiple rounds of irrigation and debridements. Vacuum-assisted closure may also be used to achieve definitive wound management.

Immediate commencement of broad-spectrum antibiotic therapy is typical, with narrowing based on intraoperative cultures and consultation with infectious disease specialists. Specifically for cervical spine procedures, 6–9 weeks of intravenous antibiotics with a longer course of oral antibiotics is often the typical regimen. In order to ensure proper resolution of infection, laboratory work including CRP and ESR levels should be followed-up. Infection of an anterior cervical wound should prompt consideration of possible esophageal injury.

OUTCOMES

Revision cervical spine surgery is complicated, technically demanding, and poses an increased risk to the patients. There are higher rates of recurrent laryngeal nerve palsy, airway complications, esophageal problems, nonunion, wound problems, and overall lower clinical success with revision surgery. Furthermore, perioperative complications are frequent but most are minor and have a limited effect on clinical outcomes. Despite these complications and increased risk, there are many reports of positive outcomes for revision cervical spine surgery.

Pseudarthrosis

As mentioned above, pseudarthrosis is one of the more common indications for revision of cervical spine surgery. A number of studies have specifically investigated repair of nonunion in the cervical spine with various techniques and outcomes.[4,72,78,82,98-101] In general, anterior revision techniques generally have lower blood loss and shorter hospital stays, however, they are associated with lower fusion rates than posterior procedures.[72,82] It is therefore generally accepted that posterior fusion procedures have better fusion rates than attempting another anterior revision fusion.[72,82,99,100] Furthermore, when fixating the spine posteriorly, the use of dual rods or domino connectors have been shown to be stronger than a single 3.5 mm rod.[102]

Prior to revision anterior approaches, a vocal fold evaluation should be obtained. Lowery et al.[82] reported a case series of 44 patients with a mean follow-up of 28 months that underwent revision cervical spine surgery for

CHAPTER 27

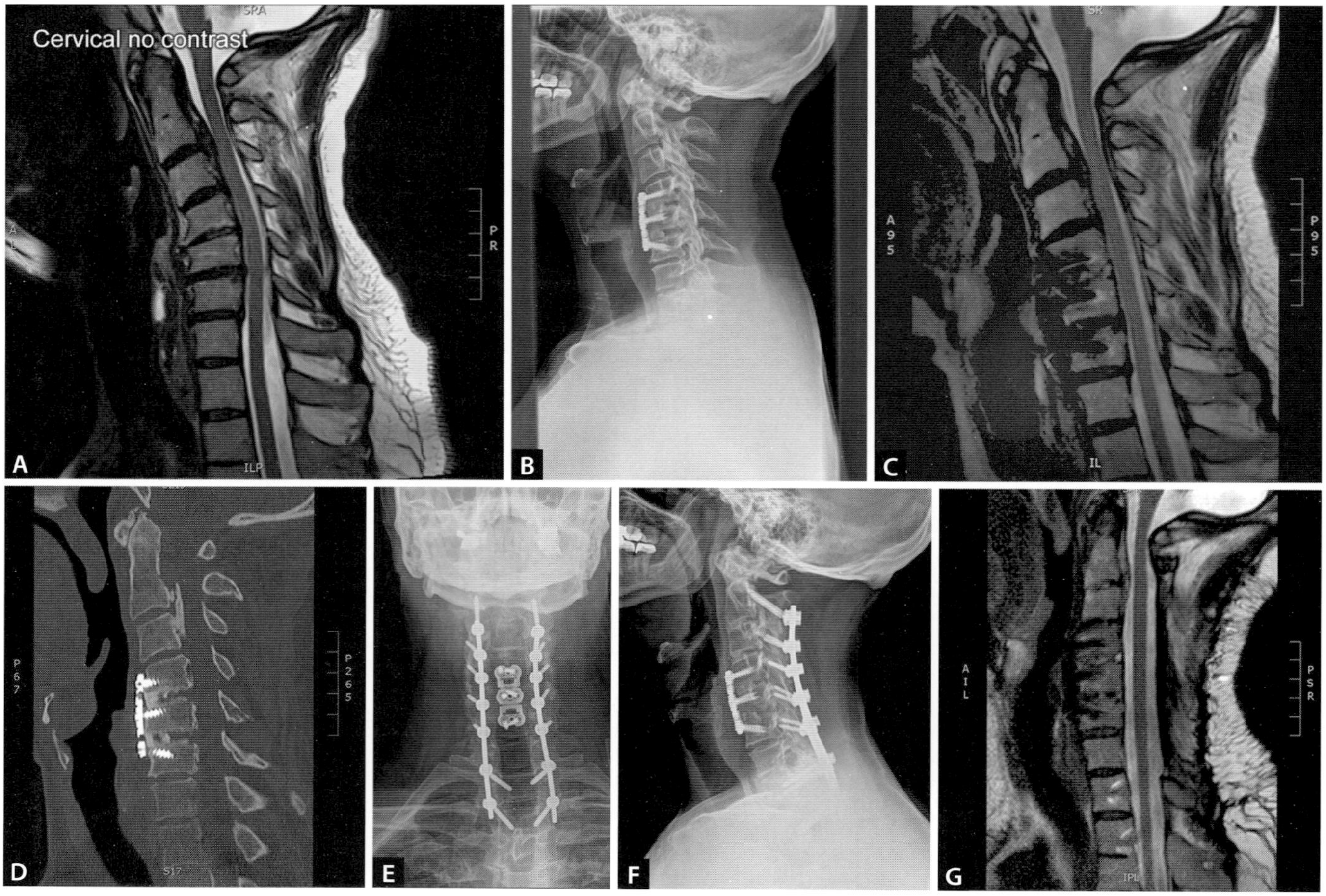

Figs. 4A to G: Incomplete decompression. (A) A 46-year-old man of Eskimo heritage was treated in Alaska for cervical myelopathy; (B) At 8 months postoperatively from 2 level, anterior cervical discectomy and fusion (ACDF) symptoms of numbness and clumsiness in the hands have not resolved; (C) Magnetic resonance imaging (MRI) demonstrates persistent stenosis and cord flattening behind the body of C3; (D) Computed tomography (CT) scan demonstrates solid fusion but severe canal stenosis due to persistent ossification of the posterior longitudinal ligament; (E and F) 2 years s/p ACDF of C2–3 and C3–4 with laminectomy from C2 to C7 and fusion from C2 to T2 patients myelopathy symptoms have completely resolved. Diskectomies did not include resection of the posterior longitudinal ligament (PLL) in order to avoid potential dural fistula. Fusion was chosen over laminoplasty due to significant axial neck pain and kyphosis from C2 to C4; (G) MRI at 4 years postoperatively demonstrates complete decompression of the spinal cord with correction of preoperative kyphosis and solid fusion.

symptomatic anterior pseudarthrosis by means of anterior surgery for 20 patients, posterior for 17, and combined for 7. The anterior surgery consisted of an incision through the previous incision, resection of the nonunion, and regrafting with anterior cervical plating. The posterior group had a posterior midline incision with fixation using lateral mass plating as a supplement to facet fusion. All the patients that received combined procedure and 16/17 patients that received the posterior procedure achieved a solid fusion at most recent follow-up.[82] A solid fusion was obtained in only 45% of the patients in the anterior group.[82]

Carreon et al.[72] specifically compared anterior and posterior fusions for the treatment of anterior cervical pseudarthrosis in 120 patients; 27 anterior and 93 posterior. The anterior group had the nonunion resected anteriorly followed by fusion with iliac crest graft while the posterior group underwent posterior wiring, lateral mass plates, and multiaxial screw/rod systems. Both procedures had similar operative times, however, the posterior group had larger blood loss, longer hospital stays, and a higher complication rate than the anterior group.[72] Despite the increase in complications for the posterior group, these patients had significantly fewer nonunions (2%) than the anterior group (44%).[72]

Kuhns et al.[99] retrospectively studied 33 patients with pseudarthrosis following ACDF and treated them with selective nerve root decompression and posterior fusion using iliac crest or local bone graft as well as posterior wiring and/or lateral mass plating. The mean follow-up was 46 months and all the patients had a solid fusion and substantial improvement in preoperative symptoms at their most recent follow-up.[99] About 72% of the patients were satisfied with their surgery and the location of the graft did not have an effect on the fusion status. This study further supports the concept of posterior fusion techniques having higher rates of fusion.

Despite these results, however, a few studies advocate for anterior fusion and report positive outcomes and fusion success.[98,101] Coric et al.[101] reported on 19 patients with pseudarthrosis following anterior cervical fusion that underwent revision with anterior cervical fusion and anterior plating. The previous nonunion was resected and an iliac allograft was used. The mean follow-up was 22.4 months and all patients demonstrated solid fusion at all levels and there were no intraoperative complications.[101] The authors report the procedure being safe and efficacious. Tribus et al.[98] investigated 16 patients with anterior pseudarthrosis that underwent anterior resection of the nonunion, autologous graft and anterior plating. 75% of the patients reported an improvement in their pain and 13/16 patients had a fusion graded as I or II.[98] These are small case series and do not compare directly to posterior procedures.

Adjacent Segment Disease

The primary techniques used to manage ASD following ACDF include repeat ACDF, anterior cervical corpectomy and fusion (ACCF), TDR, and posterior techniques such as laminectomies, laminoplasty, and laminoforaminotomy. Studies have reported on all of these techniques with varying success. Hilibrand et al.[80] retrospectively reviewed patients treated for ASD over 20 years in which they identified 38 patients treated with ACDF or corpectomy with strut grafting. Patients in either group improved equally clinically, however, the patients that received corpectomy had a higher rate of fusion than the repeat ACDF group.[80]

Chen et al.[63] recently investigated repeat ACDF for ASD in 63 patients in which the clinical symptoms significantly improved postoperatively and the clinical outcomes at 2-year follow-up were rated as excellent or good in 71.4% of the patients. Five patients developed dysphagia postoperatively and there were no implant failures at the 2-year follow-up period. The authors concluded that repeat ACDF is efficacious and does not adversely affect outcomes. Another recent study by O'Neill et al.[65] investigated the clinical outcomes of ACDF for ASD, and also included a cost analysis. The authors retrospectively reviewed 40 patients that underwent ACDF for ASD and found significant improvements in all clinical outcomes assessed including neck and arm pain, neck disability, physical and mental components of SF36, and the Zung depression score.[65] Furthermore, ACDF for the treatment of ASD was associated with a mean 2-year cost per quality-adjusted life year (QALY) gained of $ 60,526 suggesting surgery to be cost-effective.[65]

The use of disk arthroplasty in the management ASD has shown positive outcomes.[61,89,103,104] Sekhon et al.[89] reported on 15 patients who had prior cervical fusion and underwent TDR at adjacent levels. With a mean follow-up of 24.2 months, health related quality of life (HRQOL) scores significantly improved. One patient developed hypermobility with internal subluxation of the device; however, there was hypermobility at the site preoperatively. Overall, the patients did well and the authors concluded that the use of TDR in ASD is safe with good early clinical results.[89] Phillips et al.[61] prospectively investigated TDR in ASD and patients with primary radiculopathy and/or myelopathy across six different centers. One hundred fifty two patients were studied (26 ASD and 126 primary) and both groups had similar significant improvements in neck disability and neck and arm pain at 1 year postoperatively.[61] Revision was required for two patients in each of the groups. The authors concluded that TDR at adjacent levels to prior fusions are well-tolerated and offer similar clinical improvement to the outcomes after primary TDR.[61]

Finally, posterior techniques such as laminoplasty and laminectomy to address ASD have also been investigated.[74,84,105-107] Wang et al.[107] reported 24 cases in which the authors used laminoplasty for stenotic myelopathy following ACDF. Improvements in the myelopathy were observed in 83% of the patients.[107] Complications included two cases of C5 nerve root palsy and two cases of new-onset neck pain.[107] Matsumoto et al.[84] retrospectively reviewed 62 patients that underwent open-door expansive laminoplasty for ASD (31 patients) and primary myelopathy (31 patients). The mean recovery rate [difference in preoperative and postoperative Japanese Orthopedic Association (JOA) scores] in the patients who had ASD was significantly lower than the primary patients.[84] However, the mean JOA scores were statistically similar at final follow-up.

Laminectomy has also been reported to result in positive outcomes. Adogwa et al.[106] recently reported on a series of 50 patients that underwent laminectomy and extension of fusion for symptomatic ASD. The mean HRQOL scores were all significantly improved at 2 years postoperatively compared with preoperative values.[106] Adogwa and colleagues[105] expanded their previous study by investigating the cost per QALY gained from laminectomy and extended fusion for ASD. The authors found that posterior decompression and extension of the fusion for ASD resulted in a 2 year QALY gain of $ 62,995, very similar to costs for revision ACDF.

Postlaminectomy Kyphosis

As mentioned above, the primary goals are deformity correction and neural decompression when managing postsurgical cervical kyphosis. A number of studies have reported outcomes for an anterior approach.[56,57,90,93,108] Herman et al.[56] reported on a series of 20 patients treated for postlaminectomy kyphosis with anterior corpectomy, bone graft, and cervical plate. The mean preoperative kyphosis was 38° and at the final follow-up (mean 28 months), this was corrected to 16° of residual kyphosis with all patients having a solid fusion.[56] Steinmetz et al.[90] investigated 12 patients with iatrogenic cervical kyphosis treated by an anterior approach and plating. The authors achieved a mean kyphosis correction of 20° with a mean postoperative angle of 6° of lordosis, which at final follow-up was 2.2°.[90]

Park et al.[108] recently reported on 23 patients who underwent anterior reconstruction for postlaminectomy kyphosis treated with either multiple diskectomies and interbody fusions or a combination of diskectomies and corpectomies with a mean follow-up of 44.5 months. The mean preoperative kyphosis of 20° was corrected to a mean 14° of lordosis and maintained to 9.6° at final follow-up.[108] The authors also reported the HRQOL results including neck disability and VAS as well as the Nurick grades; all of which were significantly improved at final follow-up.[108] The complications included graft/implant displacement, dysphagia, wound infection, a dural tear, and pneumonia.

These procedures are not without significant complications. Riew et al.[109] specifically investigated the complications associated with anterior corpectomy and strut grafting for post-laminectomy kyphosis. The authors reported 18 patients in which 11 sustained 16 complications during the follow-up period of 2.7 years.[109] Four of the patients required a reoperations, five grafts extruded (three while in a halo vest), four developed pseudarthrosis, three patients had an increase in kyphosis compared with preoperative values by 10°, two had respiratory distress requiring reintubation, one had a small dural tear, and one had transient dysphagia.[109]

CONCLUSION

Cervical spine revision surgery is very complicated and it is of utmost importance to recognize the underlying problem and understand the failures of the initial procedure in order to guide management and avoid repeat revision. Thorough history-taking, physical examination, appropriate imaging, and other relevant studies should be employed when identifying the fundamental issues that necessitated revision. The indications for revision of cervical spine surgery are numerous and dictate the appropriate workup and management. The primary indications include pseudarthrosis, ASD, recurrent stenosis, postoperative deformity, and infection. Revision cervical spine surgery poses an increased risk to the patients. There are higher rates of recurrent laryngeal nerve palsy, airway complications, esophageal problems, nonunion, wound problems, and overall lower clinical success with revision surgery. Furthermore, perioperative complications are frequent but most are minor and have a limited effect on clinical outcomes. Despite these complications and increased risk, there are many reports of positive outcomes for revision cervical spine surgery.

REFERENCES

1. Rihn JA, Harrod C, Albert TJ. Revision cervical spine surgery. Orthop Clin North Am. 2012;43:123-36, ix-x.
2. Helgeson MD, Albert TJ. Surgery for failed cervical spine reconstruction. Spine. 2012;37:E323-7.
3. Liu G, Buchowski JM, Bunmaprasert T, et al. Revision surgery following cervical laminoplasty: etiology and treatment strategies. Spine. 2009;34:2760-8.
4. Newman M. The outcome of pseudarthrosis after cervical anterior fusion. Spine. 1993;18:2380-2.

5. Deutsch H, Haid RW, Rodts GE, et al. Postlaminectomy cervical deformity. Neurosurg Focus. 2003;15:E5.
6. Fang A, Hu SS, Endres N, et al. Risk factors for infection after spinal surgery. Spine. 2005;30:1460-5.
7. Ishihara H, Kanamori M, Kawaguchi Y, et al. Adjacent segment disease after anterior cervical interbody fusion. Spine J. 2004;4:624-8.
8. Bohlman HH, Emery SE, Goodfellow DB, et al. Robinson anterior cervical discectomy and arthrodesis for cervical radiculopathy. Long-term follow-up of one hundred and twenty-two patients. J Bone Joint Surg Am. 1993;75:1298-307.
9. Papadopoulos EC, Huang RC, Girardi FP, et al. Three-level anterior cervical discectomy and fusion with plate fixation: radiographic and clinical results. Spine. 2006;31:897-902.
10. Wang JC, McDonough PW, Endow KK, et al. Increased fusion rates with cervical plating for two-level anterior cervical discectomy and fusion. Spine. 2000;25:41-5.
11. Wang JC, McDonough PW, Kanim LE, et al. Increased fusion rates with cervical plating for three-level anterior cervical discectomy and fusion. Spine. 2001;26:643-6; discussion 6-7.
12. Hilibrand AS, Fye MA, Emery SE, et al. Impact of smoking on the outcome of anterior cervical arthrodesis with interbody or strut-grafting. J Bone Joint Surg Am. 2001;83(5):668-73.
13. Wang JC, McDonough PW, Endow K, et al. The effect of cervical plating on single-level anterior cervical discectomy and fusion. J Spinal Disord. 1999;12:467-71.
14. Bolesta MJ, Rechtine GR 2nd, Chrin AM. Three- and four-level anterior cervical discectomy and fusion with plate fixation: a prospective study. Spine. 2000;25(6):2040-4; discussion 5-6.
15. Phillips FM, Carlson G, Emery SE, et al. Anterior cervical pseudarthrosis. Natural history and treatment. Spine. 1997;22:1585-9.
16. Ploumis A, Mehbod A, Garvey T, et al. Prospective assessment of cervical fusion status: plain radiographs versus CT-scan. Acta Orthopaed Belgica. 2006;72:342-6.
17. Cannada LK, Scherping SC, Yoo JU, et al. Pseudoarthrosis of the cervical spine: a comparison of radiographic diagnostic measures. Spine. 2003;28:46-51.
18. Hilibrand AS, Robbins M. Adjacent segment degeneration and adjacent segment disease: the consequences of spinal fusion? Spine J. 2004;4:190S-4S.
19. Song KJ, Choi BW, Jeon TS, et al. Adjacent segment degenerative disease: is it due to disease progression or a fusion-associated phenomenon? Comparison between segments adjacent to the fused and non-fused segments. Eur Spine J. 2011;20:1940-5.
20. Rihn JA, Lawrence J, Gates C, et al. Adjacent segment disease after cervical spine fusion. Instr Course Lect. 2009;58:747-56.
21. Seo M, Choi D. Adjacent segment disease after fusion for cervical spondylosis; myth or reality? Br J Neurosurg. 2008;22:195-9.
22. Kepler CK, Hilibrand AS. Management of adjacent segment disease after cervical spinal fusion. Orthoped Clin North Am. 2012;43:53-62, viii.
23. Baba H, Furusawa N, Imura S, et al. Late radiographic findings after anterior cervical fusion for spondylotic myeloradiculopathy. Spine. 1993;18:2167-73.
24. Hilibrand AS, Carlson GD, Palumbo MA, et al. Radiculopathy and myelopathy at segments adjacent to the site of a previous anterior cervical arthrodesis. J Bone Joint Surg Am. 1999;81:519-28.
25. Javedan SP, Dickman CA. Cause of adjacent-segment disease after spinal fusion. Lancet. 1999;354:530-1.
26. Maldonado CV, Paz RD, Martin CB. Adjacent-level degeneration after cervical disc arthroplasty versus fusion. Eur Spine J. 2011;20(Suppl 3):403-7.
27. Eck JC, Humphreys SC, Lim TH, et al. Biomechanical study on the effect of cervical spine fusion on adjacent-level intradiscal pressure and segmental motion. Spine. 2002;27:2431-4.
28. Maiman DJ, Kumaresan S, Yoganandan N, et al. Biomechanical effect of anterior cervical spine fusion on adjacent segments. Biomed Mater Eng. 1999;9:27-38.
29. Matsunaga S, Kabayama S, Yamamoto T, et al. Strain on intervertebral discs after anterior cervical decompression and fusion. Spine. 1999;24:670-5.
30. Park DH Ramakrishnan P, Cho TH, et al. Effect of lower two-level anterior cervical fusion on the superior adjacent level. J Neurosurg Spine. 2007;7:336-40.
31. Prasarn ML, Baria D, Milne E, et al. Adjacent-level biomechanics after single versus multilevel cervical spine fusion. J Neurosurg Spine. 2012;16:172-7.
32. Ragab AA, Escarcega AJ, Zdeblick TA. A quantitative analysis of strain at adjacent segments after segmental immobilization of the cervical spine. J Spinal Disord Tech. 2006;19:407-10.
33. Schwab JS, Diangelo DJ, Foley KT. Motion compensation associated with single-level cervical fusion: where does the lost motion go? Spine. 2006;31:2439-48.
34. Pal GP, Sherk HH. The vertical stability of the cervical spine. Spine. 1988;13:447-9.
35. Djurasovic MO, Carreon LY, Glassman SD, et al. Sagittal alignment as a risk factor for adjacent level degeneration: a case-control study. Orthopedics. 2008;31:546.
36. Kumar MN, Baklanov A, Chopin D. Correlation between sagittal plane changes and adjacent segment degeneration following lumbar spine fusion. Eur Spine J. 2001;10:314-9.
37. Park P, Garton HJ, Gala VC, et al. Adjacent segment disease after lumbar or lumbosacral fusion: review of the literature. Spine. 2004;29:1938-44.
38. Rahm MD, Hall BB. Adjacent-segment degeneration after lumbar fusion with instrumentation: a retrospective study. J Spinal Disord. 1996;9:392-400.
39. Katsuura A, Hukuda S, Saruhashi Y, et al. Kyphotic malalignment after anterior cervical fusion is one of the factors promoting the degenerative process in adjacent intervertebral levels. Eur Spine J. 2001;10(4):320-4.
40. Albert TJ, Vacarro A. Postlaminectomy kyphosis. Spine. 1998;23:2738-45.

CHAPTER 27

41. Kaptain GJ, Simmons NE, Replogle RE, et al. Incidence and outcome of kyphotic deformity following laminectomy for cervical spondylotic myelopathy. J Neurosurg. 2000;93: 199-204.
42. Steinmetz MP, Stewart TJ, Kager CD, et al. Cervical deformity correction. Neurosurgery. 2007;60:S90-7.
43. Butler JC, Whitecloud TS 3rd. Postlaminectomy kyphosis. Causes and surgical management. Orthop Clin North Am. 1992;23(3):505-11.
44. O'Shaughnessy BA, Liu JC, Hsieh PC, et al. Surgical treatment of fixed cervical kyphosis with myelopathy. Spine. 2008;33:771-8.
45. Nowinski GP, Visarius H, Nolte LP, et al. A biomechanical comparison of cervical laminaplasty and cervical laminectomy with progressive facetectomy. Spine. 1993;18:1995-2004.
46. Zdeblick TA, Zou D, Warden KE, et al. Cervical stability after foraminotomy. A biomechanical in vitro analysis. J Bone Joint Surg Am. 1992;74:22-7.
47. Louis R. Spinal stability as defined by the three-column spine concept. Anat Clin. 1985;7:33-42.
48. Cattell HS, Clark GL, Jr. Cervical kyphosis and instability following multiple laminectomies in children. J Bone Joint Surg Am. 1967;49:713-20.
49. Lonstein JE. Post-laminectomy kyphosis. Clin Orthop Relat Res. 1977:93-100.
50. Yasuoka S, Peterson HA, MacCarty CS. Incidence of spinal column deformity after multilevel laminectomy in children and adults. J Neurosurg. 1982;57:441-5.
51. Shimizu K, Nakamura M, Nishikawa Y, et al. Spinal kyphosis causes demyelination and neuronal loss in the spinal cord: a new model of kyphotic deformity using juvenile Japanese small game fowls. Spine. 2005;30:2388-92.
52. Jarzem PF, Quance DR, Doyle DJ, et al. Spinal cord tissue pressure during spinal cord distraction in dogs. Spine. 1992;17:S227-34.
53. Tachibana S, Kitahara Y, Iida H, et al. Spinal cord intramedullary pressure. A possible factor in syrinx growth. Spine. 1994;19:2174-8; discussion 8-9.
54. Iida H, Tachibana S. Spinal cord intramedullary pressure: direct cord traction test. Neurol Med Chir. 1995;35:75-7.
55. Kitahara Y, Iida H, Tachibana S. Effect of spinal cord stretching due to head flexion on intramedullary pressure. Neurol Med Chir. 1995;35:285-8.
56. Herman JM, Sonntag VK. Cervical corpectomy and plate fixation for postlaminectomy kyphosis. J Neurosurg. 1994;80:963-70.
57. Stewart TJ, Steinmetz MP, Benzel EC. Techniques for the ventral correction of postsurgical cervical kyphotic deformity. Neurosurgery. 2005;56:191-5; discussion 5.
58. Elsawaf A, Mastronardi L, Roperto R, et al. Effect of cervical dynamics on adjacent segment degeneration after anterior cervical fusion with cages. Neurosurg Rev. 2009;32:215-24; discussion 24.
59. Gause PR, Davis RA, Smith PN, et al. Success of junctional anterior cervical discectomy and fusion. Spine J. 2008;8:723-8.
60. Shin DA, Yi S, Yoon do H, et al. Artificial disc replacement combined with fusion versus two-level fusion in cervical two-level disc disease. Spine. 2009;34:1153-9; discussion 60-1.
61. Phillips FM, Allen TR, Regan JJ, et al. Cervical disc replacement in patients with and without previous adjacent level fusion surgery: a prospective study. Spine. 2009;34:556-65.
62. Arnold P, Boswell S, McMahon J. Threaded interbody fusion cage for adjacent segment degenerative disease after previous anterior cervical fusion. Surg Neurol. 2008;70:390-7.
63. Chen Y, He Z, Yang H, et al. Anterior cervical diskectomy and fusion for adjacent segment disease. Orthopedics. 2013;36:e501-8.
64. Acikbas SC, Ermol C, Akyuz M, et al. Assessment of adjacent segment degeneration in and between patients treated with anterior or posterior cervical simple discectomy. Turkish Neurosurg. 2010;20:334-40.
65. O'Neill KR, Wilson RJ, Burns KM, et al. Anterior cervical discectomy and fusion for adjacent-segment disease: clinical outcomes and cost-utility of surgical intervention. Clin Spine Surg. 2016;29(6):234-41.
66. Angevine PD, Kaiser MG. Radiographic measurement techniques. Neurosurgery. 2008;63:40-5.
67. Smith JS, Shaffrey CI, Fu KM, et al. Clinical and radiographic evaluation of the adult spinal deformity patient. Neurosurg Clin N Am. 2013;24:143-56.
68. Scheer JK, Tang JA, Smith JS, et al. Cervical spine alignment, sagittal deformity, and clinical implications: a review. J Neurosurg Spine. 2013;19(2):141-59.
69. Ames CP, Smith JS, Scheer JK, et al. Impact of spinopelvic alignment on decision making in deformity surgery in adults: a review. J Neurosurg Spine. 2012;16:547-64.
70. Apfelbaum RI, Kriskovich MD, Haller JR. On the incidence, cause, and prevention of recurrent laryngeal nerve palsies during anterior cervical spine surgery. Spine. 2000;25: 2906-12.
71. Boakye M, Patil CG, Ho C, et al. Cervical corpectomy: complications and outcomes. Neurosurgery. 2008;63:295-301; discussion 2.
72. Carreon L, Glassman SD, Campbell MJ. Treatment of anterior cervical pseudoarthrosis: posterior fusion versus anterior revision. Spine J. 2006;6:154-6.
73. Brown CV, Antevil JL, Sise MJ, et al. Spiral computed tomography for the diagnosis of cervical, thoracic, and lumbar spine fractures: its time has come. J Trauma. 2005;58:890-5; discussion 5-6.
74. Baba H, Furusawa N, Imura S, et al. Laminoplasty following anterior cervical fusion for spondylotic myeloradiculopathy. Int Orthop. 1994;18:1-5.
75. Clarke MJ, Ecker RD, Krauss WE, et al. Same-segment and adjacent-segment disease following posterior cervical foraminotomy. J Neurosurg Spine. 2007;6:5-9.
76. Cho SK, Riew KD. Adjacent segment disease following cervical spine surgery. J Am Acad Orthopaed Surg. 2013;21:3-11.
77. Cunningham BW, Hu N, Zorn CM, et al. Biomechanical comparison of single- and two-level cervical arthroplasty versus arthrodesis: effect on adjacent-level spinal kinematics. Spine J. 2010;10:341-9.

78. Farey ID, McAfee PC, Davis RF, et al. Pseudarthrosis of the cervical spine after anterior arthrodesis. Treatment by posterior nerve-root decompression, stabilization, and arthrodesis. J Bone Joint Surg Am. 1990;72(8):1171-7.
79. Herkowitz HN, Kurz LT, Overholt DP. Surgical management of cervical soft disc herniation. A comparison between the anterior and posterior approach. Spine. 1990;15:1026-30.
80. Hilibrand AS, Yoo JU, Carlson GD, et al. The success of anterior cervical arthrodesis adjacent to a previous fusion. Spine. 1997;22:1574-9.
81. Liu Y, Chen L, Gu Y, et al. [Open-door laminoplasty for the treatment of failed anterior cervical spine surgery]. Zhonghua Wai Ke Za Zhi [Chin J Surg.]. 2010;48(24):1859-63.
82. Lowery GL, Swank ML, McDonough RF. Surgical revision for failed anterior cervical fusions. Articular pillar plating or anterior revision? Spine. 1995;20:2436-41.
83. Lunsford LD, Bissonette DJ, Jannetta PJ, et al. Anterior surgery for cervical disc disease. Part 1: Treatment of lateral cervical disc herniation in 253 cases. J Neurosurg. 1980;53:1-11.
84. Matsumoto M, Nojiri K, Chiba K, et al. Open-door laminoplasty for cervical myelopathy resulting from adjacent-segment disease in patients with previous anterior cervical decompression and fusion. Spine. 2006;31:1332-7.
85. Mikhael MM, Celestre PC, Wolf CF, et al. Minimally invasive cervical spine foraminotomy and lateral mass screw placement. Spine. 2012;37:E318-22.
86. Hart RA, Tatsumi RL, Hiratzka JR, et al. Perioperative complications of combined anterior and posterior cervical decompression and fusion crossing the cervico-thoracic junction. Spine. 2008;33:2887-91.
87. Hart RA, Dupaix JP, Rusa R, et al. Reduction of airway complications with fluid management protocol in patients undergoing cervical decompression and fusion across the cervico-thoracic junction. Spine (Phila Pa 1976). 2013;38(18):E1135-40.
88. Uchida K, Nakajima H, Sato R, et al. Cervical spondylotic myelopathy associated with kyphosis or sagittal sigmoid alignment: outcome after anterior or posterior decompression. J Neurosurg Spine. 2009;11:521-8.
89. Sekhon LH, Sears W, Duggal N. Cervical arthroplasty after previous surgery: results of treating 24 discs in 15 patients. J Neurosurg Spine, 2005;3:335-41.
90. Steinmetz MP, Kager CD, Benzel EC. Ventral correction of postsurgical cervical kyphosis. J Neurosurg. 2003;98:1-7.
91. Emery SE, Bohlman HH, Bolesta MJ, et al. Anterior cervical decompression and arthrodesis for the treatment of cervical spondylotic myelopathy. Two to seventeen-year follow-up. J Bone Joint Surg Am. 1998;80:941-51.
92. Vaccaro AR, Falatyn SP, Scuderi GJ, et al. Early failure of long segment anterior cervical plate fixation. J Spinal Disord. 1998;11:410-5.
93. Zdeblick TA, Hughes SS, Riew KD, et al. Failed anterior cervical discectomy and arthrodesis. Analysis and treatment of thirty-five patients. J Bone Joint Surg Am. 1997;79:523-32.
94. Herkowitz HN. A comparison of anterior cervical fusion, cervical laminectomy, and cervical laminoplasty for the surgical management of multiple level spondylotic radiculopathy. Spine. 1988;13:774-80.
95. Herkowitz HN. Cervical laminaplasty: its role in the treatment of cervical radiculopathy. J Spinal Disord. 1988;1:179-88.
96. Anderson PA, Sasso RC, Riew KD. Update on cervical artificial disk replacement. Instr Course Lect. 2007;56:237-45.
97. Thongtrangan I, Balabhadra RS, Kim DH. Management of strut graft failure in anterior cervical spine surgery. Neurosurg Focus. 2003;15:E4.
98. Tribus CB, Corteen DP, Zdeblick TA. The efficacy of anterior cervical plating in the management of symptomatic pseudoarthrosis of the cervical spine. Spine. 1999;24:860-4.
99. Kuhns CA, Geck MJ, Wang JC, et al. An outcomes analysis of the treatment of cervical pseudarthrosis with posterior fusion. Spine. 2005;30:2424-9.
100. Brodsky AE, Khalil MA, Sassard WR, et al. Repair of symptomatic pseudoarthrosis of anterior cervical fusion. Posterior versus anterior repair. Spine. 1992;17:1137-43.
101. Coric D, Branch CL Jr, Jenkins JD. Revision of anterior cervical pseudoarthrosis with anterior allograft fusion and plating. J Neurosurg. 1997;86:969-74.
102. Tatsumi RL, Yoo JU, Liu Q, et al. Mechanical comparison of posterior instrumentation constructs for spinal fixation across the cervicothoracic junction. Spine. 2007;32:1072-6.
103. Mobbs RJ, Mehan N, Khong P. Cervical arthroplasty for myelopathy adjacent to previous multisegmental fusion. J Clin Neurosci. 2009;16:150-2.
104. Sekhon L. Cervicothoracic junction arthroplasty after previous fusion surgery for adjacent segment degeneration: case report. Neurosurgery. 2005;56:E205; discussion E.
105. Adogwa O, Parker SL, Shau DN, et al. Cost per quality-adjusted life year gained of laminectomy and extension of instrumented fusion for adjacent-segment disease: defining the value of surgical intervention. J Neurosurg Spine. 2012;16:141-6.
106. Adogwa O, Parker SL, Mendenhall SK, et al. Laminectomy and extension of instrumented fusion improves 2-year pain, disability, and quality of life in patients with adjacent segment disease: defining the long-term effectiveness of surgery. World Neurosurg. 2013;80(6):893-6.
107. Wang MY, Green BA. Laminoplasty for the treatment of failed anterior cervical spine surgery. Neurosurg Focus. 2003;15:E7.
108. Park Y, Riew KD, Cho W. The long-term results of anterior surgical reconstruction in patients with postlaminectomy cervical kyphosis. Spine J. 2010;10:380-7.
109. Riew KD, Hilibrand AS, Palumbo MA, et al. Anterior cervical corpectomy in patients previously managed with a laminectomy: short-term complications. J Bone Joint Surg Am. 1999;81:950-7.

CHAPTER 28

Current Concepts and Evidence in Cervical Spinal Deformities

Michael P Kelly, Adam L Wollowick, K Daniel Riew

EPIDEMIOLOGY AND NATURAL HISTORY

Cervical spine deformity is caused by a broad spectrum of diagnoses with variable prevalences and natural histories (Table 1). Deformity of the cervical spine may affect both the pediatric and adult patient populations. This chapter will address many of the common causes of cervical deformity.

Congenital Anomalies

Failure of formation and segmentation of the vertebral column is a rare cause of deformity in the cervical spine, known as Klippel Feil (KF) syndrome. The incidence of KF is estimated to be approximately 1 in 40,000 with an estimated prevalence of 0.7%.[1] As many KF patients are asymptomatic, the reported prevalence is most likely an underestimate. KF has historically been described as the triad of: (1) short neck, (2) low posterior hairline, and (3) limited range of motion of the cervical spine, but current research defines all congenital fusions of the cervical spine as KF.[2] The cervical anomalies have been classified by Samartzis et al.[3] as:

Type 1: Single congenitally fused segment

Type 2: Multiple noncontiguous, congenitally fused segments

Type 3: Multiple contiguous, congenitally fused segments.

The authors also found that patients with Type 1 KF complained of axial neck pain more frequently, while those with Type 2 and Type 3 anomalies were more likely to develop myelopathy or radiculopathy. Patients with Type 2 and Type 3 presented with symptoms at a mean age of 17 years, but only 11% of patients in the series underwent surgery. In many cases, the cervical spine remains well aligned, and surgery is performed for decompression, rather than deformity correction. As noted previously, the prevalence of asymptomatic KF is unknown, so the true natural history is also unknown.

Iatrogenic Deformities

Instability resulting in kyphosis following multilevel cervical laminectomy is a well-known complication.[4-6] Overall rates of deformity following multilevel laminectomy approach 30–35%, with some increased risk for laminectomies performed on children and those associated with resection of intradural tumors.[4] Patients with preoperative lordotic alignment and those undergoing resection of more than 50% of the facet joint are at increased risk for the development of post-laminectomy kyphosis.[6] Resection of the dorsal elements removes the tension band and allows for lengthening of the neck extensors (particularly, the semispinalis cervicis), which can result in kyphosis. Post-laminectomy kyphosis usually follows a slow, progressive course, during which patients develop difficulty maintaining horizontal gaze and complain of muscle spasm and pain, as the extensors attempt to hold the head up. As the kyphosis progresses, patients may develop neurological complaints if ventral compression ensues.

Deformity following fusion procedures may be due to a number of factors, often including some combination of adjacent segment pathology, pseudarthrosis, infection, and/or implant failure. Deformity may also result if an anterior or posterior cervical fusion is performed in a malaligned position. Careful patient positioning at the onset of the procedure and confirming appropriate alignment of instrumentation will minimize the risk of this complication. The prevalence of iatrogenic deformity is unknown and the natural history of iatrogenic deformity

Table 1: Summary of citations regarding natural history and surgical outcomes for cervical spinal deformities.

Author, journal, year	*Design*	*LoE*	*Topic*	*F/U (m)*	*Measures*	*Main results*
Doran, Arthritis and Rheumatism, 2002	Population-based cohort	III	Trends in RA incidence	40 years	Incidence of rheumatoid arthritis (RA)	A progressive decline in incidence of RA
Pellicci, JBJS Am, 1981	Prospective cohort	II	Progression of RA	5 years	Pain, radiographic progression, neural involvement	Radiographic progression is common; pain often improves; basilar invagination portends a poor prognosis
Winfield, Annals of Rheumatic Diseases, 1983	Prospective cohort	II	Progression of spine and other joint disease in RA	9.5 years	Radiographic progression	Peripheral joint involvement predicts cervical spine involvement
Kauppi, J Rheumatology, 2009	Prospective cohort	II	DMARDs and atlantoaxial disease	5 years	Radiographic progression, physical function (HAQ)	Combination disease-modifying antirheumatic drugs (DMARD) therapy effective in preventing atlantoaxial disease
Chikuda, JBJS Am, 2012	Population-based cohort	II	Morbidity and mortality of spine surgery in dialysis patients	N/A	Death, major complication	10-fold higher risk of death for dialysis-dependent patients
Eskander, Spine, 2010	Retrospective cohort	II	Vertebral artery anatomy	N/A	Course of VA	Medial migration (8%), extraforaminal (7%) at C6, intraforaminal (1%) at C7
Langeloo, Euro Spine Journal, 2006	Retrospective case series	IV	Osteotomies for AS	Not reported	Radiographic results, perioperative complications, neurologic monitoring	Monitoring is essential; prone rather than upright positioning is a feasible technique
Etame, Spine, 2008	Literature review	III	Management of cervicothoracic kyphosis in AS	N/A	Radiographic results, complications	Restoration of horizontal gaze and satisfaction good; neurologic deficit rate of 4%
Belanger, JBJS Am, 2005	Case series	IV	Extension osteotomies for ankylosing spondylitis (AS)	4.5 years	Radiographic results, complications	Average 38° correction via extension osteotomy; procedure carries risks of death and paraplegia
Riley, Spine, 2010	Systematic review	II	Postoperative dysphagia following anterior spine surgery	N/A	Dysphagia and risk factors	Approximate rate of 20%; multilevel procedures and female gender may be risk factors
O'Shaughnessy, Spine, 2008	Case series	IV	Management of fixed kyphosis with myelopathy	4.5 years	Radiographic results, Nurick score, Odom criteria	Mean 48° improvement; Nurick scores improve; 88% excellent/good by Odom's criteria
Park, Spine J, 2010	Case series	IV	Anterior management of postlaminectomy kyphosis	3.75 years	Radiographic results, NDI, VAS, Nurick, complications	Radiographic and clinical success; 30% complication rate
Deviren, J Neurosurg Spine, 2011	Case series	IV	Cervicothoracic pedicle subtraction osteotomies	2 years	Radiographic results, NDI, SF-36, VAS	Radiographic success with improvements in quality-of-life and pain scores

Neck Disability Index (NDI), Visual Analog Scale (VAS), Short Form-36 (SF-36), Vertebral Artery (VA), Level of Evidence (LoE).

is as varied as the causes. Surgeons must have detailed knowledge of prior procedures, diagnoses, and previously placed instrumentation when planning a correction of this problem.

Inflammatory Spondyloarthropathies

There are several inflammatory spondyloarthropathies associated with cervical spine deformities. The most common is rheumatoid arthritis (RA), with an incidence of approximately 30/100,000.[7] RA is associated with basilar invagination, atlantoaxial instability, and subaxial subluxations, due to the erosive nature of the disease. The prevalence of cervical spine deformity associated with RA is nearly 50% and progression is common, including progressive deformity at other joints.[8,9] Evaluation for atlantoaxial instability should precede any surgical procedure, as iatrogenic neurological injury may result if this diagnosis is missed. The rates of cervical spine deformity due to RA are declining with the advent of disease-modifying antirheumatic drugs (DMARD).[10,11]

Ankylosing spondylitis (AS) is a less common spondyloarthropathy, with an incidence of 7/100,000.[12] AS is associated with the HLA-B27 antigen and is characterized by bridging syndesmophytes causing spontaneous spine fusion. A spontaneous fusion of the cervical spine is associated with a loss of cervical lordosis, causing difficulty with horizontal gaze. Just as the cervical spine may be affected, so may the thoracic and lumbar spine be involved. For this reason, the alignment of the entire spine must be considered when evaluating these patients with a cervical flexion deformity. These patients may suffer from hip flexion contractures, which further complicate the management of their sagittal plane malalignment.

Renal spondyloarthropathy (RSA) is a rare disorder, associated with renal failure and dialysis treatment. Older patients and those with longer durations of dialysis treatment are at increased risk of developing this disease.[13] RSA is attributed to the inflammatory response to the build-up of beta-2-microglobulin and amyloid. The disease process may mimic osteomyelitis/diskitis radiographically. Surgical management of RSA is associated with high complication rates, due to the poor bone quality and medical comorbidities of these patients.[14]

Dropped Head Syndrome

Dropped head syndrome (DHS) is a spectrum of disorders characterized by a loss of cervical extensor strength, with a passively correctable chin on chest deformity representing the end stage of the disease. DHS is uncommon and no good estimates of its prevalence exist. The disease does have a female predilection (F:M, 3:2) and patients present, on average, in the eighth decade of life.[15] Several disease processes, including myasthenia gravis and amyotrophic lateral sclerosis, are associated with flexible, kyphotic deformities. A workup should be performed to ensure that patients are not improperly diagnosed with isolated neck extensor myopathy (INEM). Radiofrequency ablation of facets has been associated with DHS and this procedure should not be performed in a single stage, bilateral fashion.[16] Other causes include postradiation myositis/osteonecrosis and inflammatory myositis, as seen in polymyositis. Myositis, as opposed to myopathy, can be treated nonoperatively with steroids and the distinction between the two pathologies must be made, using electromyography and magnetic resonance imaging (MRI) as needed.

EVALUATION

History

As with any patient, the evaluation of a cervical spine deformity patient begins with complete history. Any symptoms of radiculopathy must be thoroughly assessed, particularly with respect to duration of symptoms, location along with a dermatomal distribution, and modifying symptoms. Also, the surgeon must inquire about the signs and symptoms of cervical myelopathy, such as difficulty with fine motor tasks, numbness in fingers/hands, and/or gait disturbances. With regard to the deformity, it is critical to understand the duration of time that the deformity has been present as well as the rapidity of progression. Procedures or diagnoses that preceded the onset of the deformity may guide the surgeon in planning treatment, such as previous radiation therapy or a prior cervical laminectomy. One must carefully collect information regarding prior spine surgeries. Patients with prior anterior surgeries should be evaluated by otolaryngology for evidence of recurrent laryngeal nerve palsy prior to planned revision anterior cervical surgery. If there is no palsy, then we will approach the spine from the opposite side. If there is a deficit, then we will approach the spine from the same side as the prior surgery, to avoid a potentially devastating bilateral nerve injury. One should carefully question the patient about pain medication use, with particular interest paid to narcotic medications, as some studies suggest that outcomes in these patients may be compromised.[17]

Physical Examination

The examination begins as the patient walks into the examination room. The surgeon should watch for signs of an abnormal gait. One should note any compensatory positions that help the patient maintain horizontal gaze (e.g. a hyperlordotic lumbar spine or flexed hips). The coronal and sagittal alignment of the spine should be assessed by having the patient stand upright with the hips and knees maximally extended. In some cases, such as AS, there may be a loss of lumbar lordosis with cervical kyphosis, causing a forward sagittal alignment. In some instances, restoring normal lumbar lordosis will realign the spinal column into a position acceptable to the patient. Compensatory hip or knee flexion can minimize the deformity in the sagittal plane. With the patient standing, perform Romberg's test, which can indicate cervical myelopathy when positive.

Examine the neck for active and passive range of motion, in extension, flexion, and lateral rotation. Any prior incisions should also be examined. The posterior cervical musculature should be assessed for dehiscence or atrophy, as these conditions can create a difficult situation for wound closure following revision surgery. Soft tissue concerns may require an evaluation by a plastic surgeon. A standard, complete sensorimotor examination should be formed. As it is not uncommon for patients undergoing corrective osteotomies to develop some postoperative weakness at the level of the osteotomy, careful baseline motor examinations must be documented. Fortunately, the vast majority of neurologic deficits will resolve spontaneously within a few weeks to months. With chronic neurological changes, muscles may atrophy and the hands should be examined for signs of intrinsic wasting, possibly indicating a myelopathy hand.[18] Reflexes should be tested with attention to side-to-side asymmetry if present. Hyperreflexia may be a sign of myelopathy, and a jaw jerk should be checked as well. In some cases, this hyperreflexic response is found in normal individuals. The jaw jerk is a supratentorial response, not affected by cervical cord compression. The presence of pathologic reflexes should also be noted, including the scapulohumeral reflex, inverted radial reflex, Hoffman's reflex, and Babinski's response. All may indicate some degree of upper motor neuron disease and myelopathy.

The correction of rigid cervical deformities requires a different surgical approach than flexible deformities. One way to assess for the rigidity of the deformity is to have the patient lie supine on the examination table to assess the passive range of motion and flexibility of the deformity. Often, what appears to be a rigid severe kyphotic deformity will correct to a less dramatic deformity with the patient relaxed in a supine position for several minutes. While supine, it is helpful to assess for hip flexion contractures by performing the Thomas test. The patient is laid supine on the examination table and asked to bring one knee to their chest. A hip flexion contracture is present if the contralateral limb lifts off the examination table. In some cases, a hip flexion contracture may need to be addressed prior to a spinal realignment procedure as the patient may end up pitched forward if the contracture is severe enough.

Signs and Symptoms

Cervical deformities are often readily apparent, either because of the cervical deformity itself or the compensatory mechanisms employed by the patient. In the absence of neural compression, patients may have minimal symptoms, with muscle fatigue due to compensatory mechanisms causing most complaints. As the cervical deformity progresses or persists, however, patients may have difficulty maintaining horizontal gaze and performing activities of daily living. They may also complain of dysphagia and respiratory difficulties. The end-stage of cervical kyphosis is a chin on chest deformity. In some cases, patients may develop significant pain, although not necessarily proportional to the magnitude of deformity.

Laboratory Findings

Postinfectious cervical deformities should have a complete blood count (CBC), erythrocyte sedimentation rate (ESR), and C-reactive protein (CRP) checked prior to an instrumented deformity correction. If the patient complains of dysphagia and there is a concern for malnutrition, we will obtain preoperative nutrition markers including albumin, prealbumin, and transferrin. These values may not "normalize" with a change in the preoperative routine, but the surgeon should try to optimize them which may require the help of a nutritionist. HLA-B27 is associated with AS, though we do not order this as it will not change our management of an ankylosed cervical spine.

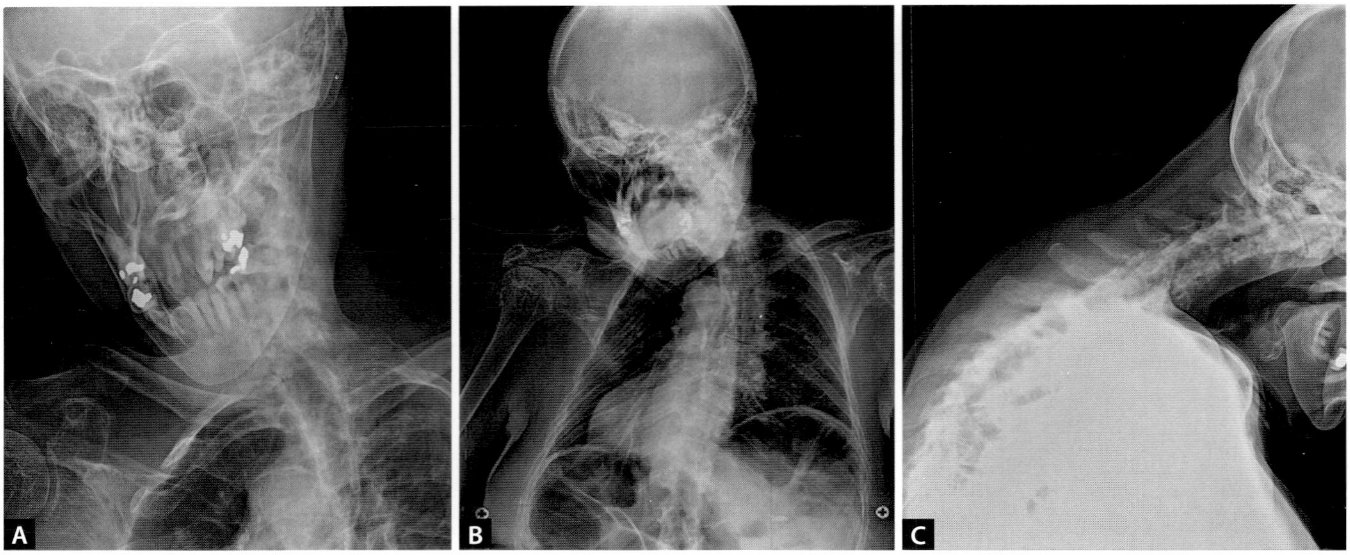

Figs. 1A to C: (A) Preoperative anteroposterior (AP) cervical radiograph of a patient with ankylosing spondylitis and a fixed cervicothoracic kyphosis. (B) Preoperative upright AP cervicothoracic radiograph. (C) Lateral radiograph of a patient with ankylosing spondylitis and a fixed cervicothoracic kyphosis.

The Tensilon test and antiacetylcholine receptor antibody test can be performed to rule out myasthenia gravis when seeing a patient with DHS. ESR and creatine kinase may be elevated in cases of myositis associated with DHS, which is sometimes amenable to steroid therapy. Most patients, though, do not have abnormal laboratory findings and should receive a routine preoperative evaluation.

Imaging

A full cervical spine radiograph series (AP, lateral, flexion, extension, and obliques) should be obtained for all patients (Figs. 1A to C). The flexion/extension films help assess the flexibility of the deformity. Full-length standing AP and lateral radiographs *are essential* for assessing global spinal alignment and planning major realignments. Compensatory deformities elsewhere (e.g. thoracolumbar spine, hips, or knees) should be evaluated *so that the major deformity is managed first*. In some cases, addressing the lumbar spine will restore horizontal gaze and avoid the need for a cervical procedure. If a thoracolumbar procedure follows a cervical realignment, the patient may be left looking above the horizon, an equally disabling position. A supine lateral radiograph also helps to assess the rigidity of the deformity.

An MRI scan should be obtained. Areas of active compression and potential compression following realignment should be noted so that an appropriate decompressive procedure can be planned if needed. In addition to the neural elements, surgeons must pay attention to the course of the vertebral artery. The course at C6 is actually quite variable.[19] The C7 transverse foramen is usually empty, although in some cases, the vertebral artery does enter here. The course of the vertebral artery should be known prior to performing an anterior approach, placing C7 pedicle screws, and performing a C7 pedicle subtraction osteotomy. In some cases, medial migration of the vertebral artery places it at risk for injury during corpectomy procedures (Fig. 2).[20] Finally, the vertebral artery may be located more cranially than usual at C2, putting it at risk during C1–C2 instrumentation and fusion procedures. With careful planning, it is possible to significantly minimize the risk of vertebral artery injury. Attention to spinal cord signal changes on MRI allows the surgeon to more appropriately counsel patients, as decreased T1 intensity with increased T2 intensity has been associated with less improvement in neurological symptoms.[21,22]

Computed tomography (CT) scans of the cervical spine with coronal and sagittal reformatted images are essential for planning reconstructions, particularly in a revision setting. One must be aware of areas of exposed dura (after laminectomy) and have knowledge of which segments are fused as compared to those with pseudarthroses. If no support is placed under the patient's head, the sagittal

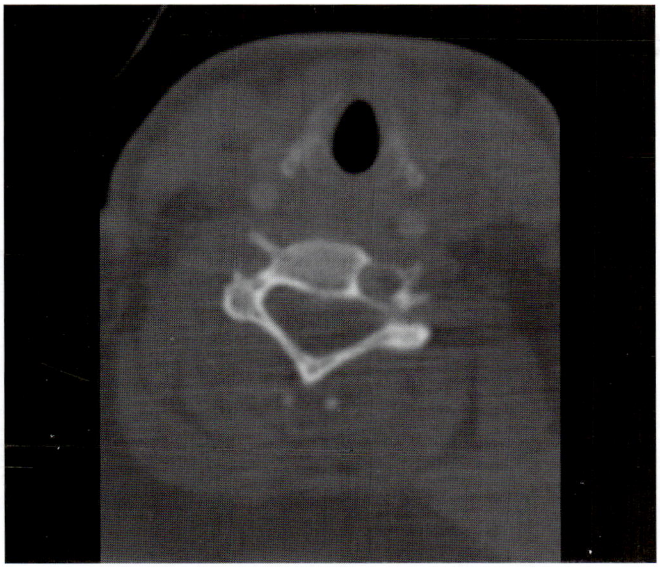

Fig. 2: Medial migration of the vertebral artery at C5.

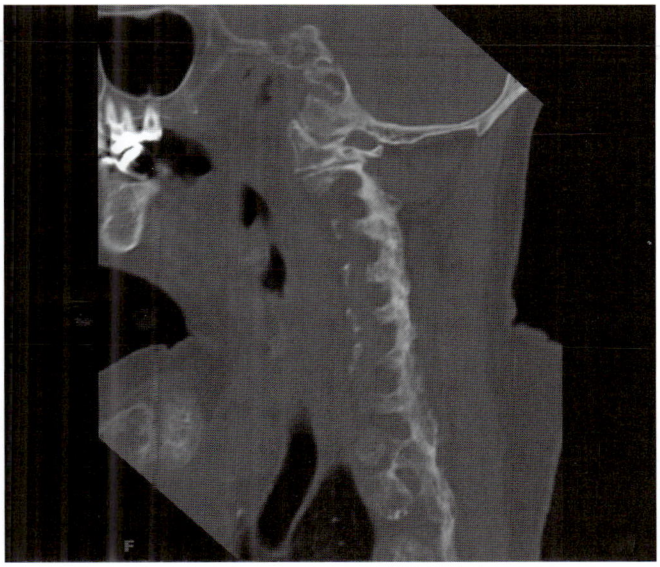

Fig. 3: Parasagittal images show ankylosis of the facet joints.

images also allow for an assessment of deformity flexibility (Fig. 3). A three-dimensional reconstruction of the cervical spine is also useful when planning a three-column realignment and will often give information not easily obtained from standard CT images. A CT myelogram is useful to evaluate areas of neural compression when the patient has a contraindication to MRI or in the setting of prior instrumentation, as artifact may render an MRI difficult to fully evaluate.

Medical Management

There are limited nonoperative options available to cervical deformity patients. Radiculopathy and myelopathy in the setting of a fixed and stable deformity should receive standard interventions, such as oral medications (preferably non-narcotic) and epidural steroid injections. Cervical deformities are not, generally, assisted by cervical collars. These may temporarily hold the head in an improved position, but the correction is not maintained after removal of the brace. Of particular concern with the use of a cervical orthosis in the setting of spinal deformity is skin breakdown, due to the high pressures and long duration of use. Constant collar use will also weaken the neck extensors, potentially exacerbating the deformity.

SURGICAL INDICATIONS AND TREATMENT

Correction of a cervical deformity is indicated when nonoperative interventions have failed to offer relief of disability or pain. Progressive myelopathy is an indication for surgery, with the goal of surgery to halt the progression of symptoms. Other indications include the inability to perform activities of daily living, including eating and swallowing (extreme cases may present with cachexia), and the inability to maintain horizontal gaze. In our practice, abnormal T2 signal intensity in the spinal cord seen on MRI is also an indication for surgery.

The preoperative imaging will help guide the location and degree of correction, as well. We have found that, if a plumb line is dropped from the clivus and falls anterior to the manubrium, the deformity is often caused by a thoracic deformity. This is ideally corrected with a thoracic level procedure. In some cases, patients may have both a thoracic deformity and an acute cervical kyphosis (e.g. AS patient with a C7 fracture). In these cases, a correction at the C7 level will often provide an excellent result. One must take care not to overcorrect patients. A goal of slight undercorrection is ideal, with the head placed in a slightly flexed position. This will allow them to see ahead, as well as down in front of their bodies. If the head is placed with a level horizontal gaze, then they cannot see their feet when descending stairs.

Neurological Monitoring

While a debate may exist for the use of neurological monitoring in degenerative spine surgery, we feel that it is essential when performing deformity correction in the cervical spine.[23] We monitor the anterior corticospinal tracts using transcranial motor-evoked potentials (tcMEP). The dorsal columns are monitored using somatosensory-evoked potentials (SSEP). To perform this type of monitoring, a total intravenous anesthetic (TIVA) must be used. In patients with severe deformity and cord compression, we obtain prepositioning baseline monitoring data, as patients may lose signals due merely to positioning. If a patient has a significant change in monitoring data, the surgeon should react promptly, which includes ensuring that mean arterial blood pressure is maintained at a level greater than 80 mm Hg. While the blood pressure is raised, the spinal cord should be inspected for areas of compression and further decompression performed as needed. Relaxation of the correction should be considered if no areas of residual compression are found and no improvement in data has occurred. If the cervical spine has been rendered unstable, then stabilization is needed to avoid potentially worsening the neurological deficit. An intraoperative wake-up test should be performed to confirm that the change in monitoring signals indicates a true neurological deficit.

Patient Positioning

Prone Procedures

We prefer to place Gardner-Wells tongs, rather than Mayfield tongs, as this allows for easier intraoperative modifications to head position. All patients are placed on a Jackson Spinal Table (Mizuho OSI, Broken Arrow, OK) with chest and iliac crest pads. In the past, we used a chest bolster, but have found fewer sensitive pressure areas postoperatively using the chest pads. In cases of severe cervical/cervicothoracic kyphosis, one may need to use the bolster and build it up with blankets and pillows. The legs are placed in a sling, to encourage venous pooling of blood. The bed is placed in the maximal reverse Trendelenburg position. This accomplishes two goals: it brings the neck into a comfortable position for the operating surgeon and encourages venous pooling in the lower extremities, which decreases blood loss and facilitates exposure of the spine. The head is placed in 15 pounds of bi-vector traction through the use of two ropes attached to the Gardner-Wells tongs (Figs. 4A and B). During exposure, we will place the head in slight flexion with one rope. When the deformity correction is performed, we switch to the second rope in order to hold the head in extension and assist with deformity correction and maintenance of cervical lordosis.

Supine Procedures

We perform supine procedures on a flat, radiolucent table. A small amount of traction is applied to the shoulders with tape to assist with obtaining adequate lateral intra-operative radiographs. Soft "ties" are placed around the wrists of the patient, so that traction may be applied if visualization of the cervicothoracic junction is inadequate on the lateral radiograph. Towels may be placed under the head in cases of fixed, kyphotic deformities. These are removed when the correction is performed. Ideally, the

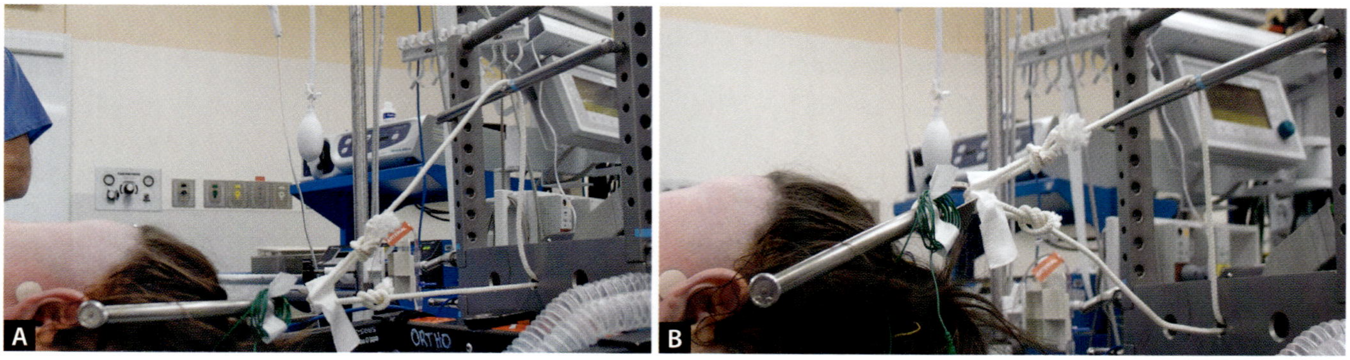

Figs. 4A and B: (A) Bi-vector traction through Gardner-Wells tongs to produce slight flexion; (B) Bi-vector traction through Gardner-Wells tongs to produce neck extension prior to fusion.

patient is positioned with the head in neutral rotation, with the nose pointing toward the ceiling, which may require the surgeon to look at the patient from the head of the bed. Once the head is properly positioned, it is gently tapped into position. One must remember that, despite the tape, the head may move during the anterior procedure. This is particularly true for high cervical approaches when some rotation is often required to perform the procedure. The surgeon should have the anesthesiologist check the position again, and be certain that the alignment is appropriate, before placing instrumentation.

Procedure Details

Preoperative Planning

Planning for the correction of a cervical deformity requires knowledge of prior procedures, where implants and fusions are found, and the distribution of symptoms. Circumferential procedures are commonly needed in deformity correction operations in order to maximize the chance of achieving a successful fusion and to minimize the possibility of deformity recurrence. The rigidity of the deformity, however, will also dictate the preferred approach for each procedure. A flexible post-laminectomy kyphosis may be treated with a circumferential fusion with multiple diskectomies, while a rigid AS kyphosis may require a pedicle subtraction procedure. Angular kyphosis will often require a combination of anterior diskectomies and/or corpectomy with posterior column osteotomies. If a pedicle subtraction osteotomy is done above C7, care should be taken with the vertebral artery, as it courses just lateral to the pedicles.

POSTLAMINECTOMY KYPHOSIS

We will usually address post-laminectomy kyphosis with an anterior procedure, followed by a posterior procedure. For these cases, posterior instrumentation helps to stabilize the spine when a corpectomy is performed. Laminectomy splits the spinal ring posteriorly. When a subsequent total corpectomy is done, it divides the ring of the spinal column completely in half, leaving only soft tissues to stabilize the two halves. This renders the segment extremely unstable to torsional forces. For corpectomies longer than a single level, the anterior instrumentation is at risk of failure if it is not supplemented with posterior fixation. Exceptions are if the patient has a multilevel hybrid construct with corpectomies and diskectomies with segmental fixation at multiple points, or with bicortical fixation into the nonosteoporotic bone. Posterior instrumentation following multilevel anterior diskectomies also increases the rigidity of the construct and improves fusion rates. Conversely, even if adequate correction of the kyphosis is achieved with positioning alone, we prefer to avoid posterior only procedures. This is because the surface area for fusion is poor with the lateral mass and facets being the only surface area for fusion in a post-laminectomy kyphosis case. We prefer to ensure that our operation is the last one that the patient needs at these same levels since these patients have already had one operation for this problem We believe that the best way to achieve this and avoid further complications such as graft collapse or extrusion, instrumentation failure, or pseudarthrosis is to perform a circumferential procedure. Most patients prefer a circumferential operation that maximizes the odds of avoiding yet another operation in such cases.

IATROGENIC DEFORMITY

In the setting of an iatrogenic deformity with an instrumented fusion, corrective options include a three-stage procedure such as posterior-anterior-posterior or anterior-posterior-anterior surgery, a two-stage procedure or a single-stage operation such as an anterior osteotomy or posterior pedicle subtraction osteotomy. Which of these options are chosen is dependent upon many factors including, surgeon experience, comfort level, type, and nature of the instrumentation, ease of approach, location of the vertebral artery, neural compression, and patient symptomatology, to name a few.

Anterior Osteotomies

For patients with an anterior fusion, without a prior posterior fusion, anterior osteotomies can provide an excellent correction. In most cases, however, the posterior facets autofuse within a few months after a solid anterior fusion. A CT scan can often be quite helpful to determine the fusion status. To perform this, we use a standard Smith-Robinson approach to the anterior spine. In some cases, identifying the old disk space can be difficult. After confirming the course of the vertebral artery (as it may be anomalously extraforaminal above C7), dissect the longus colli lateral, to expose the costal process (the anterior roof of the foramen transversarium). Penfield 4 is then used to confirm the lateral border of the uncovertebral joint,

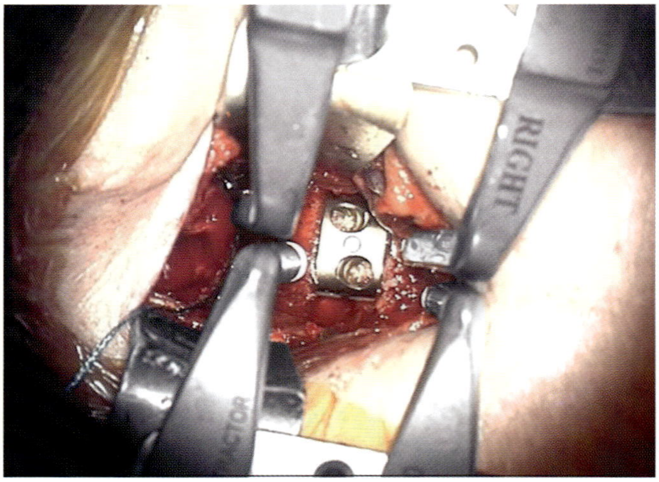

Fig. 5: Two Caspar pins are placed into each vertebral body to assist with osteoclasis of the posterior facet fusions.

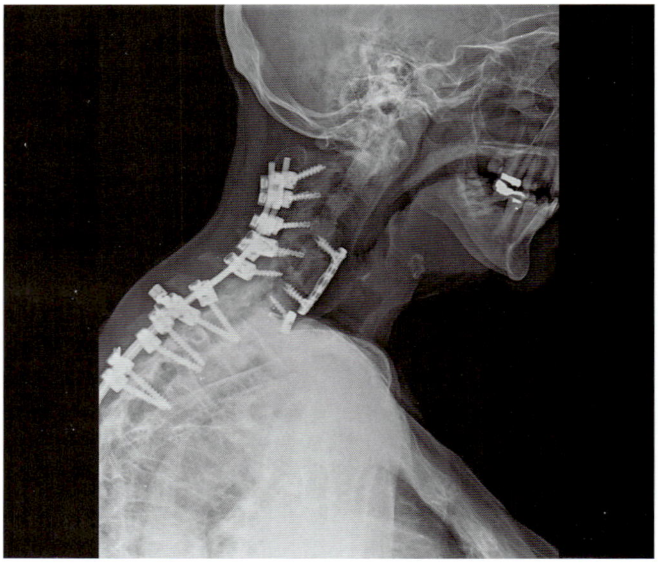

Fig. 6: Postoperative lateral radiograph of the previously shown ankylosing spondylitis patient. Correction was obtained via the anterior procedure and a posterior spinal fusion was performed to support the anterior instrumentation.

confirming the disk space. A Penfield 2 is placed lateral to the uncinate to protect the vertebral artery and define the boundaries of the disc space. A 3 mm matchstick burr resects the fusion mass back to the posterior longitudinal ligament. The resection is carried laterally, within a millimeter or two of the Penfield, thinning out the uncovertebral joint. The final portion of the joint is removed, completing the osteotomy, using a back-angled curette, working from lateral to medial. All work must be performed moving away from the vertebral artery.

If there is a noninstrumented fusion posteriorly, then correction ensues using Caspar pins to apply distraction across the osteotomy. If facet fusion exists, we place two Caspar pins into each vertebral body, applying distraction force through the facets (Fig. 5). One can also augment this with a vertebral body spreader. In addition, the patient should have been positioned with the kyphotic head and neck supported by some sheets. After performing the osteotomy, some of these are removed and the forehead is pushed posteriorly through the sterile drapes. With a combination of these techniques, one can usually plastically deform the facet fusion and restore some lordosis. A standard instrumented fusion ensues. In cases where more correction through each segment will be required during a posterior approach, a buttress plate or an interference screw is used to prevent graft extrusion. The buttress plate is better placed at the cranial end of the construct, as one placed at the caudal end will protrude into the retropharyngeal space after further posterior correction when the cranial part of the osteotomized segment moves further posteriorly. A posterior instrumented fusion is frequently performed after the anterior procedure to minimize the risk of subsidence and loss of correction (Fig. 6).

Posterior Osteotomies

In cases of a posterior fusion, with open disk spaces in the front, we will often perform posterior osteotomies alone. To position the head, bi-vector traction is applied through Gardner-Wells tongs. This allows the surgeon to move the head from a flexed/neutral position to an extended position, simply by switching the weight from one rope to the other. In cases where a prior laminectomy has been performed, one must remove as much of the scar and laminectomy membrane as possible. The dura should be soft and ballotable before proceeding with any deformity correction. If it is not, a scar can sometimes buckle into the cord and cause spinal cord compression when the spine is extended. After debridement, we perform chevron osteotomies (posterior column osteotomy, PCO) with a 3 mm matchstick burr. Soft tissue, including scar and ligamentum flavum, should be removed again to guard against neural compression. Generally, traction alone is inadequate to obtain optimal lordosis. Therefore, we use stainless steel spinous process wires or titanium cables, whichever is easier, to help induce and hold segmental lordosis, until rods are placed. If stainless steel wires are used, we often remove them, especially if we use crosslinks, since, with titanium crosslinks, there is the potential for a galvanic response if the two metals are in close proximity. If all of the arthrodesis levels have had laminectomies, one can place the wire or cable at the next cranial and caudal spinous processes and then remove them after the lordosis has been achieved.

Cases of instrumented, circumferential fusions may require a "540°" approach. This is especially necessary when 3.5 mm diameter cobalt chromium rods have been used to augment the posterior fusion since these are too stiff to deform after an anterior osteotomy alone. If 3.5 mm were used and the patient had a laminectomy, one can often do the anterior osteotomy and partial correction as described above. When performing a posterior approach (e.g. to remove implants) before anterior osteotomies, we will perform incomplete PCOs across the kyphosis. Instead of completing the osteotomy at each facet joint, however, we will leave a small, bridging fusion mass. This confers some stability to the spine while the patient is turned to the supine position for the anterior approach. When performing the anterior osteotomy and correction, the remaining bone at the facet joints will either break or plastically deform. As a second posterior procedure will be performed, we will use variable angle screws and low profile, stand-alone interbody spacers to allow for further correction during the second posterior stage of the procedure. When using a stand-alone interbody spacer, only one screw should be placed through the implant. This allows for stability during the flip but permits further compression around the implant to create segmental lordosis. Alternatively, one can use bone graft fixed with an interference screw to prevent extrusion during the posterior operation. Again, if spinous processes remain, cables can be used to obtain and hold segmental lordosis, while placing and securing the rods into lateral mass screws.

Pedicle Subtraction Osteotomy

A C7 pedicle subtraction osteotomy (PSO) may be performed for cases of fixed sagittal malalignment, as is seen in AS. Before proceeding with a PSO, one must ensure that the course of the vertebral artery is known. If a patient is fused to the occiput, the instrumentation is extended to the occiput. If there is upper cervical motion, then the upper instrumented vertebra (UIV) is usually C2. C2 can be fixed with pars, pedicle, or intralaminar screws. At the subaxial segments, lateral mass screws are placed at each level. The exception is C6 and T1. If the PSO is performed at C7, a single lateral mass screw is placed into C6, skipping the T1 pedicle on that side, and a single T1 pedicle screw is placed on the other side, skipping the C6 lateral mass. This helps to minimize implant crowding after deformity correction. T2 to T4 are instrumented with bilateral pedicle screws. After all implants are placed, AP and lateral X-rays are obtained to confirm the position of all implanted hardware. If the preoperative CT reveals facet arthrosis or fusion at T4–5, then one can add that level also.

A laminectomy of C7 is performed next, preserving the bone for use as a local bone graft. The caudal 20–30% of C6 and the cranial 10–20% of C7 laminae are also removed to make adequate room for the cord. Next, we do a total facetectomy bilaterally. The decompression is carried cranially, to the inferior aspect of the C6 pedicle (removing the inferior facet), and caudally, to the cranial aspect of the T1 pedicle (removing the superior facet). This additional bony resection is performed initially with a Leksell Rongeur, preserving the bone for autograft. The lateral mass of C7 is completely resected. We then finish removing the facet and lateral mass with a blunt-tipped, matchstick burr. The osteotomy is made in a chevron shape in order to provide rotational stability. Hemostasis of bleeding epidurals is obtained using bipolar electrocautery and/or a liquefied hemostatic collagen preparation.

The pedicle of C7 is now isolated and the C7 and C8 nerve roots should be visualized. Cotton paddies are placed to protect these two nerve roots and the dura medially. The paddies are held in place with Penfield 2 and 4 retractors. The surgeon now has free access to the pedicle. The matchstick burr is placed down the channel of the pedicle, preserving the pedicle walls. Once the pedicle is decancellated, the walls are further thinned with the bur and imploded into the central cavity with a round tamp. This provides access to the C7 body. The body is decancellated using reverse angled curettes and tamps, to create a void in the posterior portion of the C7 body. The dorsal cortex of the vertebral body wall should be thinned carefully using the curette. After the void is created on one side, it is packed with demineralized bone matrix and cotton paddies for hemostasis. The same procedure is then

CHAPTER 28

performed at the contralateral pedicle. The dorsal cortex of the vertebral body should be quite thin and should be easily impacted with a downward pushing curette. If it does not break easily, then the cortex should be thinned further. When the cortex is pushed ventrally into the void, the three-column osteotomy is complete.

Precontoured, or articulating, rods are placed into the heads of the screws distal to the osteotomy site and provisionally held with set screws. We prefer to use articulating rods, as we find them easier to use. The rods are fixed to the screws both proximal and distal to the osteotomy with loose set screws. This allows it to slide as the deformity is corrected. The surgeon takes hold of the Gardner-Wells tongs and holds the head in a stable position, while an assistant changes the weight to the extension rope. The surgeon pulls the head into extension closing the osteotomy site around the decancellated C7 body. One must check for compression of the exiting nerve roots and spinal cord. The neurological monitoring data should be assessed to ensure that there has been no change. Typically, an adequate extension is achieved when the spinous processes of C6 and T1 are nearly touching. Then, the set screw for the articulation is tightened to hold the osteotomy position and the lateral mass set screws are final tightened. Radiographs are obtained to confirm an appropriate correction in both the sagittal and coronal planes.

The intact C7 lamina is split in half along its midsagittal plane and cabled in place across the C6 and T1 spinous processes, providing additional stability and aiding the fusion. The facet joints at all unfused levels are decorticated with a high-speed burr and a locally obtained bone graft is placed from the lateral masses of C6 to the transverse processes and lamina of T1.

Wound Closure

One must pay meticulous attention to wound closure. First, we cauterize any bleeder that results when the retractors are removed and then cover the bleeding area with liquefied collagen and Surgicel (Johnson & Johnson), one of the most effective and least expensive hemostatic agents available. After final irrigation, a deep drain is placed along the spine. Vancomycin powder (0.5–1.0 g) is placed in the deep layer of the wound and sprinkled in the wound prior to every layer of closure. We place a thrombin soaked gel foam sponge in the wound on top of the drain to coagulate the muscle bleeders from the first layer of closure. This should never be placed over a laminectomy defect since it will expand after closure and can cause cord compression. The deep, paraspinal layer is closed in multiple layers taking small "bites" of the fascia. After each layer, hemostasis is aided by holding pressure. By closing the paraspinal muscle in many layers, atrophy, dehiscence, and infections can be minimized. A suprafascial drain is placed superficial to the fascia if the subcutaneous fatty layer is greater than 2 cm, and the subcutaneous tissue is also closed in multiple layers. A suture is placed every centimeter such that there is no dead space. Using the above-described techniques, we have had only 1 infection in over 1,500 posterior cervical spine cases. The skin is closed with a running subcuticular stitch. Occasionally, there is redundant skin after a corrective osteotomy. Usually, this does not pose a problem for wound closure and will smooth out over time. When redundant skin is significant, an ellipse of skin and fat may be removed to achieve proper apposition of the tissue edges.

Postoperative Care

Patients are placed in hard cervical collars postoperatively. Patient-controlled analgesia (PCA) is used immediately postoperatively but is discontinued on postoperative day 1. The drains are removed when output is less than 30 mL per 8-hour shift, which is usually on postoperative day 1 if the hemostatic techniques described above are utilized. Diet is advanced as tolerated, and the patient is encouraged to walk with physical therapy on postoperative day 1. The majority of patients are discharged home on postoperative days 1 or 2.

COMPLICATIONS

The management of cervical deformities requires expertise in less complex cervical spine procedures, as deformity correction requires the skills needed to perform several smaller procedures in one setting. In addition, complications are common. Performing anterior surgery over three levels or more must be done expeditiously. If the length of the retraction for the anterior operation exceeds 3 hours, there is a greater risk of edema causing airway compromise. Also, longer retraction times in the anterior cervical spine increase the risk of dysphagia and dysphonia. Similarly, one must be facile with posterior cervical surgical techniques. One will ideally have experience dissecting post-laminectomy membranes. This membrane must be dissected to allow for safe deformity correction. An incidental durotomy, while not devastating, adds operative time and can cause problems with wound healing if a watertight closure is not obtained. The surgeon must work with a neurophysiology team accustomed to multimodal monitoring, and the entire surgical team (anesthesia, scrub tech, circulators) should be familiar with deformity corrections so that any unanticipated events may be dealt with quickly and smoothly.[24]

Failure of instrumentation is uncommon if the appropriate techniques are used at the time of surgery. For long constructs, we will often choose T3 or T4 as the lowest instrumented vertebra (LIV), to provide several points of fixation distal to the cervicothoracic junction. Stopping closer to the junction puts the construct at risk for distal junctional kyphosis, due to screw pullout, vertebral body fracture or a combination thereof. The choice for proximal fixation is dependent upon numerous factors. In patients who are autofused to the skull, instrumenting to the skull lowers the risk of instrumentation failure. On the other hand, if there is no such autofusion, all techniques to avoid including the occiput to C2 joints should be utilized, as these are the two most important motion segments in the neck. One can utilize multiple points of fixation at the C2 level, with a combination of the pedicle or pars screws along with laminar screws. One can use a third rod attached to C2 and C7 or thoracic laminar screws, for example. Cables or wires can also augment screw fixation. While we have never found it to be necessary, if there is any doubt about the ability of the instrumentation to hold the correction, one should have a low threshold for placing the patient in a halo orthosis.

Neurologic complication rates from complex cervical spine reconstructions such as PSOs have reported neurologic injury rates as high as 23%.[25,26] These injuries are often transient deficits, with C8 neurapraxia the most common neurological complication. Delayed onset neurological complications have been reported, and the surgeon performing complex cervical reconstructions must be aware of this.[27] Pseudarthrosis is a concern, with reported rates ranging from 0% to 13%.[24,26,28] The rates of pseudarthrosis and implant failure are higher in renal dialysis patients, with rates reported to be as high as 22%.[13] Dysphagia is a common, often transient, complication of both anterior and posterior reconstructions.[29] While there have been no reported vertebral artery injuries for PSOs performed at the C7 level,[30] we have had such a case where an anomalous artery was in the foramen transversarium at C7. With the addition of vancomycin powder at wound closure, double drains for corpulent necks and meticulous closure, the infection has become a nonevent for us. The perioperative mortality of patients undergoing reconstruction for RSA has been reported to be 7%, which is high relative to other cervical spine procedures but comparable to the mortality rate for other major procedures in dialysis patients.[13]

PROGNOSIS

Results of reconstructions for cervical deformity are generally good, despite the aforementioned high complication rates.[25,26,28,30-35] As cervical deformities remain relatively rare and present in a heterogeneous population, no "best management" option exists. Several series have reported the experience with anterior only surgery for severe kyphotic deformities.[33,36] While generally considered successful, these procedures frequently left the patients in kyphosis. More recent series have reported the results of circumferential procedures for fixed kyphotic deformities.[32,35,37] Mummaneni et al. reported their experience in 30 patients with fixed kyphosis and myelopathy.[37] The majority of patients experienced an improvement in clinical symptoms (mean Nurick score improvement of 1.9 points) and radiographic parameters (average correction of 28°). Two patients died in the immediate postoperative period, emphasizing the significant risk associated with these procedures. O'Shaughnessy et al. also reviewed 20 patients with fixed kyphosis and myelopathy. Clinical (mean Nurick score improvement of 0.9) and radiographic (average correction of 48°) improvements were obtained. Their experience also underscores the magnitude of these procedures, as 25% of the patients required a temporary gastrostomy tube and 19% required a temporary tracheostomy.

Some deformities may not be so angular as to require circumferential corrections. Several recent reports have described techniques and results of performing a C7 PSO.[24,28,38] Belanger et al. and Langeloo et al. presented radiographic outcomes associated with this procedure, and both studies noted the excellent correction.[24,28] In each series, neurologic complications were common, with one patient sustaining quadriplegia. Langeloo et al. emphasized the importance of neurologic monitoring and showed that appropriate corrective maneuvers can help avoid neurologic catastrophe.[24] Deviren et al.

presented similar radiographic results and also reported preoperative and postoperative outcomes scores. Patients showed significant improvements in Neck Disability Index scores (Pre: 51.1, Post: 38.6, $P = 0.03$) and visual analog pain scores (Pre: 8.1, Post: 3.9, $P = 0.0021$).

The correction of cervical spine deformity requires an experienced surgeon, trained in the concepts of spinal deformity, and a customized surgical plan for each patient. An experienced assistant is necessary as well, as the case must move forward with efficiency, to minimize blood loss, anesthesia time, and complications related to the length of surgery. One can expect good results if the preoperative preparation is appropriate, the surgical team is experienced in managing complex cervical procedures, and meticulous surgical technique is executed.

REFERENCES

1. Brown MW, Templeton AW, Hodges FJ 3rd. The incidence of acquired and congenital fusions in the cervical spine. Am J Roentgenol Radium Ther Nucl Med. 1964;92:1255-9.
2. Klippel M, Feil A. Un cas d'absence des vertebres cervicales. Avec cage thoracique remontant jusqu'a la base du crane (cage thoracique cervicale). Nouv Iconog Salpetriere. 1912;25:223-50.
3. Samartzis DD, Herman J, Lubicky JP, et al. Classification of congenitally fused cervical patterns in Klippel-Feil patients: epidemiology and role in the development of cervical spine-related symptoms. Spine. 2006;31:E798-804.
4. Albert TJ, Vacarro A. Postlaminectomy kyphosis. Spine. 1998;23:2738-45.
5. Bell DF, Walker JL, O'Connor G, et al. Spinal deformity after multiple-level cervical laminectomy in children. Spine. 1994;19:406-11.
6. Guigui P, Benoist M, Deburge A. Spinal deformity and instability after multilevel cervical laminectomy for spondylotic myelopathy. Spine. 1998;23:440-7.
7. Doran MF, Pond GR, Crowson CS, et al. Trends in incidence and mortality in rheumatoid arthritis in Rochester, Minnesota, over a forty-year period. Arthritis Rheum. 2002; 46:625-31.
8. Pellicci PM, Ranawat CS, Tsairis P, et al. A prospective study of the progression of rheumatoid arthritis of the cervical spine. J Bone Joint Surg Am. 1981;63:342-50.
9. Winfield J, Young A, Williams P, et al. Prospective study of the radiological changes in hands, feet, and cervical spine in adult rheumatoid disease. Ann Rheum Dis. 1983;42:613-8.
10. Kauppi MJ, Neva MH, Laiho K, et al. Rheumatoid atlantoaxial subluxation can be prevented by intensive use of traditional disease modifying antirheumatic drugs. J Rheumatol. 2009;36:273-8.
11. Korpela M, Laasonen L, Hannonen P, et al. Retardation of joint damage in patients with early rheumatoid arthritis by initial aggressive treatment with disease-modifying antirheumatic drugs: five-year experience from the FIN-RACo study. Arthritis Rheum. 2004;50:2072-81.
12. Kaipiainen-Seppanen O, Aho K. Incidence of chronic inflammatory joint diseases in Finland in 1995. J Rheumatol. 2000;27:94-100.
13. Veeravagu A, Ponnusamy K, Jiang B, et al. Renal osteodystrophy: neurosurgical considerations and challenges. World Neurosurg. 2012;78:191, E23-33.
14. Chikuda H, Yasunaga H, Horiguchi H, et al. Mortality and morbidity in dialysis-dependent patients undergoing spinal surgery: analysis of a national administrative database in Japan. J Bone Joint Surg Am. 2012;94:433-8.
15. Umapathi T, Chaudhry V, Cornblath D, et al. Head drop and camptocormia. J Neurol Neurosurg Psychiatry. 2002;73:1-7.
16. Stoker GE, Buchowski JM, Kelly MP. Dropped head syndrome following multilevel cervical radiofrequency ablation: a case report. J Spinal Disord Tech. 2013;26(8):444-8.
17. Lawrence JT, London N, Bohlman HH, et al. Preoperative narcotic use as a predictor of clinical outcome: results following anterior cervical arthrodesis. Spine. 2008;33:2074-8.
18. Ono K, Ebara S, Fuji T, et al. Myelopathy hand. New clinical signs of cervical cord damage. J Bone Joint Surg Br. 1987;69:215-9.
19. Eskander MS, Drew JM, Aubin ME, et al. Vertebral artery anatomy: a review of two hundred fifty magnetic resonance imaging scans. Spine. 2010;35:2035-40.
20. Eskander MS, Connolly PJ, Eskander JP, et al. Injury of an aberrant vertebral artery during a routine corpectomy: a case report and literature review. Spinal Cord. 2009;47:773-5.
21. Yukawa Y, Kato F, Yoshihara H, et al. MR T2 image classification in cervical compression myelopathy: predictor of surgical outcomes. Spine. 2007;32:1675-8; discussion 9.
22. Zhang YZ, Shen Y, Wang LF, et al. Magnetic resonance T2 image signal intensity ratio and clinical manifestation predict prognosis after surgical intervention for cervical spondylotic myelopathy. Spine. 2010;35:E396-9.
23. Park P, Wang AC, Sangala JR, et al. Impact of multimodal intraoperative monitoring during correction of symptomatic cervical or cervicothoracic kyphosis. J Neurosurg Spine. 2011;14:99-105.
24. Langeloo DD, Journee HL, Pavlov PW, et al. Cervical osteotomy in ankylosing spondylitis: evaluation of new developments. Eur Spine J. 2006;15:493-500.
25. Etame AB, Than KD, Wang AC, et al. Surgical management of symptomatic cervical or cervicothoracic kyphosis due to ankylosing spondylitis. Spine. 2008;33:E559-64.
26. Tokala DP, Lam KS, Freeman BJ, et al. C7 decancellisation closing wedge osteotomy for the correction of fixed cervicothoracic kyphosis. Eur Spine J. 2007;16:1471-8.
27. Hojo Y, Ito M, Abumi K, et al. A late neurological complication following posterior correction surgery of severe cervical kyphosis. Eur Spine J. 2011;20:890-8.

28. Belanger TA, Milam RA 4th, Roh JS, et al. Cervicothoracic extension osteotomy for chin-on-chest deformity in ankylosing spondylitis. J Bone Joint Surg Am. 2005;87:1732-8.
29. Riley LH 3rd, Vaccaro AR, Dettori JR, et al. Postoperative dysphagia in anterior cervical spine surgery. Spine. 2010;35:S76-85.
30. Hoh DJ, Khoueir P, Wang MY. Management of cervical deformity in ankylosing spondylitis. Neurosurg Focus. 2008;24:E9.
31. Traynelis VC. Total subaxial reconstruction. J Neurosurg Spine. 2010;13:424-34.
32. O'Shaughnessy BA, Liu JC, Hsieh PC, et al. Surgical treatment of fixed cervical kyphosis with myelopathy. Spine. 2008;33:771-8.
33. Zdeblick TA, Bohlman HH. Cervical kyphosis and myelopathy. Treatment by anterior corpectomy and strut-grafting. J Bone Joint Surg Am. 1989;71:170-82.
34. Park Y, Riew KD, Cho W. The long-term results of anterior surgical reconstruction in patients with postlaminectomy cervical kyphosis. Spine J. 2010;10:380-7.
35. Abumi K, Shono Y, Taneichi H, et al. Correction of cervical kyphosis using pedicle screw fixation systems. Spine. 1999;24:2389-96.
36. Herman JM, Sonntag VK. Cervical corpectomy and plate fixation for postlaminectomy kyphosis. J Neurosurg. 1994; 80:963-70.
37. Mummaneni PV, Dhall SS, Rodts GE, et al. Circumferential fusion for cervical kyphotic deformity. J Neurosurg Spine. 2008;9:515-21.
38. Deviren V, Scheer JK, Ames CP. Technique of cervicothoracic junction pedicle subtraction osteotomy for cervical sagittal imbalance: report of 11 cases. J Neurosurg Spine. 2011;15: 174-81.

CHAPTER 29 Cervical Tumors

Mari L Groves, Ziya L Gokaslan, Jean Paul Wolinsky

EPIDEMIOLOGY AND NATURAL HISTORY

There are over 1.4 million new cases of cancer diagnosed annually in the United States.[1,2] Primary tumors to the spine are rare entities and account for only 4–13% of all primary osseous tumors,[3] approximately 7,500 new cases of primary vertebral tumors per year in the United States. Conversely, up to 90,000 new cases of spinal metastasis occur in the United States annually. Primary tumors are historically categorized by their clinical aggressiveness ranging from benign, benign but locally aggressive, and malignant tumors. The distribution and type of primary tumor vary significantly with age and location (Table 1). The vertebral body is more often associated with malignant pathologies (75%) while the posterior elements are more commonly associated with benign pathologies. Adults are more likely to be diagnosed with a malignant pathology, whereas children younger than 18 years of age are more likely to have a benign diagnosis. The cervical spine is not commonly affected by primary tumors. However, of the benign primary tumors, chondromas or osteochondromas have a predilection for the cervical spine, especially within C2. Of the benign aggressive-to-malignant primary tumors, chordomas commonly affect the sacrum and coccyx, but the skull base and upper cervical spine are affected in 35% of patients.[4] Recent analysis of the SEER cancer database analyzed 2,627 primary malignant tumors of the bone and found the most common lesions diagnosed as osteosarcoma (35.1%), chondrosarcoma (25.8%), Ewing's sarcoma (16%), chordoma (8.4%), and malignant fibrous histiocytoma (5.6%).[4] The Leeds tumor registry, which focuses on all osseous spine tumors, found that the most common malignant spine tumors were multiple myeloma and plasmacytoma.[3] This was followed by chordomas and osteosarcomas. For the purposes of this chapter, we will highlight the features of chondromas and chordomas as they are the most common primary tumors found within the cervical spine.

Metastatic lesions to the spine far outweigh primary lesions.[2] Cadaveric studies have shown that as many as 30–90% of terminal cancer patients have metastatic disease to the spine[5-7] with roughly 10% of cancer patients developing symptomatic spinal lesions.[8] The thoracic spine is most commonly affected in metastatic disease (70%), likely due to its increased number of vertebral levels in comparison to the lumbar spine (20%), cervical, or sacrum.[4] Metastatic disease to the cervical spine occurs in 8–20% of cases.[9,10] The craniovertebral junction is rare and only accounts for 0.5% of all metastatic spine lesions.[11-13] The most common primary tumor pathologies are breast, prostate, and non-small cell lung carcinoma.[13] A recent retrospective analysis found that breast cancer preferentially metastasizes to the cervical spine over other cancer pathologies.[14] Spinal metastases are more common in men compared with women and are most common among individuals in the fourth through the sixth decade of life.[4]

METASTATIC DISEASE

Workup

Symptoms and Signs

Metastatic disease to the cervical spine can present with a large spectrum of signs and symptoms.[4,10] Patients may be found incidentally during the workup of an unrelated problem, however, in those patients who present with specific complaints, pain is the most common presenting symptom and occurs in 83–95% of patients.[10,13,15,16] There are three classic pain syndromes that can affect

Table 1: Epidemiology of primary tumors.

Tumor	*% of tumors*	*Cell of origin*	*Age range*	*Location*	*CT/MRI appearance*	*Growth*	*Treatment*
Benign							
Osteoid osteoma/ osteoblastoma	10–12	Osteoblasts	1st and 2nd decades	Lumbar Cervical Posterior elements	Sclerotic, nidus	Slow	Nonsteroidal anti-inflammatory drugs Curettage Radiosurgery?
Chondroma/ osteochondroma	4	Mesenchymal/ cartilage	1st through 4th decades	Cervical Spinous/transverse process	Lytic, circumscribed, nonenhancing	Slow	Resection if symptomatic
Aneurysmal bone cyst	10	Vascular	1st through 3rd decades	Lumbar Posterior elements Vertebral bodies	Cystic/lytic Fluid-fluid level Hemosiderin	Non-neoplastic	Excision Curettage Embolization
Hemangioma	30	Vascular	4th through 6th decades	No preference	Honeycomb Cystic/lytic	Non-neoplastic	Resection if aggressive Embolization Radiation?
Fibrous dysplasia	n/a	Bone marrow stomal cells	1st decade or adulthood	No preference	Lytic, ground glass	Non-neoplastic	Resection if symptomatic
Eosinophilic granuloma	12–25	Histiocytes	1st and 2nd decades	Thoracic Lumbar	Expansile, lytic, vertebrae planae	Non-neoplastic	
Benign, locally aggressive							
Chordoma	2–4	Notochord	4th through 6th decades	Sacrum/coccyx (50%) Mobile spine (15%)	Lytic, enhancing, calcification, infiltrating disk space	Slow, but locally aggressive	En bloc Radiation Proton beam
Giant cell	5	Osteoclastic giant cells	2nd and 3rd decades	Sacrum Thoracic Lumbar	Cystic/lytic Nonsclerotic + Hemosiderin enhancing	Slow, but locally aggressive, metastasis to lung	En bloc Embolization Radiation?
Malignant							
Plasmacytoma	20–30	Plasma cells	5th and 6th decades	Thoracic	Lytic "Punched out"		Chemosensitive Radiation sensitive
Chondrosarcoma	7–12	Chondrocytes	3rd through 5th decades	Thoracic	Lytic Destructive "Ring and arc" calcification, enhancing	Malignant	En bloc Resection Chemo/radiotherapy insensitive
Osteosarcoma	< 5	Osteocytes	4th and post-6th decades	No preference	Lytic Destructive Enhancing Osteoblastic	Malignant	Chemo/radiation sensitive Surgery

Source: Adapted from Chi JH, Bydon A, Hsieh P, et al. Epidemiology and demographics for primary vertebral tumors. Neurosurg Clin N Am. 2008;19(1):1-4.

patients with metastatic disease: referred, mechanical, or nonmechanical pain. Referred pain may radiate to the shoulder or trapezial area, and is typically secondary to nerve root irritation or compression. Mechanical pain is characterized by pain that is relieved by rest and/or stabilization and exacerbated by motion or weight-bearing forces. Nonmechanical pain may occur secondary to tumor invasion of the vertebral body leading to periosteal stretching and a local inflammatory process that stimulates the pain fibers within the spinal periosteum.[17]

The vertebral body is most commonly affected by metastatic disease.[4,10] Pathologic collapse of the vertebral body can occur due to lytic or erosive lesions of the local cancellous bone.[10] Disease in the subaxial cervical spine is more likely to lead to angular kyphotic deformity. This results in mechanical pain due to flexion/extension instability from muscle, tendon, ligament, and/or joint capsule strain. At the craniovertebral junction, stability is more reliant on intact ligamentous complexes as well as the lateral articular masses, and metastatic disease to this area can result in painful rotational instability or difficulty holding the head upright unassisted.[18] Radicular pain may occur when the spinal metastasis compresses or irritates an exiting nerve root. This compression may lead to dysesthetic or neuropathic pain, or may create a sharp, shooting, or stabbing pain in a dermatomal distribution. Patients with new-onset back or neck pain with a known history of cancer should be considered to have the spinal metastatic disease until proven otherwise.[4]

Patients may also present with neurological dysfunction due to the spinal cord or nerve root compression.[9,10,13,16] Patients with metastatic epidural spinal cord compression may present with weakness up to 60–85% of the time.[4] Long tract signs can also occur and result in myelopathic symptoms including spasticity, ambulation difficulty, trouble with fine motor activity, increased deep tendon reflexes, and distal hand weakness or proximal leg weakness. Autonomic dysfunction is least common and is often a late finding that portends a poor prognosis for neurologic recovery despite decompression.[4] Spinal cord compression is more common in the subaxial spine as there is a progressive caudal narrowing of the spinal canal in comparison to the craniocervical junction prior to any spinal cord compression. Additionally, tumor or retropulsed bone is more common with a tumor in the subaxial spine vertebral bodies as the craniocervical ligaments also serve as a barrier to the invasion of the canal by containing the tumors ventrally. The posterior longitudinal ligament in the subaxial spine is typically not as robust as the craniocervical ligaments and cannot contain the tumor mass.[4]

Physical examination is an essential component of any workup and should elicit important findings that include palpable masses, pain, and neurologic dysfunction. Pain associated with flexion/extension more commonly corresponds to lesions located in the subaxial spine, whereas pain elicited by rotational movement is more commonly associated with the craniovertebral junction. Neurologic dysfunction at presentation is the most positive prognostic factor for postintervention neurologic status.[19] Common neurological findings include paraparesis, hyperreflexia, spasticity, Hoffman sign, abnormal plantar responses, and occasionally Brown-Sequard syndrome. Lesions located at the craniovertebral junction most often cause atlantoaxial subluxation and can compress the upper cervical spine and/or brainstem. Cerebellar ataxia and bulbar symptoms may occur if the neoplasm extends across the foramen magnum.[20]

The clinician should also perform a comprehensive review of the system to help determine if any constitutional symptoms or specific physiologic findings are present to suggest primary cancer. Most malignancies will present with weight loss, cachexia, and generalized fatigue. Additionally, patients with an underlying lung primary might develop some hemoptysis, chest pain, or shortness of breath. Patients with colon cancer might have noticed melena or hematochezia. Lymphoma can sometimes manifest as easy bruising. Prostate cancer can manifest as difficulty with urination or increased frequency of urination. A comprehensive review of symptoms and thorough history and physical is often the most important aid in determining a primary etiology.

Laboratory Findings

Metastatic workup for patients presenting with carcinoma of an unknown primary site dictates a wide initial workup. Basic laboratory values include a complete blood count, urinalysis, basic serum chemistries, computed tomography (CT) and magnetic resonance imaging (MRI) of the abdomen and pelvis. In women, the evaluation should include a pelvic examination and mammography. The assessment in men should also include a prostate examination and measurement of prostate-specific antigen (PSA). If there is a concern for gastrointestinal

SECTION 3

cancer, a hemoccult for occult blood in the stool in addition to colonoscopy may be indicated. Common tumor markers such as carcinoma embryonic antigen (CEA), CA 19-9, CA 15-3, and CA-125 may be useful as either diagnostic or prognostic tests. Serum alpha fetal protein (AFP) concentrations above 10,000 ng/mL exclusively occur in germ cell tumors and hepatocellular carcinoma. Beta-hCG concentrations >10,000 mIU/mL may be seen in patients with trophoblastic differentiation of a lung or gastric primary cancer.

If there is a concern for multiple myeloma or lymphoma, additional workup can be done to help make this diagnosis. Routine laboratory values might show anemia, elevated creatinine, and hypercalcemia. Urine studies and serum studies can help detect the presence of the monoclonal (M) protein, which is characteristic of multiple myeloma. Protein electrophoresis of the serum (SPEP) or a urine protein electrophoresis (UPEP) from a 24-hour collection can be analyzed using immunohistochemistry and can determine its subtype.

In men, a PSA elevation may be seen with prostate cancer. However, these levels can be nonspecific and should be interpreted cautiously without additional clinical signs. PSA levels greater than 4 have a positive predictive value of only 30%. However, a PSA value of greater than 10 has a positive predictive value of 64%.[21] Other common metastatic primaries include breast and lung cancer. However, there are no screening serum tests that are specific markers for these pathologies.[21] Other laboratory tests are specific for primary cancers but can be seen with metastatic disease. Alkaline phosphatase and lactate dehydrogenase may be higher in patients with primary tumors. However, alkaline phosphatase may be high with bony turnover and is nonspecific.

Imaging

Imaging workup for patients with osseous lesions should include plain radiographs, MRI, and CT. Plain radiographs assess alignment as well as any dynamic changes that might occur with flexion/extension. They can provide an overall evaluation of the extent of metastatic disease as well as evaluation of the disk spaces.[10] However, plain radiographs lack sensitivity in detecting lesions, as osteolytic lesions are not evident until 30–50% of the bone is demineralized.[10] CT imaging is complementary to plain film and provides a more detailed rendering of the bony spinal canal and osseous structures. Signs of spinal instability include progressive deformity, translation or angulation of the vertebral body, and/or greater than 50% involvement of the vertebral body. Retropulsed bony fragments following pathologic collapse can also be clearly visualized.[10] CT myelography is the imaging of choice to evaluate soft tissue involvement, nerve root or spinal cord impingement for any patient with a contraindication to MRI.[13]

Since its introduction in the early 1980s, MRI visualizes the bone-soft tissue interface with a highly detailed rendition of compression and/or invasion of osseous, neural, and paraspinal structures.[4,10] T2-weighted imaging (T2WI) is best used to assess spinal cord compression and the degree of spinal stenosis. Osseous invasion can also be visualized as the replacement of normal marrow fat signal with neoplastic tissue makes the tumor hypointense on T1-weighted imaging (T1WI). The tumor may also demonstrate gadolinium enhancement on T1-weighted imaging that can further enhance the visualization of tumor tissue. Due to the high-fat content of bone marrow on T1WI, fat suppression techniques are useful in evaluating osseous lesions that enhance with contrast.[22] Diffusion-weighted imaging may also help distinguish between benign and pathologic compression fracture (Figs. 1A to F).[23]

Only 11% of metastatic cervical lesions are isolated and an additional workup should commence to assess the overall disease burden of the patient.[24] Bone scintigraphy or Positron Emission Tomography with CT imaging (PET/CT) with 18F-fluorodeoxyglucose can be used to demonstrate additional areas of involvement through whole-body metastatic surveys. Bone scintigraphy is a measure of bone turnover, however, and findings are not specific to a neoplastic process as positive results may be seen in healing fractures, spondylosis, or infection. Positive findings should be correlated with MRI or CT. PET/CT can be used for whole-body metastatic surveys or as staging techniques in patients with known systemic cancer.[25] PET/CT may also be used to follow treatment response after the initiation of therapy.

Angiography should be considered in any spinal metastasis that results from a highly vascular primary tumor: renal cell carcinoma, thyroid carcinoma, angiosarcoma, leiomyosarcoma, hepatocellular carcinoma, and neuroendocrine tumors (pheochromocytoma, paraganglioma).[26] In the cervical spine, the patency of the vertebral artery as well as any collateral circulation should be

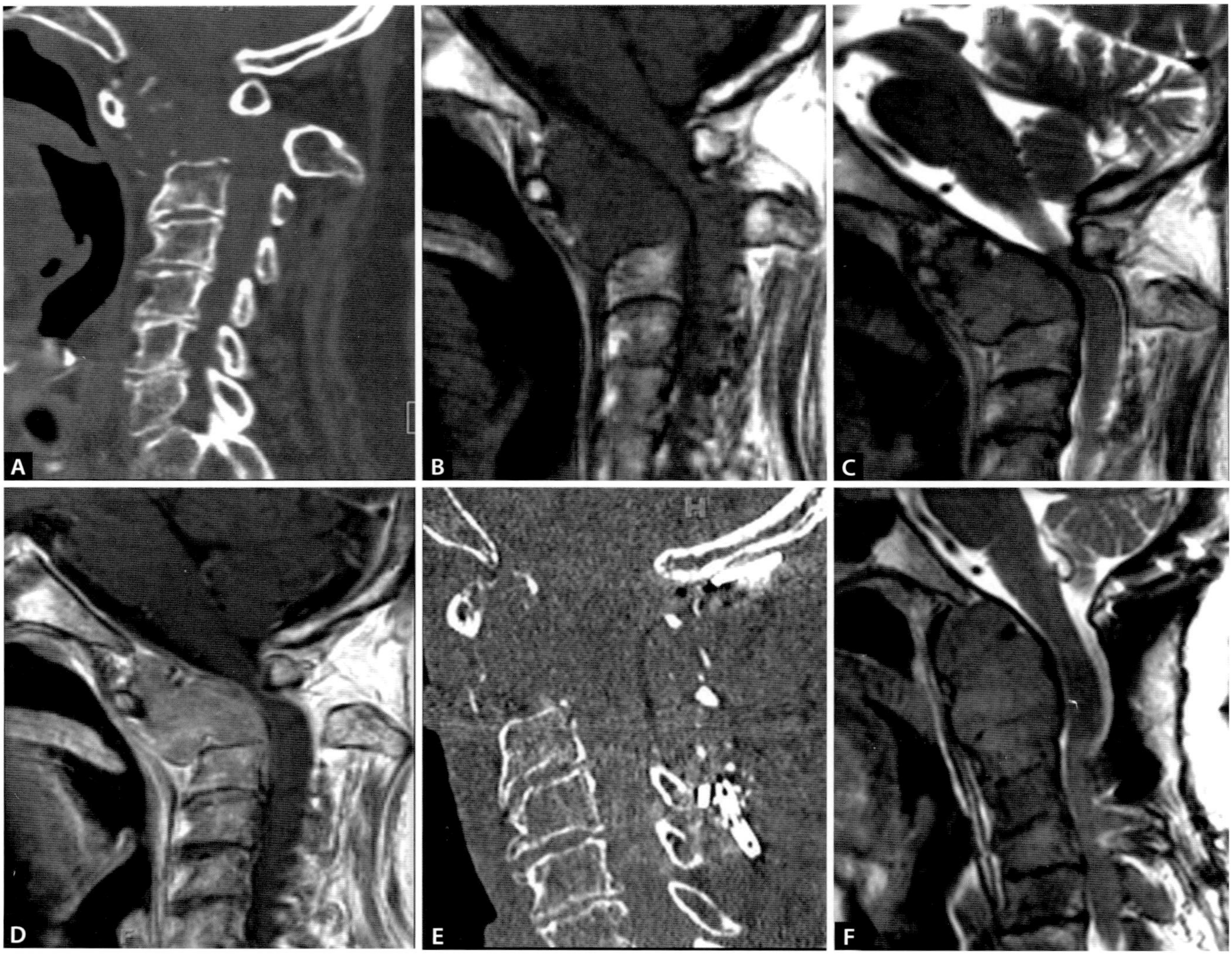

Figs. 1A to F: Spinal instability resulting from expansile metastatic C2 lesion. (A) Computed tomography (CT) scan showing a destructive, osteolytic process. (B to D) T2-weighted imaging demonstrating hyperintensity and compression of the cervical spinal cord. T1-weighted imaging with (B) and without (D) contrast demonstrating hypointensity that is diffusely contrast-enhancing. Postoperative imaging shows decompression and restoration of normal alignment immediately following posterior decompression (E). Despite growth 18 months following surgery the patient still demonstrates adequate decompression (F).

identified preoperatively as the tumor-vessel interface can sometimes be difficult to determine and inadvertent sacrifice may be necessary. At this time, preoperative embolization of any tumor feeders should also be considered to help decrease intraoperative blood loss.[26]

Nonsurgical Management

Management of metastatic disease requires a multidisciplinary approach that includes medical, surgical, and radiation oncology. Treatment in large part depends on appropriate patient selection as well as tumor pathology and can range from palliative nonoperative management to aggressive surgical intervention. Patient characteristics such as their age, current medical condition, overall life expectancy, systemic tumor burden, and prior treatments must be considered when designing an appropriate management plan. Age, although not an absolute contraindication to surgical management, is an important contributor to estimate an individual's life expectancy as well as their ability to tolerate surgery. Life expectancy is also an important consideration as those patients with a life expectancy of less than 8–12 weeks are more appropriate for nonoperative management. Rao et al. found a mean survival of all metastatic tumors to the bony cervical spine at 14.7 months,[24] however, this can vary widely based on the underlying tumor pathology, as some are associated with a poorer prognosis. Lung cancers tend to do poorly once the metastatic disease is discovered with a median survival of 7–9 months compared to patients with metastatic breast cancer who have a median survival of 30 months.[10]

Several scoring systems for spinal metastasis exist using a range of prognostic factors to assess clinical outcome and survival. Most recently, the Spinal Oncology Study Group (SOSG) defined standardized indications for surgical treatment of tumor-related spinal instability.[27] The Spinal Instability Neoplastic Score (SINS) assigns a numerical score based on the subcategories of location, pain, pathology, radiographic alignment, vertebral body collapse, and posterolateral involvement of the spinal elements. Scores predict the level of instability and are grouped into stable (SINS score 0–6), potentially unstable (SINS score 7–12), and unstable (SINS score 13–18) lesions. Based on these markers, the patient may be a candidate for surgical stabilization. Tokuhashi et al. also released updated guidelines regarding their prognostic criteria to evaluate metastatic spinal tumors prior to treatment. Their scale divides patients into three groups (0–8, 9–12, and 12–15) based on length of survival (<6 months, 6–12 months, and >12 months) and found this correlated with the goals of treatment (palliative, palliative surgery, and excisional surgery) (Table 2).[28]

In general, nonsurgical management is recommended when tumor involvement has not resulted in spinal instability, neurologic deficit, and medically refractory pain.[16] Nonsurgical management includes radiotherapy, chemotherapy, and hormonal therapy depending on the underlying pathology.

Radiation Treatment

Radiation therapy plays an important role in palliation of spinal metastasis and is effective in obtaining pain relief, preventing pathologic fracture or vertebral collapse, and avoids progression/allowing reversal of neurologic dysfunction.[4,10] Response to radiation therapy varies by tumor type with some lesions being more radiosensitive

Table 2: Surgical classification systems as indications for surgical stabilization and prognostic stratification.

Tomita (1995)[29]	• Phase I (1987–1991): Retrospective analysis of 67 patients to evaluate predictors. Hazard ratios were analyzed and standardized • Phase 2 (1993–1996): Prospective validation of 61 patients • Total score 2–10 based on: – Grade of malignancy of primary tumor: 1 slow growth, 2 moderate growth, 4 rapid growth – Visceral metastases to vital organs: 0 no mets, 2 treatable mets, 4 untreatable mets – Bone metastases: 1 solitary/isolated, 2 multiple	• 2–3 points: Long-term control (mean OS 50 m), wide, or marginal excision • 4–5 points: Middle term (mean survival 23.5 m), marginal, or intralesional excision • 6–7 points: Short-term palliation (mean survival 15 m), palliative surgery • 8–10 points: Terminal care (mean survival 6 m), supportive care/no surgery Correlation of combined score better than individual factors
Tokuhashi (2005)[28]	Evaluation system for the prognosis of metastatic spine tumors: • General condition/performance status (poor, moderate, good) • Number of extraspinal bone mets (>3, 1–2, 0) • Number of mets in the vertebral body (>3, 2, 1) • Metastases to major internal organs (unremovable, removable, none) • Primary site of cancer: – Lung, osteosarcoma, stomach, bladder, esophagus, pancreas – Liver, gallbladder, unidentified – Others – Kidney, uterus – Rectum – Thyroid, breast, prostate, carcinoid tumor • Spinal cord palsy (complete, incomplete, none)	All categories range from 0 to 2 points with exception of primary tumor pathology (maximum 5 points), which places the highest prognostic weight on primary tumor pathology. • Total score 0–8 ≤ 6 months, nonoperative or conservative treatment • 9–11 ≥ 6 months, palliative surgery or excisional surgery if single lesion without extraspinal metastases • 12–15 ≤ 1 year, excisional surgery

Contd...

Contd...

SINS (2010)[30]	Elements of SINS • Location: – Junctional – Mobile spine – Semi-rigid – Rigid • Pain relief with recumbency and/or pain with movement/loading of the spine (yes, no, pain-free) • Bone lesion (lytic, mixed, blastic) • Radiographic spinal alignment (subluxation/translation, de novo deformity, normal alignment) • Vertebral body collapse (>50%, <50%, no collapse, none) • Posterolateral involvement of spinal elements (facet, pedicle, or CV joint fracture or replacement with tumor: bilateral, unilateral none)	• 0–6: Stability • 7–12: Indeterminant (possibly impending) instability • 13–18: Instability Surgical consultation recommended for patients with SINS >7. Scoring system has not been validated but based on expert opinion
Tomita (2006)[31]	Anatomic description and local extent of tumor Intracompartmental: • Anterior or posterior lesion in situ • Extension to pedicle • Anterior-posterior development Extracompartmental: • Epidural extension • Paravertebral development • Involvement to adjacent vertebrae Multiple, skip lesion (type 7)	Types 2–5: En bloc vertebrectomy is recommended Types 1 and 6: En bloc vertebrectomy is relatively recommended Type 7: En bloc vertebrectomy is contraindicated
Weinstein-Boriani-Biagini[32]	Precise data-gathering tool that describes tumor involvement of vertebral body and adjacent tissues: Vertebrae divided into 12 sectors in a clock-face arrangement beginning at the spinous process. Six tissue layers in the cervical spine are defined: • Extraosseous soft tissues • Intraosseous superficial • Intraosseous deep • Extraosseous extradural • Extraosseous intradural • Transverse foramen/vertebral artery	Three major methods for performing en bloc excision: • Tumor confined to zones 4–8 or 5–9 with one pedicle free of tumor, 2 stages en bloc approach • Tumor occupies zones 3–5 or 8–10, eccentrically located, sagittal resection recommended • Tumor occupies zones 10 and 3, en bloc excision can be performed via posterior approach
Enneking[33]	Benign tumors: • S1, latent inactive. Asymptomatic with true capsule • S2, active slow-growing, bordered by a thin capsule • S3, aggressive benign, may not have a capsule and invades neighboring tissue Localized malignant tumors: • I: A, tumor within vertebrae or B, tumor invading paravertebral compartments • II: A/B, quick-growing lesions with epidural and paravertebral extension Metastatic high-grade malignant tumors: • III: A, intracompartmental, and B extracompartmental	Treatment strategies: • S1, no surgery necessary unless for decompression or stabilization; S2 intralesional excision; S3, marginal en bloc excision should be attempted • I A/B and IIA/B with attempted wide en bloc resection

than others (Table 3). Indications for stand-alone radiation include radiosensitive tumors, expected survival of less than 3 months, poor surgical candidate, or multilevel or diffuse spinal involvement. No randomized control studies have elucidated an optimal dosing regimen. Positive response to tumor therapy can be measured by decreased tumor size and control of local pain. In 2005, Patchell et al. conducted a randomized controlled trial comparing the relative efficacy of surgery alone, radiotherapy alone, and combined radiotherapy and surgery. While their study included patients with cervical metastasis, only 8/50 from the surgical cohort and 5/50 of the radiation cohort had

Table 3: Sensitivity of primary tumor types to radiation treatment.	
Radiosensitivity of primary tumor pathologies	
Highly radiosensitive	Multiple myelomas, lymphoma, small cell lung cancer, seminoma of testes, neuroblastoma, Ewing's sarcoma
Moderately radiosensitive	Prostate, breast, lung, and colon
Not radiosensitive	Thyroid, kidney, melanoma

cervical metastasis. The authors determined that both survival and functional outcomes were superior in the group undergoing both surgery and radiotherapy for all included patients.[34]

Conventional radiation is typically administered over a 10- to 14-day course with a total radiation dose of 25–40 Gy.[35] Traditionally, the radiation field includes the diseased level with a 5 cm margin or approximately two vertebral bodies above and below the target.[36] However, the primary limiting factor of radiation dosing to the vertebral body is the low tolerance of the spinal cord for radiation-induced myelopathy.[37] This results in below optimal therapeutic doses being delivered to the metastatic lesion with a concern for local failure and disease progression.

Stereotactic radiosurgery (SRS) is increasingly utilized for the treatment of osseous lesions with a growing body of literature supporting its use. Several large case series documents the efficacy of SRS for spinal metastatic disease, however, there is still a paucity of Class I data comparing this to conventional radiotherapy. Gerszten et al.[38] report one of the largest series of patients with spinal tumors treated with SRS with a total of 393 patients who were treated for 500 lesions involving the vertebral body. The majority of these lesions were metastatic and pain was the primary indicator of treatment. Of the patients who underwent treatment, 86% experienced long-term improvement in pain control. Certain tumor histology, breast, melanoma, renal, and lung cancer, were more likely to be associated with pain control. There was an 88% rate of local control on follow-up imaging with no tumor progression at adjacent vertebral body levels. Ryu et al. also reported on a series of 177 patients with 230 lesions in the vertebral body.[39] They reported complete or partial pain relief in 85% of the patients who underwent SRS for spinal metastasis. There was a 4% failure rate at adjacent vertebral body levels in their series. Chang et al.[40] found that the epidural space was the most common area of recurrence (47%) followed by the pedicles and posterior elements (18%). This suggests that the recurrence was along the portion of the tumor receiving the smallest dose or perhaps a marginal miss. In the literature, there is a greater than 80% local control rate although follow-up times vary among studies.[41]

A large proportion of patients (43–97%) experienced improvement in back pain after SRS, which is comparable to rates for patients undergoing standard fractionated radiotherapy. However, several Class I studies exist to determine the comparative efficacies of single-dose versus fractionated-dose radiation therapy and have not found a significant difference in pain, functional, and complication outcomes.[41] It is unclear whether SRS may reverse preexisting neurological deficits. Gerszten et al. reported patients had some improvement in radiculopathies. Wowra et al.[42] conducted a prospective case series assessing the clinical results of 102 patients who underwent CyberKnife treatment for spinal lesions. They found a significant decrease in pain. In addition, a 2% complication rate was reported which was primarily due to segmental neuropathy due to tumor hemorrhage as well as vertebral instability. Gibbs et al.[43] also prospectively analyzed outcomes in 74 patients with 102 spinal metastases treated with radiosurgery. They reported an overall 84% rate of improvement in functional outcomes with only 2% of patients demonstrating deteriorating neurological function. Only 4% of patients experienced myelopathic symptoms, which were the only reported complication. However, many studies exclude patients who have significant cord compression and median survival in some series is also quite short, suggesting a patient selection bias.

Chemotherapy

Chemotherapeutic agents are classified into two major categories: antitumor drugs and drugs that minimize the secondary effects of the tumor, such as bisphosphonates, corticosteroids, or analgesics.[44] Chemotherapy may be used in the setting of sensitive tumors for primary control of the systemic disease, however, it is not the primary treatment for spinal instability. Traditionally, breast, thyroid, and small cell lung carcinomas are sensitive to chemotherapy, whereas gastrointestinal tract, squamous cell carcinoma of the lung, and renal cell carcinomas are not.[45-49] Hormonal treatment is also commonly used for prostate and breast adenocarcinoma.[46,50-53] Estrogen agonists or antagonists such as tamoxifen and aromatase inhibitors such as letrozole have been shown to be effective against breast cancer. Prostate cancer may respond to androgen deprivation with GnRH agonists and/or flutimide.

Bisphosphonate therapy is also advocated in the setting of metastatic spine disease as they have been shown to reduce the incidence of skeletal-related events (SRE). Class I evidence has shown the efficacy of clonodrate, pamidronate, and zoledronate in decreasing the incidence of total SRE, such as fractures.[54-57] Rosen et al.[56] conducted a randomized controlled trial comparing the efficacy of zoledronate to pamidronate and found that zoledronate was more efficacious in reducing the incidence of both pathologic vertebral fractures and cord compression.

Corticosteroids are a primary component of pharmacologic therapy for pain and neuropathy associated with vertebral metastasis. They decrease tumor-associated inflammation, decrease spinal cord edema and can improve neurologic function, and may have some oncolytic effects in the case of certain tumor pathologies (lymphoma, multiple myeloma, and breast cancer).[19] Analgesics are also important to help the patient manage uncontrolled pain. Narcotics, certain anticonvulsant medications with an effect on neuropathic pain, tricyclic antidepressants, and topical treatments are all important components to helping patients with metastatic disease to help improve their functional status and quality of life.

Surgical Indications and Treatment

Once the appropriate patient has been selected for surgical management, determining the extent and surgical approach requires a staging of the lesion. Various surgical staging systems have been devised to determine the best surgical approach and to recommend whether a particular lesion is amenable to curative or palliative intervention. The Tomita[31] and Weinstein-Boriani-Biagini (WBB)[32] system provides anatomic descriptions of the tumor involvement. Both are further described later in this chapter (*Primary Tumors, Surgical Indications, and Treatment*), but neither addresses the prognosis related to surgical resection. Curative surgery is most often limited to primary spinal tumors, and a palliative approach is generally indicated in the setting of metastatic tumors.

The general indications for surgical intervention are neurologic dysfunction, spinal instability, and medically intractable pain. Metastatic disease of the upper cervical spine is more commonly attributable to spinal instability that may or may not be associated with spinal cord compression. The subaxial spine is more commonly involved than the craniovertebral junction and as a result, is more often associated with surgical stabilization.[58] However, neurologic compromise and deficits might exist given the smaller caliber of the spinal canal. This may result in earlier onset of a neurologic deficit as well as increased intersegmental mobility of the subaxial spine.

Reconstruction Options

The approach for tumor resection is determined by the location of the bone, epidural, and paraspinal tumor. Metastatic tumors causing epidural cord compression typically arise from the vertebral body and extend dorsally. In these cases, an anterior approach will provide the best ability to decompress the spinal cord. Posterior approaches are less commonly used as a primary standalone technique as most metastases are located anteriorly. However, this technique can be used as an adjunct to anterior decompression and reconstruction. The potential for failure of anterior instrumentation is significant given the poor bone quality due to cachexia, prior irradiation, and medication usage.

High cervical spine lesions at the craniocervical junction provide a unique set of challenges for decompression and fixation. While anterior decompression and instrumentation may be advocated for primary tumors, it plays a limited role in patients with metastases. Despite the presence of anterior epidural disease, decompression from an anterior approach may be associated with morbidity rates as high as 32%.[59] The vast majority of these lesions are well decompressed and instrumented posteriorly.[12,27,60] Anterior subluxation may be seen secondary to tumor erosion leading to ligamentous instability. This instability may lead to significant motion of the atlas or axis leading to compression and damage of the upper cervical cord.[13,61] The ligamentous structures (the apical, transverse, and nuchal ligaments) provide a robust barrier for extension of tumor from the vertebral body into the epidural space. Pain and neurologic compromise usually result from O to C1 or C1 to 2 instability. Therefore, treatment can be aimed at reconstituting the craniocervical junction with posterior stabilization techniques (*see* Figs. 1A to F). Reduction of the craniocervical deformity and stabilization provides decompression and relief of symptoms. Adjuvant treatment with radiation therapy or chemotherapy will be needed to treat the ventral tumor.

Determining which fusions should be extended to the occiput in cases of high cervical metastasis should be dependent on the spinal alignment. In patients with normal spinal alignment or patients who can be reduced in extension, standard instrumentation from C1 to 3 may be possible. However, in patients with spinal instability, fracture subluxations and significant osteolytic destruction of multiple vertebral levels should be considered for extension of the instrumentation to the occiput. In cases where C1 and C2 are extensively involved, fusion to the occiput could help prevent loss of fixation should there be additional disease progression.[12] Anterior subluxation due to instability at the craniocervical junction may be addressed through a posterior decompression and reduction. This technique requires laminectomies of C1 and C2 to ensure adequate space at the level of deformity. This technique is performed first by distracting against the occipital plate to allow vertical occipitocervical decompression. This is followed by compressing the rod within the occipital plate to allow anterior translation of C2, thus reducing the atlantodens interval.[61]

A recent review of the literature by Witham et al.[62] showed an evolution toward more aggressive decompressive surgery with extensive stabilization. Their review of the literature showed that patients with metastatic epidural spinal cord compression, patients who had radiation alone had a neurologic improvement in 36%, and 17% of patients worsened. Patients who underwent a laminectomy with or without radiation showed similar results, as 42% of patients demonstrated neurologic improvement and 13% with worsening function. Surgical morbidity and mortality was 6% overall. In patients who underwent spinal stability in addition to decompression and radiation, a motor improvement was seen in 64% of patients. Pain relief was also achieved in 88% of patients. Patients who had anterior decompression and stabilization in addition to XRT had an improvement in neurological function in 75% of patients although there was a slight increase in surgical mortality to 10%.[62]

Complications

Anterior approaches can be more complicated than a case of degenerative cervical spine disease. If the patient has been irradiated prior to surgery, the planes of dissection can be more difficult to find secondary to radiation-related scarring. Esophageal injury and swallowing dysfunction can lead to significant postoperative morbidity and are more common in patients with distorted anatomy secondary to an underlying tumor. In highly vascular metastasis (e.g. renal cell carcinoma), preoperative embolization may help avoid significant intraoperative hemorrhage.[26] Bone quality should also be assessed on preoperative imaging as lytic lesions may involve multiple vertebral levels and concern for hardware settling may necessitate supplemental posterior fusion.

The vertebral artery anatomy should be carefully studied on preoperative imaging since tumor involvement of the transverse foramina and encroachment of the vessel may present a potential risk of injury. Collateral cerebral circulation should be identified if the vertebral artery requires intraoperative sacrifice. Vertebral artery bleeding can generally be controlled with pressure and ligation with aneurysmal clips, however, this places the patient at risk of postoperative stroke.

Cerebrospinal fluid (CSF) leaks are potential in any cervical operation, however, the potential risk is significantly higher in tumor resections. If the patient has undergone prior irradiation, there can be significant scarring of the plane between the tumor and dura. Extensive drilling may also be required for decompression, which can put the dura at risk. Additionally, if the metastatic disease extends into the dura, durotomy can be difficult to avoid. Prolonged lumbar drainage may be indicated in patients where there is not a primary dural closure.[58]

Esophageal injury is a known risk factor with anterior surgery, and in those patients with preoperative radiation, esophageal tears can be more easily encountered. An experienced head and neck surgeon may be helpful in assisting with exposure if there is significant distortion from tumor growth or if the patient has had preoperative irradiation. If there is a tear encountered intraoperatively, they can also be helpful in primary repair or coverage of this region. Given the need for adjuvant therapy and the additional stress, it will place on the surrounding tissue, definitive therapy through tissue coverage should be considered. This may be done through free flaps from the radial forearm or omental, or potentially a rotational flap from the pectoral muscles. Additional adjuvant therapy such as radiation and chemotherapy may be delayed if the esophageal injury is not dealt with in a timely manner. The patient may need alternate sources of nutrition postoperatively either through a gastrostomy tube or parenteral nutrition until the perforation has healed.

Prognosis

Resection of cervical metastasis with reconstruction and instrumented stabilization is an efficacious means for improving patient quality of life based on high-quality evidence (Class I and II). Several studies have shown significantly decreased pain and improvement or preservation of physical functioning.[4,58]

Patchell et al.[34] performed the only Class I evidence with a 10-year multi-institutional, nonblinded randomized controlled trial that assessed the efficacy of direct decompressive surgery in the treatment of metastatic cancer. This study randomized 101 patients into surgery followed by radiotherapy compared with radiotherapy alone. Radiotherapy was delivered in Ten 3 Gy fractions for a total of 30 Gy. The study found that significantly more patients who underwent surgery with radiation were able to ambulate in comparison to the radiotherapy group (84% vs. 57%, respectively). There were also higher rates of retention of ambulation, reacquisition of ambulation, American Spinal Injury Association (ASIA) muscle strength scores, and Frankel scores in the cohort that underwent surgery plus radiotherapy. There was also a survival advantage for those patients who underwent surgery plus radiotherapy compared with radiotherapy alone (126 days vs. 100 days, respectively). Pain control was also measured as a measure of daily narcotic use and was also significantly improved in the surgical cohort. The data was not stratified to the cervical spine, but only 13 patients affected with cervical spine metastatic disease were included in the study.[34]

Two prospective studies have identified surgical efficacy in improving the quality of life in patients with spinal metastasis. Ibrahim et al.[63] conducted a multicenter prospective study that enrolled 223 patients, of which 16% had cervical spine disease. Neurologic outcomes were improved in the majority of patients and included postoperative ambulation (98%) and reacquisition of ambulation postoperatively (55%). These patients were further stratified according to the type of surgery performed and the authors found neurological outcomes were best for patients undergoing excisional surgical management.

Quan et al.[64] also performed the only prospective study that addressed surgical management and outcomes in patients with metastatic cervical spine lesions. They reported the outcomes of 26 patients who underwent surgery for symptomatic metastases in the cervical and cervicothoracic spine. A variety of approaches were performed that included palliative decompression and stabilization through anterior, posterior, and combined approaches. These patients were followed at the 1-, 3-, 6-, and 12-month interval. These patients had statistically improved pain control and global health score based on EORTC QLQ-C30 questionnaire. These patients did not experience any neurologic decline, and the authors concluded that surgical intervention in addition to adjuvant medical management had low morbidity and good symptomatic palliation to prevent further neurologic decline.

Although treatment of the metastatic disease requires a multidisciplinary approach, recent advances in medical management over the past several decades have improved outcomes and allowed more aggressive treatments. Improvement in chemotherapy regimens has led to overall increased survival and a rise in prevalence of metastatic spinal disease.[58] Improvement in spinal fixation devices allows surgeons to decompress the spine more completely, thus leading to improved functional outcomes. In combination with improved techniques in radiotherapy, patients have a greater likelihood of regaining and maintaining ambulation after treatment. The advent of SRS has allowed a more precise targeting of the malignant process while sparing the neighboring tissues.[41] Depending on the pathology and patient prognosis, oncologic cure with surgical and adjuvant therapy is pursued by medical and surgical oncologists alike.

PRIMARY SPINAL TUMORS

Osteochondromas also have a predilection for the cervical spine (greater than 50%), especially at C2. This may be associated with the greater mobility of the cervical spine, which can lead to increased stress and microtrauma on cartilaginous plates. Osteochondromas are typically found in patients less than 30 years of age and there is a 2:1 male predominance. Osteochondromas are more commonly found in the posterior elements of the vertebrae.[65] Rarely, these lesions will undergo malignant transformation to chondrosarcomas.[65]

Chordomas are one of the most common primary malignant bone tumors with an overall incidence of 0.08 per 100,000 individuals.[66] They occur more commonly in men than women and have an increased incidence in middle adulthood. These lesions arise from notochordal remnants and are one of the only primary osseous tumors that only occur in the spine. They are considered slow-growing, but locally invasive and demonstrate a propensity to metastasize in an estimated 5–40% of patients.[67-69]

Workup (Clinical Findings)

Symptoms and Signs

Patients with a primary vertebral column tumor may present similarly to those patients with metastatic disease. The most common symptom is neck pain, which is classically described as unremitting, worse in the supine position, less relieved by positional changes, unresponsive to analgesia, and more noticeable while at rest or in bed at night.[65] Similarly to metastatic disease, referred, mechanical, and nonmechanical pain may all be components of a patient's pain at presentation. Nonmechanical pain may result from tumor growth that causes the bony cortex of the vertebral body to expand and results in a pathologic fracture. This infiltration of the vertebral body and neoplastic destruction can lead to mechanical instability. Tumor growth can also lead to compression of the spinal cord and associated nerve roots leading to focal and radicular symptoms of pain, paraparesis, or paraplegia. Autonomic symptoms such as bowel and bladder dysfunction may also be present. The time course of symptoms may also suggest whether a lesion is benign, with slow onset, or malignant, with insidious onset.

Primary vertebral column neoplasms may also present as a spinal deformity with or without pain. Torticollis, scoliosis, or kyphosis can result from bony lesions that lead to bony collapse or secondarily reactive muscle spasms.[65] Pediatric patients who present with atypical scoliosis should be evaluated for an underlying pathology as part of a routine workup.

Primary cervical spine neoplasms may be locally aggressive and infiltrative and can cause symptoms related to impairment of the soft tissue surrounding the cervical spine. Patients may present with airway obstruction due to compression on the trachea. Anteriorly projecting tumors may abut the esophagus or oral palate and can cause significant dysphagia. If there is extensive soft tissue involvement of the tumor, these patients may also present with an oropharyngeal mass.[70]

Physical examination findings are similar to those patients with metastatic lesions and depend on the degree of the spinal cord or radicular impingement. Again, the most common neurological findings include paraparesis, hyperreflexia, spasticity, Hoffman sign, abnormal plantar responses, and Brown-Sequard syndrome. Bulbar symptoms may result from compression of the brainstem and cerebellar ataxia may also manifest due to compression across the foramen magnum. Radicular symptoms include dysesthetic pain in a dermatomal distribution or focal weakness.

Laboratory Findings

Please see laboratory findings for metastatic disease.

Imaging

Imaging for any cervical spine lesion is similar between primary and secondary lesions. Often, the metastatic disease must be considered given its prevalence in the general population and the rarity of primary osseous tumors. Standard imaging that should be obtained includes plain radiograph, CT or MRI imaging. Plain radiographs can be a useful screening test in patients with persistent back pain, new-onset deformity, or neurological deficits. Given the concern for limited contrast resolution and low sensitivity for vertebral bone loss, as previously mentioned, a CT scan should be obtained to cortical bone. CT imaging is also useful in identifying pathologic fractures and for characterizing the matrix of primary osseous tumors. Primary tumors may show osteolytic or osteoblastic effects dependent on their tumor pathology and are often described as "moth-eaten" in appearance (Figs. 2A and B). Chordomas show low attenuation on CT and are less often associated with calcifications. They also have a myxoid soft tissue component and vertebral collapse can be seen. Thin-cut CT imaging is the diagnostic tool of choice for osteochondromas as their pathologic hallmark is continuity of the lesion with the marrow and cortex of underlying bone.[71] Plain films may demonstrate a well-circumscribed, lytic lesion without reactive sclerosis.

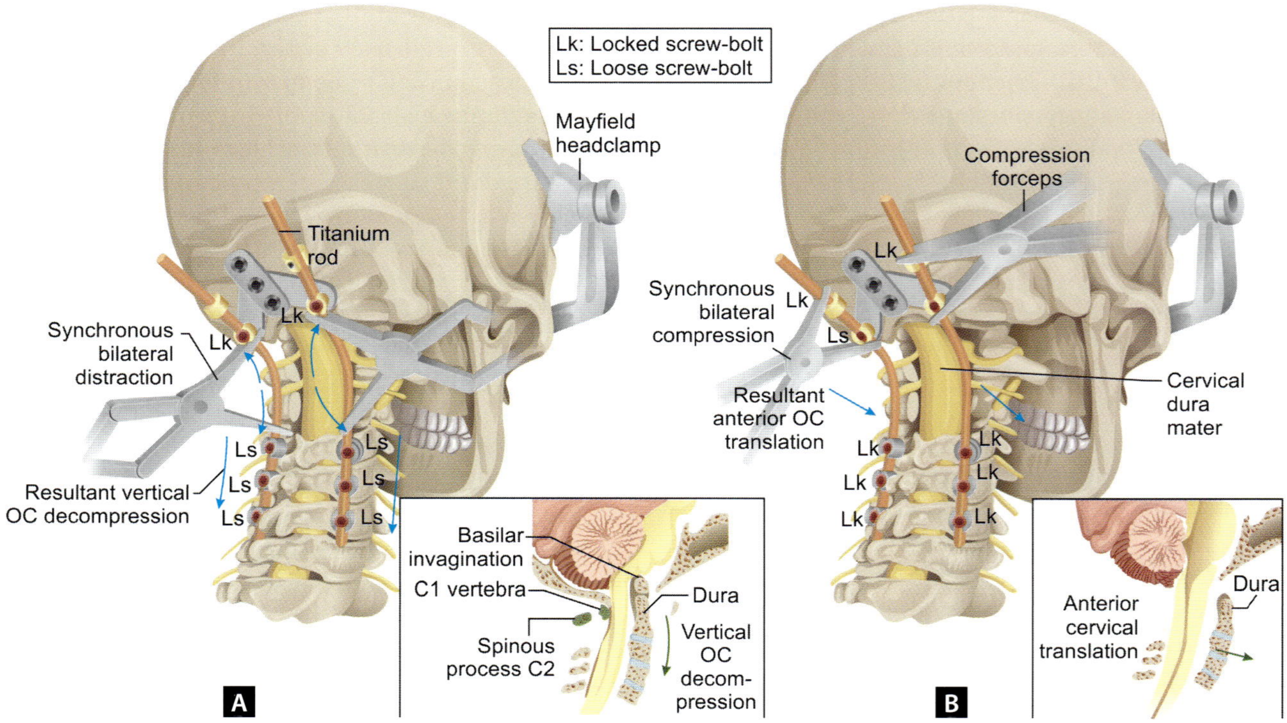

Figs. 2A and B: Technique demonstrating posterior decompression and fusion for the restoration of alignment for an unstable mass of the odontoid.

Source: Adapted from Hsu W, Zaidi HA, Suk I, et al. A new technique for intraoperative reduction of occipitocervical instability. Neurosurgery. 2010;66(6 Suppl Operative):319-23; discussion 323-4 (requested permission).

CT imaging may show a radiolucent or erosive lesion as cartilage appears with low attenuation on CT. Stippled patterns of calcification may be present.[71]

When used in conjunction with myelography, CT myelograms may be useful for evaluating impingement of the spinal canal or the relationship of a soft tissue mass to the thecal sac, especially in patients where an MRI is contraindicated. However, its role in the evaluation of spinal lesions is limited and has been largely supplanted by MRI. CT angiography may also be a useful screening study to assess the involvement of the foramen transversarium with tumor and the potential involvement of the vertebral arteries.

Magnetic resonance imaging is superior in defining the extraosseous soft tissue component of a neoplasm from the normal paraspinal soft tissue and neural structures.[72] In the case of primary tumors, different tumor pathologies have characteristic findings on MRI. Chordomas are midline lesions that can be destructive and infiltrative in paraspinal and epidural spaces. Chordomas often infiltrate the intervertebral disk space and can have an epidural extension. They will appear slightly iso- or hypointense compared with muscle on T1WI and hyperintense to muscle on T2WI. They demonstrate heterogeneous enhancement with gadolinium and often have foci of low signal attenuation in calcified areas. Cervical lesions may have prominent epidural and paravertebral components that are associated with foraminal enlargement and can mimic nerve sheath tumors.[73] MRI imaging for chondromas may be useful to distinguish between benign and malignant lesions, as an enhancing lesion may be more consistent with sarcomatous transformation.[73] Osteochondromas may also show continuity of the marrow, osseous, and cartilaginous components. The hyaline cartilaginous cap has an intermediate signal on T1WI and is hyperintense on T2WI. A cartilaginous cap of greater than 1.5 cm in thickness suggests malignant degeneration to chondrosarcoma (Figs. 3A to C).[74,75]

Angiography is important if there is any concern for occlusion of the vertebral artery or if preoperative planning suggests the potential sacrifice of this vessel. Formal

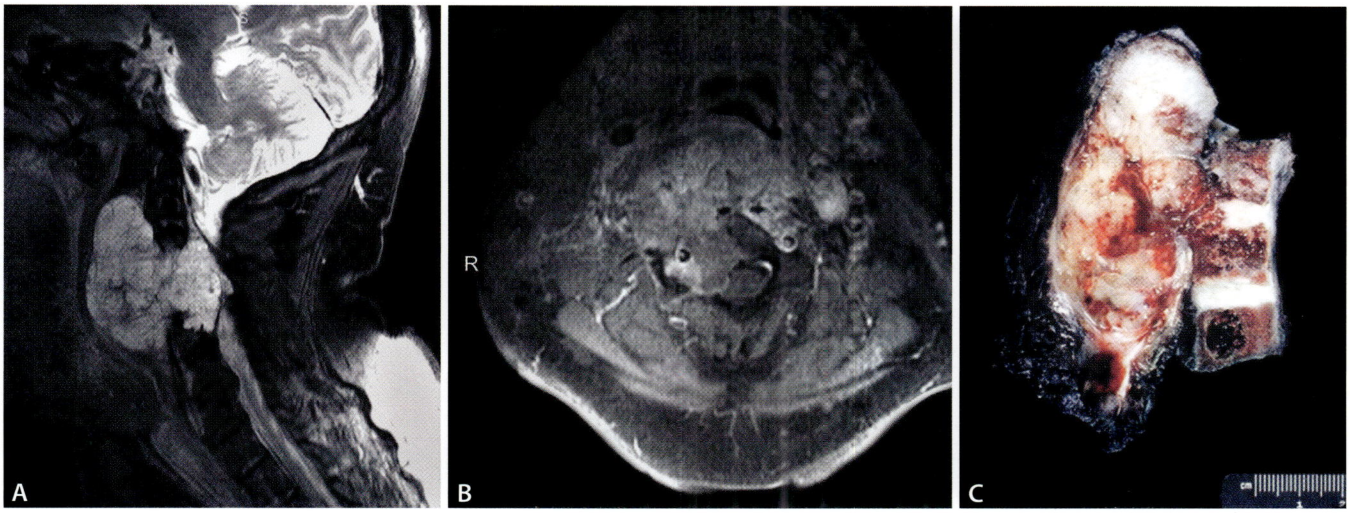

Figs. 3A to C: (A) Sagittal T2-weighted magnetic resonance imaging (MRI) demonstrating typical lobulated, physaliphorous appearing mass infiltrating C3–4 with anterior projection. (B) T1-weighted image with contrast showing heterogeneous enhancing lesion that encompasses the right vertebral artery and abuts the spinal cord and dura. (C) Showing corresponding specimen with margins intact.

digital-subtraction four-vessel cerebral angiograms help determine the patency of the involved vessel, the caliber, and patency of the contralateral vessel, and the intracranial collateral blood supply to the posterior circulation. Temporary balloon occlusion tests should be performed to determine the ability of the patient to tolerate potential vertebral artery sacrifice.[70]

Metastatic workup should also be considered for any spinal osseous tumor given the prevalence of metastatic disease over primary lesions. In addition, for highly malignant tumors, such as primary sarcomas, there is potential for metastatic spread and evaluation of the tumor's stage becomes important. This may be accomplished through either a scanning PET/CT or CT of the chest, abdomen, and pelvis with both oral and IV contrast. Chondromas have a low potential for malignant transformation and as a result, rarely metastasize. Chordomas, especially dedifferentiated chordomas, may metastasize and are most commonly found in the lungs or along the spinal column.[65]

Nonsurgical Management

Medical management has limited utility in the treatment of primary vertebral body tumors. There are several pathologies that have had increased responsiveness to chemotherapeutic regimens including Ewing's sarcoma and osteosarcoma, but these are not commonly seen in the cervical spine. However, the overwhelming majority of benign and malignant osseous tumors respond poorly to chemotherapy and conventional radiation therapy. Of those tumors, most commonly found in the cervical spine, surgical resection remains the mainstay of definitive therapy.

An important part of the medical decision-making includes obtaining a sample of tissue. Tissue-proven diagnosis is important even if the imaging is suggestive of a primary tumor as it may dictate the degree of surgical aggressiveness and help plan for any adjuvant therapy. Some primary osseous lesions are not primarily surgical lesions and tissue-proven diagnosis will help guide appropriate medical or surgical treatment. In addition, there are some primary lesions in which an *en bloc* approach is paramount to improving local disease control as well as overall survival and should be aggressively managed. *If certain tumor types are considered, such as chordomas, the biopsy tract should be carefully considered. These lesions tend to recur along a biopsy tract and biopsy needles should not transgress other body cavities (oral cavity or rectum).*[76] Modern biopsy techniques minimize this risk as the core biopsy needles retract close, and therefore, do not allow deposition of tumor cells along the biopsy tract. In the cervical spine, the resection of the biopsy tract is not commonly employed.

Radiotherapy

Most spinal tumors, including chordomas, have traditionally been thought resistant to conventional radiation as a stand-alone treatment or when coupled with debulking or palliative therapy.[77] Radiation therapy is not indicated in benign primary osseous tumors such as chondromas, as definitive surgical resection of these lesions is generally curative. However, advances in radiation technology and treatment have allowed clinicians to target the neoplasm with higher doses of radiation while sparing the adjacent critical structures. Due to the close proximity of the cervical spine to the spinal cord, brain stem, and cranial nerves, myelopathy due to radiation injury is a common adverse event.[78] Additionally, other structures such as the carotid and vertebral arteries, esophagus, and trachea limit the ability to deliver conventional radiotherapy at doses of 40–60 Gy with 5-year local control rates of 10–40%.[79-81] Traditional dosing of less than 60 Gy has not been effective in treating the gross or macroscopic disease of chordomas. There is minimal evidence examining radiotherapy for mobile cervical spine chordomas as the overall prevalence is small. However, the majority of data has been extrapolated from the treatment of skull-based or sacral chordomas.

There have been significant advances in the delivery of photon radiotherapy using the technique of intensity-modulated radiotherapy (IMRT). IMRT allows a more conformal delivery to achieve higher doses to the target and lower doses to the surrounding tissue. Proton beam therapy also allows improved sparing of the immediate critical organs due to the ballistic property of protons that can deliver precise deposition of ionizing energy due to the "Bragg peak" effect. Thus, the treatment is extremely conformal and 5-year local control rates reach 50–60% with stand-alone treatment.[82,83] Centers have started to combine therapies with both photon and proton ionizing radiation and have reported successful treatments with both local control and 5-year survival rates of 59–82% in skull base and cervical chordomas. No clinical trials have compared photon and proton beam therapy with IMRT and stereotactic delivery techniques.

Noel et al. present a case series of 100 patients with chordomas of the skull base and upper cervical spine treated with surgical resection and a combination of proton and photon beam therapy.[84] They reported a 2- and 5-year local control rate of 86.3% and 53.8% with an overall survival rate at 2- and 5-year of 94.3% and 80.5%, respectively. DeLaney et al.[85] also used a range of 50.4–77.4 Gy of neoadjuvant photon beam therapy in 50 patients with chordoma or primary sarcoma. Of these patients, 37 went on to have a surgical resection, and the 5-year local control and overall disease survival rates were 78% and 63%, respectively. Yasuda et al.[86] recently reported a series of 40 patients with chordomas of the skull base and cervical spine. The series had an extensive resection rate of 42.5% with a median follow-up of 56.5 months. Radiotherapy was performed in 75% with a mean dose of 68.9 cobalt gray equivalents. The 5-year progression-free survival and overall survival rate were 70% and 83.4%, respectively. Metastases were seen in 12.5% of patients.[86]

In patients where proton beam therapy is planned, an anterior approach through a transoral, transmandibular resection should not be considered due to the high risk of mandibular pseudoarthrosis. Osteonecrosis of the mandible may be encountered in 2–13% of patients undergoing proton beam therapy for head and neck cancers.[65] This may rise to between 30% and 50% in patients with oral cancers or pathologies that require transection of the mandible and this can require extensive debridement or resection.[70] Planned adjuvant therapy should be discussed amongst all members of the treatment team to determine the best treatment order.

Neoadjuvant treatment with SRS may also improve rates of local control and disease-free survival. A recent report from the North American Gamma Knife Consortium identified 71 patients who underwent SRS for skull-based chordomas. The mean tumor volume treated was 7.1 cm^3, but this ranged from 0.9 cm^3 to 109 cm^3 with a median dose range of 15 Gy (range 9–25 Gy).[87] These patients had a median follow-up of 5 years with an actuarial overall survival of 80%. They found that younger age, longer interval between initial diagnosis and SRS, no previous radiosurgery, smaller tumor volumes, and less than 2 cranial nerve deficits were associated with improved patient survival. The 5-year tumor control rate was 66% for the entire group. Jiang et al.[88] reported a series of 20 patients treated with CyberKnife radiotherapy and found the tumor control rate was 55%. They treated tumor volumes on average of 16.1 cm^3 (range 2.4–45.9 cm^3) and found patients who were initially presenting without prior treatment had improved outcomes. Tumor progression was seen in 45% of treated patients. Long-term outcomes are not yet well-established for this therapy in comparison to proton beam therapy. However, both the economical advantage and decreased treatment time (1–5 days vs. 6 weeks) have been raised in the literature.

One additional consideration when determining the application of adjuvant radiotherapy is intraoperative hardware placement. Spinal hardware that is used to stabilize the spine following resection can pose a significant limitation for postoperative radiation. Metal implants produce artifacts on postsurgical CT scans which can influence the calculation of the correct range of heavy charged particles.[89] Even if there are no artifacts, metal implants may lead to a range of uncertainties since they are not equivalent to biological tissue. Some centers have advocated preoperative irradiation of the chordoma to help contain tumor spillage intraoperatively as well as minimizing the artifact created by spinal hardware, but no outcome data exist to support this expert opinion.

Chemotherapy

Treatment of the most common primary tumors in the cervical spine has historically been insensitive to conventional chemotherapy. Several primary osseous tumors, namely Ewing's sarcoma and osteogenic sarcoma, have had improved survival with the advent of more effective chemotherapeutic options. However, these lesions are uncommonly found in the cervical spine.[70,90] No chemotherapeutic regimens have been described for the treatment of chondromas unless there is a concern for malignant conversion. Chordomas pathologically consist of physaliferous cells with immunoreactivity to S-100, epithelial markers, epithelial membrane antigen, and cytokeratin. In systematic reviews of the literature, chordomas were found to be insensitive to conventional chemotherapies. Case reports of anthracycline, cisplatin, alkylating agents,[91] and camptothecin analogs[92] have shown some sensitivity but overall survival remains poor. Identification of cytogenetic and proteomic markers has promoted new targeted chemotherapy trials that have shown some promise. Dedifferentiated chordomas are similar to high-grade sarcomas and are a rare subgroup. These tumors may show some response to a number of chemotherapeutic agents.[74,93]

Imatinib mesylate (Gleevec, Novartis) is a tyrosine kinase inhibitor that targets platelet-derived growth factor receptor-β (PDGFβ). A phase II clinical study by Stacchiotti et al.[94] showed that imatinib mesylate has some antitumor activity against advanced chordoma. Of the 26 patients receiving imatinib, 10 (39%) achieved a greater than 25% decrease in PET uptake 3 months after treatment initiation and there was disease stabilization in 72% of the total cases. Median survival and progression-free survivals were 34.9 and 9.2 months, respectively. One limitation of this series is a median follow-up was only 26.4 months, as the indolent nature of chordomas causes slow growth and adequate time for disease progression may not have been achieved. Additionally, 42% of these patients developed metastatic disease despite treatment.[94]

Another potential target for treatment is epidermal growth factor receptor (EGFR) and c-MET. Several in vitro analysis have demonstrated high expressivity of EGFR in chordoma pathogenesis[91,95] and that growth was markedly inhibited when given an EGFR inhibitor. Hof et al. investigated the use of a combination of cetuximab/gefitinib, two well-known drugs that inhibit the EGFR pathway in the treatment of a sacral chordoma. This patient originally presented with a sacral chordoma and pulmonary metastasis and underwent adjuvant radiotherapy. After 11 months, he had a progression of the pulmonary metastasis and at that time was treated with cetuximab/gefitinib. His pulmonary metastasis showed a partial response over a 9-month follow-up.[96]

There have been several in vitro studies that have evaluated the expressivity and promotion in the growth of chordoma cell lines and targets include: brachyury,[97] MTAP, insulin-like growth factor-1 receptor/insulin (IGF1R), PI3K/AKT/TSC1/TSC2/Mtor, multidrug resistance-associated protein 1 (MRP1), and hypoxia-inducible factor 1 alpha (HIF-1a), and signal transducer and activator of transcription 3 (STAT3).[91] Several clinical trials are underway including a phase 1 trial of nilotinib therapy (NCT01407198) and a study involving dasatinib (NCT00464620).[91] In addition, there are ongoing trials involving lapatinib and everolimus.[91]

Surgical Indications and Treatment

For the majority of osseous tumors, the primary mode of treatment is surgical. After an initial assessment, it becomes necessary to stage the tumor to assess the patient's prognosis and to determine the best therapeutic option for the patient. Several scoring systems exist that assess the patient's general status as well as the patient's prognosis and to determine the best therapeutic option for the patient. The Tomita scoring system provides an anatomic description and local extent of the tumor within the vertebra.[31] This scoring system is a modification of the

Enneking system and helps surgeons determine whether curative or palliative treatment is warranted. The vertebral body is divided into five anatomic sites (vertebral body, pedicle, lamina and spinous process, the spinal canal, and paravertebral space). The numbers denote the anatomic site and reflect the sequence of tumor progression. The authors classify lesions as intracompartmental (sites 1–3) or extracompartmental (4–6). Multiple or skip lesions are denoted as type 7. Total en bloc resection is recommended for types 2–5, relatively indicated for types 1 and 6, and contraindicated for type 7 lesions.[31]

The Weinstein-Boriani-Biagini (WBB) staging system was designated to help surgeons plan the most appropriate avenue of tumor resection.[32,33] The vertebra is divided into 12 equal zones radiating from the spinal canal that is numbered clockwise from 1 to 12. The tumor is additionally classified into one of the six concentric layers, from paravertebral extraosseous soft tissue (A) to the dura (E) and the vertebral artery (F). Traditional teaching states that en bloc excisions can be performed if the tumor is confined to WBB zones 4–8 or 5–9 with at least one pedicle free of tumor. If a tumor is isolated to zones 10 to 3, removal of only the posterior elements may be indicated. Tumors involving zones 2–5 or 7–11 should have a sagittal resection performed which is defined as an en bloc excision of a tumor arising eccentrically in the vertebral body, pedicle, or transverse process.

Enneking first described principles for surgical management of long bone tumors that has since been applied to spinal column tumors.[33] Benign tumors are divided into three stages: inactive, active, and aggressive. Malignant tumors are also staged based on tumor histology with subclassification based on anatomic compartmentalization. These lesions are then recommended for conservative, intralesional, or en bloc resection (*see* Table 2).

En Bloc Resection

En bloc resections refer to the surgical resection of a tumor in a single piece without violations of the tumor margin. A wide excisional margin will include a healthy layer of tissue completely surrounding the tumor, however, given the proximity of the spine to the dura, arteries, and surrounding nerve roots the risk of a wide resection has many technical challenges. The majority of the literature on en bloc resections in the cervical spine refers to marginal resections in which the surgeon has operated along the pseudocapsule or reactive tissue immediately surrounding the tumor.[70] En bloc resection in the cervical spine is particularly challenging given the juxtaposition of critical structures including the spinal cord, cervical roots, and vertebral artery. Achieving wide-margin resection is nearly impossible without the sacrifice of those structures, which can lead to significant morbidity or mortality to the patient. Other risks of en bloc resections include possible tumor margin violation during resection and significant operative blood loss secondary to epidural venous bleeding and bleeding from the osteotomy sites. Other obstacles include tumor size, tumor location in relation to functional elements such as the oral cavity, neck, and chest, and the inability to provide reconstruction and stabilization or soft tissue coverage of the defect. Additionally, a true wide resection cannot truly be performed if there is an epidural extension as this necessitates dural removal, which has been reported but has significant risk and challenges. Multiple case reports for resection of chordomas have shown early recurrence and death with a 5-year survival estimated at 50–70% with piecemeal resection.[31,98,99] However, 5-year survival with an en bloc resection is as high as 100%.[31,99] Malignant tumors are at significant risk for local recurrence with less than half of the patients surviving beyond 5 years.[11,32,100] Recent evidence suggests that with en bloc excision, 5-year survival can reach as high as 60–70%.

There are three distinct categories of en bloc resection based on the location and anatomic involvement of the surrounding cord, roots, and vertebral artery: high cervical lesions arising from C1 to 3, mid-cervical tumors arising from C4 to 6, and cervicothoracic tumors that involve the cervicothoracic junction at C7–T1.[101]

High-cervical en bloc resections often involve the cervical roots and vertebral arteries. The cervical nerve roots C1–2 can be sacrificed without significant neurological defects and C3–4 can generally be unilaterally sacrificed without concern for diaphragm paralysis. However, vertebral artery sacrifice can lead to strokes and other neurological injuries especially in cases of dominant vertebral artery sacrifice or if there is an absence of adequate collateral supply in the posterior circulation. En bloc removal generally requires an anterior submandibular or transmandibular approach. Reconstruction of the upper cervical spine can also be challenging, especially in cases that involve the C1–2 complex. The craniocervical junction is responsible for the transition of axial loading forces from the occiput to the spinal column. This transition allows the axial loading forces to be located entirely lateral to the spinal canal and to then distribute the forces anteriorly to the vertebral column at the C2–3 disks and posterolaterally to the C2–3 facet joints. Advanced instrumentation has allowed progressive complex reconstructions but biomechanically has been difficult to recapitulate. Pseudoarthrosis and instrumentation failures can be common in this location (Figs. 4 to 6).[101]

Mid-cervical tumors with involvement of C4–6 levels can involve the C5–6 nerve roots as well as the vertebral artery. Cervical nerve roots in this location cannot be sacrificed with impunity and will result in loss of function in proximal upper extremity muscle groups. Neurological deficits may be acceptable to the patient in exchange for improved long-term survival or cure, but a thorough discussion should be had with the patient preoperatively. Anterior approaches to this region may be accomplished with a modified Smith-Robinson approach with radical dissection of soft tissues along the anterolateral region

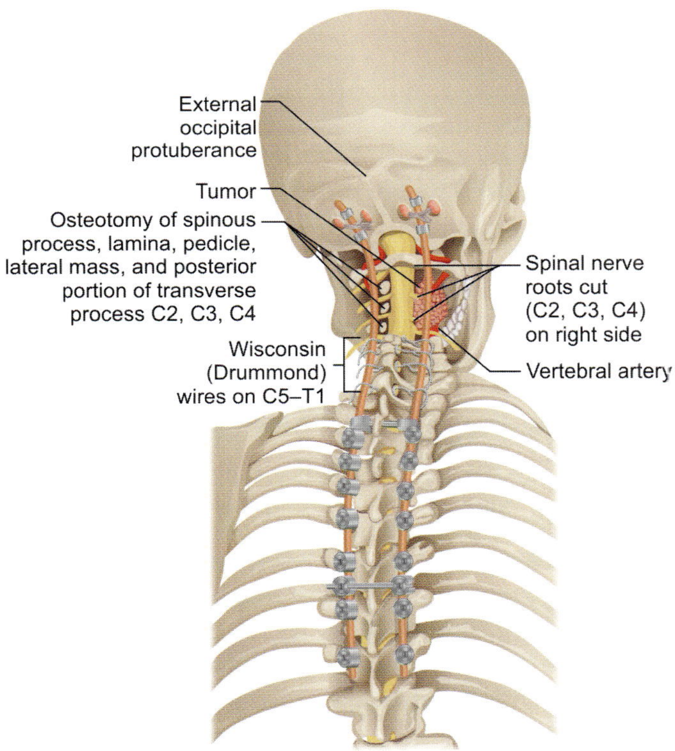

Fig. 4: Artist depiction demonstrating the posterior approach in preparation for en bloc resection of multilevel cervical chordoma.

of the cervical spine. Reconstructions in this area are more established and can be performed with an anterior strut graft or cage placement. Posterior screw and rod constructs may be constructed in a similar fashion to those used in the treatment of degenerative or traumatic cervical pathologies.

Cervicothoracic tumors at the cervicothoracic junction may involve the C7–T1 nerve roots. The neurological sacrifice of these roots will lead to weakness in the distal arms and hands and can be quite debilitating for patients. The vertebral arteries are typically anterolateral to the vertebral column and are typically not associated with the foramen transversarium at these levels.[102] Anterior approach to this region can vary from a transcervical approach to a more extended manubrial window or median sternotomy depending on the inferior extension of the tumor and its relationship to the sternum. Spinal reconstruction can be similar to the mid-cervical tumors. However, given the complete dissociation of the spinal column following an en bloc resection, there are typically increased biomechanical demands on the instrumentation that can lead to higher rates of pseudoarthrosis and instrumentation failure.

Patients with extensive anterior prevertebral tumor extension should undergo preoperative tracheostomy and gastrostomy tube as there is a significant concern for postsurgical airway obstruction and dysphagia. The goal of surgery should be to achieve a wide or marginal en bloc tumor excision while preserving the most optimal functional and neurological outcomes.

Complications

The anatomical complexity of the cervical spine precludes a high morbidity with surgical intervention. Although the cervical spine is the third most common location for chordomas, relatively few case series exist. Morbidity rates are substantially better described for skull base and high cervical chordomas and have been reported between 22.6% and 60.3% with a 2–7.8% mortality.[91] In one case series of seven patients, postoperative complications were noted in 4/7 patients. They included one wound dehiscence, two CSF leaks, and one C5 palsy. Previous reports also suggest permanent neurological morbidity in 4.1–33% of cases.[91]

Cerebrospinal fluid leak is the most frequent surgical complication for surgery at the skull base or cervical

CHAPTER 29

spine. Its incidence ranges from 4% to 35.7%.[70,91] When diagnosed, CSF diversion through lumbar drainage may be necessary for a prolonged period of time until the area has had a chance to scar and heal. Meningitis is a potential concern, especially if the approach was contaminated through dehiscence of the oral mucosa or wound leakage. Patients should be placed on broad-spectrum antibiotics as prophylaxis.

Wound breakdown is also a serious consideration, especially in the upper cervical spine. High cervical spondylectomy may include approaches that transect the posterior pharyngeal wall. Long anterior constructs can erode and promote dehiscence of the anterior approach and possible dehiscence. Also, pressure from the subluxation of the initial graft and plate into the retropharyngeal space and extensive dissection required for revision may account for eventual erosion.[103] Reinforcement at the time of initial surgery with a free muscle flap should be considered in conjunction with the other surgical teams. Once dehiscence occurs, prolonged antibiotics with meningitic coverage should be provided, as removal of hardware is not possible.

With the complete circumferential reconstruction of the spine, rigid fixation should address axial, sagittal, and torsional aspects of any applied force.[61,103] Posterior fusion may limit cervical motion, but inadequate fusion will cause a weak connection. Cervical spondylectomy may be associated with significant posterior constructs that span from the occiput to the thoracic spine. Such long constructs may have significant functional limitations for the patients. However, the risk of construct failure is high without incorporation of the junctional regions above and below the lesion.[60,61] Common teaching is that spinal instrumentation is a bridge until bony healing has occurred and long-term hardware failure is not clear for the treatment for primary tumors. In prior reports of occipitocervical thoracic fusion, bony fusion was not documented in the patient population.[101,103]

The sacrifice of a vertebral artery may be necessary intraoperatively but may be associated with significant risk given the importance and variability of the radiculomedullary branches. If there is any concern that the artery may be sacrificed as part of the operative plan or inadvertently during dissection, preoperative imaging should be obtained. CTA or formal angiography may be performed to ensure flow within the contralateral vertebral artery. Functional testing should also be considered either preoperatively with a balloon occlusion test or intraoperatively with temporary occlusion and monitoring of somatosensory-evoked potentials.[70]

Often these patients may have prolonged intubation or difficulty weaning from mechanical ventilation. In addition, high cervical approaches require preoperative tracheostomy for airway management intraoperatively. Alternative forms of enteral feeding should be considered through a gastrostomy tube as all patients will require alternative means of nutrition either during the immediate perioperative period or, in some instances, for a prolonged period of time.

Prognosis

Aggressive surgical excision is the most ideal treatment to provide patients with the hope for long-term disease-free survival and possible cure in some tumor pathologies. Chordomas are considered slowly-growing, locally aggressive lesions, however, median overall survival is estimated from 6 years to 8 years. Median overall survival rates at 5 and 10 years are 67–87% and 39–64%, respectively.[66,76,98,100] Recent publications by the Spinal Oncology Study Group strongly recommended that intralesional biopsy or resection significantly increases the risk of tumor recurrence for chordomas.[104] En bloc wide or marginal excision of chordomas and chondrosarcomas is associated with decreased recurrence and mortality rates.[99] Several clinical series with Class IV data has demonstrated treatment of chordomas through en bloc tumor resection (Table 4).[104]

Choi et al.[111] reported a multicenter case series of 132 skull base and high cervical chordomas with a 5- and 10-year survival of 55% and 36%. In this series, all patients underwent an intralesional resection with the goal of gross total resection. Meantime to tumor recurrence or progression was not reported, but they found patients who presented for revision surgery after prior resections had a worse survival than those with a primary surgical resection at the authors' centers. They concluded that patients with craniocervical chordomas should have as complete and as radical a tumor excision as possible during the first attempt and the first resection is the patient's best chance for complete excision.[111] Barrenechea et al.[109] reported a series of seven patients who underwent intralesional resection of cervical spine chordoma and

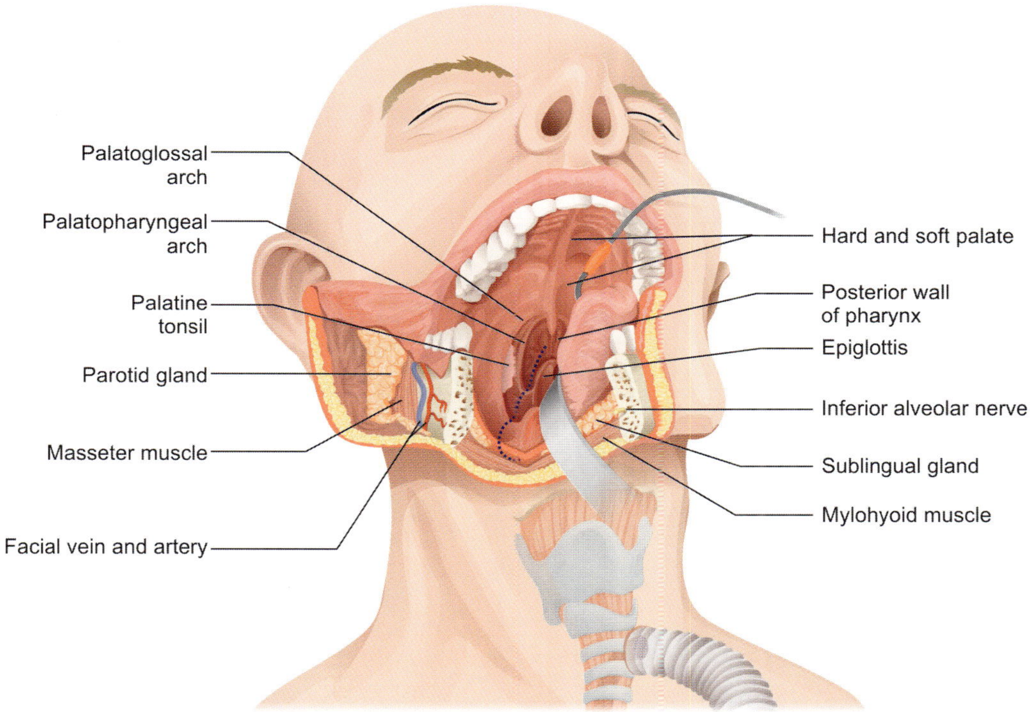

Fig. 5: Artist rendition for the anterior approach to a high cervical chordoma.
Source: Adapted from Rhines LD, Fourney DR, Siadati A, et al. En bloc resection of multilevel cervical chordoma with C2 involvement. Case report and description of operative technique. J Neurosurg Spine. 2005;2(2):199-205.

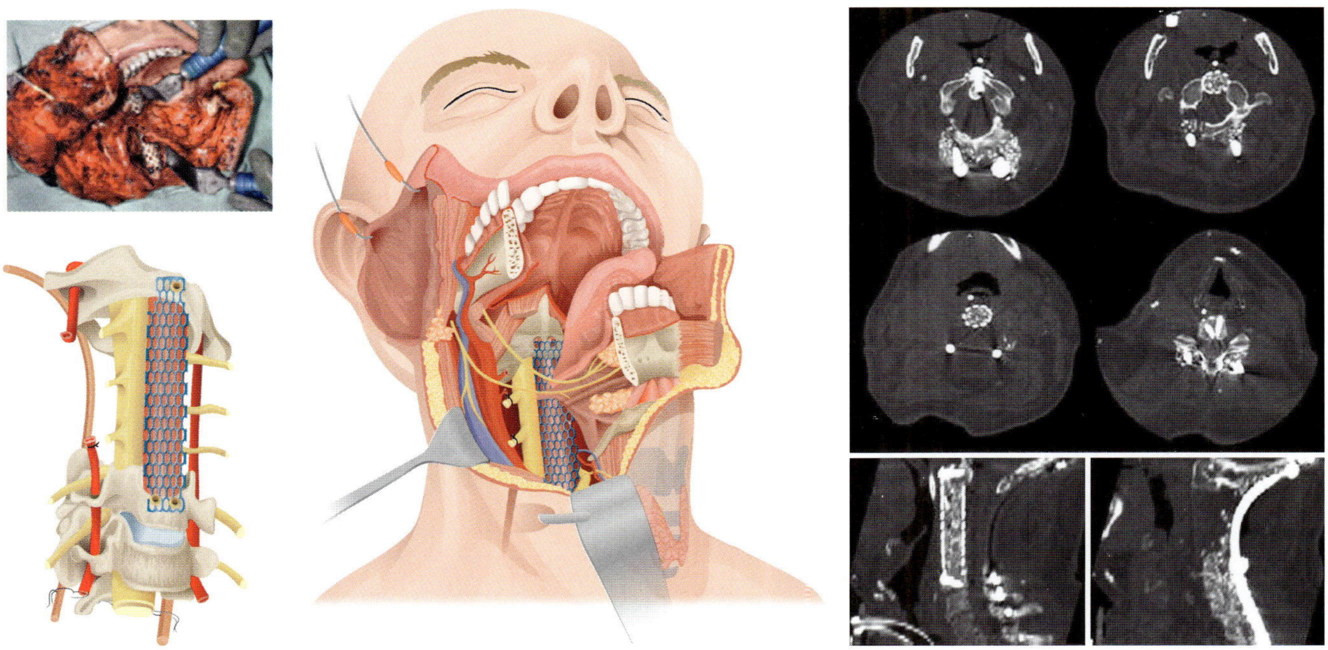

Fig. 6: Instrumentation, operative approach, and hardware.
Source: Adapted from Rhines LD, Fourney DR, Siadati A, et al. En bloc resection of multilevel cervical chordoma with C2 involvement. Case report and description of operative technique. J Neurosurg Spine. 2005;2(2):199-205.

Table 4: Prognostic indicators of en bloc versus intralesional resection for cervical chordomas.

Author (year)	*LoE*	*Patients (cerv)*	*Wide or marginal/ intralesional*	*Adjuvant*	*Morbidity*	*Survival*
Fisher (2005)[105]	II	26 (7 Chordomas, 1 cervical)	6/7 Chordomas with wide resections; 1/7 intralesional at the dural margin	NR	Massive blood loss (42%), infection (15%), nonunion (8%)	3.5 year f/u. No patient with local recurrence, one with systemic disease. SF-36 did not show a significant decline
Bjornsson (1992)[68]	II	40 (19 Cervical, 48%)	NR, but noted that most were incomplete resections	Radiation in all but 11 pts	NR	Mean survival 56 months. 65 m mean f/u. All patients who died had subtotal resection. OS at 5 years was 58%. Only 5% developed metastasis
Di Lorenzo (1992)[106]	III	38 Primary, 7 chordomas	All intralesional	All RT (40 Gy)	2 pts with transient dysphagia and dysphonia	Two patients with chordoma reoperated for recurrence
Bergh (2000)[76]	III	39 (5 Cervical)	4/5 Intralesional, 1/5 marginal	NR	Mobile spine (56%) instrumentation failure	5-, 10-, 15-, and 20-year survival, 84%, 64%, 52%, and 52%. Local recurrence associated with risk of metastasis and tumor-related death. Larger tumor size, performance of an invasive morphologic diagnostic procedures outside of tumor center, inadequate surgical margins, microscopic tumor necrosis, Ki-67>5%, local recurrence associated with a negative prognosis
Carpentier (2001)[107]	III	36 (8 Cervical)	NR	28 Underwent RT (10 proton beam)	Morbidity 4/8 pts with transient Horners, 5 pts with lower cranial nerve weakness	Average f/u 4 years. Disease mortality was 20% in the primary tumor group compared with 57% for those patients with recurrence
Boriani (2006)[108]	II and III	52 (37 Prospective, retrospective 15), 15 cervical (29%)	P: average f/u 58 m Local recurrence 32 of 48% controlled cases; 66%		Respiratory failure cause of death in 3/15 pts with cervical chordomas. Some loosening of occipital screws did not require revision	Rate of local recurrence 16/30 (53%) vs. 16/18 (89%) previously treated cases. All patients with palliative/ intralesional surgery recurred and died average 57 m following treatment. No patient died who underwent en bloc resection, but 2/10 have local disease
Barrenechea (2007)[109]	III	7 Cervical	All intralesional. All posterior, 5 anterior only	5 RT (mean 79 Gy), 2 chemo (dedifferentiated)	2/7 with CSF, 1/7 C5 palsy, 1/7 dehiscence pharyngeal incision	Median f/u 23 m. 2 Distant mets both died, 1 patient required second resection

Contd…

Contd...

Author (year)	*LoE*	*Patients (cerv)*	*Wide or marginal/ intralesional*	*Adjuvant*	*Morbidity*	*Survival*
Zileli (2007)[110]	III	35, Most common level affected C2 (14), C7 (10). 8 chordomas	6/7 Subtotal resection, 1/7 total intralesional resection	6/7 RT	1 Epidural hematoma, 1 respiratory problem, 2 graft failure (hardware/ graft extrusion), 1 trach complication (death)	Mean f/u 53.4 m. All chordomas recurred. 3 patients died during follow-up
Choi (2009)[111]	III	97 Patients, not clear how many cervicals or in clivus	NR	NR, "majority" received RT	Major complications included velopharyngeal incompetence 3.1%, vertebral artery stroke 1%, wound infection 3.1%, CSF leak 6.2%	Median survival 84 m. Mean f/u period 50.4 m. OS at 5- and 10-year were 55% and 36%. Patients who presented for revision surgery had a worse survival than those who underwent de novo surgery
Stacchiotti (2010)[112]	III (two center, retrospective)	9 Cervical tumors, 138 total	NR	42 Patients (30%) received radiotherapy with a dose of >60 Gy in 9. No difference in length of survival	10% of surgical complications	Median f/u 142 m. Total of 69 deaths. 64 related to chordoma or surgical complications. OS 5- and 10-year, 78% and 54%, median OS 131 m. Disease-free survival was better for patients who had primary tumor wide surgery, 45% at 19 years. 22% of patients with metastatic disease
Hsieh (2011)[101]	III	5 Cervical	5/5 En bloc	NR	1 wound infection, 1 radiculopathy	Mean f/u 54.7 m. 2/5 with local recurrence (25 m and 83 m)
Wang (2012)[113]	III	14 Cervical	All intralesional 5 Cases of total spondylectomy	All postop RT (44–80 Gy, mean 63.7 Gy). No chemotherapy	1 pulmonary infection (mortality), 1 weakness resolved in 2 m	Mean f/u 58.6 m. Symptom and neurological signs improved after surgery. Factors associated with high rate of tumor recurrence, age <40 or age >70 and upper cervical tumor location
Yasuda (2012)[86]	III	13 CCJ, 10 cervical (12 ps, 11 RS)	5 Extensive, 4 subtotal, 0 partial CCJ: 6 extensive, 4 STR, 3 partial	75% of cases w/ radiation, all but 3 proton beam	CSF leak 11.3%	Mean time to disease progression 30.4 m; 12.5% of patients died during follow-up with a mean interval of 45.8 m in patients receiving pure proton therapy, recurrence and death was 25/0% with a mean period of 62.3 m

(CSF: cerebrospinal fluid; f/u: follow-up; m: months; NR: not recorded; RT: radiation therapy) achieved gross total resection in six out of seven. Their average disease-free survival was 58.7 months, however, their median follow-up was only 23 months. Hseih et al. reported a series of five patients who underwent en bloc excision of cervical chordomas.[101] Their median disease-free survival was 84.2 months with disease-free progression at a mean of 43.4 months.

There is class II evidence to suggest that malignant or benign aggressive spinal tumors, such as chordomas, are best treated with aggressive margin-free excisions whenever possible.[104] Achieving an en bloc excision of chordomas in the cervical spine remains technically challenging given the proximity to vital structures. Despite a significant morbidity rate, en bloc excision can be performed with acceptable mortality rate. Given the improvement in overall survival and improved local disease control, en bloc excision should be performed whenever possible by a multidisciplinary team of surgeons who are familiar with these complex procedures. While adjuvant chemotherapy has not significantly impacted survival in these patients, there are new targeted therapies that are undergoing clinical trials.[91] Advancements in radiotherapy have also improved overall survival and local disease control when applied in a conformal manner at increased therapeutic doses. No large, prospective multicenter trials exist, but current interest in collecting a larger cohort of patients will prove beneficial for these rare disorders.

REFERENCES

1. Wu AS, Fourney DR. Evolution of treatment for metastatic spine disease. Neurosurg Clin N Am. 2004;15(4):401-11.
2. American Cancer Society, editor. Cancer Facts and Figures. Atlanta: American Cancer Society; 2005.
3. Dreghorn CR, Newman RJ, Hardy GJ, et al. Primary tumors of the axial skeleton. Experience of the Leeds regional bone tumor registry. Spine. 1990;15(2):137-40.
4. Molina CA, Gokaslan ZL, Sciubba DM. Diagnosis and management of metastatic cervical spine tumors. Orthop Clin North Am. 2012;43(1):75,87, viii-ix.
5. Cobb CA 3rd, Leavens ME, Eckles N. Indications for nonoperative treatment of spinal cord compression due to breast cancer. J Neurosurg. 1977;47(5):653-8.
6. Wong DA, Fornasier VL, MacNab I. Spinal metastases: the obvious, the occult, and the impostors. Spine. 1990;15(1):1-4.
7. Lenz M, Freid JR. Metastases to the skeleton, brain and spinal cord from cancer of the breast and the effect of radiotherapy. Ann Surg. 1931;93(1):278-93.
8. Sundaresan N, Digiacinto GV, Hughes JE, et al. Treatment of neoplastic spinal cord compression: results of a prospective study. Neurosurgery. 1991;29(5):645-50.
9. Fehlings MG, David KS, Vialle L, et al. Decision making in the surgical treatment of cervical spine metastases. Spine. 2009;34(22 Suppl):S108-17.
10. Jenis LG, Dunn EJ, An HS. Metastatic disease of the cervical spine. A review. Clin Orthop Relat Res. 1999;359(359):89-103.
11. Bilsky MH, Boland PJ, Panageas KS, et al. Intralesional resection of primary and metastatic sarcoma involving the spine: outcome analysis of 59 patients. Neurosurgery. 2001;49(6):1277,86; discussion 1286-7.
12. Bilsky MH, Shannon FJ, Sheppard S, et al. Diagnosis and management of a metastatic tumor in the atlantoaxial spine. Spine. 2002;27(10):1062-9.
13. Moulding HD, Bilsky MH. Metastases to the craniovertebral junction. Neurosurgery. 2010;66(3 Suppl):113-8.
14. Chaichana KL, Pendleton C, Sciubba DM, et al. Outcome following decompressive surgery for different histological types of metastatic tumors causing epidural spinal cord compression. clinical article. J Neurosurg Spine. 2009;11(1):56-63.
15. Marchesi DG, Boos N, Aebi M. Surgical treatment of tumors of the cervical spine and first two thoracic vertebrae. J Spinal Disord. 1993;6(6):489-96.
16. Mazel C, Balabaud L, Bennis S, et al. Cervical and thoracic spine tumor management: surgical indications, techniques, and outcomes. Orthop Clin North Am. 2009;40(1):75,92, vi-vii.
17. Gokaslan ZL. Spine surgery for cancer. Curr Opin Oncol. 1996;8(3):178-81.
18. Phillips E, Levine AM. Metastatic lesions of the upper cervical spine. Spine. 1989;14(10):1071-7.
19. Posner J. Neurological Complications of Cancer. Philadelphia: FA Davis; 1995.
20. Dickman CA, Sonntag VK. Posterior C1-C2 transarticular screw fixation for atlantoaxial arthrodesis. Neurosurgery. 1998;43(2):275,80; discussion 280-1.
21. Coley CM, Barry MJ, Fleming C, et al. Early detection of prostate cancer. Part I: Prior probability and effectiveness of tests. The American College of Physicians. Ann Intern Med. 1997;126(5):394-406.
22. Khanna AJ, Shindle MK, Wasserman BA, et al. Use of magnetic resonance imaging in differentiating compartmental location of spinal tumors. Am J Orthop. 2005;34(10):472-6.
23. Li KC, Poon PY. Sensitivity and specificity of MRI in detecting malignant spinal cord compression and in distinguishing malignant from benign compression fractures of vertebrae. Magn Reson Imaging. 1988;6(5):547-56.
24. Rao S, Badani K, Schildhauer T, et al. Metastatic malignancy of the cervical spine. A nonoperative history. Spine. 1992;17(10 Suppl):S407-12.
25. Francken AB, Hong AM, Fulham MJ, et al. Detection of unsuspected spinal cord compression in melanoma patients

by 18F-fluorodeoxyglucose-positron emission tomography. Eur J Surg Oncol. 2005;31(2):197-204.
26. Gottfried ON, Schloesser PE, Schmidt MH, et al. Embolization of metastatic spinal tumors. Neurosurg Clin N Am. 2004;15(4):391-9.
27. Fourney DR, York JE, Cohen ZR, et al. Management of atlantoaxial metastases with posterior occipitocervical stabilization. J Neurosurg. 2003;98(2 Suppl):165-70.
28. Tokuhashi Y, Matsuzaki H, Oda H, et al. A revised scoring system for preoperative evaluation of metastatic spine tumor prognosis. Spine. 2005;30(19):2186-91.
29. Tomita K, Kawahara N, Baba H, et al. Total en bloc spondylectomy for solitary spinal metastases. Int Orthop. 1994;18(5):291-8.
30. Fisher CG, DiPaola CP, Ryken TC, et al. A novel classification system for spinal instability in neoplastic disease: an evidence-based approach and expert consensus from the spine oncology study group. Spine. 2010;35(22):E1221-9.
31. Tomita K, Kawahara N, Murakami H, et al. Total en bloc spondylectomy for spinal tumors: improvement of the technique and its associated basic background. J Orthop Sci. 2006;11(1):3-12.
32. Boriani S, Weinstein JN, Biagini R. Primary bone tumors of the spine. terminology and surgical staging. Spine. 1997;22(9):1036-44.
33. Chan P, Boriani S, Fourney DR, et al. An assessment of the reliability of the Enneking and Weinstein-Boriani-Biagini classifications for staging of primary spinal tumors by the spine oncology study group. Spine. 2009;34(4):384-91.
34. Patchell RA, Tibbs PA, Regine WF, et al. Direct decompressive surgical resection in the treatment of spinal cord compression caused by metastatic cancer: a randomised trial. Lancet. 2005;366(9486):643-8.
35. Klimo P Jr, Schmidt MH. Surgical management of spinal metastases. Oncologist. 2004;9(2):188-96.
36. Leidbel S, Phillips T, editors. Textbook of Radiation Oncology. Philadelphia: WB Saunders; 1998.
37. Faul CM, Flickinger JC. The use of radiation in the management of spinal metastases. J Neurooncol. 1995;23(2):149-61.
38. Gerszten PC, Burton SA, Ozhasoglu C, et al. Radiosurgery for spinal metastases: clinical experience in 500 cases from a single institution. Spine. 2007;32(2):193-9.
39. Ryu S, Jin JY, Jin R, et al. Partial volume tolerance of the spinal cord and complications of single-dose radiosurgery. Cancer. 2007;109(3):628-36.
40. Chang EL, Shiu AS, Mendel E, et al. Phase I/II study of stereotactic body radiotherapy for spinal metastasis and its pattern of failure. J Neurosurg Spine. 2007;7(2):151-60.
41. Hsu W, Nguyen T, Kleinberg L, et al. Stereotactic radiosurgery for spine tumors: review of current literature. Stereotact Funct Neurosurg. 2010;88(5):315-21.
42. Wowra B, Muacevic A, Zausinger S, et al. Radiosurgery for spinal malignant tumors. Dtsch Arztebl Int. 2009;106(7): 106-12.
43. Gibbs IC. Spinal and paraspinal lesions: the role of stereotactic body radiotherapy. Front Radiat Ther Oncol. 2007;40:407-14.
44. Yu MK, Buys SS. Medical management of skeletal metastasis. Neurosurg Clin N Am. 2004;15(4):529,36, xi.
45. Amato RJ, Hernandez-McClain J, Henary H. Bone-targeted therapy: Phase II study of strontium-89 in combination with alternating weekly chemohormonal therapies for patients with advanced androgen-independent prostate cancer. Am J Clin Oncol. 2008;31(6):532-8.
46. Cazzaniga ME, Dogliotti L, Cascinu S, et al. Diagnosis, management and clinical outcome of bone metastases in breast cancer patients: results from a prospective, multicenter study. Oncology. 2006;71(5-6):374-81.
47. Harel R, Angelov L. Spine metastases: current treatments and future directions. Eur J Cancer. 2010;46(15):2696-707.
48. Kattan JG, Farhat FS, Chahine GY, et al. Weekly docetaxel, zoledronic acid and estramustine in hormone-refractory prostate cancer (HRPC). Invest New Drugs. 2008;26(1):75-9.
49. Lin AM, Rini BI, Derynck MK, et al. A phase I trial of docetaxel/estramustine/imatinib in patients with hormone-refractory prostate cancer. Clin Genitourin Cancer. 2007;5(5):323-8.
50. Lipton A, Steger GG, Figueroa J, et al. Extended efficacy and safety of denosumab in breast cancer patients with bone metastases not receiving prior bisphosphonate therapy. Clin Cancer Res. 2008;14(20):6690-6.
51. Nagata M, Ueda T, Komiya A, et al. Treatment and prognosis of patients with paraplegia or quadriplegia because of metastatic spinal cord compression in prostate cancer. Prostate Cancer Prostatic Dis. 2003;6(2):169-73.
52. Paridaens RJ, Dirix LY, Beex LV, et al. Phase III study comparing exemestane with tamoxifen as first-line hormonal treatment of metastatic breast cancer in postmenopausal women: The European Organisation for Research and Treatment of Cancer Breast Cancer Cooperative Group. J Clin Oncol. 2008;26(30):4883-90.
53. Amir E, Ooi WS, Simmons C, et al. Discordance between receptor status in primary and metastatic breast cancer: an exploratory study of bone and bone marrow biopsies. Clin Oncol. 2008;20(10):763-8.
54. Hortobagyi GN, Theriault RL, Porter L, et al. Efficacy of pamidronate in reducing skeletal complications in patients with breast cancer and lytic bone metastases. protocol 19 aredia breast cancer study group. N Engl J Med. 1996;335(24):1785-91.
55. Lipton A, Theriault RL, Hortobagyi GN, et al. Pamidronate prevents skeletal complications and is effective palliative treatment in women with breast carcinoma and osteolytic bone metastases: long-term follow-up of two randomized, placebo-controlled trials. Cancer. 2000;88(5):1082-90.
56. Rosen LS, Gordon D, Tchekmedyian S, et al. Zoledronic acid versus placebo in the treatment of skeletal metastases in patients with lung cancer and other solid tumors: a phase III, double-blind, randomized trial—the zoledronic acid lung cancer and other solid tumors study group. J Clin Oncol. 2003;21(16):3150-7.

57. Paterson AH, Powles TJ, Kanis JA, et al. Double-blind controlled trial of oral clodronate in patients with bone metastases from breast cancer. J Clin Oncol. 1993;11(1):59-65.
58. Sciubba DM, Gokaslan ZL. Diagnosis and management of metastatic spine disease. Surg Oncol. 2006;15(3):141-51.
59. Jones DC, Hayter JP, Vaughan ED, et al. Oropharyngeal morbidity following transoral approaches to the upper cervical spine. Int J Oral Maxillofac Surg. 1998;27(4):295-8.
60. Jackson RJ, Gokaslan ZL. Occipitocervicothoracic fixation for spinal instability in patients with neoplastic processes. J Neurosurg. 1999;91(1 Suppl):81-9.
61. Hsu W, Zaidi HA, Suk I, et al. A new technique for intraoperative reduction of occipitocervical instability. Neurosurgery. 2010;66(6 Suppl Operative):319,23; discussion 323-4.
62. Witham TF, Khavkin YA, Gallia GL, et al. Surgery insight: current management of epidural spinal cord compression from metastatic spine disease. Nat Clin Pract Neurol. 2006;2(2):87,94; quiz 116.
63. Ibrahim A, Crockard A, Antonietti P, et al. Does spinal surgery improve the quality of life for those with extradural (spinal) osseous metastases? an international multicenter prospective observational study of 223 patients. invited submission from the joint section meeting on disorders of the spine and peripheral nerves, march 2007. J Neurosurg Spine. 2008;8(3):271-8.
64. Quan GM, Vital JM, Pointillart V. Outcomes of palliative surgery in metastatic disease of the cervical and cervicothoracic spine. J Neurosurg Spine. 2011;14(5):612-8.
65. Dickman CA, Fehlings MG, Gokaslan ZL, editors. Spinal Cord and Spinal Column Tumors: Principles and Practice, 1st edition. New York: Thieme; 2006.
66. McMaster ML, Goldstein AM, Bromley CM, et al. Chordoma: incidence and survival patterns in the united states, 1973-1995. Cancer Causes Control. 2001;12(1):1-11.
67. McPherson CM, Suki D, McCutcheon IE, et al. Metastatic disease from spinal chordoma: a 10-year experience. J Neurosurg Spine. 2006;5(4):277-80.
68. Bjornsson J, Wold LE, Ebersold MJ, et al. Chordoma of the mobile spine. A clinicopathologic analysis of 40 patients. Cancer. 1993;71(3):735-40.
69. Chambers PW, Schwinn CP. Chordoma. A clinicopathologic study of metastasis. Am J Clin Pathol. 1979;72(5):765-76.
70. Sciubba DM, Chi JH, Rhines LD, et al. Chordoma of the spinal column. Neurosurg Clin N Am. 2008;19(1):5-15.
71. Murphey MD, Andrews CL, Flemming DJ, et al. From the archives of the AFIP. Primary tumors of the spine: radiologic pathologic correlation. Radiographics. 1996;16(5):1131-58.
72. Mehta RC, Marks MP, Hinks RS, et al. MR evaluation of vertebral metastases: T1-weighted, short-inversion-time inversion recovery, fast spin-echo, and inversion-recovery fast spin-echo sequences. Am J Neuroradiol. 1995;16(2):281-8.
73. Wippold FJ 2nd, Koeller KK, Smirniotopoulos JG. Clinical and imaging features of cervical chordoma. Am J Roentgenol. 1999;172(5):1423-6.
74. Fleming GF, Heimann PS, Stephens JK, et al. Dedifferentiated chordoma. Response to aggressive chemotherapy in two cases. Cancer. 1993;72(3):714-8.
75. Flemming DJ, Murphey MD, Carmichael BB, et al. Primary tumors of the spine. Semin Musculoskelet Radiol. 2000;4(3):299-320.
76. Bergh P, Kindblom LG, Gunterberg B, et al. Prognostic factors in chordoma of the sacrum and mobile spine: a study of 39 patients. Cancer. 2000;88(9):2122-34.
77. Boriani S, Chevalley F, Weinstein JN, et al. Chordoma of the spine above the sacrum. Treatment and outcome in 21 cases. Spine. 1996;21(13):1569-77.
78. Casali PG, Stacchiotti S, Sangalli C, et al. Chordoma. Curr Opin Oncol. 2007;19(4):367-70.
79. Catton C, O'Sullivan B, Bell R, et al. Chordoma: long-term follow-up after radical photon irradiation. Radiother Oncol. 1996;41(1):67-72.
80. Cummings BJ, Hodson DI, Bush RS. Chordoma: the results of megavoltage radiation therapy. Int J Radiat Oncol Biol Phys. 1983;9(5):633-42.
81. Forsyth PA, Cascino TL, Shaw EG, et al. Intracranial chordomas: a clinicopathological and prognostic study of 51 cases. J Neurosurg. 1993;78(5):741-7.
82. Austin-Seymour M, Urie M, Munzenrider J, et al. Considerations in fractionated proton radiation therapy: clinical potential and results. Radiother Oncol. 1990;17(1):29-35.
83. Suit HD, Goitein M, Munzenrider J, et al. Definitive radiation therapy for chordoma and chondrosarcoma of base of skull and cervical spine. J Neurosurg. 1982;56(3):377-85.
84. Noel G, Feuvret L, Calugaru V, et al. Chordomas of the base of the skull and upper cervical spine. One hundred patients irradiated by a 3D conformal technique combining photon and proton beams. Acta Oncol. 2005;44(7):700-8.
85. DeLaney TF, Liebsch NJ, Pedlow FX, et al. Phase II study of high-dose photon/proton radiotherapy in the management of spine sarcomas. Int J Radiat Oncol Biol Phys. 2009;74(3):732-9.
86. Yasuda M, Bresson D, Chibbaro S, et al. Chordomas of the skull base and cervical spine: clinical outcomes associated with a multimodal surgical resection combined with proton-beam radiation in 40 patients. Neurosurg Rev. 2012;35(2):171,82; discussion 182-3.
87. Kano H, Iqbal FO, Sheehan J, et al. Stereotactic radiosurgery for chordoma: a report from the North American Gamma Knife Consortium. Neurosurgery. 2011;68(2):379-89.
88. Jiang B, Veeravagu A, Lee M, et al. Management of intracranial and extracranial chordomas with CyberKnife stereotactic radiosurgery. J Clin Neurosci. 2012;19(8):1101-6.
89. Jakel O, Kramer M, Karger CP, et al. Treatment planning for heavy ion radiotherapy: clinical implementation and application. Phys Med Biol. 2001;46(4):1101-16.
90. Sciubba DM, Okuno SH, Dekutoski MB, et al. Ewing and osteogenic sarcoma: evidence for multidisciplinary management. Spine. 2009;34(22 Suppl):S58-68.
91. Walcott BP, Nahed BV, Mohyeldin A, et al. Chordoma: current concepts, management, and future directions. Lancet Oncol. 2012;13(2):e69-76.
92. Chugh R, Dunn R, Zalupski MM, et al. Phase II study of 9-nitro-camptothecin in patients with advanced chordoma or soft tissue sarcoma. J Clin Oncol. 2005;23(15):3597-604.

93. Chou WC, Hung YS, Lu CH, et al. De novo dedifferentiated chordoma of the sacrum: a case report and review of the literature. Chang Gung Med J. 2009;32(3):330-5.
94. Stacchiotti S, Longhi A, Ferraresi V, et al. Phase II study of imatinib in advanced chordoma. J Clin Oncol. 2012;30(9): 914-20.
95. Shalaby A, Presneau N, Ye H, et al. The role of epidermal growth factor receptor in chordoma pathogenesis: a potential therapeutic target. J Pathol. 2011;223(3):336-46.
96. Hof H, Welzel T, Debus J. Effectiveness of cetuximab/ gefitinib in the therapy of a sacral chordoma. Onkologie. 2006;29(12):572-4.
97. Hsu W, Mohyeldin A, Shah SR, et al. Generation of chordoma cell line JHC7 and the identification of brachyury as a novel molecular target. J Neurosurg. 2011;115(4):760-9.
98. York JE, Kaczaraj A, Abi-Said D, et al. Sacral chordoma: 40-year experience at a major cancer center. Neurosurgery. 1999;44(1):74,9; discussion 79-80.
99. Boriani S, Saravanja D, Yamada Y, et al. Challenges of local recurrence and cure in low grade malignant tumors of the spine. Spine. 2009;34(22 Suppl):S48-57.
100. Baratti D, Gronchi A, Pennacchioli E, et al. Chordoma: natural history and results in 28 patients treated at a single institution. Ann Surg Oncol. 2003;10(3):291-6.
101. Hsieh PC, Gallia GL, Sciubba DM, et al. En bloc excisions of chordomas in the cervical spine: review of five consecutive cases with more than 4-year follow-up. Spine. 2011;36(24):E1581-7.
102. Xu R, Ebraheim NA, Tang G, et al. Location of the vertebral artery in the cervicothoracic junction. Am J Orthop. 2000;29(6):453-6.
103. Rhines LD, Fourney DR, Siadati A, et al. En bloc resection of multilevel cervical chordoma with C2 involvement. Case report and description of operative technique. J Neurosurg Spine. 2005;2(2):199-205.
104. Yamazaki T, McLoughlin GS, Patel S, et al. Feasibility and safety of en bloc resection for primary spine tumors: a systematic review by the spine oncology study group. Spine. 2009;34(22 Suppl):S31-8.
105. Fisher CG, Keynan O, Boyd MC, et al. The surgical management of primary tumors of the spine: initial results of an ongoing prospective cohort study. Spine. 2005;30(16): 1899-908.
106. Di Lorenzo N, Delfini R, Ciappetta P, et al. Primary tumors of the cervical spine: surgical experience with 38 cases. Surg Neurol. 1992;38(1):12-8.
107. Carpentier A, Blanquet A, George B. Suboccipital and cervical chordomas: radical resection with vertebral artery control. Neurosurg Focus. 2001;10(3):E4.
108. Boriani S, Bandiera S, Biagini R, et al. Chordoma of the mobile spine: fifty years of experience. Spine. 2006;31(4):493-503.
109. Barrenechea IJ, Perin NI, Triana A, et al. Surgical management of chordomas of the cervical spine. J Neurosurg Spine. 2007;6(5):398-406.
110. Zileli M, Kilincer C, Ersahin Y, et al. Primary tumors of the cervical spine: a retrospective review of 35 surgically managed cases. Spine J. 2007;7(2):165-73.
111. Choi D, Melcher R, Harms J, et al. Outcome of 132 operations in 97 patients with chordomas of the craniocervical junction and upper cervical spine. Neurosurgery. 2010;66(1):59,65; discussion 65.
112. Stacchiotti S, Casali PG, Lo Vullo S, et al. Chordoma of the mobile spine and sacrum: a retrospective analysis of a series of patients surgically treated at two referral centers. Ann Surg Oncol. 2010;17(1):211-9.
113. Wang Y, Xiao J, Wu Z, et al. Primary chordomas of the cervical spine: a consecutive series of 14 surgically managed cases. J Neurosurg Spine. 2012;17(4):292-9.

CHAPTER 30

Trauma of the Cervical Spine

George Rymarczuk, Geoffrey Stricsek, James S Harrop

INTRODUCTION

Classification of injuries to the cervical spine has historically proven to be more daunting than the thoracolumbar spine. The relative uniformity of the subaxial cervical spine lends itself to relatively straightforward descriptions, however, this stands in contrast to the more complex osseous and ligamentous arrangements that characterize the upper cervical spine and the occipitocervical junction. The condyles of the occipital bone, the atlas, and the axis are highly specialized structures that allow significant freedom of movement, and consequently can be afflicted by injuries morphologically and biomechanically dissimilar to other regions of the spine.

UPPER CERVICAL INJURIES

The anatomical complexity of the region of the craniocervical junction has led to myriad, narrowly applicable, niche classification schemes that have been proposed to convey injury morphology. In an attempt to more concisely characterize the pertinent aspects of individual injuries, the AOSpine Upper Cervical Classification system broadly arranges injuries to this region into bony injuries (Type A), tension band and ligamentous injuries (Type B), and translational injuries (Type C) for the condyles and craniocervical junction (Group I), the atlas and C1–2 joint (Group II), and the axis and C2–3 joint (Group 3). This is summarized in Table 1.

For Type IA injuries, the system of Anderson and Montesano[1] can be used to further characterize the specific fracture pattern. Injuries of this nature are often without neurologic injury, although the 12th cranial nerve should be assessed. These fractures are typically amenable to immobilization. Type IC injuries encompass the atlanto-occipital dislocations (AOD), and were originally described by the system of Traynelis.[2] Atlanto-occipital dislocations can be diagnosed by the so-called "BAI-BDI" method, or by assessing the condylar gap on reformatted computer tomography.[3,4]

Group II injuries are those to the atlas and associated ligamentous complex of the C1–2 joint. Isolated C1 arch fractures can often be managed conservatively, however, injuries of increasing severity within this group are more likely to result in disruption of the transverse atlantal ligament (TAL), which is a relative indication for surgical stabilization. The Type IIC injury is defined by atlantoaxial

Table 1: The AOSpine Upper Cervical Classification system.

	I: Condyle and craniocervical junction	*II: Atlas, C1–2 joint*	*III: Axis, C2–3 joint*
Type A: Isolated bony injury	Condyle fractures	C1 arch fracture	Osseous injuries of C2 (e.g. nondisplaced Hangman's, odontoid)
Type B: Ligamentous and tension band injuries	Craniocervical ligamentous injuries	Transverse atlantal ligament disruptions (e.g. Jefferson fractures)	C2 tension band injuries
Type C: Translational or displaced injuries	Atlanto-occipital dislocations	Atlantoaxial subluxation	Translational injuries (e.g. C2–3 disc disruptions)

instability. Magnetic resonance imaging (MRI) is well suited to assess the integrity of the TAL[5] and, therefore, is indispensable in assisting in guiding therapy.

Group III injuries include all osseous injuries to the axis, as well as the C2–3 joint complex and disk. Type IIIA injuries include the odontoid fractures,[6] nondisplaced traumatic isthmic spondylolysis of the axis (the so-called "Hangman's" fractures), and the remaining miscellaneous C2 body fractures and atypical Hangman's-type injuries. With Type IIIB and IIIC injuries, there is progress tension band and C2–3 disk disruption, which may result in spondylolisthesis of the axis.[7-9] Angulation and translation of C2 with respect to C3, indicating C2–3 discoligamentous disruptions, are criteria for fixation.

SUBAXIAL CERVICAL SPINE

The immediate predecessor to the AOSpine Subaxial Cervical Injury Classification system,[10] the Subaxial Cervical Spine Injury Classification (SLIC),[11] represented a dramatic improvement over all other systems that had been iterated up to that point.[12,13] Previous schema that had been somewhat widely used before SLIC, while in many cases quite comprehensive, were notable for their cumbersomeness, lack of agreement among clinicians, difficulty conveying pertinent radiographic aspects of individual clinical scenarios and were of relatively low reproducibility and reliability.[11,14-18]

The AOSpine Subaxial Classification system is in keeping with the basic format of the thoracolumbar scheme, broadly classifying injuries into compression (Type A), tension band (Type B), and translational (Type C) injuries. Unique to the Subaxial Cervical system are modifiers specifically designed to convey injury to the facet complexes. "Type F" injuries—those to the facet joint—are graded on a continuum of severity. Type F1 facet injuries include those that involve fragments of less than 1 cm in height and less than 40% of the lateral mass overall. Injuries of this nature were first described by Spector in 2006 as being biomechanically stable.[19] Type F2 injuries are facet fractures larger than these criteria, and finally F3 and F4 injuries represent the so-called "floating lateral mass" and finally "perched" or "jumped" facets, respectively. The additional modifier "BL" denotes bilateral facet complex injury.

CASE ILLUSTRATIONS

Case 1: Complete Burst Fracture of the Subaxial Cervical Spine

A 31-year-old male patient was injured during the partial collapse of a building, in which he was pinned under a wall. He presented with left-sided hemiparesis and total ASIA motor score of 64, as well as a sensory disturbance consistent with a Brown-Sequard-type injury. His imaging revealed a sagittal-split, complete burst fracture of the C5 vertebral body (Type A4 injury) with associated fracture of the posterior elements. The intake computed tomography (CT) can be seen in Figures 1A (coronal) and B (axial). Mid-sagittal T2-weighted MRI can be seen in Figure 2. This demonstrates a large intramedullary cord contusion extending from C3 to T1, with persistent compression of the cord most notably across the C4–5 interval. The patient was taken for a circumferential decompression, stabilization, and fusion consisting of C5 corpectomy and C3–T1 posterior decompression and fusion. Postoperative lateral radiograph can be seen in Figure 3. The patient made a significant neurologic recovery, with ASIA motor score of 99 at approximately 11 months from surgery.

Case 2: Translational Injury of the Subaxial Cervical Spine

A 26-year-old male was injured during a motor vehicle accident and roll-over. He presented clinically as an ASIA Type B incomplete spinal cord injury, with no motor function distal to the triceps, however, with preserved sensation in sacral dermatomes. His ASIA motor score on admission was 35. Intake sagittal CT, shown in Figure 4, demonstrates a Type C translational injury at C6–7, with subluxation and bilateral "jumped" facets, thus the modifiers "F4" and "BL" are also applied. An initial attempt at a closed reduction with Gardner-Wells tongs was unsuccessful, thus the patient was treated with a staged open fracture reduction followed by circumferential decompression and fusion. The translational injury at C6–7 was successfully reduced via an anterior approach. Figures 5 (mid-sagittal CT) and 6 (mid-sagittal T2-weighted MRI) demonstrate the appearance after the initial procedure. On the mid-sagittal T2-weighted MRI (Fig. 6), a large cord contusion spanning the C5–7 segments is apparent, with ventral hematoma and persistent dorsal

CHAPTER 30

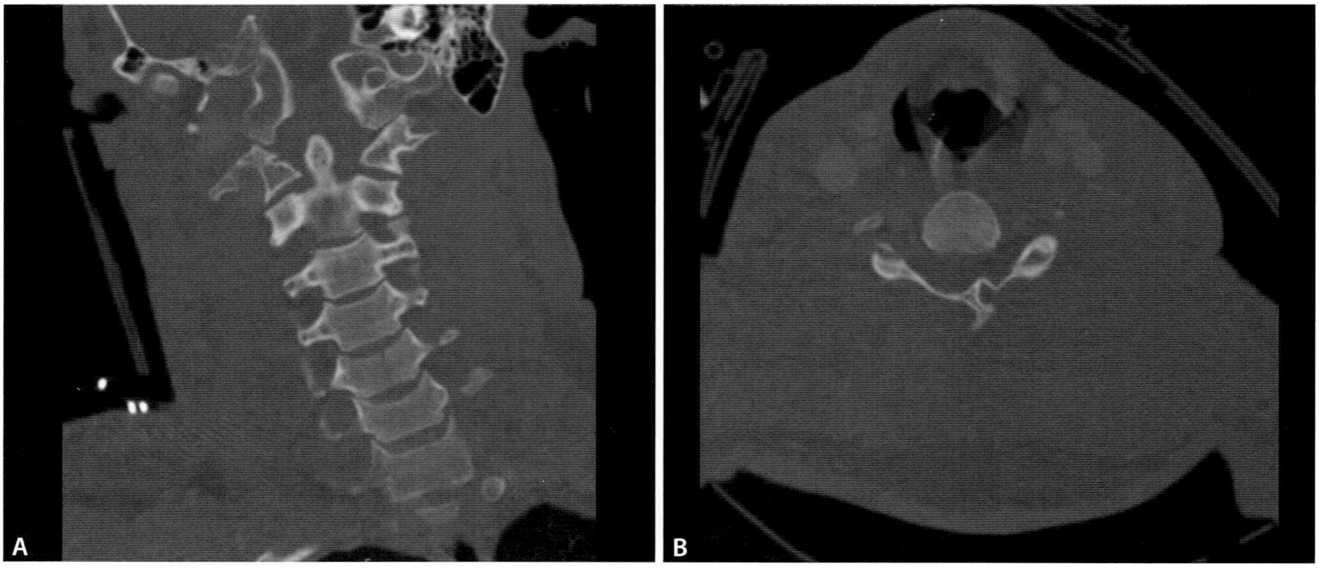

Figs. 1A and B: (A) Coronal computed tomography (CT) scan demonstrating Type A4 complete burst fracture of the C5 vertebral body. (B) Axial CT scan demonstrating the associated laminar fracture.

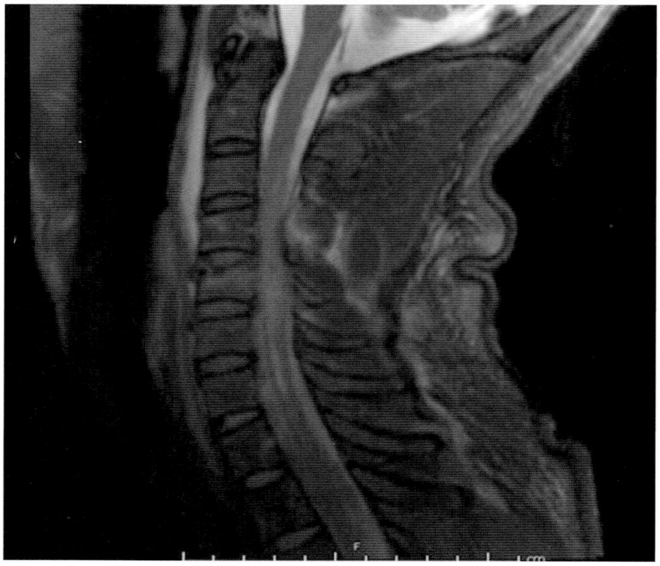

Fig. 2: Mid-sagittal T2-weighted magnetic resonance imaging (MRI) demonstrating intramedullary cord contusion extending from C3 to T1, with persistent compression of the cord.

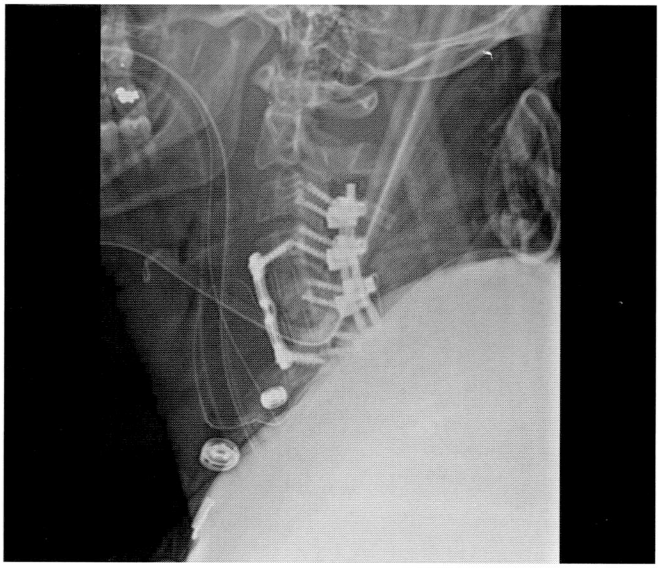

Fig. 3: Postoperative lateral radiography demonstrating C5 corpectomy and C3–T1 decompression and fusion, with C7 pedicle screws.

compression from the posterior elements apparent. The injury to the posterior ligamentous complex can also be appreciated. The patient then underwent C4–T2 posterior decompression and fusion, with postoperative parasagittal CT shown in Figure 7. At 1 year postinjury, while still nonambulatory, the patient had made a significant neurologic recovery and had transitioned to living independently.

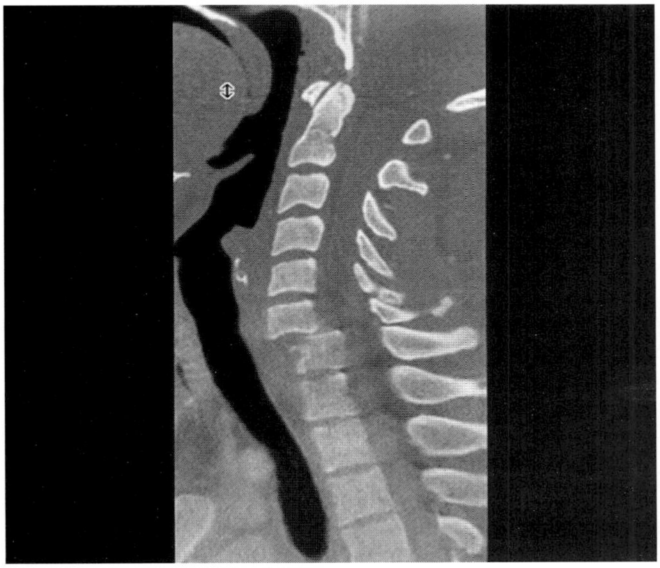

Fig. 4: Sagittal computed tomography (CT) demonstrating a Type C translational injury at C6–7, with subluxation and bilateral "jumped" facets.

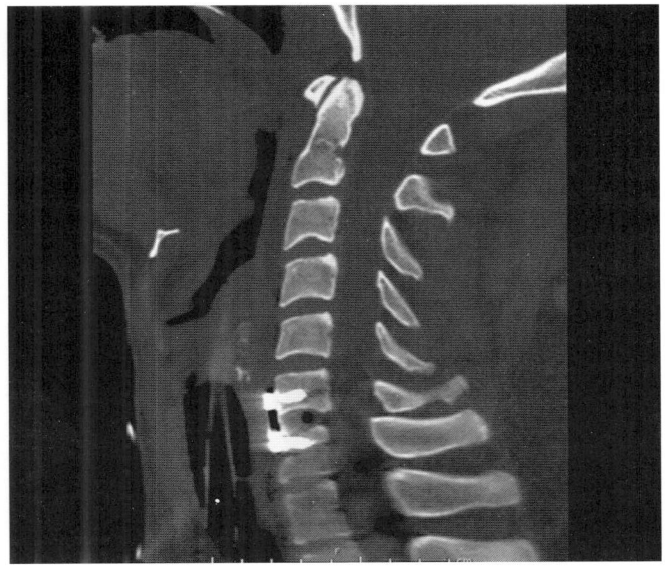

Fig. 5: Mid-sagittal computed tomography (CT) after open reduction via C6–7 anterior cervical discectomy and fusion (ACDF).

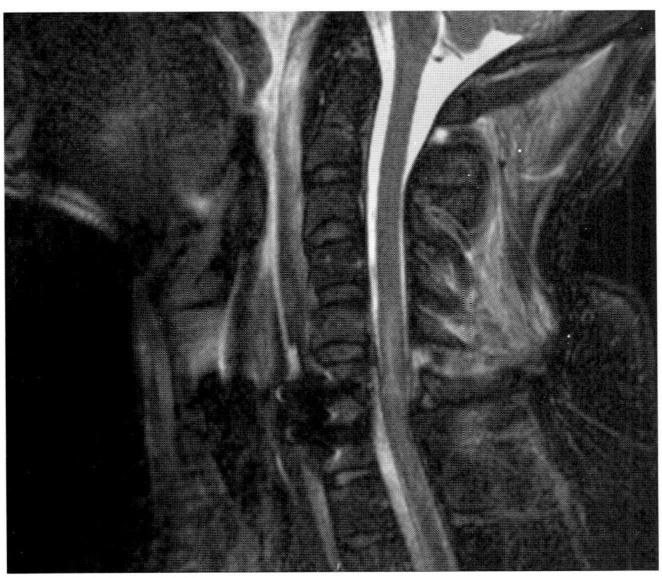

Fig. 6: Mid-sagittal T2-weighted magnetic resonance imaging (MRI) after C6–7 anterior cervical discectomy and fusion (ACDF), demonstrating a large cord contusion spanning the C5–7 segments.

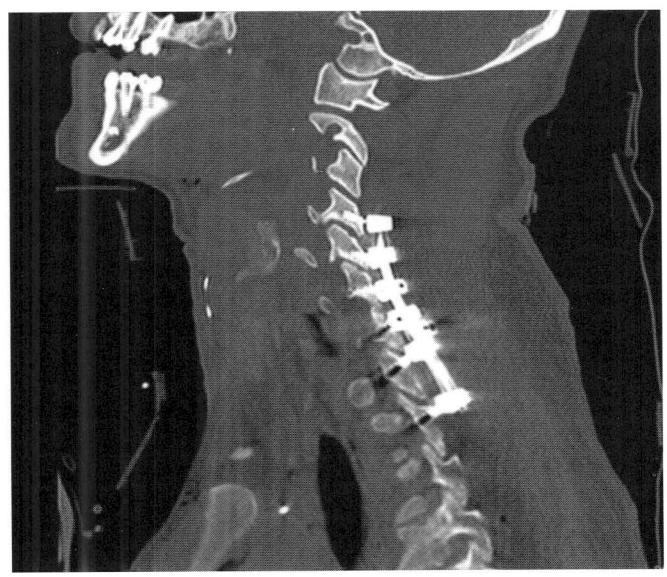

Fig. 7: Postoperative parasagittal computed tomography (CT) after C6–7 anterior cervical discectomy and fusion (ACDF) and C4–T2 posterior decompression and fusion.

Case 3: Extension Injury of the Cervical Spine in the Setting of Abnormal Bone Metabolism

A 66-year-old male patient presented to the emergency department for persistent neck pain, approximately 36 hours after a relatively innocuous fall from seated. He demonstrated a normal neurologic examination. Intake imaging can be seen in Figures 8A and B. Mid-sagittal CT (Fig. 8A) reveals the presence of diffuse osteophytosis and

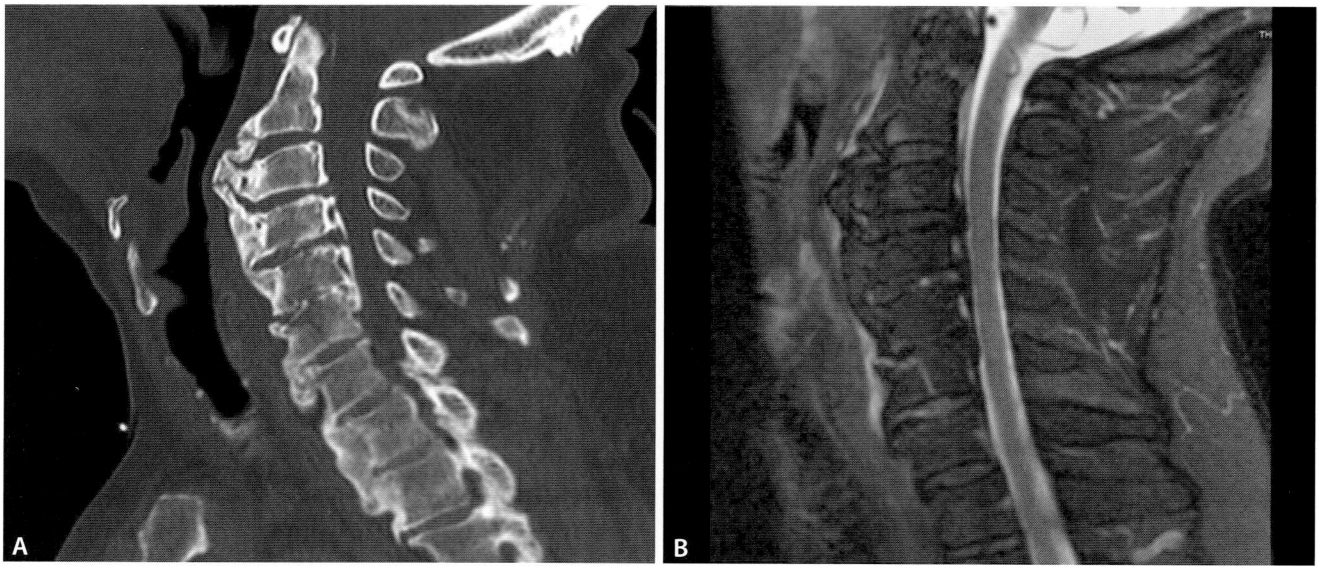

Figs. 8A and B: Mid-sagittal (A) computed tomography (CT) and (B) magnetic resonance imaging (MRI) demonstrating diffuse idiopathic skeletal hyperostosis (DISH) and Type B3 extension injury through the C6 vertebral body.

incomplete ossification of the poster longitudinal ligament consistent with a diagnosis of diffuse idiopathic skeletal hyperostosis (DISH). An atypical fracture line can be seen beginning at the osteophyte complex centered over C5–6, passing through the mid-body of C6, and coming to rest at the C6–7 disk space. This fracture is also demonstrated in the mid-sagittal STIR sequence (Fig. 8B). This injury pattern represents a Type B3 anterior tension band lesion after a hyperextension, and furthermore, the "M3" modifier for "stiffening or metabolic bone disease" is also applicable.

Conditions such as DISH and ankylosing spondylitis present unique challenges when formulating a treatment plan. Due to metabolic abnormalities of the bone and cartilage, with superimposed stress-shielding, lack of flexible ligamentous support, and long lever arms, patients with these diagnoses may be susceptible to fracture patterns of atypical and usual morphology from even the most minor of traumas, such as a fall from the seated position.[20-23] Long-segment posterior stabilization is typically indicated, and any baseline deformity should be taken into consideration when formulating a surgical plan. The patient underwent posterior stabilization of the fracture, from C3 to T1. Postoperative radiography can be appreciated in Figure 9.

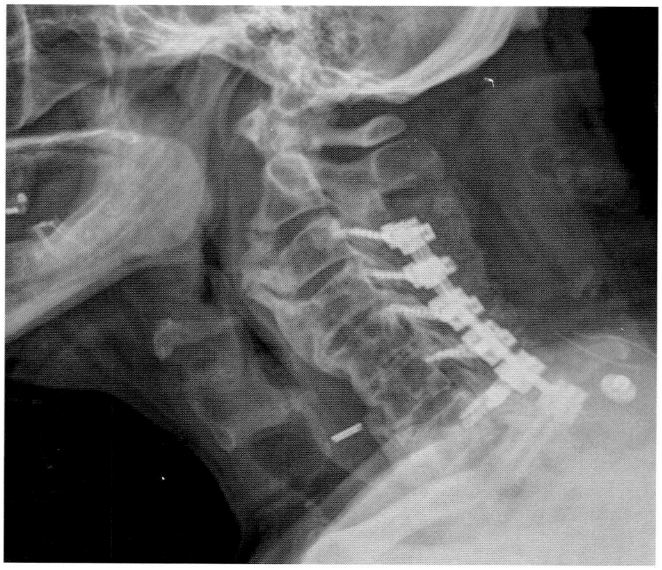

Fig. 9: Lateral postoperative radiography after C3–T1 posterior stabilization using C7 pedicle screws.

Case 4: Geriatric Odontoid Fracture

A 75-year-old female patient presented to the emergency department with several weeks of progressive axial neck pain. She had a normal neurologic examination on presentation. The patient was involved in a minor motor

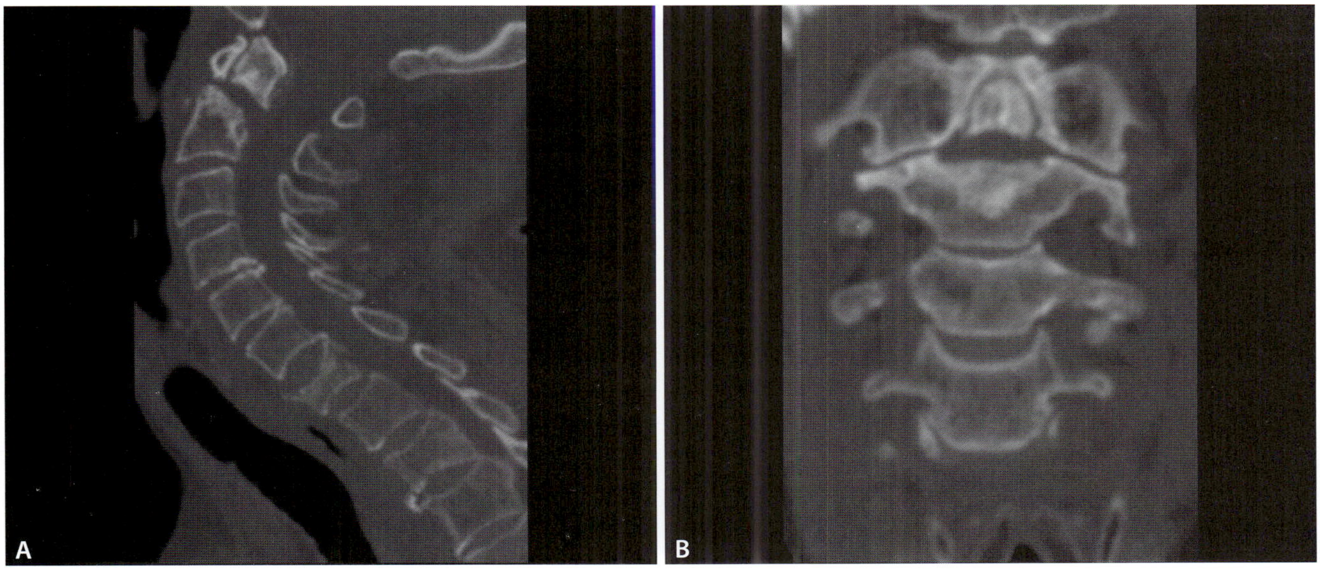

Figs. 10A and B: (A) Sagittal and (B) Coronal computed tomography (CT) scan demonstrating a Type IIIA injury: a Type II odontoid fracture.

vehicle accident 2 years prior to presentation, however, there was otherwise no history of the antecedent inciting event. Sagittal (Fig. 10A) and coronal (Fig. 10B) CT scan demonstrated a Type IIIA injury, more specifically a Type II odontoid fracture. The fracture fragment was displaced cranially and dorsally with regard to the body of the axis, with well-corticated fracture edges suggesting some degree of chronicity. Magnetic resonance imaging (Fig. 11) revealed a patent canal with some degree of T2 hyperintensity within the fracture. Management of Type II odontoid fractures has historically been somewhat controversial, however, for fractures that are significantly displaced, as well as those in the elderly, recent studies have suggested that early and aggressive intervention through fixation has been associated with improved outcome, perhaps in part due to early mobilization.[24-27] This patient was treated with posterior C1–2 fusion as described by Harms,[28] with postoperative radiography shown in Figure 12.

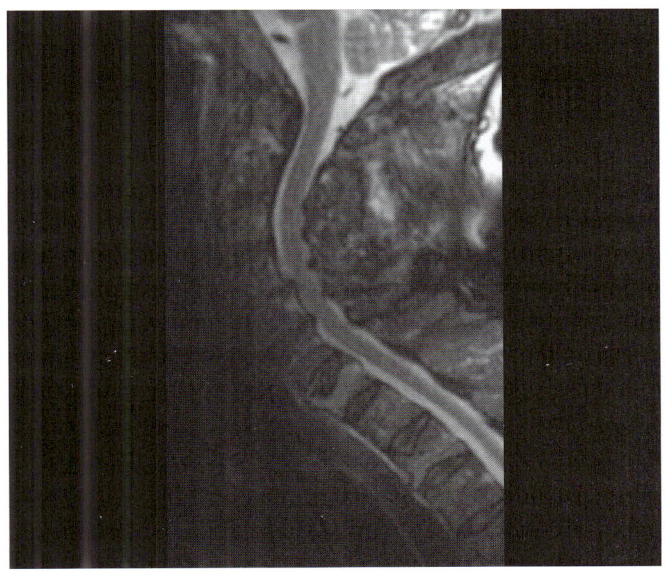

Fig. 11: Mid-sagittal T2-weighted magnetic resonance imaging (MRI) of Type II odontoid fracture.

KEY POINTS

- The cervical spine, particularly the occipitocervical junction, is an anatomically complex region with unique osseous and ligamentous structures and relationships.
- Subaxial cervical injuries are graded in a pattern similar to the thoracolumbar spine, broadly characterized into compression-type, tension band, and translational injuries. The importance of the facet complex is further underscored with specific modifiers used to characterize these injuries.
- The Upper Cervical Classification System, due to unique anatomic considerations, classifies injuries by the region involved. Condyle fractures and

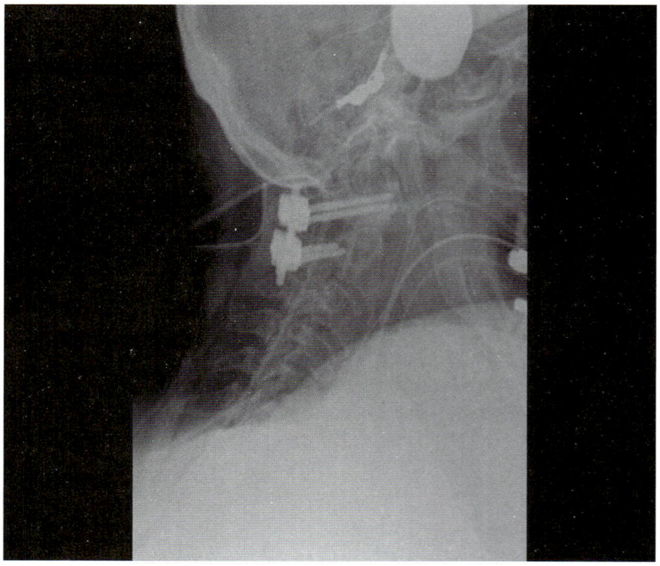

Fig. 12: Lateral radiograph after posterior C1–2 fusion.

atlanto-occipital injuries are grouped as Type A, C1–2 complex injuries as Type B, and C2–3 injuries as Type C.

- Atlanto-occipital dislocation can be assessed by the "BAI-BDI" method as well as the condylar gap.
- The integrity of the TAL is of paramount importance with regard to the treatment of C1 fractures.
- There is a general trend for fixation of displaced Type II odontoid fractures, particularly for the elderly.
- In the context of traumatic spondylolysis of the axis, angulation, and translation of C2 with regard to C3 imply a degree of discoligamentous instability necessitating fixation.
- Patients with metabolic bone diseases, such as DISH and ankylosing spondylitis, can incur fractures with even minimal trauma, and management of these injury patterns can be challenging.

REFERENCES

1. Anderson PA, Montesano PX. Morphology and treatment of occipital condyle fractures. Spine. 1988;13(7):731-6.
2. Traynelis VC, Marano GD, Dunker RO, et al Traumatic atlanto-occipital dislocation. Case report. J Neurosurg. 1986;65(6):863-70.
3. Theodore N, Aarabi B, Dhall SS, et al. The diagnosis and management of traumatic atlanto-occipital dislocation injuries. Neurosurgery. 2013;72(Suppl 2):114-26.
4. Horn EM, Feiz-Erfan I, Lekovic GP, et al. Survivors of occipitoatlantal dislocation injuries: imaging and clinical correlates. J Neurosurg Spine. 2007;6(2):113-20.
5. Ryken TC, Aarabi B, Dhall SS, et al. Management of isolated fractures of the atlas in adults. Neurosurgery. 2013;72(Suppl 2):127-31.
6. Anderson LD, D'Alonzo RT. Fractures of the odontoid process of the axis. J Bone Joint Surg Am. 1974;56(8):1663-74.
7. Francis WR, Fielding JW, Hawkins RJ. Traumatic spondylolisthesis of the axis. J Bone Joint Surg Br. 1981;63-B(3):313-8.
8. Effendi B, Roy D, Cornish B, et al. Fractures of the ring of the axis. A classification based on the analysis of 131 cases. J Bone Joint Surg Br. 1981;63-B(3):319-27.
9. Levine AM, Edwards CC. The management of traumatic spondylolisthesis of the axis. J Bone Joint Surg Am. 1985;67(2):217-26.
10. Vaccaro AR, Koerner JD, Radcliff KE, et al. AOSpine subaxial cervical spine injury classification system. Eur Spine J. 2016;25(7):2173-84.
11. Vaccaro AR, Hulbert RJ, Patel AA, et al. The subaxial cervical spine injury classification system: a novel approach to recognize the importance of morphology, neurology, and integrity of the disco-ligamentous complex. Spine. 2007;32(21):2365-74.
12. Harris JH, Edeiken-Monroe B, Kopaniky DR. A practical classification of acute cervical spine injuries. Orthop Clin North Am. 1986;17(1):15-30.
13. Allen BL, Ferguson RL, Lehmann TR, et al. A mechanistic classification of closed, indirect fractures and dislocations of the lower cervical spine. Spine. 1982;7(1):1-27.
14. Aarabi B, Oner C, Vaccaro AR, et al. Application of AOspine subaxial cervical spine injury classification in simple and complex cases. J Orthop Trauma. 2017;31(Suppl 4):S24-32.
15. Aarabi B, Walters BC, Dhall SS, et al. Subaxial cervical spine injury classification systems. Neurosurgery. 2013;72(Suppl 2):170-86.
16. Urrutia J, Zamora T, Campos M, et al. A comparative agreement evaluation of two subaxial cervical spine injury classification systems: the AOSpine and the Allen and Ferguson schemes. Eur Spine J. 2016;25(7):2185-92.
17. Stone AT, Bransford RJ, Lee MJ, et al. Reliability of classification systems for subaxial cervical injuries. Evid Based Spine Care J. 2010;1(3):19-26.
18. van Middendorp JJ, Audigé L, Hanson B, et al. What should an ideal spinal injury classification system consist of? A methodological review and conceptual proposal for future classifications. Eur Spine J. 2010;19(8):1238-49.
19. Spector LR, Kim DH, Affonso J, et al. Use of computed tomography to predict failure of nonoperative treatment of unilateral facet fractures of the cervical spine. Spine. 2006;31(24):2827-35.

20. Westerveld LA, Verlaan JJ, Oner FC. Spinal fractures in patients with ankylosing spinal disorders: a systematic review of the literature on treatment, neurological status and complications. Eur Spine J. 2009;18(2):145-56.
21. Westerveld LA, Verlaan J-J, Lam MGEH, et al. The influence of diffuse idiopathic skeletal hyperostosis on bone mineral density measurements of the spine. Rheumatology (Oxford). 2009;48(9):1133-6.
22. Chaudhary SB, Hullinger H, Vives MJ. Management of acute spinal fractures in ankylosing spondylitis. ISRN Rheumatol. 2011;2011:150484.
23. Gelb DE, Aarabi B, Dhall SS, et al. Treatment of subaxial cervical spinal injuries. Neurosurgery. 2013;72(Suppl 2): 187-94.
24. Ryken TC, Hadley MN, Aarabi B, et al. Management of isolated fractures of the axis in adults. Neurosurgery. 2013;72(Suppl 2):132-50.
25. Wagner SC, Schroeder GD, Kepler CK, et al. Controversies in the management of geriatric odontoid fractures. J Orthop Trauma. 2017;31(Suppl 4):S44-8.
26. Smith JS, Kepler CK, Kopjar B, et al. Effect of type II odontoid fracture nonunion on outcome among elderly patients treated without surgery: based on the AOSpine North America geriatric odontoid fracture study. Spine. 2013;38(26):2240-6.
27. Schroeder GD, Kepler CK, Kurd MF, et al. A systematic review of the treatment of geriatric type II odontoid fractures. Neurosurgery. 2015;77(Suppl 4):S6-14.
28. Harms J, Melcher RP. Posterior C1-C2 fusion with polyaxial screw and rod fixation. Spine. 2001;26(22):2467-71.

SECTION 4

Thoracic

CHAPTER 31 Thoracic Spine: History and Physical Examination

Alexandra Paraskos, Marzena Buzanowska, Michael P Steinmetz

INTRODUCTION

The thoracic spine evaluation is very unique due to this area's complex anatomy, unique biomechanics, and the representation of less common disorders. While distal symptoms related to the cervical spine involve the upper extremity, distal symptoms related to the thoracic spine involve the flank and chest. For that reason, the evaluation of thoracic spine must include consideration of conditions originating from the visceral structures in the thoracic and abdominal cavities. Thoracic spine serves as a source of stability to the axial skeleton and is characterized by a very limited range of motion. It has numerous articulations—the intervertebral disk, zygapophyseal joints, costovertebral and costotransverse joints, scapula-thoracic articulation and anteriorly, the sternoclavicular, sternocostal, and costochondral joints.

HISTORY

As in the cervical spine, history taking relies on the knowledge of conditions of the thoracic spine and their respective presentations. It focuses on eliciting the location and nature of patient's symptoms, type of onset, mechanism of injury, time course and duration, factors that may modify the symptoms (alleviate or exacerbate) as well as any associated findings, with special attention to "red flags." Red flag assessment is particularly important in the evaluation of thoracic spine given the likelihood of referred symptoms from visceral organs. Clinician should ask questions about systemic illness, malignancy, unexplained weight loss, fever, and night pain.

Nature

The most common type of symptom in the mid-back that patients present with is pain. The choice of descriptors points toward the possible source. Severity is important to elicit and often patients will appear uncomfortable in association with higher amounts of pain. If the patient complains of stiffness, the length of time and time of day should be obtained. Pain and stiffness have been identified in multiple studies as the most common symptoms in diffuse idiopathic skeletal hyperostosis (DISH) and have been shown to be more frequent than in healthy controls.[1] Back pain that is described as sharp and severe along with rapid onset is often described by patients with aortic dissection and is more common in patients with dissection distal to the left subclavian artery.[2] Focal tenderness and nociceptive pain descriptors (achy, throbbing, dull) point toward myofascial or articular etiology, while referred symptoms along with neuropathic pain descriptors (tingling, numb) point toward radicular or myelopathic etiologies.

Location

Unlike in the cervical spine, the precise location of pain in the thoracic spine is often possible to obtain from the patient. Common landmarks can be utilized, including T4 often at the level of the nipple line and T10 approximately the level of the umbilicus.[3] Radicular pain may move anteriorly across the chest or abdomen at the level of pathology. Special attention should be paid if symptoms are unilateral or if they cross midline. Painful syndromes such as herpes zoster will present in a dermatomal pattern with unilateral involvement prior to rash development. Pain localized to the paraspinal musculature often indicates mechanical etiology. The differential of mechanical back pain includes disk degeneration, facet arthropathy, fracture, and musculoligamentous sprain/strain. Lower extremity symptoms are most commonly due to spinal stenosis and disk herniation. Infection and neoplasm are rare, systemic causes of back pain but the thoracic spine is the most common location.[4]

Onset

The onset of symptoms can be sudden, delayed, or insidious. The type of onset may be related to the mechanism. More sudden onset with associated trauma will have a far different differential, including fracture (vertebral body or rib), than chronic pain with gradual onset which may involve facet arthropathy, myofascial pain, or costovertebral joint dysfunction especially when associated with a chronic enthesopathy such as ankylosing spondylitis.

Modifying Factors

Aggravating and relieving factors inform about the possible source of the patient's symptoms. Pain that is alleviated with laying down and sleeping is often mechanical with differential including facet arthropathy and vertebral fracture. If the symptoms include pain at night affecting sleep or pain at rest, this should raise suspicion for a more concerning diagnosis such as malignancy, inflammatory condition, or infection.[4]

Time Course

With few exceptions, patients would not be present with thoracic spine conditions immediately after the onset of pain. A more acute onset should be concerning for a more urgent diagnosis than a patient with chronic pain, especially in the setting of trauma.[5] Acute pain in an elderly patient with osteoporosis should raise suspicion for an acute vertebral compression fracture and even minor trauma may be relevant. A gradually worsening pain with acute to subacute time course may indicate infection or malignancy in the right patient.

Associated Findings

Neurologic changes are important to gather from the patient. Lower limb weakness and sensory deficit are the most common symptoms found in thoracic myelopathy.[6] Patients with severe stenosis may also present with hyperreflexia and clonus in the lower extremities as well as gait dysfunction. Descriptions of a specific dermatome by the patient can help to localize the lesion if a nerve root is affected. Always rule out symptoms indicative of significant cord compression requiring emergent intervention, including bowel/bladder incontinence and saddle anesthesia. Fevers and chills with elevated inflammatory markers increase the likelihood of diskitis or epidural abscess on the differential.

Past Medical History

A past medical history can give vital clues to the diagnosis, given that the abdominal viscera can refer to the thoracic region and mimic thoracic pain. Flank pain should be differentiated from thoracic pain and they may or may not be related but widen the differential to include conditions such as nephrolithiasis, pyelonephritis, rib fractures due to trauma, or pathologic fractures from tumors. A history of malignancy and prior spine surgeries should always be investigated. Postmortem studies have suggested up to 70% of patients with metastatic disease have metastases to the spine.[7]

PHYSICAL EXAMINATION

Physical examination of the thoracic spine follows the typical structure of a musculoskeletal examination and includes observation, palpation, range of motion, neurologic examination, and special tests. The physical examination needs to be thorough, but the clinician will confirm or reject the hypotheses that they have formulated in the history-taking portion of the evaluation. Once again, a complete examination includes an evaluation of the affected area and at least all the proximal joints.

Observation

The examination begins by observing the patient as she/he walks into the room. This includes analysis of the gait, ease of mobility, and guarding. Serious conditions of the thoracic spine, such as infections, tumors, or unstable fractures may affect the spinal cord, leading to thoracic myelopathy and may initially only manifest with subtle gait issues. Conditions such as acute compression fractures will cause excruciating pain with movement, even with deep breathing or coughing, so the patient will be very guarded and careful with functional tasks. Observation of the thoracic spine should occur with the patient in the gown and with the affected area and proximal joints exposed. The clinician evaluates for any signs of swelling, postural asymmetry, skin changes, deformity (scoliosis, kyphosis, etc.). Scoliosis and asymmetry can often be better observed with the patient in a flexed position. Thoracic kyphosis along with stiffness could raise suspicion for ankylosing spondylitis or Scheuermann's kyphosis.

Palpation

The palpation portion of the examination includes soft tissue as well as bony palpation. The examiner is looking for tenderness, swelling, rash, spasms and trigger points, and motion anomalies. The clinician will palpate soft tissues, spinous processes, costotransverse, costovertebral, and zygapophyseal joints, paraspinal muscles as well as anterior sternal, chondral, and clavicular joints. Tenderness over the ribs with a history of major trauma may be due to a rib fracture that can mimic thoracic radiculopathy. Sensitivity of 78.4% and specificity of 72.9% has been found with positive clinical examination findings including midline tenderness, deformity, pain, and neurologic deficit when evaluating for thoracolumbar spine fractures.[8]

Active Movements

Active range of motion includes flexion, extension, and rotation. Studies regarding the thoracic spine range of motion have wide variability. Since the primary movement of the thoracic spine is rotation, it can be helpful to have the patient plant their feet and rotate the shoulders 90° in both directions.[9] The examiner should look for symptom reproduction and for abnormal or asymmetric patterns of movement. Reproduction of symptoms with a specific movement may indicate a mechanical pain source, such as myofascial, joint capsule, or nerve.

Neurological Examination

Neuromuscular evaluation should be performed on every patient, even if the patient does not endorse radicular pain or neurological symptoms. This is because patients tend to under-report symptoms that are not painful and certain conditions such as thoracic myelopathy or motor neuron disease in early stages may present with subtle neurological deficits. The neurologic examination includes testing of muscle strength, muscle stretch reflexes, upper motor neuron signs (Hoffmann's sign, Babinski reflex, Lhermitte's sign, clonus), sensory examination, balance and coordination testing, and on occasion, cranial nerve examination. Pin-prick sensation testing should be examined in any cases of suspected spinal cord compression or injury as this can help identify the level of the lesion. Both upper and lower extremity strength and reflexes should be examined. Description of a detailed neurological examination is beyond the scope of this chapter.

Special Tests

Special tests are not a major part of thoracic spine evaluation, given the very limited range of motion in this region of the spine. However, there are some special tests that can be used along with the rest of the examination in order to support the differential diagnoses.

Springing of the Ribs

Springing of the ribs is a useful test to screen for rib fracture. The examiner provides a lateral compression to the chest and the test is positive if the pain is elicited.[10]

Maximal Inspiration

Pressure changes in the chest with inspiration and expiration are transmitted to the epidural and paravertebral spaces. Negative pressure in the epidural space will be increased further with deep inspiration. Increased pain with a deep breath can be considered a dural sign when the rest of the examination further suggests disk herniation.

Cough/Sneeze Test

Cough or sneeze produces a Valsalva effect and can cause a net positive pressure in the epidural space. This increase in pressure can transiently produce radicular symptoms in the thoracic spine. A patient may have noticed this phenomenon prior to the appointment and may provide increased pain with sneezing or coughing in their history.[11]

Thoracic Expansion

Thoracic expansion is determined by the difference in chest circumference at maximal inhalation compared to maximal exhalation. It is used as a measurement tool to assess for limited mobility seen in ankylosing spondylitis. There has been some debate over whether thoracic expansion should be measured at the level of the xiphoid notch or the more traditional fourth intercostal space. It has been suggested that obesity can confound measurements taken at the fourth intercostal space. The original New York Classification Criteria suggested >2.5 cm difference in thoracic expansion at the fourth intercostal space was considered normal, while newer studies have suggested that the majority of patients measured 1.9 ± 0.07 cm difference at the xiphoid notch.[12] Chest expansion less than 2.5 cm was found to have a sensitivity of 10–15% and specificity of 93–97%.[13]

SUMMARY

Mid-back pain is a fairly common condition, which most of the time originates from myofascial structures. However, given that thoracic spine is a common location of spinal metastases and the possibility of a visceral referred pain, it is thus imperative that a knowledgeable clinician performs a thorough history and physical examination prior to administering a treatment plan.

TAKE HOME POINTS

- Vast majority of the time, the clinician will have a high level of suspicion of the underlying condition of the thoracic spine based on the history of the presenting symptoms.
- The most important part of the physical examination of the thoracic spine is the neurological examination.
- Physical examination of the thoracic spine must include an examination of the neck and shoulder as well as the lumbar spine.

REFERENCES

1. Mata S, Fortin PR, Fitzcharles M, et al. A controlled study of diffuse idiopathic skeletal hyperostosis. Medicine. 1997;76(2):104-17.
2. Hagan PG, Neinaber CA, Isselbacher EM, et al. The International Registry of Acute Aortic Dissection (IRAD): new insights into an old disease. JAMA. 2000;283(7):897-903.
3. Lee MWL, McPhee RW, Stringer MD. An evidence-based approach to human dermatomes. Cin Anat. 2008;21:363-73.
4. Golob AL, Wipf JE. Low back pain. Med Clin North Am. 2014;98(3):405-28.
5. Michael ALR, Newman J, Rao AS. The assessment of thoracic pain. Orthop Trauma. 2010;24(1):63-73.
6. Hou X, Sun C, Liu X, et al. Clinical features of thoracic spinal stenosis-associated myelopathy: a retrospective analysis of 427 cases. Clin Spine Surg. 2016;29(2):86-9.
7. Guo M, Kolberg KL, Smith EC, et al. Predominance of spinal metastases involving the posterior vertebral body. World Neurosurg. 2018;119:e991-6.
8. Inaba K, Nosanov L, Menaker J, et al. Prospective derivation of a clinical decision rule for thoracolumbar spine evaluation after blunt trauma: an American Association for the Surgery of Trauma Multi-Institutional Trials Group study. J Trauma Acute Care Surg. 2015;78(3):459-67.
9. Lauerman W, Russo M. Thoracolumbar spine disorders in the adult. DeLee & Drez's Orthopaedic Sports Medicine, 4th edition. Philadelphia: Saunders; 2015. pp. 1523-41.
10. Dandy DJ, Edwards DJ. History and clinical examination. Essential Orthopaedics and Trauma, 5th edition. Cambridge: Elsevier Limited; 2009. pp. 9-31.
11. Evans DC. Lumbar spine. Illustrated Orthopedic Physical Assessment, 3rd edition. Maryland, US: Mosby; 2009. pp. 535-698.
12. Assassi S, Weisman MH, Lee M, et al. New population-based reference values for spinal mobility measures based on the 2009-2010 national health and nutrition examination survey. Arthritis Rheumatol. 2014;66(9):2628-37.
13. Moll JMH, Wright V. New York clinical criteria for ankylosing spondylitis. Ann Rheum Dis. 1973;32(4):354-63.

CHAPTER 32 Thoracic Radiculopathy and Myelopathy

Karthikeyan E Ponnusamy, Emmanuel Menga, A Jay Khanna

EPIDEMIOLOGY AND NATURAL HISTORY

Radiculopathy and myelopathy represent a continuum of diseases caused by nerve root compression and spinal cord compression, respectively. Although thoracic radiculopathy and myelopathy remain rare diagnoses, thoracic radiculopathy is a common cause of thoracic back and chest wall pain, often described as a band-like sensation of weakness, numbness, tingling, or paresthesias around the trunk in the distribution of the affected thoracic nerve root. Thoracic myelopathy, however, is often caused by central/midline spinal cord compression and results in varying symptoms relative to the degree of nerve compression, ranging from radicular symptoms of pain and paresthesia to myelopathic symptoms of gait disturbance and physical examination findings of long-tract signs.[1]

Thoracic radiculopathy and myelopathy typically result from degenerative conditions such as nerve root and spinal cord compression secondary to intervertebral disk herniation, osteophyte formation, and stenosis. However, thoracic vertebral fractures, tumors, vascular insufficiency, and infections have also been associated with thoracic radiculopathy and myelopathy.

The true incidence of thoracic radiculopathy and myelopathy secondary to primary or metastatic tumors remains unknown. However, the thoracic region is the most common site involved in spinal tumor metastasis, accounting for 70% of all spinal metastases.[2,3] Localized pain, axial spinal pain, and radicular pain are the most common early symptoms in patients presenting with spinal metastasis.[4] Similarly, the thoracolumbar spine represents the most common site of spinal trauma, accounting for 75–90% of all the spinal traumas.[5]

Intervertebral disk herniation remains a common cause of nerve root and spinal cord compression, leading to thoracic radiculopathy and myelopathy. Thoracic disk herniation represents 0.25–0.75% of all symptomatic (radiculopathy and myelopathy) disk herniations;[6] the incidence has been reported to be 1 per 1,000,000 individuals per year.[7] It is more common in males than females, with a reported 1.5:1 ratio, and it involves mostly the lower thoracic vertebra, with a 75% incidence between T8 and L1 vertebra.[6,8,9] Thoracic radiculopathy secondary to a disk herniation is most commonly associated with upper thoracic and lateral disk herniation compressing the nerve root as it exits the foramen, whereas myelopathy most commonly results from midline disk herniation compressing the spinal cord. Acute myelopathy occurs in 4% of patients with thoracic disk herniation.[10]

Brown et al.[9] reported on the natural history of thoracic disk herniation in 55 patients with radiculopathy and myelopathy. Radicular symptoms were the most common, with anterior band-like chest pain reported as the most common early symptom in patients with thoracic disk herniation. Most patients (73%) were managed nonoperatively with physical therapy and activity modification and attained good results without progression of their disease.[9]

WORK-UP (CLINICAL FINDINGS)

Symptoms and Signs

Patients presenting with thoracic radiculopathy and myelopathy show a variable clinical course with broad and extensive differential diagnoses including disk herniation, inflammatory processes, tumor, and vascular insufficiency. A thorough medical history and clinical examination must be complemented with radiographic and advanced imaging findings in the evaluation and management of patients presenting with symptoms suspicious for thoracic radiculopathy and myelopathy.

Chest wall and upper abdominal pain, numbness, and tingling that radiates along a dermatome distribution are common findings in patients with thoracic radiculopathy. Brown et al.[9] described anterior band-like chest pain as the most common early radicular symptoms in patients with radiculopathy secondary to disk herniation. Lower extremity paresthesias and weakness are common symptoms of thoracic myelopathy.[9] Vanichkachorn and Vaccaro[11] described three groups of presenting symptoms ranging from radiculopathy to myelopathy in patients with symptomatic thoracic disk herniations. The first group consisted of patients presenting with predominantly axial pain of mild-to-moderate intensity localized to the middle to lower thoracic region and sometimes circumferential. The second group consisted of patients with band-like anterior-chest discomfort on a dermatomal pattern most commonly observed at the T10 dermatome distribution irrespective of the involved thoracic nerve root level. The third group comprised patients presenting with myelopathic symptoms of muscle weakness with lower extremity symptoms of gait instability, sustained clonus, and spasticity. Bowel and bladder dysfunction (15–20% of patients) and Brown-Sequard syndrome are seen in cases of large acute midline thoracic disc herniation.[11]

Focal back pain and neck pain are also the most common symptoms in 90% of patients presenting with spinal metastasis, with radicular symptoms indicative of nerve root compression. Myelopathic symptoms of weakness, numbness, bowel/bladder dysfunction, and Brown-Sequard syndrome are likely associated with spinal canal compromise.[2,12]

Other signs that may aid in the clinical evaluation of patients presenting with symptoms concerning for thoracic radiculopathy and myelopathy include superficial abdominal reflex response, which is elicited by scratching the skin along the axis of the dermatome from the lateral abdomen toward the midline umbilicus. A normal reflex is noted with shifting of the umbilicus toward the direction of the stimulus. Absence of this reflex is common in upper motor neuron lesions, and it can serve as a proxy in the localization of the level of thoracic spinal cord lesions.[13]

Laboratory Findings

Thoracic radiculopathy and myelopathy present with variable clinical signs and symptoms. The broad differential diagnoses associated with these symptoms require appropriate laboratory examinations in conjunction with a thorough clinical history, physical examination, and imaging studies to serve as a guide toward diagnosis and patient management. The following laboratory testing should be considered: complete blood count, complete chemistry panel, erythrocyte sedimentation rate (ESR), C-reactive protein (CRP), antinuclear antibody, human leukocyte antigen B27, and blood cultures. Although laboratory findings are nonspecific, they may prove to be a valuable tool in the diagnosis of the cause of the disease considering the clinical history, physical examination, and imaging findings. Biopsy of lesions may play a role in cases of suspected infection or tumor for definitive diagnosis and management.

Elevated white blood count, ESR, and CRP are common markers of infectious causes.[14] These markers may be elevated in spinal tumors, thus emphasizing the need for a complete and thorough examination, as well as the correlation of laboratory findings with other diagnostic modalities.

Imaging

Standard conventional radiography, computed tomography (CT), CT with myelography, and magnetic resonance imaging (MRI) with and without contrast all represent imaging modalities that play a role in the diagnosis of patients with thoracic radiculopathy and myelopathy.

Standard anteroposterior and lateral conventional radiography remains the most commonly used initial imaging modality in the evaluation of patients presenting with radicular or myelopathic symptoms. Conventional radiographs play an important role but are limited to the evaluation of osseous anatomy, osseous injuries, spinal alignment, and disk space height. Ossific changes enhancing some neoplasias, osteophyte formation in spondylosis, and ossification of the posterior longitudinal ligament sometimes observed on conventional radiography may represent possible causes of a nerve root or spinal cord compression causing thoracic radiculopathy or myelopathy. These limitations, therefore, warrant more advanced imaging modalities for appropriate diagnosis and management.

A CT scan is a valuable imaging modality in the evaluation of calcification of the intervertebral disk, herniated disk calcification and osteophytes, and osseous changes from trauma or primary or metastatic spinal lesions. CT imaging can be viewed in the coronal, axial, and sagittal planes to assess the morphology and any changes in anatomy. Images can also be viewed in various "windows" that highlight osseous or soft-tissue structures. CT with myelography provides a detailed evaluation of disk herniation, ossification of the posterior longitudinal ligament and ligamentum flavum, and potential areas of a nerve root or spinal cord compression causing thoracic radiculopathy and myelopathy. CT with myelography provides superior special resolution and may be used for patients with pacemakers and other implantable devices and for patients for whom MRI is contraindicated.

Magnetic resonance imaging is the most sensitive, specific, and/or effective imaging modality for a variety of conditions. It remains the most sensitive imaging study for the evaluation of nerve root and spinal cord abnormalities. MRI provides excellent soft-tissue evaluation and plays a critical role in evaluating disk herniation, infections, and neoplastic diseases; and it is effective in delineating intradural and extradural abnormalities. MRI with contrast is especially useful for evaluating spinal infections and neoplasia. It is also the most sensitive and specific imaging modality available for the evaluation of spinal metastasis, the extraosseous extent of spinal metastasis, neural impingement, and leptomeningeal disease[3] and the most effective imaging modality in evaluating spinal infections. The use of gadolinium contrast enhancement can allow for the differentiation of infections from degenerative changes of the spine and of epidural granulation from an epidural abscess.[14]

Disk herniations typically involve the annulus fibrosis, which is represented as an area of low signal intensity on T1- and T2-weighted images. Involvement of the nucleus pulposus as seen in annular fissures or tears can be visualized as an area of high signal intensity on the T2-weighted images. The high-intensity signal of the cerebrospinal fluid seen on T2-weighted images provides a myelographic effect, which allows for size delineation and configuration of the disk herniation and of its relationship to and effects on the spinal cord and nerve roots (Figs 1 to 3).

Despite which imaging modality is used, correlation with the patient's history and clinical examination is critical and must be taken into account. Imaging findings

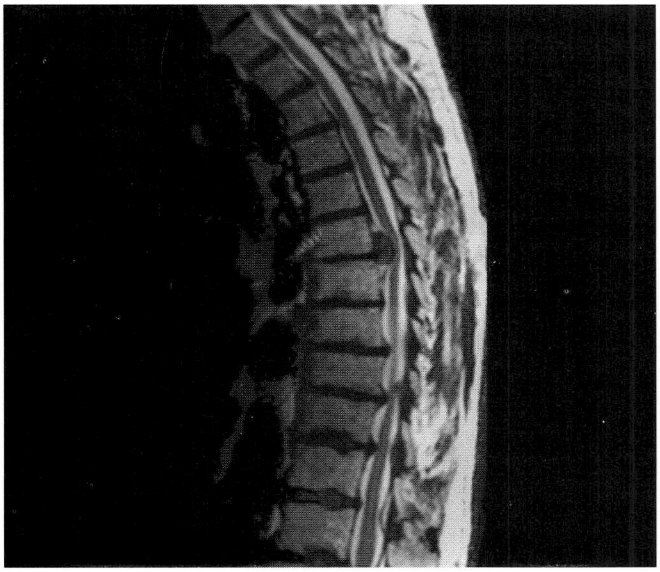

Fig. 1: T2-sagittal image of a T6–7 disk herniation impinging on the cord.
Source: Reprinted with permission from Krauss WE, Edwards DA, Cohen-Gadol AA. Transthoracic discectomy without interbody fusion. Surg Neurol. 2005;63(5):403-8, discussion 408-9; Fig. 1A, p. 404.

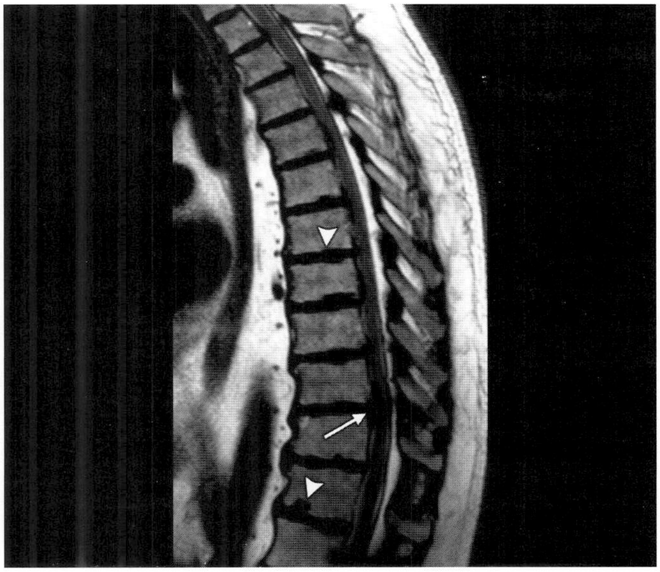

Fig. 2: T2-sagittal image of a disk herniation (arrow) and Schmorl's nodes (arrowheads) with cord impingement.
Source: Reprinted with permission from Okubadejo GO, Daftary AR, Buchowski JM, et al. The lumbar and thoracic spine. In: Khanna AJ (Ed). MRI for Orthopaedic Surgeons. New York: Thieme; 2010. pp. 269-315; Fig. 11.29A, p. 290.

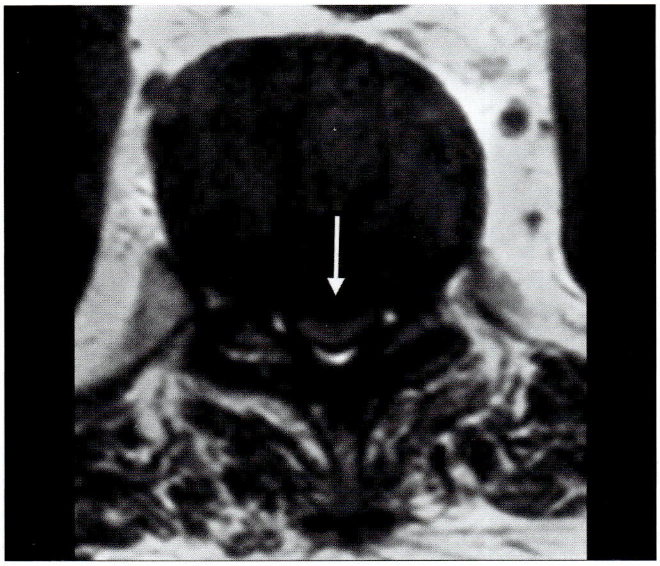

Fig. 3: T2 axial image of a central disk herniation (arrow).
Source: Reprinted with permission from Okubadejo GO, Daftary AR, Buchowski JM, et al. The lumbar and thoracic spine. In: Khanna AJ (Ed). MRI for Orthopaedic Surgeons. New York: Thieme; 2010. pp. 269-315; Fig. 11.29B, p. 290.

and diagnostic studies should serve to support clinical examination findings and patient history because changes in imaging studies do not necessarily equate to the causality of symptoms.

MEDICAL MANAGEMENT

Awareness of the broad differential diagnosis of the true cause of thoracic radiculopathic or myelopathic symptoms is critical in the decision-making process and management of thoracic abnormalities. Medical management, including anti-inflammatory medications, muscle relaxants, intravenous antibiotic therapy, chemotherapy, physical therapy, bracing, activity modification, and epidural injections, remains the mainstay for treatment for most patients with thoracic radiculopathy.

For thoracic radiculopathy, treatment starts with nonsurgical approaches. Vanichkachorn and Vaccaro[11] have suggested combinations of hyperextension bracing, physical therapy, and oral steroids. They cautioned that prolonged bracing leads to deconditioning and worsening function and should be used only temporarily in patients who have severe symptoms. Physical therapy should begin initially with passive range of motion and then can build up to an active range of motion and strengthening. Using a short 3- to 5-day course of oral steroids can help calm the acute inflammation and improve the patient's functional status. In addition, nonsteroidal anti-inflammatories are helpful in improving symptoms. Of course, the patient's medical comorbidities need to be considered before prescribing either medication. If these approaches do not help, more aggressive treatments, including intercostal or epidural corticosteroid injections, can be considered. If the patient has no improvement or worsens after 4–6 weeks of nonsurgical management, Vanichkachorn and Vaccaro[11] have suggested considering surgical options.

Thoracic myelopathy is treated more aggressively because of the combination of symptom severity and risk for progression. Many clinicians recommend that treatment of myelopathy begins with surgery.

Because of the small incidence of thoracic myelopathy and radiculopathy, there is a dearth of literature regarding the results of medical management. Brown et al.[9] performed a retrospective Level IV chart review of 55 patients with thoracic disk herniations to determine their natural history. Of these patients, only 4% had frank symptoms of myelopathy (weakness), whereas the rest had radicular or axial pain symptoms. In the management of all but one of these patients (a patient with rapid-onset paraplegia), the initial regimen was medical management with nonsteroidal anti-inflammatories and physical therapy. Of those 55 patients, 15 (27%) underwent surgery by the end of the study and 2 other patients were considering it because of continued symptoms. Among the 40 patients treated nonoperatively, 77% were able to return to their baseline activity level. These results suggest that medical management of thoracic radiculopathy and axial back pain from a thoracic disk herniation often results in a return to baseline functional level. Brown et al.[9] acknowledged that patients with long-term signs of myelopathy would benefit from surgery.

SURGICAL INDICATIONS AND TREATMENT APPROACHES

Indications

Thoracic radiculopathy and myelopathy present with variable symptoms because of the broad differential and multiple causes. Treatment is aimed at preventing additional neurologic compromise. Surgical management remains an option for patients for whom nonsurgical modalities have failed and is reserved for patients with persistent radicular symptoms despite nonoperative management, patients presenting with acute or progressive myelopathy, and patients for whom nonsurgical management will be ineffective. Infection and tumor (primary and metastatic) leading to thoracic radiculopathy and myelopathy are also well-described indications for surgical intervention. Tay et al.[14] described five surgical indications for patients with spinal infection: (1) for tissue diagnosis if percutaneous needle aspiration failed to identify the pathogen; (2) for infections causing sepsis or neurologic deficit; (3) for the treatment of patients with neurologic deficit caused by compression secondary to infection; (4) for the management of patients with structural instability or deformity secondary to infection; and (5) for the management of patients with elevated inflammatory markers for whom medical management has failed. Similarly, Rose and Buchowski[3] listed four primary surgical indications for the management of spinal metastasis: neurologic compression, spinal instability, unrelenting pain, and histologic diagnosis.

Approaches

The approach to the thoracic spine for the management of infection or tumor depends on the location of the offending entity. Compression secondary to mass effect originating from the posterior spinal elements is usually approached posteriorly, whereas mass effects originating from the anterior and middle spinal elements are usually approached from an isolated anterior or anterolateral approach or a combined anterior and posterior approaches.

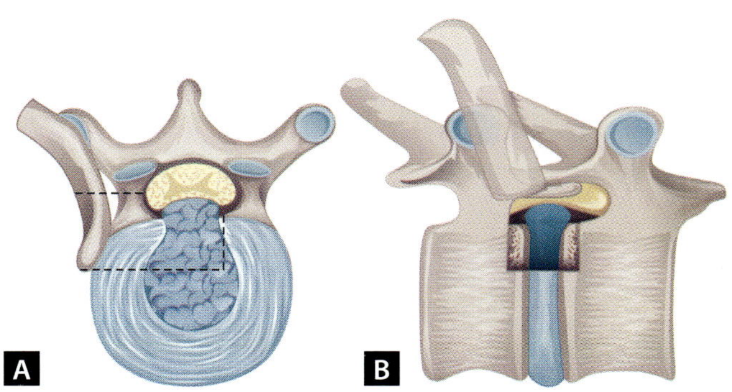

Figs. 4A and B: The bony resections necessary to access a central disk herniation via a transthoracic approach: (A) Axial view; (B) Sagittal view.
Source: Reprinted with permission from Krauss WE, Edwards DA, Cohen-Gadol AA. Transthoracic discectomy without interbody fusion. Surg Neurol. 2005;63(5):403-8, discussion 408-9; Figs. 3A and B, p. 405.

Multiple surgical approaches have been described for the management of patients with thoracic radiculopathy and myelopathy secondary to thoracic disk herniation. Nerve root and spinal cord decompression is the goal for treatment and the key to alleviating or preventing the progression of symptoms.

Anterior Approaches

The anterior transthoracic approach provides direct access to the decompression of the spinal cord and nerve root from anterior structures. The transthoracic approach is the most effective approach for the excision of central and paracentral disk herniation. It involves very little to no spinal cord manipulation with minimal risk for instability (Figs. 4 and 5). This approach provides direct visualization and excellent decompression of central and paracentral disk herniation, and direct access for interbody fusion. Various authors have reported good to excellent results with transthoracic excision of symptomatic thoracic disk herniation.[8,15] However, appropriate patient selection is critical to a successful outcome with improved morbidity, especially for patients with compromised pulmonary function. It should also be noted that the potential for wrong-level surgery is particularly high for thoracic disk

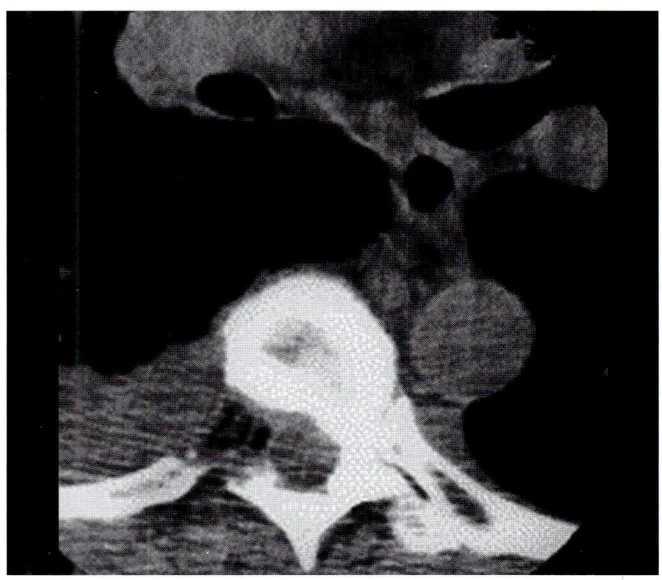

Fig. 5: Postoperative axial computed tomography (CT) scan showing the bony resections needed for a transthoracic approach.
Source: Reprinted with permission from Krauss WE, Edwards DA, Cohen-Gadol AA. Transthoracic discectomy without interbody fusion. Surg Neurol 2005;63(5):403-8, discussion 408-9; Fig. 1C, p. 404.

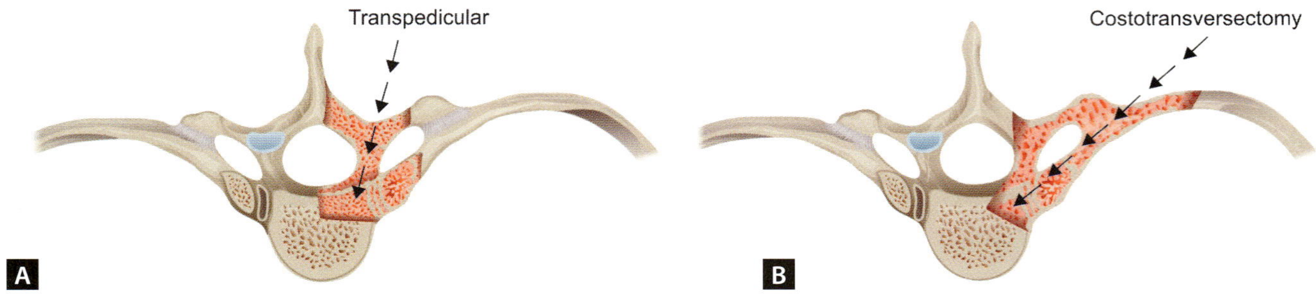

Figs. 6A and B: Two posterolateral thoracic spine approaches. (A) Transpedicular; (B) Costotransversectomy.
Source: Reprinted by permission from Fessler RG, Sturgill M. Review: complications of surgery for thoracic disc disease. Surg Neurol. 1998;49(6):609-18; Fig. 2, p. 610 and Fig. 3, p. 611.

herniations, and specific and deliberate steps should be taken to confirm the level of pathology.[11]

The utility of video-assisted thoracic surgery (VATS) or thoracoscopic procedures was first described by Regan et al.[16] for the management of thoracic spinal disorders. They reported improved postoperative pain, shorter intensive care, and shorter overall hospital stay. VATS is a minimally invasive technique and effective for disk herniation excision, anterior releases for deformity correction, osteotomies, and corpectomies.[11] The minimally invasive approach provides less morbidity than that associated with the open anterior transthoracic approach.[11,16] However, considering the steep learning curve associated with this procedure, VATS should be performed by an experienced surgeon; it has not gained widespread adoption in the United States.

Posterior/Posterolateral Approaches

Direct posterior laminectomy and variations of the posterior approach, including the transpedicular or pediculofacetectomy approach, transfacet pedicle-sparing approach, costotransversectomy, and the lateral extracavitary approach, have been described by multiple authors with successful outcomes (Figs. 6A and B).

Conventional laminectomy was the original surgical procedure of choice for the management of thoracic disk herniation. However, the narrow thoracic spinal canal, combined with the necessary spinal cord manipulation for adequate excision of a herniated disk, has been associated with a high incidence of neurologic complications.[6,17,18] Therefore, conventional laminectomy alone has no role in the treatment of thoracic disk herniation.[6,17,18] The high risk of morbidity associated with this approach has led to the development of alternative approaches that require minimal manipulation of the spinal cord.

The transpedicular or pediculofacetectomy approach involves resection of the facet and the pedicle at the level of the disk herniation and provides direct access to the lateral disk and some soft paracentral disk herniations. Le Roux et al.[19] reported significant improvement in symptoms in 20 patients after the transpedicular approach for the management of symptomatic thoracic disk herniation; 8 patients were asymptomatic at the 1-year follow-up.

The transfacet pedicle-sparing approach decreases the risk of instability associated with the pediculofacetectomy approach. Despite the six patients who required surgery for postoperative complications, Bransford et al.[20] reported improvement in preoperative symptoms at the 1-year follow-up for all 14 patients who underwent the pedicle-sparing approach combined with short segmental arthrodesis. Despite preventing destabilization, the technique is limited by poor visualization through a small bone window with especially limited access to central disk herniations.[1]

Costotransversectomy involves resection of the medial aspect of the corresponding rib, the transverse process, the facet, the pedicle, and the lamina; it is most effective for the excision of lateral and paracentral disk herniations. This approach is also useful for tumor resection and the management of spinal infection.[21,22] Simpson et al.[23] reported excellent to good results in 16 of 19 patients and fair results in the other three patients undergoing costotransversectomy for the management of thoracic disk herniation.

The lateral extracavitary approach, like the costotransversectomy approach, is also used for the management of infections, for tumor resection, and for the excision of lateral and paracentral thoracic soft and calcified disks. It involves a larger amount of rib resection relative to the costotransversectomy approach. Initially designed for the treatment of symptomatic tuberculous spondylitis, it has proven to be a valuable procedure in the management of disk herniation, thoracic and lumbar radiculopathy, and myelopathy secondary to trauma.[24,25]

Minimally Invasive Approaches

In addition to the VATS procedure detailed above, other minimally invasive techniques have been described for the decompression of symptomatic thoracic disk herniations. Uribe et al.[26] described a minimally invasive lateral approach using the extreme lateral interbody fusion technique, with excellent or good overall outcomes in 80% of patients with symptomatic thoracic disk herniation. Deviren et al.[27] reported on a minimally invasive anterolateral transthoracic transpleural approach for a single-level thoracic disk herniation, finding excellent exposure with consistent decompression and significant improvement in the visual analog pain score in a series of 12 patients treated with this approach.

COMPLICATIONS

The literature has widely varying reports of complications for VATS and open thoracotomies (Table 1).[26,28] It is difficult to compare these two procedures because a VATS approach may tend to be used for more simple cases, whereas thoracotomies may tend to be used for more difficult or complex cases. To our knowledge, there has been no study comparing the two approaches for patients with similar baseline characteristics, but it is thought that the VATS technique may lead to fewer issues with pleural effusion and neuralgia. For example, the widely reported incidental durotomy rate for thoracotomies includes studies using it for heavily calcified disk herniations.[11] More rigorous studies will be needed to truly understand the complication profile for each approach.

A minimally invasive lateral approach has recently been developed as an extension of the extreme lateral interbody fusion to the lumbar spine; its complication rate is comparable to that for VATS and open thoracotomies (Table 1).[26,28] Other approaches include transfacet pedicle sparing, transpedicular, and anterolateral transpleural. These approaches are not as frequently discussed in the literature and their detailed complication profile is unknown at this time.

OUTCOMES

Thoracotomy and Video-assisted Thoracic Surgery

In the treatment of thoracic lesions, multiple studies have tried to determine whether an open thoracotomy or a VATS approach leads to better outcomes.[28-34] However, the major limitation of these studies is that the cohorts treated with each approach did not have the same baseline characteristics. For example, Wait et al.[28] examined a series of 121 consecutive patients treated with VATS for herniated thoracic disks. This Level III study compared the complication rates with an unmatched cohort of 39 patients treated with thoracotomy during the same time. In that study, the contraindications to VATS were more difficult herniations such as giant and densely ossified disks, three or more levels, great vessels preventing access, or level above T3–T4 or below T11–T12. Patients with those contraindications were generally treated with thoracotomy instead. Of the VATS patients, 43% had radiculopathy, 28.9% had myelopathy, 27.2% had myelopathy and pain, and 2% had axial pain alone. This study used the Frankel scale, visual analog scale, and a questionnaire

Table 1: Types and rates of complications by the procedure.

Approach	*Pleural effusion requiring drainage (%)*	*Incidental durotomy (%)*	*Recurrence and incomplete discectomy requiring reoperation (%)*	*Mislocalized level (%)*	*Pneumonia (%)*	*Neuralgia (%)*	*Additional neurological deficit (%)*
VATS[28]	2–5	0–1.7	1.7–4	0.8–2	2–6	13–17	2–3
Thoracotomies[28]	0–15.4	0–27.3	0–2.6	2.6	25–27.3	5.6–75	13
Minimally invasive lateral[26]	0–1.7	7.7–11.7	1.7	--*	1.7	1.7	1.7

(VATS: video-assisted thoracic surgery)
*: not available.

regarding patient satisfaction with the surgery for an average follow-up of 2.4 years (range: 1–148 months). For the patients with myelopathy, 73.5% improved one Frankel grade, 17.6% had improvement not reaching a Frankel grade, 7.4% had no change, and 1.5% worsened but recovered to baseline. In the radiculopathy patients, 84% had a complete resolution, 14% had improvement, and 1% each had no change and worsening. For patients with back pain, 56.8% had a complete resolution, 29.7% improvement, and 13.5% no change. Compared with patients who underwent thoracotomy, those who were treated with VATS had significantly lower average intercostal neuralgia (23.1% vs 5.8%, respectively), length of hospital stay (8.6 days vs 4.9 days, respectively), chest tube duration (4.6 days vs 3.4 days, respectively), and estimated blood loss (EBL) (1,440 mL vs 311 mL, respectively). Another study by Anand and Regan[29] of 100 consecutive patients undergoing VATS had similar perioperative measures: average EBL, 261 mL (range: 50–2,500 mL); average intensive care unit stay, less than one day (0.62 day; range: 0–4 days); and average hospital stay, 4 days (range: 1–11 days). The thoracotomy group from the study by Wait et al.[28] had larger and more calcified disks and greater baseline neurological deficits. Those authors recommended VATS for disks that were less than 40% of the canal area, noncalcified, or near the center.

A complementary Level III study by Hott et al.[30] reported that giant herniated disks (more than 40% of the spinal canal) would have improved functional outcome with open thoracotomy instead of VATS. This study was limited by small numbers with only eight in the thoracotomy group and another eight in the VATS group. There were no neurological complications in the thoracotomy group, whereas the VATS group had two cases of neurological worsening: one patient returned to baseline and the second improved but not to baseline. Hott et al.[30] reported that VATS could address soft giant herniations but could not as easily address hard giant herniations.

In a Level II prospective nonrandomized study, Johnson et al.[31] used VATS for 36 patients with single- or two-level herniations and thoracotomy for eight patients with three or more levels, ossified posterior longitudinal ligament (OPLL), or adhesions after a previous VATS. Myelopathy was present in all patients in the thoracotomy group and in 53% of the VATS group; the remaining 47% had radiculopathy. The outcome measures were the Oswestry Disability Index for radiculopathy and Frankel scores for myelopathy. Patients undergoing VATS had significantly shorter chest tube durations (1.3 days vs 4.1 days) and hospital stays (3.1 days vs 5.4 days) and nonsignificantly shorter operative times (212 minutes vs 305 minutes) and EBL (225 mL vs 380 mL). Of the patients with myelopathy who underwent a VATS, Frankel grades improved in 47.4%, were unchanged in 47.4%, and worsened in 5.3%. The patients with myelopathy who underwent a thoracotomy had worse baseline Frankel scores; after surgery, Frankel scores improved in 50%, were unchanged in 37.5% and worsened in 12.5%. These results cannot be directly compared because baseline Frankel scores in 21% of the patients with myelopathy treated with VATS started at the highest Frankel score. Frankel scores for the outcome are not sensitive enough to detect changes in such patients. Those authors thought that single- or two-level lesions could be treated by VATS but that a thoracotomy would have been better for more than two levels or for OPLL.

Oskouian and Johnson[34] had comparable results in their prospective Level IV study of 47 VATS patients. They used indications similar to those of Johnson et al.[31] where patients had a VATS procedure if they had two or fewer pathologic levels and lacked an OPLL. In their patient population, the outcome measure used in the 55% with myelopathy was the Frankel grade and in the 45% with radiculopathy, it was the Oswestry Pain Scale. Of the patients with myelopathy, 39.1% had improvement, with a mean improvement of two grades (range: 1–2 grades), and 58.7% had no change; only one patient (2.2%) had a worsened Frankel grade. All patients with radiculopathy experienced improvement, with an average preoperative pain score of 60 (range: 40–80) that improved to an average of 14 (range: 0–40) after surgery. Oskouian and Johnson[34] agreed with Johnson et al.[31] that multilevel lesions, such as OPLL, would benefit from thoracotomy.

Because of the technical challenges of VATS, these studies suggest that it be selectively used for certain patients, including those with soft herniations that occupy less than 40% of the spinal canal area, have two or fewer levels, and do not have OPLL. In these cases, the use of VATS may be able to lead to less blood loss and shorter hospitalizations. For patients who do not meet these criteria, other surgical approaches, such as thoracotomy, may be better suited. These studies also suggest that patients with myelopathy and radiculopathy generally have better outcomes with surgical intervention than those treated for axial pain. Anand and Regan[29] reported that Oswestry Disability Index scores improved 60% in patients with myelopathy, 37% in patients with axial and radicular pain, 28% in patients with axial and leg pain, and 24% in patients with pure axial pain.

Many clinicians believe that arthrodesis is necessary after a thoracic discectomy. To test that assumption, Krauss et al.[32] conducted a Level IV study to determine outcomes after a transthoracic discectomy without arthrodesis. They followed 18 patients (17 with myelopathy and 1 with radiculopathy) with a mean follow-up of 28 months (±20 months SD). Of those patients, 83% had an improvement in their symptoms, 11% were unchanged, and 6% had worsened symptoms. The authors reported that these outcomes were comparable to those in the literature for thoracic discectomies with arthrodesis. Krauss et al.[32] suggested that indications for arthrodesis could include patients with a wide vertebral body and/or disk resection, multilevel discectomies, thoracic spine pain, and discectomies at the thoracolumbar junction.

Minimally Invasive Lateral

Deviren et al.[27] studied a minimally invasive anterolateral transthoracic approach that uses a table-mounted retractor system (NuVasive Inc., San Diego, CA) to access the thoracic spine for diskectomy and fusion. In their Level IV study, 12 patients, 8 of whom had myelopathy, underwent this procedure; visual analog scale and Short Form-36 data were used to assess clinical outcomes. The patients had an average operative time of 210 minutes (range: 133–298 minutes), EBL of 440 mL (range: 100–1,200 mL), and a hospital stay of 5 days (range: 2–12 days). Patients had significant improvements in visual analog scale and nonsignificant increases in Short Form-36 scores. The authors proposed that the anterolateral transthoracic approach could be an alternative to VATS with an easier learning curve.

Kasliwal and Deutsch[35] also studied the minimally invasive direct lateral approach to the thoracic spine using the same retractor system (NuVasive Inc.) and proposed an alternative method for anterior access to the thoracic spine through the retropleural space. An operative microscope was used in conjunction with the retractor system, and the authors warned that the long working channel makes bleeding and other complications more difficult to address. They treated seven patients with central disk herniations and myelopathy and did not fuse the levels. Three of seven patients had an improvement of 1 point on the Nurick scale, and no patients worsened. All four of the patients who also had radiculopathy improved.

Uribe et al.[26] conducted a Level IV retrospective multicenter study using the NuVasive retractor system (NuVasive Inc.) in 60 patients with a mean follow-up of 11 months (range: 0.5–24 months). In this patient population, 70% had myelopathy, 52% had radiculopathy, and 77% had axial back pain. Posterior arthrodesis was used if the patient showed substantial instability, and a posterior decompression was used if there was severe canal stenosis. The average EBL was 290 mL (range: 10–3,000 mL), and the average length of hospitalization of 5 days (range: 1.1–12 days). Of the myelopathy patients, 83% had improvement, whereas 91% of those with radiculopathy and 87% with axial back pain had improvement. The authors compared their results with those in the literature for other thoracic approaches and reported comparable outcomes. Of note, Uribe et al.[26] provided extensive tables summarizing many of the published studies in terms of results and complications.

Khoo et al.[36] used an alternative approach using progressive tubular dilators (e.g. METRx retractor system, Medtronic Inc., Minneapolis, MN) in an extracavitary approach. Through a paramedian oblique approach, they directed the retractor toward the junction between the transverse process and the lateral aspect of the facet. They used the approach on 13 patients and had an average operative times of 94 minutes [86.5 minutes (range: 60–120 minutes) for one level, 130 minutes (range: 120–140 minutes) for two levels], an average EBL of 33 mL (range: 10–50 mL), and an average hospitalization of 3.1 days (range: 1.5–5 days). This group was compared to a control group of 11 patients who had a thoracotomy. The thoracotomy group had an average operative time of 175 minutes, an average EBL of 295 mL, and an average hospitalization of 5.3 days. The retractor group had a significantly decreased EBL, operative time, intensive care unit stay, transfusion incidence, and overall length of stay. At a mean follow-up of 10 months, there was no difference in the assessment of neurological function in the two groups by Frankel scores.

These novel retractor-based approaches were developed with the goal of providing minimally invasive approaches to the thoracic spine without the technical demands of VATS. Other advantages of these techniques are that patients may not need postoperative chest tubes or require intraoperative lung collapse. Additional study is necessary to better compare the risks and benefits of these approaches relative to the more commonly used VATS and thoracotomy techniques (Table 2).

Posterior

Decades ago, the initial approach to the thoracic spine was a posterior approach via a laminectomy. It was a risky approach because of the narrowness of the thoracic spinal canal and its occupation by the thoracic spinal cord, and it was associated with 59% morbidity and 13% mortality from spinal cord manipulation.[36] As a result, alternative posterior approaches were developed.

Bilsky[37] studied the use of a transpedicular thoracic disk excision in 20 patients; 70% had myelopathy and 30% had radiculopathy. All patients with myelopathy improved except for one who had a transient neurological worsening but returned to normal function. Of the patients with radiculopathy, a third had a complete resolution, a third had a mild resolution, and a third had no improvement. Bilsky[37] reported that this approach would be better for lateral or centrolateral disk herniations, and it could be used for central calcified disks. However, anterior and lateral approaches have better exposure for central calcified disks, and the authors recommended using transthoracic approaches for those disks. To better approach the central disks and anterior aspect of the spinal cord, Jho[38] described a posterior transpedicular approach using a 70° endoscope for better visualization. He studied the use of this technique in 25 patients, 28% of whom had myelopathy, 24% of whom had myelopathy and radiculopathy, 40% of whom had radiculopathy, and 8% of whom axial pain. All patients with myelopathy improved, except for one whose symptoms recurred after a motor vehicle accident after surgery. Among the patients with radiculopathy, 90% had a complete resolution, whereas the remaining patients with radiculopathy and all the patients with axial pain had no improvement. Those patients were usually in the hospital overnight, and none had any surgery-associated complications.

CONCLUSION

Multiple techniques have generally shown good results when used in appropriate patients. The key factors discussed by Bransford et al.[20] include location of the abnormality, patient comorbidities, and surgeon experience. Thoracic spine pathologies are frequently attributable to disk herniations, and they can occur in a multitude of locations. More central locations are better approached via an anterior thoracotomy or VATS approach, whereas lateral or centrolateral herniations

Table 2: Summary of results for VATS vs minimally invasive vs thoracotomy.

Author, journal, year	*Design*	*LoE*	*Topic*	*F/U (m)*	*Measures*	*Main results*
Wait, Spine, 2012[28]	Retrospective comparison	III	VATS versus unmatched thoracotomy	28.2 (1–148)	Frankel, VAS, patient satisfaction, complications	Decreased complications with VATS
Anand, Spine, 2002[29]	Case series	IV	VATS	48 (24–72)	Oswestry disability scores, VAS	VATS had good long-term outcomes
Hott, J Neurosurg Spine, 2005[30]	Retrospective comparison	III	VATS versus unmatched thoracotomy versus unmatched posterolateral	31 (1–36)	Frankel	VATS for patients with giant herniations had worse short- and long-term functional outcomes
Johnson, Neurosurg Focus, 2000[31]	Prospective nonrandomized comparison	II	VATS versus thoracotomy	12	Oswestry Pain Scale Frankel	VATS can be effective but should be limited to specific indications
Uribe, J Neurosurg Spine, 2012[26]	Retrospective multicenter case series	IV	Minimally invasive lateral	11 (0.5–24)	VAS, perioperative characteristics, complications	Minimally invasive lateral approaches can have reproducible outcomes

(LoE: level-of-evidence; VAS: visual analog scale; VATS: video-assisted thoracic surgery)

can be approached via posterior techniques. In addition, ossified ligamentum flavum causing thoracic myelopathy is better addressed via posterior approaches. Another important consideration is the patient's comorbidities, especially pulmonary issues. For VATS and thoracotomy, single-lung ventilation can be necessary, and as a result, patients with chronic obstructive pulmonary disease or other respiratory illnesses may not tolerate such an approach. Lastly, not all surgeons are equally adept at all techniques. Surgeons need to use approaches with which they are comfortable to minimize the complication risks for patients.

REFERENCES

1. Bono CM. Thoracic spondylosis, stenosis, and disc herniations. In: Bono CM, Garfin SR (Eds). Spine. Philadelphia: Lippincott Williams & Wilkins; 2004. pp. 122-31.
2. Perrin RG, Laxton AW. Metastatic spine disease: epidemiology, pathophysiology, and evaluation of patients. Neurosurg Clin N Am. 2004;15(4):365-73.
3. Rose PS, Buchowski JM. Metastatic disease in the thoracic and lumbar spine: evaluation and management. J Am Acad Orthop Surg. 2011;19(1):37-48.
4. Gokaslan ZL, York JE, Walsh GL, et al. Transthoracic vertebrectomy for metastatic spinal tumors. J Neurosurg. 1998;89(4):599-609.
5. Patel AA, Vaccaro AR. Thoracolumbar spine trauma classification. J Am Acad Orthop Surg. 2010;18(2):63-71.
6. Arce CA, Dohrmann GJ. Herniated thoracic disks. Neurol Clin. 1985;3(2):383-92.
7. Carson J, Gumpert J, Jefferson A. Diagnosis and treatment of thoracic intervertebral disc protrusions. J Neurol Neurosurg Psychiatry. 1971;34(1):68-77.
8. Bohlman HH, Zdeblick TA. Anterior excision of herniated thoracic discs. J Bone Joint Surg Am. 1988;70(7):1038-47.
9. Brown CW, Deffer PA, Jr., Akmakjian J, et al. The natural history of thoracic disc herniation. Spine. 1992;17(6):S97-102.
10. Cornips EMJ, Janssen MLF, Beuls EAM. Thoracic disc herniation and acute myelopathy: clinical presentation, neuroimaging findings, surgical considerations, and outcome. J Neurosurg Spine. 2011;14(4):520-8.
11. Vanichkachorn JS, Vaccaro AR. Thoracic disk disease: diagnosis and treatment. J Am Acad Orthop Surg. 2000;8(3):159-69.
12. Perrin RG, Livingston KE, Aarabi B. Intradural extramedullary spinal metastasis: a report of 10 cases. J Neurosurg. 1982; 56(6):835-7.
13. Dick JPR. The deep tendon and the abdominal reflexes. J Neurol Neurosurg Psychiatry. 2003;74(2):150-3.
14. Tay BKB, Deckey J, Hu SS. Spinal infections. J Am Acad Orthop Surg. 2002;10(3):188-97.
15. Currier BL, Eismont FJ, Green BA. Transthoracic disc excision and fusion for herniated thoracic discs. Spine. 1994;19(3):323-8.
16. Regan JJ, Mack MJ, Picetti GD, III. A technical report on video-assisted thoracoscopy in thoracic spinal surgery: preliminary description. Spine. 1995;20(7):831-7.
17. Hulme A. The surgical approach to thoracic intervertebral disc protrusions. J Neurol Neurosurg Psychiatry. 1960;23:133-7.
18. Ridenour TR, Haddad SF, Hitchon PW, et al. Herniated thoracic disks: treatment and outcome. J Spinal Disord. 1993;6(3):218-24.
19. Le Roux PD, Haglund MM, Harris AB. Thoracic disc disease: experience with the transpedicular approach in twenty consecutive patients. Neurosurgery. 1993;33(1):58-66.
20. Bransford R, Zhang F, Bellabarba C, et al. Early experience treating thoracic disc herniations using a modified transfacet pedicle-sparing decompression and fusion. J Neurosurg Spine. 2010;12(2):221-31.
21. Ando K, Imagama S, Wakao N, et al. Single-stage removal of thoracic dumbbell tumors from a posterior approach only with costotransversectomy. Yonsei Med J. 2012;53(3): 611-7.
22. Rangel-Castilla L, Hwang SW, Whitehead WE, et al. Surgical treatment of thoracic Pott disease in a 3-year-old child, with vertebral column resection and posterior-only circumferential reconstruction of the spinal column: case report. J Neurosurg Pediatr. 2012;9(4):447-51.
23. Simpson JM, Silveri CP, Simeone FA, et al. Thoracic disc herniation: re-evaluation of the posterior approach using a modified costotransversectomy. Spine. 1993;18(13): 1872-7.
24. Larson SJ, Holst RA, Hemmy DC, et al. Lateral extracavitary approach to traumatic lesions of the thoracic and lumbar spine. J Neurosurg. 1976;45(6):628-37.
25. Maiman DJ, Larson SJ, Luck E, et al. Lateral extracavitary approach to the spine for thoracic disc herniation: report of 23 cases. Neurosurgery. 1984;14(2):178-82.
26. Uribe JS, Smith WD, Pimenta L, et al. Minimally invasive lateral approach for symptomatic thoracic disc herniation: initial multicenter clinical experience. J Neurosurg Spine. 2012;16(3):264-79.
27. Deviren V, Kuelling FA, Poulter G, et al. Minimal invasive anterolateral transthoracic transpleural approach: a novel technique for thoracic disc herniation: a review of the literature, description of a new surgical technique and experience with first 12 consecutive patients. J Spinal Disord Tech. 2011;24(5):E40-8.
28. Wait SD, Fox DJ, Jr., Kenny KJ, et al. Thoracoscopic resection of symptomatic herniated thoracic discs: clinical results in 121 patients. Spine. 2012;37(1):35-40.
29. Anand N, Regan JJ. Video-assisted thoracoscopic surgery for thoracic disc disease: classification and outcome study of 100 consecutive cases with a 2-year minimum follow-up period. Spine. 2002;27(8):871-9.

30. Hott JS, Feiz-Erfan I, Kenny K, et al. Surgical management of giant herniated thoracic discs: analysis of 20 cases. J Neurosurg Spine. 2005;3(3):191-7.
31. Johnson JP, Filler AG, Mc Bride DQ. Endoscopic thoracic discectomy. Neurosurg Focus. 2000;9(4):e11.
32. Krauss WE, Edwards DA, Cohen-Gadol AA. Transthoracic discectomy without interbody fusion. Surg Neurol. 2005;63(5):403-8; discussion 08-9.
33. Oskouian RJ, Johnson JP. Endoscopic thoracic microdiscectomy. J Neurosurg Spine. 2005;3(6):459-64.
34. Oskouian RJ, Johnson JP. Endoscopic thoracic microdiscectomy. Neurosurg Focus. 2005;18(3):e11.
35. Kasliwal MK, Deutsch H. Minimally invasive retropleural approach for central thoracic disc herniation. Minim Invasive Neurosurg. 2011;54(4):167-71.
36. Khoo LT, Smith ZA, Asgarzadie F, et al. Minimally invasive extracavitary approach for thoracic discectomy and interbody fusion: 1-year clinical and radiographic outcomes in 13 patients compared with a cohort of traditional anterior transthoracic approaches. J Neurosurg Spine. 2011;14(2):250-60.
37. Bilsky MH. Transpedicular approach for thoracic disc herniations. Neurosurg Focus. 2000;9(4):e3.
38. Jho HD. Endoscopic transpedicular thoracic discectomy. Neurosurg Focus. 2000;9(4):e4.

CHAPTER 33

Classification and Management of Thoracic Spine Trauma

Sajeel R Khan, Ankit I Mehta

INTRODUCTION

Thoracolumbar fractures are predominantly the result of high impact trauma. The incidence has steadily increased over time.[1] It is critical for spinal surgeons to identify, classify, and manage these injuries, as overall treatment and interdisciplinary communication is dependent upon a systematic algorithm.

Anatomically, the thoracic spine extends from the first (T1) to the twelfth thoracic vertebra (T12) and has a global kyphotic orientation. The cephalad thoracic spine (T1–T10) is supported by the ribcage and sternum and this caging imparts relative rigidity to this region. A significant force vector is required to cause injury. The thoracolumbar region (T10–L2), or the transition zone, is unique due to transition from the kyphotic thoracic spine to the lordotic lumbar spine, is relatively mobile and thus more prone to injury.[2] Additionally, due to a narrow spinal canal, injuries throughout T1–L2 can often result in spinal cord injury.[3] Despite their distinct anatomical location, thoracic and lumbar spine injuries are very similar in their mechanisms, morphology, and management. Thereby, we will discuss both of these entities together.

Annually, 160,000 spinal injuries occur in North America.[4] Recent meta-analysis by Katsuura et al. analyzed the epidemiology of thoracolumbar trauma. The most frequent cause of thoracolumbar injuries was found to be high-velocity trauma (36.70%) followed closely by a fall from significant height (31.70%) with L1 vertebral injury being most frequent level injured in approximately one-third (34.40%) patients.[5] Alarmingly, one-fourth of all thoracolumbar injuries result in spinal cord trauma (26.56%). The most common injury was burst fracture (AO type A3) followed by compression fracture (AO type A1). Fracture dislocations (AO type C) were found in 14.20% cases and flexion-distraction injuries (AO type B) came in low at 6.70%.

MECHANISM OF THORACIC SPINAL INJURIES

At any given time, the force vectors acting on the spinal column can be summed up as: (1) compression vector; (2) distraction vector; and (3) torsion vector.

Physiologically, all of these vectors are balanced by the ligamentous and osseous structures of the spine. The compression vector is counteracted by the intervertebral disk and vertebral bodies. The distraction vector is countered by the posterior elements including the vertebral facets and the ligamentous tension band as well as the anterior tension band, which is comprised of the anterior longitudinal ligament. The torsion vector is countered by all of the above mentioned structural components. Under traumatic conditions, these vectors are disrupted, causing structural damage to the spine.

Compression injuries result in collapsing vertebral body and disk injuries with shortening of the vertebral column, whereas distraction injuries result in the posterior column disruption and consequently lengthen the vertebral column. Torsional injuries can result in the most unstable of all injuries and a variety of injury patterns with potential circumferential discontinuation of the spinal column resulting in a fracture dislocation (Figs. 1 and 2).

Following the discussion of mechanisms of injury and the resultant spinal column disruption, it is prudent to understand the way the spinal injuries are classified. Importantly, the classification of these injuries follows from the mechanism of antecedent trauma.

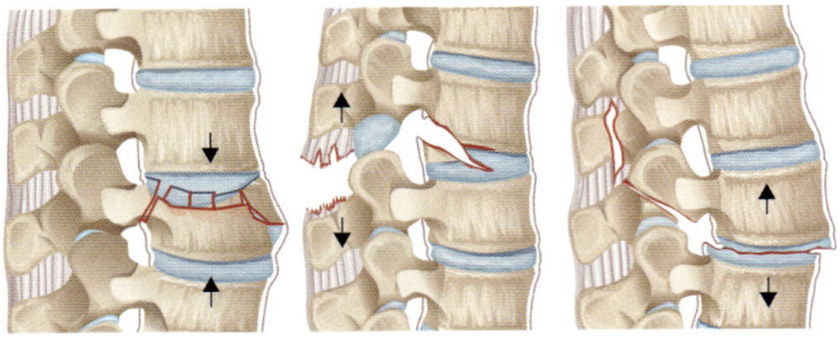

Fig. 1: Compression and distraction vectors acting on spinal column.
Source: Dr Max Aebi, et al.

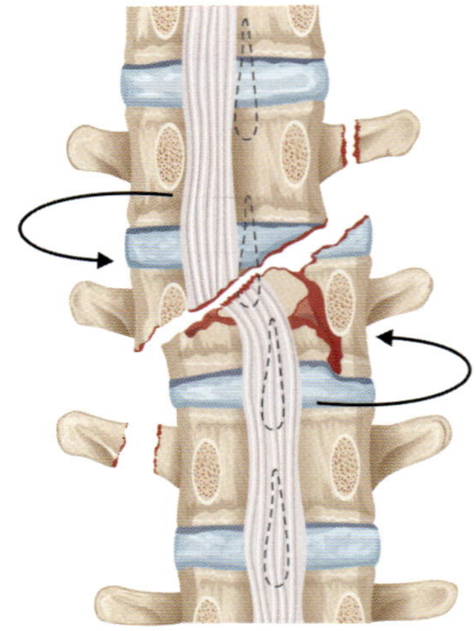

Fig. 2: Torsion vector acting on spinal column.
Source: Dr Max Aebi, et al.

CLASSIFICATION

Due to a similar mechanism and management paradigm, thoracic and lumbar injuries are usually classified as a single entity. It is useful to study the different classification strategies from a historical perspective.

Three-column Model

Spinal trauma and stability have been classified using the "Three-column model" proposed by Denis in 1983. The main paradigm of the model was based on the extent of the injury to the bony and ligamentous structures of the spine. This system divided the spine into three anatomical columns with the anterior column comprising the anterior longitudinal ligament and the anterior two-thirds of the vertebral body. The middle column comprises of the posterior one-third of the vertebral body and posterior longitudinal ligament. Lastly, the posterior column consists of the vertebral facets and posterior ligaments.[6]

This classification model was widely used as a guide for the management of spinal trauma and has gained wide acceptance. It introduced the concept of instability based on the extent of the injury and led the way to further classification systems.

Magerl Classification of Thoracolumbar Trauma

In 1994, Magerl introduced a system of classification, which comprised of a morphological assessment of the injured spine and focused on the extent of injury to the osseous and ligamentous structures. This system faced criticism, as it did not take into account the neurologic status of the patient in management.

The concept was based on the 3/3/3 model with three types: A, B, C, followed by three groups each with three subtypes. Type A represents compression injuries, type B distraction injuries, and type C torsion injuries. Altogether, this led to an exhaustive classification with more than 50 types of injuries.[7]

Thoracolumbar Injury Classification and Severity Score

Surgical decision-making was dependent mostly upon the extent of anatomical disruption of the injured spine. It became imperative to factor in the neurological status of the patient in clinical decision-making.

A new classification system was proposed with an algorithm for surgical decision-making based on the injury mechanism, fracture anatomy, as well as the neurologic status of the patient. This classification system was called the thoracolumbar injury classification and severity score (TLICS). It was devised by the Spine Trauma Study Group and was published in 2005.[8] TLICS was created to standardize decision-making in spinal injuries.

The TLICS score has gained wide traction and shows good reliability among spinal surgeons, both from the disciplines of Orthopedic Surgery and Neurosurgery.[9] Patel et al. prospectively studied interobserver reliability and concluded that it could be taught effectively and incorporated into clinical practice.[10]

Thoracolumbar Injury Classification and Severity Score Components

The score components can be broadly subdivided into two categories: (1) injury morphology and (2) neurologic

Table 1: Thoracolumbar injury classification and severity score.

TLICS components	*Point value*
Injury type:	
• Compression	1
• Burst component	1
• Translation rotaion	3
• Distraction	4
Ligamentous status:	
• Intact	0
• Indeterminate	2
• Disrupted	3
Neurological status:	
• Intact	0
• Nerve root injury	2
• Complete	2
• Incomplete (cord or cauda equina)	3

(TLICS: thoracolumbar injury classification and severity score)

status. Injury morphology and antecedent mechanism forms the first main component and can be further divided into osseous and ligamentous components.

In osseous injury, compressive forces resulting in compression or burst fracture garners one point followed by shear or torsional forces causing translational or rotational injuries scoring three points. The most points are awarded to forces causing distraction injuries, which can result in circumferential spinal separation. An attempt is made to accommodate a combination of injuries with both flexion and extension vectors, which respectively cause vertebral body fractures and fractures of the posterior elements.

The next major component is the integrity of the posterior ligamentous complex including facet ligaments, interspinous ligaments, ligamentum flavum, and supraspinous ligaments. The scoring is incremental going from no injury to obvious ligamentous disruption. Imaging, particularly magnetic resonance imaging (MRI), is helpful to discern ligamentous complex injury as suggested by Zhang et al.[11]

Next, we discuss the novel and arguably the most important addition to the spine classification systems; the neurologic status of the patient. This subdivision spans from no neurologic injury to incomplete spinal cord injury with incomplete spinal cord injury harnessing the most points.

- *TLICS at a glance*: Table 1.
- *Clinical decision-making algorithm*: The algorithm has been described in Flowchart 1.

Flowchart 1: Clinical decision-making paradigm.

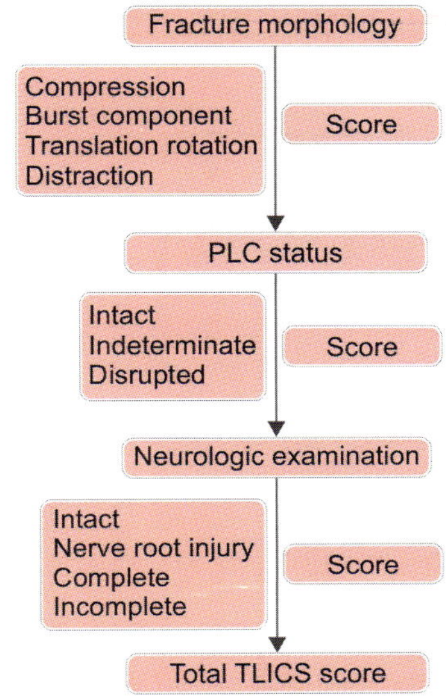

(PLC: posterior ligamentous complex; TLICS: thoracolumbar injury classification and severity score)

Validity of TLICS

The TLICS score was well received and was able to be incorporated in the day-to-day management of thoracolumbar trauma. The studies undertaken to assess the validity of the score showed consistency amongst the surgical treatment offered.

A recent retrospective multicenter study by Joaquim et al. suggested that the TLICS score matched surgical treatment in 96% (47/49) patients and correlated with the AO classification.[12] This was followed by another retrospective study comprising of more than 400 consecutive patients with thoracolumbar trauma. While the study showed an excellent correlation in 99% of patients managed conservatively, the subgroup of burst fracture within the surgical group with the intact neurologic examination, the treatment offered, and TLICS recommendation did not correlate.[13] The study hinted at and potentially identified a subgroup of burst fractures with intact neurologic examination where some of the patients may require surgical treatment based on individual fracture morphology and treating surgeon despite TLICS advocating for conservative management.

Modified AO Spine Thoracolumbar Injury Classification

The latest iteration of classification of thoracolumbar spine trauma is the modified AO thoracolumbar spine injury classification system and hereby referred to as AO thoracic and lumbar system (TLS). The need for a modified TL injury classification system arose partly because TLICS did not adequately address fracture management where scores fell between 3 and 5; including neurologically intact patients with burst fractures with a suspected posterior ligamentous complex injury. The management in such scenarios was left to individual surgeon preference. Hence, a modified AO TLS system was devised which incorporated components from both Magerl as well as TLICS classification system. This addressed fracture morphology in better detail along with the incorporation of the patient's neurologic status.

The components of the AO spine TL consist of the following:

- Fracture morphology.
- Neurologic status.
- Modifiers (injury-specific/patient-specific).

Fracture Morphology

The fracture morphology is divided into three broad types:

1. *A*: Compression fracture.
2. *B*: Tension-band injury (both anterior and posterior) without translation/distraction.
3. *C*: Disruption of the spinal column resulting in translation/distraction.

   Also includes complete disruption of soft tissue hinge even in the absence of translation/distraction.

Subtypes:

- *Subtype A (Figs. 3 to 6)*: Compression vector-mediated injuries primarily to the vertebral body:
  - *A0*: Minor injury such as transverse process/spinous process fracture.
  - *A1*: Anterior wedging-type fracture.
  - *A2*: Pincer-type fracture involving both superior and inferior endplates without posterior wall involvement.
  - *A3*: Incomplete burst fracture without involvement of posterior wall.
  - *A4*: Complete burst fracture with involvement of posterior wall.
- *Subtype B (Figs. 7 to 9)*:
  - *B1*: Osseous disruption of posterior tension band as seen in chance fracture.
  - *B2*: Ligamentous disruption of posterior tension band.
  - *B3*: Disruption of anterior tension band as seen in ankylosing spondylitis.
- *Subtype C*:
  - Involves disruption of the spinal column with translation/distraction. This also includes complete disruption of the soft tissue hinge even in the absence of any overt signs of listhesis.

Neurologic Status

- *N0*: Intact neurologic examination.
- *N1*: Transient neurologic deficit with complete recovery.
- *N2*: Nerve root injury resulting in individual muscle group weakness/radiculopathic pain.
- *N3*: Cauda equina/incomplete spinal cord injury.

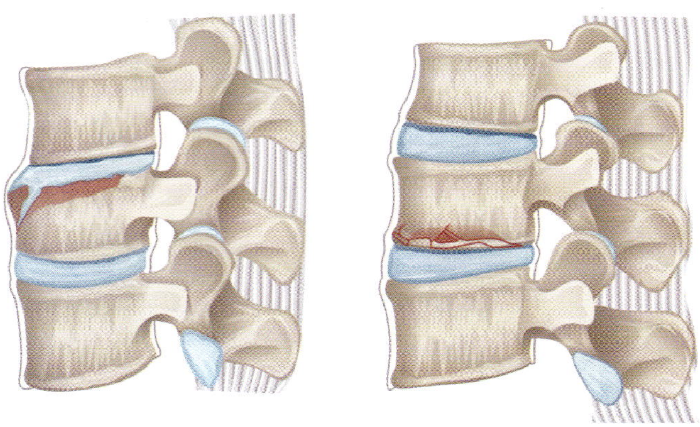

Fig. 3: A1-type fracture.
Source: AO Foundation, Switzerland. AO spine is a clinical division of the AO Foundation.

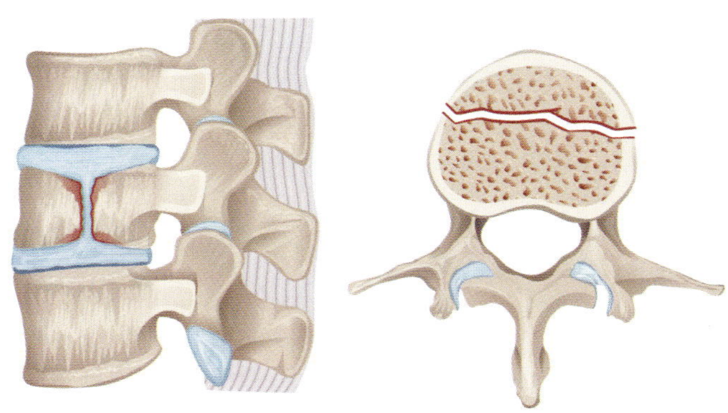

Fig. 4: A2-type fracture.
Source: AO Foundation, Switzerland. AO spine is a clinical division of the AO Foundation.

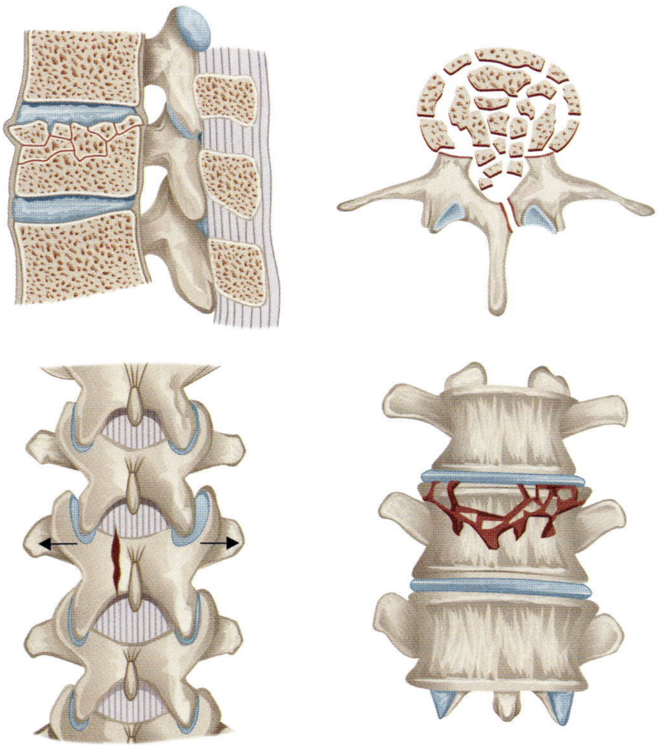

Fig. 5: A3-type fracture, incomplete burst fracture.
Source: AO Foundation, Switzerland. AO spine is a clinical division of the AO Foundation.

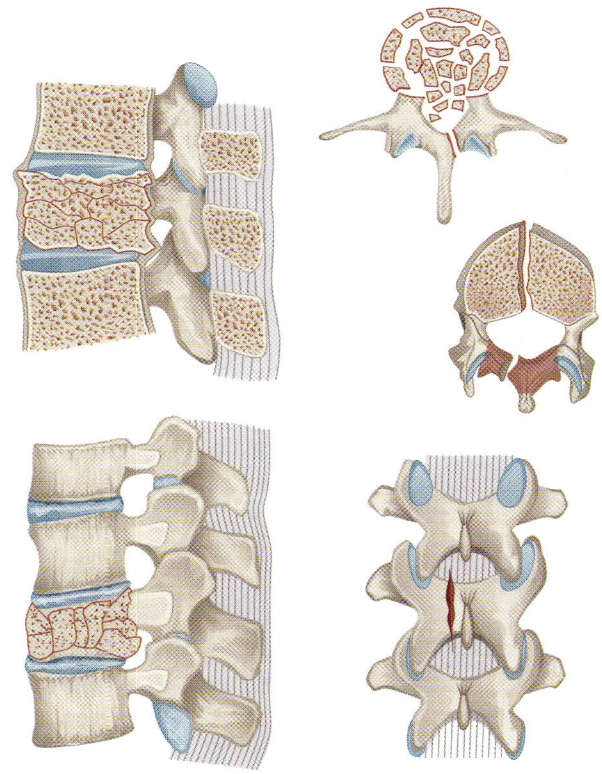

Fig. 6: A4-type fracture, complete burst fracture.
Source: AO Foundation, Switzerland. AO spine is a clinical division of the AO Foundation.

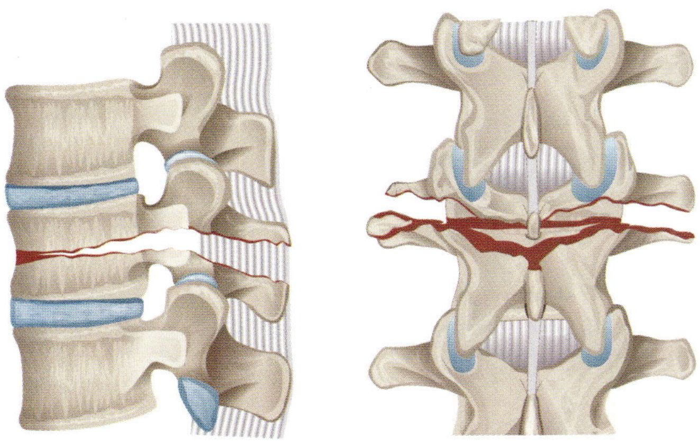

Fig. 7: Osseous-type posterior tension band disruption, e.g. chance fracture.
Source: AO Foundation, Switzerland. AO spine is a clinical division of the AO Foundation.

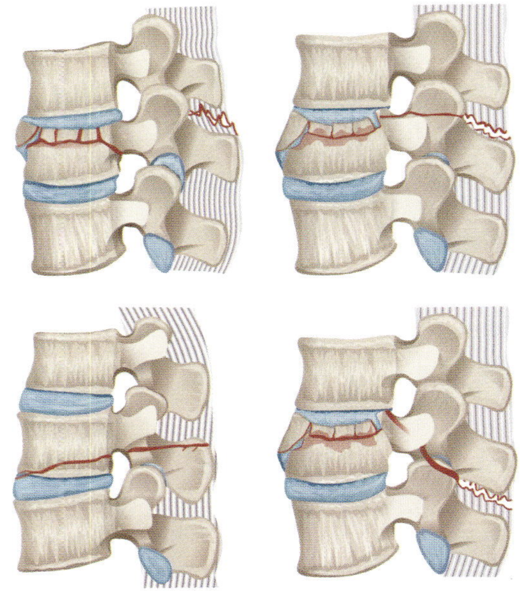

Fig. 8: Osseous and/or ligamentous-type posterior tension band injury.
Source: AO Foundation, Switzerland. AO spine is a clinical division of the AO Foundation.

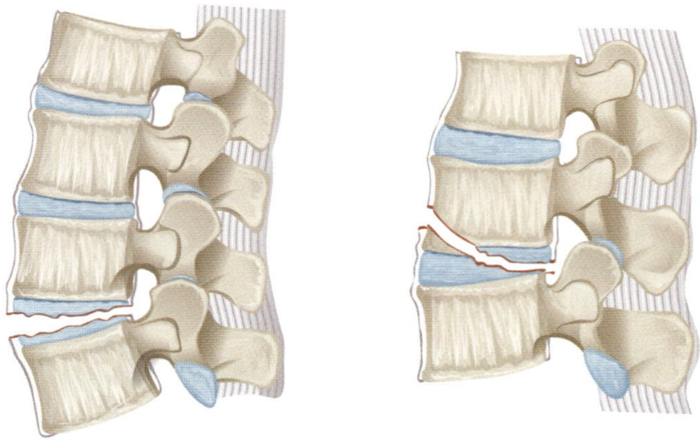

Fig. 9: Anterior tension band injury resulting in hyperextension injury. *Source:* AO Foundation, Switzerland. AO spine is a clinical division of the AO Foundation.

- *N4*: Complete spinal cord injury.
- *NX*: Neurologic examination unable to be assessed, e.g. intubated and sedated patients.

Modifiers

Modifiers were included to account and adjust for factors that could influence the surgical decision making. They can be classified into both injury- and patient-specific factors:

- *M1*: Injury-specific modifier is reserved for indeterminate tension band injury suspected on imaging.
- *M2*: Patient-specific modifier is reserved for patient characteristics complicating management such as ankylosing spondylitis, diffuse idiopathic spinal hyperostosis, burns overlying surgical site, osteoporosis, etc. that can sway the surgeon's opinion one way or the other.

The reliability of the classification system was subsequently studied. Vaccaro et al. reported that the internal reliability in the identification and classification of the injuries as substantial with a kappa value of 0.72.[14] Urrutia et al. also demonstrated similar inter and intraobserver reliability.[15]

MANAGEMENT

As discussed earlier, the management of the thoracic spine trauma is mostly dependent upon the injury morphology as well as the neurologic status of the patient. The management strategy can be broadly classified into conservative and surgical management depending upon the injury classification.

Conservative Management

Conservative management usually entails observation, pain control with supervised early ambulation, physical therapy to maintain muscle strength and tone as well as prevention of deep vein thrombosis.

Broadly speaking, conservative management, as described above, is the mainstay of management for A0–A3 type fracture morphology with an intact neurologic examination. In other words, fractures including and up to incomplete burst fracture with an intact posterior wall (no retropulsion) can be safely and routinely managed with conservative management.

Traditionally bracing or specifically thoracolumbosacral orthosis (TLSO) has been the cornerstone of conservative management of the spinal fractures. It has been extensively studied and has wide acceptance in the literature, as suggested recently by Chang et al.[16] However, the evidence is now accumulating that shows good and equivalent outcomes without bracing in groups with early mobilization as demonstrated in a retrospective analysis by Jaffrey et al.[17]

Bailey et al. also showed that no TLSO was equivalent in outcomes to TLSO in management of burst fractures without tension band injury and intact neurologic status (AO TL A0–A3 fractures).[18] This was followed by a pilot randomized controlled trial conducted by Shamji et al. The decision to forego bracing hinged on neurologically stable patients with AO Type A3 injuries with mild deformity. They demonstrated similar clinical and radiographic outcomes at 6 months for both brace and nonbrace groups.[19]

To date, there is no broad-based clinical consensus on orthoses in thoracolumbar trauma. The decision to brace is solely dependent upon the preference of the treating surgeon.

Surgical Management

Surgical management offers certain advantages including early mobilization with physical therapy and more reliable correction of the sagittal deformity. Patient-specific factors, such as patients who cannot tolerate longer periods of time in a cast/orthosis may also be suitable candidates for surgery.

Surgical management is usually reserved for patients with unstable injuries including type B injuries (anterior/posterior tension band injuries) with or without type A injuries, type C injuries (circumferential disruption) of the spinal column and type A injuries with M1 modifier (suspected tension band injury). Thoracolumbar injuries with any neurologic deficit (N1–N4) are also suitable surgical candidates.

Burst Fractures with No Neurologic Deficit

Recently, there has been a movement away from immediate surgical treatment of burst fractures with no neurologic deficit. Several studies have shown that most of these injuries can be managed conservatively, including injuries with a moderate degree of kyphosis, and even with moderate to significant spinal canal stenosis.[20-23] Alternatively, prospective randomized trials conducted by Siebanga and Wood et al. also suggest that both operative and nonoperative management of stable burst fracture without neurologic compromise have equivalent outcomes.[24-26] At the present, there is no consensus opinion regarding definitive management of this fracture morphology, however, emerging data show equivalent outcomes between surgical and nonsurgical management.

Operative Strategy

The goals of surgery should be to achieve decompression, deformity correction (if applicable), and fusion. Instrumented fusion via posterior pedicle screw construct is a safe, reliable, and well-tolerated method of management. Short segment instrumented fusion, with well-positioned screws with good triangulation, can be done one or two levels above and below the level of injury to achieve adequate stability.[27-30] Short segment instrumented fusion is associated with a significant risk of potential complications. The risks include instrumentation failures such as screw/rod breakage, intraoperative neurologic injury, cerebrospinal fluid leak, infection, and significant blood loss. Iatrogenic fracture and/or loss of kyphosis is a concern and can result in early failure of the fusion as suggested by McLain et al.[31]

Due to concerns arising from the failure of dorsal instrumentation, McCormack et al. suggested load-sharing classification. The goal of this classification was to clarify when an accompanying anterior fusion was needed to avoid dorsal instrumentation failure.[32]

Anterior Surgery

Since its inception in the 1980s, anterior surgery has now become a significant component of the spine surgeon's armamentarium. Its origins can be traced back to the need to buttress dorsal instrumentation but have since evolved as an independent stand-alone approach to treat thoracic trauma. It is a useful approach for anterior spinal decompression, restoration of the height of the spinal column, correction of kyphotic deformity, and alleviation of pain. This approach has been shown to be safe, effective, and reliable with comparable operating room time and blood loss.[33,34] The functional outcomes were also found to be similar as suggested by Wood et al.[35]

Sasso et al. demonstrated that unstable thoracolumbar burst fracture could be successfully managed via anterior only approach.[36] Currently, the decision to proceed with the anterior or posterior approach or combined anterior and posterior approach to treat spinal trauma is surgeon dependent

Minimally Invasive Surgery

The constant evolution of minimally invasive approaches has led to breakthroughs in the management of thoracolumbar trauma. Minimally invasive approaches using endoscope have been developed, studied, and increasingly used over the past decade. Video-assisted thoracoscopic surgery (VATS) offers decreased blood loss, decreased postoperative pain, decreased hospital stay, and quicker recovery while offering equivalent outcomes. Endoscopic approaches show good visualization of the entire thoracic spine and with recent advances, transdiaphragmatic approach is increasingly being used for thoracolumbar junction trauma. One of the drawbacks of these approaches is steep initial learning curves and operating times as suggested by Khoo et al. who studied 371 consecutively treated patients. The severe complication rate [aortic injury, splenic contusion, cerebrospinal fluid (CSF) leak, and neurologic deterioration] was reported to be <2%. Endoscopically treated patients required 42% less narcotics compared to open surgery.[37] Later reports suggest minimally invasive endoscopic surgery is associated with a low incidence of complications including pneumothorax, hemothorax, intercostal neuralgia, major vessel injury, or organ injury with significant improvement in average operating time compared with earlier reports.[38-40]

Percutaneous Instrumentation

Percutaneous pedicle screw placement can serve as effective means of internal bracing in patients without neurologic injury and/or tension band injury. This technique allows healing to occur and promotes early mobilization, especially in patients where casting/orthosis is not advisable in circumstances such as polytrauma, burns, obesity with a bronchopulmonary disease where orthoses would inhibit respiratory function. Percutaneous instrumentation even without fusion is suggested to be equivalent in outcomes in thoracolumbar burst fractures management as reported by Wang et al.[41]

Vertebral Augmentation

Kyphoplasty and vertebroplasty are useful techniques used as solo or adjunct methods to treat thoracolumbar trauma, particularly compression fractures and more recently in burst fractures.

Vertebroplasty entails transpedicular injection of cement in the fractured vertebral body. Kyphoplasty involves balloon elevation of the fracture site prior to injection of cement. These techniques can be used primarily or as an adjunct especially intraoperatively to elevate the fractured endplate and improve kyphotic angulation. This was demonstrated by Marco et al. who used this technique as an adjunct in their series to restore anterior column height during surgical management for unstable burst fractures.[42] These are effective techniques and result in long-lasting pain relief—thought due to stabilization at the fracture site and endplates—and correction of kyphotic deformity with low-complication rate.

These techniques are especially useful in the management of osteoporotic thoracic compression fractures, which are increasingly been seen with an aging population. The annual incidence of these fractures is estimated at 700,000 in the United States with 10% requiring hospitalization.[43] Contraindications include significant injury to the posterior wall with retropulsion into the spinal canal, rigid fracture, and severe cardiopulmonary disease. The potential complications of the procedures include extravasation of cement into the spinal canal with neurologic compromise, extravasation into the venous system resulting in pulmonary embolism and adjacent compression fractures. The risk of the adjacent compression fractures is estimated to be 10% within the first 90 days.[44]

Kyphoplasty is considered to be more effective and safer than vertebroplasty, which was suggested by Hulme et al. in their literature review.[45] All in all, vertebral augmentation is a safe and effective treatment for thoracic vertebral fractures and can be employed as an adjunct to short segment instrumented fusion for anterior column support and kyphotic deformity correction.

CONCLUSION

Thoracic and thoracolumbar traumas are significant cause of mortality and morbidity. The management of the thoracic and thoracolumbar injuries begins with correct identification and classification of injuries, taking into account ligamentous status, preoperative neurologic examination, and injury- and patient-specific modifiers. The surgeon is endowed with various strategies including conservative as well as surgical management along with auxiliary techniques such as vertebral augmentation. The goal of surgical management involves the decompression of neurologic elements, placement of instrumentation, correction of deformity, and achieving bony fusion for long-term spinal stability.

ACKNOWLEDGMENT

We would like to acknowledge the following individuals/entities for the use of copyrighted material in the compilation of this chapter:

- AO Foundation, Switzerland: AO spine is a clinical division of the AO Foundation.
- M Alvarez, AO Foundation for copy right content permission.
- Dr Max Aebi, et al.

REFERENCES

1. Doud AN, Weaver AA, Talton JW, et al. Has the incidence of thoracolumbar spine injuries increased in the United States from 1998 to 2011? Clin Orthop Relat Res. 2015;473(1):297-304.
2. Wood KB, Li W, Lebl DR, et al. Management of thoracolumbar spine fractures. Spine J. 2014;14(1):145-64.
3. Bohlman HH. Treatment of fractures and dislocations of the thoracic and lumbar spine. J Bone Joint Surg Am. 1985;67(1):165-9.
4. el-Khoury GY, Whitten CG. Trauma to the upper thoracic spine: anatomy, biomechanics, and unique imaging features. Am J Roentgenol. 1993;160(1):95-102.

5. Katsuura Y, Osborn JM, Cason GW. The epidemiology of thoracolumbar trauma: a meta-analysis. J Orthop. 2016;13(4):383-8.
6. Denis F. The three column spine and its significance in the classification of acute thoracolumbar spinal injuries. Spine (Phila Pa 1976). 1983;8(8):817-31.
7. Magerl F, Aebi M, Gertzbein SD, et al. A comprehensive classification of thoracic and lumbar injuries. Eur Spine J. 1994;3(4):184-201.
8. Vaccaro AR, Zeiller SC, Hulbert RJ, et al. The thoracolumbar injury severity score: a proposed treatment algorithm. J Spinal Disord Tech. 2005;18(3):209-15.
9. Raja Rampersaud Y, Fisher C, Wilsey J, et al. Agreement between orthopedic surgeons and neurosurgeons regarding a new algorithm for the treatment of thoracolumbar injuries: a multicenter reliability study. J Spinal Disord Tech. 2006;19(7):477-82.
10. Patel AA, Vaccaro AR, Albert TJ, et al. The adoption of a new classification system: time-dependent variation in interobserver reliability of the thoracolumbar injury severity score classification system. Spine (Phila Pa 1976). 2007;32(3):E105-10.
11. Zhang T, Feng SQ, Jiang WX. [Reliability of magnetic resonance imaging in diagnosing posterior ligament complex injury in thoracolumbar fractures]. Zhonghua Wai Ke Za Zhi. 2008;46(16):1241-4.
12. Joaquim AF, Fernandes YB, Cavalcante RA, et al. Evaluation of the thoracolumbar injury classification system in thoracic and lumbar spinal trauma. Spine (Phila Pa 1976). 2011;36(1):33-6.
13. Joaquim AF, Daubs MD, Lawrence BD, et al. Retrospective evaluation of the validity of the Thoracolumbar Injury Classification System in 458 consecutively treated patients. Spine J. 2013;13(12):1760-5.
14. Vaccaro AR, Oner C, Kepler CK, et al. AOSpine thoracolumbar spine injury classification system: fracture description, neurological status, and key modifiers. Spine (Phila Pa 1976). 2013;38(23):2028-37.
15. Urrutia J, Zamora T, Yurac R, et al. An independent interobserver reliability and intraobserver reproducibility evaluation of the new AOSpine Thoracolumbar Spine Injury Classification System. Spine (Phila Pa 1976). 2015;40(1):E54-8.
16. Chang V, Holly LT. Bracing for thoracolumbar fractures. Neurosurg Focus. 2014;37(1):E3.
17. Jaffray DC, Eisenstein SM, Balain B, et al. Early mobilisation of thoracolumbar burst fractures without neurology: a natural history observation. Bone Joint J. 2016;98-B(1):97-101.
18. Bailey CS, Urquhart JC, Dvorak MF, et al. Orthosis versus no orthosis for the treatment of thoracolumbar burst fractures without neurologic injury: a multicenter prospective randomized equivalence trial. Spine J. 2014;14(11):2557-64.
19. Shamji MF, Roffey DM, Young DK, et al. A pilot evaluation of the role of bracing in stable thoracolumbar burst fractures without neurological deficit. J Spinal Disord Tech. 2014;27(7):370-5.
20. Shen WJ, Liu TJ, Shen YS. Nonoperative treatment versus posterior fixation for thoracolumbar junction burst fractures without neurologic deficit. Spine (Phila Pa 1976). 2001;26(9):1038-45.
21. Mumford J, Weinstein JN, Spratt KF, et al. Thoracolumbar burst fractures. The clinical efficacy and outcome of nonoperative management. Spine (Phila Pa 1976). 1993;18(8):955-70.
22. Cantor JB, Lebwohl NH, Garvey T, et al. Nonoperative management of stable thoracolumbar burst fractures with early ambulation and bracing. Spine (Phila Pa 1976). 1993;18(8):971-6.
23. Shen WJ, Shen YS. Nonsurgical treatment of three-column thoracolumbar junction burst fractures without neurologic deficit. Spine (Phila Pa 1976). 1999;24(4):412-5.
24. Siebenga J, Leferink VJ, Segers MJ, et al. Treatment of traumatic thoracolumbar spine fractures: a multicenter prospective randomized study of operative versus nonsurgical treatment. Spine (Phila Pa 1976). 2006;31(25):2881-90.
25. Wood K, Buttermann G, Mehbod A, et al. Operative compared with nonoperative treatment of a thoracolumbar burst fracture without neurological deficit. A prospective, randomized study. J Bone Joint Surg Am. 2003;85(5):773-81.
26. Wood KB, Buttermann GR, Phukan R, et al. Operative compared with nonoperative treatment of a thoracolumbar burst fracture without neurological deficit: a prospective randomized study with follow-up at sixteen to twenty-two years. J Bone Joint Surg Am. 2015;97(1):3-9.
27. Singh R, Rohilla RK, Kamboj K, et al. Outcome of pedicle screw fixation and monosegmental fusion in patients with fresh thoracolumbar fractures. Asian Spine J. 2014;8(3):298-308.
28. Yue JJ, Sossan A, Selgrath C, et al. The treatment of unstable thoracic spine fractures with transpedicular screw instrumentation: a 3-year consecutive series. Spine (Phila Pa 1976). 2002;27(24):2782-7.
29. Ökten AI, Gezercan Y, Özsoy KM, et al. Results of treatment of unstable thoracolumbar burst fractures using pedicle instrumentation with and without fracture-level screws. Acta Neurochir (Wien). 2015;157(5):831-6.
30. Kanna RM, Shetty AP, Rajasekaran S. Posterior fixation including the fractured vertebra for severe unstable thoracolumbar fractures. Spine J. 2015;15(2):256-64.
31. McLain RF, Sparling E, Benson DR. Early failure of short-segment pedicle instrumentation for thoracolumbar fractures. A preliminary report. J Bone Joint Surg Am. 1993;75(2):162-7.
32. McCormack T, Karaikovic E, Gaines RW. The load sharing classification of spine fractures. Spine (Phila Pa 1976). 1994;19(15):1741-4.
33. Elzinga M, Segers M, Siebenga J, et al. Inter- and intraobserver agreement on the Load Sharing Classification of thoracolumbar spine fractures. Injury. 2012;43(4):416-22.
34. Hrabalek L, et al. [Reliability of load-sharing classification in indications for anterior vertebral body replacement in thoracolumbar spine fractures]. Rozhl Chir. 2010;89(4):223-8.
35. Wood KB, Bohn D, Mehbod A. Anterior versus posterior treatment of stable thoracolumbar burst fractures without neurologic deficit: a prospective, randomized study. J Spinal Disord Tech. 2005;(18 Suppl):S15-23.

36. Sasso RC, Renkens K, Hanson D, et al. Unstable thoracolumbar burst fractures: anterior-only versus short-segment posterior fixation. J Spinal Disord Tech. 2006;19(4):242-8.
37. Khoo LT, Beisse R, Potulski M. Thoracoscopic-assisted treatment of thoracic and lumbar fractures: a series of 371 consecutive cases. Neurosurgery. 2002;51(5 Suppl):S104-17.
38. Beisse R, Verdu-Lopez F. [Current status of thoracoscopic surgery for thoracic and lumbar spine. Part 1: general aspects and treatment of fractures]. Neurocirugia (Astur). 2014;25(1):8-19.
39. Kim DH, Jahng TA, Balabhadra RS, et al. Thoracoscopic transdiaphragmatic approach to thoracolumbar junction fractures. Spine J. 2004;4(3):317-28.
40. Kocis J, Wendsche, Muzik V, et al. [Minimally invasive thoracoscopic transdiaphragmatic approach to thoracolumbar junction fractures]. Acta Chir Orthop Traumatol Cech. 2009;76(3):232-8.
41. Wang ST, Ma HL, Liu CL, et al. Is fusion necessary for surgically treated burst fractures of the thoracolumbar and lumbar spine? A prospective, randomized study. Spine (Phila Pa 1976). 2006;31(23):2646-52; discussion 2653.
42. Marco RA, Meyer BC, Kushwaha VP. Thoracolumbar burst fractures treated with posterior decompression and pedicle screw instrumentation supplemented with balloon-assisted vertebroplasty and calcium phosphate reconstruction. Surgical technique. J Bone Joint Surg Am. 2010;92(Suppl 1 Pt 1):67-76.
43. Kim DH, Vaccaro AR. Osteoporotic compression fractures of the spine; current options and considerations for treatment. Spine J. 2006;6(5):479-87.
44. Lavelle WF, Cheney R. Recurrent fracture after vertebral kyphoplasty. Spine J. 2006;6(5):488-93.
45. Hulme PA, Krebs J, Ferguson SJ, et al. Vertebroplasty and kyphoplasty: a systematic review of 69 clinical studies. Spine (Phila Pa 1976). 2006;31(17):1983-2001.

SECTION 5

Lumbosacral

CHAPTER 34 Lumbosacral Spine: History and Physical Examination

Alexandra Paraskos, Marzena Buzanowska, Michael P Steinmetz

INTRODUCTION

The lumbosacral spine evaluation should be detailed and precise in order to produce a specific diagnosis with a structured treatment plan. Accurate diagnosis is essential in a common yet complex entity as low back pain. Low back pain is the most common cause of global disability and is associated with large economic cost.[1] A systematic approach including musculoskeletal, neurologic, and vascular assessment should be included for complete evaluation. Identifying sacroiliac joint dysfunction can be difficult as there is no gold standard for physical examination resulting in diagnosis. The close proximity of lumbar spine and sacrum require differentiation based on a careful history and physical examination. Biomechanics of the pelvis and sacroiliac joints have been studied extensively, and clinical impact of altered mechanics and age-related degeneration are not fully understood. Examiners need to include evaluation of the pelvis and hips in a comprehensive assessment, and sacroiliac joint pathology should be maintained in the differential diagnosis.

HISTORY

Similar to the cervical and thoracic spine, a comprehensive history is obtained with knowledge of the anatomy of the lumbosacral spine and understanding of both common and rare disorders and their presentation. The clinician will elicit the nature and location of the patient's symptoms including radiation, onset and time course, factors that modify (alleviate or aggravate) symptoms, associated findings, and past medical history that may be relevant to their current condition. Special attention should be paid to "red flag" symptoms with particular interest in suspected surgical emergencies including conus medullaris and cauda equina syndrome that can result in spinal cord or nerve injury.[2] As in the cervical and thoracic spine evaluation, systemic illness, unexplained weight loss, fevers, night pain, and history of malignancy are also important aspects of the evaluation.

Nature

The great majority of patients with lumbosacral pathology will present with some form of low back pain. The quality of pain can guide the clinician to the appropriate diagnosis. Descriptors including dull and aching pain that are nonradiating are typically attributed to mechanical etiology including facet-mediated or discogenic pain. Inflammatory spondyloarthropathy should be considered in the setting of dull pain identified deep in the buttocks or low back associated with stiffness in the morning and improvement with activity.[3] Pain that is sharp or burning in nature, especially in the setting of radiation into one or both lower extremities and/or paresthesia, can lead the clinician toward a diagnosis of radiculitis or radiculopathy. Lumbar vertebral fractures should be considered in patients who present with acute onset of sharp and severe midline low back pain, particularly in patients of advanced age, in the setting of trauma, or with a history of osteoporosis or malignancy.

Location

Referral patterns of lumbosacral spine pathology can be complex and consist of a large body of research. Knowing these patterns can aid the clinician with examination. Localization of radicular patterns is of particular importance because it can guide interventional and surgical treatment. The level of pathology is identified using distinct dermatomal patterns. However, recent studies have suggested that nondermatomal location is often described by patients.[4] The clinician should keep in mind that facet-mediated pain as well as sacroiliac joint dysfunction can cause referral of pain into the thigh. Pain not above L5 and pain over the posterior superior iliac spine (PSIS) with tenderness are the most reliable tests for sacroiliac joint pathology.[5] Pain referral into the lower limbs past the knee is most commonly due to disk herniation and spinal stenosis. Radiation of pain into both lower limbs can be more indicative of spinal stenosis.

Onset

Onset of pain may or may not be tied to the etiology. It can be described as insidious, delayed, or abrupt. Inciting event should be elicited, as it can indicate trauma or overuse injury and alter the differential diagnosis. Insidious onset of painis most commonly due to discogenic, facet-mediated, or myofascial pain, but can also less likely be an indication of malignancy or infection in the appropriate patient. Sudden onset of pain can indicate fracture especially when there is a history of trauma.

Modifying Factors

Exacerbating and remitting factors can provide further clues to the etiology of lumbosacral pain. Nonradicular low back pain aggravated by flexion can lead the clinician to strongly consider discogenic pain in the differential. Flexion reproducing radicular symptoms can be more indicative of spondylolisthesis with instability. Pain with rotation and oblique extension can indicate a zygapophyseal joint origin of pain. Lower limb pain with walking and standing that is improved with sitting can be suggestive of spinal stenosis.

Time Course

The majority of low back pain improves in the acute setting. Severe, acute pain especially in an elderly patient is concerning for fracture. A patient who presents with chronic pain is more likely to have a mechanical etiology including discogenic or facet-mediated pain. Radiculopathy in the setting of a large herniated disk or foraminal stenosis can also become chronic. Spinal stenosis will often present with a chronic, gradual progression of low back pain and lower extremity symptoms. Pain that is constant even at night while lying supine and does not improve with time, is concerning for a more sinister diagnosis such as malignancy or infection.

Associated Findings

Focal neurologic symptoms including weakness and sensory deficits are extremely important to elicit from the patient and should not be missed. Progressive, rapid onset of lower extremity weakness and paresthesias, especially in the setting of saddle anesthesia and/or bowel and bladder incontinence should always be considered a medical emergency, as conus medullaris and cauda equina syndrome can lead to permanent neurologic injury in a short timeframe. Discitis and epidural abscess should be considered in the setting of elevated inflammatory markers associated with fevers and chills. Occasionally, patients presenting to the authors with chief complaint of low back pain have also admitted to hand weakness and balance deficits concerning for cervical myelopathy.

PHYSICAL EXAMINATION

A comprehensive physical examination of the lumbosacral spine follows the organization of a standard musculoskeletal examination and includes observation, palpation, range of motion, neurologic assessment, and special tests. Like the cervical and thoracic spine, the clinician will confirm or reject hypotheses formulated during the history taking portion of the evaluation during the physical examination. A complete evaluation of the lumbosacral spine includes no less than evaluation of the affected area, proximal joints, and the extremities distal to the area affected. Full neurologic examination and evaluation of proximal joints are beyond the scope of this chapter.

Observation

Examination can begin before the patient enters the room by observing gait, guarding, and ease of mobility. Spastic gait pattern can be easily identified as symptoms progress indicating an upper motor neuron lesion. Antalgic gait can warrant further assessment of the distal joints but can also be seen with radiculopathy. Patients presenting with acute compression fractures may have significant guarding or even present in a wheelchair due to severe pain. Observation of the lumbosacral spine should occur with the patient in a gown with the affected area and proximal joints exposed. The clinician will evaluate for signs of swelling, skin changes, postural asymmetry, or deformity (scoliosis, loss of lordosis, etc.). Increased or exaggerated lordosis can indicate spondylolisthesis, hip flexion contracture, or weak hip extensors.[6] An abnormal tuft of hair along the skin of the lumbosacral spine can be indicative of spina bifida. Scoliosis and asymmetry of the paraspinal musculature can be assessed through observation and comparison of the shoulders, scapula, and iliac crest as well as with the spine in flexion. Severely limited flexion with stiffness grossly to the observer is highly suspicious for ankylosing spondylitis but is often not observed grossly without special testing. The lower extremities should be observed for muscle atrophy best appreciated through contrasting the opposing limb. Landmarks can be used to determine location of pain. A line connecting the most superior portion of the iliac crests should be balanced and most often identifies the level of the L4 vertebra. The anterior superior iliac spine (ASIS) and PSIS are important bony landmarks that can also be identified and compared for symmetry.

Palpation

The examiner will evaluate for bony landmarks in order to further identify asymmetry especially in obese patients where bony prominences may be difficult to observe. Palpation of the most superior portion of the iliac crests with the fingers will often direct the thumbs to the L4–L5 vertebra and allow for palpation and further appreciation for symmetry. Spinous processes should be evaluated both for pain and for step-off deformity consistent with spondylolisthesis. Vertebral percussion of tenderness can be present in vertebral fractures, malignancy or osteomyelitis. The clinician should palpate the paraspinal musculature for muscle spasm and for the presence of trigger points. Tenderness over the PSIS is sensitive for sacroiliitis and severe tenderness over the sacrum can also be found in sacral fractures. Tenderness over the greater trochanters could be an indication of greater trochanteric pain syndrome. Ischial tuberosities can also be palpated to further localize pain.

Active Movements

Active range of motion of the lumbosacral spine can help to identify restrictions in motion as well as detect etiology of pain. Motion should be evaluated in all planes including flexion, extension, lateral flexion and axial rotation. Asymmetry in motion can be identified. Range of motion can vary depending on the age and sex of the patient. Flexion is a function of both lumbar and pelvic motion. The relationship of lumbar and pelvic movement can be quantified through measurement of the distance between the patient's middle fingertip to the floor with the patient in flexion and the knees fully extended. Lateral flexion can be similarly measured by observing fingertip position on the thigh. A large systematic review and meta-analysis revealed significant variation in range of motion of subjects without low back pain due to variation in measurement methods, but did confirm decreased average range of motion in subjects with low back pain.[7] There is currently no gold standard on physical examination to measure range of motion of the lumbar spine, and radiographic analysis remains the gold standard.[8]

Neurologic Examination

Neuromuscular examination is critical to the spine evaluation, regardless of the endorsement of radicular pain or neurologic symptoms by the patient. Tandem spinal stenosis, or narrowing of the diameter of the spinal canal in two discrete areas of the spine (often cervical and lumbar), is present in up to 60% of patients with spinal stenosis.[9] A complete evaluation should include all four extremities with assessment including manual muscle testing, deep tendon reflexes, upper motor neuron testing (Babinski reflex, Hoffmann's sign, Lhermitte's sign, and clonus), sensory examination, as well as balance and coordination testing. A comprehensive neurologic examination is beyond the scope of this chapter.

Special Tests

Special tests are an important aspect of the lumbosacral physical examination and can further confirm or eliminate differential diagnoses. Identifying sacroiliac pathology can be difficult as studies have shown that provocative testing is unreliable in the diagnosis of sacroiliac joint pathology. Pain above the L5 level is extremely uncommon in sacroiliitis, and most patients localize their pain near the PSIS. It is still important to keep lumbar etiology of pain in the differential as sacroiliac pain accounts for only 15% of patients with low back pain.[5]

Schober Test

The Schober test is used to measure flexion of the lumbar spine. Two marks are made, both at the first sacral spinous process and 10 cm above with the patient standing erect. The patient is made to flex forward and the distance between the two marks is again measured. In normal flexion, the distance between the two marks should increase to 14–15 cm. Although studies have shown high inter-rater reliability, motion found on testing only weakly correlated to motion detected on imaging.[10]

Modified Schober Test

The original Schober test was eventually modified to include both a mark 10 cm above the midpoint of the intersection of the dimples of Venus at S1 and an additional mark 5 cm below S1. The patient is made to flex forward or extend and the distance between the two marks is measured. The modified Schober test was found to better represent lumbar mobility than the original Schober test, however there was still poor correlation compared to imaging measurement.[10]

Modified-Modified Schober Test

A line is created between the bilateral PSIS and a mark is made 15 cm above this line with the patient standing erect. The patient is made to flex forward or extend and the distance between the two marks is measured and compared. Similar results related to poor correlation with imaging analysis were also found.[10]

Straight-leg Raise Test (Lasègue's Sign)

The straight-leg raise test includes reproduction of pain below the knee when the patient is supine and the symptomatic leg is lifted between 30° and 70°. Numerous analyses have been performed with varying results for specificity and sensitivity of the straight-leg raise test in identifying disk herniations in the lumbar spine. Overall, data has shown high sensitivity (pooled estimate 0.92) with varying specificity (pooled estimate 0.28).[11] The maneuver can also be performed in the seated position (seated straight-leg raise test), although studies have shown a decrease in sensitivity from 0.67 for the straight-leg raise test to 0.41 for the seated straight-leg raise test.[12]

Crossed Straight-leg Raise

The crossed straight-leg raise includes the same method as the straight-leg raise test, but pain in the symptomatic leg is reproduced when raising the contralateral leg. Multiple studies have been performed regarding the validity of the crossed straight-leg raise. High specificity (pooled estimate 0.90) and low sensitivity (pooled estimate 0.28) were found in a Cochrane systematic review.[11]

Bowstring Sign

If a positive straight-leg raise test is noted, the examiner may slightly flex the leg and apply pressure to the tibial nerve in the popliteal fossa. A positive result includes reproduction of pain. Investigation has revealed a sensitivity of 69% when compared to intraoperative pathology.[13]

Slump Test

The slump test is performed with the patient sitting with legs together and arms behind the back. The patient should have both knees directly over the examination table and the sacrum should remain vertical. The patient is asked to slump forward as far as possible for full trunk flexion. The neck is then flexed and the examiner provides slight pressure. The patient then extends the knee while the examiner dorsiflexes the ankle. The test is positive if pain is reproduced with this maneuver. A study performed in 2009 found significant correlation between a positive straight-leg raise test and a positive slump test in patients with unilateral leg pain.[14]

Ankle Dorsiflexion Test (Braggard Sign)

The ankle dorsiflexion test is an extension of the straight-leg raise test. After straight-leg raise testing is performed to the point of pain provocation, the lower extremity is subsequently lowered until the pain subsides, and the ipsilateral ankle is dorsiflexed to increase dural tension. Reproduction of radicular pain that had subsided or improved after dropping the leg slightly indicates a positive test. Analyses have used the ankle dorsiflexion test to enhance the correlation found between the straight-leg raise and slump tests.[14]

Femoral Nerve Stretch Test

The femoral nerve stretch test is used to identify an upper lumbar disk herniation resulting in lumbar radiculopathy. The patient is instructed to lie prone while the clinician places a hand at the popliteal fossa while dorsiflexing the knee of the affected leg. A positive test will reproduce pain in the same distribution, whether that is the anterior thigh, groin, or hip. Cross-sectional studies found that the femoral nerve stretch test has 100% specificity and 50% sensitivity for mid-lumbar nerve root impingement (L2, L3, and L4) as well as 88% specificity and 70% sensitivity for L3 nerve root impingement confirmed with MRI findings.[15]

Crossed Femoral Nerve Stretch Test

The crossed femoral nerve stretch test consists of the same technique used in the femoral nerve stretch test on the contralateral leg. There are very few reports in the literature that show efficacy of the test. In the cross-sectional study performed by Suri et al. the femoral nerve stretch test had such high specificity for mid-lumbar nerve root impingement (L2, L3, and L4) that crossed femoral nerve stretch test did not improve specificity of the examination. It was also positive in only one participant out of 160. It was however specific, along with patellar reflex testing and medial ankle sensation, for L4 nerve root impingement.[15]

Waddell Signs

Waddell signs consist of five factors on physical examination including tenderness, distraction, simulation, regional and overreaction. Initially, at least three positive signs were considered significant in a patient with physical findings without anatomic source. Significant findings were thought to indicate psychological contribution to pain. These findings have since become controversial in the literature. Waddell signs should not be used to evaluate malingering. A recent retrospective cohort study found no statistical difference in severity of pathology in patients with low back pain with and without Waddell signs.[16]

The Hoover Test

The Hoover test has been performed in order to test the amount of effort by a patient who may be avoiding or guarding. The clinician places his hands underneath the heels of the patient while the patient individually lifts each leg. Force should be felt in the contralateral limb as the ipsilateral limb is raised if the patient is providing good effort. The Hoover test has not been studied in the literature and therefore reliability as well as specificity and sensitivity are unknown.

Standing Flexion Test

The standing flexion test can be used to evaluate symmetry of movement of the pelvis. The patient stands facing away from the evaluator with feet underneath the acetabulum, about one foot apart. The clinician places both thumbs on the inferior aspect of the PSIS. The patient flexes forward with both knees in extension and symmetry of movement of the thumbs over the PSIS is evaluated. Studies have shown no correlation with a positive standing flexion test and confirmation with injection of lidocaine into the sacroiliac joint. The test has also been found to have a high false-positive prevalence.[17]

Seated Flexion Test

The seated flexion test is theorized to test for decreased mobility of the sacrum on the ilium. The examiner begins with the patient in a seated position with both legs firmly on the floor. The patient's legs should be abducted to allow for movement of the shoulders. The clinician will place both thumbs on the bilateral PSIS. The examiner instructs the patient to flex forward until both hands reach the floor. The test is positive if one PSIS with thumb overtop moves less cephalad than the contralateral side, indicating hypomobility. Studies have provided inconsistent results regarding sensitivity and specificity, and certain studies have shown a high false-positive rate as well as poor reliability of results between different clinicians.[17]

One-leg Stork Test (Gillet Test)

The Gillet test is meant to detect sacroiliac joint dysfunction. The clinician begins the test with the patient in the same position as the standing flexion test and thumbs over the PSIS. The patient is then asked to stand on one leg while flexing the opposite hip and bringing the knee to the chest. Studies have shown mixed results regarding reliability between clinicians. As with the standing and seated flexion tests, studies have shown a high false-positive rate.[17]

Fortin Finger Test

The Fortin finger test was first described by Fortin in the 1990s as a sign on examination of sacroiliac joint dysfunction. If a patient is made to point to the region of pain with one finger, the test is considered positive if the patient indicates an area within one centimeter inferomedial to the PSIS consistently at least twice during the examination.[18] A study in 1997 by Fortin confirmed sacroiliac joint dysfunction by provoking symptoms through sacroiliac injections. A direct correlation of positive Fortin finger test and sacroiliac dysfunction was found in 16 patients.[19]

Compression Test

The sacroiliac compression test has long been taught as a maneuver to detect sacroiliac joint dysfunction.

With the patient lying supine, the examiner may exert a medial force on each ASIS on both sides. The maneuver can also be performed with the patient lying on one side and the examiner exerting a downward pressure on the anterolateral iliac crest. The compression test is considered positive if the patient reports pain near the sacroiliac joint. The majority of literature includes a small sample size and there are various reports of reliability between examiners. One study of sacroiliac joint pain confirmed by injection found the compression test to be specific (100%) but not sensitive (26%).[20] Other studies have found the test to be unreliable in diagnosis.[21]

Distraction (Gapping Test)

The distraction test, also known as the gapping test, is another test to rule out sacroiliac joint dysfunction through compression of the posterior and stretching of the anterior portion of the joint. The patient rests in a supine position while pressure is placed downward and laterally onto both ASIS. The literature has reported great variability in examiner reliability as well as sensitivity and specificity of the distraction test. Sensitivity in the majorities of studies is <21% while specificity ranges from 90% to 100%.[22]

FABERE (Patrick) Test

FABERE test, also known at the Patrick test, is an acronym for flexion, abduction, external rotation, and extension and describes the technique of the test. A positive test produces sacroiliac pain when the knee is depressed while the ankle rests above the extended knee of the opposite leg. Force can be applied to the flexed leg and the ASIS on the side of the extended leg. Numerous studies have found this test to be unreliable.[21]

Gaenslen Test

The Gaenslen test is performed with the patient in the supine position at an angle so that one leg can extend to the side of the examination table. The patient is instructed to fix the pelvis and lumbar spine by flexing the opposite knee and hip and wrapping both arms to hug the flexed leg to the chest and abdomen. The clinician then applies a force to both the extended leg and the flexed leg. This maneuver is thought to provide stress to the sacroiliac joint and is considered positive if the patient reports pain in the symptomatic sacroiliac joint. A 2002 review of the literature found an agreement on reliability for the Gaenslen test, thigh thrust test, Fortin finger test, and sacroiliac joint pain mapping.[21] A subsequent 2005 study of 48 patients confirmed with local anesthetic injection found the test had a sensitivity of 50–53% and specificity of 71–77%. Researchers found that a combination of three or more out of six positive sacroiliac provocation tests resulted in a sensitivity of 93.8% and specificity of 78.1%. However, the Gaenslen test did not add to the area under the curve and it was concluded that it may be omitted from clinical examination without compromising diagnostic value.[23]

Cranial Shear Test

The cranial shear test involves lying the patient in prone position while the clinician applies a downward pressure to the distal sacrum. The clinician also concurrently applies a traction force to the thighs directed caudally. The test is considered positive if pain is provoked. A 1994 study consisting of 51 patients found greater that 80% agreement between clinicians with a 0.61 κ coefficient.[24]

Thigh Thrust Test

The thigh thrust test is performed with the patient in supine position. The hip and knee are placed in a flexed position while the clinician provides pressure along the femur which also provides force to the ilium posteriorly. The sacrum is stabilized by the clinician with the opposite arm. Pain provocation results in a positive test. A study performed in 1996 by Dreyfuss et al. found sensitivity of 42% and specificity of 45% when confirmed by at least 90% pain reduction after diagnostic injection. It was concluded that none of the 12 tests performed, including the thigh thrust test, provided diagnostic value of sacroiliac joint pain.[25] Conversely, a 2002 review of the literature determined the test is reliable and valid when multiple studies are taken into account.[21]

Midline Sacral Thrust

The midline sacral thrust is performed with the patient relaxed in a prone position. The clinician applies a downward force onto the sacrum. The test is considered positive if pain is reproduced. As with other provocative sacroiliac joint maneuvers, Dreyfuss et al. found no correlation between the midline sacral thrust and diagnostic injection with specificity of 40% and sensitivity of 51%.[25] A 2002 review of the literature also found the test to be invalid as well as unreliable.[21]

Active Straight-leg Raise and Active Assisted Straight-leg Raise

The active straight-leg raise is performed with the patient in a supine position legs in extension and the feet apart. The patient is asked to raise each leg independently with the knee in extension 5–20 cm off of the examination table. The patient is then graded on a four-point scale:

- The patient reports no limitation
- The patient reports decreased ability to raise the leg but the clinician finds no signs of impairment on examination
- The patient reports decreased ability to raise the leg and the clinician observes impairment
- The patient is unable to raise the leg.

High inter-examiner reliability was found in one study of consisting of 25 patients. The study also described the assisted straight-leg raise, which included the straight-leg raise test while the patient wears a sacroiliac belt. They found that the score improved in 20 out of 21 patients with a sacroiliac belt.[26]

SUMMARY

Low back pain is a common entity with numerous etiologies that must be differentiated using a thorough history and physical examination. The appropriate diagnosis is necessary for an effective treatment plan. Emergencies should be quickly identified and referred for surgical opinion. Sacroiliac joint pain can be difficult to differentiate from lumbar pain due to limited validity of sacroiliac provocative maneuvers in the literature. Sacroiliac joint pain is less common and accounts for only 15% of low back pain incidence.[5]

TAKE HOME POINTS

- In the overwhelming majority, the clinician will have a high level of suspicion of lumbosacral etiology based on the history and symptoms provided by the patient.
- The most important aspects of evaluation of the lumbosacral spine are the neurological examination, hip examination, and provocative maneuvers.
- Sacroiliac dysfunction can be difficult to identify but comprises a low prevalence when compared to lumbar etiology of low back pain.

REFERENCES

1. Driscoll T, Jacklyn G, Orchard J, et al. The global burden of occupationally related low back pain: estimates from the Global Burden of Disease 2010 study. Ann Rheum Dis. 2014;73(6):975-81.
2. Seecharan DJ, Arnold PM. Spinal Cord Injuries and Syndromes. In: Shen FH, Samartzis D, Fessler RG (Eds). Textbook of the Cervical Spine. Maryland Heights, Missouri: Saunders Elsevier; 2015. pp. 192-6.
3. Taurog JD, Chhabra A, Colbert RA. Ankylosing Spondylitis and Axial Spondyloarthritis. N Engl J Med. 2016;374(26): 2563-74.
4. Furman MB, Johnson SC. Induced lumbosacral radicular symptom referral patterns: a descriptive study. Spine J. 2019;19(1):163-70.
5. Dreyfuss P, Dreyer SJ, Cole A, et al. Sacroiliac joint pain. J Am Acad Ortop Surg. 2004;12(4):255-65.
6. Woznica DN, Press JM. Physical Examination of the Lumbar Spine and Sacroiliac Joint. In: Malanga GA, Mautner K (Eds). Musculoskeletal Physical Examination: An Evidence-based Approach, 2nd edition. Philadelphia, PA: Elsevier; 2017. pp. 106-44.
7. Laird RA, Gilbert J, Kent P, et al. Comparing lumbo-pelvic kinematics in people with and without back pain: a systematic review and meta-analysis. BMC Musculoskeletal Disord. 2014;15:229.
8. Littlewood C, May S. Measurement of range of movement in the lumbar spine—what methods are valid? A systematic review Physiotherapy. 2007;93:201-11.
9. Overley SC, Kim JS, Gogel BA, et al. Tandem spinal stenosis: a systematic review. JBJS Rev. 2017;5(9):e2.
10. Rezvani A, Ergin O, Karacan I, et al. Validity and reliability of the metric measurements in the assessment of lumbar spine motion in patients with ankylosing spondylitis. Spine. 2012;37:E1189-96.
11. van der Windt DA, Simons E, Riphagen II, et al. Physical examination for lumbar radiculopathy due to disc herniation in patients with low-back pain. Cochrane Database Syst Rev. 2010;(2):CD007431.
12. Rabin A, Gerszten PC, Karausky P, et al. The sensitivity of the seated straight-leg raise test compared with the supine straight-leg raise test in patients presenting with magnetic resonance imaging evidence of lumbar nerve root compression. Arch Phys Med Rahabil. 2007;88:840-3.
13. Supik LF, Broom MJ. Sciatic tension signs and lumbar disc herniation. Spine. 1994;19:1066-9.
14. Walsh J, Hall T. Agreement and correlation between the straight leg raise and slump tests in subjects with leg pain. J Manipulative Physiol Ther. 2009;32(3):184-92.
15. Suri P, Rainville J, Katz JN, et al. The accuracy of the physical examination for the diagnosis of midlumbar and low lumbar nerve root impingement. Spine. 2011;36(1):63-73.

16. Cox JS, Blizzard S, Carlson H, et al. Lumbar magnetic resonance imaging findings in patients with and without Waddell signs. Spine J. 2017;17(7):990-4.
17. Dreyfuss P, Dryer S, Griffin J, et al. Positive sacroiliac screening tests in asymptomatic adults. Spine. 1994;19(10):1138-43.
18. Fortin JD, Dwyer AP, West S, et al. Sacroiliac joint: pain referral maps upon applying a new injection arthrography technique. 1: Asymptomatic volunteers. Spine. 1994;19:1475-82.
19. Fortin JD, Falco FJ. The Fortin finger test: an indicator of sacroiliac pain. Am J Orthop. 1997;26:477-80.
20. Werner CM, Hoch A, Gautier L, et al. Distraction test of the posterior superior iliac spine (PSIS) in the diagnosis of sacroiliac joint arthropathy. BMC Surg. 2013;13:52.
21. Cattley P, Winyard J, Trevaskis J, et al. Validity and reliability of clinical tests for the sacroiliac joint. A review of the literature. Australas Chiropr Osteopathy. 2002;10(2): 73-80.
22. Van der Wurff P, Meyne W, Hagmeijer RH. Clinical tests of the sacroiliac joint. Man Ther. 2000;5:89-96.
23. Laslett M, Aprill CN, McDonald B, et al. Diagnosis of sacroiliac Joint Pain: validity of individual provocation tests and composites of tests. Man Ther. 2005;10(3):207-18.
24. Laslett M, Williams M. The reliability of selected pain provocation tests for sacroiliac joint pathology. Spine. 1994;19(11):1243-9.
25. Dreyfuss P, Michaelsen M, Pauza K, et al. The value of medical history and physical examination in diagnosing sacroiliac joint pain. Spine. 1996;21(22):2594-602.
26. Mens JM, Vleeming A, Snijders CJ, et al. The active straight leg raising test and mobility of the pelvic joints. Eur Spine J. 1999;8(6):468-73.

CHAPTER 35

Low Back Pain Spine Surgery: Current Concepts and Evidence

David E Fish, Jason D Berk, Casey Fisher, Stephen Dechter

EPIDEMIOLOGY

One of the most common medical complaints presented to healthcare professionals such as internists, orthopedists, and physiatrists is that of low back pain , with or without associated symptoms radiating to the lower limbs. For the purposes of this chapter, low back pain will be defined as back pain with or without radiculopathy even though there is a difference in treatment and outcomes. It has been suggested that more than 80% of the population will endure a form of low back pain sometime during life.[1,2] There are a number of studies assessing the prevalence and incidence of low back pain in the population, however, these studies are difficult to compare as a result of the differences in definitions and research parameters used.[1,3-5] In a review of 12 studies available in the medical literature, Hoy et al. found that the 1-year incidence of a "first-ever" episode of low back pain ranged from 6.3% to 15.4%, while the incidence of experiencing an episode of low back pain (first-ever or recurrence) within a year ranged from 1.5% to 36% (Table 1).[6]

Similarly, assessments of 1-year prevalence are variable with values ranging from 2% to 65% dependent

Table 1: One year incidence of low back pain in the general population.[6]

Citation	*Country*	*Age range (years)*	*Inclusion criteria at baseline*	*Case definition*[a]	*Incidence (%)*	*Standard error (%)*	*Risk of bias*
Incidence of number of people who have a first-ever episode							
Biering-Sorensen	Denmark	30–60	Never had low back pain	Low back pain over past year	6.3[c]	0.8	Low
Croft et al.	United Kingdom	18–75	Never had low back pain	Low back pain over past year	15.4[c]	0.9	Moderate
Mustard et al.	Canada	21–34	Never had back pain > 1 day	Back pain > 1 day over past year	7.5[c]	0.6	High
Incidence of number of people who have any episode (first-ever or recurrent)							
Al-Awadhi et al.	Kuwait	15–99	No low back pain at baseline	Low back pain over past year	1.5[b]	0.2	High
Cassidy et al.	Canada	20–69	No low back pain for 6 months prior to baseline	Low back pain over past year	18.9[b]	2.2	Low
Croft et al.	United Kingdom	18–75	No low back pain at baseline	Low back pain over past year	36.0[c]	1.2	Moderate
Hestbaek et al.	Denmark	30–50	No low back problems over past year	Low back problems over past year	19.3[c]	1.7	Low
Jacob et al.	Israel	22–70	No activity-limiting low back pain > 1 day over past month	Activity-limiting low back pain > 1 day over past year	18.4[c]	2.7	Moderate

[a]Definition of a new episode of low back pain.
[b]Age and sex-standardized.
[c]Unadjusted.

upon the definitions employed as well as the methods in data collection,[1,6-8] with a lifetime prevalence estimated to be 60–85%.[5,9-11] Moreover, over the course of a lifetime, this prevalence increases with age until 60–65 years after which it begins to decline,[12,13] with a number of studies showing that low back pain is a common occurrence during the period of adolescence.[6,14-16]

While methodological parameters may vary between studies assessing the epidemiology of low back pain, what seems to be apparent is that this is a common condition with individuals often requiring the care of medical professionals. In those with back pain, approximately 40–70% required the evaluation and management of a physician at some time throughout the course of their lives.[17,18] What is more, trends suggest that the number of people requiring medical care to address low back pain is likely to be increasing as was shown by Freburger et al.[1] In their 2009 study, it was demonstrated that in a 14-year time-period between 1992 and 2006 in North Carolina, the prevalence of chronic low back more than doubled from 3.9% to 10.2%.[1] This significant increase was seen among all sex, age, and race/ethnic demographics. Further, occurrences of acute low back pain defined as pain that limited usual activity for at least 1 day but less than 3 months; or less than 25 episodes of low back pain that limited activity, rose from 7.3% to 10.5% in a years' time.[1] While Freburger's data is specific to the individuals residing in North Carolina, it is not unreasonable to suspect that it can likely be extrapolated to represent what is being experienced throughout the population at large.

The natural course and progression of low back pain have been seen to be widely variable, with symptoms being present only a few days for some, while years for others.[19] From the onset of the first episode of low back pain, the median length of time during which symptoms were experienced has been reported to be 42 days.[6,20] Von Korff reported that at 1-year follow-up, the median number of days affected by pain was 15.5 in those with low back pain lasting less than 3 months from baseline, and 128.5 days when low back pain lasted between 3 months and 6 months.[21] When considering the progression of this condition, one must also take into account recurrent episodes.

Often individuals with low back pain have a natural history of resolution of symptoms, however, 50% will experience a resurfacing of their low back pain within a year, 60% by 2 years, and 70% by 5 years.[22] Over the course of a lifetime, approximately 85% of people will have a recurrent episode at some point.[23] In attempting to identify factors that predispose one to have repeat episodes, recurrence rates have been seen to increase with age,[24] and women have been seen to be more at risk than men.[25] Additionally, people whose initial episode of low back pain causes limitations in daily functioning and lasts for more than 1 day, often proceed to have repeat events.[22,26]

While not an issue that is life-threatening or typically requiring of emergent medical attention, this pain complaint has been documented in the literature to be a leading cause of functional disability and missed time from work.[6,27] In a given year, low back pain accounts for approximately 149 million days lost from work,[28] with individuals who suffer recurrent episodes having longer periods of work disability than those who do not.[29] Moreover, in those under the age of 45, it represents the most frequent cause of limitation in overall physical activity.[30]

Aside from the negative impact on daily function and overall quality of life, low back pain results in significant economic costs to individuals and their families, as well as industry and government.[31-33] Those consulting a physician to address have been shown to utilize about twice as much healthcare than the general population, with individuals between the ages of 20 years and 30 years being responsible for the majority of this consumption.[7] In 1998, it was estimated that direct health expenditure related to low back pain in the United States was $90.7 billion.[34] With prevalence values having been on the rise since that time, it is safe to assume that this expenditure has seen a substantial increase as well.

Determining the risk factors that make one more susceptible to experiencing low back pain and its associated sequelae would be beneficial in better understanding this condition as well as improve the healthcare provider's ability to prevent and manage it. As described previously, age is a common risk factor, with some studies demonstrating that the highest incidence occurs between 20 years and 30 years,[35,36] while overall prevalence increases with age until 60–65 years after which it begins to decline.[12,13] In assessing gender differences, prevalence has been seen to be higher amongst women.[6] Low back pain has also been associated with lower levels of education[37,38] and social status.[39,40] As may be expected, those with occupations that are more physically demanding, involving activities such as manual handling, bending, twisting, and whole-body vibration, have a higher likelihood of developing pain in the low back.[41,42] Further, it has been indicated that a number of psychological elements, including anxiety, depression, and stress, are contributing factors that should be appreciated and managed appropriately.[43] Bodyweight and body mass index have also been shown to influence the probability of low back pain presenting itself during the course of one's lifetime.[44,45]

The epidemiologic data, as well as the relative strength of associated risk factors, varies throughout the medical literature. What remains constant throughout, however, is that low back pain is an exceedingly common condition, negatively impacting quality of life and causing significant functional limitations, resulting in both direct and indirect costs to those affected as well as society in general (Table 2).

WORKUP

There are a myriad of pathologies leading to low back, including, but not limited to, skeletal etiologies such as

Table 2: Level-of-evidence.

Author, Journal, Year	*Design*	*LoE*	*Topic*	*F/U*	*Measures*	*Main results*
Atlas, Spine, 2005	PC	II	Surgical vs. nonsurgical	10 years	MRDS MOSSF SF BI	Surgical group better function, satisfaction, and leg pain relief
Wilson-Mac Donald, JBJS, 2005	RCT	I	ESI for acute pain	2 years	Oxford Pain Chart VAS	SS reduction in acute pain, but not in long-term pain relief
Chou, Spine, 2009	Systematic review	II	ESI	1 month-3 years	VAS ODI	Some short-term benefit, inconsistent long-term benefit
Ng, Spine, 2005	RTC	I	ESI vs. local for chronic pain	3 months	ODI VAS Claudication Satisfaction	No SS difference between groups
Karppinen, Spine, 2001	RTC	I	ESI vs. saline for acute to subacute sciatica	1 year	VAS Satisfaction Sick leave Cost	SS acute benefits but not long-term benefits
Weinstein, JAMA, 2006	PC	I	Surgical vs. nonsurgical	2 years	MOSSF MODI	Improved radicular pain, no difference in disability
Pauza, Spine, 2004	RTC	I	IDET vs. sham		VAS SF-36 ODI	Improved VAS, ODI, and depression in IDET group
Chinmoy, JVIR, 2012	PC	II	RFA + steroid	1 year	VAS NRS	Sustained improvement in VAS and NRS at 1 year
Arden, Rheum, 2005	RCT	I	ESI vs. saline	1 year	ODQ	SS short-term improvement, no long-term benefits of repeated ESI
Storheim, Rehab Med, 2003	RCT	I	Exercise vs. cognitive vs. physician care for LBP	4 months	VAS RM	SS improvement in exercise and cognitive groups vs. control
Foster, Neurology, 2001	RCT	II	Botox vs. saline for chronic LBP	3 and 8 weeks	VAS OLBPQ	SS improvement in pain and disability in the botox group
North, NSGY, 2005	RCT	I	SCS vs. reoperation	3 years	VAS Opioid use ADL Work status	SS pain reduction in SCS group vs. reoperation group

(BI: Bothersome indexes; ESI: epidural steroid injections; F/U: follow-up; JOA: Japanese Orthopaedic Association score; LoE: level of evidence; MODI: modified Oswestry disability index; MOSSF: medical outcomes study short form; MRDS: modified Roland disability scale; NDI: neck disability index; NRS: numeric rating scale; OLBPQ: Oswestry low back pain questionnaire; PC: prospective cohort; R: retrospective; RCT: randomized controlled trial; RM: Roland-Morris questionnaire; SCS: spinal stimulation; SF: sciatica frequency; SS: statistically significant; VAS: visual analog scale).

vertebral fractures, spinal malalignment, facet arthropathy, and sacroiliitis; diskogenic causes like lumbar disk herniation and annular tears; neural sources from nerve root impingement; as well as muscular origins involving myofasciitis and strains. The healthcare provider then becomes challenged with the job of determining which of these numerous possibilities is responsible for producing the presenting pain symptoms. This process begins with a thorough history focusing on duration and location of pain, presence of an event that led to symptom onset, character of the pain (i.e. sharp, dull, burning, etc.) and intensity level, exacerbating and remitting factors, as well as the perception of new-onset weakness, numbness, and bowel or bladder incontinence.

Often times, the information collected in a complete history is sufficient to generate a strong impression of what the diagnosis is likely to be. In a prospective study of 100 patients by Roshan and Rao, it was shown that the collection of history by itself led to the generation of the correct diagnosis in 78.58% of the patients assessed.[46] The strength of the "history of present illness" is not only dependent on the physician's ability to ask focused nonleading questions, but also on the ability of the individual being examined to provide consistent and accurate information. Limitations to this aspect of the workup arise when one is unable to precisely describe their symptoms. Such a situation can occur when medical attention is being sought at a time when pain or associated symptoms are not actively present. Consequently, despite the relative strength of history gathering, more information through additional workup often needs to be obtained to determine the etiology of one's low back pain.

With the history collected, the focus shifts to performing a physical examination to further narrow in on the likely pathology responsible for the individual's low back pain. The examination should be focused and include not only a thorough musculoskeletal assessment but a comprehensive neurological evaluation as well. Generally, the physical examination begins with a general survey of the person including general appearance, posture, gait, muscle bulk, skin discoloration or masses over the spine, spinal alignment, as well as a range of motion. Assessment of motor strength, pinprick and light touch sensation, and reflexes can provide clues regarding affected dermatomes or myotomes, suggesting the presence of a radiculopathy. Additional investigation of neural tension signs such as straight leg raise and slump tests would offer further support for an injury affecting the level of the lumbar nerve roots. The presence of so-called "long track signs" including clonus, increased tone, Babinski sign, Hoffman sign, hyperreflexia, and inability to tandem walk would suggest pathology above the level of the nerve roots, in the central nervous system. Myofascial and bursae pain generators should be explored with a reproduction of symptoms with the palpation of such musculature as the lumbar paraspinals, quadratus lumborum, iliopsoas, piriformis, and gluteals, as well as the greater trochanteric bursa.

With pathology related to the sacroiliac joint, such as sacroiliitis and arthropathy, accounting for an estimated 10–30% of low back pain complaints,[47,48] an evaluation of this joint with palpation as well as provocative maneuvers including Patrick's and Yeoman's tests is warranted. In addition to the sacroiliac joint, the lumbar facet joints should be assessed with palpation and facet-loading techniques as inflammation or arthropathy of these small synovial joints can often be an etiology of axial low back pain.[49]

Much like with history taking, this aspect of the workup of an individual with low back pain is not without its shortcomings. The interpretation of findings on a physical examination is subjective, with results often demonstrating variation between examiners. Additionally, the validity of the physical examination is largely dependent upon the willingness or ability of one to fully participate and provide full effort. Frequently, the presenting pain inhibits an individual's ability to tolerate all aspects of a full examination. Moreover, it is not uncommon for inconsistencies in examination findings to be present, making it difficult to weigh their relative clinical significance. While the great majority of people with low back pain have an organic cause to explain their symptoms and present to a medical professional in hopes of getting relief, an examiner should maintain a level of caution for individuals falsifying examination findings for the purposes of obtaining some sort of secondary gain.

With the inherent limitations of history taking making it difficult to always be able to deduce the prevailing diagnosis, as well as the presence of doubt surrounding the ability of physical examination to elucidate the myriad of low back pain etiologies,[50-52] physicians require additional modalities to workup on this patient population. Typically, the next tool employed to generate additional information is diagnostic imaging, most commonly plain X-ray films and magnetic resonance imaging (MRI).

Plain X-ray imaging provides insight into spinal osseous architecture, alignment, presence of fractures, as well as potential degenerative changes. Obtaining lumbar flexion and extension X-rays allows one to assess for abnormal lumbar vertebral shifting when assuming these positions. While X-rays can generally be obtained quickly and can serve as a good initial study, these images do not offer clear details or allow for an assessment of soft tissues as is obtainable with MRI studies.

Magnetic resonance imaging is excellent for providing evidence of abnormalities in lumbar anatomy and architecture. One needs to be mindful, however, that these images simply provide a snapshot in time of the structure of an individual's lumbar spine, and "abnormal" findings do not necessarily correlate with an etiology for low back pain. Boden et al.[53] performed MRI studies on 67 patients without a history of low back pain, sciatica, or neurogenic claudication and found that even in people ranging from 20 years to 39 years of age, 34% had findings consistent with a herniated disk. Moreover, this investigation demonstrated a direct relationship between advancing age and the percentage of those found to have abnormal findings on MRI studies. The prevalence of coincidental abnormalities on lumbar spine MRI imaging is further demonstrated by Jensen et al. who reported on the imaging results from 98 asymptomatic subjects.[54] This investigation revealed abnormal findings in 68% of these individuals. Further analysis of the data showed that 52% of the subjects had a lumbar vertebral disk bulge at one or more levels, 27% had evidence of a disk protrusion, and 1% were found to have a disk extrusion. Additionally, abnormalities at multiple intervertebral levels were seen in the MRI examinations of 38% of study participants. Collectively, these studies clearly illustrate that findings on MRI do not necessarily equate to a diagnosis explaining symptoms in those experiencing with low back pain. The fallibility of these more conservative diagnostic techniques, including radiographic imaging, physical examination, and history taking, has lead to the emergence of more specialized and somewhat more invasive modalities.

The assessment of motor units by electromyography (EMG) can be employed to determine the presence of a lumbar radiculopathy, as well as the severity and chronicity of such pathology. The presence of electrophysiologic abnormalities in distinct muscles that share innervation by a common nerve root but different peripheral nerves is required to make the diagnosis of a radiculopathy. In a population of "definite radiculopathy" subjects, Nardin et al. demonstrated a correlation rate of 60% between abnormalities observed on EMG and abnormal findings seen on MRI evaluation.[55] This study also provided evidence regarding the specificity of EMG in the diagnosis of a radiculopathy, as abnormality rates were 72% and 29%, respectively in a comparison of subjects categorized as definite versus possible radiculopathy. Therefore, this diagnostic test serves well in ruling in the presence of a radiculopathy. Conversely, EMG lacks the sensitivity of other examination techniques. Generally, it takes 7–10 days, at times up to 3 weeks, following a nerve injury before deviations from normal are apparent on electrodiagnostic evaluation. Additionally, normal findings may be seen in the presence of nerve root irritation versus actual nerve damage, or result from simply testing an area of muscle that has not experienced denervation. Therefore, while possibly not as useful a means of screening, EMG is a valuable tool in ruling in the presence of radiculopathy and should be employed with other elements of the low back pain workup when radicular symptoms are present.

Diskography is a diagnostic technique utilized to determine if one's low back pain is being generated from pathology intrinsic to the intervertebral disk itself. Under fluoroscopic guidance, a spinal needle is inserted into the nucleus pulposus of the disk in question, and nonirritating contrast is injected. In theory, if the disk is the etiology of one's low back pain, the introduction of this contrast will cause the disk to distend with reproduction and concurrence of their symptoms. Injection of a normal disk will still cause the disk to expand, but should not result in the production of pain. A study by Holt suggested that diskography lacked specificity in the diagnosis of diskogenic low back pain.[56] Alternatively, in a sample population including 7 men without a history of low back pain and 10 men with known low back pain, Walsh et al. demonstrated a 0% false-positive rate associated diskogram evaluation.[57] A factor contributing to this issue of the specificity of diskography, not to mention its sensitivity, in the diagnosis of diskogenic low back pain, is the subjective nature of this test. Much like other techniques described in the workup of low back pain, the strength of this diagnostic tool is almost entirely dependent upon an individual's participation and feedback. Not only must they be able to determine if the pain is being experienced with the introduction of the contrast dye, but also an assessment of whether this pain is similar in nature or concordant to their normal symptomology must be accurately made. Consequently, the assessment of data obtained from a diskogram must take into account not only the abilities of the examiner conducting the study but also patient factors that could potentially affect their responses. For example, a study by Carragee et al. suggested that individuals with chronic pain, disability issues, and compensation claims have a higher probability of reporting concordant pain during diskography.[58]

It is clear that the various aspects of the low back pain workup, history taking, physical examination, and diagnostic imaging or invasive spinal procedures, are not without their individual limitations. Therefore, the strength of the evaluation of any individual resides in the use of each of these components in concert with one another to develop a comprehensive impression of them. Roshan and Rao showed that healthcare provider confidence in having reached the correct diagnosis increased from 6.36 (on a numerical scale to 10) after history taking to 7.57 following a physical examination. This confidence score increased yet further to 9.84 with the addition of diagnostic investigations. Ultimately, the ability to correctly identify the low back pain etiology is imperative for initiation of effective and appropriate treatment.

MEDICAL MANAGEMENT

Low back pain, whether axial in nature, or radicular, is a result of various processes, and as such, can be treated with various modalities and medications most often in combination. It can be treated by invasive procedures or simple topical ointments. All of this management has varying levels of success and there is no one medication or modality which has been shown to completely alleviate all forms of back pain. This section will discuss the medical management of low back pain that is not caused by the tumor, infection, congenital processes, or rheumatologic syndromes. This includes axial low back caused by pathology involving myofascial, ligamentous, joint complexes, and disk degeneration. It also includes radicular low back pain caused by pathology to nerve root complexes. Treatments for such etiologies to be discussed in this section include physical therapy, modalities, medications, and psychological treatment. Any treatment which involves spinal interventional technique or surgical technique will be discussed in the next section or subsequent chapters.

Physical Therapy

Physical therapy is a broad term which denotes the treatment of disease or dysfunction by physical means of massage, modalities, and exercise rather than with medication. This therapy is delivered by a licensed, professional therapist. For the purposes of back pain, physical therapy denotes modalities and therapeutic exercises which include stretching and strengthening which is indicated for back pain of an axial or radicular nature due to mechanical or myofascial pathology with or without primary spine pathology.

There are many therapeutic exercises available for low back pain. Exercise therapy is a very heterogeneous, widely studied, and widely used treatment for the initial presentation of low back pain of axial or radicular etiology. Unfortunately, there is very little consensus on what types of exercise to use and when these exercises should be employed. According to a 2005 Cochrane review of 61 randomized-controlled trials with 6,390 participants who had acute, subacute, and chronic low back pain, exercise therapy was effective for chronic low back pain by improved function and decreased pain.[59] Conversely, in the acute low back pain population, exercise therapy was not more effective than rest. In the subacute population, a graded or stepwise approach to activity including therapeutic exercise showed fewer days of work missed, but no other significant functional outcomes.[59] Also, when comparing types of exercise, it appears that individualized, monitored, exercises designed for stretching and strengthening are the most effective for subacute and chronic low back pain improvement of pain and function.[60] Overall, physical therapy and therapeutic exercise can be considered one of the first-line treatments for low back pain. These treatments are the least invasive options for low back pain and may have fewer complications or morbidities.

Modalities

Modalities will be defined as any nonmedication that can use physical energy for the therapeutic effect of alleviating pain. For the low back pain population, there are many of these things available which can be used in the treatment of pain. Cryotherapy, diathermy, transcutaneous electric nerve stimulation (TENS), traction, medical massage, spinal manipulation, prosthetics, bracing, and acupuncture are the most widely used modalities to treat low back pain.

Cryotherapy is the use of cold to treat localized pain. This is often accomplished using ice packs, cold baths, or vapocoolant sprays. The therapeutic effect of cold temperature is based on its ability to decrease the local temperature of the tissues which causes local vasoconstriction and decreased metabolic demand, increased nerve pain threshold, decreased inflammatory response,[61] and decreased muscle spindle activity including the decreased firing of afferent nerve fiber types Ia and II.[62] These properties can make cryotherapy very effective at relieving pain in the back related to muscle strains, ligamentous sprains, and localized joint inflammation in the acute, subacute or chronic periods of low back pain.

Diathermy is the use of deep heat to treat pain without overheating subcutaneous tissues or skin. Diathermy refers to mechanisms that can heat tissue to a depth of 3–5 cm, which is deeper than the superficial heat of a heating pad or hot pack. These mechanisms use energy conversion to achieve deep heat. The three types of energy used are therapeutic ultrasound, shortwave (radio wave) diathermy, and microwave diathermy.[63-65] Additionally, ultrasound can also be used to deliver medications to the deep tissue layers, such as corticosteroids or local anesthetic, through the skin of the back in a process called phonophoresis or sonophoresis. This allows medications to penetrate the epidermis more effectively by increasing the permeability of the epidermis by a factor of at least 10, and with some medications, a factor of 1,000.[66]

Transcutaneous electric nerve stimulation is a process by which an electric signal is delivered via electrodes attached to the skin. TENS can be effective at the relief of low back pain in part due to the pain theory of gate control that was first described by Melzack and Wall. In this theory, pain signals can be blocked by stimulation of larger, myelinated afferent fibers[67] which is what happens when applying a TENS unit to an individual. It is speculated that TENS delivers electrical signals at low frequency and may offer relief by the release of endogenous opioids because it has been shown that subjective pain relief for individuals can be reversed by naloxone.[68] Most TENS units are portable and programmable and may offer patients a relatively safe and reliable pain-relieving option.

Medical massage as a treatment for low back pain has been available for many years. The use of pressure and stretching of soft tissue in the back provides mechanical, psychological, and reflexive effects, and it has been shown to be beneficial if provided with education and exercise for subacute and chronic low back pain.[69] There are many different types of massage including effleurage, petrissage, tapotement, friction, myofascial release, acupressure, and soft tissue mobilization, but there is very little evidence that one type is more beneficial than any other. There is evidence to suggest that massage compared to sham treatment decreased pain and improved function after short- and long-term follow-up.[69]

Traction or the use of force in distraction of the vertebrae is used more often with neck pain, but it is also can be used for low back pain.[70] When used for back pain, traction can be done intermittently or continuously and it can be achieved mechanically with motorized devices or pulley systems. The use of traction for low back pain has not been very well studied although it has been shown to be effective at decreasing leg and back pain by at least 50% in a subset of low back pain sufferers in their forties who were hypolordotic, had chronic unilateral lumbosacral radiculopathy associated with L5–S1 lumbar disk prolapsed, and duration of symptoms more than 3 months.[71] In these patients, an extension-type traction provided by a computerized traction unit was used to deliver traction, which was effective at decreasing leg and back pain and improving hypolordosis.[71]

While most studies have mixed results regarding benefit for low back pain in the acute or chronic states, spinal manipulative therapy is used frequently to treat low back pain. This practice is done most often by chiropractors or doctors of osteopathy and often involves some form of manipulation and mobilization. However, mobilization should be avoided in anyone who has a progressive neurologic disorder or alteration of the anatomy of their spine due to fracture, infection, or malignancy.[72] Of note, a large 2004 Cochrane review of spinal manipulation did not show any significant results compared to general practitioner care, analgesic regimens, physical therapy, or exercises, but spinal manipulation had clinical and statistically significant results compared to sham manipulation.[73] This may mean that spinal manipulation may have more than just placebo effects on those with low back pain, but studies are needed to further investigate this therapy.

Though there is a very large commercial market for bracing using orthotics for low back pain, there has been no evidence that bracing using lumbar supports is an effective means to prevent or treat low back pain once it has occurred.[74] There is some thought that these results may be due to noncompliance in wearing the brace, but that remains to be seen as there are very few high-quality studies on the use of bracing in low back pain. There is reluctance by most practitioners to prescribe bracing for back pain because it tends to promote immobility of spinal stabilizer muscles which can lead to more weakness of those muscles and can further decondition individuals suffering from low back pain.[75] Conversely, there is a role for bracing when it comes to conservative management of fractures in the spine which cause pain. This type of management is seen most often in young athletes with spondylolysis, with the goal being immobilization of the stress fracture to the pars interarticularis so that osseous healing of the defect occurs.[76] In this case, treatment with a thoracolumbosacral orthosis for 3–6 months combined with physical therapy to decrease lumbar lordosis and hamstring contractures and without playing sports for the initial 3 months has been shown to improve pain and fracture healing.[77]

Acupuncture, a therapeutic intervention where fine needles are placed into or through the skin at specific places on the body, has been a part of traditional Chinese medicine for over 2,000 years. Although there are varying theories and mixed evidence as to what is actually occurring to treat pain when these needles are placed, studies have shown a myriad of different physiologic outcomes when acupuncture needles are placed. The various physiological changes include PET scans showing increased μ-opioid binding potentials, functional MRIs showing increased activity in areas of the brain known to be part of pain processing, and release of endogenous opioids in the brain stem.[78] While not regarded as first-line therapy, it appears to be a viable form of complementary treatment for chronic low back pain especially as a part of multidisciplinary treatment of low back pain. It does not appear to be more effective than a sham, but it is more effective than no treatment at all.[79,80]

Medications

Medical management of low back pain can also include the use of medications. Both oral and topical mediations are available to treat low back pain. Oral medications used most widely for low back pain include nonsteroidal anti-inflammatory drugs (NSAIDs), salicylates, acetaminophen, muscle relaxants, antiepileptics, tricyclic antidepressants, and opioids. Topical medications used for low back pain include local anesthetics, NSAIDs, capsaicin, and compounding medications with methyl salicylate and menthol. Each of these medications has a role in treating certain aspects of the pain that can occur with low back pain.

Nonsteroidal anti-inflammatory medications (NSAIDs) are used worldwide and are known to improve low back pain by decreasing swelling and inflammation.[81] Indications for the use of NSAIDs are mild to moderate pain and rheumatoid or osteoarthritic pain. These medications work by inhibition of predominantly type 2 cyclooxygenase (COX-2) enzymes, which inhibits prostaglandin synthesis. Inhibition of cyclooxygenase type 1 enzymes (COX-1) is what is thought to cause the side effects of NSAIDs.[82] Dyspepsia, antiplatelet activity, and increased risk of cardiovascular events are some of the more common serious side effects associated with NSAIDs. That is the reason these medications should be avoided in individuals with gastric ulcers or who are already taking blood-thinning medication or who have coronary artery disease. NSAIDs do play a role in the treatment of low back pain especially acutely after an injury or with re-exacerbation of a chronic injury. In these instances, NSAIDs and salicylates are considered one of the first-line medications and a trial can be beneficial to treating low back pain especially when the back pain is related to muscle strain, ligament sprain, or acute joint inflammation.

Salicylates, like nonsteroidal anti-inflammatory medications, help to decrease low back pain by decreasing inflammation and affecting prostaglandin production. Salicylates also have similar indications and side effect profile to NSAIDs. Acetaminophen, also commonly known as paracetamol, is another first-line medication for low back pain and is used for similar therapeutic effects to salicylates, but it lacks anti-inflammatory, antiplatelet, and gastric ulcerative effects. Acetaminophen is very commonly used, especially in combination with opioids, but can have severe effects on kidney and liver function if used in high doses for prolonged periods of time.[83,84]

Other medications that are often prescribed for initial treatment of low back pain, especially if patients are also experiencing muscle spasms and neuropathic type pain pattern, are a group of medications known as muscle relaxants. The three most common groups of muscle relaxants are the antispasmodic benzodiazepines, the nonbenzodiazepine antispasmodics, and the antispasticity class. Diazepam (Valium), alprazolam

(Xanax), and lorazepam (Ativan) tend to be the most common medications in this class of benzodiazepine medications used for low back pain. Cyclobenzaprine (Flexeril), methocarbamol (Robaxin), and tizanidine (Zanaflex) are some of the most commonly prescribed nonbenzodiazepine antispasmodics. Baclofen and dantrolene (Dantrium) are the most prescribed oral antispasticity medications used for muscle spasms. There are differing opinions about what muscle relaxants are best when they should be used, and for how long, but guidelines from the federal drug enforcement agency suggest that muscle relaxants should not be used for longer than 2 weeks to treat muscle spasms in low back pain patients. According to a large 2003 Cochrane database review of 30 studies, all of these medications are more effective than placebo for short-term treatment of nonspecific low back pain, but they carry with them increased risk of adverse effects predominantly relating to their sedating qualities on the central nervous system.[85]

There is a group of medications that have recently been utilized for the neuropathic type pain that can accompany low back pain. These medications, gabapentin (Neurontin) and pregabalin (Lyrica), are known to work as voltage-sensitive calcium channel subunit α_2-δ ligands[86] and were initially used only as antiepileptics. Currently, these medications now also have indications for postherpetic neuralgia and neuropathic pain and pregabalin (Lyrica) is also indicated for use in fibromyalgia. Compared to benzodiazepines and selective serotonin reuptake inhibitors, these medications may have fewer complications when used.[87] They do, however, need to be started at low doses due to their sedating properties, but once individuals get to a steady-state of these medications, they are fairly well-tolerated and can be titrated with higher dosing until effective pain relief is determined by the individual.

Tricyclic antidepressants, such as nortriptyline (Pamelor), amitriptyline (Elavil), and selective serotonin-norepinephrine inhibitors (SNRIs) such as duloxetine (Cymbalta), which are used as antidepression medications, have been found to be efficacious in the neuropathic component of low back pain.[87] These medications may work by selective serotonin and norepinephrine reuptake inhibition to treat neuropathic pain and are considered effective in treating neuropathic pain. In one review of 105 randomized-controlled clinic trials, the number of peripheral neuropathic pain sufferers needed to treat was shown to be 2.1–3.1.[87] These medications are considered a possible first-line treatment for neuropathic pain along with gabapentin (Neurontin) and pregabalin (Lyrica).[88] One advantage of taking an SNRI over taking a TCA is that there are fewer side effects. This is because the TCAs also block muscarinic receptors for acetylcholine, alpha receptors, and histamine receptors, which leads to anticholinergic effects including blurred vision, urinary retention, constipation, postural hypotension, and sedation.

Opioids are becoming more commonly used in the treatment of low back pain, but the use of these medications is very controversial as to when to start using, how much to give, and for how long to use. Opioid type of medications can be long- or short-acting and consist of hydrocodone, morphine, hydromorphone, oxycodone, and codeine. Caution should be given to the provider who begins opioid medications for nonmalignant back pain as the incidence of abuse, misuse, diversion, and level of effectiveness can affect outcomes. Most often these medications are prescribed in combination with acetaminophens, such as codeine and acetaminophen (Tylenol #3), hydrocodone and acetaminophen (Vicodin), or oxycodone and acetaminophen (Oxycontin, Percocet). Morphine is also prescribed often for low back pain. Other opioids that could be prescribed are oxymorphone (Opana), hydromorphone (Dilaudid), fentanyl, meperidine (Demerol), methadone (Dolophine), levorphanol, propoxyphene (Darvon), tapentadol (Nucynta), and the partial agonists and agonist-antagonists such as buprenorphine (Subutex) and pentazocine (Talwin). All of these medications have certain specific characteristics which have their advantages and disadvantages. Opioids have an indication for acute and subacute low back pain. Opioids can be prescribed for chronic low back pain even though the literature does not support the use in the chronic pain patient, especially at high doses for reasons of safety and efficacy.[89] Short-acting opioid medications can be used for patients who are opioid-naive, have acute or subacute pain, or only take pain medication intermittently. Care should be taken when prescribing opiates for a myofascial diagnosis because addiction can be common with long-term use.[89] When prescribing opioids, it is important to educate patients about safe and appropriate use, such as using only what is prescribed, not refilling medications early, avoiding the use of recreational drugs, not diverting medications to other people, and maintaining opioid management with a single provider and pharmacy. Clinicians should utilize toxicology studies to screen for inappropriate use. Conversion between opioids should take into account incomplete cross-tolerance. After calculating equianalgesic conversion, a practitioner should dose the new opioid at a lower level compared to the converted dose of its predecessor. It is recommended to reduce total dosage by approximately 25–50% when converting from one opioid to another or from immediate-release to long-acting formulation to account for incomplete cross-tolerance.[90] Strategies for diminishing tolerance and the progressive escalation of opioid doses include opioid rotation, periodic opioid holidays with the restarting of medication at lower doses, or discontinuing therapy altogether. The practitioner should always be concerned about addiction and the ceiling effect of chronic use and discuss openly with individuals on chronic medications. If the individual is on high dosing of opiates (long- or short-acting), but the pain is still significant, discontinuing the medications is strongly advised.

Lidocaine is the most commonly used topical anesthetic medication that is indicated for low back pain. It comes as a patch or a topical ointment, which can come in combination with prilocaine in a eutectic mixture of local anesthetics or EMLA cream. It may be beneficial for neuropathic pain and is considered a possible first-line treatment for the pain of nerve origin.[88] It may also be effective in the treatment of back pain as a result of postherpetic neuralgia, which will often affect a thoracic level dermatomal distribution.[91] Contact with nonintact skin, eyes, face, and mucous membranes should be avoided when using this medication because it can cause systemic effects.

Topical medications of menthol and methyl salicylate ointments, individually or in combination, capsaicin, and diclofenac are all available for percutaneous use and may be found to be beneficial for the myofascial component of low back pain. Diclofenac, a nonsteroidal anti-inflammatory medication, is also available in the topical form as a patch or ointment. Its primary indication is osteoarthritis of the peripheral joints, but it can also be effective for back pain with a myofascial component. Menthol and methyl salicylate topical ointments are available as over the counter agents to treat pain. Menthol gives the skin a sense of coldness to an individual while the methyl salicylate treats as an anti-inflammatory of the local epidermis and dermis. Capsaicin, a synthetic version of a chili pepper metabolite, can cause a sensation of burning when it comes into contact with skin and is also used as a topical pain reliever for low back pain. Capsaicin has been found to be beneficial in myofascial and neuropathic type pain at concentrations of 0.025% and 0.075% with varying degrees of efficacy.[92]

Psychological Treatment

Another important strategy in the treatment of low back pain is the use of psychiatric or psychological interventions. This is typically a component of the multi-disciplinary approach to low back pain management. The psychological process can be helpful predominantly if the individual has a history of psychiatric disorders, such as post-traumatic stress, depression, bipolar, or schizoaffective disorders, but psychological interventions can also be beneficial for personality disorders such as borderline, histrionic, or obsessive-compulsive personality disorders. It is very important to identify environmental stressors in the low back pain population and determine how outside stressors, such as job satisfaction, psychological distress, and psychosocial factors, affect those who have back pain or pain of any other kind.[93] Treatment with coping strategies and other healthy means to control environmental stressors can be a large factor in improvement of pain in the low back pain population and should be employed whenever available to the treatment provider.

INTERVENTIONAL MANAGEMENT

Surgical management of low back pain, whether axial or radicular, is often reserved for situations in which the pain is refractory to medical management. However, there are interventional procedures available for low back pain that are less invasive and can be used along with medical management to improve function and decrease pain to avoid surgery or to treat those patients who are at too high risk for surgery. When surgery is indicated, it is important to know what pathology absolutely needs to be treated immediately and what can be effectively treated with elective surgery and also what types of options exist to treat those pathologies. It is also important to know what is available for individuals who have already had surgery but continue to have low back pain. All of these topics will be covered in this section.

Interventional Procedures

Prior to the surgical evaluation, low back pain sufferers with radicular or axial low back pain will often be offered interventional procedures, especially if they have a diffuse degenerative disease such that one level diskectomy or laminectomy would not improve. For the most part, these procedures involve the use of needles to deliver medication to a particular site of interest on the back. These procedures include myofascial injections such as trigger point and prolotherapy injections, epidural steroid injections, medial branch blocks, and subsequent radiofrequency ablation, intradiskal interventions, and kyphoplasty or vertebroplasty.

Myofascial trigger point injections can provide relief for low back pain that is myofascial, cutaneous, fascial, ligamentous, or periosteal in origin. Trigger points are defined as a point on a tissue area that is irritable and radiates pain when palpated with the presence of a taut band of muscle. Options for treatment include inserting a needle without any medication and applying a repeated insertion motion to the area (dry needling), injection of local anesthetics such as lidocaine, injection of local anesthetic and corticosteroid such as triamcinolone (Kenalog), or injection of botulinum toxins. The technique and injectate vary among practitioners, but there is limited data showing that a certain medication combination has increased benefits. In fact, in one study, dry needling was found to be just as effective as using medications.[94]

Prolotherapy, or proliferative therapy, is also a technique of injecting into the peripheral tissues, namely spinal ligaments, except in this case, the thought is to try to increase inflammatory mediators, such as granulocytes, macrophages, and fibroblasts, which will, in theory, promote repair and growth of those ligaments to stabilize spinal segments. Different solutions including phenol, guaiacol, tannic acid, and pumice flour, sodium morrhuate, glycerin, and dextrose are used to produce this irritation, but dextrose appears to be the most commonly used. There has been no data to suggest that prolotherapy is better than placebo on its own, but as an adjunct to other therapies, it has shown to be efficacious for low back pain.[95,96]

Epidural steroid injections and selective nerve root blocks are interventional options for the treatment of lumbar radiculopathy or radicular type pain related to radiculitis. These injections are commonly used with fluoroscopy to guide needle location in order to avoid major blood vessels and to allow visualization of the needle tip, but ultrasound and computed tomography are also used. Some practitioners have been trained to perform injections without the use of image guidance and can be appropriate based on the level of expertise of the practitioner and the understanding of anatomical structures of the spine. There are three approaches to achieve epidural delivery of medication and they are interlaminar, caudal, and transforaminal. The interlaminar approach is the placement of the needle in between and through the lamina in the posterior aspect of the lumbar spine. This approach is typically done midline between spinous processes on the interspinous ligament or paramedian to avoid the spinous processes and ligament altogether.[97] The caudal epidural approach is the placement of the needle through the sacral hiatus and sacrococcygeal ligament to access the epidural space from the bottom in the midline.[98] The transforaminal approach is the placement of the needle just below the pedicle, transverse process, and lamina of the vertebral level of interest in order to enter the neuroforamen. With all of these approaches, the medication injected is typically a combination of local anesthetic and corticosteroid. There are many different combinations of injectate and no one combination has been found to be superior to the other. These injections are used for the relief of symptoms and improvement in function, but they can also serve a diagnostic purpose by assessing whether an individual responds to the injections to make the diagnosis of the pain generator nerve root. No relief of pain with injection may suggest that pain is secondary to another source and not a lumbar radiculopathy, but could also imply the medication was not placed near the nerve root to block the impulses. Improvement of the individual's symptoms with an epidural steroid injection or selective nerve root block may indicate that insult to the lumbar nerve roots is responsible for the individual's symptoms, but could be the development of a placebo response.

Facet joints, also known as zygapophyseal joints, can be a major contributor to axial low back pain. In the literature, it has been reported that the prevalence of pain secondary to facet joints is estimated to be 15–40%.[99,100] Facet joints are innervated by the medial branches of the dorsal rami nerves at the level of the nerve root and the level above. Injection of anesthetic agent and steroid into the facet joint capsule or around the dorsal rami medial branches can have a diagnostic purpose when done with a double block protocol. The target site is midway along the linear junction of the superior articular process and the transverse process of the lumbar vertebra or the sacral ala (dorsal rami of Lumbar 5). No relief of pain with injection suggests that pain is secondary to another source or that the medication was not placed on the nerve root. Improvement of the individual's symptoms with facet joint injection or medial branch block may suggest that facet-mediated pain is responsible for the symptoms. Once it is established that the individual's pain is facet-mediated, radiofrequency ablation of the offending medial branches may be performed so that lasting relief can be achieved. Medial branch blocks and radiofrequency ablation are valuable and effective tools in the diagnosis and treatment of facet joint-mediated pain.[101]

Other nonsurgical interventions that can be performed for low back pain are intradiskal electrothermal annuloplasty (IDET), nucleoplasty, radiofrequency annuloplasty (discTRODE), and biacuplasty. Conversely, these procedures are performed for back pain due to an internal disk disruption or contained disk protrusions. Typically, the procedure is done after a provocative diskogram determined the cause of the low back pain. A diskogram can be an important diagnostic tool to help determine if a disk is, in fact, the pain generator, especially if other causes of axial back pain such as the facet and sacroiliac joints have been ruled out. Unfortunately, there is no significant data that radiofrequency of the annulus or biacuplasty improves low back pain caused by internal disk disruption[102] and IDET is sparingly used but has been noted for pain relief with fair success in certain patient populations with diskogenic type pain proven with diskography.[102,103] The concept for IDET is to introduce an intradiskal catheter that uses a coil which causes conductive heating of the annulus, effective denaturing of collagen fibrils, cauterizing granulation tissue, and coagulating nerve fibers.[104]

Kyphoplasty or vertebroplasty is indicated for the treatment of low back pain caused by a vertebral compression fracture of the osteoporotic source. These procedures use a cement, poly-methyl-methacrylate (PMMA), placed through an introducer cannula which goes into the vertebral body. The difference between kyphoplasty and vertebroplasty is that kyphoplasty is attempted to restore the height of the collapsed vertebral body and endplate alignment, whereas a vertebroplasty attempts to stabilize the compression fracture pain. Kyphoplasty procedure uses a balloon tamp and introducer cannula in order to augment the vertebral body and raise the height and align the endplates prior to the placement of the cement. Although these procedures may be used less than they were previously due to a recent study showing no difference between sham treatment and vertebroplasty,[105] they remain a viable option for those patients who are refractory to conservative management but are not candidates for surgery if done within 3 months of onset.[106]

Surgical Procedures

If low back pain sufferers continue to be refractory to the previously mentioned procedures or medical management, surgical interventions are indicated if they have new trauma with spinal instability, bowel or bladder dysfunction, or weakness. Surgical emergent or urgent situations do occur with patients who experience back pain and the healthcare provider should be conscious of changing physical examination or symptoms to indicate the need for spine surgery. Surgical planning will vary depending on symptoms and what anatomical abnormalities are causing those symptoms. Some common indications for an urgent surgical consult include any significant or increasing neurologic deficit, including numbness or weakness, cauda equina syndrome, or trauma causing spinal instability.

Postsurgical Options

Postsurgical back pain, also known as failed back surgery syndrome, is comprised of those individuals who have undergone surgery for back pain and are still experiencing pain. The concept of failed back surgery syndrome is a misnomer because often the surgery can be successful in stabilizing and decompressing the spine as the degenerative process may continue to cause pain at other levels in the spine or due to other structures at the level with previous surgery with scaring. Options for these individuals include more surgery, conservative treatment, implantable devices, such as intrathecal pumps, or neuromodulation. In these cases, more surgery or conservative management often occurs, but placement of an intrathecal pain pump or neuromodulation generator with spinal leads can reduce pain.[107,108] The general concept with spinal cord stimulation of the dorsal columns may impede the transmission of pain signals at the level of the spinal cord to from the periphery to the brain. Neuromodulation may work on the dorsal columns in a manner presented by Melzack and Wall, known as the gate theory.[67] Intrathecal pump placement is done by placing a catheter into the intrathecal space to allow the microdosing of opioid medication for pain treatment.

COMPLICATIONS

Low back pain as a disease process is generally self-limiting and benign, however, from time to time can lead to significant disability. Prolonged pain can lead to functional changes in gait patterns, altering biomechanical stresses in nearby joints, and can influence the development of degenerative changes. Furthermore, individuals may develop neurologic compromise leading to motor and sensory loss depending on the specific etiology (spinal stenosis, spondylosis, or herniated nucleus pulposis causing neuroforaminal narrowing, etc.). It is of utmost importance that the pain physician must be vigilant and circumspect for both cancer and infectious etiologies as possible causes of the patient's symptoms—both can cause significant pain and neurological compromise and warrant a careful history, physical examination, and thorough workup. The specifics about the etiology and workup of the various causes of low back pain have been thoroughly discussed elsewhere in this chapter.

A number of complications can arise following the treatment of low back pain. Therefore, the risks and benefits of any treatment plan must be carefully considered and thoroughly discussed with the patient before initiating any form of treatment. The frequency and rate of complications vary on the type of treatment modality; however, the most worrisome is an infection, vascular or nerve trauma, or intravascular injection of medication, spinal cord injury, seizures, and death.

Myofascial and Ligamentous Interventional Complications

The most basic of interventions for low back pain are the nonspinal myofascial trigger point injections. Trigger point injections are generally considered safe, however, cases of increased pain at the injection site and transient paresthesias associated with local anesthetics have been reported in the literature.[94] Botulinum toxin type A can also be utilized for long-term relief for myofascial low back pain, however, there is a black box warning that must be thoroughly discussed with the patient including the risk of severe anaphylaxis and death due to the possible spread of botulinum toxin outside of the target muscle.[109] Prolotherapy is a treatment technique aimed at strengthening or sclerosing ligaments thought to be contributing to an individual's low back pain. The most common complication after prolotherapy injections is increased pain at the injection site, which is usually temporary.[110,111] Case reports of more serious complications have been reported infrequently in the literature such as death and paraplegia.[112]

Axial Interventional Complications

If the etiology of an individual's pain is determined to be caused by the posterior spinal elements, both intra-articular facet joint injections or medial branch blockade followed by neurolysis can be utilized. Both, when done properly under fluoroscopic guidance, are generally considered safe, however, one must be leery of the epidural or intravascular spread of the injectate which has been reported in up to 8% of patients in the literature.[113] Radiofrequency neurolysis of the medial branch of the primary dorsal rami for lumbar facet-mediated back pain also has a very low incidence of complications. In 2004, Kornick et al. reviewed 616 radiofrequency lesions in 92 individuals and found an overall 1% incidence of minor complications including transient increased localized pain and radicular pain. There were no major complications reported.[114] More recently, Manchikanti performed over 15,000 lumbar medial branch blocks, facet joint injections, and radiofrequency ablations over a 20-month period and found that the incidence of minor complications was 4% for intravascular flow with no incidence of a nerve root or spinal cord trauma, epidural hematoma, or infections.[115] Other procedures such as sacroiliac joint corticosteroid injections and piriformis injections have a similarly low-complication rate, the majority of which are infectious, neural trauma, or drug-related complications.[116] Radiofrequency neurolysis of the S1–S3 lateral branches also has been shown to be a safe and viable option for sacroiliac mediated joint pain. In one smaller randomized-controlled trial, the majority of individuals undergoing the procedure complained of a temporary worsening of pain at 10 days postprocedure and only one patient in the study reported transient gluteal paresthesias. No other major complications were noted.[117]

Intradiskal Interventional Complications

Diskography can be an important diagnostic tool to help determine if a disk is intrinsically painful. The risks associated with the procedure include infection, neural and spinal cord trauma, intravascular injection, and postprocedure diskitis. Frasier in 1987 demonstrated a 2.7% incidence of postprocedure diskitis, which reduced to 0.7% using a stiletted double-needle technique.[118] IDET has been utilized as an alternative to surgical treatment of diskogenic pain confirmed by diskography. Complications associated with this procedure occur relatively infrequently and are most commonly associated with catheter breakage, neural trauma, or postprocedure disk herniation.[119] Other more rare complications have been reported in the literature including vertebral osteonecrosis[120] and cauda equina syndrome.[121]

Epidural Interventional Complications

For radicular low back pain, the most commonly utilized interventional modality is epidural steroid injections. Epidural steroid injections are typically preformed under the utmost of sterile conditions, utilizing both fluoroscopic guidance and a radiopaque dye for confirmation of correct needle placement. There are a number of possible points of entry including transforaminal, intralaminar, and caudal approaches, however, whenever a needle is advanced into the epidural space there is a risk for significant consequences. There have been a few case reports in the literature of infection, abscess, spinal cord injury, and death. The incidence of these more serious complications is difficult to estimate due to the lack of mandatory reporting in the United States and fear of legal ramifications. More recently, there has been an outbreak of fungal meningitis after epidural steroid injection causing 664 infections and 40 deaths in 19 states at the time of this publication. A few of these individuals have gone on to develop an epidural abscess, arachnoiditis, diskitis, and vertebral osteomyelitis. According to the Center for Disease Control, these have been attributed to contaminated steroid medication acquired from a compounding pharmacy.[122]

More commonly, the preponderance of complications is typically self-limited and benign. In 2000, Botwin et al. followed 227 individuals who received 322 lumbar epidural steroid injections. He reported a rate of minor complications of 9.6% per injection, all of which resolved without significant morbidity or mortality. These complications included transient headaches in 3.1%, increased back pain in 2.4%, increased leg pain in 0.6%, facial flushing in 1.2%, vasovagal reaction in 0.3%, increased blood sugar in 0.3%, and hypertension in 0.3%. There were no other major complications noted.[123] More recently, McGrath published data on 2,000 individuals who received over 4,000 lumbar epidural steroid injections over a 7-year period. He found that the rate of minor complications was 6% for intralaminar approach versus 2.1% for transforaminal approach with an overall rate of complications of 2.4%. These complications included increased pain in 1.1%, pain at the injection site 0.33%, and persistent numbness in 0.14% without any other major complications noted.[124]

Many physicians also routinely use aspiration, nonparticulate steroids, and digital subtraction angiography (DSA) to further reduce the incidence of complications, especially those associated with the intravascular injection. However, there has yet to be a single well-designed study demonstrating the superiority or improved safety with the use of nonparticulate steroid or DSA and their overall effectiveness of improving the safety profile of these procedures remains controversial. Furman demonstrated in 2000 that 11.2% of fluoroscopically guided spinal injections result in vascular spread despite negative aspiration. Furthermore, Furman found that the specificity and sensitivity of aspiration to predict intravascular flow was 97.9% and 44.7%, respectively.[125] Okubadejo demonstrated that intravascular injection of particulate steroid has been shown to cause diffuse neurologic injury while intravascular injection of nonparticulate steroid has demonstrated no adverse sequelae.[126]

Implantable Device Complications

For the individuals who continue to have back pain despite both unsuccessful interventional and surgical treatments, implantation of a spinal cord stimulator or an intrathecal drug delivery system remains a viable option. However, the use of these treatment modalities comes with its share of potential complications. In 2005, North demonstrated that nearly one-third of individuals with spinal cord stimulator systems experienced electrode migration, infection, or problems with the stimulator lead.[127] Kumar in 2007 confirmed these findings with an overall complication rate of 32% at 12 months and documented electrode migration in 10%, infection or wound breakdown in

8%, and loss of paresthesia in 7%.[107] Intrathecal drug delivery systems (IDDS) have been used for both chronic cancer and noncancer pain. Paice in 1996 evaluated 419 individuals with intrathecal drug delivery systems and found an overall complication rate of 21.6%.[128] These complications typically include nausea, pruritus, urinary retention, and problems with the catheter itself.[129] More rare complications can include intrathecal granuloma formation and peripheral edema.[130]

PROGNOSIS

The vast majority of individuals with acute low back pain experience resolution of symptoms by 12 weeks without any residual functional deficits or long-term sequelae.[131] The rate of recurrence of low back pain is highly variable in the literature. Rossignol reported 20% reoccurrence by 1 year and 36% by year 3[132] with overall lifetime reoccurrence rates of up to 85%.[133] For the few individuals who transition into chronic pain, return to work rates are inversely proportional to the length of time off work. Less than half of the individuals will return to work after 6 months of disability, fewer than 25% by 1 year, and nearly 0% by 2 years of disability.[134]

Noninterventional Treatment Modality Prognosis

The foundation of most treatment paradigms for low back pain typically involves some form of physiotherapy. It is not within the scope of this section to discuss the outcomes of the various forms of physical therapy, but rather the goal of which is to briefly touch on the general principals. In 2003, Storheim et al. found that exercise therapy was better at reduction of pain and improvement of function than treatment by their primary care provider alone.[135] In 2005, Hayden found that an individualized supervised stretching or strengthening program can improve both pain and function in individuals with subacute or chronic low back pain.[60] Other therapeutic modalities including pillates[136] and yoga[137] have been reported to be beneficial for individuals with chronic low back pain at reducing pain and improving disability, whereas studies of acupuncture[138,139] and aerobic exercise[140] have been less favorable.

Myofascial and Ligamentous Interventional Prognosis

Trigger point injections, both with and without corticosteroids[94] have been found to be superior to placebo for short-term[141] improvement in myofascial low back pain, however, no studies have evaluated long-term outcomes based upon this modality alone.[142] Botulinum toxin injections have also been found to be superior to saline for short-term improvement in myofascial pain and Oswestry Disability Index (ODI) scores at both 3 and 8 weeks, however, these benefits subside by 4–5 months.[143] The evidence behind prolotherapy is lackluster. The majority of randomized-controlled studies in the literature found prolotherapy to be ineffective as a solo treatment of chronic low back pain and the majority of individuals have a short-term increase in their pain and stiffness following injections.[142,144]

Axial Interventional Prognosis

Therapeutic medial branch blocks and less commonly lumbar facet joint injections are utilized for the treatment of facet mediated axial low back pain; however, the actual data regarding their effectiveness is mixed. Carette in 1991 found that there was no difference between steroid and saline facet injections for chronic low back pain at 1 or 3 months, however, by 6 months, the steroid group had significant improvement in their symptoms.[145] Conversely, Mayer et al. found that intra-articular facet steroid injections and a home stretching program were no more beneficial than a home stretching program alone.[146] Recently a small, randomized-controlled trial suggested that the use of repeated intra-articular facet joint injections either with or without steroid for individuals with chronic low back pain demonstrated greater than 50% reduction in pain in individuals at 2 years.[115]

Alternatively, radiofrequency ablation of the medial branch of the primary dorsal rami appears to have more favorable evidence in the literature. Gofeld in 2007 demonstrated that nearly 70% of individuals had a 50–80% reduction in pain for 6–12 months after radiofrequency neurolysis of the medial branch.[147] More recent evidence has emerged that combining radiofrequency ablation with corticosteroid injection of the medial branch demonstrated both long-term improvement in pain and quality of life.[148] For sacroiliac-mediated joint pain either intra-articular corticosteroid injections or radiofrequency ablation of the S1–S3 lateral branches can be considered. Slipman in 2001 documented a significant reduction in pain, improvement in ODI, and return to work rates in individuals undergoing therapeutic sacroiliac joint corticosteroid injections at an average of up to 2 years postprocedure.[149] Radiofrequency ablation of the S1–S3 lateral branches also appears to be a viable option. Cohen demonstrated that 64% of patients at 3 months and 57% at 6 months post-procedure experienced greater than 50% pain relief and significant improvement in function.[117] One recent randomized-controlled trial demonstrated significant improvement in pain, disability, and function at 9 months in nearly 60% of individuals studied.[150]

Intradiskal Interventional Prognosis

For diskogenic pain in carefully selected patient population, IDET may have some utility[142] and reduce the need for surgery.[151] Pauza et al. showed a 2-point pain reduction in 56% of individuals and demonstrated a significant improvement in pain severity and back function compared to sham treatment.[152] In a smaller nonrandomized study, Bogduk reported similar findings with 20% of individuals pain-free at 2 years post-IDET.[153] However, rigorous peer-reviewed double-blind studies are lacking at this time.

Epidural Interventional Prognosis

The data behind lumbar epidural steroid injections echos that of medial branch blocks and facet injections. There have been a number of studies evaluating the effectiveness of epidural steroid injections in the treatment of low back pain which have demonstrated short-term, but not long-term, reduction in acute and subacute pain in individuals with radicular symptoms.[154-156] For chronic, nonradicular low back pain there is some evidence that epidural steroid injections can offer short-term benefits, but show a little long-term reduction in pain or improvement in function.[157,158]

Implantable Device Prognosis

When considering alternatives for reoperation, spinal cord stimulation for postback surgery pain syndrome with persistent radicular pain has been shown to have improved long-term pain relief and reduced opioid use compared to reoperation.[127] Kumar in 2007 compared spinal cord stimulation to conservative care for post back surgery pain syndrome and found that that 48.8% of individuals in the spinal cord stimulator group obtained 50% reduction in pain and experienced a significant improvement in function and treatment satisfaction at 12 months.[107] Intrathecal drug delivery systems for chronic noncancer low back pain also appear to demonstrate long-term improvements in pain, mood, and function.[108] Grider in 2011 demonstrated a significant reduction in VAS pain scores from preimplantation levels which was sustained for at least 12 months when oral opioids were tapered and a 6-week opioid-free period was used prior to implantation.[159]

REFERENCES

1. Freburger J, Holmes GM, Agans RP, et al. The rising prevalence of chronic low back pain. Arch Intern Med. 2009;169(3):251-8.
2. Rubin DI. Epidemiology and risk factors for spine pain. Neurol Clin. 2007;25(2):353-71.
3. Deyo RA, Mirza SK, Martin BI, et al. Back pain prevalence and visit rates: estimates from U.S. National Surveys, 2002. Spine. 2006;31(23):2724-7.
4. Harkness EF, Macfarlane GJ, Silman AJ, et al. Is musculoskeletal pain more common now than 40 years ago? Two population-based cross-sectional studies. Rheumatology (Oxford). 2005;44(7):890-5.
5. Elders L, Burdorf A. Prevalence, incidence, and recurrence of low back pain in scaffolders during a 3-year follow-up study. Spine. 2004;29(6):E101-6.
6. Hoy D, Brooks P, Blyth F, et al. The epidemiology of low back pain. Best Practice Res Clin Rheumatol. 2010;24:769-81.
7. Joud A, Petersson IF, Englund M. Low back pain: epidemiology of consultations. Arthritis Care Res. 2012;64(7):1084-8.
8. Rossignol M, Rozenberg S, Leclerc A. Epidemiology of low back pain: what's new? Joint Bone Spine. 2009;76:608-13.
9. Deyo RA. Nonsurgical care of low back pain. Neurosurg Clin North Am. 1991;2:851-62.
10. Burton AK, Clarke RD, McClune TD, et al. The natural history of LBP in adolescents. Spine. 1996;21:2323-8.
11. Anderson GBJ. The epidemiology of spinal disorders. In: Frymoyer JW (Ed). The Adult Spine: Principles and Practice, 2nd edition. New York: Raven Press; 1997. pp. 93-141.
12. Loney PL, Stratford PW. The prevalence of low back pain in adults: a methodological review of the literature. Phys Ther. 1999;79(4):384-96.
13. Lawrence RC, Helmick CG, Arnett FC, et al. Estimates of the prevalence of arthritis and selected musculoskeletal disorders in the United States. Arthritis Rheum. 1998;41(5):778-99.
14. Dionne CE, Dunn KM, Croft PR, et al. Does back pain prevalence really decrease with increasing age? A systematic review. Age Ageing. 2006;35(3):229-34.
15. Jeffries LJ, Milanese SF, Grimmer-Somers KA, et al. Epidemiology of adolescent spinal pain: a systematic overview of the research literature. Spine. 2007;32(23):2630-7.
16. Grimmer K, Nyland L, Milanese S, et al. Longitudinal investigation of low back pain in Australian adolescents: a five year study. Physiother Res Int. 2006;11(3):161-72.
17. Carey TS, Evans A, Hadler N, et al. Care-seeking among individuals with chronic low back pain. Spine. 1995;30:312-7.

18. Carey TS, Evans AT, Hadler NM, et al. Acute severe low back pain: a population-based study of prevalence and care-seeking. Spine. 1996;21:339-44.
19. Roland MO. The natural history of back pain. The Practitioner. 1983;227(1381):1119-22.
20. Van den Hoogen, Koes BW, van Eijk JTM, et al. On the course of low back pain in general practice: a one year follow up study. Annals Rheum Dis. 1998;57(1):13-9.
21. Von Korff M, Deyo RA, Cherkin D, et al. Back pain in primary care. Outcomes at 1 year. Spine. 1993;18(7):855-62.
22. Hestbaek L, Leboeuf-Yde C, Manniche C, et al. Low back pain: what is the long-term course? A review of studies of general patient populations. Eur Spine J. 2003;12(2):149-65.
23. van Tulder M, Koes B, Bombardier C, et al. Low back pain. Best Pract Res Clin Rheumatol. 2002;16(5):761-75.
24. Cassidy JD, Côté P, Carroll LJ, et al. Incidence and course of low back pain episodes in the general population. Spine. 2005;30(24):2817-23.
25. Chenot JF, Becker A, Leonhardt C, et al. Sex differences in presentation, course, and management of low back pain in primary care. Clin J Pain. 2008;24(7):578-84.
26. Pengel LH, Herbert RD, Maher CG, et al. Acute low back pain: systematic review of its prognosis. BMJ. 2003;327(7410):323.
27. Lidgren L. The bone and joint decade 2000-2010. Bull World Health Organization. 2003;81(9):629.
28. Guo HR, Tanaka S, Halperin WE, et al. Back pain prevalence in US industry and estimates of lost workdays. Am J Public Health. 1999;89(7):1029-35.
29. Wasiak R, Kim J, Pransky G. Work disability and costs caused by recurrence of low back pain: longer and more costly than in first episodes. Spine. 2006;31(2):219-25.
30. Bigos S, Bowyer O, Braen G, et al. Acute Low Back Problems in Adults. Clinical Practice Guideline No. 14. AHCPR Publication No. 95-0642. Rockville, MD: Agency for Health Care Policy and Research, Public Health Service, U.S. Department of Health and Human Services; 1994.
31. Steenstra IA, Verbeek JH, Heymans MW, et al. Prognostic factors for duration of sick leave in patients sick listed with acute low back pain: a systematic review of the literature. Occup Environ Med. 2005;62(12):851-60.
32. Kent PM, Keating JL. The epidemiology of low back pain in primary care. Chiropr Osteopat. 2005;13:13.
33. Thelin A, Holmberg S, Thelin N. Functioning in neck and low back pain from a 12-year perspective: a prospective population-based study. J Rehabil Med. 2008;40(7):555-61.
34. Luo X, Pietrobon R, Sun SX, et al. Estimates and patterns of direct health care expenditures among individuals with back pain in the United States. Spine. 2004;29(1):79-86.
35. Kopec JA, Sayre EC, Esdaile JM, et al. Predictors of back pain in a general population cohort. Spine. 2004;29(1):70-7.
36. Waxman R, Tennant A, Helliwell P, et al. A prospective follow-up study of low back pain in the community. Spine. 2000;25(16):2085-90.
37. Reisbord LS, Greenland S. Factors associated with self-reported back-pain prevalence: a population-based study. J Chronic Dis. 1985;38(8):691-702.
38. Dionne CE, Von Korff M, Koepsell TD, et al. Formal education and back pain: a review. J Epidemiol Commun Health. 2001;55(7):455-68.
39. Heistaro S, Vartiainen E, Heliövaara M, et al. Trends of back pain in eastern Finland, 1972-1992, in relation to socioeconomic status and behavioral risk factors. Am J Epidemiol. 1998;148(7):671-82.
40. Croft PR, Rigby AS. Socioeconomic influences on back problems in the community in Britain. J Epidemiol Commun Health. 1994;48(2):166-70.
41. Matsui H, Maeda A, Tsuji H, et al. Risk indicators of low back pain among workers in Japan: association of familial and physical factors with low back pain. Spine. 1997;22(11):1242-8.
42. Hoogendoorn WE, van Poppel MN, Bongers PM, et al. Systematic review of psychosocial factors at work and private life as risk factors for back pain. Spine. 2000;25(16):2114-25.
43. Linton SJ. Occupational psychological factors increase the risk for back pain: a systemic review. J Occup Rehabil. 2001;11(1):53-66.
44. Vogt MT Lauerman WC, Chirumbole M, et al. A community-based study of postmenopausal white women with back and leg pain: health status and limitations in physical activity. J Gerontol Ser A Biol Sci Med Sci. 2002;57(8):M544-50.
45. Webb R, Brammah T, Lunt M, et al. Prevalence and predictors of intense, chronic, and disabling neck and back pain in the UK general population. Spine. 2003;28(11):1195-202.
46. Roshan M, Rao AP. A study on relative contributions of the history, physical examination and investigations in making medical diagnosis. J Assoc Phys India. 2000;48(8):771-5.
47. Forst SL, Wheeler MT, Fortin JD, et al. The sacroiliac joint: anatomy, physiology and clinical significance. Pain Physician. 2006;9(1):61-7.
48. Hansen HC, McKenzie-Brown AM, Cohen SP, et al. Sacroiliac joint interventions: a systematic review. Pain Physician. 2007;10(1):165-84.
49. Stone JA, Bartynski WS. Treatment of facet and sacroiliac joint arthropathy: steroid injections and radiofrequency ablation. Tech Vasc Interv Radiol. 2009;12(1):22-32.
50. White AA 3rd, Gordon SL. Synopsis: workshop on idiopathic low-back pain. Spine. 1982;7(2):141-9.
51. Boden SD, Wiesel SW. Lumbar spine imaging: role in clinical decision making. J Am Acad Orthop Surg. 1996;4(5):238-48.
52. Boden SD. The use of radiographic imaging studies in the evaluation of patients who have degenerative disorders of the lumbar spine. J Bone Joint Surg Am. 1996;78(1):114-24.
53. Boden SD, Davis DO, Dina TS, et al. Abnormal magnetic-resonance scans of the lumbar spine in asymptomatic subjects. A prospective investigation. J Bone Joint Surg. 1990;72-A:403-8.
54. Jensen MC, Brant-Zawadzki MN, Obuchowski N, et al. Magnetic resonance imaging of the lumbar spine in people without back pain. New Engl J Med. 1994;331(2):69-73.

55. Nardin RA, Patel MR, Gudas TF, et al. Electromyography and magnetic resonance imaging in the evaluation of radiculopathy. Muscle Nerve. 1999;22(2):151-5.
56. Holt EP Jr. The question of lumbar discography. J Bone Joint Surg Am. 1968;50(4):720-6.
57. Walsh TR, Weinstein JN, Spratt KF, et al. Lumbar discography in normal subjects. A controlled, prospective study. J Bone Joint Surg Am. 1990;72(7):1081-8.
58. Carragee EJ, Tanner CM, Khurana S, et al. The rates of false-positive lumbar discography in select patients without low back symptoms. Spine. 2000;25(11):1373-80, discussion 1381.
59. Hayden JA, van Tulder MW, Malmivaara A, et al. Exercise therapy for treatment of non-specific low back pain. Cochrane Database Syst Rev. 2005;(3):CD000335.
60. Hayden JA, van Tulder MW, Tomlinson G. Systematic review: strategies for using exercise therapy to improve outcomes in chronic low back pain. Ann Intern Med. 2005;142(9):776-85.
61. Swenson C, Swärd L, Karlsson J. Cryotherapy in sports medicine. Scand J Med Sci Sports. 1996;6(4):193-200.
62. Knutsson E, Mattsson E. Effects of local cooling on monosynaptic reflexes in man. Scand J Rehabil Med. 1969;1(3):126-32.
63. Lehman JF, Silverman DR, Baum BA, et al. Temperature distributions in the human thigh, produced by infrared, hot pack and microwave applications. Arch Phys Med Rehabil. 1966;47(5):291-9.
64. Lehman JF, DeLateur BJ, Sonebridge JB, et al. Therapeutic temperature distributions produced by ultrasound as modified by dosage and volume of tissue exposed. Arch Phys Med Rehabil. 1967:48(12):662-6.
65. Lehman JF, Guy AW, DeLateur BJ, et al. Heating patterns produced by shortwave diathermy using helical induction coil applicators. Arch Phys Med Rehabil. 1968;49(4):193-8.
66. Mitragotri S, Blankschtein D, Langer, R. Transdermal drug delivery using low-frequency sonophoresis. Pharm Res. 1996;13:411-20.
67. Melzack R, Wall PD. Pain mechanisms: a new theory. Science. 1965;50:971-9.
68. Cheng RS, Pomeranz B. Electroacupuncture analgesia could be mediated by at least two pain relieving mechanisms; endorphin and non-endorphin systems. Life Sci. 1979;25(23):1957-62.
69. Furlan AD, Imamura M, Dryden T, et al. Massage for low-back pain. Cochrane Database Syst Rev. 2008;(4):CD001929.
70. Judovich BD. Lumbar traction therapy: elimination of physical factors that prevent lumbar stretch. JAMA. 1955;159:549-50.
71. Moustafa IM, Diab AA. Extension traction treatment for patients with discogenic lumbosacral radiculopathy: a randomized controlled trial. Clin Rehabil. 2013;27(1):51-62.
72. Farabaugh RJ, Dehen MD, Hawk C. Management of chronic spine-related conditions: consensus recommendations of a multidisciplinary panel. J Manipulative Physiol Ther. 2010;33(7):484-92.
73. Assendelft WJ, Morton SC, Yu EL, et al. Spinal manipulative therapy for low back pain. Cochrane Database Syst Rev. 2004;(1):CD000447.
74. Jellema P, van Tulder MW, van Poppel MN, et al. Lumbar supports for prevention and treatment of low back pain: a systematic review within the framework of the Cochrane Back Review Group. Spine. 2001;26:377-86.
75. Lantz SA, Schultz AB. Lumbar spine orthosis wearing. II. Effect on trunk muscle myoelectric activity. Spine. 1986;11(8):838-42.
76. Blanda J, Bethem D, Moats W, et al. Defects of pars interarticularis in athletes: a protocol for nonoperative treatment. J Spinal Disord. 1993;6:406-11.
77. Steiner ME, Micheli LJ. Treatment of symptomatic spondylolysis and spondylolisthesis with the modified Boston brace. Spine. 1985;10:937-43.
78. Berman B, Langevin HM, Witt CM, et al. Acupuncture for chronic low back pain. New Engl J Med. 2010;363:454-61.
79. Yuan J, Purepong N, Kerr DP, et al. Effectiveness of acupuncture for low back pain: a systematic review. Spine. 2008;33:E887-900.
80. Rubinstein SM, van Middelkoop M, Kuijpers T, et al. A systematic review on the effectiveness of complementary and alternative medicine for chronic non-specific low-back pain. Eur Spine J. 2010;19(8):1213-28.
81. Singh G, Ramey D, Morfeld D, et al. Gastrointestinal tract complications of nonsteroidal anti-inflammatory drug treatment in rheumatoid arthritis. A prospective observational cohort study. Arch Intern Med. 1996;156:1530-6.
82. Cashman JN. The mechanisms of action of NSAIDs in analgesia. Drugs. 1996;52(l5):13-23.
83. Larsen AM, Polson J, Fontana RJ, et al. Acute liver failure study group. Acetaminophen-induced acute liver failure: results of a United States multicenter, prospective study. Hepatology. 2005;42(6):1364-72.
84. Curhan GC, Knight EL, Rosner B, et al. Lifetime nonnarcotic analgesic use and decline in renal function in women. Arch Intern Med. 2004;164(14):1519-24.
85. van Tulder MW, Touray T, Furlan AD, et al. Muscle relaxants for nonspecific low back pain: a systematic review within the framework of the cochrane collaboration. Spine. 2003;28(17):1978-92.
86. Thorpe AJ, Offord J. The alpha2-delta protein: an auxiliary subunit of voltage-dependent calcium channels as a recognized drug target. Curr Opin Investig Drugs. 2010;11(7):761-70.
87. Finnerup NB, Otto M, Jensen TS, et al. An evidence-based algorithm for the treatment of neuropathic pain. Med Gen Med. 2007;9(2):36.
88. Dworkin RH, O'Connor AB, Audette J, et al. Recommendations for the pharmacological management of neuropathic pain: an overview and literature update. Mayo Clin Proc. 2010;85(Suppl 3):S3-14.
89. Ballantyne JC, Mao J. Opioid therapy for chronic pain. New Eng J Med. 2003;349:1943-53.

90. Pasternak GW. Incomplete cross tolerance and multiple mu opioid peptide receptors. Trends Pharmacol Sci. 2001;22(2):67-70.
91. Rowbotham MC, Fields HL. Topical lidocaine reduces pain in post-herpetic neuralgia. Pain. 1989;38(3):297-301.
92. Mason L, Moore RA, Derry S, et al. Systematic review of topical capsaicin for the treatment of chronic pain. BMJ. 2004;328(7446):991.
93. Nahit ES, Hunt IM, Lunt M, et al. Effects of psychosocial and individual psychological factors on the onset of musculoskeletal pain: common and site-specific effects. Ann Rheum Dis. 2003;62:755-60.
94. Garvey T, Marks M, Wiesel S. A prospective, randomized, double-blind evaluation of trigger-point injection therapy for low-back pain. Spine. 1989;14:962-4.
95. Klein RG, Eek BC, DeLong WB, et al. A randomized double-blind trial of dextrose-glycerine-phenol injections for chronic, low back pain. J Spinal Disord. 1993;6(1):23-33.
96. Ongley MJ, Klein RG, Dorman TA, et al. A new approach to the treatment of chronic low back pain. Lancet. 1987;2(8551):143-6.
97. Manchikanti L, Singh V, Cash KA, et al. The role of fluoroscopic interlaminar epidural injections in managing chronic pain of lumbar disc herniation or radiculitis: a randomized, double-blind trial. Pain Pract. 2013;13(7):547-58.
98. Murakibhavi VG, Khemka AG. Caudal epidural steroid injection: a randomized controlled trial. Evid Based Spine Care J. 2011;2(4):19-26.
99. Schwarzer AC, Aprill CN, Derby R, et al. Clinical features of patients with pain stemming from the lumbar zygapophysial joints. Is the lumbar facet syndrome a clinical entity? Spine. 1994;19:1132-7.
100. Schwarzer AC, Wang S, Bogduk N, et al. Prevalence and clinical features of lumbar zygapophysial joint pain: a study in an Australian population with chronic low back pain. Ann Rheum Dis. 1995;54:100-66.
101. Cohen SP, Huang JH, Brummett C. Facet joint pain-advances in patient selection and treatment. Nat Rev Rheumatol. 2013;9(2):101-16.
102. Helm IS, Deer TR, Manchikanti L, et al. Effectiveness of thermal annular procedures in treating discogenic low back pain. Pain Physician. 2012;15(3):E279-304.
103. Kapural L, Hayek S, Malak O, et al. Intradiscal thermal annuloplasty versus intradiscal radiofrequency ablation for the treatment of discogenic pain: a prospective matched control trial. Pain Med. 2005;6(6):425-31.
104. Kloth DS, Fenton DS, Andersson GB, et al. Intradiscal electrothermal therapy (IDET) for the treatment of discogenic low back pain: patient selection and indications for use. Pain Physician. 2008;11(5):659-68.
105. Buchbinder R, Osborne RH, Ebeling PR, et al. A randomized trial of vertebroplasty for painful osteoporotic vertebral fractures. New Engl J Med. 2009;361(6):557-68.
106. Alexandru D, So W. Evaluation and management of vertebral compression fractures. Perm J. 2012;16(4):46-51.
107. Kumar K, Taylor RS, Jacques L, et al. Spinal cord stimulation versus conventional medical management for neuropathic pain: a multicentre randomized controlled trial in patients with failed back surgery syndrome. Pain. 2007;132(1):179-88.
108. Thimineur MA, Kravitz E, Vodapally MS. Intrathecal opioid treatment for chronic non-malignant pain: a 3-year prospective study. Pain. 2004;109(3):242-9.
109. Li M, Goldberger BA, Hopkins C. Fatal case of BOTOX-related anaphylaxis? J Forensic Sci. 2005;50:169-72.
110. Hunt WE, Baird WC. Complications following injections of sclerosing agent to precipitate fibro-osseous proliferation. J Neurosurg. 1961;18:461-5.
111. Kim SR, Stitik TP, Foye PM, et al. Critical review of prolotherapy for osteoarthritis, low back pain, and other musculoskeletal conditions: a physiatric perspective. Am J Phys Med Rehabil. 2004;83(5):379-89.
112. Schneider RC, Williams JL, Liss L. Fatality after injection of sclerosing agent to precipitate fibro-osseous proliferation. JAMA. 1959;170:1768-72.
113. Dreyfuss P, Schwarzer A, Lau P, et al. Specificity of lumbar medial branch and L5 dorsal ramus blocks: a computed tomography study. Spine. 1997;22(8):895-902.
114. Kornick C, Kramarich S, Lamer T, et al. Complications of lumbar facet radiofrequency denervation. Spine. 2004;29(12):1352-4.
115. Manchikanti L, Singh PV, Falco FJ, et al. Evaluation of lumbar facet joint nerve blocks in managing chronic low back pain: a randomized, double-blind, controlled trial with a 2-year follow-up. Int J Med Sci. 2010;7(3):124-35.
116. Manchikanti L, Staats PS, Singh PV, et al. Evidence-based practice guidelines for interventional techniques in the management of chronic spinal pain. Pain Physician. 2003;6(1):3-81.
117. Cohen SP, Hurley RW, Buckenmaier CC 3rd, et al. Randomized placebo-controlled study evaluating lateral branch radiofrequency denervation for sacroiliac joint pain. Anesthesiology. 2008;109(2):279-88.
118. Fraser RD, Osti OL, Vernon-Roberts B. Discitis after discography. J Bone Joint Surg. 1987;69(1):26-35.
119. Saal JA, Wetzel FT, Saal JS, et al. IDET related complications: a multi-center study of 1,675 treated patients with a review of the FDA MDR data base. Proceedings of the North American Spine Society, 16th Annual Meeting, Seattle; 2001. pp. 187-9.
120. Scholl BM, Theiss SM, Lopez-Ben R, et al. Vertebral osteonecrosis related to intradiscal electrothermal therapy: a case report. Spine. 2003;28(9):161-4.
121. Hsia AW, Isaac K, Katz JS. Cauda equina syndrome from intradiscal electrothermal therapy. Neurology. 2000;55:320.
122. Centers for Disease Control and Prevention. (2012). Multistate Fungal Meningitis Outbreak Investigation. [online] Available from https://www.cdc.gov/hai/outbreaks/meningitis.html [Last Accessed August 2019].

123. Botwin KP, Gruber RD, Bouchlas CG, et al. Complications of fluoroscopically guided transforaminal lumbar epidural injections. Arch Phys Med Rehabil. 2000;81:1045-50.
124. McGrath JM, Schaefer MP, Malkamaki DM. Incidence and characteristics of complications from epidural steroid injections. Pain Med. 2011;12(5):726-31.
125. Furman MB, O'Brien EM, Zgleszewski TM. Incidence of intravascular penetration in transforaminal lumbosacral epidural steroid injections. Spine. 2000;25:2628-32.
126. Okubadejo GO, Talcott MR, Schmidt RE, et al. Perils of intravascular methylprednisolone injection into the vertebral artery. An animal study. J Bone Joint Surg Am. 2008;90:1932-8.
127. North RB, Kidd DH, Farrokhi F, et al. Spinal cord stimulation versus repeated lumbosacral spine surgery for chronic pain: a randomized, controlled trial. Neurosurgery. 2005; 56:98-107.
128. Paice J, Penn R, Shott S. Intraspinal morphine for chronic pain: a retrospective, multicenter study. J Pain Symptom Manage. 1996;11:71-80.
129. Turner JA, Sears JM, Loeser JD. Programmable intrathecal opioid delivery systems for chronic noncancer pain: a systematic review of effectiveness and complications. Clin J Pain. 2007;23(2):180-95.
130. Patel VB, Manchikanti L, Singh V, et al. Systematic review of intrathecal infusion systems for long-term management of chronic non-cancer pain. Pain Physician. 2009;12(2):345-60.
131. Andersson GBJ, Svensson HO, Oden A. The intensity of work recovery in low back pain. Spine. 1983;8:880-4.
132. Rossignol M, Suissa S, Abenhaim L. Working disability due to occupational back pain: three-year follow-up of 2300 compensated workers in Quebec. J Occup Med. 1988;30:502-5.
133. Valkenburg HA, Haanen HCM. The epidemiology of low back pain. In: White AA, Gordon SL (Eds). Symposium on Idiopathic Low Back Pain. St Louis: Mosby; 1982. pp. 9-22.
134. Spitzer WO, LeBlanc FE, Dupuis M, et al. Scientific approach to the assessment and management of activity-related spinal disorders: a monograph for clinicians. Report of the Quebec Task Force on Spinal Disorders. Spine. 1987;12:S1-59.
135. Storheim K, Brox JI, Holm I, et al. Intensive group training versus cognitive intervention in sub-acute low back pain: short-term results of a single-blind randomized controlled trial. J Rehabil Med. 2003;35(3):132-40.
136. Rydeard R, Leger A, Smith D. Pilates-based therapeutic exercise: effect on subjects with nonspecific chronic low back pain and functional disability: a randomized controlled trial. J Orthop Sports Phys Ther. 2006;36(7):472-84.
137. Sherman KJ, Cherkin DC, Erro J, et al. Comparing yoga, exercise, and a self-care book for chronic low back pain. Ann Intern Med. 2005;143(12):849-56.
138. Cherkin DC, Eisenberg D, Sherman K, et al. Randomized trial comparing traditional Chinese medical acupuncture, therapeutic massage, and self-care education for chronic low back pain. Arch Intern Med. 2001;161(8):1081-8.
139. Cherkin DC, Sherman KJ, Avins AL, et al. A randomized trial comparing acupuncture, simulated acupuncture, and usual care for chronic low back pain. Arch Inter Med. 2009;169(9):858-66.
140. Chan CW, Mok NW, Yeung EW. Aerobic exercise training in addition to conventional physiotherapy for chronic low back pain: a randomized controlled trial. Arch Phys Med Rehabil. 2011;92(10):1681-5.
141. Sonne M, Chirstensen K, Hansen S, et al. Injection of steroids and local anaesthetics as therapy for low-back pain. Scand J Rheum. 1985;14:343-5.
142. Chou R, Loeser J, Owens D. Interventional therapies, surgery, and interdisciplinary rehabilitation for low back pain an evidence-based clinical practice guideline from the American Pain Society. Spine. 2011;34(10)1066-77.
143. Foster L, Clapp L, Erickson M, et al. Botulinum toxin A and chronic low back pain: a randomized, double-blind study. Neurology. 2001;56:1290-3.
144. Dechow E, Davies RK, Carr AJ, et al. A randomized, double-blind, placebo-controlled trial of sclerosing injections in patients with chronic low back pain. Rheumatology. 1999;38:1255-9.
145. Carette S, Marcoux S, Truchon R, et al. A controlled trial of corticosteroid injections into facet joints for chronic low back pain. N Engl J Med. 1991;325:1002-7.
146. Mayer TG, Gatchel RJ, Keeley J, et al. A randomized clinical trial of treatment for lumbar segmental rigidity. Spine. 2004;29:2199-205.
147. Gofeld M, Michael J, Faclier G. Radiofrequency denervation of the lumbar zygapophysial joints: 10-year prospective clinical audit. Pain Physician. 2007;10(2):291-300.
148. Chinmoy R, Nilay C, Sudeshna G, et al. Efficacy of combined treatment with medial branch radiofrequency neurotomy and steroid block in lumbar facet joint arthropathy. J Vasc Interv Radiol. 2012;23(12):1659-64.
149. Slipman CW, Lipetz JS, Plastaras CT, et al. Fluoroscopically guided therapeutic sacroiliac joint injections for sacroiliac joint syndrome. Am J Phys Med Rehabil. 2001;80(6): 425-32.
150. Patel N, Gross A, Brown L, et al. A randomized, placebo-controlled study to assess the efficacy of lateral branch neurotomy for chronic sacroiliac joint pain. Pain Med. 2012;13(3):383-98.
151. Andersson GBJ, Mekhail NA, Block JE. Treatment of intractable discogenic low back pain: a systematic review of spinal fusion and intradiscal electrothermal therapy (IDET). Pain Physician. 2006;9(3):237-48.
152. Pauza KJ, Howell S, Dreyfuss P, et al. A randomized, placebo-controlled trial of intradiscal electrothermal therapy for the treatment of discogenic low back pain. Spine. 2004;4:27-35.

153. Bogduk N, Karasek M. Two-year follow-up of a controlled trial of intradiscal electrothermal anuloplasty for chronic low back pain resulting from internal disc disruption. Spine. 2002;2:343-50.
154. Karppinen J, Malmivaara A, Kurunlahti M, et al. Periradicular infiltration for sciatica: a randomized controlled trial. Spine. 2001;26:1059-67.
155. Arden NK, Price C, Reading I, et al. A multicenter randomized controlled trial of epidural corticosteroid injections for sciatica. Rheumatology. 2005;44:1399-406.
156. Wilson-MacDonald J, Burt G, Griffin D, et al. Epidural steroid injection for nerve root compression. A randomized, controlled trial. J Bone Joint Surg Br. 2005;87:352-5.
157. Resnick D, Choudhri T, Dailey A, et al. Guidelines for the performance of fusion procedures for degenerative disease of the lumbar spine. Part 13: injection therapies, low-back pain, and lumbar fusion. J Neurosurg Spine. 2005;2:707-15.
158. Ng L, Chaudhary N, Sell P. The efficacy of corticosteroids in periradicular infiltration for chronic radicular pain. A randomized, double-blind, controlled trial. Spine. 2005;30:857-62.
159. Grider JS, Harned ME, Etscheidt MA. Patient selection and outcomes using a low-dose intrathecal opioid trialing method for chronic nonmalignant pain. Pain Physician. 2011;14(4):343-51.

CHAPTER 35

CHAPTER 36 Lumbar Disk Herniation

Perry Dhaliwal, Ajit A Krishnaney

INTRODUCTION

Within the spectrum of degenerative disk changes, lumbar disk herniations represent fragments of nucleus pulposus, cartilage, osteophytes or annulus that have escaped beyond the confines of the disk space. These fragments may remain in continuity with the remainder of the disk or they may be seen as completely separate fragments within the spinal canal. Given their location in the spinal canal, lumbar disk herniations may cause a constellation of symptoms. Many patients will be asymptomatic, some will present with back or leg pain and some will present with severe chronic pain syndromes. Here we review the presentation, natural history, and management of lumbar disk herniations.

EPIDEMIOLOGY AND NATURAL HISTORY

Though lumbar disk herniations account for significant pain and disability, there is very limited data on the incidence and prevalence of the disease. It is estimated that the lifetime prevalence of lumbar radiculopathy in both males and females is approximately 3–5%.[1] The etiological factors that predispose patients to acute lumbar disk herniations are also not clear. In one study, common factors thought to be related to precipitation of degenerative disk disease were assessed in twins.[2] Factors such as occupation, exercise, sitting, lifting, twisting, trauma, and smoking were assessed. None of these factors seemed to be associated with significantly increased disk degeneration. This study suggested that genetic factors may play a significant role in the development of degenerative disk disease. Similarly, a Danish study that assessed genetic predisposition to developing low back pain suggested that in later life, genetic factors are more important than environmental factors in the development of back pain and degenerative disk diseases.[3] However, in several other studies,[4-6] examining the role of occupational exposures, there is conflicting evidence whether individuals with jobs requiring repetitive heavy lifting were more likely to have symptomatic lumbar disk herniations. Needless to say, there is a complex interplay between environmental and genetic factors that may predispose certain individuals to symptomatic lumbar disk herniations.

There have been many retrospective and prospective studies that have examined the natural history of lumbar disk herniations. In very early studies, radiological and autopsy studies confirmed the presence of degenerative disk disease in both symptomatic and asymptomatic adult patients.[7,8] Indeed, degenerative disk disease was seen in over 90% of patients over 40 years of age and was very clearly associated with increasing age. Early studies also alluded to the fact that the majority of patients will have resolution of their pain symptoms over time without any surgical intervention. In one study,[9] 165 patients with lumbar radiculopathy secondary to a lumbar disk herniation were followed over time. Each patient received aggressive conservative therapy with epidural steroid injections. Of these, only 23 patients required surgery whereas the majority of patients made a successful recovery over time. Similarly, another study[10] involving 64 patients with confirmed lumbar disk herniation and clinical signs and symptoms of lumbar radiculopathy were followed over time. Of these patients, 90% recovered over the course of the study. Weber et al.[11] performed serial evaluations on 208 patients who presented within 2 weeks of having symptomatic lumbar radiculopathy. Patients were placed on bed rest for 1 week after which they were allowed to resume activity. The patients were evaluated for pain and functional outcomes. Interestingly, they noted that 70% of patients would have resolution of their symptoms within 4 weeks without any intervention. Early studies such as these suggested that many patients, whether symptomatic or asymptomatic, have disk herniations and of those that are symptomatic, the majority will go on to recover without surgical intervention. These studies also reinforce the need for at least 4 weeks of observation in these patients given that most patients will have spontaneous resolution of their symptoms within the first month.

WORKUP

Symptoms and Signs

A thorough history and physical examination are crucial in establishing a diagnosis of acute radiculopathy secondary to a lumbar disk herniation. A complete history strives to exclude common mimics such as osteoarthritis of the hip, hip bursitis, iliotibial band syndrome, piriformis syndrome, and peripheral neuropathies as well as more concerning pathology such as traumatic or pathologic fractures and diskitis or osteomyelitis.

A patient with lumbar radiculopathy secondary to lumbar disk herniation will commonly present with an acute episode of sharp lancinating pain that radiates down the lower extremity. The pain is often exacerbated by sitting or standing and is often relieved by lying in a recumbent position. In contrast, patients with an underlying neoplastic or infectious process will often have exacerbation of their radiculopathy when recumbent. In those patients with lumbar disk herniation, the patient may have felt the pain with flexion and rotational movements though the onset may be completely spontaneous. In addition to pain, patients may develop numbness and weakness in a particular dermatome (Fig. 1) and myotome. The location

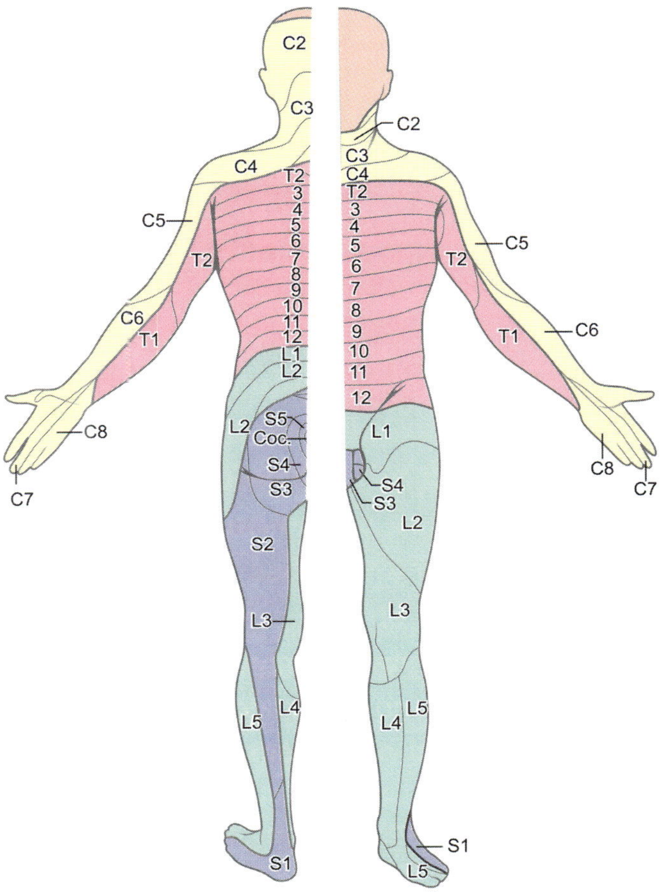

Fig. 1: Map of human dermatomes.

of the pain, numbness or weakness will depend on which nerve root is under compression (Table 1). It should be noted that the nerve root may be compressed at any point along its path from the conus medullaris down through the thecal sac and as it exits out the foramen. This has bearing on the radiological diagnosis since one must consider the possibility that the nerve root may be compressed by a

Table 1: Clinical examination findings in single nerve root radiculopathies.

Root	*Pain*	*Motor weakness*	*Sensory changes*	*Reflexes*
L1	Inguinal region	Hip flexors	Scrotum	-
L2,3,4	Anterior or medial thigh, medial leg	Knee extension	Anterior or medial thigh, medial leg	Patellar tendon
L5	Back, buttock, lateral thigh, lateral leg, dorsum of foot, great toe	Foot dorsiflexion, EHL extension	Lateral leg, dorsal web space between first and second toe	Semitendinosus (internal hamstring)
S1	Back, buttock, posterior aspect of thigh and calf, sole of foot	Hip extension, knee flexion, plantar flexion of foot	Posterior calf, lateral or plantar surface of foot	Achilles tendon
S2,3,4	Sacral or buttock pain, perineal region	Fecal and urinary incontinence	Medial buttock, perineal region	Bulbocavernosus reflex

(EHL: extensor hallucis longus)

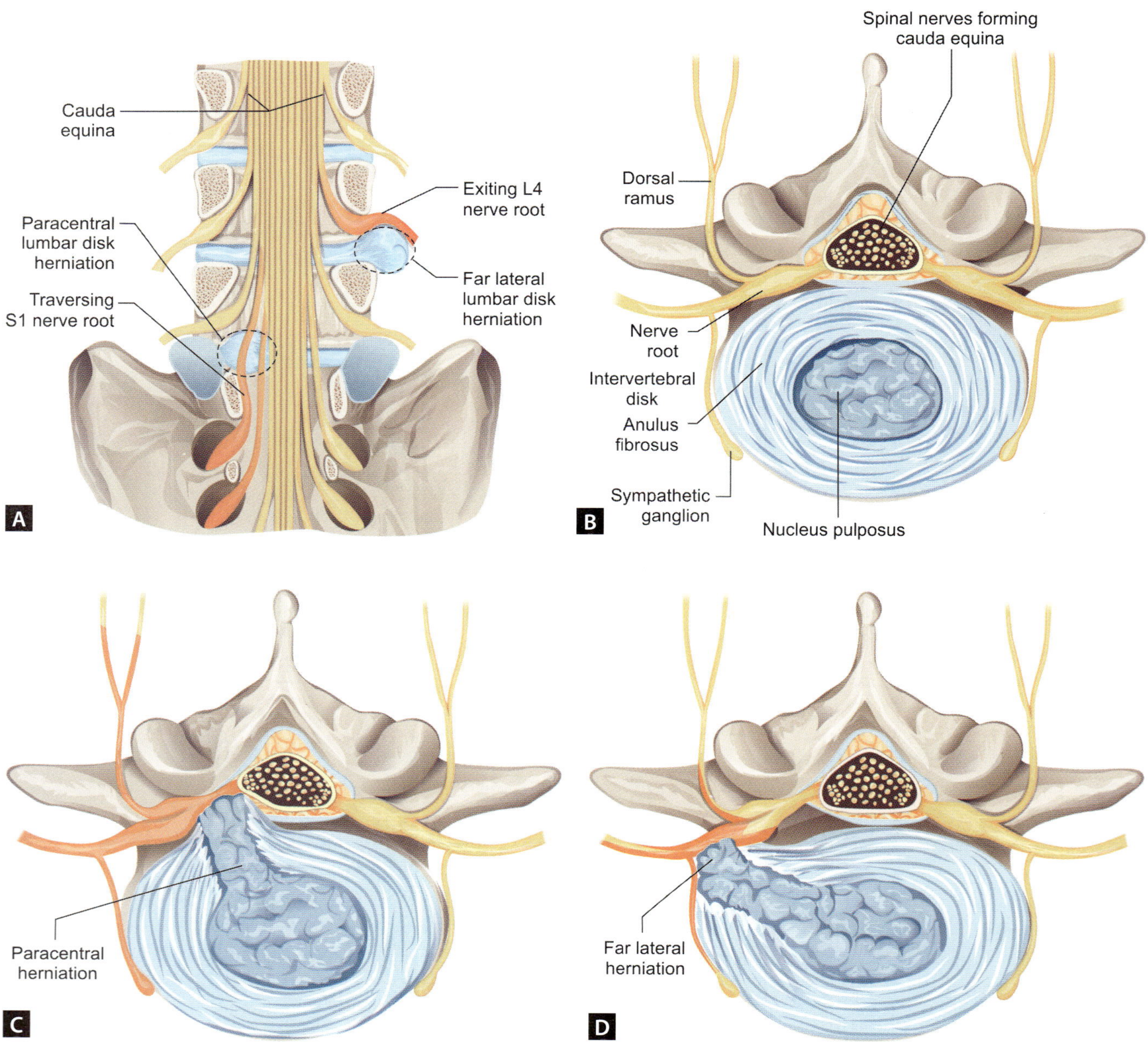

Figs. 2A to D: (A) Coronal view of nerve roots with dura removed. Note that the nerve root may be compressed by either a paracentral disk herniation or a far lateral disk herniation. Thus, when nerve root compression is suspected, one must carefully evaluate the radiological imaging to elucidate the cause of compression. Cross-section of spine at the level of the lumbar intervertebral disk demonstrating normal anatomy (B), paracentral (C), and far lateral (D) disk herniations with resultant nerve root compression.

paracentral disk herniation or a far lateral disk herniation (Figs. 2A to D).

Albeit rare, if a disk herniation involves either the L1 or L2 nerve root, the patient may present with pain in the inguinal area. The patient may also have objective hip flexor weakness though this can be difficult to establish. It should be noted that pain in this distribution may also be associated with osteoarthritis of the hip. Therefore, in the examination of a patient where L1 or L2 nerve root involvement is suspected, it is critical to perform maneuvers to elucidate hip pathology.

Disk herniations involving L2 or L3 nerve roots may be difficult to distinguish. Patients with involvement of these nerve roots may have pain radiating into the anterior thigh. They may present with numbness in the anterior thigh as well and weakness in knee extension and hip adduction. A useful physical examination sign that points to nerve root tension is the femoral stretch test. Due to the distribution of pain, one must also consider hip pathology for this presentation.

A patient with an L4 radiculopathy will often present with pain radiating down the thigh and along the medial aspect of the leg to the medial malleolus. There may also be weakness in foot dorsiflexion (which must be distinguished from an L5 radiculopathy). A patient with an L2, L3, or L4 radiculopathy may also have a diminished patellar reflex.

An L5 radiculopathy typically presents with pain radiating down the lateral aspect of the thigh down to the lateral calf and lateral malleolus. Pain may also extend into the dorsum of the foot. The patient may have signs of numbness but due to the overlap from the L4 nerve root, the most specific location for numbness is on the dorsum of the foot between the first and second digits. A patient with an L5 radiculopathy may also have weakness in dorsiflexion but more specifically will have weakness in extension of the first digit of the foot. It is also critical to distinguish an L5 radiculopathy from neuropathy of the peroneal nerve. This can be done by testing hip abduction as an L5 radiculopathy will cause weakness of the gluteus medius and minimus. Moreover, a patient with peroneal neuropathy will have normal foot inversion whereas a patient with an L5 radiculopathy will have weak foot inversion.

Finally, an S1 radiculopathy will present with a patient experiencing pain and numbness from the buttock, down the posterior aspect of the thigh and leg, and into the plantar surface of the foot. The patient may also have weakness in plantar flexion though this may only be demonstrated with the patient standing and attempting to stand on his or her toes. The patient may also have an absent Achilles reflex.

Though many patients with lumbar radiculopathy will present in a subacute fashion, there is one concerning presentation that may present acutely. The findings of unilateral or bilateral lower extremity weakness in multiple myotomes, pain, urinary retention, perineal sensory loss, urinary or bowel incontinence constitute cauda equina syndrome. These patients will often present acutely to the emergency room with some combination of the aforementioned findings and require urgent attention. However, it should be mentioned that many patients will present acutely with concerns of urinary or bowel incontinence without pain, weakness, or numbness in the lower extremities. In such circumstances, where incontinence is present without any other radicular symptoms, lumbar disk herniation is not a likely cause of incontinence, and other causes must be sought.

A very important part of the history is that of the presence or absence of night pain. Patients with lumbar radiculopathy often do not have pain that awakens them from sleep. In cases where patients do have pain while asleep, there are several very important possibilities that must be considered. Firstly, though night pain is not common with lumbar radiculopathy, it can often be seen in patients with chronic pain issues. Patients with chronic pain often have issues with depression, anxiety, and insomnia, all of which may be related to the pain experience. Thus, further questions regarding their mood, energy level, and other psychosocial factors should be asked in order to complete the diagnosis of a chronic pain disorder. This is important to assess given that a multidisciplinary approach may be necessary in order to manage that patient's pain issues and surgical intervention in isolation may not be successful. Another cause for night pain in patients with lumbar radiculopathy is the presence of a malignant process. Classically, patients with neoplastic disease involving the spine have pain at night and pain that is mechanical in nature. The pain presumably arises due to instability of the spine or compression of spinal nerve roots from a neoplastic process or pathological fracture. Finally, night pain may also indicate the presence of hip pathology. Patients with osteoarthritis of the hip will often have pain at night, pain with forward flexion, and pain with weight bearing on the affected side. Thus, the presence of night pain is an important feature of the history which may help to pinpoint different causes for pain, and each of these possibilities must be considered in turn.

Investigations

Having taken a complete history and physical examination from a patient with lumbar radiculopathy, one must correlate the findings with the appropriate investigations. There are numerous different modalities that may help in identifying the nerve root involved and the location of the disk herniation. Magnetic resonance imaging (MRI), computed tomography (CT) scanning, and X-rays are commonly employed in the evaluation of a patient with lumbar radiculopathy.

Before delving into the role of each of these modalities for the diagnosis of lumbar radiculopathy, it should be made clear that imaging outside of the context of a patient history and physical examination may be very misleading. The presence of degenerative changes on imaging is very common. A study[12] of lumbar spine CT in asymptomatic patients demonstrated degenerative changes in 50% of patients over 40 years of age. When 148 asymptomatic adult volunteers underwent MRI of the lumbar spine,[13] 83% of patients had moderate to severe disk desiccation, 64% had bulging disks, and 32% had at least one disk protrusion. These findings were confirmed in another study[14] where 32% of asymptomatic patients had degenerative disk changes at more than one level. In another study,[15] baseline MRI in 200 asymptomatic patients at risk for low back pain were compared with MRI obtained in the same cohort of patients after they experienced an episode of back pain. Interestingly, they noted that 25% of patients went on to have back pain within 5 years, and of these, 84% had no significant change in their MRI as compared to the baseline study. Thus, had the patients not had baseline studies, their symptoms may have been attributed to these degenerative changes and may have gone on to receive surgical intervention.

Of the different modalities employed in the diagnosis of lumbar radiculopathy, X-ray has the least utility in securing a diagnosis of lumbar disk herniation. Though this imaging technique may be useful to assess for the quality of bone, the presence of fractures, and general spinal alignment, a plain X-ray film has limited ability to assess intervertebral disk pathology. One may see clues of degenerative disk disease through the presence of narrowed disk spaces or vacuum phenomena though these findings do not necessarily equate with lumbar disk herniation. Thus, X-ray is most useful where one suspects that a patient has signs and symptoms consistent with instability or sagittal imbalance. It may also be useful in the preoperative planning phases where the presence of spondylolisthesis or scoliosis may substantially change the scope of the surgical procedure for the management of a lumbar disk herniation.

Computed tomography scanning may be as useful as MRI scanning in the identification of a lumbar disk herniation.[16,17] CT scanning is most useful to evaluate cortical and trabecular bone though one may also assess soft tissues and lumbar disk herniations using this modality. Comparatively, CT scans are more useful in the identification of osteophytes whereas MRI is more useful to assess the spinal cord, thecal sac, and nerve roots in relation to the intervertebral disks. CT myelography remains a useful tool to evaluate the neural elements in circumstances where the patient may not have an MRI performed.

With respect to MRI of the spine, a series of changes occur in the spine that affect both the vertebral bone marrow and the intervertebral disk. These changes were first described by Modic et al.[18] Type 1 changes are seen as a hypointensity within the vertebral body adjacent to the disk space on T1 weighted images and a hyperintensity on T2 weighted images. These changes are seen in approximately 4% of the general population and in 8% after diskectomy procedures.[19,20] Histopathologically, these changes are seen as fissuring within the endplates and fibrous changes to the vertebral bone marrow. Type 2 changes are seen as slight hyperintensities in the adjacent vertebral marrow on T1 weighted images and iso- to hyperintensity seen on T2 weighted images. These changes reflect the replacement of bone marrow with lipid in the fibrous areas of the bone marrow. Finally, type 3 changes are felt to represent sclerotic changes to the bone and are seen as hypointensities on both T1 weighted and T2 weighted images. In trying to correlate these bone marrow findings with degenerative spinal conditions, MRI was performed on 670 patients that presented with low back pain and sciatica.[21] Interestingly, in those patients that had resolution of symptoms, the type 1 changes had converted to type 2 changes. In those patients with persistent symptoms the type 1 changes had indeed worsened. Similarly, it has been noted that patients with type 1 changes tend to respond better to lumbar spinal fusion procedures for back pain than patients with other types of changes.[22] Similarly, persistence of type 1 changes after spinal fusion is associated with worse outcomes whereas resolution of these changes is associated with better outcomes in those patients with lumbar spinal fusions.[23]

In addition to CT and MRI scans, there are several other tests that can be useful in the diagnosis and evaluation of a patient with lumbar disk herniation. In patients with back pain, some authors have proposed the use of provocative testing in the form of diskography to identify disks that may be the cause of low back pain. With this technique, the lumbar disk is injected with saline and it is determined whether pressure within the specified lumbar disk reproduces the patient's pain. If the findings are concordant, then it is proposed that the degenerative disk is the cause of pain and surgical intervention may be warranted. However, pain may also be elicited in asymptomatic patients and, therefore, it is difficult to differentiate false positive findings in a patient with multiple degenerative lumbar disks. The breadth of data and controversies around diskography has been reviewed elsewhere.[24] Electromyography (EMG) and nerve conduction studies (NCS) may also be useful in the diagnosis of lumbar radiculopathy. Though less useful in the absence of motor weakness (i.e. in those patients presenting with pain or sensory findings only), these studies may be very useful to identify true motor weakness from reduced effort secondary to pain. These studies may also help identify specific nerve root pathology in cases where the neurological examination is not diagnostic. Finally, EMG and NCS may be very useful to distinguish lumbar radiculopathy from mononeuropathies or polyneuropathies. In patients with longstanding pain syndromes, EMG and NCS can help to distinguish chronic demyelination from conduction block. This may be particularly useful in patients presenting with recurrent pain in the distribution of a nerve that has been previously decompressed with surgery. Despite the utility of EMG and nerve conduction testing, there are important limitations to the use of this technique. Firstly, EMG and NCS are less useful in patients without motor weakness (i.e. in those patients presenting with pure sensory symptoms or pain). EMG and NCS may also not provide any useful information within 3 weeks of the clinical diagnosis due to the fact that Wallerian degeneration must occur before manifestation of any electrical findings.

In the setting of cauda equina syndrome, patients often present with urinary retention. Thus, in the acute setting, measurement of post-void residual volume in the bladder is valuable in establishing a diagnosis. Normal post-void residual volume is typically <100 mL whereas higher post-void residual volumes are felt to be diagnostic. Indeed, in a recent study,[25] post-void residual volume of >500 mL, alone or in combination with any two of the following findings—bilateral sciatica and urinary incontinence or bowel incontinence, was most predictive of true cauda equina syndrome secondary to a lumbar disk herniation. As mentioned previously, MRI is an important diagnostic tool to diagnose lumbar disk herniation and this remains true in the setting of cauda equina syndrome.

Medical Management

Prior to considering surgery in any patient with a lumbar disk herniation, an adequate trial of conservative therapy should be attempted. There are several therapeutic modalities that may be employed in attempting conservative treatment. These include aerobic activity, physical therapy, chiropractic manipulation, massage, analgesics, acupuncture, and cognitive behavioral therapy.

Given the significant pain issues that patients may experience early in their presentation, adequate pain management is of utmost importance. According to WHO guidelines, management of acute pain entails an escalation of medications depending on the needs of the patient. The patient should first be started on non-opioid analgesics such as acetaminophen or nonsteroidal anti-inflammatories. Analgesics can then be increased in escalating doses and potency through the use of mild opioids such as codeine, stronger opioids (e.g. morphine, hydromorphone), and IV analgesics such as opioids and nonsteroidal anti-inflammatories (e.g. ketorolac). Adjuvant analgesics such as tricyclic antidepressants and antiepileptic medications (e.g. gabapentin, pregabalin, and topiramate) have also been shown to be effective in the multimodality treatment of pain. Adjuvant analgesics may be started at any point during the escalation of opioids. Though management of pain is of utmost importance, it should be noted that opioids should be used sparingly due to issues with addiction and drug dependency.

Having administered adequate analgesia, the patient should undertake means to strengthen the back musculature and increase aerobic capacity. Though the evidence for commonly prescribed therapies such as physical therapy, chiropractic manipulation, and massage are limited, the non-invasive nature of these therapies permits aggressive use and is often tolerated by patients. If, despite all efforts, the patient cannot tolerate physical maneuvers during the trial of conservative therapy, then it may be reasonable to consider surgical intervention.

In general terms, 4–6 weeks is generally considered an adequate duration of time for conservative therapy, and surgical intervention prior to this period of time may result in a large proportion of unnecessary surgical procedures given that a large number of patients will have resolution of their symptoms within the first 4 weeks of presentation *(see Epidemiology and Natural History section)*. It should be noted that even very large disk herniations can be treated without surgical intervention as they have been shown to resolve spontaneously over time.[26] The presence of a large disk fragment is not an indication for surgical intervention. It should be noted that the size, location or behavior of lumbar disk herniations did not correlate with outcome in patients that were followed prospectively over time with serial MR imaging.[27]

Though there is certainly a role for conservative therapy in patients with lumbar radiculopathy, one must not employ this strategy in the setting of cauda equina syndrome. In those patients with cauda equina syndrome, urgent surgical intervention is necessary to allow for recovery of bowel and bladder function. Failure to intervene surgically acutely may result in serious adverse consequences for the patient including weakness of the lower extremity, neuropathic pain as well as loss of bowel and bladder control. As such, current guidelines advocate against observation in these patients and emergent surgical intervention is generally recommended *(see Surgical Indications section for a complete discussion)*.

Surgical Indications

Though the majority of patients will do well with conservative treatment of lumbar radiculopathy following a lumbar disk herniation, there is still a certain percentage of patients that will require surgery to get relief of their pain syndrome. Over the past three decades, there have been three separate randomized controlled trials that have examined the role of surgery against conservative treatment in the setting of lumbar disk herniations. Also, the surgical technique has also evolved over time where minimally invasive approaches are becoming more popular.

Results from the first randomized controlled trial to compare surgery against conservative management for lumbar disk herniation were published in 1983.[28] In this study, 126 patients with lumbar disk herniation were randomized to either surgery or conservative management if it was unclear to the treating physician which strategy would be best. The surgical procedure consisted of a lumbar diskectomy and the conservative treatment consisted of 2 weeks of bed rest followed by gradual increase in activity and back strengthening exercises. These patients were then followed at intervals of 1, 4, and 10 years. At each examination, a physical examination was performed and a questionnaire was administered to judge patient satisfaction. An intention-to-treat analysis was performed which demonstrated better outcomes with surgery after 1 year, but at the 4-year and 10-year follow-up, there was no significant difference amongst the groups. Regardless of treatment, patients with motor weakness had a good prognosis but only 50% of patients with sensory symptoms recovered.

In a similar study, Osterman et al.[29] conducted a prospective randomized controlled trial where 56 patients were randomized to surgery or isometric exercises. The patients were followed for 2 years but no significant difference was seen between the two groups. It was suggested that surgical patients recovered sooner than those treated conservatively.

Buttermann et al.[30] compared lumbar diskectomy to epidural steroid injection in 169 patients that were randomized to either treatment following failure of 6 weeks of conservative therapy. The patients that underwent surgery had rapid relief of their symptoms but nearly half of the patients that received epidural steroid injections also had relief of their symptoms. Of those patients that crossed over to the surgical arm, there was no harm from delayed treatment.

The most recent, and largest, randomized controlled trial was published in 2006.[31,32] In this trial, patients that failed 6 weeks of conservative therapy were randomized to either lumbar diskectomy or ongoing conservative treatment. Conservative treatment was not standardized across groups. A total of 501 patients were randomized and were followed for 2 years. Primary treatment outcomes included changes in the SF-36 patient questionnaire, bodily pain and physical function scales as well as changes in the Oswestry disability index (ODI). At the end of follow-up, 50% of the surgical group did not undergo surgery and 30% of the medical group underwent surgery. There was no statistical difference in primary outcomes between the surgical and conservative treatment groups in the intention to treat analysis, though in the as-treated analysis the results strongly favored surgical management.

The high rates of crossover between the two study arms may lead to bias in the interpretation of the results. The study authors also enrolled 743 patients that were unwilling to participate in the randomization process into an observational study. In this study, patients that underwent surgery had a statistically significant improvement in bodily pain scores, ODI scores and in physical function. In a recent update on the study,[33] the authors reported 4 years outcomes on a combined as-treated analysis on the patients from the aforementioned trial. At 4 years, patients that underwent surgery had better outcomes than those treated conservatively for all primary outcome measures.

Cauda equina syndrome is commonly regarded as a surgical emergency.[34] However, there is ongoing debate about the urgency of surgery. In a meta-analysis, the authors found that patients that had surgical decompression in the setting of cauda equina within 48 hours of presentation had better postoperative outcomes. However, the results should be interpreted with caution as the study involves a meta-analysis of case reports as opposed to prospective data with comparison groups. Others have argued that the severity of neurological injury (i.e. presence or absence of urinary retention) may be more important than timing of surgery.[35] In the largest prospective series[36] of patients with cauda equina syndrome, 33 patients were followed and assessed at 3 months and 12 months following the initial onset of cauda equina syndrome. Of these patients, 12 had surgery within 48 hours whereas 21 patients had decompressive surgery greater than 48 hours from symptom onset. Of those patients that presented with urinary incontinence, there were higher rates of back and leg pain, higher rates of bowel leakage at 3 months follow-up, and greater dissatisfaction with bowel and bladder function. In this prospective series, there was no significant correlation of neurological outcome with time to surgery.

Based on these studies, it is clear that patients that undergo conservative management will recover to equivalent functional outcomes over the long-term as the patients that undergo surgery (Table 2). Moreover, delaying surgery to allow for spontaneous resolution of lumbar radiculopathy does not seem to reduce the chance of recovery should the patient eventually require surgery. A common theme in these trials is to ensure that the patient undergoes 4–6 weeks of conservative therapy prior to initiating surgical intervention. Also, it would seem that motor weakness may improve at equal rates in conservatively and surgically treated patients and, therefore, may not be an absolute indication for surgery in the setting of lumbar disk herniation. Thus, surgical intervention should be offered to those patients with acute, rapidly progressive neurological deterioration, or in those

Table 2: Evidentiary table.

Author, journal, year	*Design*	*Topic*	*Follow-up*	*Outcome measures*	*Results*	*Level-of-evidence*
Weber et al., Spine, 1983	RCT	Standard microdiscectomy vs. conservative treatment for lumbar disk herniation	1, 4 and 10 years	Independent observer rating	Surgical arm had statistically significant improvement at 1 year, but no differences seen between both groups at 4 and 10 years	II
Buttermann et al., JBJS, 2004	RCT	Standard diskectomy vs. epidural steroid injections	3 years	Back and leg pain, ODI, need for 2nd procedure	96–98% of patients who had a diskectomy had improvement in outcome whereas only 46–52% of patients that had epidural steroid injection had positive outcomes	II
Osterman et al., Spine, 2006	RCT	Standard diskectomy vs. isometric back exercises	2 years	Leg pain, health related quality-of-life score, Oswestry low back disability score	No difference between surgical and conservative therapy over 2 years though there was initial rapid recovery in the surgical group	II
Weinstein et al., JAMA, 2006	RCT and observational cohort	Standard diskectomy vs. conservative treatment	2 years	SF-36, bodily pain and function assessment, ODI	Patients treated with surgery had faster recovery initially but no difference between two groups at final follow-up	II

(ODI: Oswestry disability index; RCT: randomized controlled trial)

patients that have had an adequate trial of conservative therapy but remain symptomatic.

Surgical Treatment

For patients requiring surgical intervention for lumbar disk herniation, there are two commonly performed procedures that allow for removal of the disk herniation—lumbar microdiscectomy and minimally invasive diskectomy.

The traditional microdiscectomy is a procedure that entails a midline incision, dissection through the fascia, subperiosteal mobilization of muscle off of the spinous processes and lamina followed by a laminotomy at the site and side of interest. After the laminotomy is performed, the ligamentum flavum is removed, the traversing nerve root is identified, and the disk herniation is removed. This procedure involves an open incision and the use of a microscope for better visualization. The minimally invasive, or muscle-splitting, approach involves a parasagittal incision and dissection *through* the muscles in order to access the lamina using a series of tubes which progressively dilate the opening through the muscle. Thereafter, the approach to disk removal is similar to that described for the traditional microdiscectomy. The impetus for the muscle-splitting approach is the thought that subperiosteal dissection deinnervates the muscle generating more muscle injury and atrophy and thereby more pain resulting in longer recovery for the patient. It is also often argued that the tubular retractor systems allow for a smaller incision and less blood loss than the traditional open microdiscectomy.

Though there has been much enthusiasm for minimally invasive techniques, there is very limited evidence that these techniques indeed result in better outcomes for patients undergoing surgery for lumbar disk herniation.[37] One randomized controlled trial involving 40 patients demonstrated smaller incisions and shorter hospital stays with minimally invasive approaches though the small sample size prevents one from making firm conclusions regarding the merits of these techniques. There is also significant concern that the use of minimally invasive techniques results in greater radiation exposure to healthcare personnel.[38] Others have also argued that the minimally invasive approaches may limit the extent of decompression that can be obtained especially as one is learning the technique.

Overall, both open microdiscectomy and minimally invasive approaches are widely used to remove lumbar disk herniations and further studies with large numbers of patients and longer follow-up will be required to determine if there is indeed any significant difference between the two techniques.

Complications

Though surgery for lumbar disk herniation is a commonly performed and well-tolerated procedure, there are invariably complications associated with standard microdiscectomy. In the Spine Patient Outcomes Research Trial (SPORT),[33] the most common complications included—dural tears (10%), recurrent disk herniations (15%), and wound infection (2%). Vascular and neurological events were rare in this trial. These findings are similar to those of older studies.

Some have postulated that recurrent disk herniations may be related to the extent to which the intervertebral disk is removed. Carragee et al.[39] examined this issue in their case control study where they compared 30 patients undergoing subtotal diskectomy to a cohort of historical controls where limited diskectomy (i.e. removal of extruded disk fragment alone) was performed. Though there was no statistically significant difference, there was a recurrence rate of 9% in patients undergoing subtotal diskectomy and 18% in those that underwent limited diskectomy.

The rate of wound infections in older studies is also similar to those seen in the SPORTstudy. In one series[40] of 984 patients, the rate of wound infections was less than 3%. Similarly, in a larger study[41] where both a retrospective and prospective series of patients were evaluated, the rate of infection was approximately 2%.

The rates of neurological injury in previous study were also very similar to those of the SPORT study with two studies reporting neurological injury in less than 1% of patients undergoing lumbar diskectomy.[40,41]

Other rarely reported complications include injury to the aorta or iliac arteries, intestinal perforation, injury to the ureter, and death.

SUMMARY

Lumbar disk herniation is a common cause of pain and disability in the general population. Spine surgeons must often make important decisions regarding the timing and extent of investigations and treatment for these patients. As discussed, a thorough history and physical examination are crucial as first steps to identify the site and side of nerve root compression and to rule out other more insidious medical conditions. Neuroimaging is then performed which may confirm the findings of the physical examination. Thereafter, the literature would support a trial of conservative therapy lasting at least 4–6 weeks as the natural history of lumbar disk herniation is that the majority of patients will indeed improve. Those patients that remain symptomatic after an adequate trial of conservative therapy may require surgical intervention to relieve pain. Both standard open microdiscectomy and minimally invasive techniques may be employed in the surgical treatment of lumbar disk herniation. Patients should be warned of common complications of the procedure which include incidental durotomy, recurrent disk herniations, wound infections, and rarely, neurological injury.

REFERENCES

1. Tarulli AW, Raynor EM. Lumbosacral radiculopathy. Neurol Clin. 2007;25(2):387-405.
2. Battié MC, Videman T, Gibbons LE, et al. 1995 Volvo Award in clinical sciences. Determinants of lumbar disc degeneration. A study relating lifetime exposures and magnetic resonance imaging findings in identical twins. Spine (Phila Pa 1976). 1995;20(24):2601-12.
3. Hestbaek L, Iachine IA, Leboeuf-Yde C, et al. Heredity of low back pain in a young population: a classical twin study. Twin Res. 2004;7(1):16-26.
4. Heliövaara M. Occupation and risk of herniated lumbar intervertebral disc or sciatica leading to hospitalization. J Chronic Dis. 1987;40(3):259-64.
5. Kelsey JL. An epidemiological study of the relationship between occupations and acute herniated lumbar intervertebral discs. Int J Epidemiol. 1975;4(3):197-205.
6. Seidler A, Bolm-Audorff U, Siol T, et al. Occupational risk factors for symptomatic lumbar disc herniation; a case-control study. Occup Environ Med. 2003;60(11):821-30.
7. Hult L. The Munkfors investigation; a study of the frequency and causes of the stiff neck-brachialgia and lumbago-sciatica syndromes, as well as observations on certain signs and symptoms from the dorsal spine and the joints of the extremities in industrial and forest workers. Acta Orthop Scand Suppl. 1954;16:1-76.
8. Hult L. Cervical, dorsal and lumbar spinal syndromes: a field investigation of a non-selected material of 1200 workers in different occupations with special reference to disc degeneration and so-called muscular rheumatism. Acta Orthop Scand Suppl. 1954;17:1-102.
9. Bush K, Cowan N, Katz DE, et al. The natural history of sciatica associated with disc pathology. A prospective study with clinical and independent radiologic follow-up. Spine (Phila Pa 1976). 1992;17(10):1205-12.
10. Saal JA, Saal JS. Nonoperative treatment of herniated lumbar intervertebral disc with radiculopathy. An outcome study. Spine (Phila Pa 1976). 1989;14(4):431-7.
11. Weber H, Holme I, Amlie E. The natural course of acute sciatica with nerve root symptoms in a double-blind placebo-controlled trial evaluating the effect of piroxicam. Spine (Phila Pa 1976). 1993;18(11):1433-8.
12. Wiesel SW, Tsourmas N, Feffer HL, et al. A study of computer-assisted tomography. I. The incidence of positive CAT scans in an asymptomatic group of patients. Spine (Phila Pa 1976). 1984;9(6):549-51.
13. Jarvik JJ, Hollingworth W, Heagerty P, et al. The Longitudinal Assessment of Imaging and Disability of the Back (LAIDBack) Study: baseline data. Spine (Phila Pa 1976). 2001;26(10):1158-66.
14. Jensen MC, Brant-Zawadzki MN, Obuchowski N, et al. Magnetic resonance imaging of the lumbar spine in people without back pain. N Engl J Med. 1994;331(2):69-73.
15. Carragee E, Alamin T, Cheng I, et al. Are first-time episodes of serious LBP associated with new MRI findings? Spine J. 2006;6(6):624-35.
16. Bischoff RJ, Rodriguez RP, Gupta K, et al. A comparison of computed tomography-myelography, magnetic resonance imaging, and myelography in the diagnosis of herniated nucleus pulposus and spinal stenosis. J Spinal Disord. 1993;6(4):289-95.
17. Jarvik JG, Deyo RA. Diagnostic evaluation of low back pain with emphasis on imaging. Ann Intern Med. 2002;137(7):586-97.
18. Modic MT, Steinberg PM, Ross JS, et al. Degenerative disk disease: assessment of changes in vertebral body marrow with MR imaging. Radiology. 1988;166(1 Pt 1):193-9.
19. Ross JS, Obuchowski N, Zepp R. The postoperative lumbar spine: evaluation of epidural scar over a 1-year period. AJNR Am J Neuroradiol. 1998;19(1):183-6.
20. Ross JS, Robertson JT, Frederickson RC, et al. Association between peridural scar and recurrent radicular pain after lumbar discectomy: magnetic resonance evaluation. ADCON-L European Study Group. Neurosurgery. 1996;38(4):855-61; discussion 861-3.
21. Mitra D, Cassar-Pullicino VN, McCall IW. Longitudinal study of vertebral type-1 end-plate changes on MR of the lumbar spine. Eur Radiol. 2004;14(9):1574-81.
22. Vital JM, Gille O, Pointillart V, et al. Course of Modic 1 six months after lumbar posterior osteosynthesis. Spine (Phila Pa 1976). 2003;28(7):715-20;discussion 721.
23. Buttermann GR, Heithoff KB, Ogilvie JW, et al. Vertebral body MRI related to lumbar fusion results. Eur Spine J. 1997;6(2):115-20.
24. Resnick DK, Malone DG, Ryken TC. Guidelines for the use of discography for the diagnosis of painful degenerative lumbar disc disease. Neurosurg Focus. 2002;13(2):E12.
25. Domen PM, Hofman PA, van Santbrink H, et al. Predictive value of clinical characteristics in patients with suspected cauda equina syndrome. Eur J Neurol. 2009;16(3):416-9.

26. Benson RT, Tavares SP, Robertson SC, et al. Conservatively treated massive prolapsed discs: a 7-year follow-up. Ann R Coll Surg Engl. 2010;92(2):147-53.
27. Modic MT, Obuchowski NA, Ross JS, et al. Acute low back pain and radiculopathy: MR imaging findings and their prognostic role and effect on outcome. Radiology. 2005;237(2):597-604.
28. Weber H. Lumbar disc herniation. A controlled, prospective study with ten years of observation. Spine (Phila Pa 1976). 1983;8(2):131-40.
29. Osterman H, Seitsalo S, Karppinen J, et al. Effectiveness of microdiscectomy for lumbar disc herniation: a randomized controlled trial with 2 years of follow-up. Spine (Phila Pa 1976). 2006;31(21):2409-14.
30. Buttermann GR. Treatment of lumbar disc herniation: epidural steroid injection compared with discectomy. A prospective, randomized study. J Bone Joint Surg Am. 2004;86(4):670-9.
31. Weinstein JN, Tosteson TD, Lurie JD, et al. Surgical vs nonoperative treatment for lumbar disk herniation: the Spine Patient Outcomes Research Trial (SPORT): a randomized trial. JAMA. 2006;296(20):2441-50.
32. Weinstein JN, Lurie JD, Tosteson TD, et al. Surgical vs nonoperative treatment for lumbar disk herniation: the Spine Patient Outcomes Research Trial (SPORT) observational cohort. JAMA. 2006;296(20):2451-9.
33. Weinstein JN, Lurie JD, Tosteson TD, et al. Surgical versus nonoperative treatment for lumbar disc herniation: four-year results for the Spine Patient Outcomes Research Trial (SPORT). Spine (Phila Pa 1976). 2008;33(25):2789-800.
34. Ahn UM, Ahn NU, Buchowski JM, et al. Cauda equina syndrome secondary to lumbar disc herniation: a meta-analysis of surgical outcomes. Spine (Phila Pa 1976). 2000;25(12):1515-22.
35. Gleave JR, MacFarlane R. Prognosis for recovery of bladder function following lumbar central disc prolapse. Br J Neurosurg. 1990;4(3):205-9.
36. Qureshi A, Sell P. Cauda equina syndrome treated by surgical decompression: the influence of timing on surgical outcome. Eur Spine J. 2007;16(12):2143-51.
37. German JW, Adamo MA, Hoppenot RG, et al. Perioperative results following lumbar discectomy: comparison of minimally invasive discectomy and standard microdiscectomy. Neurosurg Focus. 2008;25(2):E20.
38. Mariscalco MW, Yamashita T, Steinmetz MP, et al. Radiation exposure to the surgeon during open lumbar microdiscectomy and minimally invasive microdiscectomy: a prospective, controlled trial. Spine (Phila Pa 1976). 2011;36(3):255-60.
39. Carragee EJ, Spinnickie AO, Alamin TF, et al. A prospective controlled study of limited versus subtotal posterior discectomy: short-term outcomes in patients with herniated lumbar intervertebral discs and large posterior anular defect. Spine (Phila Pa 1976). 2006;31(6):653-7.
40. Davis RA. A long-term outcome analysis of 984 surgically treated herniated lumbar discs. J Neurosurg. 1994;80(3):415-21.
41. Wiese M, Krämer J, Bernsmann K, et al. The related outcome and complication rate in primary lumbar microscopic disc surgery depending on the surgeon's experience: comparative studies. Spine J. 2004;4(5):550-6.

CHAPTER 37

Spinal Stenosis

Sandeep N Gidvani, Michael D Daubs

EPIDEMIOLOGY AND NATURAL HISTORY

Spinal stenosis is defined as a narrowing of the volume of the central spinal canal, the lateral recesses of the spinal canal, or the neural foramina, that results in compression of either the thecal sac or the exiting nerve roots, respectively. The general incidence of this disease ranges from 1.7% to 8%.[1]

There are various causes of spinal stenosis. Generally, spinal stenosis is grouped into congenital and acquired etiologies. With congenital narrowing of the canal caused by anatomically short pedicles and lamina, the diameter can be reduced, and patients are more likely to become symptomatic. For the majority of patients with this diagnosis, the condition is a result of a degenerative process. Disk degeneration in the anterior spinal column with age results in a loss of disk height and bulging of the disk. In turn, there is an increased load transfer to the facet joints and with this an increased wear of the cartilage within the facet joints, increased bony contact, hypertrophy of the joints, and osteophyte formation. The loss of the height of the disk space also results in infolding of the ligamentum flavum and increased endplate contact with resultant posterior vertebral body osteophyte formation. Together disk bulging, facet hypertrophy, ligamentum flavum infolding and hypertrophy, and posterior osteophyte formation encroach on the central spinal canal and impinge the exiting nerve root as it courses through the foramen bordered by the disk and the facets (Figs. 1 and 2). As the capsules of the facets are attenuated and joint integrity is compromised, there is a cyclic transfer to the annulus, which is already degenerated. Thus, dynamic subluxation can exist within the facets resulting in degenerative spondylolisthesis, and additional narrowing of the spinal canal.[2]

Other causes of spinal stenosis are varied. Adjacent segment disease after fusion, postlaminectomy kyphosis, and tumor or infectious process encroachment are a few diagnoses that are more commonly responsible for narrowing of the diameter of the canal. Essentially, any process, whether biomechanical, metabolic, or traumatic, that changes the dimensions of the canal can be responsible for the symptoms of spinal stenosis.

Animal studies have examined the effects of increasing degrees of spinal stenosis.[3] Cortical evoked potentials were found to be highly sensitive to compression and demonstrated changes long before neurological deficits were discoverable. Venous congestion and arterial constriction were present around the nerve roots and the dorsal root ganglion. From a histological standpoint, the increasing stenosis resulted in blockage of axoplasmic flow, edema, and demyelination within the nerve roots, and Wallerian degeneration of motor and sensory fibers. The latter of these fibers were more susceptible to direct pressure and slower to recover. This may explain why subjective sensory deficits are sometimes relayed by patients during the history in the absence of frank motor deficits on clinical examination.

The natural history of spinal stenosis is variable and does not necessarily follow a progressive deteriorating course.[4] It is present within 20–25% of the population and risk of development increases with age greater than 50. Johnsson performed a retrospective review of patients with spinal stenosis and found that though symptoms remain unchanged in 70% of the patient population, no patient experienced severe deterioration over the course of a 4-year follow-up.[4]

In more recent studies that have been performed in a prospective fashion with 8–10 years follow-up, specific

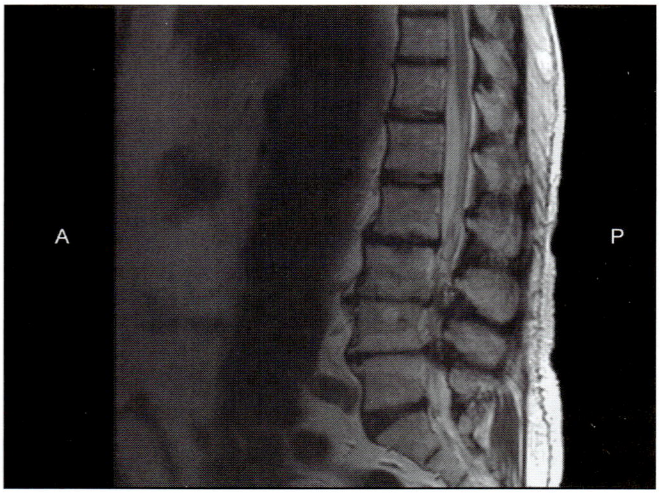

Fig. 1: Magnetic resonance imaging sagittal T2 weighted image demonstrating multilevel spinal stenosis secondary to the degenerative cascade—degenerative disk disease, disk bulging, ligamentum infolding, and facet hypertrophy.

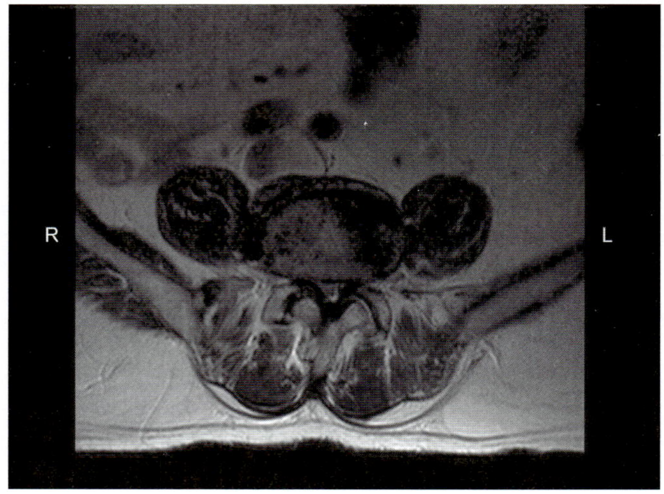

Fig. 2: MRI axial T2 weighted image demonstrating significant spinal stenosis at the level of the lateral recess. Facet hypertrophy, gapping, ligamentum flavum hypertrophy—all result in significant narrowing of the central spinal canal.

outcomes were evaluated to determine whether there is a significant difference between those treated surgically and nonsurgically.[5] This provides further insight to the natural course of the disease. Low back pain, predominant symptom improvement, and satisfaction with the current state of the patient were no different in those treated with surgery versus those managed nonoperatively. However, leg pain relief and back-related functional status were improved in those who received surgical treatment.[6-8]

In the Spine Patient Outcomes Research Trial (SPORT), the nonsurgical arm of patients with spinal stenosis improved only moderately within 2 years in all outcome measures. However, similar to the prior retrospective studies discussed there was no evidence of sudden or severe deterioration.[9,10]

As the quality of studies improves with respect to spinal stenosis, a clearer picture of the true natural history will evolve. At the present time, it appears that there is potential for symptoms to worsen over time, however, the speed of decline is unpredictable.

WORKUP (CLINICAL FINDINGS)

Symptoms or Signs

From a symptom standpoint, patients present with lower extremity pain, numbness, and weakness in this order and frequency.[11] Approximately 70% of the time symptoms are bilateral. There is a variable degree of associated low back pain usually based on the presence of other degenerative pathology such as disk degeneration, facet arthritis, and spondylolisthesis.

Patients with spinal stenosis may present either with radicular symptoms if the majority of their pathology occurs within the lateral recess or neural foramina or neurogenic claudication. In particular, nerve root symptoms can be a predominant part of the clinical picture if the spinal stenosis is secondary to degenerative spondylolisthesis. Neurogenic claudication is manifested as diminished standing tolerance or reduced walking ability and tolerance secondary to fatigue. The commonly described pattern is that of being able to walk a limited distance, sitting for a short period of time, and then being able to get up and walk again. Symptoms are typically recreated with extension and therefore discomfort is experienced with standing erect. Patients may have a positive shopping cart sign, indicating that a position of forward flexion that opens the canal improves their symptoms. Likewise, a sitting position is better tolerated than standing.

It is important when eliciting symptoms from patients presenting for evaluation to differentiate between neurogenic and vascular claudication (Table 1). Those with the latter have a limited walking distance secondary to cramping of the lower extremity muscles with exertion

Table 1: Differentiating between neurogenic and vascular claudication.

Findings	*Neurogenic claudication*	*Vascular claudication*
Low back pain	May be present	Usually absent
Sensory symptoms	Usually present	Absent
Muscle weakness	Usually present	Absent
Reflexes	Diminished or absent	Normal
Arterial pulses	Normal	Absent or diminished
Skin or trophic changes (shiny skin, loss of hair)	Absent	Present
Stationary bike	Able to perform exercise longer	Not able to perform
Postural dependency	Yes	No
Relief with rest	Yes	No

and this typically is a fixed distance. The duration of ambulation cannot be improved with postural changes, e.g. walking in a flexed forward position or leaning forward on an ambulatory aid. Symptoms cannot be differentiated between riding a stationary bike (assuming a flexed position) and walking. Usually, those with vascular claudication also have diminished pulses and trophic changes such as shiny skin and hair loss. Neurogenic claudication is more frequently associated with low back pain and reflex changes.[12]

On physical examination, patients may have decreased sensation in a dermatomal distribution or specific motor deficits if pathology results in nerve root impingement. Peroneal or Extensor Hallucis Longus (EHL) weakness consistent with L5 nerve root impingement is most common in the setting of spinal stenosis.[4] Evaluation of gait is pertinent to assess for compensatory flexion or development of the "simian" posture in which the shoulders are anterior to the pelvis. Reflexes are usually diminished or absent. Range of motion will often be restricted secondary to degeneration, and may be manifested as stiffness and rigidity in all three planes. As mentioned above, pain may be recreated with extension, and thus standing in an extended position for 30 seconds or greater may result in thigh pain. This is referred to as the sustained lumbar extension provocation test.[12] Straight leg raise testing is not commonly positive as it is in the case of lumbar disk herniation. Only about 10% of patients with spinal stenosis will have a positive straight leg test.[13] It is also important to evaluate peripheral pulses and lower extremity appearance in distinguishing neurogenic from vascular claudication. A thorough physical examination should also be performed to differentiate from other potential differential diagnoses. For example, the examiner should assess hip range of motion and impingement signs to rule out intra-articular pathology as well as perform complete neurologic testing to ensure there is no component of cervical myelopathy or central nervous system pathology responsible for disturbed gait pattern or walking tolerance or balance.

Laboratory Findings

There are no specific laboratory abnormalities that are associated with spinal stenosis. Blood parameters such as complete blood count (CBC), erythrocyte sedimentation rate (ESR), and C-reactive protein (CRP) have not been shown to be elevated in this condition. Of course, if one is suspicious based on MRI findings and a clinical history for an associated infection or malignancy being responsible for the spinal stenosis, then appropriate laboratory workup can be obtained to confirm or deny this.

A useful adjunct to MRI in the setting of spinal stenosis is electromyography (EMG) or nerve conduction studies. If there are confounding results from the standpoint of radiographic compression and nerve root symptoms, an EMG can be obtained to help pinpoint the source of the radiculopathy (i.e. specific nerve root and central vs. peripheral pathology). In addition, if the examiner is suspicious for peripheral nerve root entrapment, such as with the peroneal nerve as it crosses the head of the fibula or the tibial nerve in tarsal tunnel syndrome, electrodiagnostic studies can identify the location of nerve conduction delay. In postsurgical settings, electrodiagnostic studies can also help confirm the acuity or chronicity of nerve radiculopathy and thereby aid the physician in offering a prognosis regarding the patient's symptoms.

Imaging

Evaluation of patients with spinal stenosis must begin with a basic set of lumbar radiographs including anteroposterior (AP), lateral, flexion, and extension films. Sagittal alignment should be assessed on the lateral film, taking note of spondylolisthesis if present and what percentage of slippage has occurred of one vertebral body with respect to another. This finding can explain specific nerve root symptoms. Disk space height, osteophyte presence at the anterior and posterior vertebral bodies, and end plate sclerosis should be noted to determine amount of degeneration present and assess the level of stability afforded by reactive osteophyte formation. The AP X-ray can be used to look for the presence of adult degenerative scoliosis which should be weighed in surgical decision making, lateral listhesis of one body on another, and asymmetric disk collapse which can again explain specific nerve root symptoms, and facet hypertrophy that can create encroachment on the central canal. Flexion/extension films allow for evaluation of dynamic instability and the potential need for fusion in addition to decompression if surgical intervention is warranted.

Generally if neurologic symptoms have been persistent, an MRI is a necessary part of the evaluation for diagnosis and treatment of spinal stenosis. The sagittal T2 images can be used to assess disk hydration, disk height, end plate changes, disk bulging, foraminal stenosis (loss of epidural fat around the exiting nerve root), ligamentum flavum infolding, and importantly, constriction of the cauda equina as the nerve roots course distally.[14] The axial T2 images allow for evaluation of the AP and transverse diameter of the canal, facet hypertrophy/lateral recesses stenosis, ligamentum hypertrophy, disk bulging and resulting compression of central canal versus exiting nerve root, foraminal narrowing, gapping or subluxation of facet joints with fluid within the facets indicating the potential for dynamic instability.[15] It is crucial to correlate the findings on magnetic resonance imaging (MRI) with clinical symptoms, as it is not uncommon to find radiographic changes in patients that are asymptomatic, especially as patient age climbs over 60.[16] Boden found that up to 57% of asymptomatic patients within a population examined had abnormal MRIs with 20% of them demonstrating spinal stenosis.[16]

A computed tomography (CT) myelogram can be used in those patients for whom it is not possible to obtain an MRI. For example, a patient may have a pacemaker or prior instrumentation that may create significant artifact thereby decreasing the accuracy of interpretation. A CT myelogram is a procedure in which a needle is used to puncture the dura and contrast dye is injected to highlight the contours of the thecal sac. Nerve root entrapment in the lateral recess or foramina or central canal stenosis is demonstrated by the cutoff of contrast material. The disadvantages of this test include its invasiveness with postinjection spinal headache being common and it has been shown to have inferior accuracy in comparison to MRI.[17] Prior studies have used CT myelography to obtain a cutoff for symptomatic lumbar spinal stenosis to be an anteroposterior (AP) diameter of 10 mm.[18] A complete cutoff of the dye has also been found to better correlate with surgical outcomes.[19]

Medical Management

Medical or nonsurgical management is aimed at controlling the symptoms such that patients can return to their daily activities of living and maintain baseline function prior to the onset of their disease.

Low back pain secondary to degenerative disk disease or facet arthritis can be associated with the symptoms of spinal stenosis and is often effectively managed with the use of anti-inflammatories, such as nonsteroidal anti-inflammatory drugs (NSAIDs). The use of narcotic medication should be avoided especially in an elderly population as their side effects are numerous and can be deleterious. Neuropathic pain can be treated with γ-aminobutyric acid (GABA) agonists such as gabapentin (Neurontin) and pregabalin (Lyrica). Initiation of such medications and dosage adjustments are often best made by a pain management specialist for long-term pain control. The patient should understand that spinal stenosis is an ongoing compression of the nerves within the thecal sac or as they exit the neural foramina. Though symptoms may be manageable with medication and other nonoperative modalities, the anatomical narrowing that is present will not change.

The mainstays of nonoperative management for spinal stenosis remain physical therapy and the use of epidural steroid injections.[20] These have been repeatedly shown to offer symptomatic relief of pain, numbness, and weakness sometimes associated with spinal stenosis but in varying degrees depending on the individual patient and the number of levels and degree of stenosis present.[2]

Physical therapy should focus on core strengthening including the abdominal musculature and the paraspinal extensors. In turn, this allows for improved range of motion, functional status, and decrease in axial loading of the anterior vertebral column. Comprehensive nonoperative treatments consisting of flexion exercises, manual therapy, and treadmill exercises are more beneficial in reducing symptoms than less vigorous programs.[21] It is also important for patients to focus on active strengthening rather than passive modalities to manage their symptoms.

Epidural steroid injections are invasive and involve administering localized steroid injections to the epidural space under fluoroscopic guidance. They serve both a diagnostic purpose and therapeutic means of providing short-term relief for patients of varying duration. They are given via different routes depending on the pain specialists' assessment—interlaminar, transforaminal, and caudal. Botwin looked at specific outcomes following transforaminal epidural injections including pain scores, walking tolerance, and standing tolerance at 1-year follow-up and found all to have increased.[22] Manchikanti showed significant pain relief and functional status improvement with caudal epidural injections in patients with spinal stenosis regardless of whether they received local anesthetic or anesthetic plus steroid.[23] This study was performed in randomized and double blinded controlled fashion. There can be notable downsides to epidural injections. Radcliff analyzed a subgroup of the SPORT spinal stenosis population and found that those patients that did have epidural steroid injections preoperatively had increased operative time, longer duration of stay, and overall significantly less improvement in outcomes at 4 years.[24] This may be due to scarring and adhesions that result in the epidural space in the area of prior injections, making surgical dissection of the dura from surrounding lamina and facet borders difficult. Other concerns include temporary elevation of blood glucose levels in diabetics and localized effects on bone quality. If temporary relief of symptoms associated with spinal stenosis is desired, epidural injections can be used with attention paid to long-term effects. From a diagnostic standpoint, epidural injections can help target which levels of stenosis to address surgically, in particular, when there are varying degrees of stenosis at different levels. They may also be used to perform selective nerve root blocks to elucidate which neural foramen requires decompression. Careful attention to relief of symptoms is essential on the part of the patient following this procedure.

Surgical Indications and Treatment

With the exception of the onset of cauda equina syndrome, surgery for spinal stenosis is an elective decision that should be made by the patient. The main considerations in the discussion should include intractable pain, progressive neurologic deficit or progressively diminished walking ability and tolerance, significantly altered quality of life and functional status, all within the setting of failed nonoperative management. The goal of surgery is to alleviate radicular pain if this appears to be a component and mostly the symptoms of neurogenic claudication. Patients should be made aware that simply addressing the stenosis will not necessarily affect their low back pain as it is difficult to predict what amount of this pain is attributed to degenerative disk disease, arthritis, and subtle or gross instability.[25]

Open and Minimally Invasive Options

As has been previously mentioned, it is important to correlate clinical symptoms with radiographic findings. Once this process has been completed and epidural steroid injections have been used as an adjunct to confirm the location of the pathology, surgical intervention can be planned. Relative stability, including spondylolisthesis, lateral listhesis, or hypermobile facets may need to be addressed with in situ posterolateral arthrodesis or instrumented fusion. The goal of surgery is to alleviate all areas of symptomatic compression, inclusive of the central canal, the lateral recess, and the neuroforamina. The standard means of achieving this decompression is to perform a combination of a laminectomy, partial medial facetectomy, and foraminotomy. Essentially, the lamina is removed in order to gain access to the central canal. The patient is positioned in a prone position on a Jackson table with bony prominences well-padded and a midline incision is made after using fluoroscopy to confirm the levels of intervention. Soft tissue dissection is carried down alongside the spinous processes and lamina out to the facet, with care taken to preserve the facet capsules so as not to create instability in the functional spinal unit.[26] The pars interarticularis is also exposed so as to identify the lateral most border of the decompression. The interspace to be addressed is then entered by releasing the ligamentum flavum from the underside of the superior lamina or the dorsal surface of the inferior lamina. Once the level of the dura has been identified, Kerrison Rongeurs in combination with a high-speed burr are used to remove the ligamentum as well as the desired lamina. It is safer to remove the lamina in a cephalad direction starting at the inferior aspect of the superior lamina as the ligamentum is present underneath to protect the dura. The lateral recess should then be identified, decompressed, and any additional hypertrophic osteophytes from the facet joint can also be taken down to follow the course of the traversing nerve root out of the caudal foramen. The canal surrounding the nerve root is also decompressed, ensuring that a Woodson or ball-tipped probe can be freely passed through the foramina. Every attempt is made to preserve the integrity of the pars to maintain stability.[11]

Is this surgery effective? The SPORT study was a prospective randomized multicenter study that evaluated patients with spinal stenosis without spondylolisthesis who had symptoms for at least 12 weeks and failed conservative management. The patients were assigned into two groups, and underwent either decompressive surgical management as described above or nonsurgical management inclusive of anti-inflammatories and physical therapy. Surgical treatment showed substantial decreases in pain and physical function improvement, with statistically significant differences in SF-36 scores and modified Oswestry Disability Index (ODI) both at 2 years and 4 years out from surgery.[9,10]

The Maine Lumbar Study referenced above also evaluated the outcomes of surgery for spinal stenosis with up to 8–10 years of follow-up. Leg or back pain was substantially improved at 1-year follow-up with a comparative difference of 55–28%, with surgery outweighing nonsurgical management. Over time this difference in outcomes narrowed. This study was not randomized and degree of stenosis was variable amongst the population with some patients also undergoing fusion.[6-8]

Other studies have confirmed these results in favor of surgical intervention but their data is confounded by patients who underwent concomitant fusion.[27] As the inclusion of a fusion can significantly affect back pain and functional status, it is difficult to isolate the improvement of outcomes in these patients to the effects of the decompressive surgery.

Another open surgical option to treat spinal stenosis, especially in cases isolated to a single level or unilateral symptoms, is to perform a microdecompression with laminotomy/hemilaminotomy or hemilaminectomy and assistance of the microscope. The difference between these two procedures is the amount of lamina removed on only one side. In the more limited laminotomy/hemilaminotomy, resection of the distal half of the superior lamina on one side as well as the proximal half of the inferior lamina if necessary is used to address unilateral symptoms. If there are contralateral symptoms, one can use the microscope to visualize and decompress the contralateral side through the same laminotomy defect. This is technically demanding in terms of visualizing and decompressing the contralateral lateral recess and foramen as the medial structures of the spinous process and interspinous ligaments make obtaining the correct angle with the Kerrison Rongeurs difficult and decompression is performed via palpation rather than visualization. If necessary, the operating table may also be tilted. The hemilaminectomy version involves take down of the entire lamina on the affected side instead of portions of the superior and inferior lamina to gain access to the laminotomy window. The decision of which technique to use should be guided by where the majority of the compression is located with respect to known anatomical landmarks.[28]

A final open option is to perform a lumbar laminoplasty, which is similar in concept to a cervical laminoplasty. The lamina is hinged open on one side and the resected spinous process is secured to the lamina on the other side to maintain patency of the canal. The goal of this technique is to decompress the central canal by expanding the diameter of the bony circumference. Lumbar laminoplasty is best indicated in young and active patients with primarily central stenosis as it is difficult to address the lateral recess with this technique.[29] Initial studies demonstrated an increase in canal diameter by approximately 20% with a 70% improvement rate of preoperative Japanese Orthopedic Association (JOA) score at a mean of 3-year follow-up.[30] Matsui has also reported marked recovery of clinical symptoms as assessed by pre- and postoperative JOA scores and 80% good or excellent results at 5-year follow-up when expansive lumbar laminoplasty is combined with stabilization procedures and a relatively small risk of repeat surgery.[13] Longer term follow-up of laminoplasty alone (without fusion) has been performed by Kawaguchi, again with assessment of JOA scores. They found satisfactory neurological recovery within 1 year and maintenance of recovery at 5 years for most patients. Three patients with lateral stenosis in the setting of scoliosis had poor recovery. Beyond 5 years, seven patients had late functional deterioration with adjacent segment disease. Five developed spondylolisthesis and therefore this should be screened for postoperatively. Interlaminar fusions did occur in approximately 40% of patients, though recovery was not affected by this.[29] Overall, laminoplasty remains an option in carefully selected patients with predominantly central stenosis.

Minimally invasive options to address spinal stenosis include endoscopic laminotomy with the use of a tubular retractor and fiberoptic endoscopic systems. There is a steep learning curve associated with this procedure and during the initial learning curve visualization of the ipsilateral lateral recess without significant resection of the facet joint can be difficult.[31] Studies have shown significant improvement in ODI scores validating the technique.[32] When compared to open procedures there is a higher rate of complications such as incidental durotomy and transient neuralgia thought to be due to excessive retraction on nerve roots and central thecal sac for visualization. More recent studies looking at tubular endoscopic decompression have modified the original techniques used. A series of dilators is used to visualize the spinolaminar junction. The tubular retractor is then aimed medially and the contralateral lateral recess and foramen are addressed first. This allows for improved visualization of ipsilateral side, which is thought to reduce the durotomy rate fourfold.[33] Proposed advantages of endoscopic decompression include reduced blood loss, shorter length of stay, and diminished use of narcotics with equivalent outcomes to open decompression.[33,34]

An additional means of treating spinal stenosis is the use of interspinous process devices. These devices are thought to function by expanding the canal diameter by blocking extension and increasing the foraminal height. The induced flexed position is thought to allow for symptomatic improvement of neurogenic claudication and nerve root impingement. This device is placed with the patient in the lateral decubitus position with their lumbar spine slightly flexed. A proposed advantage is the ability to insert these devices under local anesthetic. This creates an option for surgical management of spinal stenosis in elderly patients with significant medical comorbidities who may not tolerate administration of general anesthesia well. Zucherman et al. performed a multicenter prospective randomized study comparing patients with spinal stenosis treated with the X STOP device to those who managed nonoperatively and used the Zurich Claudication Questionnaire (ZCQ) as the primary outcome measure. The ZCQ's components include physical function, symptom severity, and patient satisfaction. At 1 year, operative versus nonoperative patients had a success rate of 59% and 12%, respectively.[35] 2-year follow-up for this same patient population showed maintained improvement over the nonsurgical group in all three domains of ZCQ assessment.[36] The concern for use of these devices is the high rate of revision (up to 30% at 3.5 years follow-up)[37] and the potential for the device to erode through poor quality bone in the spinous processes and thus prevent significant improvement in symptoms. Long-term follow-up studies in the near future should shed light on the utility of such devices and will likely govern their availability and use.[35,36]

Complications

There are several potential complications associated with spinal stenosis, most of which can occur during or following surgical management. The main complication of nonsurgical management can be the onset of cauda equina syndrome. Severe compression can result in acute neurologic sensory or motor deficit in the lower extremities, urinary retention (detrusor weakness), post-void incontinence, fecal incontinence, sexual dysfunction, and saddle anesthesia. This should be considered a surgical emergency and managed with immediate decompression. Interestingly, there are case reports of epidural steroid injections also causing cauda equina syndrome There are various mechanisms postulated by which transient neurologic symptoms may occur. These include inadvertent intrathecal injections, neurotoxicity of agents administered, compromise of blood supply to the cord, and loculation of injected fluids. It is important to be vigilant in screening postoperative patients who report concerns of neurologic symptoms, although symptoms may be carefully monitored before proceeding directly to surgical intervention.[38]

During surgical decompression of spinal stenosis, scarring, adherence, or calcification can result in dural tears with resultant leakage of cerebrospinal fluid.[39] The incidence in the literature of dural tears in the setting of spinal stenosis ranges from 8% to 10%,[40] and of course, is higher in the revision setting. Management includes complete exposure of the tear and repair whenever possible with either a running locked stitch or interrupted stitches. A watertight seal resistant to an intraoperative-induced Valsalva maneuver should be attained. Adjuvant fibrin glue or collagen matrices can be used to seal the defect. If excessive tension is felt to be present across the repair, fat, fascial, or muscle grafts can be used to patch the defect. Attention should be paid to obtain a watertight fascial closure as well, and use of a drain is both optional and controversial for fear of creation of a fistula or pseudomeningocele in the subcutaneous tissue.[41] If a dural leak is refractory to primary and possibly revision repair, then a drain may be used to shunt fluid proximal to the repair to allow for healing or epidural blood patches may be used. In rare cases of a persistent dural leak, meningitis can occur with an incidence of 0.18%.[11] In any case, the goal is to repair the durotomy and prevent or treat symptoms associated with traction on the structures of the brain such as postoperative spinal headache, photophobia, phonophobia, tinnitus, vertigo, nausea, and vomiting.[42]

Postoperatively, infection can occur with a reported rate of approximately 2% of deep infection after surgical management of lumbar spinal stenosis. Perioperative antibiotic treatment and strict adherence to sterile protocol is always imperative. Infection rates can be expected to increase with comorbidities such as diabetes mellitus, smoking, increased body mass index, and history of infection.[11]

Epidural hematoma formation after decompression can occur but is relatively rare. Meticulous hemostasis throughout the surgical case and prior to closure are keys to prevention. A thorough postoperative examination is a key to avoid missing the onset of a new neurologic deficit, and exploration of the wound is necessary if there is concern for development of a significant hematoma in association with a progressive change in examination. MRI can be used in the postoperative period to aid surgical decision-making.

Postlaminectomy instability is another complication that can occur after decompressive surgery for spinal stenosis. Prior biomechanical studies have shown that stability should be maintained so long as at least 50% of the facet joint is preserved and the pars interarticularis is not violated.[43] Careful dissection should allow for preservation of facet capsules. Postoperative X-rays should be obtained to ensure maintenance of stability at the level that was decompressed.

During surgical decompression, manipulation of the central thecal sac and decompression of the foramina and lateral recess can potentially result in nerve root injury. Postoperatively, this may manifest as temporary neuralgia or frank neurologic deficit that will usually recover over time.

The SPORT study, the Maine Lumbar Spine Study, and Malmivaara all looked at reoperation rate for recurrent stenosis on the patients who underwent surgical management of stenosis. They all quoted extremely low rates of 1.3%, 1.2%, and 2% at 1 year, respectively.[8,10,27] Symptoms may recur in patients as there is potential for bony regrowth of lamina. Postacchini et al. assessed AP radiographs postoperatively and found that 40% of patients had greater than 40% of regrowth, while only 12% showed no regrowth at all.[44] The amount of bony regrowth has in turn been correlated with clinical outcomes, and as expected, the less regrowth the better the outcomes.[44,45]

Prognosis

Sigmundsson et al. surveyed the Swedish Spine registry for those patients who were treated for central spinal stenosis with decompression without fusion. They considered various outcome scores including ODI, self-estimated walking distance, leg and back pain levels via visual analog scale (VAS) and the EuroQol-5D (EQ-5D). They found that several factors could predict the outcome of operative intervention for spinal stenosis. Duration of leg pain exceeding 2 years preoperatively predicted inferior outcomes in terms of leg and back pain and function. Those patients who had documented higher use of preoperative analgesics had higher levels of back pain postoperatively. Low preoperative function predicted low function and dissatisfaction at follow-up. Finally, narrow dural sac area predicted more gains in terms of back pain and absolute leg pain at follow-up. Thus, this group was able to identify several factors that can be assessed and used to predict outcome and educate patients on prognostic expectations postoperatively.[46]

Previous sections have discussed outcome studies of surgical versus nonsurgical management of spinal stenosis. Most studies have shown that over time results do deteriorate after surgical intervention, however, a greater proportion of patients treated surgically have sustained relief with long-term follow-up. This has been documented for up to 4 years in the SPORT study with a specific patient population suffering from spinal stenosis without spondylolisthesis treated with decompressive surgery only.[9,10] Subgroup analysis of the SPORT patient population has identified that spinal stenosis patients with predominant leg pain over low back pain improved significantly more than patients with predominant low back pain.[47] Another interesting finding in a separate subanalysis of the SPORT spinal stenosis population was that if surgery was performed, the number of levels did not affect the outcome; multilevel stenosis did not demonstrate worse baseline symptoms or worse treatment outcomes than isolated spinal stenosis. If degenerative spondylolisthesis was also present, however, those with a single level of stenosis did better than those with multilevel stenosis.[48] Ragab has shown that expected outcomes are not affected by advanced age as in over 100 patients between the ages of 70 and 101; there was no further morbidity of surgical intervention compared to a younger population.[49] To enhance outcomes, it is recommended that a more extensive decompression be performed at the time of intervention. This ensures a higher chance of addressing symptomatic pathology and avoiding early revision surgery. Comorbidities should be optimized preoperatively. The role of fusion in combination with decompressive procedures remains controversial. In the absence of instability, arthrodesis is not justified; however, it is difficult to predict what proportion of those with back pain associated with their symptoms from spinal stenosis will require reoperation. The natural history of spinal stenosis has been shown to be favorably altered with surgical intervention and does result in improved functional status, walking ability, and quality of life measures.

REFERENCES

1. Patel C, Truumees E. Spinal stenosis: pathophysiology, clinical diagnosis, and differential diagnosis. In: Rothman RH, Simeon FA (Eds). The Spine, 6th edition. Vol. 2. Philadelphia, PA: W.B. Saunders; 2011. p. 1064.
2. Daffner SD, Wang JC. The pathophysiology and nonsurgical treatment of lumbar spinal stenosis. Instr Course Lect. 2009;58:657-68.
3. Delamarter RB, Bohlman HH, Dodge LD, et al. Experimental lumbar spinal stenosis. Analysis of the cortical evoked potentials, microvasculature, and histopathology. J Bone Joint Surg Am. 1990;72(1):110-20.
4. Johnsson KE, Rosén I, Udén A. The natural course of lumbar spinal stenosis. Clin Orthop Relat Res. 1992;(279):82-6.
5. Amundsen T, Weber H, Nordal HJ, et al. Lumbar spinal stenosis: Conservative or surgical management? A prospective 10-year study. Spine (Phila Pa 1976). 2000;25(11):1424-35;discussion 1435-6.
6. Atlas SJ, Deyo RA, Keller RB, et al. The Maine Lumbar Spine Study, Part III. 1-year outcomes of surgical and nonsurgical management of lumbar spinal stenosis. Spine (Phila Pa 1976). 1996;21(15):1787-94;discussion 1794-5.
7. Atlas SJ, Keller RB, Robson D, et al. Surgical and nonsurgical management of lumbar spinal stenosis: four-year outcomes from the maine lumbar spine study. Spine (Phila Pa 1976). 2000;25(5):556-62.
8. Atlas SJ, Keller RB, Wu YA, et al. Long-term outcomes of surgical and nonsurgical management of lumbar spinal stenosis: 8 to 10 year results from the maine lumbar spine study. Spine (Phila Pa 1976). 2005;30(8):936-43.
9. Weinstein JN, Tosteon TD, Lurie JD, et al. Surgical versus nonoperative treatment for lumbar spinal stenosis four-year results of the Spine Patient Outcomes Research Trial. Spine (Phila Pa 1976). 2010;35(14):1329-38.
10. Weinstein JN, Tosteon TD, Lurie JD, et al. Surgical versus nonsurgical therapy for lumbar spinal stenosis. N Engl J Med. 2008;358(8):794-810.
11. Su BW, Rihn J, Byers R, et al. Surgical management of lumbar spinal stenosis. In: Rothman RH, Simeon FA (Eds). The Spine, 6th edition. Vol. 2. Philadelphia: WB Saunders; 2011. p. 1083.
12. Thomas SA. Spinal Stenosis: history and physical examination. Phys Med Rehabil Clin N Am. 2003;14(1):29-39.
13. Matsui H, Kanamori M, Ishihara H, et al. Expansive lumbar laminoplasty for degenerative spinal stenosis in patients below 70 years of age. Eur Spine J. 1997;6(3):191-6.
14. Fortin JD, Wheeler MT. Imaging in lumbar spinal stenosis. Pain Physician. 2004;7(1):133-9.
15. Schinnerer KA, Katz LD, Grauer JN. MR findings of exaggerated fluid in facet joints predicts instability. J Spinal Disord Tech. 2008;21(7):468-72.
16. Boden SD, Davis DO, Dina TS, et al. Abnormal magnetic-resonance scans of the lumbar spine in asymptomatic subjects. A prospective investigation. J Bone Joint Surg Am. 1990;72(3):403-8.
17. de Schepper EI, Overdevest GM, Suri P, et al. Diagnosis of lumbar spinal stenosis: an updated systematic review of the accuracy of diagnostic tests. Spine (Phila Pa 1976). 2013;38(8):E469-81.
18. Bolender NF, Schönström NS, Spengler DM. Role of computed tomography and myelography in the diagnosis of central spinal stenosis. J Bone Joint Surg Am. 1985;67(2):240-6.
19. Herno A, Airaksinen O, Saari T, et al. The predictive value of preoperative myelography in lumbar spinal stenosis. Spine (Phila Pa 1976). 1994;19(12):1335-8.

20. Mazanec, D. Nonoperative management of lumbar spinal stenosis. In: Rothman RH, Simeon FA (Eds). The Spine, 6th edition. Vol. 2. Philadelphia: WB Saunders; 2011. p. 1078.
21. Whitman JM, Flynn TW, Childs JD, et al. SPORT Investigators. A comparison between two physical therapy treatment programs for patients with lumbar spinal stenosis: A randomized clinical trial. Spine. 2006;31(22):2541-9.
22. Botwin KP, Gruber RD, Bouchlas CG, et al. Fluoroscopically guided lumbar transformational epidural steroid injections in degenerative lumbar stenosis: An outcome study. Am J Phys Med Rehabil. 2002;81(12):898-905.
23. Manchikanti L, Cash KA, McManus CD, et al. Results of 2-year follow-up of a randomized, double-blind, controlled trial of fluoroscopic caudal epidural injections in central spinal stenosis. Pain Physician. 2012;15(5):371-84.
24. Radcliff K, Kepler C, Hilibrand A, et al. Epidural steroid injections are associated with less improvement in patients with lumbar spinal stenosis: a subgroup analysis of the Spine Patient Outcomes Research Trial. Spine (Phila Pa 1976). 2013;38(4):279-91.
25. Johnsson KE, Udén A, Rosén I. The effect of decompression on the natural course of spinal stenosis. A comparison of surgically treated and untreated patients. Spine (Phila Pa 1976). 1991;16(6):615-9.
26. Hansraj KK, Cammisa FP Jr, O'Leary PF, et al. Decompressive surgery for typical lumbar spinal stenosis. Clin Orthop Relat Res. 2001;(384):10-7.
27. Malmivaara A, Slätis P, Heliövaara M, et al. Finnish Lumbar Spinal Research Group. Surgical or nonoperative treatment for lumbar spinal stenosis? A randomized controlled trial. Spine (Phila Pa 1976). 2007;32(1):1-8.
28. Toyoda H, Nakamura H, Konishi S, et al. Clinical outcome of microsurgical bilateral decompression via unilateral approach for lumbar canal stenosis: Minimum five-year follow-up. Spine (Phila Pa 1976). 2011;36(5):410-5.
29. Kawaguchi Y, Kanamori M, Ishihara H, et al. Clinical and radiographic results of expansve lumbar laminoplasty in patients with spinal stenosis. J Bone Joint Surg Am. 2004;86(8):1698-703.
30. Matsui H, Tsuji H, Sekido H, et al. Results of expansive laminoplasty for lumbar spinal stenosis in active manual workers. Spine (Phila Pa 1976). 1992;17(Suppl 3):S37-40.
31. Rahman M, Summers LE, Richter B, et al. Comparison of techniques for decompressive lumbar laminectomy: The minimally invasive versus the "classic" open approach. Minim Invasive Neurosurg. 2008;51(2):100-5.
32. Pao JL, Chen WC, Chen PQ. Clinical outcomes of microendoscopic decompressive laminotomy for degenerative lumbar spinal stenosis. Eur Spine J. 2009;18(5):672-8.
33. Azgarzadie F, Khoo LT. Minimally invasive operative management for lumbar spinal stenosis: overview of early and long-term outcomes. Orthop Clin North Am. 2007;38(3):387-99; abstract vi-vii.
34. Khoo LT, Fessler RG. Microendoscopic decompressive laminotomy for the treatment of lumbar stenosis. Neurosurgery. 2002;51(Suppl 5):S146-54.
35. Zucherman JF, Hsu KY, Hartjen CA, et al. A prospective randomized multi-center study for the treatment of lumbar spinal stenosis with the X STOP interspinous implant: 1-year results. Eur Spine J. 2004;13(1):22-31.
36. Zucherman JF, Hsu KY, Hartjen CA, et al. A multicenter, prospective, randomized trial evaluating the X STOP interspinous process decompression system for the treatment of neurogenic intermittent claudication: two-year follow-up results. Spine (Phila Pa 1976). 2005;30(12):1351-8.
37. Tuschel A, Chavanne A, Eder C, et al. Implant survival analysis and failure modes of the X-STOP interspinous distraction device. Spine (Phila Pa 1976). 2013;38(21):1826-31.
38. Bilir A, Gulec S. Cauda equina syndrome after epidural steroid injection: a case report. J Manipulative Physiol Ther. 2006;29(6):492.e1-3.
39. Desai A, Ball PA, Bekelis K, et al. Surgery for lumbar degenerative spondylolisthesis in Spine Patient Outcomes Research Trial: does incidental durotomy affect outcome? Spine (Phila Pa 1976). 2012;37(5):406-13.
40. Takahashi Y, Sato T, Hyodo H, et al. Incidental durotomy during lumbar spine surgery: risk factors and anatomic locations: clinical article. J Neurosurg Spine. 2013;18(2):165-9.
41. Wang JC, Bohlman HH, Riew KD, et al. Dural tears secondary to operations on the lumbar spine: Management and results after a two-year minimum follow-up of eighty-eight patients. J Bone Joint Surg Am. 1998;80(12):1728-32.
42. Campbell PG, Hanna A, Harrop J, et al. Spinal dural injuries. In: Rothman RH, Simeon FA (Eds). The Spine, 6th edition. Vol. 2. Philadelphia, PA: Saunders; 2011. p. 1720.
43. Lee CK. Lumbar spinal instability (olisthesis) after extensive posterior spinal decompression. Spine (Phila Pa 1976). 1983;8(4):429-33.
44. Postacchini F, Cinotti G. Bone regrowth after surgical decompression for lumbar spinal stenosis. J Bone Joint Surg Br. 1992;74(6):862-9.
45. Chen Q, Baba H, Kamitani K, et al. Postoperative bone re-growth in lumbar spinal stenosis. A multivariate analysis of 48 patients. Spine (Phila Pa 1976). 1995;19(19):2144-9.
46. Sigmundsson FG, Kang XP, Jönsson B, et al. Prognostic factors in lumbar spinal stenosis surgery. Acta Orthop. 2012;83(5):536-42.
47. Pearson A, Blood E, Lurie J, et al. Predominant leg pain is associated with better surgical outcomes in degenerative spondylolisthesis and spinal stenosis: results from the Spine Patient Outcomes Research Trial (SPORT). Spine (Phila Pa 1976). 2011;36(3):219-29.
48. Park DK, An HS, Lurie JD, et al. Does multilevel stenosis lead to poorer outcomes? A subanalysis of the Spine Patient Outcomes Research Trial (SPORT) lumbar stenosis study. Spine (Phila Pa 1976). 2010;35(4):439-46.
49. Ragab AA, Fye MA, Bohlman HH. Surgery of the lumbar spine for spinal stenosis in 118 patients 70 years of age or older. Spine (Phila Pa 1976). 2003;28(4):348-53.

CHAPTER 38 Degenerative Spondylolisthesis

Gabriel Widi, Faiz Ahmad, Jason I Liounakos, Yi Lu, Michael Y Wang

INTRODUCTION

Spondylolisthesis refers to the forward slippage of one vertebra relative to adjacent vertebrae. It is estimated to affect approximately 5% of the general population.[1-3] Spondylolisthesis was first described by an obstetric surgeon named Herbinaux in 1772 as a boney prominence anterior to the sacrum resulting in pelvic outlet narrowing and difficult delivery. Junghanns first described degenerative spondylolisthesis in 1930, separating the pathology from isthmic spondylolisthesis. He described this entity as a "pseudospondylolisthesis." This anterior translation of one vertebral body in relation to the next often results in significant central/lateral recess stenosis, which can manifest symptomatically with lower back pain, radiculopathy, and/or neurogenic claudication as a result of central and foraminal stenosis. Since then, much has been uncovered regarding the pathophysiology/etiology of the various forms of lumbar spondylolisthesis.[1] The etiology of degenerative spondylolisthesis is multifactorial and related to other under the umbrella of lumbar spondylosis.

In comparison with other medical disciplines, the evidence base for surgical management of lumbar spondylolisthesis remains relatively sparse, and clear-cut guidelines for optimal management are not presently available. This is likely due to a variety of reasons, including the inherent ethical/logistic challenges involved in designing and executing a proper blinded and randomized trial in surgical cohorts. The presence of several distinct subtypes of lumbar spondylolisthesis and the heterogeneity of this patient population precludes the derivation of widely applicable therapeutic conclusions/guidelines. Since the majority of the available literature is disproportionately related to degenerative lumbar spondylolisthesis, it will form the basis of this chapter, with selective references on isthmic spondylolisthesis contributing to a lesser extent.

EPIDEMIOLOGY AND NATURAL HISTORY

Degenerative spondylolisthesis, further referred to as spondylolisthesis, is a disease of the aging spine with most people afflicted over the age of 50 years. It is characterized by a posterior slip of one vertebra on another. L4–L5 is the most commonly affected level. If L5 is sacralized the risk of developing spondylolisthesis at L4–L5 increased four-fold. Less commonly affected is L5–S1 because of strong iliolumbar ligaments keeping L5 relatively fixed, anatomically. Postmortem studies have revealed an occurrence rate of 4% overall and 10% in women older than 60 years. Male to female ratio is 1:5–6. Black women are three times more likely to develop than condition than white females.[4,5] Other associated conditions include diabetes and curiously a history of oophorectomy; however, the role of estrogen in the development of spondylolisthesis remains unclear.[6,7]

In terms of mechanical factors contributing to development the actual orientation of the facet joints has been implicated. It is hypothesized that exaggerated sagittal orientation of the facet joints may be instrumental in the development of a slip. Conversely, others have argued that this exaggerated facet joint orientation may just be the result of bony remodeling.[8-11] Relative height of the intercrestal line, inherent strength of the supporting ligaments, degree of degenerative disk disease, and lumbar lordosis are also likely involved.[7,12]

Jacobsen et al.[7] reviewed 4,151 participants of the Copenhagen Osteoarthritis study to identify prevalence and individual risk factors for degenerative lumbar spondylolisthesis and found that, for women, increased body mass index (BMI), age, and degree of lordosis were risk factors for spondylolisthesis. In men only increased age was identified as a predisposing factor (level III evidence).

With regard to its natural history, conservative management is usually effective, at least initially, for the management of symptomatic low-grade spondylolisthesis without neurological deficit. Repetitive spinal flexion may lead to worsening of spondylolisthesis. Significant disk space collapse (greater than 80%) with evidence of autofusion, including intervertebral osteophytosis, understandably reduces the risk of progression.[13] Another study by the same group[14] found that the majority of patients presenting without evidence of neurologic deficit do well with conservative care, providing level II support for conservative management of patients without neurologic deficit. In addition, patients that present with sensory changes, muscle weakness, or cauda equina syndrome are more likely to develop progressive functional decline without surgery. This work also supports the notion that progression of the slip does not correlate with progression of clinical symptoms.

Degenerative lumbar spondylolisthesis was studied in a more focused population by Vogt et al.[5] in 788 white south central Pennsylvanian women over 65 years of age. Anterolisthesis was noted in 29% of this very specific population and 90% of cases involved only one level. The incidence of slip was not affected by smoking, diabetes mellitus or oophorectomy and not associated with presence of back symptoms.

Similarly, Kauppila et al.[15] detailed a population-based, retrospective, cohort study of 217 men and 400 women in which 12% of men and 25% of women developed some degree of spondylolisthesis over a period of approximately 20 years. Patients with acquired spondylolisthesis reported more daily back symptoms, but did not disability compared to controls. This study provides level III evidence that in an elderly population, back pain is correlated with the presence of spondylolisthesis; however, in only one-third of these cases is the spondylolisthesis symptomatic. Therefore, degenerative spondylolisthesis can be acquired in an asymptomatic population, with a higher incidence in females (4:1).

Current evidence, based on largely level II and III studies, indicate that lumbar degenerative spondylolisthesis presenting with neurologic deficit generally do worse with conservative measures. Future prospective studies on untreated patients with degenerative lumbar spondylolisthesis generating level I evidence may change practice paradigms and possibly lead to better outcomes.

SIGNS AND SYMPTOMS

An accurate history and focused physical examination are essential to the formulation of a plan for treatment of patients with degenerative lumbar spondylolisthesis. Degenerative lumbar spondylolisthesis may be asymptomatic or associated with symptoms of radiculopathy or neurogenic claudication with or without concomitant back pain. Furthermore, signs and symptoms of mechanical instability associated with degenerative lumbar spondylolisthesis without neurological symptoms have not been well characterized. That being said, a diagnosis of spondylolisthesis should be considered in patients presenting with radiculopathy and neurogenic intermittent claudication and is easily ruled in or out with plain radiographs.

Cauchioux et al.[16] presented a diagnostic evaluation of 26 patients with degenerative spondylolisthesis. Of these patients, 80% reported back pain, 46% reported radiculopathy, and 54% reported neurogenic claudication as their primary symptom. Sciatica tended to occur in the older patients and neurogenic claudication in the younger patients (level III evidence). Others studies conclude that while often asymptomatic, when symptomatic, radiculopathy and neurogenic claudication secondary to the associated stenosis are most common (level III evidence).[17,18]

DIAGNOSTIC IMAGING

The most fundamental tool for non-invasive detection of degenerative lumbar spondylolisthesis is the lateral radiograph. A retrospective study by Brown et al.[19] examined a number of different parameters including diagnostic features on plain radiographs during the 1980s. These patients were selected from 2,348 consecutive patients with low back pain; of which 132 (5.6%) had radiographic evidence of degenerative spondylolisthesis. Eighty eight of these patients were female and 44 were male with mean age of 63 years in the female and 65 years in the male group. These data offer level III evidence that plain radiographs are a useful test for identifying patients with degenerative spondylolisthesis (level III evidence).

In symptomatic patients, the use of plain or computed tomography (CT) myelography has proven extremely useful in the assessment of spinal stenosis in patients with degenerative lumbar spondylolisthesis. Rosenberg et al.[18] reviewed a group of 200 consecutive patients retrospectively with degenerative lumbar spondylolisthesis. Thirty nine of these patients had unremitting symptoms and 29 of them underwent myelography, which showed an hourglass constriction of the dura at the level of the slippage while seven patients also had a disk herniation. In the presence of neurological symptoms, myelography has thus proven an effective diagnostic too! (level III evidence).

The use of dynamic films has little support though some level III studies showed that flexion-extension films are predictive of instability.[20] Kanayama et al. reviewed a case series of 19 patients with dynamic imaging who were candidates for instrumented lumbar arthrodesis and decompression. Their findings indicated that disk angle in flexion and range of motion highly correlated with intraoperative distraction stiffness. The validity of intraoperative stiffness is in of itself questionable and the clinical application of such test is unknown (level IV evidence).

A CT is a useful non-invasive test for patients who have a contraindication to magnetic resonance imaging (MRI), have an inconclusive MRI, or for whom MRI findings poorly correlate with symptoms and CT myleogram is deemed inappropriate. Pathologic findings evident on CT include canal stenosis, facet hypertrophy, and foraminal stenosis.[21] In patients without contraindication; however, MRI remains the gold standard for evaluation of neural elements compression in degenerative lumbar spondylolisthesis. MRI is more superior in detecting hypertrophy of the facet joint capsule, ligament flavum hypertrophy or buckling and nerve roots compression.

Axial-loaded MRI has been shown to demonstrate a larger change compared to conventional MRI of the thecal sac cross-sectional area in patients with degenerative spondylolisthesis compared to patients with spinal stenosis without spondylolisthesis, suggesting axial-loaded MRI could be a useful diagnostic adjunctive for patients with spondylolisthesis.[22]

MEDICAL MANAGEMENT

A paucity of evidence exists addressing medical treatment for degenerative lumbar spondylolisthesis. Patients can be asymptomatic, present exclusively with axial back pain or present with neurogenic claudication and/or radicular pain with or without accompanying axial back pain. The Spine Patient Outcomes Research Trial (SPORT) was designed to compare the effectiveness of surgical and nonsurgical treatment among participants with confirmed diagnoses of intervertebral disk herniation,[23,24] spinal stenosis, and degenerative spondylolisthesis[12] (level I evidence). The study failed to find a significant advantage of surgery compared to conservative care; however, these initial conclusions were significant limited due to treatment crossover. When an as-treated analysis was performed, it was found that surgery was indeed superior to nonsurgical treatment. The somewhat greater improvement in the SPORT compared to previous studies may be related to the nonsurgical treatments received. SPORT participants had higher rates of epidural steroid injections than did the Main Lumbar Spine Study (MLSS) participants (44% vs. 18%), and less activity restriction (16% vs. 29%).[25]

SURGICAL INDICATIONS AND TREATMENT

Currently, there is a lack of strong clinical evidence demonstrating a clear therapeutic benefit for surgical intervention in degenerative spondylolisthesis. Until recently, favorable outcomes following surgical intervention for spondylolisthesis were largely limited to anecdotal experience, personal case reports, and various low-level retrospective studies. This is despite the general consensus opinion among spine surgeons that symptomatic spondylolisthesis responds well to surgical management.

In an early retrospective analysis of 32 adolescent patients with Meyerding grade III to IV spondylolisthesis, Harris et al.[26] reported 57% of patients treated with in situ posterior arthrodesis were clinically asymptomatic at mean follow-up of 24 years, as opposed to 36% of patients who were managed nonoperatively (level III evidence). This was consistent with a similar study, which also demonstrated that adolescent spondylolisthesis patients treated with in situ fusion had better clinical results and less pain than those treated conservatively with bed rest, followed by a core stabilizing exercise regimen[27] (level III evidence).

Several contemporary randomized control trials (RCTs) have evaluated the efficacy of surgery in the management of lumbar spondylolisthesis.[25,28-32] The results of these trials have proven difficult to interpret for several reasons. Diagnostically speaking, the failure to discern patients with lumbar spondylolisthesis from those with lumbar stenosis and/or degenerative disk disease contributes to the issue. In a well-designed RCT comparing surgery versus nonoperative treatment for degenerative lumbar stenosis, Malmivaara et al.[25] performed a subgroup analysis on 10 surgically treated patients with lumbar stenosis and concomitant degenerative spondylolisthesis who demonstrated more favorable functional outcomes based on Oswestry Disability Index (ODI) scale scores, as well as more alleviation of leg and back pain at 2-year follow-up, in comparison with stenosis patients who also underwent surgery (level I evidence). All 10 patients underwent laminectomy plus posterior pedicle screw arthrodesis, as opposed to the surgically treated stenosis patients who underwent decompression alone. The surgical group as a whole did better than the nonoperative cohort in terms of functional outcome and leg/back pain scores at 2-year follow-up; however, the subgroup analysis lacked sufficient power to explain the small outcome difference in favor of instrumented lumbar fusion in patients with concomitant degenerative spondylolisthesis.[25] This was similar to previous findings reported by Möller et al.[30] who demonstrated improved functional outcome based on the Disability Rating Index (DRI) and less pain in patients with adult isthmic spondylolisthesis treated with posterolateral fusion (PLF) compared to matched cohorts enrolled in a structured exercise program (level I evidence). Interestingly, in a follow-up report re-evaluating outcome at 9 years postenrollment, the degree of functional and pain improvement in the surgical cohort seemed to diminish over time; however, the surgical patients still classified their global outcome as clearly better than conservatively treated patients[30] (level I evidence). Carreon et al.[28] recently published an extensive systematic review of the ODI and Medical Outcomes Study Short Form 36 (SF-36) outcomes in fusion (unspecified) and nonsurgical treatment for symptomatic lumbar degenerative disease (level I evidence). As a whole, the fusion patients exhibited greater improvement in ODI scores, and patients with degenerative spondylolisthesis demonstrated the greatest ODI improvement following fusion, regardless of the fusion technique employed.

Recently, the 4-year follow-up results of the SPORT were made available (level I evidence). In the initial study, Weinstein et al.[23] conducted a multicenter, prospective, RCT comparing surgery, and medical/interventional treatment for neurogenic claudication from spinal stenosis and degenerative spondylolisthesis. Surgical treatment included laminectomy with or without fusion. Although the study was powered sufficiently (n = 607) to detect significant statistical trends, the high crossover rate between study groups negated some of this. In fact, nearly half of those patients assigned to conservative management had undergone surgery at 2-year follow-up. Meanwhile, 64% of those assigned to surgery actually had it performed. Importantly, the as-treated analysis for both cohorts combined demonstrated a significant advantage for surgery at 3 months and 1 year postoperatively, which only diminished slightly at 2-year follow-up[31] (level I evidence). This outcome advantage in surgically treated patients with degenerative spondylolisthesis was maintained at the 4-year follow-up.[32] Although initially designed as an RCT, the SPORT trial essentially provides level I evidence in support of surgery for the management of degenerative spondylolisthesis on the basis of as-treated analysis. Despite the noted shortcomings, the SPORT trial represents the first organized effort to specifically address the efficacy of surgery in patients with degenerative spondylolisthesis, and as such has provided valuable insight and direction for future research on the matter.

Overall, much of the available high-level evidence demonstrate a clear benefit of surgery over conservative management for lumbar spondylolisthesis with regards to functional outcome and pain alleviation, particularly at early postoperative time points. The degree of improvement appears to diminish over time; however, surgical patients tend to convey improved global outcome and satisfaction, compared to patients who are treated conservatively.

Decompression Alone versus Decompression/Arthrodesis

The role of arthrodesis for promotion of bony fusion has been debated when performing surgical decompression in the management of lumbar spondylolisthesis. In the past, various authors[16,33-37] have reported successful results with decompressive laminectomy alone, while others[4,19,38-44] have argued the utility of decompression augmented with fusion, with or without instrumentation. Overall, high quality evidence supporting one intervention over the other is lacking.

Of the available studies, many do conclude that significant benefit exists for patients undergoing decompression and fusion as opposed to decompression alone. In their landmark 1991 prospective trial, Herkowitz et al.[4] were the first to demonstrate a clear benefit in patients treated with decompression plus intertransverse noninstrumented arthrodesis versus decompression alone, with regards to relief of back and leg pain (level II evidence). The relatively high pseudarthrosis rate (36%) did not translate into poor clinical outcome, similar to previously reported results.[27] Although plagued by many significant limitations including pseudorandomization, broad pain outcome measures, and a lack of functional outcome assessment, it laid the foundation for adjunctive arthrodesis in the surgical management of lumbar spondylolisthesis. Ghogawala et al.[45] showed in a relatively small (n = 34) prospective and nonrandomized trial a significant difference in the degree of ODI improvement over baseline in favor of patients treated with decompression and fusion, as opposed to decompression alone (mean ODI difference 27.5 vs. 13.6, respectively; p = 0.02) (level II evidence). Notably, of the 20 patients treated with laminectomy alone, 15% underwent a second operation at 1 year to fuse the level of the spondylolisthesis for delayed-onset instability. Providing higher quality evidence, Martin et al.[46] performed a systematic review and meta-analysis aiming to compile the aggregate knowledge of studies comparing fusion and decompression alone, and between instrumented and noninstrumented fusion for the treatment of degenerative spondylolisthesis. The authors concluded there is moderate evidence that fusion may lead to a better clinical outcome compared with decompression alone. There was also moderate evidence that the utilization of instrumentation leads to improved fusion rates (level I evidence).

Responding to a need for higher quality RCTs regarding this subject, the recent Swedish Spinal Stenosis Study (SSSS) and Spinal Laminectomy versus Instrumented Pedicle Screw (SLIP) trial.[47,48] The SSSS provides considerable level I evidence that for the surgical management of spinal stenosis, with or without spondylolisthesis, the addition of fusion does not result in superior clinical outcomes. The study was sufficiently powered to detect significant differences in ODI at 2 years between the two primary groups and stratified subgroups (presenting with or without spondylolisthesis). In addition, two-thirds of the randomized patients completed follow-up at 5 years and the lack of any significant difference between the groups persisted through this time. Moreover the presence of spondylolisthesis had no bearing on clinical outcome and fusion surgery was associated with significantly higher cost compared to decompression alone. Conversely the SLIP trials published RCT of 66 patients (compared to 247 in the SSSS) found improved quality of life (via SF-36 scores) at 2, 3, and 4 years after surgery with clinically meaningful but not significantly different reductions in ODI scores. Importantly, reoperation rate was significantly higher in the laminectomy only group (34%) compared to 14% in the laminectomy and fusion group. Limitations of this study include the small overall sample size with a high dropout rate reducing the sample to 45 patients at 4 years follow-up as well as the significant (34%) revision rate for patients undergoing laminectomy alone, which may have affected the reported SF-36 scores.

In conclusion there still exists uncertainly as to whether decompression alone or decompression with fusion is the optimal treatment for lumbar spondylolisthesis. Further high-quality RCTs with large sample sizes are necessary to explore this further.

Instrumented versus Noninstrumented Posterolateral Fusion

The advent of pedicle screw instrumentation has helped change the practice of lumbar spine surgery despite the early lack of evidence showing superiority over PLF in terms of strength of fusion and cost-effectiveness. Studies with questionable methodologies were among the earliest reports of improved outcome with instrumentation. Chang et al.[49] retrospectively reviewed 85 cases of lumbar spondylolisthesis (57 degenerative and 28 isthmic) treated with instrumented fusion, and found that patients with degenerative spondylolisthesis had an improved clinical outcome and fusion rate with instrumentation, with 60% of patients reporting they were completely pain free at most recent follow-up (level III evidence). Interestingly, patients with isthmic spondylolisthesis also demonstrated an improved fusion rate; however, this did not translate to an improved clinical outcome with regards to pain relief and disability.

In another retrospective comparative study of 57 patients with grade I or II L4–L5 degenerative lumbar spondylolisthesis, Kimura et al. assess PLF with and without instrumentation.[50] Noninstrumented fusion cases reported a 72.4% satisfaction rate, with an 82.8% fusion rate. Patients undergoing an instrumented fusion reported an 82.1% satisfaction rate, with a 92.8% fusion rate. The only significant difference between groups was that the instrumented fusion group did have a lower incidence of back pain (level III evidence). Hence, a trend toward improved satisfaction and fusion rates with instrumentation was not powered to reach a significant difference. Lack of randomization and varying duration of follow-up between the groups limit this study.

Several RCTs have been conducted to further elucidate the potential role of instrumentation in lumbar fusion surgery.[51-54] The data heterogeneity unfortunately makes the results of several of these studies difficult to interpret in the setting of lumbar spondylolisthesis. Mélot[55] suggests that patients undergoing instrumented fusion have superior pain relief compared to the noninstrumented cohort in a meta-analysis of RCTs evaluating instrumented fusion of the degenerative lumbar spine; however, no definite conclusion could be drawn due to small sample size and inherent heterogeneity within the treatment group (level I evidence). Ekman et al.[29] were unable to demonstrate any significant difference between instrumented and noninstrumented fusion with regard to pain relief and disability in their RCT assessing instrumented fusion in adult isthmic spondylolisthesis with a follow-up of 9 years,[30,56] (level I evidence) consistent with previous accounts in the literature.[53] Likewise, Christensen et al. reported no significant difference in overall outcome in patients treated with either instrumented or noninstrumented fusion, but did note an increased reoperation rate in patients with pedicle screw instrumentation[51,52] (level I evidence). A subgroup analysis suggested that degenerative spondylolisthesis patients tended to improve significantly with pedicle screw instrumentation, whereas patients with adult isthmic spondylolisthesis (grades I and II) had superior long-term outcomes with noninstrumented fusion.[52] These findings are consistent with Martin's et al. meta-analysis, which concluded that the use of adjunctive instrumented fusion significantly increased the probability of attaining solid fusion, without any significant associated impact on clinical outcome[46] (level I evidence).

Bridwell et al. described a prospective, comparative study of 44 surgically treated patients with degenerative lumbar spondylolisthesis followed for at least 2 years[57] (level II evidence). The authors found higher fusion rates associated with the usage of instrumentation and also noted significant increases in the incidence of spondylolisthesis progression in those undergoing either laminectomy alone or laminectomy with *in situ* fusion (level II evidence).

Gibson et al.[58] performed a systematic review of 31 RCTs looking at all forms of surgical treatment for degenerative lumbar spondylosis (level II evidence). While instrumentation was associated with higher fusion rates, the clinical impact of this is less clear and instrumentation is also associated with a higher complication rate. Similar results were found by Fischgrund et al.[53] in a prospective and randomized comparative study of 76 consecutive patients with symptomatic spinal stenosis associated with degenerative lumbar spondylolisthesis (level I evidence).

Mardjetko et al.[59] conducted a meta-analysis of primarily level III studies addressing degenerative spondylolisthesis with radicular leg pain or neurogenic claudication from 1970 to 1993 (level III evidence). With regard to patient reported clinical outcome, satisfaction was significantly higher in the decompression with in situ fusion compared to the decompression only group (90% vs. 69%). Adding instrumentation did not result in a statistical difference compared to decompression and in situ fusion. The overall conclusion was that spinal fusion, with instrumentation or without, significantly improves patient satisfaction. Limitations include that only three level II studies were reviewed and the data was very heterogeneous.

Despite the findings of available, level I evidence suggesting a higher probability of achieving solid fusion with instrumented fusion, no compelling evidence at the current time suggest improved functional outcome or pain relief with the addition of instrumentation. An apparent trend for improved outcome with instrumented fusion in patients with a diagnosis of degenerative lumbar spondylolisthesis is only shown with subsequent subanalyses. Improved clinical outcomes in patients with symptomatic spinal stenosis and degenerative lumbar spondylolisthesis treated with surgical decompression with fusion and thusly recommended over decompression alone.

Lumbar Interbody Fusion versus Instrumented Posterolateral Fusion

Although first described by Briggs and Milligan in 1944, the posterior lumbar interbody fusion (PLIF) technique was later popularized by Cloward.[60,61] Over the next

50 years, the technique further evolved to include posterior pedicle screw fixation, and more recently, intersomatic porous spacers as proposed by Steffe and Brantigan.[62,63] In Yu's et al.[64] retrospective study of 76 patients comparing PLIF with mixed autogenous/allogenic bone chips versus PLIF utilizing artificial cages packed with morselized bone chips, they found that artificial cages provide better functional outcomes (ODI) and radiographic improvement (with regards to maintained disk height, slip ratio, segmental lordosis, and fusion status) than PLIF with bone chips alone (level III evidence). The theoretical advantages in favor of PLIF over PLF include maintenance of disk height, anterior column support, indirect foraminal decompression, circumferential fusion, and restoration of segmental lordosis. Like the rise of popularity in pedicle screw fixation, PLIF has also enjoyed a precipitous rise in popularity over the past 20 years despite a general lack of high quality outcome data supporting its use. Ha et al.[65] failed to demonstrate any significant difference between PLIF and PLF with regards to pain relief, ODI functional outcome, or fusion rates in 40 retrospectively studied patients (level III evidence). Dehoux et al.[66] reported a significant difference in functional outcome in favor of PLIF in patients with higher grade (Meyerding III and IV) slips, which was not evident in patients with grade I and II spondylolisthesis (level II evidence). They also reported a higher overall fusion rate in patients undergoing PLIF, though without any significant associated improvement in functional outcome. In a nonrandomized and prospective study of 60 patients with adult spondylolisthesis (isthmic and degenerative), Dantas et al.[1] reported no statistically significant difference in both the ODI and Roland-Morris scale between PLF and PLIF (level II evidence), similar to results in adult patients with isthmic spondylolisthesis published elsewhere by Ekman et al.[56] (level III evidence). In a small RCT of 20 patients, Inamdar et al.[6] showed improved radiographic reduction of spondylolisthesis with PLIF; however, PLF appeared to achieve better subjective clinical outcomes (level I evidence). In perhaps the best designed RCT on the subject, Cheng et al.[67] reported a superior fusion rate with PLIF (92.6% vs. 80.3%), without any statistical difference in clinical/functional outcome between the two groups (level I evidence). Interestingly, they noted a higher rate of complications relating to hardware biomechanics in the PLF group. Similarly, a subgroup analysis of the SPORT trial demonstrated no consistent differences in clinical outcomes among patients with degenerative spondylolisthesis treated with either noninstrumented PLF, instrumented PLF, or 360° (instrumented PLF + interbody fusion) fusion[68] (level II evidence). In another RCT by Fei et al.[69] comparing instrumented PLF with PLIF in the treatment of lumbar stenosis with low-grade lumbar spondylolisthesis, 45 patients were divided into two groups (A and B) at random (level I evidence). The patients in group A (n = 24, average age 54 years old) had a decompression with PLF and instrumentation while patients in group B (n = 21, average age 53 years old) also had a PLIF. Follow-up ranged from 12 months to 72 months. Their findings did not show any significant difference in follow-up, clinical outcome, and anatomical reduction rate though a higher number of infections and neurologic complications occurred in the PLIF group. Hence, they recommended the use of an interbody device (specifically a cage) should conform to strict use.

Currently, no level I evidence exists in favor of PLIF over instrumented PLF in the surgical management of degenerative lumbar spondylolisthesis though recent RCTs have shown promising results in isthmic spondylolisthesis.[52,67,69-72] Although there is moderate evidence to conclude that PLIF may indeed result in a higher fusion rate than instrumented PLF alone, the implicit clinical significance of this possibility is unclear. Adequately powered RCTs are needed to further document the potential role of interbody fusion in the surgical treatment of lumbar spondylolisthesis.

Anterior Lumbar Interbody Fusion versus Posterolateral Fusion and Posterior Interbody Fusion

The anterior approach to the lumbosacral spine offers the advantages of improved slip reduction, re-establishment of near anatomic coronal balance, and unimpeded access to the intervertebral disk space, permitting the use of larger grafts, and thus increasing the potential graft to endplate surface contact for enhanced anterior column arthrodesis. A retrospective analysis of 56 patients undergoing combined anterior lumbar interbody fusion (ALIF)/instrumented PLF versus instrumented PLF alone, showed almost identical fusion rates between the two groups, with less loss of postoperative slip reduction over the 2-year follow-up in the ALIF/instrumented PLF group. Despite this radiographic advantage, no significant difference in functional/clinical outcome was apparent[73] (level III evidence). These findings are similar to various other retrospective analyses in the literature evaluating clinical outcome in patients undergoing either ALIF or instrumented PLF/PLIF[74-77] (level III evidence). onversely, Remes et al.[78] reported better functional outcome as measured by ODI in patients undergoing circumferential fusion (ALIF/noninstrumented PLF), versus PLF alone[78] (level III evidence). Along the same lines, Christensen et al.[52] conducted an RCT analyzing the effects of circumferential fusion in which 148 patients were randomly selected for PLF versus ALIF with posterior instrumentation (level I evidence). Both groups had significant improvement in quality of life outcome measures and back and leg pain. Circumferential lumbar fusion though did restore lordosis ($p < 0.01$), lessen leg pain ($p < 0.03$), and back pain ($p < 0.04$) at the 1-year follow-up, and provide a higher union rate (92% vs. 80%, $p < 0.04$), with significantly fewer repeat operations (7% vs. 22%, $p < 0.009$) (level I evidence). The clinical perspective of this study implies favoring circumferential fusion as the definitive surgical procedure in complex lumbar pathology involving major instability, flat-back, and previous disk surgery in younger patients, as compared with PLF with posterior instrumentation.[52] In another study analyzing the long-term (8–13-year follow-up), clinical impact on anterior column support on sagittal balance after anterior lumbar surgery, 92 patients with severe chronic low back pain were randomly selected for PLF plus anterior support (PLF + ALIF) or PLF.[79] Their findings showed similar sagittal balance parameters between randomization groups while lumbar lordosis and type of lordosis correlated with outcome (level I evidence).

In comparing transforaminal lumbar interbody fusion (TLIF) and ALIF for low-grade isthmic spondylolisthesis, Kim et al.[74] showed in their retrospective review that TLIF at the L4–L5 level produced superior ODI scores while ALIF at L5–S1 produced superior radiographic results with regards to restoration of disk height, whole lumbar lordosis, and the sacral slope (level III evidence). These findings prompted the authors to recommend the differing techniques at the respective levels. Yan et al.[80] found no significant difference in patient outcome in a retrospective analysis of 87 patients with degenerative spondylolisthesis who underwent single level decompression/fusion with either PLIF or TLIF (level III evidence). These results are consistent with those reported by Suh et al. in their RCT evaluating PLIF using either one or two cages[81] (level I evidence).

Currently, no level I evidence is available to support ALIF over PLIF/TLIF or PLIF over TLIF for the surgical management of lumbar spondylolisthesis. However, ALIF with PLF versus PLF with instrumentation seems to provide a higher fusion rate, superior restoration of lumbosacral mechanics, and reduction in back and leg pain. The limited evidence comparing differing interbody techniques ascribes similar fusion rates and functional outcome in patients undergoing circumferential fusion, regardless of the technique utilized. There is moderate evidence to suggest superior radiographic outcome with ALIF; however, this does not appear to correlate with any associated clinical benefit.

Open versus Minimally Invasive Options

Both open and minimally invasive surgery (MIS) are used to treat patients with symptomatic degenerative spinal pathologies. Open lumbar fusion is the tried and true approach and while MIS offers a relatively excellent safety profile, the long-term durability of the fusion construct has yet to be fully validated. Rouben et al.[82] sought to evaluate the clinical efficacy of MIS-TLIF for one compared to two level fusions. The results were very encouraging with significant and sustained improvements in ODI at long-term follow-up in both groups without a significant difference between the two. In addition, excellent fusion rates were found and approached 100% for both groups at 1-year follow-up (level III evidence). Multiple other studies have demonstrated the efficacy and benefits of MIS with reduced blood loss, shortened hospital length of stay, reduced narcotic use, and accelerated return to work.[83,84] While the benefits of MIS appear clear, longer follow-up RCT studies are needed to make definitive statements regarding clinical and radiographic outcomes.

Instrumented Slip Reduction versus In Situ Fusion

Among the most controversial topics in the surgical management of lumbar, spondylolisthesis is the potential role of operative slip reduction. Whereas slip reduction provides the theoretical advantages of improving biomechanical conditions to facilitate arthrodesis, providing indirect neurological dectompression, correcting lumbosacral kyphosis, and restoring sagittal lumbosacral

SECTION 5

alignment, it comes at the cost of increased risk of neurological deficit (typically temporary or partial L5 nerve palsies) and increased procedural time and procedural blood loss. The percentage of patients with lytic spondylolisthesis in whom reduction of the slip was performed doubled from 22% to 44% over a 6-year period (1996 to 2002) despite rates of associated neurological complications ranging from 10% to 50% in the literature.[3] Early techniques for slip reduction involved noninstrumented PLF (with or without decompression), followed by staged manipulative reduction and placement in a spica cast 10–14 days postoperatively for up to 3 months.[85] Currently, the most common technique for slip reduction utilizes interbody structural grafts (placed anteriorly or posteriorly) in conjunction with posterior pedicle screw reduction/fixation. No RCTs have been conducted to directly compare functional/clinical patient outcomes between instrumented reduction and in situ fusion; therefore the available evidence regarding the benefit of operative reduction of high-grade (Meyerding grade—III/IV) spondylolisthesis is low level. In pediatric patients with high-grade isthmic spondylolisthesis undergoing reduction, no significant differences were found when compared with in situ fusion with regards to functional outcome or clinical findings concerning pain relief whereas radiographic outcome appeared superior in pediatric patients[86] (level III evidence). This is consistent with findings published by Transfeldt et al.[87] in their systematic review on the subject, leaving the authors unable to formulate clear guidelines due to the paucity of high level evidence supporting the use of instrumented slip reduction in pediatric patients with high-grade spondylolisthesis (level III evidence).

Currently, the spine literature is devoid of sufficient level I evidence to support the use of instrumented slip reduction in the surgical management of lumbar spondylolisthesis. As the risk of neurologic compromise may indeed be higher following reduction maneuvers, RCTs comparing the functional/clinical outcome in comparison with in situ fusion need to be carried out, in order to elucidate whether any clinical benefit justifies the inherent associated risks of reduction.

Motion Preservation Devices for Symptomatic Lumbar Spondylolisthesis

Recently, motion preservation devices have been advanced as viable adjuncts to decompression in the surgical management of degenerative lumbar stenosis associated with spondylolisthesis. Reduced adjacent segment degeneration (ASD) and avoidance of donor site morbidity associated with fusion have served to foster increasing interest in this emerging technology. Khoueir et al.[88] have devised a useful classification scheme of posterior dynamic stabilization. Interspinous decompression with the X STOP system (IGEA Brain, Spine & Orthopedics. Union, NJ) has been shown to provide significantly better outcomes in each domain of the Zurich Claudication Questionnaire (ZCQ) compared to medically treated controls[90] (level I evidence). Anderson et al.[89] reported a subgroup analysis data from a large RCT in 75 patients with spinal stenosis low-grade spondylolisthesis who were treated either with an X STOP or with medical/interventional treatment (level I evidence). At the 2-year follow-up, there were significant improvements in the ZCQ score and patient satisfaction in those treated with X STOP with no significant improvement in the group managed with conservative therapy. Recently, the durability of these results have come into question as surgical reintervention rates as high as 58% have been reported in patients with degenerative lumbar spondylolisthesis implanted with X STOP[91] (level III evidence).

Of the available pedicle-based dynamic stabilization systems, Dynesys (Zimmer Spine, Minneapolis, MN) has been the most extensively studied in patients with symptomatic degenerative lumbar spondylolisthesis. In a prospective multicenter trial, Dynesys was found to represent a safe and effective alternative to decompression/fusion in the surgical management of degenerative spondylolisthesis[92] (level II evidence). Schnake et al. also reported clinical results with Dynesys similar to those seen in established protocols using decompression and pedicle screw fixation; however, they also observed a relatively high implant failure rate of 17% over a minimum follow-up of 2 years with the Dynesys system[93] (level II evidence). Their long-term follow-up study at 4 years showed no further implant failure; however, radiographic evidence of ASD was seen in 39% of patients. Despite these findings, patient satisfaction remained high as 95% indicated they would undergo Dynesys implantation again[94] (level III evidence). On the other hand, Fakhil-Jerew et al.[95] reported a 45% reoperation rate within 2 years in a retrospective analysis of 55 patients who underwent Dynesys implantation for symptomatic lumbar spondylolisthesis (level III evidence).

Table 1: Evidence level and recommendation grade.	
Recommendation	*Evidence level*
• Surgical intervention for lumbar spondylolisthesis results in significantly improved pain relief and functional outcome versus nonoperative management	Ia/A
• Decompression + arthrodesis is superior to decompression alone in the surgical management of lumbar spondylolisthesis	Ia/A
• The addition of instrumentation to PLF results in a higher rate of fusion, without significant difference in functional/clinical outcome in comparison to noninstrumented fusion	Ia/A
• There is no significant difference in clinical outcomes between PLF, PLF with instrumentation, and circumferential (PLF + interbody fusion) for lumbar spondylolisthesis	II/B
• Subgroup analysis demonstrates a trend toward improved clinical outcome for instrumented PLF in patients with the diagnosis of degenerative lumbar spondylolisthesis	III/B
• MIS techniques reduce soft-tissues injury, narcotic use postoperative, and hospitalization time with no significant difference in fusion rates compared to open techniques in short-term follow-up studies	III/B
• Instrumented slip reduction does not confer any outcome benefit over in situ fusion, and adds additional risk of neurologic complication	III/B
• Dynamic stabilization demonstrates early outcome benefit comparable to that observed for decompression + fusion, but these results do not appear to be as durable as those seen with instrumented fusion	II/B

(MIS: minimally invasive surgery; PLF: posterolateral fusion)

While there is marginal level I evidence equating functional outcomes in dynamic stabilization versus the more traditional combined decompression/pedicle-screw arthrodesis procedures, the durability of these results is questionable. Additionally, the relatively high rates of device failure and ASD reported in the literature warrant further investigation. Well-designed RCTs evaluating existing dynamic stabilization devices and emerging facet replacement/resurfacing technologies are needed. It should also be emphasized that these studies focused on relatively stable low-grade degenerative spondylolisthesis associated with spinal stenosis. Dynamic devices are currently contraindicated in the presence of mobile or higher-grade slips.

CONCLUSION

Symptomatic degenerative lumbar spondylolisthesis is a relatively disabling condition with potentially far-reaching medical-economic implications related to associated secondary losses. Whereas conservative management may result in a modest improvement of pain symptoms over time, the natural history of the disease tends to be progressive, with complete spontaneous resolution of symptoms unlikely. Surgical intervention in the form of decompression and arthrodesis, results in significant improvement in pain relief and functional outcome, especially at early postoperative time points. Patients undergoing decompression/fusion tend to report a satisfactory global outcome in comparison to nonsurgical cohorts. Pedicle screw fixation and interbody fusion have both been associated with higher fusion rates, but this radiographic improvement has not translated into a demonstrable clinical benefit. The role of instrumented slip reduction remains controversial, as the inherent risk of neurological injury may not be justified by any improvements in favorable outcome. Table 1 summarizes current evidence-based recommendations regarding the treatment of symptomatic degenerative spondylolisthesis.

REFERENCES

1. Dantas FL, Prandini MN, Ferreira MA. Comparison between posterior lumbar fusion with pedicle screws and posterior lumbar interbody fusion with pedicle screws in adult spondylolisthesis. Arq Neuropsiquiatr. 2007;65(33):764-70.
2. Goyal N, Wimberley DW, Hyatt A, et al. Radiographic and clinical outcomes after instrumented reduction and transforaminal lumbar interbody fusion of mid and high-grade isthmic spondylolisthesis. J Spinal Disord Tech. 2009;22(5):321-7.
3. Hakato J, Wroński J. The role of reduction in operative treatment of spondylolisthesis. Neurologia i Neurochirurgia Polska. 2008;42:345-52.
4. Herkowitz HN, Kurz LT. Degenerative lumbar spondylolisthesis with spinal stenosis. A prospective study comparing decompression with decompression and intertransverse process arthrodesis. J Bone Joint Surg Am. 1991;73(6):802-8.
5. Vogt MT, Rubin D, Valentin RS, et al. Lumbar olisthesis and lower back symptoms in elderly white women. The Study of Osteoporotic Fractures. Spine (Phila Pa 1976). 1998;23(23):2640-7.

6. Imada K, Matsui H, Tsuji H, et al. Oophorectomy predisposes to degenerative spondylolisthesis. J Bone Joint Surg Br. 1995;77(1):126-30.
7. Jacobsen S, Sonne-Holm S, Rovsing H, et al. Degenerative lumbar spondylolisthesis: an epidemiological perspective: the Copenhagen Osteoarthritis Study. Spine (Phila Pa 1976). 2007;32(1):120-5.
8. Grobler LJ, Robertson PA, Novotny JE, et al. Etiology of spondylolisthesis. Assessment of the role played by lumbar facet joint morphology. Spine (Phila Pa 1976). 1993;18(1):80-91.
9. Love TW, Fagan AB, Fraser RD, et al. Degenerative spondylolisthesis. Developmental or acquired? J Bone Joint Surg Br. 1999;81(4):670-4.
10. McAfee PC, Yuan HA. Computed tomography in spondylolisthesis. Clin Orthop Relat Res. 1982;(166):62-71.
11. Nagaosa Y, Kikuchi S, Hasue M, et al. Pathoanatomic mechanisms of degenerative spondylolisthesis. A radiographic study. Spine (Phila Pa 1976). 1998;23(13):1447-51.
12. Birkmeyer NJ, Weinstein JN, Tosteson AN, et al. Design of the Spine Patient outcomes Research Trial (SPORT). Spine (Phila Pa 1976). 2002;27(12):1361-72.
13. Matsunaga S, Sakou T, Morizono Y, et al. Natural history of degenerative spondylolisthesis. Pathogenesis and natural course of the slippage. Spine. 1990;15(11):1204-10.
14. Matsunaga S, Ijiri K, Hayashi K. Nonsurgically managed patients with degenerative spondylolisthesis: a 10- to 18-year follow-up study. J Neurosurg. 2000;93(Suppl 2):194-8.
15. Kauppila LI, Eustace S, Kiel DP, et al. Degenerative displacement of lumbar vertebrae. A 25-year follow-up study in Framingham. Spine. 1998;23(17):1868-73.
16. Cauchoix J, Benoist M, Chassaing V. Degenerative spondylolisthesis. Clin Orthop Relat Res. 1976;(115):122-9.
17. Postacchini F, Perugia D. Degenerative lumbar spondylolisthesis. Part I: Etiology, pathogenesis, pathomorphology, and clinical features. Ital J Orthop Traumatol. 1991;17(2):165-73.
18. Rosenberg NJ. Degenerative spondylolisthesis. Predisposing factors. J Bone Joint Surg Am. 1975;57(4):467-74.
19. Brown MD, Lockwood JM. Degenerative spondylolisthesis. Instr Course Lect. 1983;32:162-9.
20. Kanayama M, Hashimoto T, Shigenobu K, et al. Intraoperative biomechanical assessment of lumbar spinal instability: validation of radiographic parameters indicating anterior column support in lumbar spinal fusion. Spine. 2003; 28(20):2368-72.
21. Rothman SL, Glenn WV Jr, Kerber CW. Multiplanar CT in the evaluation of degenerative spondylolisthesis. A review of 150 cases. Comput Radiol. 1985;9(4):223-32.
22. Ozawa H, Kanno H, Koizumi Y, et al. Dynamic changes in the dural sac cross-sectional area on axial loaded MR imaging: is there a difference between degenerative spondylolisthesis and spinal stenosis? AJNR Am J Neuroradiol. 2012;33(6): 1191-7.
23. Weinstein JN, Lurie JD, Tosteson TD, et al. Surgical vs nonoperative treatment for lumbar disk herniation: the Spine Patient Outcomes Research Trial (SPORT) observational cohort. JAMA. 2006;296(20):2451-9.
24. Weinstein JN, Tosteson TD, Lurie JD, et al. Surgical vs nonoperative treatment for lumbar disk herniation: the Spine Patient Outcomes Research Trial (SPORT): a randomized trial. JAMA. 2006 296(20):2441-50.
25. Malmivaara A, Slätis P, Heliövaara M, et al. Surgical or non-operative treatment for lumbar spinal stenosis? A randomized controlled trial. Spine (Phila Pa 1976). 2007;32(1):1-8.
26. Harris IE, Weinstein SL. Long-term follow-up of patients with grade-III and IV spondylolisthesis. Treatment with and without posterior fusion. J Bone Joint Surg Am. 1987;69(7):960-9.
27. Seitsalo S. Operative and conservative treatment of moderate spondylolisthesis in young patients. J Bone Joint Surg Br. 1990;72(5):908-13.
28. Carreon LY, Glassman SD, Howard J. Fusion and nonsurgical treatment for symptomatic lumbar degenerative disease: a systematic review of Oswestry Disability Index and MOS Short Form-36 outcomes. Spine J. 2008;8(5):747-55.
29. Ekman P, Möller H, Hedlund R. The long-term effect of posterolateral fusion in adult isthmic spondylolisthesis: a randomized controlled study. Spine J. 2005;5(1):36-44.
30. Möller H, Hedlund R. Surgery versus conservative management in adult isthmic spondylolisthesis—a prospective randomized study: part 1. Spine (Phila Pa 1976). 2000;25(13):1711-5.
31. Weinstein JN, Lurie JD, Tosteson TD, et al. Surgical versus nonsurgical treatment for lumbar degenerative spondylolisthesis. N Engl J Med. 2007;356(22):2257-70.
32. Weinstein JN, Lurie JD, Tosteson TD, et al. Surgical compared with nonoperative treatment for lumbar degenerative spondylolisthesis. Four-year results in the Spine Patient Outcomes Research Trial (SPORT) randomized and observational cohorts. J Bone Joint Surg Am. 2009;91(6): 1295-304.
33. Dall BE, Rowe DE. Degenerative spondylolisthesis. Its surgical management. Spine (Phila Pa 1976). 1985;10(7):668-72.
34. Dupuis PR, Yong-Hing K, Cassidy JD, et al. Radiologic diagnosis of degenerative lumbar spinal instability. Spine (Phila Pa 1976). 1985;10(3):262-76.
35. Epstein JA, Epstein BS, Lavine L. Nerve root compression associated with narrowing of the lumbar spinal canal. J Neurol Neurosurg Psychiatry. 1962;25:165-76.
36. Herkowitz HN, Garfin SR. Decompressive surgery for spinal stenosis. Sem Spine Surg. 1989;1:163-7.
37. Spengler DM. Degenerative stenosis of the lumbar spine. J Bone Joint Surg Am. 1987;69(2):305-8.
38. Bolesta MJ, Bohlman HH. Degenerative spondylolisthesis: the role of arthrodesis. Orthop Trans. 1989;13:564.
39. Feffer HL, Wiesel SW, Cuckler JM, et al. Degenerative spondylolisthesis. To fuse or not to fuse. Spine (Phila Pa 1976). 1985;10(3):287-9.
40. Hanley EN. Decompression and distraction-derotation arthrodesis for degenerative spondylolisthesis. Spine. 1986; 11:269-76.
41. Kaneda K, Kazama H, Satoh S, et al. Follow-up study of medial facetectomies and posterolateral fusion with instrumentation in unstable degenerative spondylolisthesis. Clin Orthop. 1986;203:159-67.

CHAPTER 38

42. Lombardi JS, Wiltse LL, Reynolds J, et al. Treatment of degenerative spondylolisthesis. Spine. 1985;10:821-7.
43. Reynolds JB, Wiltse LL. Surgical treatment of degenerative spondylolisthesis. Spine. 1979;4:148-9.
44. Wiltse LL. Common problems of the lumbar spine. Degenerative spondylolisthesis and spinal stenosis. J Contin Ed Orthop. 1979;7:17-30.
45. Ghogawala Z, Benzel EC, Amin-Hanjani S, et al. Prospective outcomes evaluation after decompression with or without instrumented fusion for lumbar stenosis and degenerative Grade I spondylolisthesis. J Neurosurg Spine. 2004;3(1):267-72.
46. Martin CR, Gruszczynski AT, Braunsfurth HA, et al. The surgical management of degenerative lumbar spondylolisthesis. A systematic review. Spine. 2007;32:1791-98.
47. Forsth P, Olafsson G, Carlsson T, et al. A Randomized, Controlled Trial of Fusion Surgery for Lumbar Spinal Stenosis. N Engl J Med. 2016;374(15):1413-23.
48. Ghogawala Z, Dziura J, Butler WE, et al. Laminectomy plus Fusion versus Laminectomy Alone for Lumbar Spondylolisthesis. N Engl J Med. 2016;374(15):1424-34.
49. Chang P, Seow KH, Tan SK. Comparison of the results of spinal fusion for spondylolisthesis in patients who are instrumented with patients who are not. Singapore Med J. 1993;34:511-4.
50. Kimura I, Shingu H, Murata M, et al. Lumbar posterolateral fusion alone or with transpedicular instrumentation in L4-L5 degenerative spondylolisthesis. J Spinal Disord. 2001;14:301-10.
51. Anderson T, Videbaek TS, Hansen ES, et al. The positive effect of posterolateral lumbar spinal fusion is preserved at long-term follow-up: a RCT with 11-13 year follow-up. Eur Spine J. 2008;17:272-80.
52. Christensen FB, Hansen ES, Laursen M, et al. Long-term functional outcome of pedicle screw instrumentation as a support for posterolateral spinal fusion. Randomized clinical study with a 5-year follow-up. Spine. 2002;27:1269-77.
53. Fischgrund JS, Mackay M, Herkowitz HN, et al. Degenerative lumbar spondylolisthesis with spinal stenosis: a prospective, randomized study comparing decompressive laminectomy and arthrodesis with and without spinal instrumentation. Spine. 1997;22:2807-12.
54. Möller H, Hedlund R. Instrumented and noninstrumented posterolateral fusion in adult spondylolisthesis. A prospective randomized study: part 2. Spine. 2000;25:1716-21.
55. Mélot C. Instrumented fusion of the degenerative lumbar spine: state of the art, questions, and controversies. Clinical Trends in Surgery: Methodologic and Statistical Criteria of Validity, with an Example of Meta-analysis of Randomized Trials in Spine Surgery. Philadelphia: Lippincott-Raven; 1996. pp. 281-9.
56. Ekman P, Möller H, Tullberg T, et al. Posterior lumbar interbody fusion versus posterolateral fusion in adult isthmic spondylolisthesis. Spine. 2007;32(20):2178-83.
57. Bridwell KH, Sedgewick TA, O'Brien MF, et al. The role of fusion and instrumentation in the treatment of degenerative spondylolisthesis with spinal stenosis. J Spinal Disord. 1993;6(6):461-72.
58. Gibson JN, Waddell G, Grant IC. Surgery for degenerative lumbar spondylosis. Cochrane Database Syst Rev. 2000;(3):CD001352.
59. Mardjetko SM, Connolly PJ, Shott S. Degenerative lumbar spondylolisthesis. A meta-analysis of literature 1970-1993. Spine. 1994;19(Suppl 20):2256S-65S.
60. Briggs DS, Milligan PR. Chip fusion of the low back following exploration of the spinal canal. J Bone Joint Surg Am. 1944;26:125-30.
61. Cloward RB. The treatment of ruptured lumbar intervertebral disc by vertebral body fusion: indications, operative technique, after care. J Neurosurg. 1953;10:154-68.
62. Brantigan JW, Steffee AD, Lewis M, et al. Lumbar interbody fusion using Brantigan I/F cage for PLIF and VSP pedicle screw system: Two year clinical results of the FDA clinical trial. Montpellier: Sauramps; 1996. pp. 239-69.
63. Steffe AD, Sitkowski DJ. Posterior lumbar interbody fusions and plates. Clin Orthop. 1988;227:99-102.
64. Yu CH, Wang CT, Chen PQ. Instrumented posterior lumbar interbody fusion in adult spondylolisthesis. Clin Orthop Relat Res. 2008;466:3034-43.
65. Ha KY, Na KH, Shin JH, et al. Comparison of posterolateral fusion with and without additional posterior lumbar interbody fusion for degenerative lumbar spondylolisthesis. J Spinal Disord Tech. 2008;21:229-34.
66. Dehoux E, Fourati E, Madi K, et al. Posterolateral versus interbody fusion in isthmic spondylolisthesis: functional results in 52 cases with a minimum follow-up of 6 years. Acta Orthop Belg. 2004;70:578-82.
67. Cheng L, Nie L, Zhang L. Posterior lumbar interbody fusion versus posterolateral fusion in spondylolisthesis: a prospective controlled study in the Han nationality. Int Orthop (SICOT). 2009;33:1043-7.
68. Abdu W, Lurie JD, Spratt KF, et al. Degenerative spondylolisthesis. Does fusion method influence outcome? Four-year results of the spine patient outcomes research trial. Spine. 2009;34:2351-60.
69. Fei Q, Wang YP, Xu HG, et al. Comparison of instrumented posterior fusion with instrumented circumferential lumbar fusion in the treatment of lumbar stenosis with low degree lumbar spondylolisthesis. Zhonghua Wai Ke Za Zhi. 2005;43(8):486-90.
70. Farrokhi MR, Rahmanian A, Masoudi MS. Posterolateral versus posterior interbody fusion in isthmic spondylolisthesis. J Neurotrauma. 2012;29(8):1567-73.
71. Inamdar DN, Alagappan M, Shyam L, et al. Posterior lumbar interbody fusion versus intertransverse fusion in the treatment of lumbar spondylolisthesis. J Orthop Surg. 2006;14:21-6.
72. Musluman AM, Yilmaz A, et al. Posterior lumbar interbody fusion versus posterolateral fusion with instrumentation in the treatment of low-grade isthmic spondylolisthesis: midterm clinical outcomes. J Neurosurg Spine. 2011;14(4):488-96.
73. Suk KS, Jeon CH, Park MS, et al. Comparison between posterolateral fusion with pedicle screw fixation and anterior interbody fusion with pedicle screw fixation in adult spondylolytic spondylolisthesis. Yonsei Med J. 2001;42:316-23.

74. Kim JS, Kang BU, Lee SH, et al. Mini-transforaminal lumbar interbody fusion versus anterior lumbar interbody fusion augmented by percutaneous pedicle screw fixation. A comparison of surgical outcomes in adult low-grade isthmic spondylolisthesis. J Spinal Disord Tech. 2009;22:114-21.
75. Kim JS, Lee KY, Lee SH, et al. Which lumbar interbody fusion technique is better in terms of level for the treatment of unstable isthmic spondylolisthesis? J Neurosurg Spine. 2010;12:171-7.
76. Kim NH, Lee JW. Anterior interbody fusion versus postero-lateral fusion with transpedicular fixation for isthmic spondylolisthesis in adults. A comparison of clinical results. Spine. 1999;24:812-7.
77. Min JH, Jang JS, Lee SH. Comparison of anterior- and posterior-approach instrumented lumbar instrumented fusion for spondylolisthesis. J Neurosurg Spine. 2007;7:21-6.
78. Remes V, Lamberg T, Tervahartiala P, et al. Long-term outcome after posterolateral, anterior, and circumferential fusion for high-grade isthmic spondylolisthesis in children and adolescents. Magnetic resonance imaging findings after average of 17-year follow-up. Spine. 2006;31:2491-9.
79. Videbaek TS, Bunger CE, Henriksen M, et al. Sagittal spinal balance after lumbar spinal fusion: the impact of anterior column support results from a randomized clinical trial with an eight- to thirteen-year radiographic follow-up. Spine (Phila Pa 1976). 2011;36(3):183-91.
80. Yan DL, Pei FX, Li J, et al. Comparative study of PLIF and TLIF treatment in adult degenerative spondylolisthesis. Eur Spine J. 2008;17:1311-6.
81. Suh KT, Park WW, Kim SJ, et al. Posterior lumbar interbody fusion for adult isthmic spondylolisthesis. A comparison of fusion with one or two cages. J Bone Joint Surg Br. 2008;90:1352-6.
82. Rouben D, Casnellie M, Ferguson M. Long-term durability of minimal invasive posterior transforaminal lumbar interbody fusion: a clinical and radiographic follow-up. J Spinal Disord Tech. 2011;24(5):288-96.
83. Adogwa O, Parker SL, Cheng J, et al. Comparative effectiveness of minimally invasive versus open transforaminal lumbar interbody fusion: 2-year assessment of narcotic use, return to work, disability, and quality of life. J Spinal Disord Tech. 2011;24(8):479-84.
84. Dhall SS, Wang MY, Mummaneni PV. Clinical and radiographic comparison of mini-open transforaminal lumbar interbody fusion with open transforaminal lumbar interbody fusion in 42 patients with long-term follow-up. J Neurosurg Spine. 2008;9(6):560-5.
85. Burkus JK, Lonstein JE, Winter RB, et al. Long-term evaluation of adolescents treated operatively for spondylolisthesis. A comparison of in situ arthrodesis only with in situ arthrodesis and reduction followed by immobilization in a cast. J Bone Joint Surg Am. 1992;74:693-704.
86. Poussa M, Schlenzka D, Seitsalo S, et al. Surgical treatment of severe isthmic spondylolisthesis in adolescents. Reduction or fusion in situ. Spine. 1993;18:894-901.
87. Transfeldt EE, Mehbod AA. Evidence-based medicine analysis of isthmic spondylolisthesis treatment including reduction versus fusion in situ for high-grade slips. Spine. 2007;32:S126-S129.
88. Khoueir P, Kim KA, Wang MY. Classification of posterior dynamic stabilization devices. Neurosurg Focus. 2007;22:1-8.
89. Anderson PA, Tribus CB, Kitchel SH. Treatment of neurogenic claudication by interspinous decompression: application of the X STOP device in patients with lumbar degenerative spondylolisthesis. J Neurosurg Spine. 2006;4:464-71.
90. Zucherman JF, Hsu KY, Hartjen CA, et al. A multicenter, prospective, randomized trial evaluating the X STOP interspinous process decompression system for the treatment of neurogenic intermittent claudication: Two-year follow-up results. Spine. 2005;30:1351-8.
91. Verhoof OJ, Bron JL, Wapstra FH, et al. High failure rate of the interspinous distraction device (X STOP) for the treatment of lumbar spinal stenosis caused by degenerative spondylolisthesis. Eur Spine J. 2008;17(2):188-92.
92. Stoll T, Gilles D, Schwarzenbach O. Dynamic stabilization of degenerative lumbar spondylolisthesis. Spine J. 2004;4:72S-3S.
93. Schnake KJ, Schaeren S, Jeanneret B, et al. Dynamic stabilization in addition to decompression for lumbar spinal stenosis with degenerative spondylolisthesis. Spine. 2006;31:442-50.
94. Schaeren S, Broger I, Jeanneret B. Dynesys stabilization in degenerative lumbar spondylolisthesis: 4 years follow-up. J Bone Joint Surg Br. 2009;91:108.
95. Fakhil-Jerew F, Haleem S, Shepperd J. Functional outcome following dynamic neurtralisation system for the treatment of spondylolisthesis without adjunct decompression. J Bone Joint Surg Br. 2009;91:463.

CHAPTER 39

Spine Surgery: Current Concepts and Evidence Isthmic Spondylolisthesis

Douglas Orr, Perry Dhaliwal

INTRODUCTION

In 1782, Dr Herbinaux, a Belgian obstetrician, described a bony prominence in the birth canal that impeded vaginal delivery. This was later found to be related to a slip of a lumbar vertebral body and was termed isthmic spondylolisthesis. Isthmic spondylolisthesis was more completely defined[1] as a defect in the pars interarticularis resulting in loss of communication of the inferior facet with the remainder of the posterior elements, and anterior translation of the more rostral vertebral body (and its associated pedicles, transverse processes, and superior articular facets) relative to the more caudal vertebral body (Fig. 1). This forward translation of the vertebral body may result in compression of the exiting and traversing nerve roots leading to symptoms of severe radiculopathy and/or neurogenic claudication. Numerous strategies have evolved over time to attempt to minimize or prevent this forward translation. Here we summarize the key aspects of the clinical findings, investigations, and management of this condition (Tables 1 to 3).

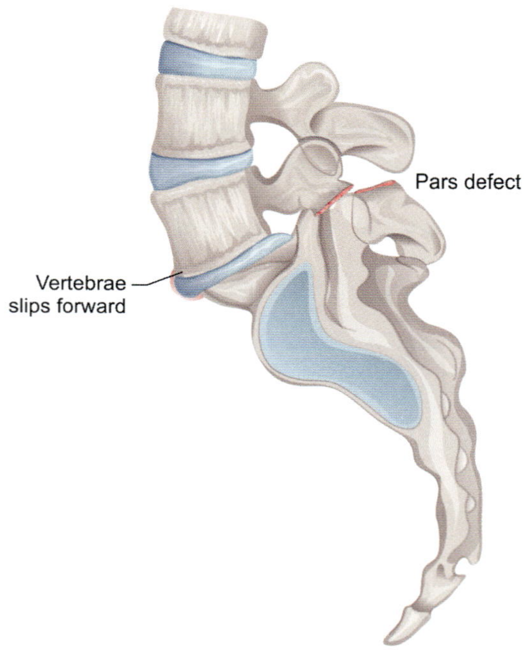

Fig. 1: Isthmic spondylolisthesis. Disruption of the pars interarticularis bilaterally resulting in anterior translation of the L5 vertebral body relative to the S1 vertebral body.

EPIDEMIOLOGY AND NATURAL HISTORY

The natural history of isthmic spondylolisthesis was well defined in many early studies.[1-3] It is generally believed that isthmic spondylolisthesis is not a congenital defect since such defects of the pars interarticularis are not seen in dissection of fetuses. Moreover, these lesions are rarely, if ever, seen in children under the age of 5. However, after the age of 5, there is a prevalence of approximately 5% of isthmic spondylolisthesis.[4] It is generally believed that isthmic spondylolisthesis may be the cumulative result of mechanical stresses placed on an aberrantly developed pars interarticularis. It is postulated that abnormal ossification of the pars interarticularis during growth predisposes the pars interarticularis to fractures in the setting of repeated trauma or stress particularly with extension of the lumbar spine.[5]

Over time, approximately half of patients with isthmic spondylolysis will go on to develop spondylolisthesis.[1] It is not clear why certain patients develop instability though it is proposed that injury to both facet joints may increase susceptibility to instability. With injury to the pars interarticularis bilaterally, the only remaining

Table 1: Evidentiary table.

Author, journal, year	*Design*	*Level-of-evidence*	*Topic*	*Duration of follow-up*	*Measures*	*Main results*
Möller, Spine, 2000	RCT	1	Surgery vs. conservative management	2 years	Disability rating index, visual analog score	Functional outcome and pain reduction were significantly greater in patients undergoing surgery
Möller, Spine, 2000	RCT	1	Instrumented vs. non-instrumented fusion	2 years	Disability rating index, visual analog score	No significant difference in outcomes between the two surgical groups
Thomsen, Spine, 1997	RCT	1	Instrumented vs. non-instrumented fusion	2 years	Dallas pain questionnaire	No significant difference in outcomes between the two surgical groups
McGuire, Spine, 1993	RCT	2	Instrumented vs. non-instrumented fusion	2 years	Fusion rates, overall outcomes graded as "Excellent", "Fair", "Good" or "Poor"	No significant difference in outcomes or fusion rates between the two surgical groups
France, Spine, 1999	RCT	2	Instrumented vs. non-instrumented fusion	2 years	Fusion rates, overall subjective outcomes, visual analog scores	No statistically significant difference between surgical groups in overall outcomes but trend toward higher fusion rates with instrumented fusion
Carragee, J Bone Joint Surg Am, 1997	RCT	2	Posterior instrumented fusion with decompression vs. without decompression	Average 4.5 years of follow-up	Pain, activity level, patient satisfaction, use of medication	No significant difference between 2 surgical arms for all outcomes assessed
Christensen, Spine, 2002	RCT	2	Posterior instrumented fusion vs. posterior instrumented fusion + ALIF	2 years	Dallas pain questionnaire, low back pain rating scale, fusion rates	Statistically significant difference in back pain, leg pain, and fusion rates favoring circumferential fusion
Musulman, J Neurosurg Spine, 2011	RCT	2	Posterior instrumented fusion vs. posterior instrumented fusion and PLIF	Average 3.3 years of follow-up	VAS, ODI, SF-36	Statistically significant difference in pain scores and functional status in patients undergoing supplementary PLIF
Farrokhi, J Neurotrauma, 2012	RCT	2	Posterior instrumented fusion vs posterior instrumented fusion and PLIF	1 year	VAS, ODI	No significant difference in outcomes between the two surgical groups
Lee, Spine J, 2004	Retro-spective case series	4	Percutaneous pedicle screw fixation + ALIF	Average follow-up was 16 months	Subjective overall outcomes, hospital stays, fusion rates	"Excellent" outcome in 35.6% of patients, "Good" outcome in 58.9% of patients, fusion rate of 97%, average hospital stay 4.1 days

(ALIF: anterior lumbar interbody fusion; ODI: Oswestry Disability Index; PLIF: posterolateral lumbar interbody fusion; RCT: randomized controlled trial; VAS: visual analog score)

Table 2: Level-of-evidence: Noninstrumented fusion.

Author, journal, year	*Design*	*LoE*	*Topic*	*F/U (m)*	*Measures*	*Main results*
Möller, Spine, 2000	RTC	II	Posterior non-instrumented fusion vs. posterior instrumented fusion	24	Disability rating index, VAS	No significant difference in fusion rates, functional outcome or pain scores between the two groups

(VAS: visual analog score; F/U: follow-up; LoE: level-of-evidence; RTC: randomized controlled trial)

Table 3: Level-of-evidence: Instrumented fusion.

Author, journal, year	*Design*	*LoE*	*Topic*	*F/U (m)*	*Measures*	*Main results*
Swan, Spine Journal, 2006	RTC	II	Posterior instrumented fusion vs. anterior and posterior instrumented fusion	24	Oswestry Disability Index (ODI), VAS, AAOS	Better clinical outcomes with combined anterior-posterior approaches at end of follow-up but between group differences were marginal at 6 months follow-up
Musulman, J Neurosurg Spine, 2011	RTC	II	Posterior lumbar interbody fusion vs. posterolateral instrumented fusion for low grade isthmic spondylolisthesis	18 months in all patients, average follow-up 3.3 years	ODI, SF-36, VAS, radiographic measurements	Reduced back pain over long-term follow-up in patients undergoing PLIF, no difference in ODI over the long term, better fusion rates with PLIF
Farrokhi, J Neurosurg Spine, 2005	RTC	II	Posterior lumbar interbody fusion vs. posterolateral instrumented fusion for low grade isthmic spondylolisthesis	12	ODI, VAS, fusion rate	Higher fusion rates and lower incidence of back pain seen with posterolateral instrumented fusion
Lee, Spine Journal, 2004	R	IV	ALIF with posterior percutaneous pedicle screws	Average follow-up 16 months	Modified MacNab criteria	Clinical outcome was excellent in 35.6%, good in 58.9%, fair in 4.1% and poor in 1.4%
Wang, Eur Spine J 2010	R	III	Minimally invasive TLIF vs. open TLIF	Average follow-up 26.3 months	ODI, VAS, fusion rates, blood loss, operative time, radiation time	Lower rates of blood loss, hospital stay, lower rates of back pain on POD#3 in minimally invasive group

(AAOS: American Academy of Orthopedic Surgery; ALIF: anterior lumbar interbody fusion; PLIF: posterolateral lumbar interbody fusion; R: retrospective; RTC: randomized controlled trial; VAS: visual analog score; LoE: level-of-evidence; F/U: follow-up)

structure preventing forward slip of the vertebrae is the intervertebral disk. When and how this disk fails is the subject of debate. One theory that serves to explain the morphological changes seen in the L5 and S1 vertebral bodies is based on Delpech's principle. It is suggested that the degree of slip is, at least in part, dependent on the contact between the L5 and S1 vertebral bodies as well as the possibility of further growth. Thus, as a child grows, vertical stresses are centered over the point of contact between the L5 and S1 vertebral bodies. In turn, those areas that are under less stress, namely the anterior inferior portion of the L5 vertebral body and the posterior superior portion of the S1 vertebral body, are able to grow out of proportion to the areas of contact. This results in a characteristic trapezoidal shape of the L5 vertebral body and a dome shape of the S1 vertebral body. In light of these changes, the L5 vertebral body becomes wedged over the superior end plate of the S1 vertebral body allowing for maintenance, and perhaps progression, of the slip. Should the spondylolisthesis develop after growth, these morphological changes do not occur and, therefore, the degree of forward translation and wedging are far less severe than in those cases where the spondylolisthesis developed during growth.

It is estimated that a defect in the pars interarticularis occurs at the L5 vertebral body in 90% of cases and at L4 in ~5% of cases.[6] However, the incidence does not seem to vary based on gender.

SYMPTOMS AND SIGNS

Patients with isthmic spondylolisthesis may present with a variety of symptoms. Just as the progression of the spondylolisthesis is not predictable, the symptoms associated with forward translation are also equally difficult to predict and are not related to the degree of spondylolisthesis.[7] Typically, patients with isthmic spondylolisthesis will present with back pain, buttock pain, and pain radiating down the lower extremities in a radicular fashion. The radicular symptoms are described by approximately 62–77% of patients who present for evaluation.[8] The patient may have sensory deficits in a radicular distribution and may also have weakness. Typically, the symptoms are worse with activity and are relieved when the patient rests. Forward flexion and lying recumbent also often relieve the pain. Patients will often discuss the significant impact on their quality of life due to their inability to ambulate. Patients with high-grade spondylolisthesis will often have characteristic posture and gait. With high-grade spondylolisthesis, patients may have retroverted pelvis in an attempt to restore sagittal balance. The patient may also have a compensatory hyperlordosis, which is manifested as protrusion of the lower abdomen and flattening of the buttocks. On inspection, one may also note that the spinous process is shifted anteriorly relative to the caudal level. Patients with high-grade isthmic spondylolisthesis may also develop a characteristic wide-based gait with flexed knees. The stride length is also much shorter than normal due to stiffness in the hamstrings and a retroverted pelvis.[9]

As mentioned previously, the onset and degree of symptoms are difficult to predict. However, age does seem to be an important factor in the clinical presentation. In general terms, symptoms of radicular pain or neurogenic claudication tend to present in adulthood. In childhood, these symptoms are indeed rare with a reported 13% of children with known spondylolysis having clinical signs or symptoms of nerve root compression.[7] In addition to age, trauma also appears to be an important factor in the precipitation of symptoms. In several series, trauma was commonly reported prior to the onset of symptoms.[8-10]

IMAGING

Having completed a thorough history and physical examination, thorough radiological investigations are necessary to characterize the spondylolisthesis. In the current management of isthmic spondylolisthesis, X-rays, computed tomography (CT) scans, and magnetic resonance imaging (MRI) studies may all provide important information.

Conventional Radiography

Routine X-ray imaging can provide important information in the evaluation of a patient with isthmic spondylolisthesis. Typically, anteroposterior (AP), lateral, and oblique views are performed and each adds different information that may be useful to the surgeon. The AP view is useful to evaluate the coronal alignment of the spine and may also help to identify disk-osteophyte complexes. It is also useful to view the position of the iliac crests with respect to the spinal levels (an important consideration in more complex cases where one is considering the possibility of a multilevel procedure with multiple interbody implants). The lateral view provides information about the degree of anterolisthesis and also gives important information about the alignment of the spine. Important parameters such as the pelvic incidence, pelvic tilt, sacral slope, and lumbar lordosis can be calculated off of this projection (Figs. 2A to C) Finally, oblique views are also important to verify the presence of an isthmic defect at the affected level as approximately 20% of pars defects may not be seen on plain lateral films especially in the circumstance where there may only be a unilateral pars defect.[11] It is also important to note that weight-bearing films should be obtained whenever possible as the X-rays may demonstrate movement of the L5 vertebral body.

Computed Tomography

Computed tomography scanning can also be a useful adjunct in the assessment of a patient with isthmic spondylolisthesis. In addition to having better visualization of the osseous anatomy, CT scanning can provide information about the degree of calcification across disk spaces or the presence of air within the disk spaces. CT scanning can also provide information about the size of the pedicles and the presence or absence of dysplasia or sclerosis within the pedicles. This is important when considering surgery as placing pedicle screws into

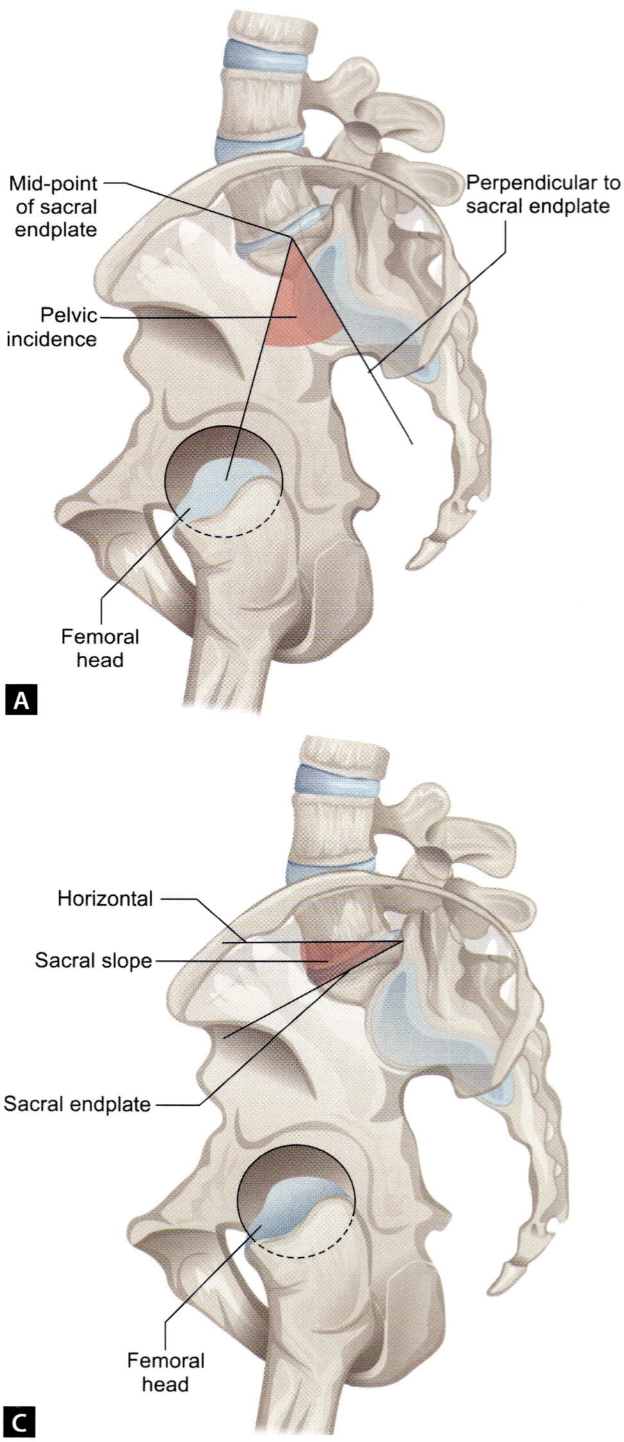

Figs. 2A to C: (A) Pelvic incidence—angle calculated by drawing line from mid-sacral point to midpoint of femoral head and a line perpendicular to the sacral end-plate; (B) Pelvic tilt—angle calculated by drawing a line from mid-sacral point to midpoint of femoral head and a vertical line; (C) Sacral slope—angle calculated by drawing line parallel to sacral end-plate and a horizontal line.

dysplastic or sclerotic pedicles may require different strategies from when placing a pedicle screw into a normal pedicle.

Magnetic Resonance Imaging

Magnetic resonance imaging is another imaging modality that is employed in the management of patients with isthmic spondylolisthesis. Though MRI is not as useful to examine the osseous anatomy, it can provide important information about which neural elements are compressed. It can also serve to exclude other compressive pathology that may cause similar neurologic findings.

CONSERVATIVE MANAGEMENT

As discussed, adult patients with isthmic spondylolisthesis may present with a constellation of signs and symptoms that might include pain, sensory disturbance, weakness, sagittal imbalance, and an altered gait. However, the onset of these symptoms is unrelated to the degree of anterolisthesis and also occurs unpredictably over the duration of a lifetime.[9] In those patients with minor symptoms, it is possible to use nonsurgical measures to help alleviate a patient's symptoms. Nonsurgical methods may also be used in patients with high-grade spondylolisthesis as even these patients have been shown to respond favorably if they have minor symptoms.[12] Such strategies may include prevention (by avoiding movements that strain the lumbar spine), exercise and strengthening of the abdominal muscles as well as paraspinal muscles, and the use of medications to help alleviate pain. In the pediatric population, symptoms may be alleviated through activity restriction particularly if the symptoms worsen with involvement in sporting activity.

SURGICAL INDICATIONS AND TREATMENT

Surgery is indicated for patients with isthmic spondylolisthesis if they have intractable pain, progressive neurological deficits, or failure of conservative measures.[8,13] It is postulated that patients with greater than 25% of anterolisthesis are more likely to progress over time though this has not been demonstrated definitively. Many surgical options have been proposed in the treatment of this condition. These include:

- Repair of the pars interarticularis
- Noninstrumented techniques:
  - Posterior decompression with laminectomy and facetectomy
  - Noninstrumented fusion
- Instrumented techniques:
  - Posterior instrumented fusion with or without decompression
  - Posterior instrumented fusion with reduction of the slipped vertebrae
  - Posterior instrumented fusion with supplementary interbody fusion
  - L5 vertebrectomy
  - Minimally invasive pedicle screw and rod insertion.

Though the options are many, the evidence for each of these options is relatively limited. Below, we discuss the various surgical options and evaluate the quality of evidence available for each of these approaches.

Noninstrumented Procedures

There are several techniques for repair of the pars defects and noninstrumented options that have been used in the management of isthmic spondylolisthesis. Though these procedures have generally been replaced by more modern instrumented techniques, they do deserve mention in the rare event where a patient may not be eligible for an instrumentation procedure. Historically, three different types of procedures have been used in this context.

Repair of Pars Defect

The primary goal of this procedure is to attempt to reconstruct the normal anatomy of the pars. The original description of this technique advocates for removal of the fibrous tissue within the area of the defect and then placing bone graft into the remaining gap to allow for fusion over time. Others have described pars screws that are placed into the lamina and across the defect.[14] A wire construct has also been proposed that involved looping of wire cables around each transverse process of the affected vertebral body and fixing the other end of the wire loop over the corresponding spinous process.[15] Though these techniques were used to stabilize the mobile segments in patients with isthmic spondylolysis, there were several limitations to each of these techniques. Namely, they required long-term bracing or bed rest following the procedure and the construct often led to an altered relationship between the facet joint and lamina. Though many authors have reported their experience with each of these techniques, the evidence is limited to small case series with no consistent methodology for evaluating postoperative outcomes. In the modern era, these techniques are reserved for younger patients, with a normal intervertebral disk, no anterolisthesis, and evidence of active defect on a bone scan or signal change on an MRI scan.

Laminectomy and Nerve Root Decompression

Surgeons performed laminectomy and nerve root decompression on patients with isthmic spondylolisthesis with the aim of decompressing the neural elements and relieving pain. The procedure traditionally involves a full laminectomy as well as removal of the fibrous tissue that is filling the defect. This allows for aggressive central and foraminal decompression. The outcome data for this technique is limited to retrospective case series and authors have reported 55–86% "good" results and 2–20% rate of worsening anterolisthesis.[16,17] This remains an accepted technique in instances where medical concerns make instrumented fusion unsafe and where disk-osteophyte complexes are present and are felt to render stability to the spinal segment in question. It remains unclear whether patients that undergo a posterior decompression will progress to a greater degree of spondylolisthesis over time and under what circumstances this might occur.

Noninstrumented Fusion

Noninstrumented lumbar fusion has also been used in an attempt to provide additional stability to the mobile segment. Various forms of the technique have been described including posterior interlaminar fusion,[18] posterolateral fusion,[8,19-22] and interbody fusion.[23,24] The most widely used technique is the posterolateral fusion where rates of pseudoarthrosis range from 19.5% to 40% in retrospective case series.[8,19,20,22] This technique typically involves the standard subperiosteal exposure of the lumbar spine including visualization of the spinous process, laminae, facet joints, and transverse processes. The fusion procedure typically involves meticulous removal of soft tissue from these structures followed by careful decortication of the facet joints and transverse processes. Care is taken to avoid damage to the adjacent facet joints and violation of the facet capsule. Morselized autograft or allograft is placed lateral to the facet joints and between the exposed transverse processes.

Though this technique has been used extensively, the high rates of pseudoarthrosis have made more modern posterior transpedicular instrumented techniques much more attractive. However, in one study,[25,26] 111 patients with lumbar isthmic spondylolisthesis of any grade, with signs and symptoms of back pain or sciatic over the previous year, were randomized to either posterior non-instrumented fusion, posterior instrumented fusion, or exercise therapy. Patients were followed over the course of 2 years and evaluated for pain and functional outcome. Over the course of 2 years, a significant reduction in pain and increase in function was noted in the two surgical groups. However, amongst the surgical groups, there was no significant difference in fusion rates, pain scores or functional outcomes in the noninstrumented versus the instrumented groups. Based on this randomized trial, it would seem that the addition of instrumentation does not appear to alter outcomes.

Instrumented Fusion

In the modern era, posterior instrumented fusion has become the treatment of choice for isthmic spondylolisthesis. Typically, this involves identification of landmarks for the insertion of the pedicle (based on anatomy or fluoroscopy), tapping of the pedicle to prevent fracture of the cortical bone, and insertion of the pedicle screw. Care is taken to prevent damage to the adjacent facet joints and to ensure that the trajectory of the pedicle screws allows for triangulation of the pedicle screw construct to avoid hardware failure. Once the pedicle screws are in place, rods are placed to lend stability to the mobile segment. Bone graft is then placed around the instrumentation to allow for fusion of the bone.

As mentioned previously, several retrospective studies have demonstrated high pseudoarthrosis rates in the absence of rigid posterior fixation. Similarly, two landmark randomized controlled trials examining fusion rates with either non-instrumented fusion, semirigid fusion or pedicle screw fixation techniques have demonstrated higher fusion rates with rigid fixation.[27,28] Thus, by extrapolation, rigid posterior fixation is considered a very important element in the surgical treatment of isthmic spondylolisthesis. In addition to the posterior instrumentation, there are three additional considerations in the management of isthmic spondylolisthesis—(1) whether or not to place an interbody implant, (2) whether or not to decompress the neural elements, and (3) whether or not to perform maneuvers to correct the sagittal alignment through a variety of reduction techniques.

Posterior instrumented fusion techniques typically involve pedicle screw and rod constructs that allow for fixation of the mobile segment. Fusion rates of 80% or greater have been reported using this technique in several case series.[29,30] There have also been small randomized controlled trials that have examined this issue.[31-33] In these studies, fusion rates range from 84% to 93% with stand-alone posterior fusions.

With recent technological advances, it has also become possible to insert interbody cages in an attempt to enhance fusion. These may be placed via an anterior, posterior or transforaminal approach. The merits of placing an interbody cage have been examined in several controlled trials.[31-33] In one study,[31] sequential cohorts of patients underwent surgery for isthmic spondylolisthesis first with posterior instrumented fusion and then a second cohort with posterior instrumented fusion supplemented with interbody implants. Patients were followed for a 2-year period of time and were evaluated for disability, pain, narcotic use, work status, and complications. Overall, patients who underwent anterior and posterior fusions had better outcomes in all measures relative to the group that had posterior instrumentation alone. A more recent study[33] showed the opposite findings with better outcomes in patients with posterior instrumented fusion alone. The current evidence is unfortunately insufficient to help determine whether interbody fusion is of any additional benefit.

Traditionally, surgeons have decompressed the exiting nerve roots, believing that compression of these nerve roots by the fibrous mass filling the pars defect was partly responsible for producing pain experienced by the patient.[34] However, in one randomized study,[35] the authors examined postoperative outcomes for posterior arthrodesis with decompression against posterior arthrodesis with decompression in patients with low-grade spondylolisthesis. In this study, trends toward better outcomes in patients that underwent posterior arthrodesis without decompression were seen. However, this study was limited by small numbers (42 patients divided amongst four subgroups), variable duration of follow-up and lack of standardized validated methodology for following functional outcomes. Also, there was significant variability in the method of fusion with 22 of 42 patients in the study undergoing noninstrumented fusion. Thus, despite this single randomized study, most spine surgeons continue to perform neural decompression in patients with isthmic spondylolisthesis who present with radicular symptoms.

Surgical Management of Patients with High-grade Isthmic Spondylolisthesis

Patients with high-grade isthmic spondylolisthesis present a particularly challenging problem for spine surgeons. By definition, these patients have greater than 50% anterolisthesis in the setting of a pars defect. This results in significant narrowing of the spinal canal and neural foramina. However, in addition to compression of the neural elements, these patients often have abnormal sagittal balance as a result of the oblique trajectory of the lumbar spine from the sacrum. The importance of sagittal balance and its relation to functional outcome has been well established[36-38] (Fig. 3). Thus, a revised classification and management scheme has been proposed that is

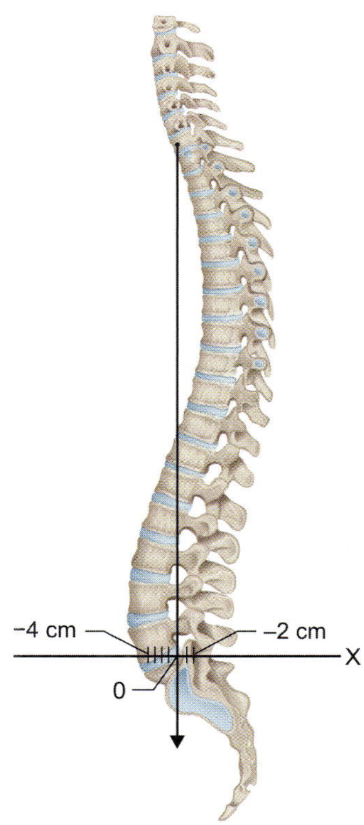

Fig. 3: Sagittal balance—note that sagittal balance is generally defined as a plumb-line drawn from the C7 vertebral body down through the sacral end-plate. With normal sagittal balance, this line should cross the posterior-superior corner of the S1 vertebral body.

Table 4: Spinal deformity study group classification of spondylolisthesis.

Type	*Definition*
Low-grade spondylolisthesis:	
Type 1	Pelvic incidence <45°
Type 2	Pelvic incidence 45–60°
Type 3	Pelvic incidence >60°
High-grade spondylolisthesis:	
Type 4	Balanced pelvis and spine
Type 5	Retroverted pelvis with balanced spine
Type 6	Unbalanced spine

based on consideration of sagittal balance (Table 4). Based on this classification, those patients that have sagittal imbalance in the setting of high-grade spondylolisthesis (types 5 and 6) should have reduction and internal fixation of the mobile segment. A detailed understanding of spinopelvic biomechanics is requisite in order to employ this classification in the management of isthmic spondylolisthesis (*see* Figs. 2A to C).

A variety of techniques have been proposed to reduce the mobile segment and to regain sagittal balance. Some surgeons advocate for a procedure performed entirely from a posterior approach. One such technique requires a sacral dome osteotomy to remove the bone overgrowth at the posterior-superior corner of the sacrum. This then allows for reduction of the translated vertebral body into normal alignment through the use of pedicle screws and rods. Another technique involves reduction of the mobile segment through the use of a temporary pedicle screw placed in the L1 pedicle and a second pedicle screw placed in the sacrum. A spondylolisthesis reduction screw is placed into the mobile segment and a rod is placed such that it spans the distance between L1 and S1. The mobile segment is then pulled up to the rod while tightening a nut down into the reduction screw. The L1 screws are then removed and rods are placed into the L5 and S1 pedicle screws. Direct visualization of the nerve roots is mandatory to avoid stretch injury to the exiting nerve roots. An interbody cage may also be placed in order to facilitate fusion in the reduced position. The interbody cage may be placed via a transforaminal approach or through an anterior approach.

Other surgeons advocate for a staged anterior-posterior procedure. Though many variations in the technique exist, the premise is to fuse the L5–S1 segment together with a large screw or fibular graft with a trajectory beginning at the anterior superior corner of L5, through the L5–S1 intervertebral disk space and into the S1 vertebral body. If this is performed under distraction, the mobile segment will eventually reduce and can be secured in place using this construct. The anterior procedure is then reinforced with a typical posterior decompression and instrumented fusion.

Finally, in cases where there is complete spondyloptosis or where the majority of the L5 vertebral body lies anterior and inferior to the sacral promontory, one may consider complete resection of the calisthenics vertebra. The procedure, as described by Gaines and Nichols,[39] involves an anterior retroperitoneal approach to complete an L5 vertebrectomy followed by posterior instrumented fusion of L4–S1 with gentle reduction of the L4 vertebral body onto the sacrum. The advantage of this technique is that it prevents L5 nerve root injury, which is common when attempts are made to reduce the L5 vertebral body in cases of spondyloptosis.

Overall, there is a significant paucity of data to provide a clear management algorithm for patients with high-grade spondylolisthesis. The available data is limited to case series with no randomized trials or prospective studies that have assessed this particular problem.[40] Moreover, there is considerable controversy as to whether reduction of the mobile segment is needed and whether it improves functional outcomes. This is particularly important in light of the numerous complications (*see* the *Complications* portion of this chapter) that are seen during attempts to reduce the mobile segment.

Minimally Invasive Options

Recently, minimal access surgery has become an important tool in the armamentarium of the spinal surgeon. As technology has progressed, the ability to access and instrument the spine with minimal tissue dissection has allowed for the treatment of very complex surgical problems. These techniques have also been used in the setting of isthmic spondylolisthesis[41-43] though the data remains limited to patients with low-grade isthmic spondylolisthesis.

In the largest series[41] examining the use of minimal access surgery for the management of symptomatic isthmic spondylolisthesis, the authors reviewed their experience with minimally invasive anterior lumbar interbody fusion followed by percutaneous pedicle screw insertion. In their 73 patients, over 90% of patients had an excellent or good outcome with reported fusion rates of 97.3%. It should be noted that these authors did not perform posterior lumbar decompression as part of their surgical technique. Though the retrospective nature of this series makes comparative analysis challenging, the results are certainly encouraging.

In another nonrandomized series,[43] 83 patients with either isthmic or degenerative spondylolisthesis underwent either a traditional open transforaminal interbody fusion or a minimally invasive transforaminal lumbar interbody fusion in addition to percutaneous pedicle screw and rod insertion. Based on this study, patients who underwent minimally invasive transforaminal lumbar interbody fusion had less blood loss, less postoperative back pain, and shorter hospital stays compared to the open group. No attempts were made to reduce the mobile segment prior to fixation.

Though no randomized controlled trials have examined the use of minimal access surgery in the setting of isthmic spondylolisthesis, it can be concluded from these retrospective series that percutaneous pedicle screw insertion with interbody fusion may be an option for management of these patients. The aforementioned studies demonstrate a trend toward shorter hospital stays, less blood loss, and reduced back pain in those patients undergoing these minimal access procedures. However, long-term follow-up data with validated functional outcome scores is still lacking. Furthermore, it remains unclear whether an anterior or posterior approach for interbody cage insertion affects patient outcomes in the setting of symptomatic isthmic spondylolisthesis.

Prognosis

Many studies have examined outcomes with both conservative and surgical management of isthmic spondylolisthesis. Though there are many published studies, reporting of data limits the conclusions that can be made about the various strategies for management.

In patients with symptomatic isthmic spondylolisthesis, there is very little data examining nonsurgical treatments for pain. In one large retrospective study,[13] patients who underwent nonsurgical management had comparable outcome to those patients who underwent lumbar spinal fusion over an average follow-up of 13 years. The authors commented that the patients who were treated without surgical intervention eventually had fusion of the mobile segment secondary to disk degeneration and osteophyte formation. However, it should also be mentioned that patients who underwent conservative management also did not have the same pain profile as those who underwent surgical intervention. Thus, the inherent bias in patient selection in this study limits the conclusions that can be made about the use of conservative management in patients with symptomatic isthmic spondylolisthesis. A more robust study[26] examining the issue of conservative versus surgical management in symptomatic isthmic spondylolisthesis demonstrated significantly better outcomes for pain and function in patients who underwent surgery over a 2-year follow-up. Patients with symptomatic isthmic spondylolisthesis typically present with such severe pain and dysfunction that conservative measures are rarely effectual.

As mentioned previously, non-instrumented fusion of the mobile segment has been a viable option in isthmic spondylolisthesis. There have been four randomized controlled trials that have examined this issue[25,44-46] though only two provide information regarding clinical outcome.[25,44] In the study by France et al. they reported "good to excellent" outcomes in 63% of patients that had instrumented fusion and 62% of patients who had a stand-alone posterior fusion. In the study by Möller et al. there were also no significant differences seen in functional outcomes between patients who underwent a posterior instrumented fusion and those who underwent a non-instrumented fusion.

Finally, in patients who had interbody fusion performed in addition to pedicle screw fixation, the data is conflicting. In one study, patients who underwent instrumentation with a pedicle screw construct had better outcomes than when a posterior interbody fusion technique was used. However, in a separate study, greater fusion rates and functional outcomes were seen in patients who had a posterior interbody fusion in addition to a pedicle screw construct. Needless to say, there is conflicting data as to whether the addition of an interbody implant makes a significant difference to patient outcomes in the setting of isthmic spondylolisthesis.

Complications

As with most lumbar spinal procedures, there are specific sets of complications associated with the surgical management of isthmic spondylolisthesis. These include pseudoarthrosis, neurological injury, infection, deep vein thrombosis, cerebrospinal fluid leak, and adjacent segment disease. Several studies provide data on the frequency of these complications as related to isthmic spondylolisthesis.

In patients undergoing instrumented posterolateral fusion, a systematic review[47] found ~2% rate of instrumentation failure amongst those patients undergoing instrumented posterolateral fusion. In the same study, it was estimated that the overall complication rate for neurological injury, dural tears, and infections was ~12% though individual complication rates were not reported.

In those patients where an interbody fusion was also performed, the overall complication rates were higher amongst those patients who had a posterolateral interbody fusion (24%) versus those who had an anterior lumbar interbody fusion (20%).[47] It should be noted, however, that the complication rates with any interbody technique appear to be higher than when pedicle screw instrumentation was used in isolation.

In a more recent randomized trial,[32] instrumented posterolateral fusion was compared to posterior lumbar interbody fusion and pedicle screw fixation. In this series of 50 patients, the authors report a 16% pseudoarthrosis rate for the patients who underwent instrumented posterolateral fusion with no failure of fusion in the group that underwent a posterior lumbar interbody fusion. The rate of deep infection was higher in the group undergoing instrumented fusion (8% vs. 4%) though the rate of neurological injury was the same in both groups (4%). In another randomized study[33] comparing instrumented posterolateral fusion versus posterior lumbar interbody fusion and pedicle screw fixation, the authors reported no significant differences in the incidence of cerebrospinal fluid leak (4.3% vs. 5%), motor impairment (4.3 vs. 5%) or infection (2.1 vs. 2.5%).

In the setting of high-grade spondylolisthesis, nerve root injury has commonly been cited as a reason not to attempt reduction of the calisthenics vertebra. The available data would suggest a 5–10% incidence of nerve root palsy where a reduction is achieved.[40]

In addition to nerve root impairment, cauda equina syndrome is a recognized complication of reduction of a mobile segment particularly in high-grade spondylolisthesis. Though the rate of this complication is difficult to ascertain, it is thought that posterior migration of the intervertebral disk, excessive stretch on nerve roots or hyperextension of the lumbosacral junction may result in cauda equina syndrome.[48]

Retrograde ejaculation is another complication that may be encountered in the management of male patients undergoing anterior lumbar interbody fusion. This complication is thought to be related to damage to the superior hypogastric plexus, which is intimately related to the common iliac vein. Excessive retraction or the use of monopolar cautery of the anterior lumbar spine may contribute to the frequency of this complication. Rates of 2–6% of retrograde ejaculation using the mini-open anterior interbody fusion technique have been reported.[49,50] The incidence of retrograde ejaculation with anterior lumbar interbody fusion is felt to be independent of the type of spondylolisthesis.

CONCLUSION

Isthmic spondylolisthesis is a condition that results from a discontinuity in the pars interarticularis, which results in separation of the inferior facet from the remainder of the posterior elements of the vertebral body. This may result in pain syndromes including neurogenic claudication or radiculopathy and patients may also have significant back pain. The available evidence suggests that patients with symptomatic isthmic spondylolisthesis should have surgical intervention to help alleviate their symptoms. The type of intervention remains controversial with conflicting evidence for decompression, noninstrumented fusion, and instrumented fusion. There is no clear evidence supporting the need for interbody fusions or minimally invasive approaches at this time. Further research should focus on delineating appropriate patient populations for each of these interventions.

REFERENCES

1. Taillard W. Le Spondylolisthésis. Paris: Masson; 1957.
2. Wiltse LL, Widell EH Jr, Jackson DW. Fatigue fracture: the basic lesion is inthmic spondylolisthesis. J Bone Joint Surg Am. 1975;57(1):17-22.
3. Wiltse LL, Newman PH, Macnab I. Classification of spondylolisis and spondylolisthesis. Clin Orthop Relat Res. 1976;(117):23-9.

4. Baker DR, McHollick W. Spondyloschisis and spondylolisthesis in children. J Bone Joint Surg. 1956;37:878-80.
5. Wiltse LL. The etiology of spondylolisthesis. J Bone Joint Surg Am. 1962;44-A:539-60.
6. Wiltse LL, Winter RB. Terminology and measurement of spondylolisthesis. J Bone Joint Surg Am. 1983;65(6):768-72.
7. Fredrickson BE, Baker D, McHolick WJ, et al. The natural history of spondylolysis and spondylolisthesis. J Bone Joint Surg Am. 1984;66(5):699-707.
8. Boxall D, Bradford DS, Winter RB, et al. Management of severe spondylolisthesis in children and adolescents. J Bone Joint Surg Am. 1979;61(4):479-95.
9. Hensinger RN. Spondylolysis and spondylolisthesis in children and adolescents. J Bone Joint Surg Am. 1989;71(7):1098-107.
10. Bradford DS, Iza J. Repair of the defect in spondylolysis or minimal degrees of spondylolisthesis by segmental wire fixation and bone grafting. Spine (Phila Pa 1976). 1985;10(7):673-9.
11. Libson E, Bloom RA, Dinari G, et al. Oblique lumbar spine radiographs: importance in young patients. Radiology. 1984;151(1):89-90.
12. Harris IE, Weinstein SL. Long-term follow-up of patients with grade-III and IV spondylolisthesis. Treatment with and without posterior fusion. J Bone Joint Surg Am. 1987;69(7):960-9.
13. Seitsalo S. Operative and conservative treatment of moderate spondylolisthesis in young patients. J Bone Joint Surg Br. 1990;72(5):908-13.
14. Buck JE. Direct repair of the defect in spondylolisthesis. Preliminary report. J Bone Joint Surg Br. 1970;52(3):432-7.
15. Nicol RO, Scott JH. Lytic spondylolysis. Repair by wiring. Spine (Phila Pa 1976). 1986;11(10):1027-30.
16. Gill GG, Manning JG, White HL. Surgical treatment of spondylolisthesis without spine fusion; excision of the loose lamina with decompression of the nerve roots. J Bone Joint Surg Am. 1955;37-A(3):493-520.
17. Amuso SJ, Neff RS, Coulson DB, et al. The surgical treatment of spondylolisthesis by posterior element resection. J Bone Joint Surg Am. 1970;52(3):529-36.
18. Bosworth DM, Fielding JW, Demarest L, et al. Spondylolisthesis; a critical review of a consecutive series of cases treated by arthrodesis. J Bone Joint Surg Am. 1955;37-A(4):767-86.
19. DeWald RL, Faut MM, Taddonio RF, et al. Severe lumbosacral spondylolisthesis in adolescents and children. Reduction and staged circumferential fusion. J Bone Joint Surg Am. 1981;63(4):619-26.
20. Laurent LE, Osterman K. Spondylolisthesis in children and adolescents: a study of 173 cases. Acta Orthop Belg. 1969;35(3):717-27.
21. Peek RD, Wiltse LL, Reynolds JB, et al. In situ arthrodesis without decompression for Grade-III or IV isthmic spondylolisthesis in adults who have severe sciatica. J Bone Joint Surg Am. 1989;71(1):62-8.
22. Turner RH, Bianco AJ Jr. Spondylolysis and spondylolisthesis in children and teen-agers. J Bone Joint Surg Am. 1971;53(7):1298-306.
23. Cloward RE. Spondylolisthesis: treatment by laminectomy and posterior interbody fusion. Clin Orthop Relat Res. 1981(154):74-82.
24. Wiltberger BR. Intervertebral body fusion by the use of posterior bone dowel. Clin Orthop Relat Res. 1964;35:69-79.
25. Möller H, Hedlund R. Instrumented and noninstrumented posterolateral fusion in adult spondylolisthesis—a prospective randomized study: part 2. Spine (Phila Pa 1976). 2000;25(13):1716-21.
26. Möller H, Hedlund R. Surgery versus conservative management in adult isthmic spondylolisthesis—a prospective randomized study: part 1. Spine (Phila Pa 1976). 2000;25(13): 1711-5.
27. Zdeblick TA. A prospective, randomized study of lumbar fusion. Preliminary results. Spine (Phila Pa 1976). 1993; 18(8):983-91.
28. Fischgrund JS, Mackay M, Herkowitz HN, et al. 1997 Volvo Award winner in clinical studies. Degenerative lumbar spondylolisthesis with spinal stenosis: a prospective, randomized study comparing decompressive laminectomy and arthrodesis with and without spinal instrumentation. Spine (Phila Pa 1976). 1997;22(24):2807-12.
29. Kim NH, Lee JW. Anterior interbody fusion versus posterolateral fusion with transpedicular fixation for isthmic spondylolisthesis in adults. A comparison of clinical results. Spine (Phila Pa 1976). 1999;24(8):812-6;discussion 817.
30. Deguchi M, Rapoff AJ, Zdeblick TA. Posterolateral fusion for isthmic spondylolisthesis in adults: analysis of fusion rate and clinical results. J Spinal Disord. 1998;11(6):459-64.
31. Swan J, Hurwitz E, Malek F, et al. Surgical treatment for unstable low-grade isthmic spondylolisthesis in adults: a prospective controlled study of posterior instrumented fusion compared with combined anterior-posterior fusion. Spine J. 2006;6(6):606-14.
32. Müslüman AM, Yilmaz A, Cansever T, et al. Posterior lumbar interbody fusion versus posterolateral fusion with instrumentation in the treatment of low-grade isthmic spondylolisthesis: midterm clinical outcomes. J Neurosurg Spine. 2011;14(4):488-96.
33. Farrokhi MR, Rahmanian A, Masoudi MS. Posterolateral versus posterior interbody fusion in isthmic spondylolisthesis. J Neurotrauma. 2012;29(8):1567-73.
34. Wenger M, Sapio N, Markwalder TM. Long-term outcome in 132 consecutive patients after posterior internal fixation and fusion for Grade I and II isthmic spondylolisthesis. J Neurosurg Spine. 2005;2(3):289-97.
35. Carragee EJ. Single-level posterolateral arthrodesis, with or without posterior decompression, for the treatment of isthmic spondylolisthesis in adults. A prospective, randomized study. J Bone Joint Surg Am. 1997;79(8):1175-80.

36. Glassman SD, Berven S, Bridwell K, et al. Correlation of radiographic parameters and clinical symptoms in adult scoliosis. Spine (Phila Pa 1976). 2005;30(6):682-8.
37. Glassman SD, Bridwell K, Dimar JR, et al. The impact of positive sagittal balance in adult spinal deformity. Spine (Phila Pa 1976). 2005;30(18):2024-9.
38. Schwab F, Lafage V, Farcy JP, et al. Surgical rates and operative outcome analysis in thoracolumbar and lumbar major adult scoliosis: application of the new adult deformity classification. Spine (Phila Pa 1976). 2007;32(24):2723-30.
39. Gaines RW, Nichols WK. Treatment of spondyloptosis by two stage L5 vertebrectomy and reduction of L4 onto S1. Spine (Phila Pa 1976). 1985;10(7):680-6.
40. Kasliwal MK, Smith JS, Kanter A, et al. Management of high-grade spondylolisthesis. Neurosurg Clin N Am. 2013;24(2):275-91.
41. Lee SH, Choi WG, Lim SR, et al. Minimally invasive anterior lumbar interbody fusion followed by percutaneous pedicle screw fixation for isthmic spondylolisthesis. Spine J. 2004;4(6):644-9.
42. Park P, Foley KT. Minimally invasive transforaminal lumbar interbody fusion with reduction of spondylolisthesis: technique and outcomes after a minimum of 2 years' follow-up. Neurosurg Focus. 2008;25(2):E16.
43. Wang J, Zhou Y, Zhang ZF, et al. Comparison of one-level minimally invasive and open transforaminal lumbar interbody fusion in degenerative and isthmic spondylolisthesis grades 1 and 2. Eur Spine J. 2010;19(10):1780-4.
44. France JC, Yaszemski MJ, Lauerman WC, et al. A randomized prospective study of posterolateral lumbar fusion. Outcomes with and without pedicle screw instrumentation. Spine (Phila Pa 1976). 1999;24(6):553-60.
45. McGuire RA, Amundson GM. The use of primary internal fixation in spondylolisthesis. Spine (Phila Pa 1976). 1993;18(12):1662-72.
46. Thomsen K, Christensen FB, Eiskjaer SP, et al. 1997 Volvo Award winner in clinical studies. The effect of pedicle screw instrumentation on functional outcome and fusion rates in posterolateral lumbar spinal fusion: a prospective, randomized clinical study. Spine (Phila Pa 1976). 1997;22(24):2813-22.
47. Ogilvie JW. Complications in spondylolisthesis surgery. Spine (Phila Pa 1976). 2005;30(Suppl 6):S97-101.
48. Schoenecker PL, Cole HO, Herring JA, et al. Cauda equina syndrome after in situ arthrodesis for severe spondylolisthesis at the lumbosacral junction. J Bone Joint Surg Am. 1990;72(3):369-77.
49. Escobar E, Transfeldt E, Garvey T, et al. Video-assisted versus open anterior lumbar spine fusion surgery: a comparison of four techniques and complications in 135 patients. Spine (Phila Pa 1976). 2003;28(7):729-32.
50. Kaiser MG, Haid RW Jr, Subach BR, et al. Comparison of the mini-open versus laparoscopic approach for anterior lumbar interbody fusion: a retrospective review. Neurosurgery. 2002;51(1):97-103;discussion 103-5.

CHAPTER 40

Spine Surgery: Current Concepts and Evidence Adult Scoliosis

Caglar Yilgor, Ahmet Alanay

INTRODUCTION

The umbrella term "adult spinal deformity" (ASD) includes diverse conditions that may cause pain, functional impairment, cosmetic concerns, and/or neurologic compromise. The most common underlying pathologies are abnormality of physiologic spinal alignment, degeneration, stenosis, and instability. This chapter summarizes the clinical workup, medical and surgical management as well as the complications and prognosis of ASD.

EPIDEMIOLOGY AND NATURAL HISTORY

Adult spinal deformity is a chronic disease that has an impact on health-related quality of life (HRQoL). When compared to self-reported chronic conditions such as arthritis, chronic lung disease, diabetes, and congestive heart failure in the general population of eight industrialized countries, the global burden of ASD was huge.[1]

Adult scoliosis can be divided into two main categories: (1) Progression of adolescent onset scoliosis and (2) degenerative (de novo) scoliosis. It is estimated that the prevalence of both are 6% over the age of 50.[2] Yet, a study on elderly volunteers reported the prevalence of adult scoliosis as high as 68%.[3] Although some aspects may intersect, the terms adult scoliosis and adult spinal deformity in this chapter will be generally used to refer to de novo scoliosis.

Adult spinal deformity differs from the adolescent counterpart in patterns of deformity, degenerative component, natural history, and clinical symptoms. Unlike adult idiopathic scoliosis, de novo scoliosis usually occurs in the lumbar spine and typically has smaller magnitudes. The incidence of central canal and foraminal stenosis are higher.

The main step in the pathophysiology of ASD is the degeneration of facet joints and disks followed by instability in the spinal column leading to lateral and/or rotatory listhesis. Osteoporosis can contribute to the deformity with vertebral body compression fractures. Impingement of the canal or nerve roots by pedicles, hypertrophic bone, or soft tissues may accompany.

The natural history of ASD is not fully delineated but some risk factors have been described. In general, the curves are expected to progress 1–6°/year with an average of 3.3°.[4] A Cobb angle >30°, lateral vertebral translation >6 mm, a grade 3 apical rotation, and prominent or deeply-seated L5 are predictors of curve progression.[4] A more recent natural history study of progressive adult scoliosis confirms the linear progression of the disease, acknowledging the rotatory subluxation as the initial element of progression. In this study where the mean delay between the first and last radiograph was 27 years, menopause constituted a period of deterioration.[5]

WORKUP

Clinical presentation of ASD varies greatly from patients who remain asymptomatic with radiographic findings alone to those with severe pain with neurogenic claudication and radiculopathy. Patient assessment requires a complete history (including comorbidities), physical examination, and appropriate imaging. It is important to perform hip, knee, and leg length examination to better understand the global sagittal profile of the patient.

Comorbidities related to cardiac, respiratory, endocrine, renal, gastrointestinal, hematopoietic, and genitourinary systems should be carefully questioned as well as history of smoking and malignancy. Treadmill or chemical stress test or dobutamine stress echocardiography may be used for further evaluation of the cardiopulmonary function.

The patient should then be classified to ensure common language, predict natural history, and guide treatment. Since ASD has a marked impact on HRQoL, it is reasonable to use clinical impact classification systems that regard disability as well as radiographic findings.

The typical workup should also include assessment for osteoporosis, since the presence and extent of osteopenia and/or osteoporosis may alter the treatment.

Symptoms and Signs

The common signs and symptoms are back pain, radiculopathy, claudication, neurological deficit, and unfavorable cosmesis. Patients with positive sagittal imbalance will tend to use compensatory mechanisms such as hip extension, knee flexion, and pelvic retroversion to counterbalance the loss of lumbar lordosis.

Back pain is the most frequent clinical complaint.[6,7] The muscle-based pain is rather diffuse, while bony and facet joint pain may be more localized. A pain, that occurs only when the patient is upright or only during certain movements, suggests instability. Diagnostics blocks may be used to better identify the pain generator(s).

The back pain can be accompanied by radicular leg pain and/or claudication. The radicular pain can be present both in the concavity and convexity since both compression and traction may evoke pain. The stenosis may occur centrally or in the lateral recesses, and such may present as claudication or radicular pain, respectively.

Neurological deficit may involve an individual root or several roots. The cauda equina may also be compromised presenting with bladder and sphincter symptoms.

Although cosmesis plays a minor role when compared to adolescents, it may present as a mental health issue for adults, reflecting their concerns whether their curves will progress or not and whether they will face the potential risk of disability in the future. This goes along with the fact that the elderly today have more active lifestyles than did the elderly of previous generations and are more resistant to the notion that disability and deformity are a part of the aging process.

Laboratory Findings

There is no specific blood test that might help in the diagnosis or follow-up of ASD patients. Electromyography (EMG) may be performed with nerve conduction studies to aid with the diagnosis of nerve compression.

Imaging

Full-length posterior-anterior and lateral views of the spine should be obtained including the shoulders, iliac crests, and hip joints. The patients should be standing with their knees fully extended. Static films demonstrate alignment, rotation, lateral listhesis, spondylolisthesis, and retrolisthesis. Supine bending or bolster films help to assess the rigidity of the curve. Dynamic standing lateral X-rays may help identify focal instability.

Oblique films can be used to identify the presence of pars defects. Likewise, diskograms were formerly used to evaluate the morphology and pain response of the disks. The use of both have fallen out of favor with the widespread use of magnetic resonance imaging (MRI) and computed tomography (CT).

Following plain radiographic evaluation, MRI should be the second-line radiographic tool with its excellent ability in assessing the disks, facet joints, ligaments, spinal cord, nerves, spinal canal, foramen, and bone marrow.

Computed tomography may be used when further evaluation of the rotational deformity, bony anatomy, and reconstruction in different planes is required.

Grading scales from X-rays, dual-energy X-ray absorptiometry (DEXA), quantitative CT, and microdensitometry can be used to diagnose and quantify osteoporosis. The DEXA values acquired from the femoral neck should be interpreted with caution because the bone density in the spine decreases earlier than in other skeletal sites in the early postmenopausal years due to turnover in this highly trabecular bone. DEXA acquired from the vertebrae may be falsely elevated due to degenerative changes.

A thorough radiographic assessment starts with defining and measuring the scoliotic curves. The central sacral vertical line (CSVL) that passes through the center of the sacrum will help analyze deviations from the vertical axis. Lateral radiographs possess more significant information regarding the treatment of ASD. First, lumbar lordosis and thoracic kyphosis should be measured. Any focal areas with a bigger Cobb angle than the global kyphosis should be noted. C7 plumb line that starts from the center of C7 vertebral body and drops straight downward in the vertical axis should be drawn. The horizontal distance from this line to the posterosuperior corner of S1 gives the sagittal alignment [sagittal vertical axis (SVA)]. Spinopelvic measurements of pelvic incidence (PI), sacral slope (SS), and pelvic tilt (PT) should be

SECTION 5

measured. SS is the angle between the horizontal line and the line that is tangential to the S1 end plate. PT is the angle between the vertical line and the line that connects the center of the femoral head to the middle of the S1 end plate. PI is the angle between the line that connects the center of the femoral head to the middle of the S1 end plate and a line that is perpendicular to the S1 end plate. From a geometric point of view PI equals to the sum of PT and SS. These spinopelvic alignment parameters, however, are affected by postural compensation mechanisms. T1 pelvic angle and global tilt (GT) incorporate the spinal and pelvic sagittal parameters and are less affected by patient positioning. The T1 pelvic angle is the angle between the line from the center of femoral heads to the center of T1 vertebral body and the line from the center of femoral heads to the middle of the S1 end plate.[8] It can be useful in preoperative planning with a target angle of <14°. GT is the angle between the line from C7 to the middle of S1 end plate and the line from the center of femoral heads to the middle of S1 endplate.[9] From a geometrical point of view, GT equals the sum of the pelvic tilt and the spinal tilt angle, which makes its calculation very easy. Plus, these two parameters do not require calibrated radiographs since they are angular and not linear measurements.

Radiographic parameters were assessed for their correlation with the visual analog scale (VAS) reported pain.[10] L3 or L4 tilt angle, olisthesis, thoracolumbar kyphosis, and loss of lordosis were found to correlate more with pain. Cobb angle, sagittal pelvic tilt index, and plumb line offset were not found to correlate with pain. The correlation of sagittal and pelvic parameters with the HRQoL parameters will be discussed in more detail later in this chapter under goals of surgery and alignment objectives.

When evaluating radiographs and their measurements, it should be kept in mind that the normative values vary with age. Aging results in an increase in thoracic kyphosis and PT, decrease in lumbar lordosis and sacral slope,[11] the sacrum is more posteriorly displaced and the mean SVA shifts forward.[12] Furthermore, the age and gender adjusted HRQoL scores show that clinical tolerance to sagittal imbalance varies with age.[13] Severe sagittal imbalance has a greater impact on HRQoL in younger patients; however, in older patients HRQoL does not markedly differ in relation to the severity of the deformity.

Disease Specific Outcome Measures

Health-related quality-of-life analysis plays a crucial role in the assessment of ASD. Baseline HRQoL values are of paramount importance to track the results of medical or surgical treatments. VAS, Oswestry Disability Index (ODI), and Scoliosis Research Society 22 (SRS-22) questionnaires are commonly used outcome instruments validated for adult deformity population.

These parameters also correlate with radiographic findings. Sagittal balance is the dominant predictor of HRQoL in ASD.[14] All HRQoL measures showed poorer results with increase in SVA.[15] Substantial coronal imbalance is a moderate negative factor in nonoperated patients.[14] ODI scores correlate with the region of greatest kyphosis. A more distal region of maximal kyphosis generates higher disability on ODI.[15]

Classification

Simmons[16] was probably the first to attempt to classify ASD patients and influence their treatment by dividing the patients into two categories based on rotation.

Aebi classified adult degenerative scoliosis based on primary causes of the deformity.[7] Although this four-category classification helps predict the natural history, it cannot be used to influence surgical treatment. On the other hand, the Faldini classification system divides the patients into two main and eight subgroups, and primarily aims to direct the surgical treatment proposing an algorithm for each subtype on the basis of decompression and fusion strategies.[17]

Spine Deformity Study Group classification,[18] Schwab classification,[19] and SRS Adult Deformity Classification[20] aimed to distinguish different curve types and used several modifiers to come up with a reliable and reproducible classification system that has the ability to categorize the patients according to the severity of the disability. The SRS-Schwab ASD classification,[21] which is the end product of this work, is to date, the most reliable clinical impact classification system for ASD. The SRS-Schwab classification has a significant impact on surgical rates and operative strategies such as the approach, fusion to sacrum, and the use of osteotomies. It reflects patient-reported pain and disability. Plus, in combination with baseline HRQoL scores, it relates to complication rates. Yet, it lacks evaluation of instability such as spondylolisthesis and lateral subluxation, which are known to have significant clinical impact in adult deformity patients.

NONSURGICAL MANAGEMENT

The classical approach is to offer nonsurgical management as the first-line therapy. Formerly, the patients were made to believe that they had to adjust their lives accordingly and assimilate to live with this condition. Because major surgeries in this age group were associated with very high complication rates and bone quality and instrumentations were considered to be poor to allow major corrections. Failure of all conservative measures was a prerequisite to surgery.

However, a standard of care for the conservative therapy is not present and the efficacy of nonsurgical management is not well-supported in the literature. Very weak evidence exists for any nonoperative treatment option for ASD.[22] Yet, since the complication rates are high, nonsurgical management can be an alternative to surgery in mild and moderate cases, especially in the absence of neurological deficit or instability. However, it should also be kept in mind that nonsurgical management is not complication-free and that it might be reasonable to operate patients before their symptoms get more severe and chronic, tailoring the treatment for every single patient.

Medical treatment options consist of pain medication, nonsteroidal anti-inflammatory drugs, and muscle relaxants. Gabapentin and pregabalin may be used for neuropathic pain. Antidepressants and anticonvulsants can also be considered. Narcotic pain medicine may have a role in an acute aggravation of back or leg pain.

Physical therapy, conditioning exercises, stretching, and core strengthening exercises may help decrease the pain in the absence of cardiovascular contraindications. Swimming, walking, cycling, and weight lifting may be viable options. Epidural, nerve root or trigger point injections as well as facet joint blocks may help for temporary pain control. Bracing may aid temporary pain relief in a small number of patients. Complementary modalities such as Yoga, Pilates, acupuncture, and chiropractic care may be other therapeutic options.

These nonsurgical treatment options may be used alone or in any combination. The goal should not be to postpone surgery as much as possible. Instead, the goal of nonsurgical treatment is to enable the patient to manage the pain and to maintain functional abilities.

SURGICAL MANAGEMENT

Goals of Surgery and Alignment Objectives

The main goal of surgery is to relieve the back and the radicular pain and neurogenic claudication. Stability should be preserved as much as possible while performing decompression. Then the coronal and more importantly sagittal plane corrections are made. If possible, preserving the facet joints while performing decompression will aid fusion by adding facet fusion to the posterolateral fusion.

The main alignment objectives for adult deformity surgery are related to the sagittal and pelvic parameters. The main goals are set to make the postoperative SVA < 5 cm, T1 tilt $< 0°$, PT $< 25°$ and LL = PI $\pm 9°$.[23,24] Among all coronal and sagittal parameters PI minus LL correlates best SRS-22 SI, function and total scores, ODI and SF 12 PCS.[23] The lumbar lordosis index (LLI), which is the ratio between LL and PI (LL/PI), correlates similarly with spinal malalignment, and is highly predictive of a spinal osteotomy performance.[25] The global sagittal parameters of SVA and T1 tilt are the second most important parameters with T1 tilt having a greater correlation with HRQoL compared to SVA; and the PT is the third.[23]

When trying to reach these goals, surgeons should be aware that intraoperative prone positioning itself and the amount of hip flexion/extension affects the lumbar lordosis. In a retrospective evaluation, patients with preoperative hypolordosis had an enhanced lumbar lordosis via prone positioning alone compared with their preoperative upright radiographs. Contrariwise, ASD patients with preoperative normal lordosis remained unchanged with prone positioning.[26]

The Big Dilemma: To Operate or not to Operate

The information on evidence-based decision-making process of ASD patients and surgeons in the selection of surgical versus nonsurgical treatment is lacking. The surgical approach to ASD is complex and exhibits a high incidence of complications. Yet, a significant number of patients still prefer operative treatment.

Surgery offers reduction/relief of pain and increased quality of life, but comes along with possibility of several surgical complications including death. Likewise, nonintervention is not harmless. It has negative implications for general health, carries the risk of decreased mobility and increased debilitating pain and/or neurologic deficits. So, the big question is: "Do benefits of ASD surgery overcome the risks related to it?"

Akbarnia et al.[27] reported 56–75% incidence of major surgical complications and 18–58% chance of unplanned reoperation rates with unproven benefits regarding improvement of HRQoL. Mok et al.[28] reported 25.8% reoperation due to infection, adjacent segment problems, implant failure, pseudarthrosis, and painful implant in their consecutive series of 89 patients with minimum 2-year follow-up. Cho et al.[29] reported similarly for their 47 degenerative lumbar scoliosis patients with an average age of 66. The overall complication rate was 68%; 30% occurring within the first 30 days. Ten patients (21%) were reoperated within an average of 3.8 years follow-up. A large series of 867 patients revealed an 8.2% unplanned hospital readmission in 30 days and 12.1% in 90 days.[30] Multivariate Cox Proportional Hazards analysis revealed that the medical comorbidities such as depression, diabetes, peripheral vascular disease, pulmonary circulatory disorder, and cardiac valvular disease contribute significant risk of unplanned readmission.[30] Long and medium length fusions when compared to short-time from discharge to rehabilitation or skilled nursing facilities are also found to be independent risk factors for readmission.

In summary, the complications and reoperation rates are high in ASD surgery. But, is surgical treatment effective for symptomatic patients? Bridwell et al.[31] compared 2-year follow-up HRQoL outcomes for surgical and nonsurgical adult scoliosis cases. In both matched and unmatched cohorts, operatively treated ASD patients outperformed nonoperatively treated patients. Furthermore, a systematic review revealed no substantial evidence for any nonsurgical treatment in adult scoliosis.[22] Similarly, Glassman et al.[32] attempted to quantify the relative costs and benefits of nonoperative treatment for ASD. In spite of its substantial recurring costs, they concluded that there was no clear target population for any specific treatment modality and that there was no apparent HRQoL benefit with nonoperative treatment. In a comparison of SRS-22, SF-12, and ODI outcomes between 83 operated and nonoperated ASD patients over 65 years of age, authors concluded that operatively treated patients had less pain and better HRQoL.[33]

Based on these studies, surgical treatment of ASD seems effective. But, what about the patients who experience minor or major perioperative and/or follow-up complications. Do they still benefit from surgery despite complications? Glassman et al.[34] performed a case-control analysis to compare major, minor, and no-complication groups based on SRS-22, SF-12, ODI, back and leg pain scales. There were 46 patients in each group and the groups were matched for age, diagnosis, preoperative SRS scores, fusion levels, and postoperative sagittal balance. Some deterioration in SF-12 General Health occurred with major complications, whereas minor complications had no effect. No deterioration in disease-specific outcome measures was observed with either major or minor complications.[34] A longer term follow-up study of 113 primary treatment ASD patients showed no deterioration in mean radiographic or clinical outcomes between 2- and 5-year follow-up.[35] About 10% of the patients experienced a new complication during the course of the follow-up period and this negatively affected the outcome.[35] Similar results were also reported for revision cases. Cho et al.[36] reported 35% major complication rates with 19 3% perioperative and 18.7% follow-up complications. Perioperative complications had no negative impact on outcome, whereas follow-up complications had negative impact.[36]

In a series of 317 adult scoliosis patients who experienced back pain, surgical treatment was found to demonstrate a significantly better improvement in Numerical Rating Scale and ODI.[37]

A retrospective risk-benefit assessment based on patient age was conducted for a prospective and multicenter ASD database of 25–85 years of age to analyze the impact of complications on outcomes.[38] The 65–85 years group had nearly 4 times the number of minor complications and nearly 5 times the number of major complications compared to the 25–44 years group. In this report, outcome measures at 2-year follow-up improved significantly for all age groups compared with baseline measures. Elderly patients had the greatest degree of improvement. The authors concluded that despite facing the greatest risk of complications, the elderly might stand to gain a disproportionately greater improvement in disability and pain with surgery compared to younger patients.[38] This data demonstrates the potential benefits of surgical treatment for ASD.

Therefore, the former belief that the failure of all appropriate conservative care is a prerequisite for surgical intervention for an ASD patient is not necessarily true. Today, it is important to understand the decision-making process of adult deformity patients and how or why they choose operative versus nonoperative treatment. Nonsurgical patients were reported to have greater preoperative medical risk factor, whilst, surgical patients had more frequent leg pain, a higher mean level of daily back pain, and more frequent moderate-to-severe back pain.[39] Pekmezci et al.[40] reported that deterioration in the functional status is a significant factor that leads the ASD patient to seek surgical treatment. Similarly, Fu et al.[41] reported for a series of 156 operative and 341 nonoperative patients that poor HRQoL uniformly determined operative treatment for ASD. This assumption is based on the fact that operative patients reported greater baseline pain and disability than nonoperative patients for all age groups.

Surgical Procedures

Posterior-only surgery including decompression with or without fusion, anterior surgery or combined anterior and posterior procedures may be applied for ASD patients.

Decompression Alone

Decompression alone can be performed to relieve the complaints of radicular pain and neurologic claudication that corresponds to neural compression. This procedure may be considered in the absence of instability and when the complaints of radiculopathy surpass the back pain. Yet, decompression alone carries the risk of resulting in increase in postoperative deformity or iatrogenic postsurgical spinal instability.[42] In cases where the predictors of worsening in static X-rays are present, fusion may be considered. These predictors, described by Prichett,[4] are lateral listhesis >6 mm, spondylolisthesis, or rotation and moderate scoliosis of >30°.

Even when the facet joints are preserved, decompression alone eliminates the stability provided by the posterior column ligaments and bony structures. Yet, there is no specific threshold that dictates to perform fusion. The total number of laminectomies that can be performed without fusion depends on the quality of the bone, magnitude of the curve, magnitude of the rotary or lateral listhesis, presence of osteophytes, and preservation of facet joints. The patient should be evaluated together with clinical and radiographic findings. For example, patients who report activity-related back pain may indicate instability and may require fusion to augment decompression.

Liu et al.[43] reported improved patient-reported outcomes in their series of 112 patients with a mean follow-up of 5.7 years, demonstrating that decompression alone or with fusion is sufficient in treating pain associated with deformity. A retrospective analysis that compares decompression alone with decompression and fusion reported lower complication rates with decompression alone (10% compared to 56%).[44] Yet, in the same report, patient-reported outcomes indicated that the decompression and fusion patients were more satisfied than the patients who underwent decompression alone.[44]

Decompression + Posterior Instrumented Fusion

Correction of the sagittal as well as coronal plane deformities via posterior instrumented fusion together with osteotomies, decompression, and interbody fusion has been the mainstay of surgical treatment for ASD patients for many years. Interbody fusion may be performed as posterior lumbar interbody fusion (PLIF) or transforaminal lumbar interbody fusion (TLIF). Several controversies, difficulties, and challenges exist when choosing and applying this complex group of procedures, which will be further detailed later in this chapter.

Anterior Surgery

Anterior instrumentation and fusion can be used to correct coronal and sagittal deformity and restore disk and foraminal height. Traditional approach is to perform anterior lumbar interbody fusion (ALIF) with anterior instrumentation.

Anterior-alone surgery has several advantages. Considering the amount of degeneration and status of the adjacent segments to the planned fusion, anterior-alone surgery may provide additional motion segment preservation. The disk space can be completely visualized and larger structural grafts may be placed to provide anterior column support, as well as achieving and maintaining lordosis correction. Additional stability is provided by the preservation of the posterior spinal elements and musculature.

Several potential complications are also associated with anterior surgery. Pseudarthrosis, graft displacement, subsidence, vascular damage, ileus and iliac artery thrombosis, ilioinguinal and iliohypogastric nerve injuries, ureteral and/or bladder damage, abdominal hernia, and retrograde ejaculation in male patients.[2]

In a report of a retrospective analysis of 62 patients who had anterior thoracolumbar deformity correction, the overall satisfaction rate was 82.2%.[45] However, 32.3%

reported pain over the thoracolumbar scar area and 43.5% reported a bulging appearance. Nearly one-fourth of the patients reported experiencing functional disturbance with daily activities due to the anterior incision and 48.4% were poorly satisfied with their appearance.[45]

A report that compares the 3-year clinical and radiographic outcomes of ALIF versus PLIF reported no significant difference in VAS, ODI scores, and complication rates.[46]

Besides the traditional approach, more recently, lateral interbody fusion with the minimal invasive lateral transpsoas approach was described.[47] This approach omits the need for mobilization of the vessels, thus the major complication rate is lower. Decreased blood loss and shortened hospital stay is reported in comparison with traditional anterior approaches.[48] Yet, access to L5–S1 and occasionally to L4–L5 can be complicated by the iliac crest.[47] Patients reported significant VAS and ODI improvements.[47,48] However, 30% of patients reported groin/thigh paresthesia and 27% reported groin/thigh pain.[47] It further has potential complications related to manipulation of the lumbar plexus.

Anterior + Posterior Surgery

Coronal and/or sagittal imbalance with a large curve may necessitate decompression and a combined anterior and posterior fusion. Performing the anterior release and interbody fusion by using cages prior to posterior surgery makes the posterior decompression easier by improving the foraminal height from the restoration of disk space height and by realigning the canal with reduction of the lateral listhesis. Yet, the added operative time and medical stress of combined procedures can lead to increased complication and morbidity rates.[49]

Several studies reported higher degree of deformity correction, higher rates of fusion, and improved patient outcomes.[49,50] A more recent study,[51] however, concluded that posterior-only surgery provided the same deformity correction as anterior + posterior fusion. Clinical outcomes and complications were equivalent at over 2-year follow-up. Combined approach resulted in higher pseudarthrosis rates and lower adjacent segment degeneration, but these were not statistically significant.[51]

A combined minimal invasive procedure by posterior percutaneous fixation together with the previously discussed minimal invasive lateral interbody fusion may be an alternative for patients when an anterior-posterior fusion is planned.[52] A retrospective report demonstrated a 97% fusion rate with this combined approach on a mean follow-up of 13.4 months.[53]

Controversies, Difficulties, and Challenges

In adults, the spine is more rigid anteriorly. This is due to the degeneration and narrowing of the disks and osteophytes that frequently bridge on the concavity. The spine is also more rigid posteriorly owing to the degenerated and narrow facet joints and osteophytes.

The fusion rates are lower in adults. In a long-term follow-up study of 232 patients the pseudarthrosis rate was 17%.[54] The most common places for pseudarthrosis were the thoracolumbar junction (58%) and the lumbosacral junction (25%). The challenge for the fixation is that the rods have to be able to survive until the fusion takes place. Yet, 42% of the nonunions did not show up until more than 3 years postoperative.[54] In this report, the risks for pseudarthrosis were smoking, >55 years of age, fusion >13 segments, and thoracolumbar kyphosis >20°.[54]

Osteopenia and osteoporosis are also factors in many ASD patients that further complicate the surgical treatment. Therefore, posterior instrumented fusion has to be specifically tailored for each patient.

The main controversies, difficulties, and challenges that will be discussed in this chapter regarding posterior surgery are—selection of fusion levels, whether to fuse to sacrum or not, determining the need for interbody fusion, determining the need for osteotomy, and how to instrument the osteoporotic spine safely and effectively.

Selection of Fusion Levels

The rules for selection of fusion levels for adolescent idiopathic scoliosis are rather set. Relatively, upper instrumented vertebra (UIV) and lower instrumented vertebra (LIV) selection for ASD is more vague. The decision-making in adults is more difficult due to the associated degenerative changes, back and leg pain, relative inflexibility, and listhetic deformities. Nonetheless, certain biomechanical and radiographic principles can be applied to maximize surgical and clinical outcomes.

First, the structural and compensatory curves should be identified since all the structural curve/curves should be included in the fusion. Stable and neutral vertebrae within Cobb levels should be chosen as UIV or LIV if it fits the rest of the criteria. Ending a fusion in the physiological apex of the kyphosis should be avoided.

The one basic principle that applies both for the selection of UIV and LIV is that fusion should not be stopped adjacent to a degenerated segment. The two main criteria for the determination of proximal instrumentation and fusion level are—(1) a centralized and neutral vertebra which usually is the upper-end vertebra of the upper structural curve or one level above it should be chosen; and (2) the UIV should not be a level that possesses high risk for development of proximal junctional kyphosis (PJK).

The general aim is to avoid ending a fusion in the thoracolumbar junction. However, there is no consensus on which vertebrae at the thoracolumbar or lower thoracic level to stop. Choosing L1 or T10 as the UIV reveals no significant difference.[55] A similar study revealed that results of choosing T9, T11 or L1 as the UIV reveals no significant difference in radiographic and clinical outcomes or revision prevalence.[56] Therefore, when trying to choose between T9-T10-T11 and L1, the more distal proximal fusion level at a neutral and stable vertebra should be satisfactory.

When trying to determine between an upper and lower thoracic UIV, one should always remember that no spinal region is immune to proximal junctional problems. UIV should be selected as T2 in patients with osteoporosis that is accompanied with hyperkyphosis. Similarly, UIV should be selected as T2 in patients with severe sagittal plane deformity in thoracolumbar transition zone and in the thoracic spine. UIV should also be selected as T2 in patients with concordant thoracic spinal stenosis due to the compression of the ligamentum flavum demonstrated by MRI. In general, choosing a UIV at the more proximal thoracic level may result in longer operative durations, greater blood loss, and higher rates of nonunion. Adversely, the rate of PJK and revision surgery is lower.[57]

A very recent study[58] that compares upper and lower thoracic UIV in fusions to sacrum/pelvis reported that clinical and radiographic outcomes at minimum 2-year follow-up were similar. Upper thoracic UIV patients had a higher rate of total complications, but major complications requiring revision surgery were similar. In this multicenter series of 198 patients, PJK was similar between the groups.[58] A similar study[57] concluded that upper thoracic UIV results in more perioperative complications, a higher pseudarthrosis rate, and probably more revision surgery. In their series, lower thoracic UIV resulted in a more PJK, but rarely required revision surgery.[57]

Fusion to Sacrum (L5 vs. S1)

The challenge in choosing the LIV to be L5 or S1 (or pelvis) is that fusion to L5 frequently leads to L5–S1 disk degeneration, whereas fusion to S1 is associated with more complications and pseudarthrosis.

Bridwell et al.[59] suggested that one should never stop at L5 in osteoporotic spines. Typically, the findings that suggest fusing to sacrum are:

- Previous L5–S1 laminectomy
- L5–S1 facet joint arthrosis, lateral recess, and foraminal stenosis
- UIV being T5 or higher
- Oblique takeoff of L5
- L5–S1 instability such as spondylolisthesis and spondylolysis.

Edwards et al.[60] reported a 61% L5–S1 disk degeneration after stopping at L5 with only 12% requiring extension of fusion to sacrum with a minimum 2-year follow-up. The same group reported 72% disk degeneration with 23% revision rate in a similar cohort with a minimum 5-year follow-up.[61]

When the fusion is extended to sacrum, the S1 screws should always be placed in a tricortical manner, directed toward the promontory. Additional interbody fusion may also be considered in the setting of severe preoperative L5–S1 disk degeneration and/or instability to increase the fusion rate at L5–S1 segment.

S1 screws alone may be inadequate in providing stable fixation for long constructs, especially in the osteoporotic spine. Besides anterior structural support, iliac screws, alar screws, S2 screws, intrasacral rods (Jackson technique), and Galveston technique are fixation options to supplement the S1 screws.[49] Adding anterior support decreased the strain on S1 screw approximately 30%, whereas adding S2 screws or iliac fixation provided a decrease of approximately 70%.[62]

Need for Interbody Fusion

Patient factors that necessitate the use of interbody fusion are severe osteoporosis, segmental instability, and having risk for pseudarthrosis. Performing wide decompressions and extension of fusion to sacrum also needs consideration of using interbody fusion. PLIF, TLIF, ALIF, lateral transpsoas interbody fusion, oblique lumbar interbody fusion (OLIF), and axial lumbar interbody fusion (AxiaLIF) are current approaches that may be used.

A meta-analysis that included four prospective randomized clinical trials compared posterolateral-only fusion with circumferential fusion.[63] Although amount of blood loss and complication rates were higher with circumferential fusion, using interbody fusion also provided better fusion rates and lower reoperation rates. A cost-utility evaluation of 135 patients at 5-year follow-up revealed similar results.[64] Physical and psychosocial summary scores were better with circumferential than posterolateral fusion. Net utility gain with posterolateral and circumferential fusion was 0.13 and 0.24, respectively. Reoperation rates were 38% for posterolateral fusion whereas only 15% of the circumferential fusion patients were reoperated.[64]

Once the surgeon decides to use an interbody fusion, the next challenge is to choose which technique to use. Familiarity with the technique is probably the most important determinant; however, some specific patient factors may dictate the use or avoidance of a particular technique.

- TLIF or PLIF may be used when decompression is done.
- TLIF or PLIF may be used for male patients in L5–S1 level.
- ALIF may be used for female patients in L5–S1 level.
- TLIF and PLIF should be avoided in severe osteoporosis, when epidural scarring is present and L5–S1 disk is wedge-shaped.
- ALIF may be used in osteoporotic, wedge-shaped L5–S1 disks.
- ALIF may be used in severe hypolordotic patients.
- Lateral transpsoas approach may be a better alternative in osteoporotic patients.
- Lateral transpsoas approach may be used for upper lumbar levels.
- OLIF may be a psoas-sparing alternative using an anterior oblique retroperitoneal approach.

Posterior lumbar interbody fusion was reported to improve ODI scores and coronal Cobb and lumbar lordosis angles with a 76.9% patient satisfaction rate.[65] Similarly TLIF resulted in improved patient reported outcomes and coronal Cobb and lordosis angles[66,67] with an 81% satisfaction rate.[66]

A study that compared the 3-year results of TLIF and ALIF found no difference in clinical outcomes or curve correction.[46] The ALIF and TLIF groups, however, were not the same regarding curve severity, number of levels of interbody fusion, and spinal imbalance. ALIF was more often used in cases of severe sagittal imbalance and hypolordosis.[46]

Although lateral transpsoas interbody fusion alone may provide less correction, its combination with posterior percutaneous pedicle screw instrumentation provided 40–75% correction of coronal curves, with modest increase of lordosis.[68] Lateral transpsoas interbody fusion in combination with minimally invasive fixation may result in lower complication rates than open circumferential fusion; however, it is not complication-free. Permanent neural deficit and visceral complications have been reported with this technique.[68]

Oblique lumbar interbody fusion that provides a monosegment transdiskal fixation was described as an alternative to lateral transpsoas interbody fusion.[69,70] OLIF may allow for less invasion of the psoas muscle and lumbar plexus, direct visualization of sensory nerves, ureter, and synthetic trunk.[70] This technique offers an indirect decompression of spinal stenosis.

Axial lumbar interbody fusion is also a relatively safe procedure that provides good clinical outcomes in both short and long constructs for adult scoliosis patients, which also is not complication-free.[71] It is generally recommended for use in combination with posterior instrumentation. Rectal injury and intrapelvic hematoma are possible complications related to this approach.[71]

Need for Osteotomy

In general, an osteotomy is necessary if the deformity cannot be corrected by diskectomy and/or facetectomy and soft tissue releases. In ASD, osteotomies are most commonly used for loss of lumbar lordosis and fixed kyphosis. Osteotomy options are Ponte osteotomy, Smith-Petersen osteotomy (SPO), pedicle subtraction osteotomy (PSO), bone-disk-bone osteotomy (BDBO), and vertebral column resection (VCR). Recently, Schwab et al. classified these osteotomies into six categories based on anatomical grades of resection.[72]

Grade 1: Osteotomies involve the resection of the joint capsule and inferior facet. Anterior column mobility is a prerequisite for this procedure that has limited deformity correction ability. SPO and Chevron osteotomies are examples for grade 1 resections.

Grade 2: Osteotomies involve removal of all posterior ligaments (supraspinous, intraspinous, and ligamentum flavum) and facet joints. It can be performed at several levels and can provide up to 10–15° of correction per level based on the amount of cone resected. They are relatively safer procedures and were reported to provide 86% satisfaction rates.[73] Ponte osteotomy may be an example of grade 2 resections.

Grade 3: Osteotomies involve the removal of the pedicles and partial body. They can provide up to 15°–20° and 30°–40° of focal sagittal correction at each segment in thoracic and lumbar spine, respectively. It can also be performed asymmetrically to achieve coronal correction in combination with sagittal. Although complication rates were high, patients reported improved ODI and SRS scores at 2-year follow-up.[74] PSO may be an example of grade 3 resections.

Grade 4: Osteotomies can be performed in different ways to provide different amounts of correction rates ranging from 35° to 60°. They involve the removal of the pedicles, partial body and disk. Grade 4 osteotomies may be an alternative to grade 5 osteotomies in patients with severe and rigid thoracolumbar and lumbar deformities, particularly when the apex of the deformity is at a disk level. BDBO may be an example of grade 4 resections.

Grade 5: Osteotomies involve the removal of whole vertebral body and disks. They provide the greatest amount of correction and play an important role in the treatment of severe deformities that cannot be acceptably corrected by less aggressive methods. Single level VCR may be an example of grade 5 resections. En block resections and multilevel VCRs are examples for grade 6 resections.

Varied clinical and radiological scenarios necessitate different grades or types of osteotomies. All the osteotomy types are technically demanding and result in high rates of complications. The appropriate selection of the grade of the osteotomy depends on the surgeons' experience, type of the deformity, and magnitude of the curve:

- If the surgeon is less experienced with osteotomies and/or the patient is in poor medical condition, intraoperative halo-femoral traction and grade 1 osteotomies may be performed.
- If the kyphosis is gradual or sweeping, the degree of sagittal imbalance is moderate and the disk space is mobile, then grade 2 osteotomies should be sufficient.
- Fixed disk space and/or severe sagittal imbalance generally necessitate grade 3 or grade 4 osteotomies.
- Sharp and focal kyphotic deformities in the lumbar region are also addressed with grade 3 and grade 4 osteotomies.
- Thoracic sharp and focal kyphosis may be corrected with grade 5 and grade 6 osteotomies.

Figures 1A and B demonstrate the preoperative coronal and sagittal MRI views of the lumbosacral spine of a 71-year-old female patient who displays adult degenerative scoliosis with stenosis. The patient was operated in another institute. Decompression and posterior instrumented fusion was applied from T9 to ilium (Figs. 1C and D). First revision surgery was performed 4 months later and iliac screws were removed. Figures 1E and F demonstrate the radiographic situation of the patient when she first applied to our clinic 3 years after the second surgery. Post-fusion flat back and pseudarthrosis with rod breakage, fracture of the UIV, and PJK was diagnosed. The flat back was addressed with L4 PSO. T8–9 and T12–L1 Chevron osteotomies were applied to the pseudarthrosis and PJK sites. T3-iliac instrumentation and fusion was applied with the double rod technique at the PSO site. Second stage surgery was performed 1 week later. Anterior T12–L1 diskectomy, ALIF, and instrumented fusion were applied. Figures 2A and B show the 2-year follow-up radiographs of the patient.

Osteopenia/Osteoporosis

In patients with low bone mineral density (BMD), spinal implants cannot be placed as securely as in patients with normal BMD, and thus application of corrective forces through the weak bone-implant interface is difficult. To avoid failure in such situations, it is important to understand the biomechanics of the osteoporotic spine and to recognize that osteoporosis is a systemic disease. A complete review of osteoporosis and its medical management is beyond the scope of this chapter.

In general, the two most common surgical problems in the osteoporotic spine are failure of the fixation and

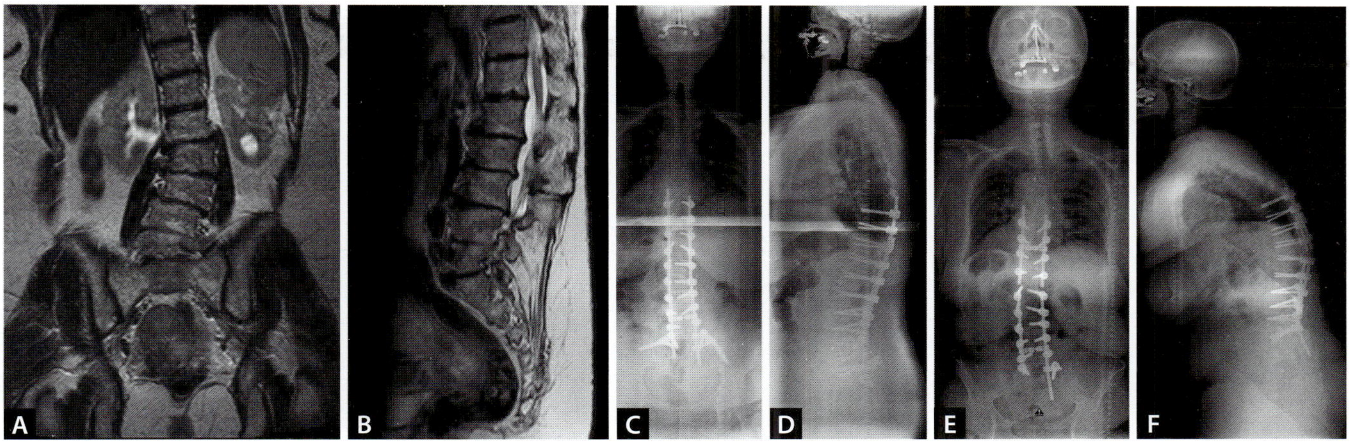

Figs. 1A to F: (A and B) Preoperative coronal and sagittal MRI slices; (C and D) X-rays 6 weeks after the first operation. SVA: slightly negative (non-calibrated X-ray); lumbar lordosis: 38°; PT: 27.5°; SS: 16.1°; PI: 43.6°; and angle between UIV and UIV+2: 9°; (E and F) X-rays 3 years after the second operation. SVA: +14 cm; lumbar lordosis: 23°; PT: 26.1°; SS: 17°; PI: 43.1°; and angle between UIV and UIV+2: 32°.
(SVA: sagittal vertical axis; PT: pelvic tilt; PI: pelvic incidence; SS: sacral slope; UIV: upper instrumented vertebra)

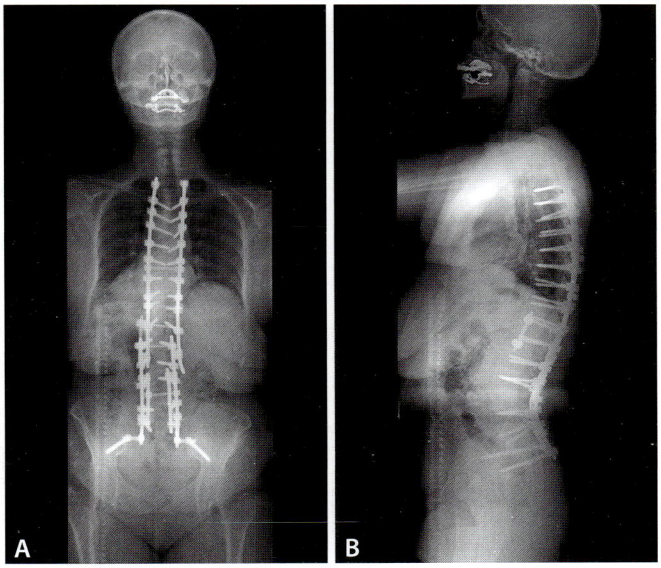

Figs. 2A and B: X-rays 2 years after the revision surgery was applied. SVA: –0.5 cm; lumbar lordosis: 45°; PT: 18.4°; SS: 25°; PI: 43.4°; and angle between UIV and UIV+2: 10°.

adjacent segment failure, either of which may result in pseudarthrosis and/or loss of correction.

No consensus has yet been reached on the optimal screw diameter, length, thread design, and shape for fixation in the osteoporotic bone. However, several pedicle screw characteristics, together with the whole preparation and screw insertion tactics, may be used to achieve a better fixation. Pedicle screw tract augmentation may be done by preparing the hole, injecting polymethylmethacrylate (PMMA) bone cement into the hole, and inserting the screw afterward. It may also be done using fenestrated pedicle screws. Bioactive cements, calcium phosphate, and calcium sulfate may also be used for augmentation. Coating the pedicle screw with hydroxyapatite is a time-dependent augmentation technique that increases osteointegration.

Starting point, insertion angle, and trajectory are other important factors that determine the strength of fixation. Resistance to pullout of parallel screws depends on the volume of cancellous bone between the threads, whereas triangulated screws provide better pullout strength because the construct is contributed by the volume of bone within the trapezoid area formed by the screws.[75]

In osteoporotic cancellous bone same size tapping results in removal of bone within the pedicle track and prevents bone compression around the screw threads. Undertapping by 0.5 mm and 1.0 mm increases the insertional torque by 47% and 93%, respectively, when compared with same-size tapping.[76]

Load sharing by multilevel fixation, use of cross-links, and taking advantage of the relatively stronger cortical bone with hooks, wires, cables, and bands are important to enhance anchor points in the osteoporotic spine. Prophylactic vertebroplasty that entails the cement augmentation of the proximal and distal adjacent noninstrumented levels decreases the revision arthrodesis rates due to adjacent vertebrae fractures.[77] Preservation of the supraspinous ligament, intraspinous ligament, and ligamentum flavum between the cranial fused level and the adjacent segment, as well as between the cranial levels of fusion to create a segment of high posterior tension. This may prevent the development of junctional instability. Furthermore, supra- and infra-adjacent facets should be preserved and the cranial disk space should not be violated with pedicle screws.

In the setting of osteoporosis, L5–S1 diskectomy and interbody fusion should be considered if the instrumentation starts above L2. Care should be given to place the cage in contact with the peripheral apophyseal ring where the cortical bone is stronger to avoid subsidence of the cage into the end plates, which may lead to collapse of the anterior column.

Effective release of spinal column may help eliminating the need for forceful manipulation of rigid curves which may result in implant failure. Confining to a lesser degree of deformity correction may also be important to prevent failure of the bone–implant interface intraoperatively.

Postoperative brace used for at least 3 months may also help to prevent implant failure and junctional problems.

Minimally Invasive Surgery

When compared with traditional approaches, minimally invasive approaches may reduce procedure-related morbidity, although a recent 1-year follow-up study of 30 patients revealed a 23% major complication rate.[78] A literature review of the minimally invasive lateral approach for interbody fusion revealed promising preliminary patient-reported outcomes.[48] However, the magnitude of radiographic correction and degree of clinical improvement with minimally invasive techniques for ASD remain unclear.[79] Yet, in a population predisposed to comorbidity, careful patient selection is critical to achieve the best surgical and clinical outcomes.[80]

COMPLICATIONS

Complications in the management of ASD can be summarized as follows:

- Complications of nonsurgical treatment:
  - Disease progression
  - Residual pain
  - Side effects related to drugs
- Complications of surgery:
  - Intraoperative complications:
    - Bleeding
    - Vascular injury
    - Neurologic injury
    - Visual loss
    - Dural tear
    - Implant failure
    - Mortality
  - Postoperative complications:
    - Fracture, implant failure
    - Infection
    - Pseudarthrosis
    - PJK-DJK (distal junctional kyphosis)
    - Loss of correction
    - Flat back deformity
    - Cerebrospinal fluid leak
    - Residual pain
    - Mortality
  - Medical complications:
    - Cardiac
    - Pulmonary
    - Thromboembolic
    - Mental status
    - Genitourinary
    - Gastrointestinal.

It is well-documented that ASD is associated with a high rate of complications. The exact rate for each type and overall complications is unclear due to variety of etiologies in the reported series.

The Scoliosis Research Society morbidity and mortality database revealed a mortality rate of 0.2%.[81] About 79% of the death occurred prior to hospital discharge. Mortality rate increased with age, reaching a rate of 3.43% for patients 90 years or older.[81]

The Scoliosis Research Society morbidity and mortality of adult scoliosis surgery revealed an overall complication rate of 13.4%.[82] They reported higher complication rates with osteotomies, revisions, and combined anterior and posterior surgeries.[82] A multicenter retrospective ASD study of 306 patients aged 50 years or older reported an overall complication rate of 39%.[83] Number of instrumented segments, fusion to the sacrum, PSO, and a preoperative PT of 26° or more was associated with increased risk of complications.[83] An age-based analysis of complications revealed rates of 17%, 42%, and 71% for age groups of 25–44, 45–64, and 65–85 years, respectively.[38]

The prevalence of infection after ASD was reported as high as 8%.[84] Deep wound infections are rare, but may lead to substantial consequences. Pseudarthrosis and need for surgery are common after deep wound infections. Urinary tract infections are the most common minor complications with prevalence up to 34%.[38]

Charosky et al. reported a 7.5% rate of neurological complications, which are mostly radicular.[83] Others reported this prevalence to be 2.9% for primary and 3.8% for revision cases, and 7% for long constructs.[85] Almost half of these deficits fully recover with nonoperative treatment especially when postoperative imaging does not display an identifiable cause. The rest of the neurological deficits will show no or partial recovery.

The prevalence of proximal junctional problems after ASD was reported as high as 26%.[86] Obesity, older age, severe sagittal imbalance, and low BMD was found to increase the risk of acute adjacent segment fractures.[87,88] In a minimum of 5-year follow-up, 76% of PJK occurred within 3 months after surgery.[89] The SRS and ODI outcome scores, however, were not different in PJK and non-PJK groups.[89] Although it is less common, distal adjacent segment is not immune to developing kyphosis, which is known as DJK.

Pseudarthrosis is the main cause of failure. Broken spinal implants suggest a nonunion unless proven otherwise and necessitate revision posterior instrumentation and fusion, and/or an anterior fusion. Pseudarthrosis rates have been reported as high as 50%.[83] Infection, older age, pedicle subtraction osteotomy, and fusion to sacrum are associated with higher rates. In a consecutive series of 171 patients who had PSO, the 2-year follow-up pseudarthrosis rate was 10.5% with 61% occurring at the actual PSO site.[89] In their series, all pseudarthrosis patients required revision surgery due to loss of sagittal alignment and pain. Although it is true that osteotomies and fusion to sacrum yield higher complication and nonunion rates, these cannot be totally avoided by not performing the osteotomy or stopping at L5. These higher rates of complications are probably the consequence of a more difficult preoperative state of the patient's deformity that makes the surgeon choose to perform an osteotomy or include the sacrum in the fusion.

There are conflicting reports in the literature about the association between the presence of comorbidities and rates of complications. High body mass index, diabetes, pulmonary disjunction, renal dysfunction, peripheral vascular disease, and osteopenia/osteoporosis are associated with higher rates of pseudarthrosis, implant loosening/failure, adjacent segment, and sagittal balance problems.[28,83,86] Yet, others concluded that the presence of comorbidity had no association with complication rates.[90,91]

Several actions can be taken to minimize, if not to prevent, complications in adult deformity surgery. The first step is to realize that an undeniable number of complications occur due to improper case selection, incorrect diagnosis, incorrect indication, incorrect level selection, or incorrect surgery. Therefore, awareness and careful planning is the crucial first step.

Proper preoperative patient evaluation should include—identifying the pain generator/generators, assessment of physiologic age, assessment of comorbidities, mental health and nutritional status, identifying the risk factors for deep vein thrombosis, prior surgeries and secondary gains if present. Careful spinal column and deformity assessment includes—instability, flexibility, coronal balance, sagittal balance, stenosis, and listhesis analysis. Bone quality should also be assessed. Prophylactic vena cava inferior filter may help decreasing thromboembolic complications.

When planning the surgery and choosing fusion levels, one should always try to find the minimum acceptable procedure with realistic surgical goals. Patient education is very important for better results. Surgical and clinical goals, realistic expectations, and possible complications should be discussed in detail with the patients.

Operative measures that can be taken are—proper positioning, reducing the anesthetic time, implementing strategies to limit blood loss, and having an effective neuromonitoring.

Although discussion is ongoing, intra-wound vancomycin application may help decreasing infection rates. When correcting the sagittal and coronal imbalance, it is reasonable to try to achieve the best correction, but the surgeon should know his/her and the spine's limits. It may always be a wise idea to stage the surgery if the patient's and/or the surgeon's status is inappropriate to carry on with the long surgery.

Perioperative monitoring in intensive care unit, consultation with geriatricians whenever feasible, and judicious use of pain medications are also factors that may help minimize the complications. Early and aggressive mobilization as well as early respiratory support and rehabilitation are essential.

PROGNOSIS

The burden of ASD is huge. Yet, it is probable that many ASD patients never seek treatment. Among the ones that seek treatment and are candidates of surgery there is a controversy in the literature on what extend surgery benefits these patients.

Infection, sagittal imbalance, post-fusion flat back, inadequate decompression in the initial surgery, recurrence of stenosis above the previous decompression, postoperative neurologic deficit, PJK, and pseudarthrosis are common scenarios that may require revision surgery.

Mok et al.[28] reported a reoperation rate of 26% at 2-year follow-up. In the series of Charosky et al.[83] the 2-year reoperation rate was also 26%, and the 6-year reoperation rate was 44%. Although long fusions and fusion to sacrum were more often reoperated for mechanical or neurological complications, the authors concluded that the long-term survival of long fusions seemed better than that of short fusions.

A very recent single institute report of 815 cases with an average of 6.4 years follow-up reported a relatively low reoperation rate of 7.61%.[92] The most common reasons for revision were implant breakage, deformity progression, and infection. This low rate may be related to the relatively lower mean age in this series, which was 30.5 years.

A report on 455 consecutive revision ASD surgeries yielded a repeat revision rate of 21%.[93] Pseudarthrosis, adjacent segment disease, infection, and implant prominence were the most common indications for reoperation. Yet, significant improvements in SRS outcome scores were observed in re-revised ASD patients.

Transfeldt et al.[44] reported results of three different surgical treatments on 85 ASD patients with radiculopathy. Complication rates for decompression alone, decompression and limited fusion, and decompression and full curve fusion were 10%, 40%, and 56%, respectively. Yet, satisfaction rates were lower with decompression alone and highest with full curve fusion.[44] Kleinstueck et al.[94] made a similar comparison and reported further surgical intervention requirement of 7% after the decompression alone, 15% after short fusion, and 28% after long fusions at 2-year follow-up. The satisfaction rates were 69%, 74%, and 76%, respectively.[94] The bottom line is that, despite the complexity of the disease and the treatment, patients benefit from surgery despite high complication and reoperation rates. This most likely reflects careful and appropriate patient selection.

On the other hand, Glassman et al.[34] concluded in their retrospective analysis of a prospective multicenter patient series that major complications adversely affect patient-reported general health outcomes at 1 year after surgery. However, major complications did not adversely affect outcome parameters for pain and function. Despite the extensive consideration of surgical complications and their prevention, complications are an inevitable risk of ASD surgery. Furthermore, results of some major complications may be irreversible. Therefore, it is critical that ASD patients understand the relative frequency and potential complications of surgery. Patient education and shared decision-making may further increase satisfaction rates and HRQoL outcomes.

In a recent review, nonsurgical treatment was not found to be cost-effective and was not shown to have a positive impact on quality-of-life.[95] An incremental cost-effectiveness analysis revealed that surgical treatment for ASD is cost-effective after a 10-year period based on predicted deterioration in HRQoL without surgery.[96] In a projected cost-effectiveness analysis of ASD patients at 5-year follow-up, the factors associated with reaching $100,000/QALY threshold were greater preoperative disability, diagnosis of idiopathic scoliosis, poor preoperative HRQoL scores, and fewer fusion levels.[97]

SUMMARY

Adult spinal deformity is a chronic disease that negatively affects HRQoL. Abnormality of physiologic spinal alignment, degeneration, stenosis, and/or instability result in back pain, radiculopathy, claudication, neurological deficit, and/or cosmetic issues. The SRS-Schwab ASD classification is a reliable clinical impact classification system. A typical patient assessment should include a complete history (including comorbidities), physical examination, appropriate imaging, and assessment for osteoporosis. Alignment, rotation, listhesis and coronal, sagittal and pelvic measurements are evaluated and several alignment objectives are set for surgeries that may vary with age. Yet, the main goal of surgery is to relieve the back and radicular pain and neurogenic claudication. Surgical procedures that may be applied are posterior-only surgery including decompression with or without fusion, anterior surgery or combined anterior and posterior procedures. The ASD surgery comes along with various controversies and difficulties. Selecting the fusion levels, determining whether to fuse to sacrum or not, determining the need for interbody fusion, and determining the need for osteotomy are commonly faced challenges. Plus, the fusion rates are lower and the complications and reoperation rates are higher in adult deformity surgery. Although follow-up complications may have a negative impact, in general, disease-specific outcome measures do not show deterioration with either major or minor complications. Furthermore, despite facing the greatest risk of complications, the elderly might stand to gain a disproportionately greater improvement in disability and pain with surgery compared with younger patients. Hence, surgical treatment of ASD seems effective. On the other hand, in spite of its substantial recurring costs, no specific treatment modality of nonoperative treatment was able to display an apparent HRQoL benefit. Plus, nonsurgical treatment is not complication-free. Therefore, the former belief that the failure of all appropriate conservative care is a prerequisite for surgical intervention for an ASD patient is not necessarily true. Careful and appropriate patient selection is the key for success. Nonetheless, several pre- and perioperative actions may be taken to minimize complications in adult deformity surgery. Patient education and shared decision-making may further increase satisfaction rates.

REFERENCES

1. Pellisé F, Vila-Casademunt A, Ferrer M, et al. European Spine Study Group, ESSG. Impact on health related quality of life of adult spinal deformity (ASD) compared with other chronic conditions. Eur Spine J. 2015;24(1):3-11.
2. Youssef JA, Orndorff DO, Patty CA, et al. Current status of adult spinal deformity. Global Spine J. 2013;3(1):51-62.
3. Schwab F, Dubey A, Gamez L, et al. Adult scoliosis: prevalence, SF-36, and nutritional parameters in an elderly volunteer population. Spine (Phila Pa 1976). 2005;30(9):1082-5.
4. Pritchett JW, Bortel DT. Degenerative symptomatic lumbar scoliosis. Spine (Phila Pa 1976). 1993;18(6):700-3.
5. Marty-Poumarat C, Scattin L, Marpeau M, et al. Natural history of progressive adult scoliosis. Spine (Phila Pa 1976). 2007;32(11):1227-35.
6. Winter RB, Lonstein JE, Denis F. Pain patterns in adult scoliosis. Orthop Clin North Am. 1988;19(2):339-45.
7. Aebi M. The adult scoliosis. Eur Spine J. 2005;14(10):925-48.
8. Protopsaltis T, Schwab F, Bronsard N, et al. International Spine Study Group. TheT1 pelvic angle, a novel radiographic measure of global sagittal deformity, accounts for both spinal inclination and pelvic tilt and correlates with health-related quality of life. J Bone Joint Surg Am. 2014;96(19):1631-40.
9. Boissière L, Obeid I, Vital JM, et al. Global tilt: a single parameter incorporating the spinal and pelvic sagittal parameters and least affected by patient positioning. Eur Spine J. 2014;23(Suppl 5):S469-96.
10. Schwab FJ, Smith VA, Biserni M, et al. Adult scoliosis: a quantitative radiographic and clinical analysis. Spine (Phila Pa 1976). 2002;27(4):387-92.
11. Roussouly P, Nnadi C. Sagittal plane deformity: an overview of interpretation and management. Eur Spine J. 2010; 19(11):1824-36.
12. Vedantam R, Lenke LG, Keeney JA, et al. Comparison of standing sagittal spinal alignment in asymptomatic adolescents and adults. Spine (Phila Pa 1976). 1998;23(2): 211-5.
13. Urquiza FP, Vila-Casademunt A, Domingo-Sabat M, et al. Clinical tolerance to sagittal imbalance varies with age. Eur Spine J. 2014 23(Suppl 5):S469-96.
14. Glassman SD, Berven S, Bridwell K, et al. Correlation of radiographic parameters and clinical symptoms in adult scoliosis. Spine (Phila Pa 1976). 2005;30(6):682-8.
15. Glassman SD, Bridwell K, Dimar JR, et al. The impact of positive sagittal balance in adult spinal deformity. Spine (Phila Pa 1976). 2005;30(18):2024-9.
16. Simmons ED Jr, Simmons EH. Spinal stenosis with scoliosis. Spine (Phila Pa 1976). 1992;17(Suppl 6):S117-20.
17. Faldini C, Di Martino A, De Fine M, et al. Current classification systems for adult degenerative scoliosis. Musculoskelet Surg. 2013;97(1):1-8.
18. Schwab F, Bridwell K, Berven S, et al. A comprehensive clinical impact classification of Adult Scoliosis. Spinal Deformity Study Group Meeting; San Diego, CA; 2005.
19. Schwab F, Farcy JP, Bridwell K, et al. A clinical impact classification of scoliosis in the adult. Spine (Phila Pa 1976). 2006;31(18):2109-14.
20. Lowe T, Berven SH, Schwab FJ, et al. The SRS classification for adult spinal deformity: building on the King/Moe and Lenke classification systems. Spine (Phila Pa 1976). 2006;31(Suppl 19):S119-25.
21. Terran J, Schwab F, Shaffrey CI, et al. International Spine Study Group. The SRS-Schwab adult spinal deformity classification: assessment and clinical correlations based on a prospective operative and nonoperative cohort. Neurosurgery. 2013;73(4):559-68.
22. Everett CR, Patel RK. A systematic literature review of nonsurgical treatment in adult scoliosis. Spine (Phila Pa 1976). 2007;32(Suppl 19):S130-4.
23. Lafage V, Schwab F, Patel A, et al. Pelvic tilt and truncal inclination: two key radiographic parameters in the setting of adults with spinal deformity. Spine (Phila Pa 1976). 2009;34(17):E599-606.
24. Schwab F, Ungar B, Blondel B, et al. Scoliosis Research Society-Schwab adult spinal deformity classification: a validation study. Spine (Phila Pa 1976). 2012;37(12):1077-82.

25. Boissière L, Vital JM, Aunoble S, et al. Lumbo-pelvic related indexes: impact on adult spinal deformity surgery. Eur Spine J. 2015;24(6):1212-8.
26. Harimaya K, Lenke LG, Mishiro T, et al. Increasing lumbar lordosis of adult spinal deformity patients via intraoperative prone positioning. Spine (Phila Pa 1976). 2009;34(22):2406-12.
27. Akbarnia BA, Ogilvie JW, Hammerberg KW. Debate: degenerative scoliosis: to operate or not to operate. Spine (Phila Pa 1976). 2006;31(Suppl 19):S195-201.
28. Mok JM, Cloyd JM, Bradford DS, et al. Reoperation after primary fusion for adult spinal deformity: rate, reason, and timing. Spine (Phila Pa 1976). 2009;34(8):832-9.
29. Cho KJ, Suk SI, Park SR, et al. Complications in posterior fusion and instrumentation for degenerative lumbar scoliosis. Spine (Phila Pa 1976). 2007;32(20):2232-7.
30. Schairer W, Carrer A, Deviren V, et al. 90-Day Readmission Rate after Spine Fusion for Adult Deformity. 47th Annual Meeting of the Scoliosis Research Society. Chicago, IL, USA: The Scoliosis Research Society; 2001.
31. Bridwell KH, Glassman S, Horton W, et al. Does treatment (nonoperative and operative) improve the two-year quality of life in patients with adult symptomatic lumbar scoliosis: a prospective multicenter evidence-based medicine study. Spine (Phila Pa 1976). 2009;34(20):2171-8.
32. Glassman SD, Carreon LY, Shaffrey CI, et al. The costs and benefits of nonoperative management for adult scoliosis. Spine (Phila Pa 1976). 2010;35(5):578-82.
33. Li G, Passias P, Kozanek M, et al. Adult scoliosis in patients over sixty-five years of age: outcomes of operative versus nonoperative treatment at a minimum two-year follow-up. Spine (Phila Pa 1976). 2009;34(20):2165-70.
34. Glassman SD, Hamill CL, Bridwell KH, et al. The impact of perioperative complications on clinical outcome in adult deformity surgery. Spine (Phila Pa 1976). 2007;32(24):2764-70.
35. Bridwell KH, Baldus C, Berven S, et al. Changes in radiographic and clinical outcomes with primary treatment adult spinal deformity surgeries from two years to three- to five-years follow-up. Spine (Phila Pa 1976). 2010;35(20):1849-54.
36. Cho SK, Bridwell KH, Lenke LG, et al. Major complications in revision adult deformity surgery: risk factors and clinical outcomes with 2- to 7-year follow-up. Spine (Phila Pa 1976). 2012;37(6):489-500.
37. Smith JS, Shaffrey CI, Berven S, et al. Spinal Deformity Study Group. Improvement of back pain with operative and nonoperative treatment in adults with scoliosis. Neurosurgery. 2009;65(1):86-934.
38. Smith JS, Shaffrey CI, Glassman SD, et al. Risk-benefit assessment of surgery for adult scoliosis: an analysis based on patient age. Spine (Phila Pa 1976). 2011;36(10):817-24.
39. Glassman SD, Schwab FJ, Bridwell KH, et al. The selection of operative versus nonoperative treatment in patients with adult scoliosis. Spine (Phila Pa 1976). 2007;32(1):93-7.
40. Pekmezci M, Berven SH, Hu SS, et al. The factors that play a role in the decision-making process of adult deformity patients. Spine (Phila Pa 1976). 2009;34(8):813-7.
41. Fu KM, Bess S, Shaffrey CI, et al. International Spine Study Group. Patients with adult spinal deformity treated operatively report greater baseline pain and disability than patients treated nonoperatively; however, deformities differ between age groups. Spine (Phila Pa 1976). 2014;39(17):1401-7.
42. Matsumura A, Namikawa T, Terai H, et al. The influence of approach side on facet preservation in microscopic bilateral decompression via a unilateral approach for degenerative lumbar scoliosis. Clinical article. J Neurosurg Spine. 2010;13(6):758-65.
43. Liu W, Chen XS, Jia LS, et al. The clinical features and surgical treatment of degenerative lumbar scoliosis: a review of 112 patients. Orthop Surg. 2009;1(3):176-83.
44. Transfeldt EE, Topp R, Mehbod AA, et al. Surgical outcomes of decompression, decompression with limited fusion, and decompression with full curve fusion for degenerative scoliosis with radiculopathy. Spine (Phila Pa 1976). 2010;35(20):1872-5.
45. Kim YB, Lenke LG, Kim YJ, et al. The morbidity of an anterior thoracolumbar approach: adult spinal deformity patients with greater than five-year follow-up. Spine (Phila Pa 1976). 2009;34(8):822-6.
46. Crandall DG, Revella J. Transforaminal lumbar interbody fusion versus anterior lumbar interbody fusion as an adjunct to posterior instrumented correction of degenerative lumbar scoliosis: three year clinical and radiographic outcomes. Spine (Phila Pa 1976). 2009;34(20):2126-33.
47. Bergey DL, Villavicencio AT, Goldstein T, et al. Endoscopic lateral transpsoas approach to the lumbar spine. Spine (Phila Pa 1976). 2004;29(15):1681-8.
48. Mundis GM, Akbarnia BA, Phillips FM. Adult deformity correction through minimally invasive lateral approach techniques. Spine (Phila Pa 1976). 2010;35(Suppl 26):S312-21.
49. Gupta MC. Degenerative scoliosis. Options for surgical management. Orthop Clin North Am. 2003;34(2):269-79.
50. McPhee IB, Swanson CE. The surgical management of degenerative lumbar scoliosis. Posterior instrumentation alone versus two stage surgery. Bull Hosp Jt Dis. 1998;57(1):16-22.
51. Good CR, Lenke LG, Bridwell KH, et al. Can posterior-only surgery provide similar radiographic and clinical results as combined anterior (thoracotomy/thoracoabdominal)/posterior approaches for adult scoliosis? Spine (Phila Pa 1976). 2010;35(2):210-8.
52. Dakwar E, Cardona RF, Smith DA, et al. Early outcomes and safety of the minimally invasive, lateral retroperitoneal transpsoas approach for adult degenerative scoliosis. Neurosurg Focus. 2010;28(3):E8.
53. Wang MY, Mummaneni PV. Minimally invasive surgery for thoracolumbar spinal deformity: initial clinical experience with clinical and radiographic outcomes. Neurosurg Focus. 2010;28(3):E9.

54. Kim YJ, Bridwell KH, Lenke LG, et al. Pseudarthrosis in adult spinal deformity following multisegmental instrumentation and arthrodesis. J Bone Joint Surg Am. 2006;88(4):721-8.
55. Simmons ED. Surgical treatment of patients with lumbar spinal stenosis with associated scoliosis. Clin Orthop Relat Res. 2001;(384):45-53.
56. Kim YJ, Bridwell KH, Lenke LG, et al. Is the T9, T11, or L1 the more reliable proximal level after adult lumbar or lumbosacral instrumented fusion to L5 or S1? Spine (Phila Pa 1976). 2007;32(24):2653-61.
57. O'Shaughnessy BA, Bridwell KH, Lenke LG, et al. Does a long-fusion "T3-sacrum" portend a worse outcome than a short-fusion "T10-sacrum" in primary surgery for adult scoliosis? Spine (Phila Pa 1976). 2012;37(10):884-90.
58. Kim HJ, Boachie-Adjei O, Shaffrey CI, et al. International Spine Study Group. Upper thoracic versus lower thoracic upper instrumented vertebrae endpoints have similar outcomes and complications in adult scoliosis. Spine (Phila Pa 1976). 2014;39(13):E795-9.
59. Bridwell KH, Edwards CC 2nd, Lenke LG. The pros and cons to saving the L5-S1 motion segment in a long scoliosis fusion construct. Spine (Phila Pa 1976). 2003;28(20):S234-42.
60. Edwards CC 2nd, Bridwell KH, Patel A, et al. Thoracolumbar deformity arthrodesis to L5 in adults: the fate of the L5-S1 disc. Spine (Phila Pa 1976). 2003;28(18):2122-31.
61. Kuhns CA, Bridwell KH, Lenke LG, et al. Thoracolumbar deformity arthrodesis stopping at L5: fate of the L5-S1 disc, minimum 5-year follow-up. Spine (Phila Pa 1976). 2007;32(24):2771-6.
62. Alegre GM, Gupta MC, Bay BK, et al. S1 screw bending moment with posterior spinal instrumentation across the lumbosacral junction after unilateral iliac crest harvest. Spine (Phila Pa 1976). 2001;26(18):1950-5.
63. Han X, Zhu Y, Cui C, et al. A meta-analysis of circumferential fusion versus instrumented posterolateral fusion in the lumbar spine. Spine (Phila Pa 1976). 2009;34(17):E618-25.
64. Soegaard R, Bünger CE, Christiansen T, et al. Circumferential fusion is dominant over posterolateral fusion in a long-term perspective: cost-utility evaluation of a randomized controlled trial in severe, chronic low back pain. Spine (Phila Pa 1976). 2007;32(22):2405-14.
65. Wu CH, Wong CB, Chen LH, et al. Instrumented posterior lumbar interbody fusion for patients with degenerative lumbar scoliosis. J Spinal Disord Tech. 2008;21(5):310-5.
66. Li F, Chen Q, Chen W, et al. Posterior-only approach with selective segmental TLIF for degenerative lumbar scoliosis. J Spinal Disord Tech. 2011;24(5):308-12.
67. Burneikiene S, Nelson EL, Mason A, et al. Complications in patients undergoing combined transforaminal lumbar interbody fusion and posterior instrumentation with deformity correction for degenerative scoliosis and spinal stenosis. Surg Neurol Int. 2012;3:25.
68. Berjano P, Lamartina C. Far lateral approaches (XLIF) in adult scoliosis. Eur Spine J. 2013;22(Suppl 2):S242-53.
69. St Clair S, Tan JS, Lieberman I. Oblique lumbar interbody fixation: a biomechanical study in human spines. J Spinal Disord Tech. 2012;25(4):183-9.
70. Fujibayashi S, Hynes RA, Otsuki B, et al. Effect of indirect neural decompression through oblique lateral interbody fusion for degenerative lumbar disease. Spine (Phila Pa 1976). 2015;40(3):E175-82.
71. Boachie-Adjei O, Cho W, King AB. Axial lumbar interbody fusion (AxiaLIF) approach for adult scoliosis. Eur Spine J. 2013;22(Suppl 2):S225-31.
72. Schwab F, Blondel B, Chay E, et al. The comprehensive anatomical spinal osteotomy classification. Neurosurgery. 2014;74(1):112-20.
73. Chang KW, Cheng CW, Chen HC, et al. Closing-opening wedge osteotomy for the treatment of sagittal imbalance. Spine (Phila Pa 1976). 2008;33(13):1470-7.
74. Rose PS, Bridwell KH, Lenke LG, et al. Role of pelvic incidence, thoracic kyphosis, and patient factors on sagittal plane correction following pedicle subtraction osteotomy. Spine (Phila Pa 1976). 2009;34(8):785-91.
75. Hadjipavlou AG, Nicodemus CL, al-Hamdan FA, et al. Correlation of bone equivalent mineral density to pull-out resistance of triangulated pedicle screw construct. J Spinal Disord. 1997;10(1):12-9.
76. Kuklo TR, Lehman RA Jr. Effect of various tapping diameters on insertion of thoracic pedicle screws: a biomechanical analysis. Spine (Phila Pa 1976). 2003;28(18):2066-71.
77. Chiang CK, Wang YH, Yang CY, et al. Prophylactic vertebroplasty may reduce the risk of adjacent intact vertebra from fatigue injury: an ex vivo biomechanical study. Spine (Phila Pa 1976). 2009;34(4):356-64.
78. Scheufler KM, Cyron D, Dohmen H, et al. Less invasive surgical correction of adult degenerative scoliosis. Part II: Complications and clinical outcome. Neurosurgery. 2010;67(6):1609-21.
79. Bach K, Ahmadian A, Deukmedjian A, et al. Minimally invasive surgical techniques in adult degenerative spinal deformity: a systematic review. Clin Orthop Relat Res. 2014;472(6):1749-61.
80. Mummaneni PV, Tu TH, Ziewacz JE, et al. The role of minimally invasive techniques in the treatment of adult spinal deformity. Neurosurg Clin N Am. 2013;24(2):231-48.
81. Smith JS, Saulle D, Chen CJ, et al. Rates and causes of mortality associated with spine surgery based on 108,419 procedures: a review of the Scoliosis Research Society Morbidity and Mortality Database. Spine (Phila Pa 1976). 2012;37(23): 1975-82.
82. Sansur CA, Smith JS, Coe JD, et al. Scoliosis research society morbidity and mortality of adult scoliosis surgery. Spine (Phila Pa 1976). 2011;36(9):E593-7.
83. Charosky S, Guigui P, Blamoutier A, et al. Study Group on Scoliosis. Complications and risk factors of primary adult scoliosis surgery: a multicenter study of 306 patients. Spine (Phila Pa 1976). 2012;37(8):693-700.

84. Bradford DS, Tay BK, Hu SS. Adult scoliosis: surgical indications, operative management, complications, and outcomes. Spine (Phila Pa 1976). 1999;24(24):2617-29.
85. Pateder DB, Kostuik JP. Lumbar nerve root palsy after adult spinal deformity surgery. Spine (Phila Pa 1976). 2005;30(14):1632-6.
86. DeWald CJ, Stanley T. Instrumentation-related complications of multilevel fusions for adult spinal deformity patients over age 65: surgical considerations and treatment options in patients with poor bone quality. Spine (Phila Pa 1976). 2006;31(Suppl 19):S144-51.
87. O'Leary PT, Bridwell KH, Lenke LG, et al. Risk factors and outcomes for catastrophic failures at the top of long pedicle screw constructs: a matched cohort analysis performed at a single center. Spine (Phila Pa 1976). 2009;34(20):2134-9.
88. Watanabe K, Lenke LG, Bridwell KH, et al. Proximal junctional vertebral fracture in adults after spinal deformity surgery using pedicle screw constructs: analysis of morphological features. Spine (Phila Pa 1976). 2010;35(2):138-45.
89. Yagi M, King AB, Boachie-Adjei O. Incidence, risk factors, and natural course of proximal junctional kyphosis: surgical outcomes review of adult idiopathic scoliosis. Minimum 5 years of follow-up. Spine (Phila Pa 1976). 2012;37(17):1479-89.
90. Daubs MD, Lenke LG, Cheh G, et al. Adult spinal deformity surgery: complications and outcomes in patients over age 60. Spine (Phila Pa 1976). 2007;32(20):2238-44.
91. Carreon LY, Puno RM, Dimar JR 2nd, et al. Perioperative complications of posterior lumbar decompression and arthrodesis in older adults. J Bone Joint Surg Am. 2003; 85(11):2089-92.
92. Zhu F, Bao H, Liu Z, et al. Unanticipated revision surgery in adult spinal deformity: an experience with 815 cases at one institution. Spine (Phila Pa 1976). 2014;39(26 Spec No.):B36-44.
93. Kelly MP, Lenke LG, Bridwell KH, et al. Fate of the adult revision spinal deformity patient: a single institution experience. Spine (Phila Pa 1976). 2013;38(19):E1196-200.
94. Kleinstueck FS, Fekete TF, Jeszenszky D, et al. Adult degenerative scoliosis: comparison of patient-rated outcome after three different surgical treatments. Eur Spine J. 2016; 25(8):2649-56.
95. Paulus MC, Kalantar SB, Radcliff K. Cost and value of spinal deformity surgery. Spine (Phila Pa 1976). 2014;39(5):388-93.
96. McCarthy I, O'Brien M, Ames C, et al. International Spine Study Group. Incremental cost-effectiveness of adult spinal deformity surgery: observed quality-adjusted life years with surgery compared with predicted quality-adjusted life years without surgery. Neurosurg Focus. 2014;36(5):E3.
97. Terran J, McHugh BJ, Fischer CR, et al. Surgical treatment for adult spinal deformity: projected cost effectiveness at 5-year follow-up. Ochsner J. 2014;14(1):14-22.

CHAPTER 41 Revision Lumbar Surgery

Michael J Lee, Jens R Chapman

INTRODUCTION

Revision lumbar surgery carries with it additional diagnostic challenge, technical requirements, greater morbidity, poorer clinical outcomes, and a higher financial burden. The rate of lumbar surgery has risen exponentially over the past decade with financial cost increases of over 500%. There are expected concordant increases in reoperations procedures with meta-analysis studies showing that 10–23% of patients require reoperation procedures in 5 years.[1] Reoperation surgery entails revision surgery at the prior surgical site and surgery at a level different from the prior surgical site, such as adjacent segment pathology.

Indications for revision lumbar surgery are largely the same as indication for primary lumbar surgery, with the exception of nonunion. The goals of revision lumbar surgery are—(1) decompression of neurocompressive pathology, (2) stabilization of unstable segments, ideally in form of a solid fusion, and (3) correction of deformity.

REASONS FOR REVISION LUMBAR SURGERY

The indication for revision lumbar surgery generally falls into the following categories—(1) recurrence of underlying pathology, (2) the development of postoperative instability, (3) the development of postoperative deformity, (4) failure of the index surgery, and (5) adjacent segment pathology.

Recurrence of Underlying Pathology

The most common recurrence of spinal pathology necessitating revision surgery is lumbar herniated nucleus pulposus (HNP) (Figs. 1A and B). Rates of recurrent disk herniation of around 10% have been reported with rates of repeat surgery ranging from 5% to 10%.[2,3] While clinical outcomes for revision microdiscectomy have been

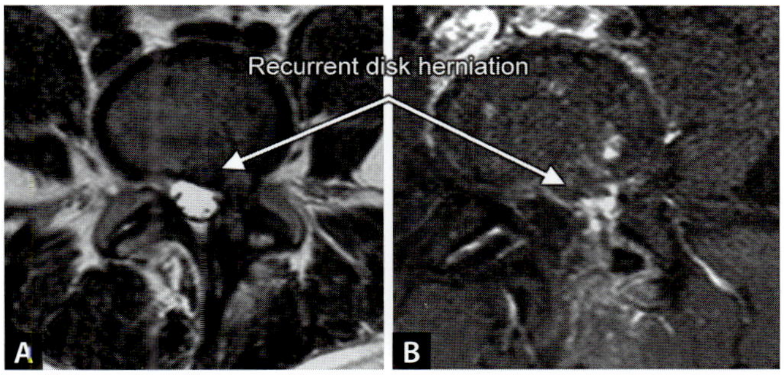

Figs. 1A and B: Recurrent herniated nucleus pulposus (HNP). (A) T2 axial image demonstrating left-sided paracentral HNP; (B) T1 postcontrast axial image demonstrating the present scar tissue at the laminotomy site as well as the left-sided paracentral HNP.

reported to be comparable to primary microdiscectomy, a higher likelihood of complication has been associated with the revision procedure.[4,5]

The recurrence of lumbar stenosis without instability has been known to occur (Figs. 2A and B), though less commonly than recurrent disk herniation. This is somewhat intuitive as HNP is more likely to be an acute process whereas the development of spondylotic stenosis can be a gradual degenerative process. The incidence of recurrent lumbar stenosis after laminectomy is poorly defined in the literature.

Development of Postoperative Instability

Lumbar stenosis was initially described by Verbiest in 1954.[6] Surgical treatment in that era often entailed radical laminectomy or the so-called "Christmas Tree Laminectomy." The radical laminectomy entailed the complete resection of the spinous process, lamina, pars, and bilateral facets. While this strategy was effective in

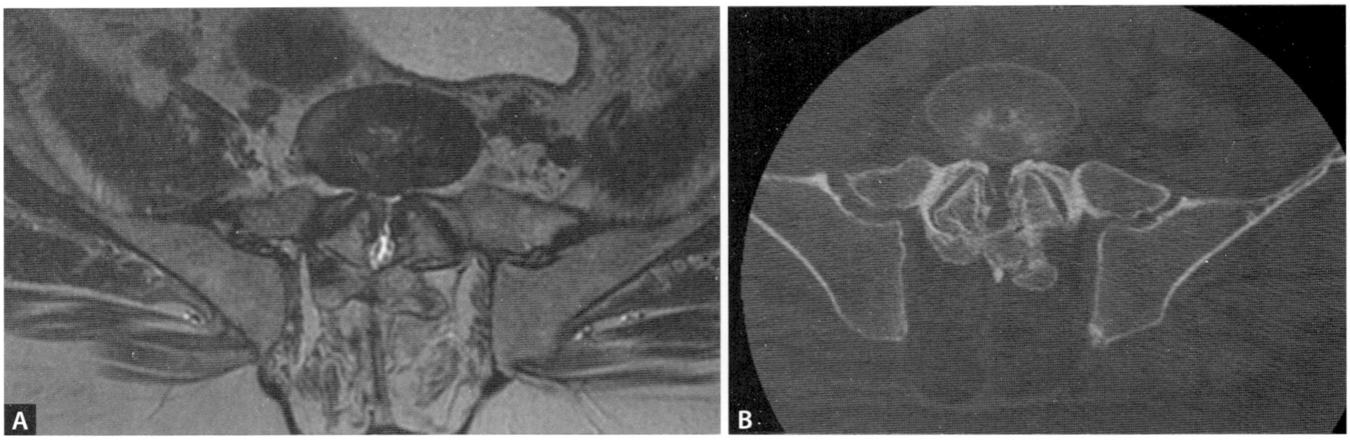

Figs. 2A and B: Recurrent lumbar stenosis after prior laminectomy. (A) Magnetic resonance imaging T2 axial image demonstrating significant stenosis; (B) Computed tomography axial image desmontrated bony overgrowth.

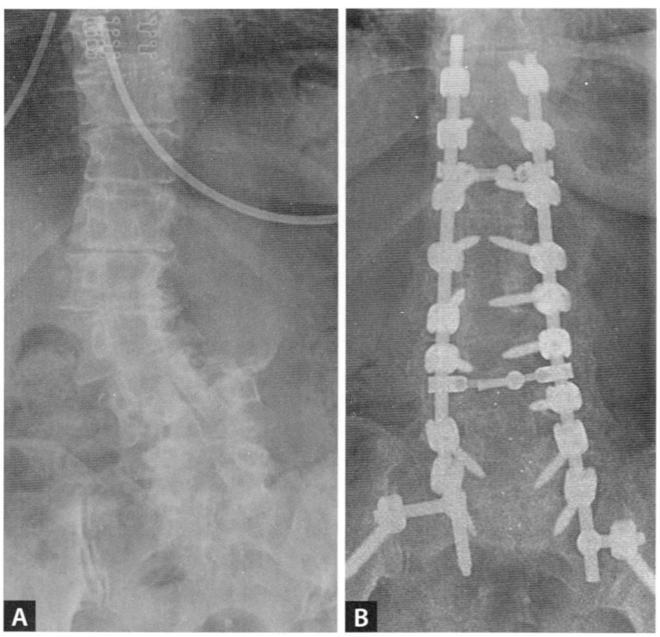

Figs. 3A and B: (A) Post-radical laminectomy instability with significant deformity and lateral listhesis; (B) Stabilization of the same patient with thoracic-lumbar-pelvic instrumented arthrodesis.

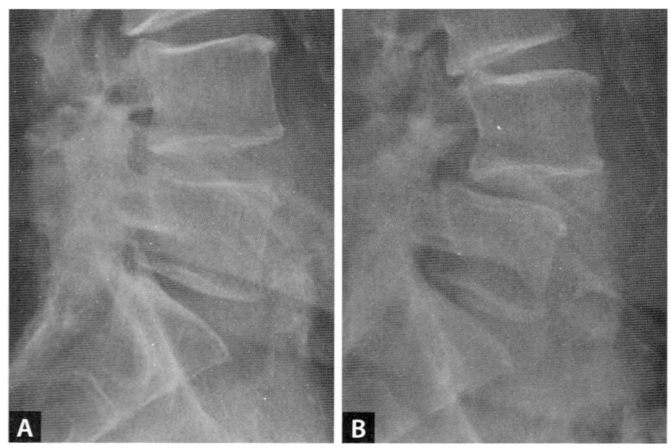

Figs. 4A and B: (A) Pre- and (B) postoperative lateral X-ray images of the lumbar spine after facet-sparing laminectomy demonstrating the development of the spondylolisthesis after the surgery.

treating neurocompressive pathology, at least in the short term, reports of postoperative instability and resultant nerve compression and mechanical pain became more frequent[7-9] (Figs. 3A and B).

In 1990, Abumi et al. published their biomechanical study entitled "Biomechanical evaluation of Lumbar Spinal Stability after graded facetectomies." From this study it has long been taught that maintenance of at least 50% of each facet is required to maintain stability.[10] However, even in the context of an appropriately done facet sparing laminectomy maintaining at least 50% of the facet and sufficient pars, the development of instability may still occur as frequently as 8–31% of the time[11,12] (Figs. 4A and B). While a post-facet sparing laminectomy spondylolisthesis does not universally result in a revision lumbar surgery, these patients are at high risk for requiring revision laminectomy and arthrodesis for stabilization.

Development of Postoperative Deformity

The development of kyphosis or a positive sagittal balance has been known to occur either through or adjacent to

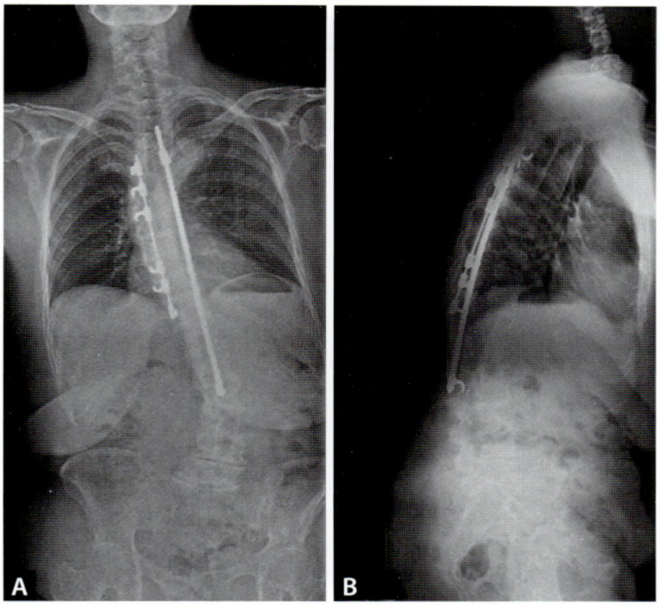

Figs. 5A and B: (A) Anteroposterior and (B) Lateral full spine standing X-rays in a patient who underwent Harrington rod fusion 30 years prior with a resultant flatback syndrome and severe positive sagittal balance.

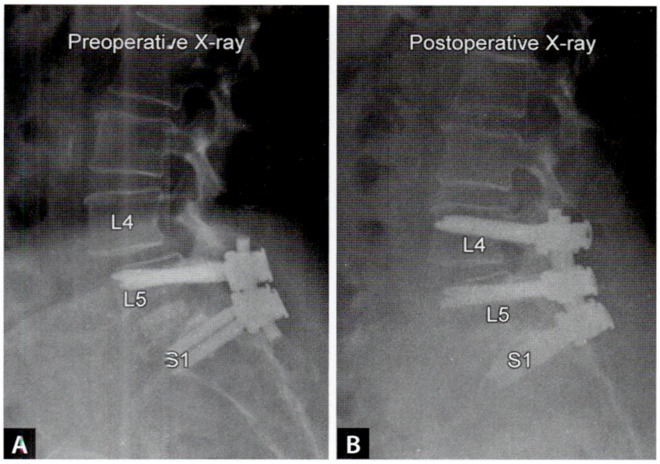

Figs. 6A and B: (A) Lateral X-ray of a patient with a previous L5–S1 posterior lateral and interbody fusion who developed adjecent segment pathology and spondylolisthesis at L45; (B) Postoperative lateral X-ray of the same patient treated with L45 laminectomy and extention of fusion to L4.

a fusion construct. Perhaps the most notable example is the development of a flatback syndrome years after the placement of Harrington rods for the treatment of scoliosis. While these rods may have been effective in the treatment of coronal deformity, the lack of lordosis in the instrumentation is now understood to have contributed to the development of positive sagittal balance (Figs. 5A and B). Often these patients may require extension of fusion with restoration of sagittal balance through osteotomy. Positive sagittal balance may occur also in the setting of subsidence through a fusion construct, or nonunion. While a single lumbar segment fused in neutral may not necessarily result in global kyphosis or positive sagittal balance, multiple lumbar levels fused without maintenance of lordosis can certainly increase the likelihood of the development of positive sagittal balance.

Failure of the Index Surgery

The large majority of lumbar spine surgeries entail decompression of compressed neural elements, or arthrodesis for stabilization. When the goals of surgery are not achieved, this may necessitate revision surgery. In the case of microdiscectomy or lumbar laminectomy, a retained disk fragment or residual lumbar stenosis causing symptoms may necessitate an early revision laminectomy or microdiscectomy procedure. Failure of fusion is also a notable cause of reoperation. However, whereas failure of neurodecompression is generally noted in the early postoperative period, failure of fusion may be observed in the perioperative period or several years after the index procedure. Hardware failure in the perioperative period may manifest as screw pullout or disengagement, whereas nonunion often manifests with screw loosening or hardware fracture, loosening, disengagement or subsidence into surrounding bone structures. In the event of a nonunion, the possibility of infection should be considered and this may alter revision strategy.

Reoperation at the index level can also be done for perioperative complication such as hematoma formation, surgical site infection, errant hardware placement, or persistent cerebrospinal fluid (CSF) leak. However, these fall outside the scope of this chapter.

Adjacent Segment Pathology

Adjacent segment pathology (ASP) of the lumbar spine requiring reoperation has been reported by Ghiselli and others to occur at a rate of 16.5% within 5 years and 36.1% within 10 years[13] (Figs. 6A and B). Since this report in 2004, multiple other studies have reported similar rates of reoperation. It is not yet known if the etiology of ASP is the fusion itself, or a natural progression of degenerative disease that would have occurred in absence of a fusion, or a combination of the two.[14] Regardless of the true etiology of ASP, it has been observed to occur. Patients undergoing arthrodesis should be counseled on the possible need for reoperation.

While the focus reoperation for ASP is not technically revision surgery as the adjacent level has theoretically not been treated surgically, accounting for and incorporating the prior fusion and decompression does add elements of revision surgery. The presence of the prior fusion may affect surgical approach and strategy.

RISKS OF REVISION LUMBAR SURGERY

While outcomes of revision lumbar surgery are arguably comparable to outcomes of primary surgery, the risks of complication are significantly higher with revision surgery. Altered anatomy, extensive scar tissue, previous fusion mass, and bony overgrowth—all contribute to the complexity of revision lumbar surgery. Longer operating times, higher blood loss, and longer hospital stays can be expected in revision lumbar procedures.[15] Inherent to greater operating room times and blood loss are higher likelihood of medical complications and surgical site infections.

Dural Tear

In a revision lumbar laminectomy, the process of separating scar tissue from native dura can be challenging. With scar tissue adherent to the dura, even in the most careful of all surgeries, a dural tear may still occur. Several studies have reported the increased likelihood of dural tear in revision surgery. In our multivariate analysis, we reported that the likelihood of dural tear in revision surgery was almost two-and-half times that of primary surgery (Relative Risk ratio, RR = 2.21).[16] Patients undergoing revision laminectomy should be counseled on the increased likelihood of unintended durotomy.

Infection

Numerous studies have examined risk factors for surgical site infection recently. Kurtz et al. reported that revision status to be significantly associated with surgical site infection using the Medicare database.[17] Conversely, much of the current literature does not statistically link surgical site infection and revision surgery after multivariate analysis,[18-27] however, this is likely to be a result of insufficient power. Revision surgery continues to be regarded as a risk factor for surgical site infection by many surgeons. In our own analysis of risk factors for surgical site infection, revision status was significantly associated with infection in our univariate analysis, but not in our multivariate analysis. This observation was felt to be secondary to insufficient power to demonstrate the relationship after multivariate analysis, despite more than 1,500 patients examined.[19] The prolonged OR times, increased blood loss, and increased need for transfusion associated with revision surgery—all indirectly suggest that revision may be associated with a higher risk of infection. In our own practices, we continue to regard revision status as a risk factor for surgical site infection.

Medical Complication

As revision surgery is inherently more complex, one can expect a greater blood loss, longer operating time and longer anesthetic exposure. As such, the risks innate to surgery are intuitively likely to be amplified with revision procedures. We previously reported that revision surgery was a significant risk factor for cardiac, gastrointestinal, hematological, and neurological medical complications in our univariate analysis.[28] While this was not born out in our multivariate analysis, this was likely a function of insufficient power as these conclusions are somewhat intuitive. Although the link between revision surgery and higher likelihood of medical complication may not be robustly supported in the literature (after multivariate analysis), due to its association with longer OR times and greater blood loss, we continue to regard revision status as a risk factor for medical complication.

OUTCOME OF REVISION LUMBAR SURGERY

Revision microdiscectomy outcomes, in more recent literature, generally have been reported to comparable to primary microdiscectomy, however, revision microdiscectomy has been associated with longer OR times and higher complications rates.[4,5,29] Morgan-Hough et al. reported an 8.7% incidence of complication in their primary microdiscectomy group and a 19.1% complication rate in the revision microdiscectomy group.[4] Dural tear was observed in 5.4% of primary microdiscectomies whereas they were observed in 14.3% of revision surgeries.

Outcomes of revision lumbar surgery for recurrent stenosis vary within the literature. Djurasovic et al.

reported health related quality-of-life (HRQoL) scores in patients undergoing revision surgery after prior decompression.[30] They reported that post decompression patients had a moderate improvement in HRQoL scores. In their study, 46% of the revision fusion patients achieved minimally important clinical difference (MICD) in the short form-36 (SF-36) physical component score (PCS) at 2-year follow-up. Only 49% of these patients achieved a minimum clinically important difference (MCID) in Oswestry Disability Index (ODI) at 2-year follow-up. However Adogwa et al. reported significant improvement in HRQoL scores in revision surgery for recurrent lumbar stenosis.

Revision lumbar spine fusion outcomes also vary in the literature and in some part have likely been affected by technological advances. In 1992, Kim and Michelson reported revision fusion of pseudarthrosis to have a failure rate as high as 45%.[31] It should be noted that the technique utilized appears to be largely a noninstrumented revision posterior lateral arthrodesis with corset immobilization. In 2011, Djurasovic et al. reported that revision lumbar fusion yielded only modest improvement in HRQoL scores. In their study, only 24% of the revision fusion patients achieved MICD in the SF-36 PCS score at 2-year follow-up. Only 29% of these patients achieved MCID in ODI at 2-year follow-up.[30] Similar to the Kim study, it should be noted that posterior lateral fusion was the technique of choice in the Djurasovic study. Albert et al. reported on 37 patients with lumbar nonunion treated with a combined anterior and posterior approach, which led to a 90% fusion rate and 65% functional improvement rate.[32] Similarly, Adogwa et al. reviewed 2 years HRQoL scores on patients undergoing revision lumbar fusion and concluded revision fusion to be viable treatment option for nonunion.[33] Conversely, Geisler et al. reported outcomes for revision anterior lumbar interbody fusion (ALIF) to be significantly lower than those without revisions surgery.

Outcomes for reoperation for ASP were recently assessed in a systematic review, which reported only eight case-series studies examining outcomes for the treatment of ASP.[34] While it may be intuitive to conclude that outcomes for reoperation for ASP mimic those of primary surgery, this hypothesis is only weakly supported with the literature.

While further study is always ideal and specifically further study of comparative effectiveness of revision lumbar surgery compared to nonsurgical treatment is needed, contemporary studies suggest that revision surgery after decompression or fusion can have improved HRQoL scores.[35]

SURGICAL STRATEGIES FOR REVISION LUMBAR SURGERY

As with any revision surgery, it is advisable to proceed from "known anatomy" to "unknown anatomy". This may entail extending the previous incision to identify an unaltered landmark. Identification and understanding bony anatomy is particularly important during revision surgery and a preoperative computed tomography (CT) scan is likely to be of benefit if the altered anatomy is not clearly understood on meganetic resonance imaging (MRI) or plain films.

Revision Decompression

Extensive study of advanced imaging is crucial prior to revision laminectomy or microdiscectomy. The obvious concern in revision laminectomy is iatrogenic nerve injury and thus it is of paramount importance to understand the location of the thecal sac relative to all surrounding posterior vertebral structures. The key to safe exposure if a revision surgery is a full understanding of the bony elements of the posterior column, and for this a preoperative CT scan can be very helpful. One should be aware of all possible defects within the residual bony column, such as pars defects, or complete facetectomies. Exposure of an adjacent virgin level can provide a reference of depth of the spinal column relative to the skin. It can also provide a starting point for exposure of posterior bony elements of the spinal column.

When exposure has been obtained and the laminectomy site is directly visible with a layer of scar directly over it, the surgeon may access the spinal canal in a number of ways.

- After identification of the bone edge-laminectomy junction, separation of the scar/dura off the medial border of the bony wall with micro-curette sharp dissection can be done to create a plane for additional lateral recess decompression. As the dura may be adherent to the medial bony wall, inadvertent durotomy may occur. Once this plane is defined, additional lateral recess decompression can allow for more space and maneuverability.
- Alternatively, a "virgin" plane may be created by creating a longitudinal trough with a high-speed burr. This trough is made lateral to the previously defined

bone edge-laminectomy junction and all the way down to the canal. When the anterior cortex is penetrated, this trough can be completed either with the burr, or with angled micro-curettes or small Kerrison Rongeurs. Once this trough has been completed, additional lateral recess decompression can be done through this trough. Resection of the medial bony fragment should be done carefully as this may be adherent to underlying dura.

As the canal is accessed, identification of the pedicle is the key for orientation. Intraoperative imaging can also assist in orientation. Mobilization of the dura from scar tissue can be time-consuming and challenging as there is a clear risk of CSF egress.

In the course of revision decompression, additional lateral recess and facet resection will likely be required. If substantial facet resection and resultant iatrogenic instability is anticipated, concurrent arthrodesis is recommended. In cases where it is unclear how much facet will need to be resected to adequately decompress the neural structures, the surgeon should prepare for the possibility of concurrent arthrodesis.

Revision Arthrodesis

Arthrodesis is a function of biology, carpentry, and mechanical stability. In the setting of nonunion, the reason for the failure to fuse should be specifically addressed in the revision. The radiographic presence of hardware failure strongly indicates a high likelihood of failure of fusion. In the absence of bony fusion, all hardware is likely to fail with enough time and loading cycles. Lucency around fixation points or frank pullout of screws or hooks indicates insufficient bony purchase, motion of the spinal column, and a high likelihood of nonunion. Hardware failure (fractured screws, rods, and cross-connectors) as well as subsidence into the adjacent vertebrae can occur even years after an arthrodesis if sufficient bony fusion has not consolidated.

Strategies for revision arthrodesis depend largely on what technique previously failed. If a nonunion occurs in an uninstrumented arthrodesis, the addition of mechanical stability through instrumentation and appropriate bone graft material may be sufficient. Identifying virgin bony surfaces for fusion can decrease the difficulty of the revision arthrodesis. If a prior posterior lateral fusion failed, then anterior interbody fusion may be considered and vice versa. For any revision fusion, a 360° fusion should be strongly considered to maximize the bony surface area for fusion potential.

Meticulous exposure and preparation of bony surfaces is required for successful fusion. Overlying or interposing soft tissue or scar should be removed and bony surface area exposure should be maximized. For posterior lateral fusion, in addition to adequate exposure of the transverse processes, pars, facets, and prior fusion mass, the creation of a posterior lateral gutter for bone graft placement is essential. Extensive decortication of these structures down to bleeding subcortical bone is recommended to optimize the likelihood of fusion. If pedicle screws are placed prior to bone graft placement, the heads of the screws can prevent optimal placement of bone graft material over decorticated bony structures. It is the author's preference to impact bone graft material over the decorticated posterior lateral structures and in the gutter prior to pedicle screw placement (through previously cannulated pedicles) so as to maximize the contact of bone graft material to decorticated native bone structures. For interbody fusion extensive diskectomy and endplate preparation are recommended.

Optimal fixation should be achieved. In the setting of screw fixation failure, larger and longer pedicle screws may be needed to achieve adequate fixation. In osteoporotic bone, a number of fixation augmentation techniques are being investigated including cement augmentation and expandable screws.

Instrumentation provides temporary mechanical stability; however, a sufficient biological healing must be mounted to achieve successful bony fusion. Autologous iliac crest bone graft remains the gold standard biological substrate to achieve fusion; however, allograft, bone graft substitute materials, and supplemental materials have been gaining increasing use. Bone morphogenetic protein 2 (BMP-2) is a potent bone-forming agent; however, has been the topic of much discussion recently regarding safety profile. BMP-2 has been suggested in the literature to be associated with inflammation, ectopic bone formation, retrograde ejaculation, and possible association with the development of neoplasia, although this warning has been largely refuted by longer term follow-up.[36] To date, BMP-2 has been Food and Drug Administration (FDA) approved for the use in an ALIF and any other use of this is considered "off label".

The author's preference of bone graft material for revision arthrodesis is autologous iliac crest bone graft when available. If not available, BMP-2 is often recommended for revision arthrodesis. An extensive discussion of the risks and benefits of BMP-2 and the aforementioned complications, is held with the patient preoperatively, and the off label use of BMP-2 is specifically consented for.

Controllable patient factors should be optimized preoperatively as well. If the patient is a smoker, it is our practice to have patients quit nicotine use and this is confirmed with serial urine cotinine tests. Optimization of nutrition is also encouraged to improve general healing.

Adjacent Segment Pathology

Surgical strategies for the treatment of ASP depend on the nature of the ASP and the prior approach used, and the goals of the reoperation surgery. In general, strategies favor avoidance of scar tissue if possible while satisfactorily achieving the goals of surgery (decompression and/or arthrodesis). For example, if a patient underwent a prior L5–S1 anterior lumbar interbody fusion (ALIF) and later develops ASP at L4-5, it may be preferable to approach L4-5 posteriorly to access virgin tissue and avoid the risks of a revision anterior approach.

It is also essential to understand the extent of the prior surgery and where one may or may not encounter scar tissue. Consider a patient with a prior L4-5 laminectomy and fusion and developed an L3-4 spondylolisthesis with stenosis. If the prior L4 level was partially laminectomized and the superior half of the L4 lamina was retained, then decompression of the cephalad L3-4 level should theoretically encounter minimal scar tissue over the dura. However, if in the prior surgery, the entire L4 lamina was resected, then in the course of the L3-4 exposure, scar tissue is likely to be encountered, and a more difficult decompression can be anticipated.

CONCLUSION

Though the goals of revision lumbar surgery are no different than the goals of primary lumbar surgery, revision surgery is undoubtedly technically more difficult and with higher likelihood of complication. Outcomes of revision surgery vary for a spectrum of reasons, but good clinical outcome after revision decompression and revision arthrodesis have been reported. A detailed understanding of preoperative anatomy, extensive preoperative counseling of risks and benefits and expectation to the patient are essential with revision lumbar spine surgery.

REFERENCES

1. Malter AD, McNeney B, Loeser JD, et al. 5-year reoperation rates after different types of lumbar spine surgery. Spine (Phila Pa 1976). 1998;23(7):814-20.
2. Carragee EJ, Han MY, Yang B, et al. Activity restrictions after posterior lumbar discectomy. A prospective study of outcomes in 152 cases with no postoperative restrictions. Spine (Phila Pa 1976). 1999;24(22):2346-51.
3. McGirt MJ, Eustacchio S, Varga P, et al. A prospective cohort study of close interval computed tomography and magnetic resonance imaging after primary lumbar discectomy: factors associated with recurrent disk herniation and disk height loss. Spine (Phila Pa 1976). 2009;34(19):2044-51.
4. Morgan-Hough CV, Jones PW, Eisenstein SM. Primary and revision lumbar discectomy. A 16-year review from one center. J Bone Joint Surg Br. 2003;85(6):871-4.
5. Papadopoulos EC, Girardi FP, Sandhu HS, et al. Outcome of revision discectomies following recurrent lumbar disk herniation. Spine (Phila Pa 1976). 2006;31(13):1473-6.
6. Verbiest H. A radicular syndrome from developmental narrowing of the lumbar vertebral canal. J Bone Joint Surg Br. 1954;36-B(2):230-7.
7. Natelson SE. The injudicious laminectomy. Spine (Phila Pa 1976). 1986;11(9):966-9.
8. Johnsson KE, Redlund-Johnell I, Udén A, et al. Preoperative and postoperative instability in lumbar spinal stenosis. Spine (Phila Pa 1976). 1989;14(6):591-3.
9. Lee CK. Lumbar spinal instability (olisthesis) after extensive posterior spinal decompression. Spine (Phila Pa 1976). 1983;8(4):429-33.
10. Abumi K, Panjabi MM, Kramer KM, et al. Biomechanical evaluation of lumbar spinal stability after graded facetectomies. Spine (Phila Pa 1976). 1990;15(11):1142-7.
11. Fox MW, Onofrio BM, Onofrio BM, et al. Clinical outcomes and radiological instability following decompressive lumbar laminectomy for degenerative spinal stenosis: a comparison of patients undergoing concomitant arthrodesis versus decompression alone. J Neurosurg. 1996;85(5):793-802.
12. Fu YS, Zeng BF, Xu JG. Long-term outcomes of two different decompressive techniques for lumbar spinal stenosis. Spine (Phila Pa 1976). 2008;33(5):514-8.
13. Ghiselli G, Wang JC, Bhatia NN, et al. Adjacent segment degeneration in the lumbar spine. J Bone Joint Surg Am. 2004;86(7):1497-503.
14. Lee MJ, Dettori JR, Standaert CJ, et al. The natural history of degeneration of the lumbar and cervical spines: a systematic review. Spine (Phila Pa 1976). 2012;37(Suppl 22):S18-30.

CHAPTER 41

15. Zheng F, Cammisa FP Jr, Sandhu HS, et al. Factors predicting hospital stay, operative time, blood loss, and transfusion in patients undergoing revision posterior lumbar spine decompression, fusion, and segmental instrumentation. Spine (Phila Pa 1976). 2002;27(8):818-24.
16. Baker GA, Cizik AM, Bransford RJ, et al. Risk factors for unintended durotomy during spine surgery: a multivariate analysis. Spine J. 2012;12(2):121-6.
17. Kurtz SM, Lau E, Ong KL, et al. Infection risk for primary and revision instrumented lumbar spine fusion in the Medicare population. J Neurosurg Spine. 2012;17(4):342-7.
18. Abdul-Jabbar A, Takemoto S, Weber MH, et al. Surgical site infection in spinal surgery: description of surgical and patient-based risk factors for postoperative infection using administrative claims data. Spine (Phila Pa 1976). 2012;37(15):1340-5.
19. Cizik AM, Lee MJ, Martin BI, et al. Using the spine surgical invasiveness index to identify risk of surgical site infection: a multivariate analysis. J Bone Joint Surg Am. 2012;94(4):335-42.
20. Kang BU, Lee SH, Ahn Y, et al. Surgical site infection in spinal surgery: detection and management based on serial C-reactive protein measurements. J Neurosurg Spine. 2010;13(2):158-64.
21. Lonjon G, Dauzac C, Fourniols E, et al. Early surgical site infections in adult spinal trauma: a prospective, multicenter study of infection rates and risk factors. Orthop Traumatol Surg Res. 2012;98(7):788-94.
22. Olsen MA, Mayfield J, Lauryssen C, et al. Risk factors for surgical site infection in spinal surgery. J Neurosurg. 2003;98(Suppl 2):149-55.
23. Olsen MA, Nepple JJ, Riew KD. Risk factors for surgical site infection following orthopaedic spinal operations. J Bone Joint Surg Am. 2008;90(1):62-9.
24. Pull ter Gunne AF, Hosman AJ, Cohen DB, et al. A methodological systematic review on surgical site infections following spinal surgery: part 1: risk factors. Spine (Phila Pa 1976). 2012;37(24):2017-33.
25. Pull ter Gunne AF, van Laarhoven CJ, Cohen DB. Incidence of surgical site infection following adult spinal deformity surgery: an analysis of patient risk. Eur Spine J. 2010;19(6): 982-8.
26. Schwarzkopf R, Chung C, Park JJ, et al. Effects of perioperative blood product use on surgical site infection following thoracic and lumbar spinal surgery. Spine (Phila Pa 1976). 2010;35(3):340-6.
27. Watanabe M, Sakai D, Matsuyama D, et al. Risk factors for surgical site infection following spine surgery: efficacy of intraoperative saline irrigation. J Neurosurg Spine. 2010; 12(5):540-6.
28. Lee MJ, Hacquebord J, Varshney A, et al. Risk factors for medical complication after lumbar spine surgery: a multivariate analysis of 767 patients. Spine (Phila Pa 1976). 2011;36(21):1801-6.
29. Suk KS, Lee HM, Moon SH, et al. Recurrent lumbar disk herniation: results of operative management. Spine (Phila Pa 1976). 2001;26(6):672-6.
30. Djurasovic M, Glassman SD, Howard JM, et al. Health-related quality of life improvements in patients undergoing lumbar spinal fusion as a revision surgery. Spine (Phila Pa 1976). 2011;36(4):269-76.
31. Kim SS, Michelsen CB. Revision surgery for failed back surgery syndrome. Spine (Phila Pa 1976). 1992;17(8):957-60.
32. Albert TJ, Pinto M, Denis F. Management of symptomatic lumbar pseudarthrosis with anteroposterior fusion. A functional and radiographic outcome study. Spine (Phila Pa 1976). 2000;25(1):123-9;discussion 130.
33. Adogwa O, Carr RK, Kudyba K, et al. Revision lumbar surgery in elderly patients with symptomatic pseudarthrosis, adjacent-segment disease, or same-level recurrent stenosis. Part 1. Two-year outcomes and clinical efficacy: clinical article. J Neurosurg Spine. 2013;18(2):139-46.
34. Chou D, Dekutoski M, Hermsmeyer J, et al. The treatment of lumbar adjacent segment pathology after a previous lumbar surgery: a systematic review. Spine (Phila Pa 1976). 2012;37 (Suppl 22):S180-8.
35. Adogwa O, Parker SL, Shau D, et al. Long-term outcomes of revision fusion for lumbar pseudarthrosis: clinical article. J Neurosurg Spine. 2011;15(4):393-8.
36. Dettori JR, Chapman JR, DeVine JG, et al. Longer follow-up continues to reveal no increased risk of cancer with the use of recombinant human bone morphogenetic protein in spine fusion. Spine J. 2019 May 17. pii: S1529-9430(19)30186-X. doi: 10.1016/j.spinee.2019.05.005. [Epub ahead of print] PubMed PMID: 31108234.

CHAPTER 42

Trauma of the Thoracolumbar Junction, Lumbar, and Sacral Spine

George Rymarczuk, Geoffrey Stricsek, Kevin Hines, James S Harrop

LUMBAR TRAUMA

There have been numerous schemes and nomenclature used to define spinal trauma. The AOSpine Thoracolumbar Injury Classification schema represents the culmination of a more than 80-year journey to streamline and simplify the manner in which we convey the pertinent aspects of spinal injury patterns. While perhaps not as disparate and overlapping as the schemes that have previously been devised for application to the cervical spine and occipitocervical junction, the history of nomenclature of injuries to the thoracolumbar spine is nonetheless long and circuitous, with refinements introduced gradually as our knowledge of spinal biomechanics increased.[1] This process was facilitated in no small part by the technological improvements in radiology that resulted in widespread availability and use of first computed tomography (CT) and subsequently magnetic resonance imaging (MRI).

Watson-Jones' initial schema in 1938[2] was based on clinical evaluations and morphology as assessed by plain radiography alone. Gradually over the ensuing decades, notions of the relative "stability" or "instability" of fracture patterns began to enter the lexicon, the importance of the posterior elements and capsuloligamentous complex was recognized, and the spine began to be viewed as consisting of various "columns", each of which had a specific biomechanical role.[3-6] In 1994, Magerl et al.[7] proposed a rather comprehensive but somewhat unwieldy AO classification system. Eleven years later, in 2005, the Spine Trauma Study Group presented the Thoracolumbar Injury Classification and Severity (TLICS) Scale.[8] This system successfully incorporated the patient's neurologic status into the decision algorithm, alongside fracture morphology and the integrity of the ligamentous complex.

The most recent AOSpine classification system represents the most recent refinement in understanding and classifying spinal trauma.[9-12] It is a system that is comprehensive, however, is also easily applicable at the bedside and derived scores are reliably reproducible between and among observers. This system uses the morphology of the injury pattern to broadly distinguish between compression-type injuries (Type A), tension band injuries caused by distracting forces (Type B), and the most severe translation- and dislocation-type injuries (Type C).[9] A point-system is then applied to the injury morphology on a continuum of increasing severity, and to this value are added qualifiers identifying the patient's neurologic status as well as other patient-specific factors that may influence the decision to operate versus manage nonoperatively.[11] In particular, metabolic bone diseases such as ankylosing spondylitis and diffuse idiopathic skeletal hyperostosis (DISH) factor significantly into the surgical decision-making process. Relative contraindicators to surgery, as pointed out by the authors of the schema, include burns or other soft tissue defects overlying the fracture that may preclude acceptable healing.[11] These three categories and their relative assigned points can be seen in Table 1, adapted from Kepler et al. 2016.[11] The summation of these variables allows one to arrive at the AOSpine Injury Score (AOSIS). For injury patterns with AOSIS of three or less, conservative management is typical. Injury patterns with AOSIS of five or greater are best managed surgically. And finally, in instances of injury patterns with scores of

Table 1: Components of the AOSpine thoracolumbar injury classification system.

Morphology	*Score*	*Neurologic status*	*Score*
A0	0	N0–no deficit	0
A1	1	N1–transient deficit no longer present	1
A2	2	N2–nerve root injury	2
A3	3	N3–incomplete SCI	4
A4	5	N4–complete SCI	4
B1	5	Nx 0–unknown	3
B2	6	*Modifier*	*Score*
B3	7	M1	1
C	8	M2	0

(SCI: spinal cord injury)

Table 2: AOSpine injury score.

AOSIS	*Therapy*
3 or less	Conservative management
4 or 5	Surgeon's discretion
6 or greater	Surgery

(AOSIS: AOSpine injury score)

4 or 5, the decision to operate is left to the discretion of the surgeon. This is summarized in Table 2.[11]

SACRAL TRAUMA

Sacral fractures require a significant amount of force, and, therefore, only rarely occur unassociated with other systemic injury.[13] Such injuries may concomitantly involve the spine, the remainders of the pelvic ring, abdominal or pelvic viscera, or other soft tissues; thus these pathologies are complex and can be life-threatening. From a treatment perspective, sacral fractures often bridge the gap between orthopedic traumatology and spinal neurosurgery. While neurosurgeons routinely instrument the ilium, the first and second sacral pedicles, and the sacroiliac joint, the remainder of the sacrum can be unfamiliar territory, and, therefore, injuries to this structure may require an integrated and multidisciplinary team in order to be addressed satisfactorily.[14]

There are many different classification schemes that have been used to categorize sacral injuries. Further complicating efforts to obtain a comprehensive understanding of sacral fractures, authors had variously lumped discussions of these sacral injuries into schemes designed to communicate the sacral injury's implied effect on the whole, be it the stability of the pelvic ring,[15-17] the spino-pelvic unit,[18-20] or simply injuries isolated to the sacrum itself.[21] There was no agreed-upon nomenclature currently used to concisely express the pertinent clinical aspects of sacral fractures as they pertained to neurosurgeons, orthopedic traumatologists, and joint specialists. Perhaps the most well-known and utilized schema was proposed by Denis in 1988,[21] however, critics argue that this system is too simplistic and not prognostic.[22] The AOSpine Sacral Fracture classification scheme was designed to address specifically these concerns, and convey pertinent points regarding the stability of the pelvis and spine in a format that follows the algorithmic format of the previous proposed AOSpine classification schemes.

The AOSpine Sacral Classification System organizes sacral fractures into three broad categories: Type A, Type B, and Type C.[22] Type A fractures are typified by lower sacral or coccygeal avulsions or other transversely-oriented fractures that are found below the level of the sacroiliac joint. Fractures of this nature have no effect on biomechanical stability, although are not necessarily without risk of neurologic deficit. These fractures typically do not require treatment or fixation. The Type B fractures broadly encompass the schema denoted by Denis[21] and can have implications regarding overall pelvic stability. Finally, the Type C fractures have implications regarding spino-pelvic instability and morphologically assume the configurations of the so-called "U", "H", and "T" type fractures that have variously been described by multiple authors, as well as fractures through the superior articular process of S1 as described by Isler.[18] It is those Type C pattern injuries that are of foremost concern to spinal surgeons due to their high rate of neurologic injury and instability.

CASE ILLUSTRATIONS

Case 1: Transosseous Tension Band Disruption

A 19-year-old man fell from height with immediate onset of axial back pain as well as radiating right flank pain consistent with lower thoracic radiculopathy. The patient demonstrated an otherwise normal motor examination as well as digital rectal examination. CT and subsequent MRI revealed 13 rib-bearing vertebrae, with a Type A3 incomplete burst fracture of the T12 vertebra which spared the inferior end plate, and an associated Type B2 transosseous disruption of the posterior tension band involving both pedicles. The radiographic findings can be seen in Figures 1A to C. The Type B2 transosseous

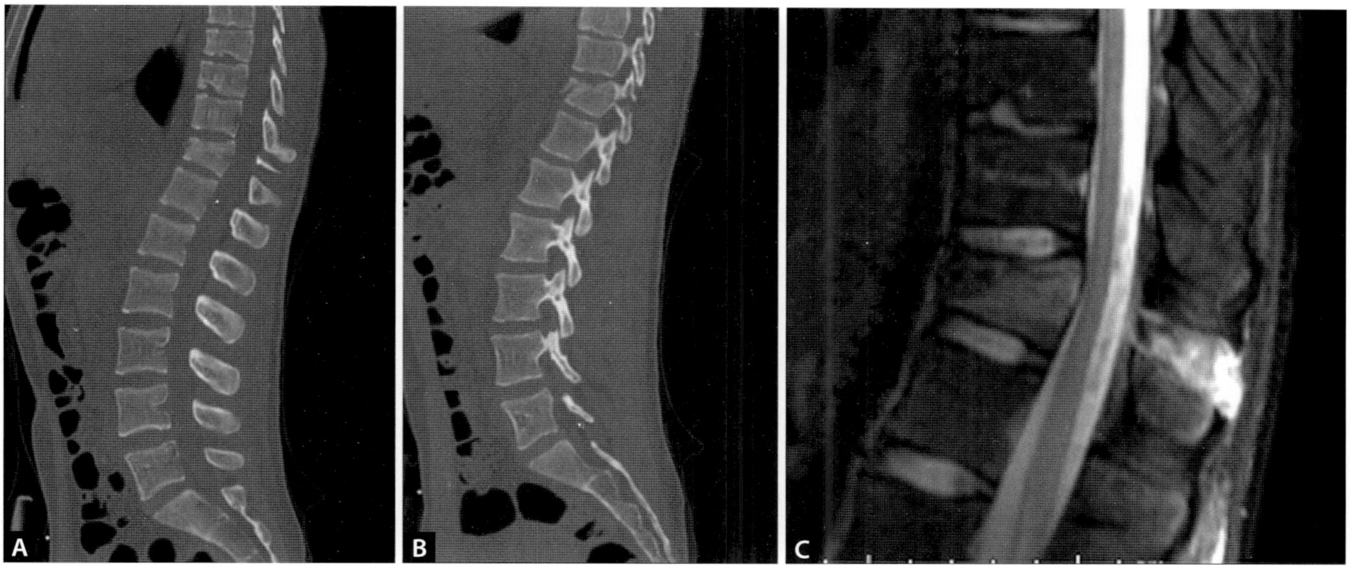

Figs. 1A to C: Midsagittal (A) and parasagittal; (B) Computed tomography (CT), as well as midsagittal T2-weighted MR; (C) Demonstrating Type A3 incomplete burst fracture of the T12 vertebra and an associated Type B2 transosseous disruption of the posterior tension band involving both pedicles. Note that the patient has 13 rib-bearing vertebrae.

tension-band injury with clinical radiculopathy yields an AOSIS of 8, recommending surgery as the preferred treatment. The patient underwent posterior decompression and stabilization from T10–L1, including a completed right-sided facetectomy at T11–12. The patient tolerated the procedure well, with resolution of radiculopathy. The postoperative anteroposterior (AP) radiograph can be seen in Figure 2.

Case 2: Transosseous Tension Band Disruption

A 24-year-old male fell from height, with immediate onset of axial back pain. His neurologic examination was normal. Imaging revealed six lumbar-type, non-rib-bearing vertebrae. He has suffered a Type A4 complete burst at the L1 level, with concomitant fracture through the left pars, pedicle, and articular process on the left side (Type B2 transosseous tension-band disruption). Sagittal and coronal CT of the lumbar spine can be seen in Figures 3A and B. Sagittal T2-weighted MRI of the lumbar spine can be seen in Figure 4. The AOSIS for this injury pattern is 6. The patient underwent T11–L3 decompression and fusion. The procedure was tolerated well. Postoperative lateral radiography can be seen in Figure 5.

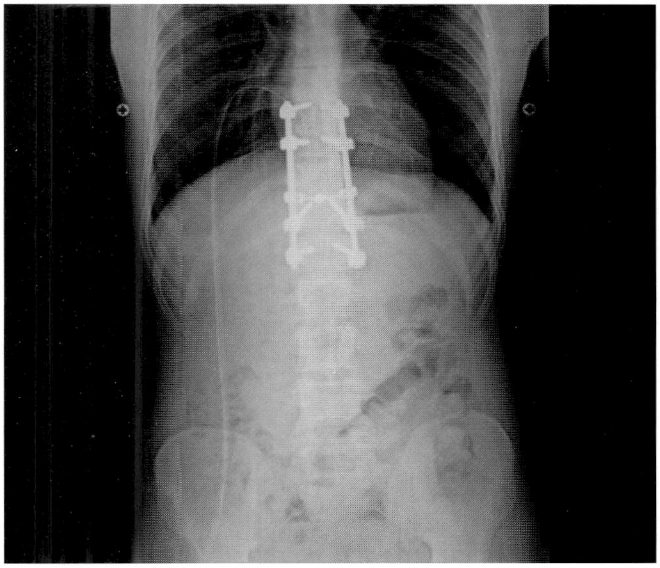

Fig. 2: Plain postoperative radiography after posterior decompression and stabilization from T10–L1. Note that the patient has 13 rib-bearing vertebrae.

Case 3: Transligamentous Tension Band Disruption

A 19-year-old male was involved in a weightlifting accident while at the gym and noted the immediate onset of axial

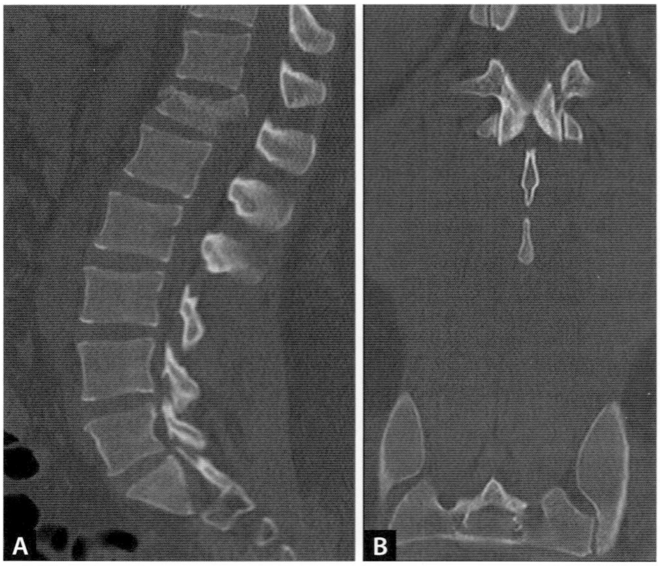

Figs. 3A and B: Sagittal (A) and coronal (B) Computed tomography (CT) of the lumbar spine demonstrating a Type A4 complete burst at the L1 level, with concomitant fracture through the left pars, pedicle, and articular process on the left side (Type B2 transosseous tension band disruption). Note that the patient has six lumbar-type, non-rib-bearing vertebrae.

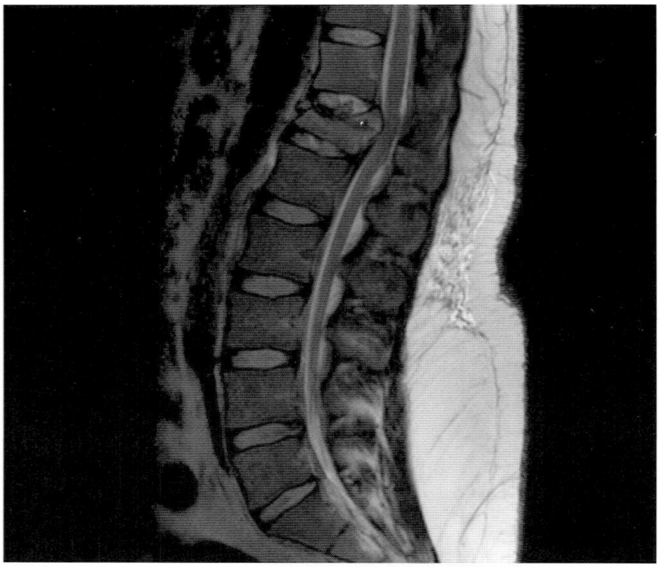

Fig. 4: Sagittal T2-weighted magnetic resonance imaging (MRI) of the lumbar spine demonstrating combination A4/B2 injury at L1. The AOSpine injury score (AOSIS) for this injury pattern is 6.

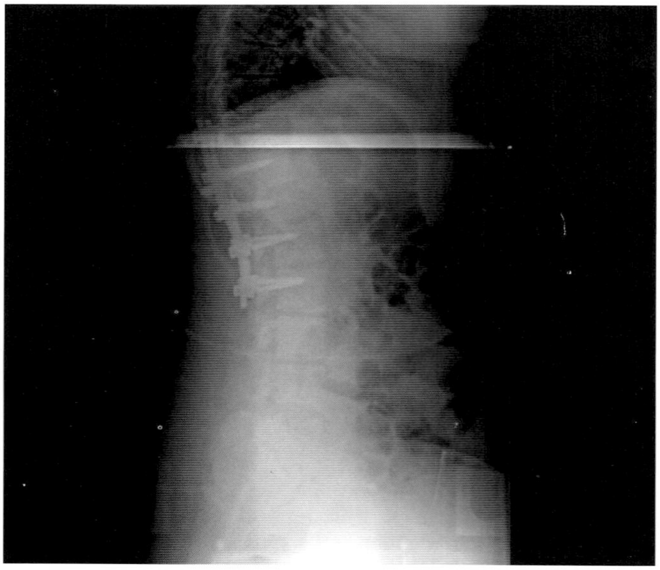

Fig. 5: Postoperative lateral radiography after T11–L3 decompression and fusion.

lower back pain. Physical examination revealed a clearly palpable step-off about the thoracolumbar junction. He has normal strength and digital rectal examination. CT revealed a Type A1 compression deformity of the T12 vertebra, with widely splayed spinous processes at T11–12, and subluxation of the facet joints at this level to a degree such that they assumed a near-perched appearance bilaterally. These findings on CT are highly suggestive of capsuloligamentous injury, and can be appreciated in Figures 6A and B. MRI demonstrated a concomitant Type B2 transligamentous tension band failure, with complete disruption of the supraspinous and interspinous ligaments, as well as the ligamentum flavum. This can be seen in Figure 7. The AOSIS for this injury totals to 6, and the patient was treated with posterior decompression, reduction, and stabilization from T10–L2. The patient tolerated the procedure without ill effect. Postoperative radiography can be seen in Figure 8.

Case 4: Penetrating Spinal Trauma

A 36-year-old man was the victim of a military-grade gunshot wound to the left flank. The bullet wound resulted in a left-sided pneumothorax and diaphragmatic laceration, as well as injuries to the left spleen and kidney, before traversing the spinal canal at L1–2, and exiting through the right flank. The patient was taken to the operating room for laparotomy and hemorrhage control, as well as splenectomy, distal pancreatectomy and left

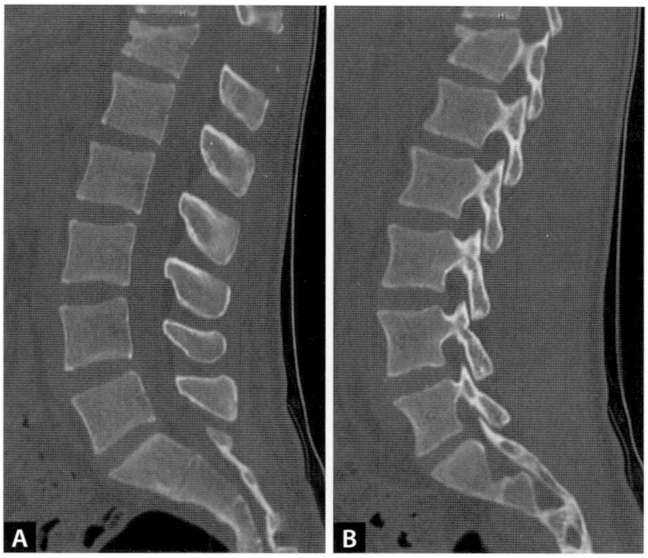

Figs. 6A and B: Midsagittal (A) and parasagittal (B) lumbar CT demonstrating Type A1 compression deformity of the T12 vertebra. Note the widely splayed spinous processes at T11–12, and subluxation of the facet joints at this level to a degree such that they assumed a near-perched appearance bilaterally. These findings on CT are highly suggestive of capsuloligamentous disruption.

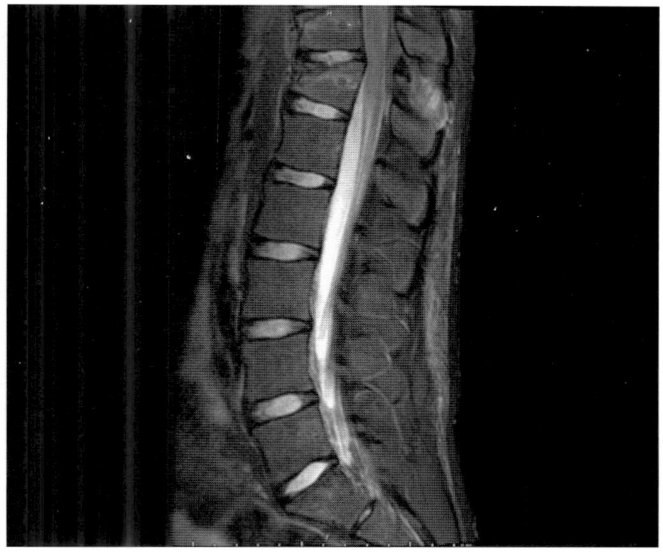

Fig. 7: Sagittal T2-weighted MRI demonstrating a concomitant Type B2 transligamentous tension band failure, with complete disruption of the supraspinous and interspinous ligaments, as well as the ligamentum flavum.

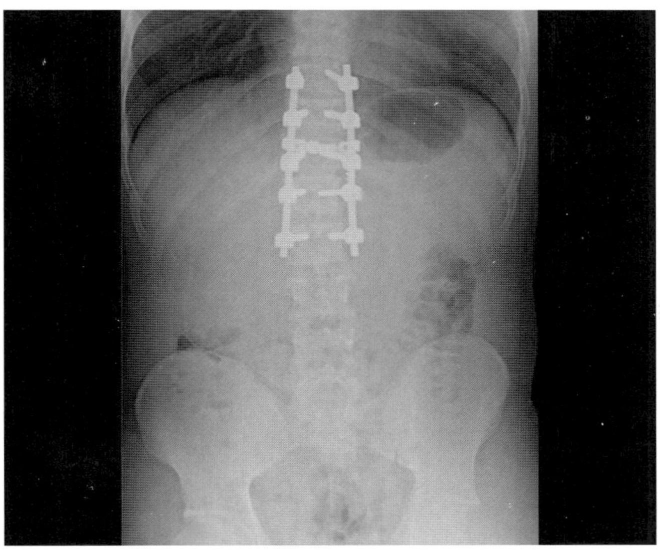

Fig. 8: Postoperative radiography after posterior decompression, reduction, and stabilization from T10–L2.

nephrectomy, and diaphragm repair. Once stabilized hemodynamically, his neurologic examination was notable for patchy sensory preservation below the level of the inguinal area, with greater sparing on the left side, which was felt to be most consistent with American Spinal Injury Association (ASIA) B, with a T12 level, clinically which makes this situation different from most penetrating injuries. Fragmentation injury from the projectile precluded the safe utilization of MRI. CT imaging can be seen in Figures 9A (axial) and B (sagittal). The path of the projectile can be seen crossing the spinal canal at the tL1-2 level, disrupting the L2 pedicles, the L1-2 facet complexes, and the remainder of the posterior elements at this level.

Penetrating spinal trauma can defy conventional classification systems and in the great majority does not require operative treatment. In this rare patient, the injury pattern is most consistent with a pure transosseous tension band disruption without concomitant Type A injury (therefore termed "Type B1"). The goal of surgery for complete spinal cord injured patients is generally stabilization of the spine and early mobilization. In the context of his presenting neurologic examination, the injury pattern yields an AOSIS of 9. The patient was taken for posterior decompression and stabilization from T11–L4. Figure 10 is an intraoperative image taken at the time of surgery. For purposes of orientation, the patient is

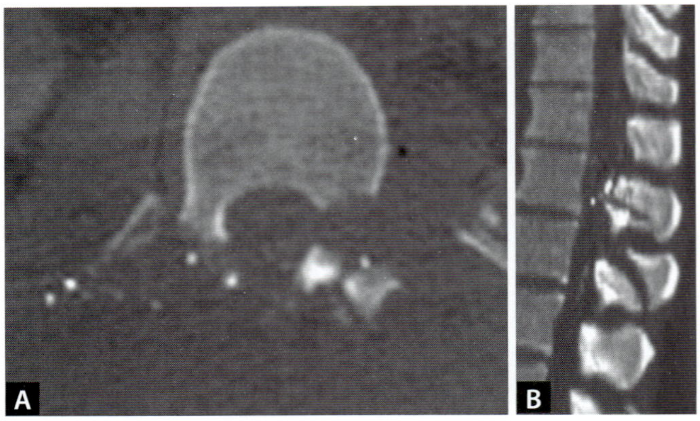

Figs. 9A and B: Axial (A) and sagittal (B) lumbar CT at the level of L1–2, demonstrating the path of the projectile crossing at the L1–2 level, with disruption of the L2 pedicles and the L1–2 facet complexes.

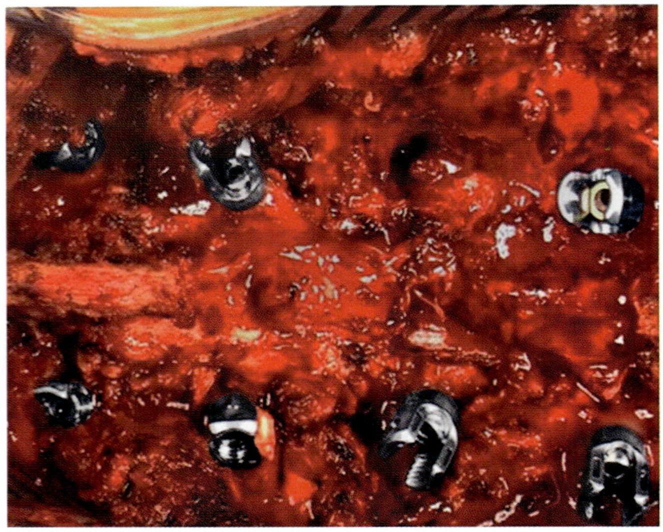

Fig. 10: Intraoperative photography. The left L2 pedicle has been omitted. Note the disrupted thecal sac with exposed neural elements.

positioned prone; the right side of the image represents the cephalad direction and the top of the image represents the patient's left flank. The left L2 pedicle screw has been omitted, as the pedicle and neurocentral junction were badly damaged by the projectile. What had remained of the posterior elements at L2 were removed, and visible in the center of the image is the transected thecal sac, with exposed neural elements, including what appeared to be the distal conus medullaris and roots of the cauda equina. Interestingly, partial preservation of somatosensory evoked potentials (SSEPs) to the lower extremities, as well as the presence of motor evoked potentials (MEPs) to the external anal sphincter, was appreciated from the intraoperative neurophysiologic monitoring data. The dural defect was too significant to be repaired primarily. The exposed neural elements were enveloped with a dural on-lay and biological glue was applied to the periphery of the repair. A postoperative radiograph can be seen in Figure 11.

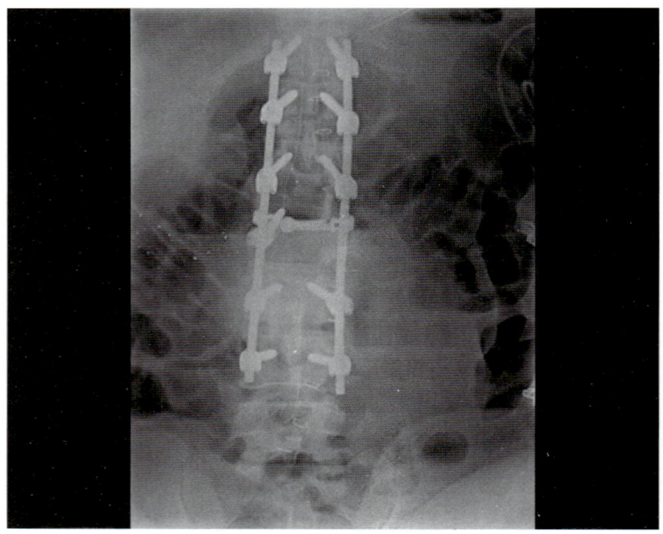

Fig. 11: Postoperative radiograph after posterior decompression and stabilization from T11–L4.

Case 5: Multiple Noncontiguous Fractures

A 21-year-old man was involved in a motor vehicle roll-over. He presented clinically with significant left distal lower extremity weakness, but otherwise normal neurologic examination, including digital rectal examination. His intake imaging revealed an incomplete burst fracture of the T7 as well as the L1 vertebrae, with associated transosseous tension band injuries at these levels. The tension band injury at L1 was characterized by a fracture of the left L1 pars and facet complex. At T7, there was a minimally displaced and horizontally-oriented fracture running the length of the posterior osseous ligamentous complex, through the pars bilaterally. The patient's CT can be appreciated in Figures 12A (mid-sagittal lumbar spine), B (coronal reconstruction and lumbar spine), and C (mid-sagittal thoracic spine). MRI revealed a large retropulsed fragment at L1 compressing the distal cord and conus medullaris, with abnormal intrinsic T2 signal apparent within the parenchyma, consistent with a contusion

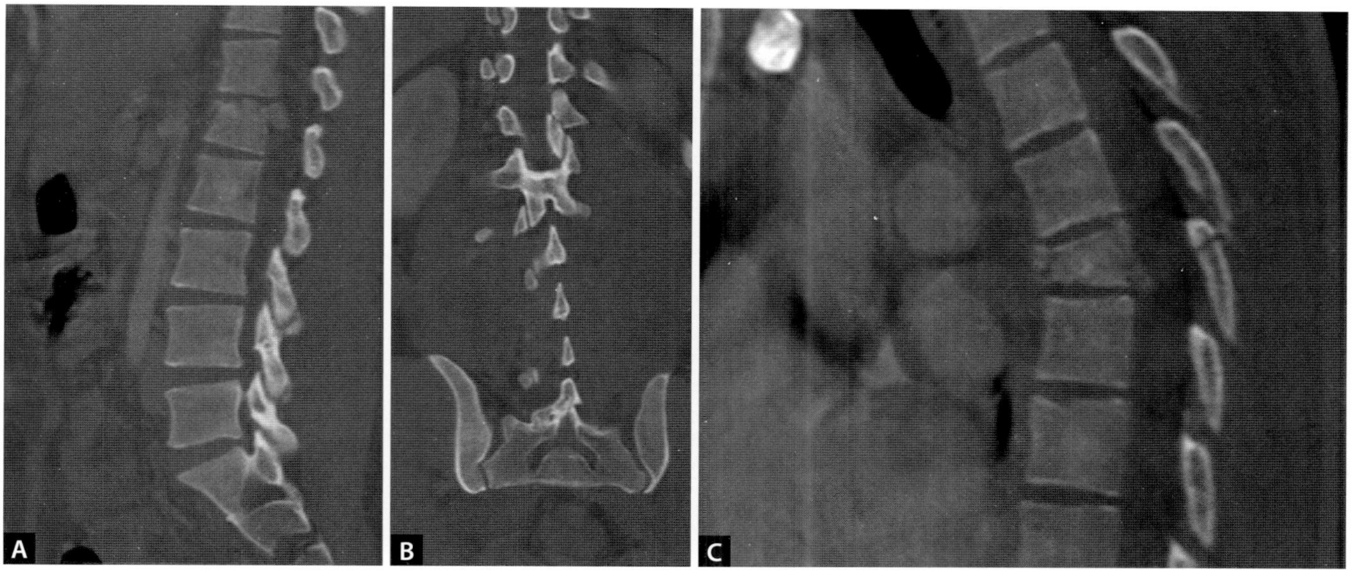

Figs. 12A to C: Sagittal (A) and coronal; (B) Lumbar CT, as well as sagittal thoracic CT; (C) Demonstrating incomplete burst fractures of the T7 as well as the L1 vertebrae, with associated transosseous tension band injuries at these levels. The tension band injury at L1 was characterized by a fracture of the left L1 pars and facet complex. At T7, there was a minimally displaced, horizontally-oriented fracture running the length of the posterior osseous ligamentous complex, through the pars bilaterally.

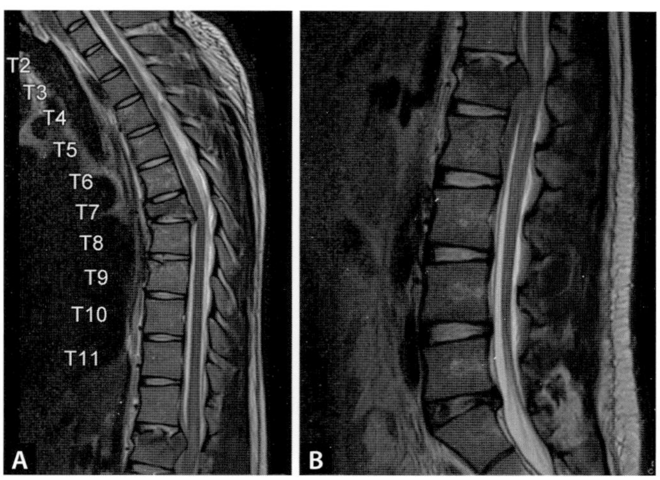

Figs. 13A and B: Sagittal T2-weighted thoracic (A) and lumbar (B) MRI demonstrating a large retropulsed fragment at L1 compressing the distal cord and conus medullaris, with abnormal intrinsic T2 signal apparent within the parenchyma, consistent with a contusion. The canal at T7 is patent.

(Fig. 13B). There was a clinically insignificant degree of retropulsed material at T7 (Fig. 13A). An incomplete spinal cord injury in the context of a Type B2 injury yields an AOSIS of 10. The patient was taken for T5–L3 posterior decompression and fusion, with improvement of left lower extremity function to near-normal postoperatively.

Case 6: Sacral Fracture Dislocation

A 68-year-old female with Parkinson's disease experienced an orthostatic fall from standing at home. She noted the immediate onset of low back pain, lower extremity weakness, and bladder incontinence. Upon neurological assessment, she was found to have a right-sided foot drop, loss of rectal tone, and diminished perianal sensation concerning for cauda equina syndrome. Midsagittal CT (Fig. 14A) and T2-weighted MRI (Fig. 14B) revealed overall osteopenic bone and an angulated distal sacral fracture, with narrowing of sacral canal and compression of subarticular S2 nerve roots bilaterally. The injury represents a Type C3 displaced sacral U-type fracture, with the following associated modifiers—N3 for cauda equina syndrome and M2 for osteoporosis. The patient was, therefore, taken to the operating room for percutaneous pelvic fixation with a sacroiliac fixation screw for stabilization and then posterior decompression and fusion L5-pelvis with pedicle screws bilaterally at L5 and S1 with fusion construct connected to S2AI screws bilaterally. A

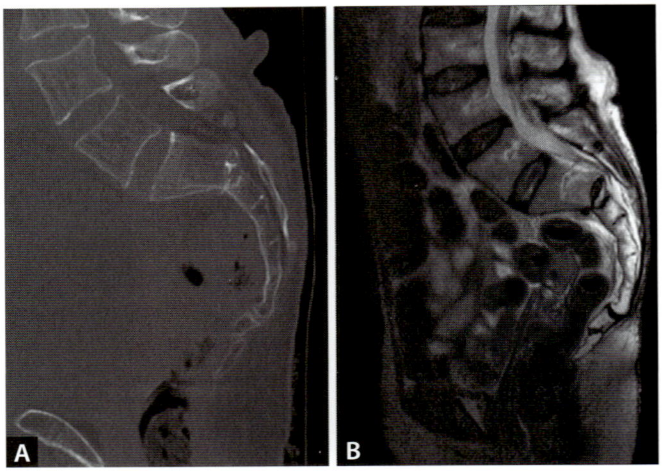

Figs. 14A and B: Mid-sagittal CT (A) and T2-weighted MRI (B) demonstrating a Type C3 displaced sacral U-type fracture with narrowing of sacral canal and compression of subarticular S2 nerve roots bilaterally.

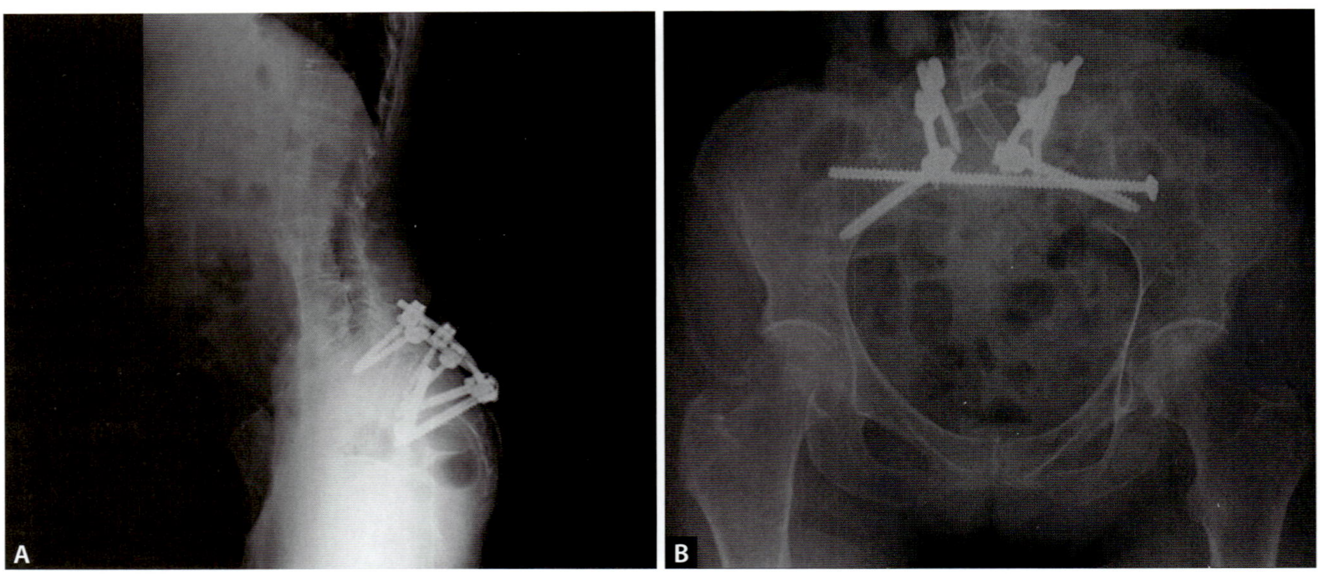

Figs. 15A and B: Postoperative lateral (A) and anteroposterior; (B) Radiography after the patient underwent L5-ilium decompression and fusion.

postoperative radiograph can be seen in Figures 15A and B showing anteroposterior and lateral views, respectively.

KEY POINTS

- Classification systems for spinal injuries have been in evolution for over 80 years. The AOSpine system is predicated on the morphology of the injury, the patient's neurologic status, and the existence of patient-specific modifying factors.
- The morphology of thoracolumbar injuries is broadly distinguished between compression-type injuries (Type A), tension band injuries (Type B), and translational injuries (Type C).
- In general, Type C injuries are to be considered highly unstable and in need of fixation. Type A injuries, in the neurologically intact pattient, can often be managed conservatively, provided that the patient is neurologically intact and there is no concomitant injury to the tension band.

- Penetrating trauma to the spine can be difficult to classify, and most frequently can be managed nonsurgically.
- The morphology of sacral injuries is classified as stable low sacral and coccygeal avulsions and transverse fractures below the SI joint (Type A), vertically-oriented fractures expounded by Denis that may affect pelvic stability (Type B), and spinopelvic disassociations (Type C).
- Sacral and pelvic fractures require significant force, and are often associated with systemic injuries. Management of these injuries often requires a multidisciplinary team of spine surgeons and orthopedic traumatologists.

REFERENCES

1. Harrop JS, Rymarczuk GN, Vaccaro AR, et al. Controversies in spinal trauma and evolution of care. Neurosurgery. 2017;80(3S):S23-32.
2. Watson-Jones R. The results of postural reduction of fractures of the spine. J Bone Joint Surg Am. 1938;20(3):567-86.
3. Nicoll EA. Fractures of the dorso-lumbar spine. J Bone Joint Surg Br. 1949;31B(3):376-94.
4. Kelly RP, Whitesides TE Jr. Treatment of lumbodorsal fracture-dislocations. Ann Surg. 1968;167(5):705-17.
5. McAfee PC, Yuan HA, Fredrickson BE, et al. The value of computed tomography in thoracolumbar fractures. An analysis of one hundred consecutive cases and a new classification. J Bone Joint Surg Am. 1983;65(4):461-73.
6. Denis F. The three column spine and its significance in the classification of acute thoracolumbar spinal injuries. Spine (Phila Pa 1976). 1983;8(8):817-31.
7. Magerl F, Aebi M, Gertzbein SD, et al. A comprehensive classification of thoracic and lumbar injuries. Eur Spine J. 1994;3(4):184-201.
8. Vaccaro AR, Lehman RA Jr, Hurlbert RJ, et al. A new classification of thoracolumbar injuries: the importance of injury morphology, the integrity of the posterior ligamentous complex, and neurologic status. Spine (Phila Pa 1976). 2005;30(20):2325-33.
9. Vaccaro AR, Oner C, Kepler CK, et al. AOSpine thoracolumbar spine injury classification system: fracture description, neurological status, and key modifiers. Spine (Phila Pa 1976). 2013;38(23):2028-37.
10. Vaccaro AR, Schroeder GD, Kepler CK, et al. The surgical algorithm for the AOSpine thoracolumbar spine injury classification system. Eur Spine J. 2016;25(4):1087-94.
11. Kepler CK, Vaccaro AR, Schroeder GD, et al. The thoracolumbar AOSpine injury score. Global Spine J. 2016;6(4):329-34.
12. Vaccaro AR, Oner C, Kepler CK, et al. AOSpine thoracolumbar spine injury classification system: fracture description, neurological status, and key modifiers. Spine (Phila Pa 1976). 2013;38(23):2028-37.
13. Rodrigues-Pinto R, Kurd MF, Schroeder GD, et al. Sacral fractures and associated injuries. Global Spine J. 2017;7(7):609-16.
14. Lindtner RA, Bellabarba C, Firoozabadi R, et al. Should displaced sacral fractures be treated by an orthopedic traumatologist or a spine surgeon? Clin Spine Surg. 2016;29(5):173-6.
15. Burgess AR, Eastridge BJ, Young JW, et al. Pelvic ring disruptions: effective classification system and treatment protocols. J Trauma. 1990;30(7):848-56.
16. Young JW, Burgess AR, Brumback RJ, et al. Pelvic fractures: value of plain radiography in early assessment and management. Radiology. 1986;160(2):445-51.
17. Tile M. Pelvic ring fractures: should they be fixed? J Bone Joint Surg Br. 1988;70(1):1-12.
18. Isler B. Lumbosacral lesions associated with pelvic ring injuries. J Orthop Trauma. 1990;4(1):1-6.
19. Roy-Camille R, Saillant G, Gagna G, et al. Transverse fracture of the upper sacrum. Suicidal jumper's fracture. Spine (Phila Pa 1976). 1985;10(9):838-45.
20. Strange-Vognsen HH, Lebech A. An unusual type of fracture in the upper sacrum. J Orthop Trauma. 1991;5(2):200-3.
21. Denis F, Davis S, Comfort T. Sacral fractures: an important problem. Retrospective analysis of 236 cases. Clin Orthop Relat Res. 1988;227:67-81.
22. Schroeder GD, Kurd MF, Kepler CK, et al. The Development of a Universally Accepted Sacral Fracture Classification: A Survey of AOSpine and AOTrauma Members. Global Spine J. 2016;6(7):686-94.

CHAPTER **43**

Thoracic, Lumbar, and Sacral Tumors

Paul E Kaloostian, Jean Paul Wolinsky, Ziya L Gokaslan

EPIDEMIOLOGY AND NATURAL HISTORY

The axial skeleton is a common site for oncologic disease. A wide variety of tumors may grow within the spinal column. These tumors may be primary or metastatic in nature. Depending on location, size, and histology, these tumors may produce a variety of neurological symptoms and deficits, and may affect patient quality of life and survival. In this chapter we extensively review the myriad tumors associated with the thoracic, lumbar, and sacral spine. Each of these tumors has its own specific epidemiological, histopathological, radiological, and treatment characteristics that are important to recognize for physicians and surgeons treating patients with these oncologic pathologies. While tumoral disease within the spine was once thought of as the terminal stage for that patient, advances in stereotactic radiosurgery, vertebroplasty, and more aggressive surgical techniques such as en bloc vertebrectomy with reconstruction have recently revolutionized the field of spine surgery and has brought new life back to these patients. The differential diagnosis of thoracic, lumbar, and sacral tumors of the spine is quite diverse. It includes pathologies such as—multiple myeloma, chordomas, giant cell tumors, hemangiomas, osteosarcomas, chondrosarcomas, aneurysmal bone cysts, hemangiomas, eosinophilic granulomas, osteoid osteomas, osteoblastomas, and metastatic tumors. The epidemiology and natural history of each of these tumors will be discussed in great detail in this chapter.

MULTIPLE MYELOMA

Workup

Multiple myeloma is a common malignant primary tumor of the spine. It accounts for over 40% of primary spinal tumors. Myeloma cells are malignant plasma cells that are described to arise from an overexpansion of a single clone of cells.[1]

Patients with multiple myeloma are commonly in their 50s–60s and may present with a variety of symptoms depending on location of lesion(s). Spinal metastasis typically presents with focal back pain at the site of the lesion. Patients may present with acute pathological fracture due to tumor that may produce acute onset focal back pain. Radicular symptoms may or may not be present depending on amount of vertebral body collapse and consequent foraminal compromise. Patients may present with bony pain at other parts of the body where tumor may be located, such as the arm or leg. Patients may present with symptoms related to associated anemia, thrombocytopenia, and renal failure from involvement of the bone marrow and kidneys.[1]

Patients with multiple myeloma have classic "punched-out" lesions on X-ray without surrounding virgin bone growth. X-rays may demonstrate focal or diffuse osteopenia as well. Computed tomography (CT) scans and magnetic resonance imaging (MRI) scans may demonstrate pathological fracture of the spine with associated foraminal compromise. Other lesions may be noted throughout the spinal axis. Bone scans may show increased activity at the site of fracture or may be normal. Skeletal survey is very useful to display multiple areas of myeloma involvement throughout the entire skeleton.[1]

Multiple myeloma is typically diagnosed through history, physical examination, and radiographic imaging findings. Classically bone marrow aspiration will yield abnormal plasma cell distribution that clinches the diagnosis. CT-guided biopsy of the spinal lesion is rarely indicated, unless diagnosis is still unclear. Hypercalcemia may be noted on the blood work in 40% of patients.[1] Multiple myeloma displays a unique histological picture. This tumor involves a clonal expansion of a single clone of plasma cells. Thus, cells are typically plasma cells that are hypercellular. The extent of plasma cells on the slides is crucial for the diagnosis. For example, the presence of over 20% plasma cells in the bone marrow provides clear evidence of myeloma tumor, while 10–20% content of plasma cells may imply multiple myeloma. Immunohistochemistry is important to identify lambda and kappa heavy chain and light chain distributions.[1]

Medical/Surgical Management

A combination of treatment modalities exists for multiple myeloma that is specific for the particular presentation. Patients with stable spinal disease without deformity or spinal cord compromise may be managed nonoperatively. This would include chemotherapy if disease is systemic and/or radiotherapy if disease if focal. Radiotherapy has been shown to improve focal bony symptoms. A patient with pathological fracture with severe kyphotic deformity, spinal instability, and spinal cord compression will benefit from surgical treatment. Surgical treatment depends on location along the spinal axis. Cervical vertebral body tumors may be approached anteriorly for corpectomy and fusion. Thoracic vertebral body tumors may be preferentially approached posteriorly via a transpedicular approach for corpectomy and posterolateral instrumentation with fusion. Lumbar vertebral body tumors may be approached anteriorly or posteriorly for either corpectomy or posterolateral instrumentation and fusion, respectively.[1]

Complications

Complications of surgical management include infection, bleeding, and instrumentation failure.

Prognosis

Despite the above treatment modalities, prognosis remains poor. The 5-year survival remains less than 30%.[1]

CHORDOMAS

Workup

Chordomas are rare benign tumors of the axial skeleton that are the most common primary malignant tumors of the spine in adults. They typically occur in middle-aged adults.[2] Common locations include the clival skull base and sacrum, but they may occur along the cervical, thoracic, or lumbar spine as well.[3] This tumor is derived from undifferentiated notochord remnants that are found to reside within the developing axial skeleton, hence the name "chordoma".[3] These notochordal cells have been shown to be the precise neoplastic cells responsible for transformation and tumor development.[4] Though their slow growth pattern enables distortion of surrounding structures and high recurrence rate, they are classified as malignant tumors.[2]

Patients may present with a variety of different symptoms depending on the site of tumor growth. For example, tumors in the presacral and sacrococcygeal region may reach such significant growth that they may distort surrounding neural structures. Patients may present with neurological compromise such as weakness of dorsiflexion, perineal numbness, bowel and bladder incontinence, and sexual dysfunction. Alternatively, cervical and thoracic tumors may present with focal back pain or if larger may present with signs of myelopathy from spinal cord compression. Lumbar chordomas may present with focal back pain or if larger may present with radicular symptoms and associated weakness or numbness or cauda equina syndrome.[2,3]

Typically, CT and MRI are used to diagnose this pathology (Fig. 1). CT scans of the spine will demonstrate a large heterogeneous, sometimes calcified, mass with distortion of surrounding architecture. Classically, chordomas may remodel the existing bony architecture due to their slow growth, rather than invasion and destruction of bone. MRI may demonstrate a heterogeneously enhancing mass with consequent neural or foraminal compromise.[2]

Chordomas are diagnosed based on imaging findings as well as a CT-guided biopsy.[2]

Chordomas display unique cellular architecture that distinguishes them from other tumors. For example, they display pathognomonic physaliferous cells, which have an unusually vacuolated cytoplasm. Microscopically, chordoma cells react intensely for S-100 and other epithelial markers such as cytokeratins and epithelial membrane.[5,6]

Medical/Surgical Management

Treatment paradigm has shifted over the last decade to a more aggressive surgical approach. These lesions are classically radioresistant to conventional fractionated

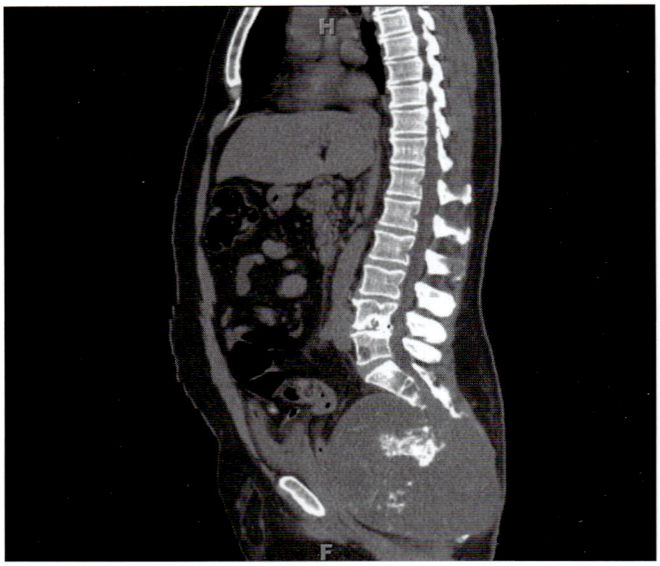

Fig. 1: Preoperative CT scan demonstrated a large sacrococcygeal mass.
Source: The Johns Hopkins Hospital.

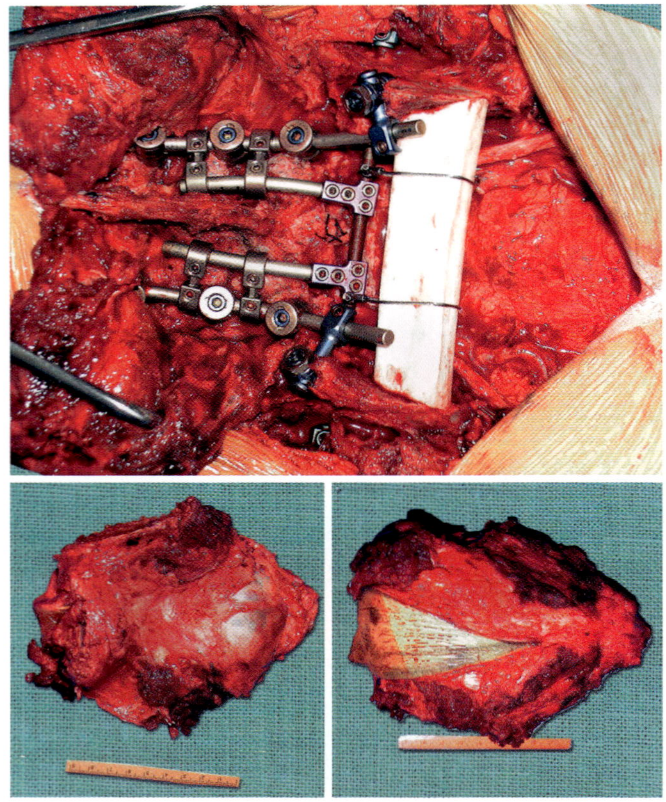

Fig. 2: En bloc sacrectomy for chordoma with postoperative instrumentation noted.
Source: With permission from Ian Suk, The Johns Hopkins Hospital.

radiotherapy. Proton beam therapy has gained momentum in the adjunctive treatment of chordomas with decreasing tissue injury and local control of tumor volume with 5-year local control rate of 50–60%.[7] The typical chemotherapeutic agents have been shown in multiple reviews to be a minimal clinical significance in the treatment of spinal chordomas.[8]

The surgical approach will vary depending on location along the spine. However, the main tenet of chordoma surgery remains the same. En bloc resection without violation of the tumor capsule remains critical toward advancing progression free survival and lowering the recurrence rate. Cervical tumors are further classified into high cervical, mid-cervical, and cervicothoracic. The location within the cervical will guide appropriate staged surgical treatment, based on ability of nerve root sacrifice and vertebral artery sacrifice. Thoracic, lumbar, and sacrococcygeal are managed in multiple staged posterior and anterior instrumentation and fusion procedures with en bloc resection of tumor without violation of tumor capsule.[9-11]

Generally, the current recommendations are en bloc surgical resection along with postoperative proton beam radiotherapy, especially in patients with primary chordomas as opposed to recurrent tumors.[12]

Complications

Complications of surgical management include infection, bleeding, and instrumentation failure. Additionally, patients who undergo aggressive en bloc thoracolumbar and sacral vertebrectomy may have complications such as esophageal perforation, pleural tears, bowel/bladder incontinence, and spinal cord injury.

Prognosis

Spinal chordoma surgery outcomes are highly correlated with en bloc resection without violation of tumor capsule (Fig. 2). If tumor capsule is violated during en bloc resection, a twofold higher rate of local recurrence is seen.[13] If subtotal resection is performed, recurrence rate is at 8 months as opposed to over 2 years with en bloc resection.[14] Typically, survival after en bloc resection without violation of tumor capsule is over 60% at 5 years' time.[14] Metastases can occur but are quite rare and studies have demonstrated survival to be closely linked to local disease rather than metastatic disease.[15]

When performing sacrectomies, recent evidence suggests that salvaging the sacral 2 nerve root is a key to restoring a 50% chance of normal bowel and bladder function postoperatively. Sacral 3 root preservation will provide additional guarantee of bowel and bladder function. It has been shown that bilateral sacral 2 nerve root sparing along with unilateral sacral 3 root sparing is associated with normal bowel and bladder function.[11]

GIANT CELL TUMORS

Workup

Giant cell tumors of the spine are typically lytic and expansile lesions that occur in mostly female patients 20–50 years of age.[16] Thus, although classified as a predominantly benign tumor, the locally aggressive behavior gives it the appearance of a more malignant tumor.[16]

Patients may present with focal back pain due to tumor causing pathological fracture. Degree of resulting kyphotic deformity may produce foraminal stenosis causing radicular symptoms as well.[17] There is no clear predilection within the spine.[16]

X-rays and CT scans help to determine extent of bony destruction associated with the vertebral body. MRI can be used to determine extent of tumor within and outside of the vertebral body, along with any neural compromise. T1 MRI will show clear demarcation between tumor and fatty marrow. A radionuclide bone scan may be used and will show decreased uptake in the center of the lytic process and high uptake along the surrounding.[17]

Diagnosis is based on imaging findings and CT-guided biopsy showing the unique histologic properties of giant mononuclear cells.[17]

Giant tumor cells display unique histology. The hallmarks are the numerous mononuclear stromal cells and giant cells throughout.[17]

Medical/Surgical Management

Giant cell tumors are placed into three stages.[17] The first stage is latent activity; second stage is slightly increased lytic activity on scans; third stage is highly aggressive lytic component within the vertebral body. For tumors involving the spinal canal, typical intralesional curettage and burning with bone cement packing cannot be done due to the tumoral infiltration and compression of the neural elements. Thus, attempts at en bloc resection have been performed. Some published data has demonstrated a decreased recurrence rate and acceptable morbidity after en bloc spondylectomy, while other studies have demonstrated an unacceptable complication rate postoperatively.[18,19] En bloc resection generally will involve a multiple staged posterior then anterior reconstruction with instrumentation and fusion.[19] While radiotherapy has been conventionally avoided due to possibility of malignant transformation of cells, studies have demonstrated adequate response that is comparable to surgical resection in patients without impending neural compromise.[20]

Complications

Complications of surgical management include infection, bleeding, and instrumentation failure.

Prognosis

Local recurrence rates are noted to be at 41–66.7% within the mobile spine.[16,17] 5–13% of patients will have pulmonary metastases, which may require surgical resection.[17,21] Pathology of the pulmonary lesions will determine benign versus malignant histology.[17]

HEMANGIOMA

Workup

Hemangiomas are generally benign lesions within the axial spine that are seen in 10% of patients postmortem. They are common and often asymptomatic lesions that can become symptomatic through increase in size and formation of pathological fracture.[22] There exists a syndrome of multiple hemangiomas of the spine where these tumors are seen within the bony elements throughout the entire neuraxis.[23] The predilection is for the lower thoracic spine.[22]

Patients are often asymptomatic at the time of diagnosis. Lesions that increase in size may cause acute pathological fracture and subsequent focal back pain with or without neural injury. Only 1% of vertebral hemangiomas are symptomatic.[24]

X-rays will show vertical striations at the site of tumor. CT scans will demonstrate the "spikes of bone" appearance within the vertebral body. MRI will show an enhancing tumor with hemorrhage and thrombosis on T1 imaging.[22]

Diagnosis is made based on history and imaging findings.

Hemangiomas typically are unencapsulated collections of thin-walled capillaries with an endothelial lining. They may have thrombosed lumens with occasional hemosiderin deposition from vessel rupture.[25]

Medical/Surgical Management

Typically, in asymptomatic patients, observation is recommended, especially if lesion(s) are small without surrounding neurological compromise or instability.[24] If patient has persistent pain associated with the spinal hemangioma, radiation therapy may be offered for symptomatic control with adequate results.[24] For lesions with hypertrophy or ballooning of the posterior cortex of the vertebral body into the spinal canal causing neurologic compromise or intractable pain from deformity, studies have demonstrated acceptable results from either an anterior approach, posterolateral approach, or posterior approach.[24] Surgical treatment will depend on location within the spinal axis. Anterior approach would involve corpectomy and tumor resection with placement of appropriate reconstructive plates. A posterolateral approach would entail a transpedicular corpectomy with appropriate reconstructive instrumentation and fusion posteriorly. A pure posterior approach would entail posterior decompression and instrumentation with fusion.[24]

Complications

Complications of surgical management include infection, bleeding, and instrumentation failure.

Prognosis

Vertebral hemangiomas that are asymptomatic rarely cause symptoms. Surgical treatment of symptomatic hemangiomas of the spine due to neurological compromise and instability has reported adequate outcomes.[24] No metastatic disease has been noted with vertebral hemangiomas.

EOSINOPHILIC GRANULOMA

Workup

Eosinophilic granulomas of the spine are benign lesions that are the localized form of Langerhans histiocytosis X. Vertebral location is noted to be around 8–25%.[26] The thoracic spine is the most common site within the spine.[27]

Patients classically are asymptomatic and these tumors are diagnosed incidentally. Granulomas that are large and/or causing pathological fracture or deformity with neurological compromise may present with severe neck pain, radicular pain, and/or signs of myelopathy from spinal cord compression.[27]

X-ray and CT scans may demonstrate vertebral flattening which precedes eventual vertebral collapse. CT and MRI may demonstrate additional lesions elsewhere within the spinal axis.[27]

Eosinophilic granulomas of the spine are diagnosed based on imaging and/or prior history of Langerhans histiocytosis systemically. A biopsy is indicated if diagnosis is not clear.

Eosinophilic granulomas demonstrate classic Langerhans cells, which are mononuclear histiocytic cells with oval nuclei and Birbeck granules on electron microscopy. Additionally, lipid-laden foam cells and lack of nuclear atypia characterize this tumor.[28,29]

Medical/Surgical Management

Typically, eosinophilic granulomas are self-limiting. Appropriate bracing is recommended for symptomatic relief of back pain and prevention of kyphosis. Chemotherapy is recommended for systemic form of Langerhans histiocytosis X. Low dose conventional radiotherapy is recommended for symptomatic lesions without neurological compromise and/or patients who are not operative candidates. If lesions are causing progressively worse intractable pain and instability and/or deformity with neurological compromise, then surgical intervention is warranted.[27] Surgical approach would depend on the level along the spine, with either an anterior corpectomy with fusion or posterior or posterolateral approach for corpectomy with instrumentation.[29]

Complications

Complications of surgical management include infection, bleeding, and instrumentation failure.

Prognosis

Granulomas generally remain stable without causing symptoms. Patients that require surgical or radiation/chemotherapy generally recover without significant morbidity.[29]

ANEURYSMAL BONE CYST

Workup

Aneurysmal bone cysts (ABC) are defined as benign expansile lesions of bone composed of blood filled cavities separated by septa of osteoclastic cells. They are seen along the spine 25% of the time. They are seen predominantly in patients younger than 20 years of age. They can be locally destructive within the spinal axis.[30] They are characterized by a central region of cystic hemorrhage surrounded by vascular proliferation tissue.

Typically, patients are asymptomatic with the cyst being found incidentally. Cysts may produce pathological fractures causing focal back pain. Larger cysts may occupy a significant portion of the spine and canal causing associated symptoms such as focal back pain, radicular pain or weakness, or even paraplegia if large enough along the posterior elements.

CT and/or MRI can demonstrate a lytic lesion surrounded by a thin shell of cortical bone with areas of cortical disruption causing a blown-out appearance.[31] Lobulated appearance, septations, and fluid-fluid levels are very suggestive. CT scan is helpful to determine the bony anatomy and invasion of bone by tumor in order to decide on required stabilization procedures. MRI is helpful to determine the relationship of the tumor from the adjacent neural structures.[31]

Typically, diagnosis is made on the basis of imaging. Rarely is there a need for biopsy, though the histology is the definitive diagnostic modality.[31]

ABC display cavernous spaces with blood filled centers without endothelial lining separated by fibrous septa composed of fibroblasts and osteoclasts.[31]

Medical/Surgical Management

The literature describes a combination of treatments, ranging from curettage, subtotal excision, en bloc resection, embolization, intralesional injection, and radiation.[31] For lesions that are asymptomatic, conservative treatment with or without bracing is indicated. For larger lesions with neurological compromise, surgical treatment is recommended. No definitive studies exist demonstrating optimal surgical management but most studies recommend en bloc resection, which is associated with higher intraoperative blood loss and requirement for transfusion, but decreases recurrence rate dramatically.[31] En bloc resections will require a multiple stage approach with instrumentation and fusion.[31] Preoperative embolization may play a role in management.[32]

Complications

Complications of surgical management include infection, bleeding, and instrumentation failure.

Prognosis

Indolent lesions may resolve spontaneously over months.[30] No documented cases of malignant transformation have been recorded. Overall recurrence rate is 28% and they are generally within the first 2 years. Therefore, continued follow-up with imaging studies is recommended.[31]

OSTEOBLASTOMA

Workup

Osteoblastomas are rare benign tumors of the spine that are very similar to osteoid osteomas, but are larger than 2 cm in size. It is seen in young adults and adolescents, and usually does not cause localized night pain, unlike osteoid osteomas. Additionally, pain is typically not controlled with aspirin use. 36% of osteoblastomas occur in the spine.[33,34]

Patients typically complain of focal pain that is not controlled with use of nonsteroidal anti-inflammatory medication. Large spinal lesions may present with acute pathological fracture and/or spinal cord compression with evidence of myelopathy on physical examination.

X-rays and CT scans demonstrate the predilection for the posterior elements and show a radiolucent lesion with surrounding reactive bone with or without expansion. Bone scan will show intense isotope uptake at the site of tumor.[33]

Diagnosis is based on history and imaging. If the diagnosis is not clear, biopsy should be performed.[33]

On histology, these tumors are similar to osteoid osteomas, with production of surrounding osteoid and primitive woven bone, with areas of fibrovascular connective tissue nearby. Osteoblasts are seen in great numbers.[33]

Medical/Surgical Management

Typically, these tumors do not resolve spontaneously. For tumors that are small, conservative treatment and observation is warranted. For tumors that increase in

CHAPTER 43

size, cause mass effect upon nearby neural structures, or cause progressive spinal instability and deformity, surgical treatment is recommended. However, no definitive surgical treatment exists for these particular tumors of the spine. Some advocate intralesional excision while others recommend en bloc resection.[35] For larger lesions and en bloc resections, a multiple-staged procedure is performed with both anterior and posterior approach, along with instrumentation and fusion.[34,35] Similar to chordoma surgery, intracapsular extension of resection will increase likelihood of recurrence.[33,34] For patients with intralesional resection, radiation therapy can be used as an adjunct for local control[35] with good results, though it is typically not radiosensitive.

Complications

Complications of surgical management include infection, bleeding, and instrumentation failure.

Prognosis

These tumors have a capacity for malignant transformation of 12–25%.[35]

CHONDROSARCOMA/OSTEOSARCOMA

Workup

Osteosarcomas are malignant tumors of the bone. It is of mesenchymal origin.[36] Osteosarcomas are generally seen in adolescents or patients in their 20s. They rarely affect the spine.[36] Chondrosarcomas are malignant tumors of the cartilage that are seen in patients between ages 30 and 70.[37] They are locally aggressive with a high recurrence rate.[37] The thoracic spine is the most common site of involvement of the spine.[38]

Osteosarcomas typically cause pain during both day and night.[36] They may grow large enough to cause neurological symptoms such as focal back pain or radicular pain.[36] Chondrosarcomas may present with focal pain or with neurological symptoms such as weakness, perineal numbness, and bowel/bladder dysfunction if the mass is large and extends into the spinal canal. Cervical or thoracic chondrosarcomas may cause myelopathy.

X-rays and CT scans for osteosarcomas demonstrate a destructive lytic lesion with evidence of new bony formation and periosteal reaction. There may or may not be an associated soft tissue mass.[36] X-rays and CT scans for chondrosarcomas demonstrate irregularly mottled calcification with bony destruction and invasion. MRI will demonstrate a heterogeneously enhancing mass with hypointensity on T1 and hyperintensity on T2 imaging.

Imaging and history are used to make the diagnosis. However, in cases where the diagnosis is not clear, a biopsy may be performed.[36]

Osteosarcomas demonstrate pleomorphic giant and atypical cells with mitotic figures. They produce osteoid with eosinophilic trabecula with occasional areas of calcification. The tumor cells are within the osteoid matrix. Chondrosarcomas demonstrate undifferentiated cartilaginous cells with mitotic figures and atypia.[36,37]

Medical/Surgical Management

Sarcomas of the spine are quite complex but in cases of neurological compromise from compression and/or instability, surgical treatment is warranted. A recent meta-analysis done for Ewings sarcoma demonstrated a strong recommendation with moderate quality evidence for neoadjuvant (before surgery) chemotherapy for local control and long-term survival. Additionally, there is a weak recommendation with very low evidence for an en bloc surgical resection followed by conventional radiotherapy for improved local control without improvement in overall survival. En bloc resection may be performed and typically involves a multistage anterior and posterior reconstruction with instrumentation and fusion.[37,38] For osteogenic sarcomas, there is a strong recommendation with moderate evidence for neoadjuvant (before surgery) chemotherapy in offering significant improvements in local control and long-term survival. Also, there is a strong recommendation with very low evidence for en bloc resection in providing improved local control and improved overall survival.[37,38]

Complications

Complications of surgical management include infection, bleeding, and instrumentation failure.

Prognosis

Most patients with osteosarcomas present with advanced stages. 70% of patients with detectable metastases will remain disease-free with surgical resection and chemotherapy. Metastatic disease is the most important factor for survival in patients with osteosarcoma. With adjunctive therapy such as chemotherapy, osteosarcoma survival is 50% over 5 years. Osteosarcomas are radioresistant. Surgical treatment is reserved for lesions that are causing neurologic compression and/or instability.

Chondrosarcomas, on the other hand, have recently undergone advances in surgical treatment that has dramatically affected patient progression-free survival.[37,38] En bloc resection without violation of tumor capsule has increased progression-free survival dramatically over 5 years. Outcome for chondrosarcomas is based on histology, patient age, and en bloc resection.[37,38]

OSTEOID OSTEOMA

Workup

Osteoid osteomas are benign tumors of the posterior elements of the spine that are less than 2 cm in size. They comprise 11% of all bone tumors and are most commonly seen in males between 4 and 25.[39]

Patients typically have intense pain at night that is relieved by aspirin.[39] Alcohol may precipitate a pain crisis. Often it is incidentally found.

X-rays and CT demonstrate areas of reactive bony formation with low attenuation nidus and sclerotic border.[40] Technetium bone scans may demonstrate intense uptake.[39-41] MRI demonstrates T1 nidus with intermediate signal intensity and T2 hypointensity with heterogeneous enhancement.[40]

Osteoid osteomas are diagnosed based on imaging studies.[40]

Osteoid osteomas demonstrate yellowish to red areas of osteoid and woven bone with interconnected trabeculae, amidst a background of vascularized, fibrous connective tissue.[39]

Medical/Surgical Management

Osteomas are typically self-limiting. Small lesions can be treated conservatively. Pain from these lesions typically responds to nonsteroidal anti-inflammatory drugs such as aspirin.[39,41] When pain is intractable or patient's tumor is causing instability or neural compromise, surgery is indicated. Surgical treatment generally involves instrumentation and fusion for tumors that are large and near neural structures.[41]

Complications

Complications of surgical management include infection, bleeding, and instrumentation failure.

Prognosis

No cases of malignant progression have been described.[39] Pain is usually well controlled with aspirin.[41]

FIBROUS DYSPLASIA

Workup

Fibrous dysplasia is a predominantly osteolytic disorder that affects young children and adolescents. It affects males and females equally.[42]

Fibrous dysplasia of the spine is quite rare but patients may present with focal back pain. Most of the time, patients are asymptomatic.[43]

X-rays, CT, and MRI demonstrate a ground-glass appearance with definite sclerotic margins. CT may show an expansile lesion with a blown-out cortical rim. McCune-Albright syndrome is a severe form of polyostotic fibrous dysplasia combined with an endocrinopathy and café-au-lait spots.[43]

Fibrous dysplasia is diagnosed based on imaging studies.

Classically, areas of curvilinear trabecular woven bone with a background of fibroblasts are seen. Foamy macrophages may also be seen.[43]

Medical/Surgical Management

Patients should undergo metabolic and endocrinological evaluation to treat an underlying vitamin D deficiency, phosphate wasting, and/or hyperparathyroidism. Oral bisphosphonates are effective for relief of pain in fibrous dysplasia.[44] Surgery is indicated in cases of neural compromise and/or instability. Surgical approach would depend on the location along the spinal axis. In some cases, a combined anterior and posterior approach with instrumentation and fusion may be indicated with an attempt to complete resection if possible.[45]

Complications

Complications of surgical management include infection, bleeding, and instrumentation failure.

Prognosis

Patients respond well to medical therapy with no evidence of malignant transformation reported.[44,45]

METASTATIC DISEASE

Workup

Approximately 70% of patients diagnosed with cancer have evidence of metastatic disease at the time of autopsy.[46] The spine is the most common osseous site of metastatic disease, with the thoracic spine being the most likely location. The most common metastatic tumors to the spinal column are—breast, lung, and prostate.[47] Other metastatic tumors that are commonly seen within the spine are renal cell carcinoma, gastrointestinal cancer, sarcoma, thyroid cancer, melanoma, and multiple myeloma. Common tumor types that cause metastatic spinal cord compression include breast cancer at 22%, lung cancer at 15%, and prostate cancer at 10%.[48]

Patients with metastatic spine disease can have a variety of presentations depending on location of metastasis and extent of tumor burden near adjacent neurological structures. Patients may complain of only focal back pain, or may present with acute paraplegia/quadriplegia from spinal cord compression.[46,47]

CT and MRI with contrast will demonstrate enhancing tumor either within the bony elements of the spine or extending into the epidural space. MRI is very useful to determine extent of tumor compression upon adjacent neural structures such as the spinal cord and nerve roots. Additionally, MRI is useful to look for any other lesions elsewhere. CT of the chest/abdomen/pelvis may reveal an underlying primary tumor.[46]

Typically the imaging modalities mentioned above are all that is required to obtain a diagnosis. In cases where the diagnosis is unclear, a CT-guided biopsy or open surgical biopsy may be obtained.

Surgical Management

Surgery for metastatic disease has gained momentum over the last few years. In the past, surgery for tumors of the vertebral columns was largely unsuccessful with laminectomy being the predominant procedure performed. Additionally, due to the failure of surgery at that time, alternative treatments such as radiotherapy were becoming popular to treat a variety of metastatic tumors. In recent years, more studies have been performed demonstrating an increase in quality of life and life expectancy in patients with metastatic spine disease.[49] Studies demonstrating the advantages of surgery were marked by the assumption that the operative patients had to be chosen wisely. In other words, preoperative prognostic factors are critical toward ultimate surgical success. Such factors include neurological compromise and preoperative adjunctive therapy, along with the general health of the patient and tumor histology. The role of preoperative embolization has reduced intraoperative blood loss, especially in cases of renal cell carcinoma. Additionally, the role of stereotactic radiosurgery and radiotherapy for metastatic spine disease revolutionized treatment paradigms. Many studies have demonstrated a benefit of radiation therapy with or without surgery in patients with metastatic spine pathology. For example, patients with documented myeloma with or without spinal cord compression have been shown to benefit from focused radiation therapy in the absence of acute surgical intervention. Other studies have demonstrated the safety and efficacy of radiosurgery, even in the presence of prior radiotherapy, in the treatment of patients with spinal metastatic disease.[49] Additionally, the role of vertebroplasty in palliative treatment of spinal metastases has helped in symptomatic control of pain for these patients affected.[50]

Complications

Complications of surgical management of metastatic tumors of the spine include infection, bleeding, and instrumentation failure, which may be caused by adjacent level tumor infiltration causing weakening of the fusion construct.

Prognosis

According to the most recent randomized clinical trial comparing surgery alone to surgery plus radiation for spinal metastatic disease, the surgical group alone demonstrated a remarkable postoperative ambulatory capacity and sphincter function significantly longer than the patients in the radiation group. Length of survival was not significantly affected.[49] Overall survival is based on extent of metastatic disease.

CONCLUSION

The primary and metastatic bony tumors of the spine are a diverse and heterogeneous group of tumors. They display specific pathophysiological mechanisms that are important to recognize when making decisions on patient management. Recent advances in radiosurgery and surgical technique have altered the mentality of mere palliative treatment for spinal oncologic disease to a more aggressive longer progression-free survival with good quality of life.

REFERENCES

1. Palumbo A, Anderson K. Multiple myeloma. N Engl J Med. 2011;364(11):1046-60.
2. Healey JH, Lane JM. Chordoma: a critical review of diagnosis and treatment. Orthop Clin North Am. 1989;20(3):417-26.
3. Bjornsson J, Wold LE, Ebersold MJ, et al. Chordoma of the mobile spine. A clinicopathologic analysis of 40 patients. Cancer. 1993;71(3):735-40.
4. Vujovic S, Henderon S, Presneau N, et al. Brachyury, a crucial regulator of notochordal development, is a novel biomarker for chordomas. J Pathol. 2006;209(2):157-65.
5. Bergh P, Kindblom LG, Gunterberg B, et al. Prognostic factors in chordoma of the sacrum and mobile spine: a study of 39 patients. Cancer. 2000;88(9):2122-34.
6. Schwab JH, Boland PJ, Agaram NP, et al. Chordoma and chondrosarcoma gene profile: implications for immunotherapy. Cancer Immunol Immunother. 2009;58(3):339-49.
7. Suit HD, Goitein M, Munzenrider J, et al. Definitive radiation therapy for chordoma and chondrosarcoma of base of skull and cervical spine. J Neurosurg. 1982;56(3):377-85.
8. Azzarelli A, Quagliuolo V, Cerasoli S, et al. Chordoma: natural history and treatment results in 33 cases. J Surg Oncol. 1988;37(3):185-91.
9. Hsieh PC, Gallia GL, Sciubba DM, et al. En bloc excisions of chordomas in the cervical spine: review of five consecutive cases with more than 4-year follow-up. Spine (Phila Pa 1976). 2011;36(24):E1581-7.
10. Sciubba DM, Gokaslan ZL, Black JH 3rd, et al. 5-Level spondylectomy for en bloc resection of thoracic chordoma: case report. Neurosurgery. 2011;69(2 Suppl Operative):onsE248-55; discussion onsE255-6.
11. Samson IR, Springfield DS, Suit HD, et al. Operative treatment of sacrococcygeal chordoma. A review of twenty-one cases. J Bone Joint Surg Am. 1993;75(10):1476-84.
12. Park L, Delaney TF, Liebsch NJ, et al. Sacral chordomas: impact of high-dose proton/photon-beam radiation therapy combined with or without surgery for primary versus recurrent tumor. Int J Radiat Oncol Biol Phys. 2006;65(5): 1514-21.
13. Kaiser TE, Pritchard DJ, Unni KK. Clinicopathologic study of sacrococcygeal chordoma. Cancer. 1984;53(11):2574-8.
14. Fuchs B, Dickey ID, Yaszemski MJ, et al. Operative management of sacral chordoma. J Bone Joint Surg Am. 2005;87(10):2211-6.
15. Chambers PW, Schwinn CP. Chordoma: a clinicopathologic study of metastasis. Am J Clin Pathol. 1979;72(5):765-76.
16. Balke M, Henrichs MP, Gosheger G, et al. Giant cell tumors of the axial skeleton. Sarcoma. 2012;2012(410973):1-10.
17. Sanjay BK, Sim FH, Unni KK, et al. Giant cell tumors of the spine. J Bone Joint Surg Br. 1993;75(1):148-54.
18. Filder MW. Surgical treatment of giant cell tumors of the thoracic and lumbar spine: report of nine patients. Eur Spine J. 2001;10(1):69-77.
19. Liljenqvist U Lerner T, Halm H, et al. En bloc spondylectomy in malignant tumors of the spine. Eur Spine J. 2008;17(4):600-9.
20. Chakravarti A, Spiro IJ, Hug EB, et al. Megavoltage radiation therapy for axial and inoperable giant-cell tumor of bone. J Bone Joint Surg Am. 1999;81(11):1566-73.
21. Donthineni R, Boriani L, Ofluoglu O, et al. Metastatic behavior of giant cell tumor of the spine. Int Orthop. 2009;33(2):497-501.
22. Ng VW, Clifton A, Moore AJ. Preoperative endovascular embolisation of a vertebral hemangioma. J Bone Joint Surg Br. 1997;79(5):808-11.
23. Karlin CA, Brower AC. Multiple primary hemangiomas of bone. Am J Roentgenol. 1977;129(1):162-4.
24. Jankowski R, Nowak S, Zukiel R, et al. Surgical treatment of symptomatic vertebral hemangiomas. Neurol Neurochir Pol. 2011;45(6):577-82.
25. Kumar V, Abbas A, Fausto N, et al. Robbins and Cotran Pathologic Basis of Disease, 8th edition. Philadelphia: Saunders; 2010. pp. 520-1.
26. Yeaom JS, Lee CK, Shin HY, et al. Langerhans' cell histiocytosis of the spine. Analysis of twenty-three cases. Spine (Phila Pa 1976). 1999;24(16):1740-9.
27. Seimon LP. Eosinophil granuloma of the spine. J Pediatr Orthop. 1981;1(4):371-6.
28. Katz RL, Silva EG, deSantos LA, et al. Diagnosis of eosinophilic granuloma of bone by cytology, histology, and electron microscopy of transcutaneous bone-aspiration biopsy. J Bone Joint Surg Am. 1980;62(8):1284-90.
29. Chen SY, Chao SC, Kao TH, et al. Surgical treatment using mesh cage and plate fixation in a 9-year-old child with solitary histiocytosis lesion in the cervical spine. Eur J Pediatric Surg. 2011;21(3):189-91.
30. Papagelopoulos PJ, Choudhury SN, Frassica FJ, et al. Treatment of aneurysmal bone cysts of the pelvis and sacrum. J Bone Joint Surg Am. 2001;83(11):1674-81.
31. Zenonos G, Jamil O, Governale LS, et al. Surgical treatment for primary spinal aneurysmal bone cysts: experience from Children's Hospital Boston. J Neurosurg Pediatr. 2012;9(3):305-15.
32. Ameli NO, Abbassioun K, Saleh H, et al. Aneurysmal bone cysts of the spine. Report of 17 cases. J Neurosurg. 1985;63(5):685-90.

33. Boriani S, Capanna R, Donati D, et al. Osteoblastoma of the spine. Clin Orthop Relat Res. 1992;278:37-45.
34. Boriani S, Amendola L, Bandiera S, et al. Staging and treatment of osteoblastoma in the mobile spine: a review of 51 cases. Eur Spine J. 2012;21(10):2003-10.
35. Marsh BW, Bonfiglio M, Brady LP, et al. Benign osteoblastoma: range of manifestations. J Bone Joint Surg Am. 1975;57(1):1-9.
36. Shives TC, Dahlin DC, Sim FH, et al. Osteosarcoma of the spine. J Bone Joint Surg Am. 1986;68(5):660-8.
37. Sciubba DM, Okuno S, Dekutoski MB, et al. Ewing and osteogenic sarcoma: evidence for multidisciplinary management. Spine (Phila Pa 1976). 2009;34(Suppl 22): S58-68.
38. Hsieh PC, Xu R, Sciubba DM, et al. Long term clinical outcomes following en bloc resections for sacral chordomas and chondrosarcomas: a series of twenty consecutive patients. Spine (Phila Pa 1976). 2009;34(20):2233-9.
39. Cohen MD, Harrington TM, Ginsburg WW. Osteoid osteomas: 95 cases and a review of the literature. Semin Arthritis Rheum. 1983;12(3):265-81.
40. Ropper AE, Cahill KS, Hanna JW, et al. Primary vertebral tumors: a review of epidemiologic, histological, and imaging findings, Part I: benign tumors. Neurosurgery. 2010;69(6):1171-80.
41. Lisbona R, Rosenthall L. Role of radionuclide imaging in osteoid osteomas. Am J Roentgenol. 1979;132(1):77-80.
42. Harris WH, Dudley HR Jr, Barry RJ. The natural history of fibrous dysplasia: an orthopaedic, pathological, and roentgenographic study. J Bone Joint Surg Am. 1962;44-A:207-33.
43. Kumar V, Abbas AK, Fausto N, et al. Robbins Basic Pathology. 8th edition. Philadelphia, PA: Elsevier Health Sciences; 2007. pp. 1-960.
44. Chapurlat RD. Medical therapy in adults with fibrous dysplasia of bone. J Bone Miner Res. 2006;21(Suppl 2):P114-9.
45. Medow JE, Agrawal BM, Resnick DK. Polyostotic fibrous dysplasia of the cervical spine: case report and review of the literature. Spine J. 2007;7(6):712-5.
46. Metastatic tumors of the spine: diagnosis and treatment. J Am Acad Orthop Surg. 1993;1(2):76-86.
47. Böhm P, Huber J. The surgical treatment of bony metastases of the spine and limbs. J Bone Joint Surg Br. 2002;84(4):521-9.
48. Gerszten PC, Welch WC. Current surgical management of metastatic spinal disease. Oncology (Williston Park). 2000;14(7):1013-24; discussion 1024, 1029-30.
49. Patchell R, Tibbs P, Regine W, et al. A randomized trial of direct decompressive surgical resection in the treatment of spinal cord compression caused by metastasis. J Clin Oncol. 2003;21:237.
50. Fourney DR, Schomer DF, Nader R, et al. Percutaneous vertebroplasty and Kyphoplasty for painful vertebral body fractures in cancer patients. J Neurosurg. 2003;98(Suppl 1): 21-30.

SECTION 6

Future Trends in Spine Surgery

CHAPTER 44 Future of Spine Surgery

Shaleen Vira, Jacob Enders, Ghaith Habboub, Michael P Steinmetz, Edward C Benzel

INTRODUCTION

The future of spine surgery is bright! The quest our profession has is to deliver affordable care in a reliable and reproducible manner. Spine surgeons today are able to improve the lives of their patients like never before, and are enabled by the ever-increasing influx of resources and technological development dedicated to better understand spinal pathologies. Innovations in both care delivery and surgical technologies have enabled us to better achieve this lofty goal and present numerous challenges as to when to appropriately deploy each innovation.

OUTPATIENT SURGERY AND THE GROWTH OF AMBULATORY SURGERY CENTERS

As medical care in the United States increasingly emphasizes value-based care, ambulatory surgery centers (ASCs) have begun to grow due to their potential benefits including smaller size, specialization, and cost containment.[1,2] Indeed, rates of outpatient surgery have increased 40% in the last 10 years among Medicare beneficiaries.[3] As technology continues to improve and surgical techniques have become less invasive, spine surgery in particular has started to shift toward utilizing ASCs to deliver care.[1,4] ASCs have the benefit of reduced costs compared to inpatient settings, with a recent study by Purger et al. showing that the cost of ambulatory anterior cervical discectomy and fusion (ACDF) was less than half that of inpatient ACDFs.[5] Similarly, for lumbar diskectomy, Bekelis et al. found that outpatient charges were approximately $11,000, while inpatient charges for the same procedure were approximately $24,000.[6]

It is also important to consider the safety of procedures performed in an outpatient setting. Chin and coauthors reported their criteria for selecting patients for ambulatory spine surgery and noted that inpatients with body mass index (BMI) of less than 42, and in the absence of cancer, major trauma, deformity, or infection, outpatient spine surgery was associated with good outcomes and similar complication rates were seen in the inpatient setting.[4] The authors also limited their outpatient spine surgery to two or fewer vertebral levels due to the decreased risk of blood loss and the shorter operation time.[4] Kamson et al. reported the results of 178 patients undergoing lumbar decompressive surgery in an ASC and noted complication rates and reoperation rates similar to or lower than those reported previously in the literature.[7]

Long-term efficacy and reoperation rates are additional components to consider with outpatient spine surgery. Pendharkar and coauthors reviewed studies on lumbar laminectomy and diskectomy, lumbar fusion, ACDF, and cervical disk arthroplasty, and found that lumbar decompression had the largest amount of data supporting its safety in the outpatient setting.[3] However, they noted that ACDF may be associated with higher reoperation rates if surgery was performed in an ASC instead of a hospital.[3] More level I and II evidence along with longer-term follow-up studies are needed on patient outcomes in ASCs because most studies are retrospective analyses of comparatively small patient cohorts. Yet, ASCs seem to be safe and effective for spine surgery provided patients have limited comorbidities and undergo surgery on one or a few spinal levels. In the future, utilization of these novel delivery environments will continue to increase.

ROBOTS AND NAVIGATION IN SPINE SURGERY

Technology will likely play an even larger role than care setting in the coming years. Robot-assisted surgery, for instance, continues to make important advances across many specialties. The field of urology has made use of robots, in particular the da Vinci Surgical System, in prostatectomies and partial nephrectomies for many years.[8] Surgical robots have arms that are more maneuverable than human hands or laparoscopic instruments, and offer increased stability and fine manipulation capabilities not always possible with other image-guided or open approaches.[8,9] In the field of spine surgery, robots such as the Mazor robot are seeing increased use for pedicle screw placement.[9] The Mazor robot is bone-mounted and relies on intraoperative fluoroscopy for proper screw placement, and studies have shown the Mazor robot to be accurate, with proper screw placement rates above 90%.[10,11] Real-time intraoperative imaging with devices such as the O-arm by Medtronic, Inc., that reduce the need for repetitive X-ray shots has allowed for increased accuracy in pedicle screw placement while also decreasing radiation exposure to the operative team.[12] Radiation reduction may also be beneficial for better long-term health outcomes in radiosensitive pediatric patients.

Additional improvements in robotic imaging and navigation have been made with the ExcelsiusGPS system developed by Globus Medical Inc. The system is novel due to its ability to monitor navigation integrity in real-time, the ability to attach to the operating room floor, and its incorporation of a rigid end effector for drilling and screw placement by the surgeon.[13] Ahmed et al. reported the case of a 69-year-old female who underwent L4–L5 decompression with pedicle screw fixation using the ExcelsiusGPS system.[13] The surgical team used a 3D cone beam computed tomography (CT) scan from an O-arm, and the images were transferred to the ExcelsiusGPS system for screw planning. The robot successfully facilitated screw placement and the patient was only exposed to 8 mSv of radiation total from the O-arm and fluoroscopic imaging.[13] The patient also had remarkable improvement in her back and lower extremity pain at 6 weeks postoperation.

Despite the enthusiasm in the literature, it is important to consider that robotic surgery is still in its infancy. Sample sizes in published reports are often small, and concerns have been raised about soft tissue, nerve, and vascular injury caused by robotic surgery. Further, problems with image registration and inappropriate sliding of the drill guide can cause robot failure.[9] In addition, there is additional time added to surgical procedures when robots are used due to the time required for docking the robot in the operative field and registering patient images. In an era where cost, quality, and efficiency are becoming increasingly important in medicine, robots will need to be objectively improve value in order for institutions to justify their high costs.

Artificial Intelligence/Machine Learning

Like robotics, artificial intelligence (AI) is exploding in many fields in healthcare and spine surgery is just one of them. Machine learning (ML) is a branch of AI that is currently attracting a lot of attention due to its capabilities in linking complex interactions between data variables. ML is shining in many healthcare specialties including dermatology, ophthalmology, radiology, genomics and other specialties.[14-16] ML's major difference to traditional AI algorithms is that we write the rules in general AI; while in ML, the algorithm defines the rules through learning from data as described in Figure 1. Several studies in spine surgeries are using ML to link unseen correlations between variables and outcome in several areas including degenerative spine, spinal deformity, epidural abscess and others.[17-19] All these studies are trying to accomplish precision personalized care for patients as opposed to the current general binning methods used. Another field in spine surgery where ML will soon play a major role is robotics. ML excels in optimizing action selection in robotics.[20] Recent advances in ML algorithms are granting robots capabilities of autonomous actions to perform complex tasks which can be translated into the robot performing part of the surgeon job autonomously.

Natural language processing is another field of ML which is dedicated on the study of language and AI. It has been heavily utilized in the unstructured healthcare data including notes, radiology reports, pathology reports and others to link notes to outcomes.[21] Mobile devices are an excellent platform where all these ML algorithms can directly interact with patients. Chatbots (Chat robots) can directly communicate with patients, collect information, communicate with ML algorithms running on either the device or at host services, and then provide meaningful results back to patients.[22] These platforms can be used for monitoring our patients in between office visits and

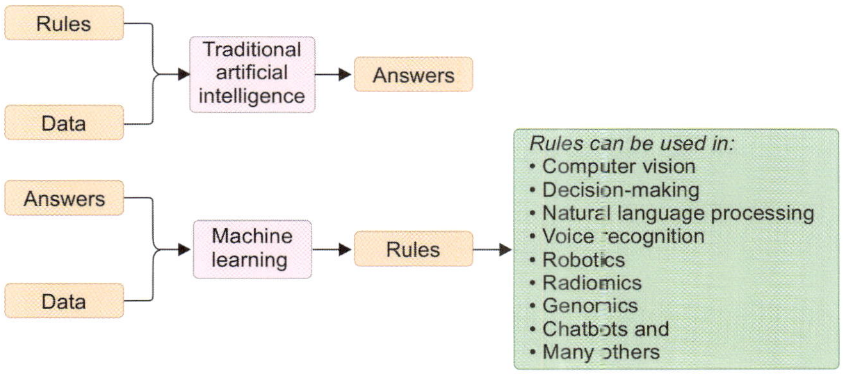

Fig. 1: Differences between traditional artificial intelligence and machine learning.

thus providing continuous healthcare to our patients. As more improvements are made, AI, ML, and robotics will likely continue to see increased use in a variety of surgical settings due to the benefits they can provide.

Continued Expansion of Minimally Invasive Surgery

Minimally invasive surgery has seen rapid growth across surgical specialties in the last two decades. Laparoscopic surgery is now commonplace for bariatric and urological procedures, and arthroscopy is often used in the surgical treatment of orthopedic conditions. Minimally invasive spine surgery may offer the benefits of decreased blood loss, lower rates of infection and neurological injury, and earlier patient ambulation following the procedure.[23,24] For instance, partial hemilaminectomy involves leaving the laminae and interspinous ligaments intact while pathologic lesions are removed, helping preserve spinal stability and integrity postoperatively.[25] Other techniques including unilateral laminotomy for bilateral decompression and split laminotomy may be used depending on the location of pathology to maintain at least partial muscle and facet integrity.[25]

Endoscopic techniques have been developed to reduce incision size while allowing for three-dimensional visualization and larger working space compared to earlier devices.[26] By reducing tissue trauma through the use of small working channels, recovery time and healing are improved compared to open surgery, and long-term follow-up studies at 5 years and 10 years have shown that patients achieve reductions in disability and back pain comparable to traditional surgical methods.[27,28]

Current limitations of minimally invasive spine procedures include a steep learning curve that usually requires advanced fellowship training and the variety of techniques with overlapping clinical uses. Instruments may also break or malfunction, and problems with working-space visualization can lead to complications including dural tears or nerve injury. Minimally invasive spine surgery may become more commonplace as endoscopic training is incorporated into orthopedic and neurosurgical residency programs and additional studies identify superior techniques for a given clinical condition.

Motion Preservation Technologies

Important advances are being made in spine technologies as well. A well-known complication of interbody fusion surgery is adjacent segment disease (ASD) where vertebral levels above and below the site of fusion begin to degenerate causing problems with spinal stability.[29] Fusion also results in increased stiffness, and as a result new technologies are being developed to preserve motion and native loading conditions to prevent additional degeneration. For instance, one-level anterior cervical diskectomy and fusion (ACDF) can reduce neck motion by about 7°, and two-level ACDF can significantly decrease range-of-motion and impair quality of life.[30,31] Cervical disk arthroplasty (CDA) is one promising motion preservation technology that involves removing a patient's damaged or herniated intervertebral disk and replacing it with a device consisting of metal endplates that attach to adjacent vertebral bodies and are connected by a flexible linker.[32]

In their 2018 systematic review, Laratta et al. examined randomized controlled trials, biomechanical studies, and case series comparing ACDF to CDA.[33] They found that ACDF patients had higher rates of reoperation and higher average costs than CDA, and that CDA was associated with increased range-of-motion compared to ACDF. Importantly, they found only moderate evidence that CDA was associated with decreased rates of adjacent-segment disease over ACDF, and that CDA had slightly higher rates of revision surgery.[33] As technology continues to improve and more long-term evidence is gathered on two-level or greater CDA, cervical motion preservation will likely continue to see increased use to help patients maintain greater quality of life.

Posterior dynamic stabilization of the lumbar spine has gathered interest in recent years because of the ability to limit ASD in the lumbar spine. Devices such as the X-stop by Medtronic and the CoFlex system by Paradigm Spine, LLC, hold the spine in slight flexion, and in doing so help decompress the spinal cord and adjacent nerve roots.[32] The Dynesys system by Zimmer similarly helps to control spine extension and flexion by combining a compressible tube with a tension-resistant polyester cord.[32] These devices help to preserve motion while also reducing spine loading responsible for disk degeneration and instability.[34] The future of these devices will lie in their ability to match native range-of-motion and ensure osseointegration through the use of materials technology. They may also continue to see increased use as longer-term follow-up studies provide evidence of efficacy.

Surface Technologies to Promote Fusion

Fusion surgery often involves the placement of interbody spacers or cages that maintain disk height and distribute load to promote bone growth and fusion. These cages have traditionally been made of titanium alloys or polyetheretherketone (PEEK), each of which has its own advantages and disadvantages. Titanium alloys such as Ti-6Al-4V are often used because they form a nonreactive TiO_2 surface layer that can facilitate bone ongrowth.[35] Surface modifications to titanium cages such as increased roughness and porosity induce growth factor expression to further increase implant osseointegration.[35-37] However, titanium has a high elastic modulus of about 110 GPa that can cause stress-shielding effects that lead to degeneration of the surrounding bone, and the radiopacity of titanium may make radiographic fusion assessment difficult in the clinic.[38-40] PEEK offers solutions to some of these challenges due to its much lower elastic modulus of about 3–4 GPa and radiolucency.[41,42] However, PEEK is a chemically inert and hydrophobic material that results in decreased bone apposition at the implant surface, leading to what has been termed the “PEEK-halo” effect.[43-45] Therefore, recent work has focused on the development of surface modifications and coatings to both titanium and PEEK to improve upon these materials’ drawbacks.

One method to increase the osseointegration of PEEK that has recently been developed is the application of a titanium coating to a PEEK cage. Two recent studies describe the use of vacuum plasma-spraying and electron-beam deposition for the application of titanium coatings to PEEK, demonstrating the feasibility of this technique.[46,47] A study by McGilvray et al. in 2017 also notes the superiority of Ti-coated PEEK in measures of stiffness and range-of-motion compared to uncoated PEEK.[40] However, a 2016 article by Kienle et al. describes potential wear-debris associated with Ti-coated PEEK interbody cages when these cages were impacted into vertebral body substitutes.[48] The authors note that over half of the wear particles were of a size large enough to be phagocytosed, raising potential concerns about postoperative chronic inflammation.[48]

An alternative strategy has been to fabricate and utilize porous PEEK, which has recently been shown to increase bone apposition relative to titanium-coated PEEK.[49,50] In their study, Torstrick and coauthors cultured mouse preosteoblast cells on smooth, porous, and Ti-coated PEEK disks cultured for 14 days after cells were confluent on the surface, and found that porous PEEK had increased levels of bone markers such as osteocalcin and VEGF compared to smooth or Ti-coated PEEK.[49] The authors also performed pullout testing on plugs inserted into rat tibias for all three materials, and found porous PEEK implants had the highest pullout strength, demonstrating superior osseointegration of this material design.[49] Using porous PEEK may serve to reduce the PEEK-halo effect discussed previously and serve to improve bone integration and fusion relative to other material designs. It is important to note, however, that many of these studies have been done in vitro or in animal models; therefore, large-scale randomized clinical trials may be needed to confirm or refute these experimental findings.

3D Printing

In recent years, 3D printing has seen an exponential increase in use across many different disciplines including the aeronautical industry,[51] dentistry,[52] and medicine.[53] Through the use of computer-aided design (CAD) software, unique shapes can be designed and printed using a variety of materials at a fraction of the cost of traditional manufacturing techniques such as milling or injection molding. While early methods used a nozzle to extrude heat-softened plastic onto a moving platform, newer methods may use laser sintering where layers are created from metal powders and are subsequently fused together, or may use stereolithography where a light source hardens resin in layers from a moving container of fluid.[54] The newer techniques of sintering and stereolithography offer more precision and are able to create models that can withstand sterilization.[54] In the field of spine surgery, recent work has focused on the application of 3D printing for surgical planning and creating customizable implants for a patient's individual anatomy.[55]

For instance, Goel et al. reported the use of thin CT sections for the creation of 3D printed models for surgical planning in 11 cases of craniovertebral anomalies.[56] The authors used the 3D models prepared preoperatively to choose rod and screw sizes and had access to those models intraoperatively to use as a guide.[56] Similarly, Guo and coauthors reported the use of 3D printed templates for pedicle screw placement in the cervical spine.[57] Placement of pedicle screws in the cervical spine is accompanied by risks such as vertebral artery injury, and thus pedicle screws must be placed with care. In this study, Guo et al. showed that the use of 3D printed models decreased operative time and significantly increased rates of acceptable pedicle screw fixation compared to traditional methods involving intraoperative CT scanning, demonstrating the efficacy of 3D printed templates for surgical guidance.[57] The reduced use of X-rays by using a physical model as a guide is also safer for patients and operating room staff alike.

However, 3D printing does carry drawbacks including the technological challenges of getting personnel accustomed to computer design software, the costs in purchasing 3D printers and necessary software, and the development time required to create unique models for a given patient's anatomy.[57,58] Indeed, it may be challenging from a financial perspective for hospitals to justify these costs, and many patients may not be able to shoulder the expenses either. As a result, the utility of 3D printed models in routine spinal surgery cases may be limited until models can be produced cheaply and quickly, and larger cost-controlled analyses are likely needed to justify widespread adoption of 3D printing technology in spine fusion.

CONCLUSION

We foresee an ever-increasing focus on utilizing care delivery innovations with technological advancements in surgical implants and instrumentation in the way we deliver spine care. With these advances come many unknowns. Under what situations is a given technology cost-effective? What care delivery models improve the level efficacy while maintaining safety? What are going to be the indications for utilizing each of these advancements? In summary, we know less about our own profession than physicians in other medical specialties know about their respective fields! This conclusion is both humbling and inspiring—the future of spine surgery will be a delightful journey as we navigate through these challenges and make the best of every opportunity possible to improve the lives of our patients.

REFERENCES

1. Gologorsky Y. Outpatient spine surgery: transition to the Ambulatory Surgery Center. World Neurosurg. 2018;114:369-70.
2. Best MJ, Buller LT, Eismont FJ. National trends in ambulatory surgery for intervertebral disc disorders and spinal stenosis: A 12-year analysis of the National Surveys of Ambulatory Surgery. Spine (Phila Pa 1976). 2015;40(21):1703-11.
3. Pendharkar AV, Shahin MN, Ho AL, et al. Outpatient spine surgery: defining the outcomes, value, and barriers to implementation. Neurosurg Focus. 2018;44(5):E11.
4. Chin KR, Pencle FJ, Coombs AV, et al. Eligibility of outpatient spine surgery candidates in a single private practice. Clin Spine Surg. 2017;30(10):E1352-8.
5. Purger DA, Pendharkar AV, Ho AL, et al. Outpatient vs inpatient anterior cervical discectomy and fusion: a population-level analysis of outcomes and cost. Neurosurgery. 2018;82(4):454-64.
6. Bekelis K, Missios S, Kakoulides G, et al. Selection of patients for ambulatory lumbar discectomy: results from four US states. Spine J. 2014;14(9):1944-50.
7. Kamson S, Trescot AM, Sampson PD, et al. Full-endoscopic assisted lumbar decompressive surgery performed in an outpatient, ambulatory facility: report of 5 years of complications and risk factors. Pain Physician. 2017;20(2):E221-31.
8. Honda M, Morizane S, Hikita K, et al. Current status of robotic surgery in urology. Asian J Endosc Surg. 2017;10(4):372-81.

CHAPTER 44

9. Joseph JR, Smith BW, Liu X, et al. Current applications of robotics in spine surgery: a systematic review of the literature. Neurosurg Focus. 2017;42(5):E2.
10. Kim HJ, Jung WI, Chang BS, et al. A prospective, randomized, controlled trial of robot-assisted vs freehand pedicle screw fixation in spine surgery. Int J Med Robot. 2017;13(3).
11. Hyun SJ, Kim KJ, Jahng TA, et al. Minimally invasive robotic versus open fluoroscopic-guided spinal instrumented fusions: a randomized controlled trial. Spine (Phila Pa 1976). 2017;42(6):353-8.
12. Shin MH, Hur JW, Ryu KS, et al. Prospective comparison study between the fluoroscopy-guided and navigation coupled with O-arm-guided pedicle screw placement in the thoracic and lumbosacral spines. J Spinal Disord Tech. 2015;28(6):E347-51.
13. Ahmed AK, Zygourakis CC, Kalb S, et al. First spine surgery utilizing real-time image-guided robotic assistance. Comput Assist Surg (Abingdon). 2019:1-5.
14. Esteva A, Kuprel B, Novoa RA, et al. Dermatologist-level classification of skin cancer with deep neural networks. Nature. 2017;542(7639):115-8.
15. Gulshan V, Peng L, Coram M, et al. Development and validation of a deep learning algorithm for detection of diabetic retinopathy in retinal fundus photographs. JAMA. 2016;316(22): 2402-10.
16. Poplin R, Varadarajan AV, Blumer K, et al. Prediction of cardiovascular risk factors from retinal fundus photographs via deep learning. Nat Biomed Eng. 2018;2(3):158-64.
17. Ames CP, Smith JS, Pellisé F, et al. European Spine Study Group, International Spine Study Group. Development of deployable predictive models for minimal clinically important difference achievement across the commonly used health-related quality of life instruments in adult spinal deformity surgery. Spine (Phila Pa 1976). 2019.
18. Mroz TE, Habboub G. Artificial Intelligence can Redefine Value-Based Spine Care. It's Already Starting To. ConsultQD. 2018. [online] Available from: https://consultqd.clevelandclinic.org/artificial-intelligence-can-redefine-value-based-spine-care-its-already-starting-to/. [Last accessed July 2019].
19. Shah AA, Ogink PT, Nelson SB, et al. Nonoperative management of spinal epidural abscess: development of a predictive algorithm for failure. J Bone Joint Surg Am. 2018;100(7):546-55.
20. Bousmalis K, Irpan A, Wohlhart P, et al. Using Simulation and Domain Adaptation to Improve Efficiency of Deep Robotic Grasping. 2018 IEEE International Conference on Robotics and Automation (ICRA). Brisbane, QLD: IEEE; 2018. pp. 4243-50.
21. Rajkomar A, Oren E, Chen K, et al. Scalable and accurate deep learning with electronic health records. NPJ Digit Med. 2018;1:18.
22. Habboub G, Mroz TE. Healthcare at your fingertips. AANS Neurosurgeon. 2018;27(4):5.
23. Uribe JS, Beckman J, Mummaneni PV, et al.; MIS-ISSG Group. Does MIS surgery allow for shorter constructs in the surgical treatment of adult spinal deformity? Neurosurgery. 2017;80(3):489-97.
24. Liu G, Liu S, Zuo YZ, et al. Recent advances in technique and clinical outcomes of minimally invasive spine surgery in adult scoliosis. Chin Med J (Engl). 2017;130(21):2608-15.
25. Banczerowski P, Czigléczki G, Papp Z, et al. Minimally invasive spine surgery: systematic review. Neurosurg Rev. 2015;38(1):11-26.
26. Oppenheimer JH, DeCastro I, McDonnell DE. Minimally invasive spine technology and minimally invasive spine surgery: a historical review. Neurosurg Focus. 2009;27(3):E9.
27. Casal-Moro R, Castro-Menéndez M, Hernández-Blanco M, et al. Long-term outcome after microendoscopic diskectomy for lumbar disk herniation: a prospective clinical study with a 5-year follow-up. Neurosurgery. 2011;68(6):1568-75.
28. Wang M, Zhou Y, Wang J, et al. A 10-year follow-up study on long-term clinical outcomes of lumbar microendoscopic discectomy. J Neurol Surg A Cent Eur Neurosurg. 2012; 73(4):195-8.
29. Wu JC, Hsieh PC, Mummaneni PV, et al. Spinal motion preservation surgery. Biomed Res Int. 2015;2015:372502.
30. Fay LY, Huang WC, Tsai TY, et al. Differences between arthroplasty and anterior cervical fusion in two-level cervical degenerative disc disease. Eur Spine J. 2014;23(3):627-34.
31. Kim SW, Limson MA, Kim SB, et al. Comparison of radiographic changes after ACDF versus Bryan disk arthroplasty in single and bi-level cases. Eur Spine J. 2009;18(2):218-31.
32. Serhan H, Mhatre D, Defossez H, et al. Motion-preserving technologies for degenerative lumbar spine: The past, present, and future horizons. SAS J. 2011;5(3):75-89.
33. Laratta JL, Shillingford JN, Saifi C, et al. Cervical disk arthroplasty: a comprehensive review of single-level, multi-level, and hybrid procedures. Glob Spine J. 2018;8(1):78-83.
34. Erbulut DU, Zafarparandeh I, Ozer AF, et al. Biomechanics of posterior dynamic stabilization systems. Adv Orthop. 2013;2013:451956.
35. Rao PJ, Pelletier MH, Walsh WR, et al. Spine interbody implants: material selection and modification, functionalization and bioactivation of surfaces to improve osseointegration. Orthop Surg. 2014;6(2):81-9.
36. Gittens RA, Olivares-Navarrete R, Schwartz Z, et al. Implant osseointegration and the role of microroughness and nanostructures: Lessons for spine implants. Acta Biomater. 2014;10(8):3363-71.
37. Olivares-Navarrete R, Hyzy SL, Gittens RA 1st, et al. Rough titanium alloys regulate osteoblast production of angiogenic factors. Spine J. 2013;13(11):1563-70.
38. Wu SH, Li Y, Zhang YQ, et al. Porous titanium-6 aluminum-4 vanadium cage has better osseointegration and less micro-motion than a poly-ether-ether-ketone cage in sheep vertebral fusion. Artif Organs. 2013;37(12):E191-201.
39. Wang Z, Fu S, Wu ZX, et al. Ti2448 pedicle screw system augmentation for posterior lumbar interbody fusion. Spine (Phila Pa 1976). 2013;38(23):2008-15.
40. McGilvray KC, Waldorff EI, Easley J, et al. Evaluation of a polyetheretherketone (PEEK) titanium composite interbody spacer in an ovine lumbar interbody fusion model: biomechanical, microcomputed tomographic, and histologic analyzes. Spine J. 2017;17(12):1907-16.

41. Pelletier MH, Cordaro N, Punjabi VM, et al. PEEK versus Ti interbody fusion devices: resultant fusion, bone apposition, initial and 26-week biomechanics. Clin Spine Surg. 2016;29(4):E208-14.
42. Schimmel JJP, Poeschmann MS, Horsting PP, et al. PEEK cages in lumbar fusion: mid-term clinical outcome and radiologic fusion. Clin Spine Surg. 2016;29(5):E252-8.
43. Walsh WR, Bertollo N, Christou C, et al. Plasma-sprayed titanium coating to polyetheretherketone improves the bone-implant interface. Spine J. 2015;15(5):1041-9.
44. Sagomonyants KB, Jarman-Smith ML, Devine JN, et al. The in vitro response of human osteoblasts to polyetheretherketone (PEEK) substrates compared to commercially pure titanium. Biomaterials. 2008;29(11):1563-72.
45. Phan K, Hogan JA, Assem Y, et al. PEEK-Halo effect in interbody fusion. J Clin Neurosci. 2016;24:138-40.
46. Han CM, Lee EJ, Kim HE, et al. The electron beam deposition of titanium on polyetheretherketone (PEEK) and the resulting enhanced biological properties. Biomaterials. 2010;31(13):3465-70.
47. Hoppe S, Albers CE, Elfiky T, et al. First results of a new Vacuum Plasma Sprayed (VPS) Titanium-Coated Carbon/PEEK Composite Cage for lumbar interbody fusion. J Funct Biomater. 2018;9(1). pii: E23.
48. Kienle A, Graf N, Wilke HJ. Does impaction of titanium-coated interbody fusion cages into the disc space cause wear debris or delamination? Spine J. 2016;16(2):235-42.
49. Torstrick FB, Lin ASP, Potter D, et al. Porous PEEK improves the bone-implant interface compared to plasma-sprayed titanium coating on PEEK. Biomaterials. 2018;185:106-16.
50. Carpenter RD, Klosterhoff BS, Torstrick FB, et al. Effect of porous orthopedic implant material and structure on load sharing with simulated bone ingrowth: A finite element analysis comparing titanium and PEEK. J Mech Behav Biomed Mater. 2018;80:68-76.
51. Joshi SC, Sheikh AA. 3D printing in aerospace and its long-term sustainability. Virtual Phys Prototyp. 2015;10(4):175-85.
52. Dawood A, Marti Marti B, Sauret-Jackson V, et al. 3D printing in dentistry. Br Dent J. 2015;219(11):521-9.
53. Christensen A, Rybicki FJ. Maintaining safety and efficacy for 3D printing in medicine. 3D Print Med. 2017;3(1):1.
54. Garg B, Mehta N. Current status of 3D printing in spine surgery. J Clin Orthop Trauma. 2018;9(3):218-25.
55. Wilcox B, Mobbs RJ, Wu AM, et al. Systematic review of 3D printing in spinal surgery: the current state of play. J Spine Surg. 2017;3(3):433-43.
56. Goel A, Jankharia B, Shah A, et al. Three-dimensional models: an emerging investigational revolution for craniovertebral junction surgery. J Neurosurg Spine. 2016;25(6):740-4.
57. Guo F, Dai J, Zhang J, et al. Individualized 3D printing navigation template for pedicle screw fixation in upper cervical spine. PLos One. 2017;12(2):e0171509.
58. Hsu MR, Haleem MS, Hsu W. 3D printing applications in minimally invasive spine surgery. Minim Invasive Surg. 2018;2018:4760769.

Index

Page numbers followed by *b* refer to box, *f* refer to figure, and *t* refer to table

A

D

E

J

K

L

M

N

Q

R

T

U

V

W

X

Y

Z